Comprehensive Dermatologic Drug Therapy

Comprehensive Dermatologic Drug Therapy

Editor

Stephen E. Wolverton, M.D.

Clinical Associate Professor of Dermatology
Indiana University School of Medicine;
Chief of Dermatology
Roudebush VA Medical Center
Indianapolis, Indiana

W.B. SAUNDERS COMPANY
A Harcourt Health Sciences Company
Philadelphia   London   Montreal   Sydney   Tokyo   Toronto

W.B. SAUNDERS COMPANY
A Harcourt Health Sciences Company

The Curtis Center
Independence Square West
Philadelphia, Pennsylvania 19106

Acquisitions Editor: Liz Fathman
Editorial Assistant: Paige Mosher Wilke
Project Manager: Carol Sullivan Weis
Production Editor: Rachel E. Dowell
Designer: Rokusek Design
Design Coordinator: Mark A. Oberkrom

Library of Congress Cataloging-in-Publication Data

Comprehensive dermatologic drug therapy / editor, Stephen E. Wolverton.
    p. ; cm.
Includes bibliographical references and index.
ISBN 0-7216-7728-2 (alk. paper)
    1. Dermatopharmacology. I. Wolverton, Stephen E.
    [DNLM: 1. Skin Diseases—drug therapy. WR 650 C7375 2001]
RL801 .C66 2001
616.5'061—dc21

                                                    00-064105

COMPREHENSIVE DERMATOLOGIC DRUG THERAPY   ISBN 0-7216-7728-2

Printed in the United States of America

Last digit is the print number: 9   8   7   6   5   4   3   2

This book is dedicated to the following individuals:

To our sons Jay Edward (age 14) and Justin David (age 12)
. . . for continually inspiring me by helping me see the wonders of the world through their eyes.

To my wife Cheryl
. . . for her ongoing support through the rigorous task of editing this book.

To my parents Elizabeth Ann* and Dr. George M. Wolverton, Sr.
. . . for continuing to be superb role models by living principled lives, always with a strong work ethic.

And in memory of my older brother Dr. George M. Wolverton, Jr. (1951-1996)
. . . although he was blessed with exceptional talents, his life ended way too soon by his own hands due to the imposing "two-edged sword" known as OCD.

---

*Just as I finished proofing the last chapter in the final phase of editing on 11/25/00, I received word that my mother died suddenly. Her passion for life, energy, encouragement, generosity, and gratitude will inspire me always.

NOTICE

CONTRIBUTORS

Stephanie Badalamenti, M.D., Ph.D.
Department of Dermatology
University of Miami School of Medicine
Miami, Florida

Jennifer L. Baumbach, B.S., M.D.
Resident in Dermatology
University Hospital
University of Cincinnati College of Medicine
Cincinnati, Ohio

Susan Baur, M.D.
Staff Physician
Departments of Dermatology
University of Frankfurt
Frankfurt, Germany

Saqib J. Bashir, B.Sc. (HONS), M.B., Ch.B.
Research Fellow
University of California School of Medicine
San Francisco, California

Brian Berman, M.D., Ph.D.
Professor
Departments of Dermatology and Cutaneous Surgery
    and Internal Medicine
University of Miami School of Medicine
Miami, Florida

Verity Blackwell, M.R.C.P.
Specialist Registrar in Dermatology
Middlesex Hospital
University College London Hospitals Trust
London, United Kingdom

Crystal S. Blankenship, Pharm. D.
Affiliate Assistant Professor
Purdue University School of Pharmacy and Pharmacal
    Sciences
West Lafayette, Indiana;
Adjunct Assistant Professor
Butler University
College of Pharmacy and Health Sciences;
Clinical Pharmacist
Drug Information Coordinator
Clarian Health Partners
Indianapolis, Indiana

Jessica Boyce, Pharm. D. Candidate
Purdue University
West Lafayette, Indiana

Robert T. Brodell, M.D.
Professor of Internal Medicine,
Clinical Professor of Dermatopathology,
Head, Dermatology Section,
Master Teacher,
Northeastern Ohio University College of Medicine
Rootstown, Ohio;
Associate Clinical Professor of Dermatology
Case Western Reserve University School of Medicine
Cleveland, Ohio;
Staff Physician
Trumbull Memorial Hospital,
Warren, Ohio

David G. Brodland, M.D.
Private Practice;
University of Pittsburgh Medical Center—Shadyside
Pittsburgh, Pennsylvania

Jeffrey P. Callen, M.D., F.A.C.P.
Professor of Medicine in Dermatology
Chief, Division of Dermatology
University of Louisville School of Medicine
Louisville, Kentucky

Charles Camisa, M.D.
Associate Professor of Internal Medicine
Ohio State University College of Medicine
Columbus, Ohio;
Vice Chairman, Department of Dermatology
Head, Section of Clinical Dermatology
Cleveland Clinic Foundation
Cleveland, Ohio

Soni Carlton, M.D.
Dermatology Resident
University of Texas Medical Branch
Galveston, Texas

Daniel A. Carrasco, M.D.
Post Doctoral Fellow
Department of Dermatology, Microbiology/Immunology,
    and Internal Medicine
University of Texas Medical Branch
Galveston, Texas

Kevin D. Cooper, M.D.
Professor, Dermatology
Chairman, Dermatology
Case Western Reserve University;
President, University Hospital Dermatology Associates;
Director, University Hospitals of Cleveland
Cleveland, Ohio

Julio C. Cruz-Ramon, M.D.
Chief Resident
Division of Dermatology
Ohio State University
Columbus, Ohio

Mark Alan Darst, M.D., A.B.F.P., A.A.F.P.,
   A.C.E.P.
Teaching Faculty
Indiana University School of Medicine
Department of Family Medicine
Indianapolis, Indiana

Loretta S. Davis, M.D.
Associate Professor
Section of Dermatology
Department of Medicine
Medical College of Georgia
Augusta, Georgia

Pauline M. Dowd, B.Sc., M.D., F.R.C.P.
Professor of Dermatology
Middlesex Hospital
University College London Hospitals Trust
London, England

Zoe Diana Draelos, M.D.
Clinical Associate Professor
Department of Dermatology
Wake Forest University School of Medicine
Winston-Salem, North Carolina;
Primary Investigator
Dermatology Consulting Services
High Point, North Carolina

Thomas J. Eads, M.D.
Staff Physician
St. Vincent Hospital
Carmel, Indiana

William H. Eaglstein, M.D.
Professor and Chairman
Department of Dermatology and Cutaneous Surgery
University of Miami School of Medicine
Miami, Florida

Tanya Y. Evans, M.D.
Dermatology Resident
University of Illinois
Chicago, Illinois

Francisco Flores, M.D.
Dermatology Resident
Department of Dermatology and Cutaneous Surgery
University of Miami School of Medicine
Miami, Florida

Mark S. Fradin, M.D.
Adjunct Clinical Associate Professor of Dermatology
University of North Carolina
Chapel Hill, North Carolina

Michael Girardi, M.D.
Assistant Professor
Department of Dermatology
Yale University School of Medicine
New Haven, Connecticut

Kenneth B. Gordon, M.D.
Assistant Professor of Dermatology
Northwestern University Medical School;
Chief, Section of Dermatology
Chicago Veteran's Affairs Medical Center
Lakeside Division
Chicago, Illinois

Malcolm W. Greaves, M.D., Ph.D., F.R.C.P.
Emeritus Professor of Dermatology
St. John's Institute of Dermatology
St. Thomas' Hospital
London, England

Aditya K. Gupta, M.D., M.A. (Cantab),
   F.R.C.P.(C)
Associate Professor
Division of Dermatology
Department of Medicine
Sunnybrook and Women's College Health Sciences
   Centre
Toronto, Ontario

Russell P. Hall III, M.D.
Professor and Chief,
Division of Dermatology
Department of Medicine
Duke University Medical Center;
Chief, Dermatology
Durham VA Medical Center
Durham, North Carolina

Peter W. Heald, M.D.
Associate Professor
Department of Dermatology
Yale University School of Medicine
New Haven, Connecticut

Adam B. Hessel, M.D.
Assistant Professor of Clinical Medicine (Dermatology
   and Pathology)
Division of Dermatology
The Ohio State University
College of Medicine and Public Health
Columbus, Ohio

Sylvia Hsu, M.D.
Associate Professor of Dermatology
Baylor College of Medicine
Houston, Texas

Michael J. Huether, B.A., M.D.
Mohs Micrographic Surgeon/Dermatologic Surgeon
Northwest Medical Center
Tucson, Arizona

Kristen Hummer, Pharm. D. Candidate
Butler University
Indianapolis, Indiana

Sewon Kang, M.D.
Associate Professor of Dermatology
University of Michigan Medical School;
Director of Clinical Research Unit
Department of Dermatology
University of Michigan Medical Center
Ann Arbor, Michigan

Marshall Kapp, J.D., M.P.H.
Director, Office of Geriatric Medicine
Department of Community Health
Wright State University School of Medicine
Dayton, Ohio

Sonya J. Keinath, Pharm. D. Candidate
Butler University
Indianapolis, Indiana

Francisco A. Kerdel, M.D., M.B.B.S., B.Sc.
Professor of Clinical Dermatology
University of Miami School of Medicine;
Director, Dermatology Inpatient Services
Cedars Medical Center
Miami, Florida

Heather Klinge, Pharm. D. Candidate
Butler University
Indianapolis, Indiana

Alfred L. Knable, Jr., M.D.
Assistant Professor of Dermatology
Wright State University
Dayton, Ohio;
Assistant Professor of Dermatology
Uniformed Services University of the Health Sciences
Bethesda, Maryland;
Member
Associates in Dermatology
Louisville, Kentucky

Sandra R. Knowles, B.Sc.Phm.
Lecturer, Faculty of Pharmacy
University of Toronto;
Drug Safety Pharmacist
Sunnybrook and Women's College Health Sciences
    Centre
Toronto, Ontario

John Y. M. Koo, M.D.
Associate Clinical Professor;
Vice Chairman, Department of Dermatology;
Director, Psoriasis Treatment Center
University of California, San Francisco Medical Center
San Francisco, California

Carol L. Kulp-Shorten, M.D.
Associate Professor of Medicine (Dermatology)
University of Louisville School of Medicine
Louisville, Kentucky

Andrea K. LaRoche, Pharm. D. Candidate
Purdue University
West Lafayette, Indiana

Chai Sue Lee, M.D.
Fellow
Department of Dermatology
University of California, San Francisco
School of Medicine
San Francisco, California

Stanley B. Levy, M.D.
Clinical Professor of Dermatology
University of North Carolina School of Medicine at
    Chapel Hill
Chapel Hill, North Carolina;
Clinical Associate in Medicine
Duke University Medical School
Durham, North Carolina

Amy B. Lewis, M.D.
Assistant Clinical Professor
Director of Dermatologic Surgery;
Attending Physician
SUNY HSC;
Attending Physician
Kings County Hospital
Brooklyn, New York

Andrew N. Lin, M.D.
Associate Professor
University of Alberta
Edmonton, Alberta

Howard I. Maibach, M.D.
Professor of Dermatology
Dermatology Department
University of California Hospital
San Francisco, California

Jack E. Maloney, M.D.
Resident
Department of Dermatology
University of Texas Health Science Center
Houston, Texas

Charles J. McDonald, B.S., M.S., M.D.
Professor of Medical Science
Chairman, Department of Dermatology
Brown University School of Medicine;
Physician in Chief
Department of Dermatology
Rhode Island Hospital
Providence, Rhode Island

Ginat Wintermeyer Mirowshi, D.M.D., M.D.
Assistant Professor
Department of Oral Surgery Medicine Pathology
Indiana University Dental School;
Assistant Professor
Department of Dermatology
Indiana University School of Medicine
Indianapolis, Indiana

Warwick L. Morison, M.B., B.S., M.D., FRCP
Professor
Johns Hopkins University
Baltimore, Maryland

Ethan-Quan H. Nguyen, M.D., M.S.
Physician
Kaiser Permanente
Department of Dermatology
Riverside, Cailfornia

Teddy D. Pan, M.D.
Resident
Brown University;
Resident
Rhode Island Hospital
Providence, Rhode Island

Rhea M. Phillips, M.D.
Professor of Dermatology
Baylor College of Medicine
Houston, Texas

Janet Hill Prystowsky, M.D., Ph.D.
Associate Clinical Professor of Dermatologic Surgery
Columbia University College of Physicians and Surgeons;
Associate Attending
New York Presbyterian Hospital
New York, New York

Long Thang Quan, M.D., Ph.D.
Resident
Baylor College of Medicine
Houston, Texas

James E. Rasmussen, M.D.
Professor of Dermatology
Professor of Pediatrics
Department of Dermatology
University of Michigan Health System
Ann Arbor, Michigan

Barbara R. Reed, M.D.
Associate Clinical Professor
University of Colorado Health Sciences Center
Denver, Colorado

Kathleen A. Remlinger, M.D.
Associate Professor of Dermatology
Rush-Presbyterian St. Lukes Medical Center
Chicago, Illinois

Theodore Rosen, M.D.
Professor of Dermatology
Baylor College of Medicine;
Chief, Dermatology Science
Veterans Affair Medical Center
Houston, Texas

Dana Sachs, M.D.
Clinical Assistant
Memorial Sloan-Kettering Cancer Center
New York, New York

Neil S. Sadick, M.D., F.A.C.P.
Clinical Associate Professor
Department of Dermatology
Cornell University Medical College;
Attending Physician
New York Presbyterian Hospital
New York, New York

Marty E. Sawaya, M.D., Ph.D.
Dermatologist and Principal Investigator
Clinical Research
ARATEC Clinics
Ocala, Florida;
Adjunct Professor
University of Miami School of Medicine
Miami, Florida

Lori E. Shapiro, M.D.
Assistant Professor
Department of Medicine
University of Toronto Medical School;
Staff, Divisions of Dermatology and Clinical
    Pharmacology
Glaxo Wellcome-Sunnybrook Drug Safety Clinic
Sunnybrook and Women's College Health Science Centre
Toronto, Ontario

Neil H. Shear, M.D., F.R.C.P.C., F.A.C.P.
Professor of Medicine and Pharmacology
Director, Drug Safety Research Group and Drug Safety
    Clinic
University of Toronto Medical School
Toronto, Ontario

Pranav B. Sheth, B.A., M.D.
Clinical Instructor
University of Cincinnati College of Medicine
Cincinnati, Ohio

Stephen K. Tyring, M.D., Ph.D.
Professor of Dermatology, Microbiology/Immunology,
    and Internal Medicine
University of Texas Medical Branch
Galveston, Texas

Melody R. Vander Straten, M.D.
Post Doctoral Fellow
University of Texas Medical Branch
Galveston, Texas

Michael Warner, M.D.
Fellow
Dermatologic Surgery and Cutaneous Oncology
Cleveland Clinic Foundation
Cleveland, Ohio

Dennis P. West, Ph.D.
Professor of Dermatology
Northwestern University Medical School
Chicago, Illinois

Stephen E. Wolverton, M.D.
Clinical Associate Professor of Dermatology
Indiana University School of Medicine;
Chief of Dermatology
Roudebush VA Medical Center
Indianapolis, Indiana

Herschel S. Zackheim, M.D.
Clinical Professor
Department of Dermatology
University of California, San Francisco
San Francisco, California

PREFACE

I am neither a researcher nor a fellowship-trained pharmacologist. I am, however, an academic clinician who has a fascination with three challenges of central importance to this book, *Comprehensive Dermatologic Drug Therapy*. These areas include (1) the challenge of simplifying and summarizing broad and complicated topics, (2) the challenge of demonstrating clinical relevance of concepts derived from the basic scientific underpinnings of dermatology, and (3) the challenge of maximizing the safety and efficacy of dermatologic drug therapy. The blend of all three challenges provides the motivation for and the mission of this book. This current book is the offspring of *Systemic Drugs for Skin Disease*, published in 1991 by W.B. Saunders. Growing the 17 chapters dedicated to systemic drugs (and related topics) in the prior book to the 50 chapters that cover all routes of drug administration and a wide variety of related topics in this book was a tremendous challenge, albeit a most interesting journey.

I was blessed with the assistance of 75 authors who responded to the structured chapter format and my highly involved editorial style. I worked with a diverse and talented group of distinguished authors from the United States, Canada, and the United Kingdom. Overall, I had tremendous cooperation from these contributors in addressing important questions and issues for the various chapters that are very important to both the physicians seeking prescribing information and patients who receive the drugs discussed in this book.

Comprehensive Dermatologic Drug Therapy is designed to be both a streamlined quick reference for busy clinicians and a thorough reference for residents in training and life-long learners, who seek in-depth information about drugs with cutaneous applications.

The numerous tables in this book are designed for clinicians in need of quick "how-to" information in managing patients suffering from a wide variety of cutaneous disorders. Some of the most valuable tables include the following:

✓ Specific-chapter drug tables list trade names, generic availability, tablet/capsule/tube sizes, standard dosage range, and cost information.

✓ Key pharmacologic concepts tables list important data on absorption, bioavailability, metabolism, and excretion for most drugs.

✓ Indications and contraindications tables list FDA-approved and off-label indications (with reference citations) for a wide variety of drugs, accompanied by contraindications and pregnancy prescribing status for the drugs.

✓ Monitoring guidelines tables provide details on baseline and follow-up tests and examinations that maximize safety for the systemic drugs with a significant element of risk.

✓ Drug interactions tables provide the most important drug interactions for various drugs, generally listed by drug category while grouping drugs and drug categories with a similar type of interaction.

A number of other tables cover adverse effects, drug mechanisms, comparisons of treatment regimens, and other issues relevant to the full spectrum of drugs for cutaneous disorders.

Individuals seeking in-depth information on selected drugs should refer to the following additional features:

✓ Drug structures are provided for 87 of the most commonly used drugs.

✓ Each chapter contains text discussions about drug history, pharmacology, indications, adverse effects, and drug interactions, frequently supplemented with background information on monitoring and therapeutic guidelines for the highest priority drugs in the book.

✓ Liberal use of section headings and subheadings facilitates easy retrieval and categorization of important information.

✓ Chapters are thoroughly referenced with a bibliography preceding the reference section, which lists a number of recent review articles and textbook chapters pertaining to each chapter in this book.

✓ Thorough references are provided for FDA-approved indications and off-label uses for drugs in the various chapters, with chapter references carefully grouped for easy retrieval.

Another special feature pertains to drug-cost information presented in two settings. For the great majority of chapters discussing systemic drugs, there is a five-tiered price index system for the major drugs covered in the chapters. In two appendices, detailed price information for systemic and topical drugs based on average wholesale price from the *Red Book on Drugs and Therapeutics* (June 2000 edition) is presented. Given the current national interest in controlling drug costs, these features provide an important information source for clinicians in all fields.

In addition to major sections on systemic drug therapy (20 chapters) and topical drug therapy (18 chapters), a number of related topics of interest are presented. An introductory section contains two chapters that provide background information on pharmacology concepts and principles to maximize the safety of drug therapy. A subsequent section addresses major potential complications such as hematologic toxicity, hepatotoxicity, drugs in pregnancy and lactation, drug interactions, and drug hypersensitivity syndromes. The book concludes with novel topics such as pharmacoeconomics, drug testing and development, medicolegal issues, the FDA, and new biotechnology/biologic therapies. The full package of topics is thorough and provides a variety of vantage points important to therapeutics.

This book has significant potential to benefit physicians in all primary care fields. The vast majority of drugs discussed in this book are indicated for conditions involving a variety of organ systems beyond the skin. In addition, management of common disorders frequently presenting to primary physicians, such as poison ivy, acne, rosacea, seborrheic dermatitis, and many others, is discussed in the Clinical Use sections under the appropriate drugs. A disease-based index streamlines the retrieval of this therapeutic information. Furthermore, drug interactions and monitoring guidelines are reasonably consistent for systemic drugs discussed, regardless of who prescribes the drug.

Dermatology, as with all fields of medicine, is continually evolving and expanding as new information is published. In spite of this reality, basic principles of therapeutics that maximize the safety and efficacy of drugs discussed in this book remain reasonably constant. Three sources of information that complement this book include (1) *The Medical Letter of Drugs and Therapeutics*, which presents balanced information on all major new drugs released in the future; (2) *CliniSphere 2.0 CD ROM* (Facts & Comparisons) is particularly helpful on the complicated, evolving subject of drug interactions; and (3) drug information pharmacists available in most hospitals and medical centers.

I sincerely hope that readers find *Comprehensive Dermatologic Drug Therapy* practical, understandable, and well organized. The clinician should be able to anticipate, prevent, diagnose early, and manage important adverse effects to maximize safe prescribing of all drugs with cutaneous applications. It is my most sincere hope that numerous patients will benefit from the therapeutic wisdom presented in this book.

Stephen E. Wolverton

ACKNOWLEDGMENTS

I would like to express my most sincere appreciation to the following individuals who went the extra mile to help me complete *Comprehensive Dermatologic Drug Therapy.*

Four students from the classes of 2002 and 2003 at the Indiana University School of Medicine responded to an advertisement asking for administrative and computer-related help toward completion of this book. Mike Thieken, Stephanie Jeske, Doug Heintzelman, and Ryan Venis were of tremendous assistance for a wide variety of special information-gathering projects.

Phil Wilson, a medical illustrator from the IU Medical Center Department of Pharmacology, provided all the drug structures used in this book, with backup from department chair Henry Besch, Ph.D. The consistency of style throughout 87 structures is greatly appreciated.

I owe a debt of gratitude to Michael Bangert, assistant automation librarian at the IU Medical Center with in-depth knowledge on all aspects of computers, who helped me survive two major computer crashes during the book preparation.

Four of the faculty from the Department of Dermatology provided frequent coverage for resident clinics I routinely staff, enabling me to free up adequate time for my very hands-on approach to editing. I am grateful to Ginat Mirowski, D.M.D., M.D., Jeff Travers, M.D., Ph.D., Charles Lewis, M.D., and Tsu-Yi Chuang, M.D. for their kindness in providing this coverage.

Finally, I worked with a very thorough, efficient, and personable staff at Harcourt Health Sciences, which oversees the editorial staff at both W.B. Saunders and Mosby. Judy Fletcher (Acquisitions Editor in the formative stages of the book project), Liz Fathman (final Acquisitions Editor), Paige Mosher (Editorial Assistant), and Rachel E. Dowell (Production Editor) were all instrumental in helping this project march on to completion in a very reasonable timeframe. To all these individuals, I am most grateful.

CONTENTS

Comprehensive Dermatologic Drug Therapy

PART I

Introduction

CHAPTER 1

Stephen E. Wolverton

Basic Pharmacologic Principles

This chapter describes and illustrates the pharmacologic principles that enable the clinician to maximize efficacy and minimize the risk (e.g., adverse effects, drug interactions) of dermatologic drug therapy. This chapter provides a broad foundation for true understanding of pharmacology that enables (1) easier assimilation of new information on medications, (2) adaptability to the many unpredictable responses of patients to medications, and (3) better long-term retention of important information on all aspects of drug therapy. The primary focus of the chapter is on pharmacologic principles related to systemic drugs. A brief section on percutaneous absorption concludes the chapter. The reader is encouraged to pursue further details and references (cited in the respective chapter for specific drugs) for drug examples used to illustrate pharmacologic principles in this chapter.

Traditionally, discussions on basic pharmacology divide the topic into two domains—pharmacokinetics (what the body does to the drug) and pharmacodynamics (what the drug does to the body) (Table 1-1). As a relatively novel way of presenting this information, topics are discussed in sequence as seen through the "eyes" of the drug as it progresses through the human body. The sequence is (1) pharmacokinetics (part I: absorption, distribution, and bioavailability), the drug must enter the body, travel to, and be "available" at the site of desired pharmacologic action; (2) pharmacodynamics, the drug interacts with a receptor/effector mechanism, producing both desirable and undesirable effects; and (3) pharmacokinetics (part II: metabolism and excretion), the drug must depart from the body. Each of these steps has a number of variables (with both predictable and unpredictable components) for which the clinician should have at least a baseline working knowledge. These variables are presented and illustrated under each chapter heading that follows.

PHARMACOKINETICS: PART I

Table 1-2 describes the major components of pharmacokinetics. Table 1-3 contains definitions and concepts central to understanding pharmacokinetics.

Drug Absorption

The routes of drug administration most pertinent to dermatology in order of descending frequency of use are—topical, oral, intramuscular, and intralesional administration. Intravenous administration is ordered infrequently by the dermatologist. Typically, drugs must be relatively lipophilic (nonionized and nonpolar) to enter the body by topical or oral routes, whereas

■ Table 1-1   Two "Entry Level" Definitions

Term	Definition
Pharmacokinetics	*What the body does to the drug*—from entry into the body until excretion of the drug or its metabolites
Pharmacodynamics	*What the drug does to the body*—once at site of action; from receptor binding through the definitive effect (desired or adverse)

■ Table 1-2   Pharmacokinetics—Major Components*

Component	Most Important Issues
Absorption	Lipophilic drugs are most optimally absorbed through the GI tract; lipophilic or hydrophilic drugs overall equal for parenteral absorption
Distribution	Body locations to which the drug is dispersed; important subcomponents include fatty tissues and blood-brain barrier
Bioavailability	Percentage of administered drug reaching circulation; also relates to free (active) versus protein bound drug
Metabolism	Lipophilic drugs get converted to more hydrophilic metabolites to enable excretion
Excretion	The above conversion to hydrophilic metabolites allows renal or biliary excretion; other synonyms—clearance, elimination

*These components relate to oral (enteral) or parenteral administered drugs.

■ Table 1-3   Definitions and Concepts Central to Understanding Pharmacokinetics

Term	Definition
Bioactivation	Either (1) conversion of prodrug to any active drug or (2) conversion of the active drug to a reactive, electrophilic metabolic intermediate
Bioequivalence*	Generally referring to overall "equal" bioavailability between two comparable drugs, usually between generic and trade name formulations of a drug
Biotransformation	In general, the metabolic change of a lipophilic drug to a more hydrophilic metabolite allowing renal excretion
Blood-brain barrier	Protective mechanism for brain neurons; due to tight junctions (and lack of inter-cellular pores) in brain capillaries; highly lipophilic drugs may "overcome" this barrier
Detoxification	The metabolic conversion of a reactive, electrophilic intermediate to a more stable, usually more hydrophilic compound
Enteral	GI administration of a drug
Enterohepatic recirculation	Sequence of initial GI absorption of drug followed by hepatic excretion into bile and small bowel, followed by subsequent GI absorption
First-pass effect	Drugs that have significant metabolism in the liver, before widespread systemic distribution; occurs after GI absorption via portal vein to liver
Half-life	Duration of time for 50% of the absorbed and bioavailable drug to be metabolized and excreted

*The US FDA definition for "bioequivalence" requires that the proposed generic drug bioavailability must have a 95% confidence interval between 80% and 120% of the trade name drug bioavailability.

Continued

▆ Table 1-3   Definitions and Concepts Central to Understanding Pharmacokinetics—cont'd

Term	Definition
Parenteral	Literally "around enteral"; either intravenous, intramuscular, or subcutaneous administration
Pharmacogenetics	The study of inherited aspects of drug metabolism that alter the likelihood of various pharmacologic effects (positive or negative)
Prodrug	A pharmacologically inactive metabolic precursor of the biologically active drug
Steady state	A balance between the amount of drug being absorbed and the amount being excreted; in general the time to reach steady state is 4 to 5 half-lives
Terminal elimination	Elimination/clearance of drug from all body compartments to which drug was distributed
Therapeutic index	The ratio of the drug dose required to give a desired pharmacologic response, to the dose that leads to significant adverse effects
Therapeutic range	Range of circulating drug levels deemed to give optimal efficacy and minimal adverse effects
Tissue reservoirs	Body locations to which a given drug is distributed, from which the drug is very slowly released—includes sites such as fatty tissues and stratum corneum

relatively hydrophilic (ionized and polar) drugs can still enter by intramuscular and intravenous routes. On absorption, drugs still must traverse other cell membranes to reach the intended destination(s). Again, a drug with lipophilic qualities is rewarded by the ability to traverse these lipid bilayers to arrive at the site of pharmacologic action.

Several other variables may affect the absorption of drugs by oral administration. Certain drugs are absorbed less efficiently in the presence of food. In descending order, the impact of food on drug absorption is as follows: tetracycline > doxycycline > minocycline. Divalent and trivalent cations in milk (calcium), various traditional antacids (aluminum-, magnesium-, calcium-containing), and iron-containing products can reduce the absorption of tetracyclines, as well as fluoroquinolone antibiotics. Gastric pH is another variable that influences drug absorption. An example would be the necessity for a relatively low gastric pH for ketoconazole and itraconazole to be optimally absorbed, whereas the gastric pH is not a critical determinant for fluconazole absorption. These absorption variables are the basis for a number of drug interactions that do not involve the cytochrome P (CYP)-450 system.

Some drugs have negligible absorption with oral administration, yet can have a pharmacologic value in the gastrointestinal (GI) tract. Several examples would be the use of oral cromolyn sodium (Gastrochrome) for the GI manifestations of mastocytosis, as well as the use of nystatin for reduction of intestinal candidal levels. The addition of a vasoconstrictor (epinephrine) to local anesthetics slows absorption and therefore prolongs the duration of anesthesia after intralesional injection of the anesthetic. Finally, a number of medications are available in sustained-release preparations, in which the drug vehicle is modified to allow a steady, slow rate of drug absorption.

Distribution

There are several issues regarding drug distribution that apply to dermatologic therapeutics. A drug can be distributed orally by the following four methods:

1. Circulation: important to widespread effects, both desirable and adverse
2. Cutaneous: logically of central importance to desired pharmacologic effects
3. Fatty tissue: both cutaneous and distant sites, very important to highly lipophilic drugs, creating a reservoir for prolonged release of the drug (as with etretinate)

4. Past the "blood-brain barrier": of importance to dermatology primarily for lipophilic drugs with the potential for sedation or other central nervous system adverse effects (first generation H_1 antihistamines cause sedation; minocycline causes dizziness)

Fortunately, there are alternative drugs to the previously mentioned drugs that do not readily cross the blood-brain barrier (second generation H_1 antihistamines, doxycycline, and tetracycline).

Many systemic drugs discussed in this book have dosages based on body weight, including drugs with doses calculated per kg of body weight (isotretinoin and etretinate) and doses calculated per m^2 (bexarotene). The question arises regarding what to do with dosage calculations for very obese patients. There are both cost and potential adverse effect implications for very high doses, thus calculating dosages based more on "ideal weight" has several reasons. Aside from treatment of panniculitis, there are virtually no indications for which the site of desired pharmacologic effect is in fatty tissue. Highly lipid-soluble drugs are readily distributed to fatty tissues, but when a steady state is reached, there is steady release back into circulation. When considering efficacy, risk, and cost, all three point towards leveling off the dosage at or near ideal body weight, perhaps allowing for a small error margin on the high side for very heavy patients who do not respond to traditional doses.

Conceptually, there are three drug reservoirs of significant interest to dermatology. The first is in systemic circulation, in the form of drug protein binding. The bound drug is pharmacologically inactive, while the unbound drug = free drug = pharmacologically active drug. Acidic drugs are most commonly bound to albumin, whereas basic drugs bind preferentially to α-1 acidic glycoprotein. There are noteworthy exceptions regarding lipophilic drugs with intracellular physiologic receptor-effector systems such as corticosteroids and retinoids. There is a large circulatory reservoir for highly protein bound drugs such as methotrexate. Sudden increases in free drug levels due to displacement of methotrexate from circulatory protein binding sites by aspirin, nonsteroidal antiinflammatory drugs, and sulfonamides can markedly increase the risk for pancytopenia. The second drug reservoir of interest is in various fatty tissues (including but not limited to subcutaneous fat) for highly lipophilic drugs as discussed in the preceding paragraph. The third drug reservoir (the stratum corneum) pertains just to percutaneous absorption for topically applied medications. In all three settings, the free drug and the drug in the reservoir are in equilibrium. As the free drug is metabolized and excreted, corresponding amounts of the drug in these tissue and circulatory reservoirs are released into the free/active drug fraction.

Bioavailability
Bioavailability is expressed as the percentage of the total drug dose administered that reaches circulation. For selected drugs taken orally, the "first-pass effect" of hepatic metabolism decreases bioavailability. The bioavailability calculations include both free and bound forms of the drug. A systemic drug with a relatively low bioavailability is acyclovir; the prodrug for acyclovir, valacyclovir, has at least three times greater bioavailability. At the other end of the spectrum are the fluoroquinolones for which oral absorption (and resultant bioavailability) is so complete that the oral and intravenous doses for many members of this drug group are identical. A more optimal method (if it were more practical) would be to calculate bioavailability at the site of intended action; for drugs discussed in this book, it would be based on tissue levels at the sites of intended action and the various skin structures. Currently, such ideal bioavailability calculations are not routinely available.

Most chapters in this book that discuss systemic drugs contain tables that present data for the following: (1) percent of bioavailability and (2) percent of protein binding. The percent of bioavailability is typically factored into ideal oral drug dosage calculations, which will produce circulating drug levels in a reasonably safe and effective "therapeutic range." The percent of protein binding is important to the subject of drug interactions; methotrexate is an important example. Changes in albumin levels in disease states, such as severe liver or renal disease, often necessitate drug dosage reductions for drugs that are highly protein bound.

Creating drug formulations with a more optimal bioavailability is a daunting task for the pharmaceutical industry. In the past two decades there have been updated formulations of older drugs with a higher percent of bioavailability, more predictable bioavailability, or both. For drugs with a relatively narrow therapeutic index (e.g., cyclosporine and methoxsalen), improved predictability of the drug absorption and resultant bioavailability is very important. The release of Neoral (in place of the prior cyclosporine formulation, Sandimmune) is an example for both improved percentage and more predictable bioavailability of the newer formulation. Likewise, Oxsoralen Ultra demonstrates improvement in both of these parameters. In a separate example, the need for improved efficacy from griseofulvin led to the progression from the original griseofulvin formulations to microsize formulations to ultramicrosize formulations. Each step of this progression resulted in improved bioavailability and reduced griseofulvin dosages required for an adequate therapeutic response.

PHARMACODYNAMICS

The subject of pharmacodynamics is very complicated. In essence this topic is the "science" behind drug mechanisms of action. Considering all of the diverse mechanisms of actions that drugs discussed in this book have (let alone the diversity of drug mechanisms in all of medicine), it is not possible to summarize general principles behind all of these drug mechanisms. In contrast, it is possible to cover a few important areas for understanding pharmacodynamics, including the concepts of drug receptors, enzyme inhibition by drugs, signal transduction, and transcription factors.

Definitions

Table 1-4 contains definitions and concepts central to pharmacodynamics. In general, the definitions utilized in pharmacodynamics are less familiar to most clinicians than the comparable terms in pharmacokinetics. These terms overall relate to factors that (1) address aspects of drug binding to receptor (ligand, affinity), (2) relay the drug "signal" to the definitive effector mechanism (signal transduction, second messenger), (3) increase the desired pharmaco-

logic response (drug agonists, partial agonists), (4) decrease an undesirable physiologic or pharmacologic response (drug antagonists or receptor blockers), or (5) lose a desirable or undesirable pharmacologic response through repeated drug use (tolerance, cross-tolerance, refractoriness, down regulation, tachyphylaxis). Only a portion of these concepts can be realistically addressed in the remaining paragraphs of this section on pharmacodynamics.

Drug Receptors

The broadest definition of a drug receptor is listed in Table 1-4. In this definition, any molecule to which a drug binds, thus initiating an effector mechanism leading to a specific pharmacologic response, is a drug receptor. In contrast, proteins involved in drug protein binding are merely drug storage or transportation sites and thus are not receptors.

The subtype of drug receptors that are easiest to characterize are cell surface receptors for endogenous neurohormonal ligands. Similar receptors are operant for various growth factors and other cytokines. Such drug receptors are common targets in current therapeutics and in drug development. In addition, lipophilic drugs, which are easily absorbed through cellular membranes, may have cytosolic drug receptors. Common examples using these cytosolic physiologic receptors include both systemic and topical versions of corticosteroids and retinoids. The "catch" with receptors for these two drug categories is that both desirable (therapeutic effects) and undesirable (adverse effects) effects are mediated through the same physiologic receptor. A dissociation of the drug receptors for the therapeutic antiinflammatory benefits (such as methionine synthetase) and adverse effects (dihydrofolate reductase, [DHFR]), of methotrexate is of interest. Folic acid/folate supplementation can competitively antagonize the DHFR inhibition of methotrexate and minimize the adverse effects of methotrexate without compromising therapeutic benefits. A few examples of drugs that are either antagonists or agonists at well-defined cellular receptors are listed in Table 1-5.

Few drugs are ideally specific for a given drug receptor molecule. The ability of both tricyclic antidepressants (such as doxepin) and first generation H_1 antihistamines (such as diphen-

■ Table 1-4 Definitions and Concepts Central to Understanding Pharmacodynamics

Term	Definition
Affinity (binding)	A physical measurement that reflects the attraction of the drug ligand to a given receptor molecule
Agonist	Drug that binds to a given receptor initiating an effector mechanism → pharmacologic response
Antagonist	Drug that binds to a receptor, but fails to activate the effector mechanism
Cross tolerance	Reduced pharmacologic effect when exposed to a new, chemically related drug (see tolerance)
Down regulation	Reduced receptor numbers/availability, presumably due to a negative feedback mechanism
Ligand	Any molecule (drug) that binds to the drug receptor; binding can be by hydrogen bonds, ionic or covalent forces
Partial agonist	Drug that binds to a receptor and weakly initiates an effector mechanism and resultant pharmacologic response
Receptor	The molecule to which the drug (ligand) binds to initiate its effector response; location can be cell membrane, cytosolic, intranuclear
Refractoriness	Temporary lack of responsiveness to a drug (synonym desensitization)
Second messenger	Biochemical mediator (most commonly calcium or cAMP) that serves to relay the signal initiated by the receptor/effector in signal transduction
Signal transduction	Cellular biochemical pathways that relay a second messenger signal from the receptor to the effector mechanism (including DNA)
Tachyphylaxis	A diminished pharmacologic response after repeated drug administration; can be due to down regulation or receptor sequestration (unavailable to the drug)
Tolerance	Diminished effect (beneficial or adverse) after repeated drug administration (most common example is tolerance to sedating drugs such as antihistamines)

■ Table 1-5 Pharmacodynamics—Selected Receptor Antagonists and Agonists

Drug	Receptor Affected	Biologic Outcome
RECEPTOR ANTAGONISTS (RECEPTOR "BLOCKERS")		
H_1 antihistamines	H_1 histamine receptor	Antagonize histamine effects via receptor—vasodilation, increased vascular permeability, etc
H_2 antihistamines	H_2 histamine receptor	Antagonize histamine effects via receptor—gastric acid secretion, suppressor T-cell effects
Spironolactone, flutamide	Androgen receptor*	Antagonize testosterone and dihydrotesterone effects via receptor—variable hair effects depending on scalp location, sebum secretion
Selective serotonin reuptake inhibitors	Serotonin transport protein	Antagonize serotonin reuptake mechanism (net effect increased persistence of serotonin as neurotransmitter)
RECEPTOR AGONISTS		
Corticosteroids	Corticosteroid receptor	Augment both the desirable pharmacologic effects and the adverse effects mediated through same receptor
Calcipotriene	Vitamin D_3 receptor	Augment vitamin D_3 effects via receptor—keratinocyte and fibroblast differentiation
Retinoids	Retinoic acid receptor (RAR), Retinoid × receptor (RXR)	Augment various vitamin A–mediated effects via gene response elements

*Primary pharmacologic (diuretic) effects of spironolactone are mediated through the mineralocorticoid receptor; antiandrogen effects are mediated via the androgen receptor for dihydrotestosterone and testosterone.

hydramine and hydroxyzine) to also bind muscarinic anticholinergic receptors can produce objectionable anticholinergic adverse effects such as dry mouth, blurred vision, and orthostatic hypotension. Relatively selective drug receptor binding was achieved in later generations of related drug groups. Selective serotonin reuptake inhibitors (such as fluoxetine and sertraline) and second-generation H_1 antihistamines (such as fexofenadine and loratadine) have a significant improvement of the adverse effect profile due to much more selective drug receptor binding. It is of interest to note that tolerance to sedative adverse effects can occur with prolonged use of the first generation H_1 antihistamines.

Enzyme Systems Inhibited by Drugs
For comparison purposes, a number of specific examples for drugs that selectively inhibit an enzyme system are listed in Table 1-6. Drugs

◼ Table 1-6   Pharmacodynamics—Selected Examples of Enzymes That Specific Drugs Inhibit

Drug	Enzyme Inhibited	Biologic Outcome
ENZYMES IMPORTANT TO DNA SYNTHESIS		
Methotrexate	Dihydrofolate reductase	Reduced formation of fully reduced folate precursors for purine and thymidylate synthesis
Mycophenolate mofetil	Inosine monophosphate dehydrogenase	Inhibition of de novo pathway for purine (guanosine) nucleotide synthesis, preferentially affects various WBC subsets (other cells can utilize salvage pathway)
ENZYMES IMPORTANT TO MICROBIAL GROWTH AND SURVIVAL		
Sulfonamides, dapsone	Dihydropteroate synthetase	Affects bacterial version of this enzyme far more readily than the mammalian enzyme; first step of two-enzyme pathway essential for folate reduction
Trimethoprim, methotrexate	Dihydrofolate reductase	Affects bacterial version of this enzyme far more readily than the mammalian enzyme; second step of two-enzyme pathway essential for folate reduction
Itraconazole, fluconazole	Lanosterol 14-α demethylase	Triazole inhibition of this enzyme inhibits formation of ergosterol, an essential component of fungal cell wall
Terbinafine, naftifine	Squalene epoxidase	Allylamine inhibition of this enzyme decreases ergosterol, and increases squalene accumulation
Acyclovir, valacyclovir, famciclovir	DNA polymerase	Triphosphorylated forms of these drugs preferentially inhibit viral DNA polymerase over human enzyme
OTHER ENZYMES OF IMPORTANCE TO INFLAMMATORY RESPONSE		
Retinoids	Ornithine decarboxylase	This is rate-limiting enzyme in polyamine pathway, which is initiated by PKC activation
Dapsone	Myeloperoxidase	This enzyme in neutrophils and macrophages is essential to microbial killing by these cells
Cyclosporine, tacrolimus	Calcineurin	This calcium-dependent signal transduction enzyme is key to increased IL-2 production dependent on NFAT*
Corticosteroids	Phospholipase A_2	Inhibition probably mediated through lipomodulin-1; net effect is reduced prostaglandins, leukotrienes, and other eicosanoids important to inflammatory responses

WBC, White blood cell count; *PKC*, protein kinase C; *NFAT*, nuclear factor–activated T cells.
*NFAT is a transcription factor essential to T-cell production of IL-2 and IL-2 receptors.

that inhibit enzyme systems of importance to nucleotide synthesis have significant potential for use in neoplastic diseases or as immunosuppressive drugs in autoimmune dermatoses. A number of drugs that serve as antimicrobial agents for bacterial, viral, and fungal infections capitalize on vital enzyme systems, which are more readily inhibited in the infectious organism than in the human host. Finally, a number of drugs inhibit enzyme systems that contribute important downstream mediators to an inflammatory response. For all three categories of enzymes listed in this table, the drug receptor may be the enzyme itself (methotrexate and DHFR) or work indirectly through another receptor/effector mechanism (as with corticosteroid inhibition of phospholipase A_2, which is probably mediated through lipomodulin-1).

Signal Transduction and Transcription Factors

Signal transduction and transcription are two aspects of pharmacodynamics that have a number of conceptual similarities, albeit with very distinctive mechanisms of action. Signal transduction is a series of intermediary steps in relaying a drug-initiated signal or message to the definitive effector mechanism. This definitive effector mechanism is commonly accomplished through DNA transcription and subsequent new protein translation. In many cases the signal transduction passes through a DNA transcription factor. This sequence and resultant overlap of topics is best illustrated by the "signal one" in activated T cells on T-cell receptor binding to antigen and is amplified by subsequent IL-2 binding to the IL-2 receptor. The rough sequence of steps is as follows: (1) T-cell receptor binding to antigen, (2) CD3 molecule–based T-cell activation, and (3) calcineurin-based activation of NFAT, a DNA transcription factor important to IL-2 upregulation. Cyclosporine and tacrolimus both interfere with this signal transduction pathway through inhibition of calcineurin activity, with a resultant decrease in activity of the transcription factor, NFAT.

Second messengers are important to this discussion as well. Probably the two most important second messengers pertinent to pharmacology are calcium and cyclic AMP (cAMP). Calcium is an important component of this T-cell signal transduction system in two locations; calcineurin is a calcium-dependent enzyme, with a calcium-binding protein (calmodulin) playing an important role as well. Although not directly related to dermatology, cAMP's role as a second messenger in the beneficial effects of β-agonists in therapy of asthma should be noted. The concept of tachyphylaxis as defined in Table 1-4 has been well characterized for β-agonists used in this setting.

Two more examples of important drugs and their effects on signal transduction (retinoids) and transcription factors (corticosteroids) are presented. The polyamine pathway creates a process known as inflammatory hyperplasia, which is important to the pathogenesis of both psoriasis and various malignancies. Retinoids inhibit the activity of ornithine decarboxylase, the rate-limiting enzyme in the polyamine pathway. This signal transduction enzyme inhibition is important to the benefits of systemic retinoids in both psoriasis therapy and for retinoid chemoprevention of cutaneous malignancies in transplantation patients.

Corticosteroids inhibit the actions of the transcription factor, nuclear factor κB (NFκB) by two mechanisms. Corticosteroids both increase production of the inhibitor of NFκB (known as IκB) and directly bind and inactivate NFκB. This transcription factor is pivotal in the upregulation of a multitude of cytokines, which are important to the inflammatory response to a wide variety of stimuli. There is tremendous amplification potential of the inflammatory response through this NFκB pathway. Likewise, a major portion of the corticosteroid (topical or systemic) antiinflammatory benefits are probably accomplished through the inhibition of this important transcription factor. It is unclear whether the relatively common tachyphylaxis noted with class I topical corticosteroids relates to down regulation of receptors involved with this particular pathway.

PHARMACOKINETICS: PART II
Metabolism

Metabolism is extensively discussed in Chapter 41. Most drugs are metabolized by phase I (oxidation reactions) and phase II (conjugation and detoxification reactions). The initial oxidation reactions in phase I are accomplished by various CYP-450 isoforms, which are largely in the liver. The result of these enzymes is a somewhat more hydrophilic/water-soluble metabolite, which may provide a binding site for subsequent conjugation reactions. To complicate matters, reactive electrophilic intermediates are often created, which in the absence of adequate phase II detoxification systems may induce important metabolic or immunologic complications (Table 1-7). Phase II conjugation reactions (i.e., glucuronidation, sulfonation, and acetylation) and detoxification systems (i.e., glutathione and epoxide hydrolase) generally accomplish production of both significantly increased hydrophilicity of the drug metabolites and stabilization of the aforementioned reactive intermediates. Many drug metabolites retain the parent drug's pharmacologic activity; for example, the itraconazole metabolite, hydroxyitraconazole, has significant antifungal activity.

Pharmacogenetics largely addresses genetically based variations in metabolic enzyme systems. At times these genetic alterations can explain idiosyncratic adverse effects of medications. Examples pertinent to phase I and II metabolic systems include the following genetic polymorphisms: (1) CYP 2D6 polymorphisms with up to fiftyfold variation in activity of this important isoform—the result is unexpected profound sedation from various antidepressants and other sedating medications; (2) "slow acetylators"—the result is more frequent occurrence of drug-induced lupus erythematosus, and (3) glutathione depletion (which in part may be acquired due to malnutrition or HIV infections)—the result is markedly increased risk of hypersensitivity to sulfonamide medications. The key research agenda for this important topic is the development of predictive tests to anticipate which patients are at increased risk for important adverse effects from drugs; these tests would be analogous to the baseline G-6-PD determinations for dapsone patients and thiopurine methyltransferase determinations for azathioprine patients.

The most important numeric parameter is the drug half-life. The discussion of the multiple subtypes of drug half-lives, such as terminal elimination half-life, is beyond the scope of this chapter. Data on a given drug's half-life are important to the determination of the time to

Table 1-7 Definitions Related to Adverse Effects

Term	Definition
Toxicity	Undesirable effects expected from a drug due to excessive doses and/or drug levels
Pharmacologic effect	Positive or negative effect from a drug, expected at normal doses and/or drug levels
Adverse effect	Negative or undesirable effect from a drug (either toxic or pharmacologic effect)
Side effect	Synonym for adverse effect (prefer to use "adverse effect" to address undesirable quality of drug effect)
Idiosyncratic	Unexpected adverse effect from a drug
Metabolic idiosyncrasy	Unexpected adverse effect from a drug occurring due to a metabolic abnormality
Immunologic idiosyncrasy	Unexpected adverse effect from a drug occurring on an immunologic basis (usually due to hypersensitivity)*

*Immunologic hypersensitivity may occur due to excessive quantities of a reactive metabolite, rendering immunogenic a previously normal endogenous protein (see Chapter 41).

reach a steady state as drug therapy is initiated (4 to 5 half-lives) and the time for complete drug clearance after drug therapy is discontinued (likewise 4 to 5 half-lives).

One flaw of this linear model presented here for discussing pharmacodynamics between the two sections on pharmacokinetics relates to prodrugs (Table 1-8). These prodrugs are pharmacologically inactive until metabolic conversion to the active drug. The conversion of prednisone (prodrug) to prednisolone (active form) is dependent on a hepatic-based enzyme, which in end-stage liver disease may not produce adequate quantities of prednisolone. Once the drug is metabolized to the active drug, the principles of interest follow through the distribution, bioavailability, and pharmacodynamics sections as with other drugs that are already in active form once absorbed.

■ **Table 1-8** Some Examples
of Prodrugs Important
to Dermatology

Prodrug	Active Drug
ANTIVIRAL AGENTS	
Valacyclovir	Acyclovir
Famciclovir	Penciclovir
CORTICOSTEROIDS	
Prednisone	Prednisolone
Cortisone	Hydrocortisone
OTHER IMMUNOSUPPRESSANTS	
Azathioprine	6-Mercaptopurine
Mycophenolate mofetil	Mycophenolic acid
MISCELLANEOUS DRUGS	
Terfenadine	Fexofenadine

Excretion

Conceptually, there are three common routes by which systemically administered medications leave the body. These routes are (1) renal excretion, (2) biliary excretion through the GI tract, or (3) excretion through the GI tract after failing to be absorbed (orally administered medications). The excreted drug can be the parent drug, drug metabolites, or combinations of both. Relatively hydrophilic drugs can be excreted unchanged through the kidney. An example would be fluconazole, which due to its relatively hydrophilic properties has a significant portion of the administered drug excreted through the kidney unchanged. Relatively lipophilic drugs commonly must be rendered more hydrophilic by the aforementioned phase I and II metabolic steps before excretion is possible through renal or biliary routes. In particular, greater hydrophilicity favors renal excretion, which has a much larger overall capacity for drug excretion than via the hepatobiliary route.

In reality, the drugs discussed in this book are frequently excreted by several of these routes, both as free drugs and as a variety of metabolites. Refer to the various pharmacology key concepts tables used for systemic drugs in this book for illustrations of this point. The reader should also be aware that many drugs

that are conjugated in the liver and excreted into bile will subsequently undergo hydrolysis in the small intestine and be reabsorbed (enterohepatic recirculation) through many cycles; eventually the definitive excretion may be through the kidney.

Disease-induced or age-dependent reduction in renal function should prompt the clinician to significantly reduce drug dosages in drugs with significant renal clearance. An example would be the increased risk for methotrexate pancytopenia and other complications from this drug when standard methotrexate doses are administered to patients with either disease- or age-related reduction in renal function. Likewise, drugs that have significant liver metabolism and excretion should have dosage reductions with advanced liver disease.

PERCUTANEOUS ABSORPTION
General Principles

There is a wealth of scientific and practical information in Tables 1-9 and 1-10. Measures that increase percutaneous absorption can always be considered a "two-edged" sword. The desired pharmacologic result is enhanced by these measures. For instance, use of a high-potency topical corticosteroid in an ointment base, after skin hydration and with total body occlusion, will do wonders for extensive psoriasis. The counterpoint is that all of these measures will markedly increase systemic absorption of the topical corticosteroid, giving a net prednisone-like effect from the topical medication. For a short period of time there will be relatively few trade-offs. After 2 to 3 weeks or more, important systemic adverse effects, such as weight gain, fluid retention, hypertension, hypokalemia, and cushingoid changes, are all possible with topical administration. It is important to note here that all topical drug absorption occurs via passive diffusion.

Topical medications applied in several clinical settings can produce immediate hypersensitivity (Gell and Coombs type I) reactions. In particular, topical application to ulcerated skin can give the applied medication almost immediate access to systemic circulation. There have been reports of anaphylactic reactions to topical bacitracin or neomycin in this setting. Likewise,

▨ Table 1-9   Percutaneous Absorption Variables

Variable	Biologic Result
DRUG VARIABLES	
Concentration	PCA is directly related to concentration and not volume of topical medication applied to a specific skin site
Lipophilicity	Most topically effective drugs are at least somewhat lipophilic
Molecular size	Most effective topical medications have a molecular weight < 1000 (tacrolimus versus poor cyclosporine topical absorption)
VEHICLE VARIABLES (SEE TABLE 1-10)	
Lipid content	Ointment is strongest vehicle due to most optimal partition coefficient in transferring drug to stratum corneum lipids (solution typically weakest vehicle)
Irritancy	Irritating vehicles will alter skin barrier function and ↑ PCA
INNATE SKIN VARIABLES	
Stratum corneum thickness	Rate limiting site for PCA; thickness of stratum corneum is inversely related to PCA
Cutaneous vasculature	Increased cutaneous vasculature can increase both local and systemic drug effects
Area of absorptive surface	Increased surface area to which drug applied will ↑ PCA total overall, but not ↑ PCA at a specific site (concentration most important variable at a specific site)
Mucosal surfaces	Far less innate barrier function, generally less well developed stratum corneum; consider that any mucosal route of administration can produce systemic drug effects
DISEASED SKIN VARIABLES	
Inflamed skin	Overall ↑ PCA, due both to altered barrier function and increased vasodilation
Ulceration	Topical application responds as if systemic administration of medication (bacitracin anaphylaxis risk after application to a leg ulcer)
OTHER VARIABLES	
Additional skin hydration	Hydrating skin (by various means) before application of topical medication ↑ PCA
Occlusion of medication	Topical occlusion locally (food wrap) or widespread ("sauna suit") with marked ↑ PCA; conceptually transdermal application of systemic medications utilizes a similar process
Age of patient	Increased total body surface area to body volume ratio in young children; therefore increased risk of systemic effects due to relatively high absorptive surface

PCA, Percutaneous absorption.

mucosal applications of medications (such as eye drops, vaginal suppositories, rectal foam, or rectal suppositories) can result in significant systemic levels of various drugs. Although the risk from topical application of medications to these sites is usually small, the clinician should always be mindful of this systemic absorption potential.

Vehicles
Much of the art and science of dermatology revolves around choosing the appropriate vehicle for topical medications (see Table 1-10). In general, the choice of vehicle is just as important as choosing the proper active ingredient. There are two common consequences of certain vehi-

■ Table 1-10   Clinical Comparisons of Various Vehicles—Generalities

	Ointments	Creams	Gels	Lotions/Solutions
Composition	Water in oil emulsion	Oil in water emulsion	Semisolid emulsion in alcohol base	Powder in water (some with oil)
Relative potency	Strong	Moderate	Strong	Low
Hydration or drying properties	Hydrating	Some hydration	Drying	Drying (variable)
Variability of generic versus trade name	Relatively low	Very significant	Very significant	Very significant
Stage of dermatitis treated	Chronic	Acute to subacute	Acute to subacute	Acute
Sensitization risk	Very low	Significant	Significant	Significant
Irritation risk	Very low	Very low	Relatively high	Moderate
Body sites where most useful	Nonintertriginous	Virtually all sites	Oral, scalp	Scalp, intertriginous
Body sites to avoid	Face, hands, groin	Sites with maceration	Fissures, erosions; also macerated	Fissures, erosions
Patient preference	Often dislike greasiness	High rate acceptance	Variable	High rate acceptance

cles. The first consequence is irritancy, most notably from high concentrations of propylene glycol; other "alcohols" or certain acidic vehicle ingredients may be irritants, particularly when applied to diseased skin. The second consequence is contact allergy/sensitization, which is common with preservatives in various water-based topical products. Common preservatives that may be sensitizers include various parabens, along with formalin releasers (such as quaternium-15, imidazolidinyl urea, and diazolidinyl urea). The astute clinician will be mindful of the potential adverse effects of the vehicle, particularly if the patient fails to improve or worsens with topical therapy. The simplest and safest way to minimize the risk of these vehicle-induced adverse effects is to choose topical products that lack the most common irritants and allergens. See Chapter 27 for additional information on this topic.

Tachyphylaxis
Tachyphylaxis is a relatively common clinical event with very high potency (class I) topical corticosteroids. The measures previously discussed, which can produce excessive systemic absorption, also predispose to diminished therapeutic benefit from the topical drug over time. The clinician should be aware that a continual daily or twice daily application of a class I topical corticosteroid to minimally inflamed skin (without any other maneuvers to increase percutaneous absorption) commonly leads to tachyphylaxis after 2 to 4 weeks of continuous therapy. The good news is that this is an easily reversible process, particularly if the clinician is mindful of the potential for tachyphylaxis. Weekend-only or alternate-day applications of these high-potency products typically prevent tachyphylaxis; a week off therapy altogether allows up regulation of the corticosteroid receptor molecules and resultant return of the desired therapeutic benefit.

Transdermal Medication Formulations
One final topic that is tangentially related to dermatology deserves mention here. The potential for certain drugs to have reduced bioavailability through excessive hepatic first-pass metabolism can be circumvented through transdermal administration of these drugs. An excellent example would be transdermal estrogen administration, which allows the drug to be absorbed directly into systemic circulation. This allows avoidance of the significant first-pass metabolism typical for orally administered estrogens with resultant improved drug bioavailability. There are numerous other medications that

can be administered in various patches for steady, continuous transdermal delivery of the active ingredient.

Given the central importance of understanding percutaneous absorption, the interested reader is encouraged to pursue further information on this subject from articles and books listed in the bibliography. The tables and clinical examples presented on this subject can help readers understand the central principles of percutaneous absorption and the importance of the drug vehicle to the optimal clinical response. Chapters 23 to 38 expand on these principles of percutaneous absorption.

Bibliography

Systemic Drugs

Benet LZ, Kroetz DL, Sheiner LB: Pharmacokinetics: the dynamics of drug absorption, distribution, and elimination. In Hardman JC, Limbird LE, Molinoff PB, et al, editors: *Goodman and Gilman's the pharmacologic basis of therapeutics,* ed 9, New York, 1996, McGraw-Hill, pp 3-28.

Ross EM: Pharmacodynamics: mechanisms of drug action and the relationship between drug concentration and effect. In Hardman JC, Limbird LE, Molinoff PB, et al, editors: *Goodman and Gilman's the pharmacologic basis of therapeutics,* ed 9, New York, 1996, McGraw-Hill, pp 29-42.

Percutaneous Absorption

Guzzo C, Lazarus GS, Werth VP: Dermatologic pharmacology. In Hardman JC, Limbird LE, Molinoff PB, et al, editors: *Goodman and Gilman's the pharmacologic basis of therapeutics,* ed 9, New York, 1996, McGraw-Hill, pp 1593-1616.

Wester RC, Maibach HI: Percutaneous absorption of drugs. *Clin Pharmacokin* 23:253-266, 1992.

CHAPTER 2

Stephen E. Wolverton

Principles for Maximizing the Safety of Dermatologic Drug Therapy

This chapter is unique in the context of the entire book. The principles that follow are a blend of science, personal experience, and common sense. Rather than provide references for comments made in this chapter, the reader is encouraged to selectively pursue detailed information and literature references pertaining to drug examples cited in the various chapters devoted to the respective drug or drug category. Most of the examples provided deal with systemic drug therapy in dermatology because the systemic drugs pose a significantly greater potential risk to the patient compared with topical or intralesional therapeutic options.

Compared with many fields of medicine, dermatologists in general must take greater precautions with systemic drug therapy. Systemic drugs utilized in this field have typically been developed for specific specialties such as rheumatology, oncology, infectious diseases, and transplantation surgery. These specialties have patients with more serious, possibly life-threatening, illnesses than the majority of conditions for which dermatologists use various systemic drugs. The clinician in any field is obligated to avoid creating a greater risk with drug therapy than the innate risk of the underlying disease to be treated.

This statement is the underlying principle behind the need for careful monitoring of systemic drug therapy: to maximize the safety and minimize the risk of therapy is essential.

Four principles summarize the proactive approach for maximizing the safety of dermatologic drug therapy. These principles are anticipation, prevention, diagnosis, and management. The goals of these principles are to (1) *anticipate* which patients and which drug regimens are at risk for various important adverse effects, (2) take appropriate measures to *prevent* adverse effects of potential concern, (3) *diagnose* any adverse effects at an early reversible stage, and (4) *manage* the adverse effect in an effective manner. These general principles can maximize the safety and efficacy of systemic drug therapy. In the following sections, each principle is illustrated by several drugs.

Anticipating, preventing, diagnosing, and managing drug-specific adverse effects maximizes drug safety; this is a broader viewpoint than merely "monitoring" for adverse effects. The goals of this broader approach are to (1) maximize safety for the patient, (2) improve the "comfort" of systemic drug therapy for the patient and physician, and (3) follow the appropriate "standards of care" to minimize medicolegal risk. These overlapping goals are interdependent. For example, when appropriate standards of care are followed, the patient's safety is the focus of these standards. In addition, if the patient's safety and comfort during drug therapy are truly of central importance to the physician, the medicolegal risk is negligible. This is particularly true if the patient assumes an active role in all aspects of systemic drug therapy, in essence forming a "therapeutic partnership" with the prescribing physician.

It is somewhat challenging to define the definitive source of these so-called standards of care. In general, such standards come from one or more of the following sources: (1) specialty-based formal guidelines such as the American Academy of Dermatology "Guidelines of Care," including guidelines recently released on systemic corticosteroids; (2) individual pharmaceutical company guidelines for specific drugs, such as the guidelines and informed consent packet for isotretinoin in females of childbearing potential; (3) FDA Advisory Committee recommendations, such as those guidelines proposed in the early 1980s for monitoring dapsone's hematologic complications; (4) consensus conference publications, such as the consensus guidelines published in 1998 for cyclosporine therapy in psoriasis patients; and (5) "Dear Doctor" letters from the FDA that update physicians nationally regarding recent findings on specific adverse effects, such as a letter in the late 1990s detailing updated isotretinoin-related pregnancy prevention and detection measures. The reality is that the standard of care for a given drug may be a blend of several of these sources, with a certain amount of ambiguity as expected from such a blend.

Historically, these standards of care were based on local practices in the "community" in which the physician practiced. Currently the realities of the "information age" tend to create a trend toward more national, if not global, standards of care. These standards should be considered guidelines and not mandates, with room for flexibility as the patient's individual circumstances and scientific "evidence" justify.

Special effort must always be given to ensure that the most serious adverse effects *never* occur. The most serious adverse effects should include several of the following characteristics: (1) sudden, precipitous onset, (2) no early warn-

ing symptoms, (3) no predictive laboratory tests, (4) potentially irreversible, and (5) potentially serious outcome. Examples of such high priority adverse effects include hematologic complications (pancytopenia from azathioprine or methotrexate, agranulocytosis from dapsone), isotretinoin teratogenesis, and corticosteroid osteonecrosis. The four principles to minimize the likelihood of these and other complications follow in the four major sections of this chapter.

No matter how careful a physician is, bad things can happen to a patient from drug therapy sooner or later. No medical risk reduction system is perfect, given the unpredictabilities of the human body. If the patient and physician have previously formed the therapeutic partnership, and if the physician continues to work with the patient to promptly diagnose and manage the drug-induced complication, there are a number of more positive results. The patient's medical outcome is optimized, the physician's ethical obligation is met, and the medicolegal risk is minimized. Either way, the physician must take a "lifelong learner" approach to the complication, carefully analyzing the events leading to the complication and learning how to minimize the likelihood of a similar adverse therapeutic outcome in the future.

ANTICIPATION

The physician anticipates adverse effects by carefully monitoring the following: (1) patient selection, (2) patient education, (3) baseline laboratory and related tests, (4) concomitant drug therapy—drug interactions, and (5) evolving guidelines—risk factors.

Patient Selection
PRINCIPLE
Carefully compare the risk of the disease to be treated with the risk of the drug regimen planned (in that particular patient)—thus a risk-risk assessment.

- The risk of high-dose systemic corticosteroids in severe pemphigus vulgaris versus the same corticosteroid regimen in patients with either pemphigus foliaceus or localized epidermolysis bullosa acquisita.

- The risk of 6 to 12 months of cyclosporine for a patient with limited plaque type psoriasis versus the same regimen in a patient with debilitating and extensive pyoderma gangrenosum.

PRINCIPLE

Choose patients who can comprehend and comply with important instructions for preventing and monitoring the most serious complications of systemic drug therapy. The following are examples where this is most important.

- The importance of avoiding abrupt cessation of long-term, high-dose prednisone therapy—risk of hypothalamic-pituitary-adrenal (HPA) axis complications such as addisonian crisis.
- The pregnancy prevention measures, which are of central importance in isotretinoin therapy for women of childbearing potential.
- Comprehending the importance of avoiding significant amounts of alcohol with long-term methotrexate therapy for severe psoriasis.

PRINCIPLE

All patients are not "created equal" regarding the risk for various adverse effects. Examples of patients who are at significantly increased risk for the following adverse effects (beyond the specifics of the drug regimen) include:

- Methotrexate hepatotoxicity—obesity, alcohol abuse, diabetes mellitus, renal insufficiency.
- Corticosteroid osteoporosis—postmenopausal women, who are thin and inactive.
- Corticosteroid osteonecrosis—recent significant local trauma, alcohol abuse, cigarette smoking, and presence of underlying hypercoagulable conditions.

Patients must be carefully matched with the various drug regimens that can be offered for any given dermatosis. This match hinges on the various risk factors and demographic variables with which a specific patient presents. Perhaps the best example is the lesson provided by the specialty of rheumatology regarding the apparent lesser risk of methotrexate in rheumatoid arthritis patients compared with the risk of the same methotrexate therapy in psoriasis patients.

This risk reduction was accomplished largely through very careful patient selection (regarding the previously mentioned risk factors) concerning who would be eligible to receive methotrexate in various studies.

Patient Education

The multiple variables regarding a given course of systemic drug therapy are often very difficult for physicians to understand. Thus it should come as no surprise that the drug regimens and risks of various therapies are much more difficult for patients (typically without a medical background) to understand. The patient needs to understand at least the following: (1) how to take the medication, regarding dose and timing, (2) expected adverse effects, (3) what symptoms to report, and (4) monitoring required. When significant risks to important organs or body systems are discussed, the understandable emotional reaction of most patients makes long-term retention most difficult. These points and others form the basis of the next principles.

PRINCIPLE

Proper and thorough patient education is essential to truly "*informed*" consent (see Chapter 47).

- Patients need to be active participants in therapeutic decision-making, requiring presentation of the information in an understandable fashion.
- In addition, the patient must be given the chance to ask questions and be given the necessary time to ponder the options.

PRINCIPLE

Use patient handouts, written at a very understandable level, to reinforce important information and instructions. Corollaries to this principle include the following:

- The physician must explain and emphasize the key points contained in the handout—such handouts are never a substitute for appropriate physician-patient communication.
- The patient should be reminded to notify the physician regarding any questions pertinent to the handout given, or for any new symp-

toms that may develop subsequently (even if the patient is not sure these new findings are due to the drug).

- Sources for these handouts include the National Psoriasis Foundation (methotrexate, cyclosporine, and many others), various pharmaceutical companies (acitretin/Soriatane), and the American Medical Association (corticosteroids and many others). Consider creating your own personalized handouts.

PRINCIPLE

Educate your patients regarding groups or clusters of symptoms, which together are important for the detection of potentially serious drug-induced complications. The grouping of these symptoms may not be emphasized in the previously mentioned handouts.

- Corticosteroid osteonecrosis—focal, significant joint pain (especially hip, knee, and shoulder) with decreased range-of-motion of the affected joint.
- Isotretinoin pseudotumor cerebri—headache, visual change, nausea, and vomiting.
- Dapsone hypersensitivity syndrome—fever, fatigue, sore throat, and morbilliform rash.

Open communication between the patient and physician is essential in maximizing the safety of systemic drug therapy. Any extra time the physician spends in this communication process typically pays great dividends in regards to improved therapeutic outcomes.

Baseline Laboratory and Related Tests

Any organ system with potential for drug-induced complications needs a baseline assessment before initiating therapy. Exceptions to this principle are few and far between. Pre-existing pathology in an organ or body system, for which a given drug has the potential to induce problems, will increase the likelihood of further injury to this same organ.

PRINCIPLE

Assess the baseline status of any potential target organ or site of excretion for a given drug. Similarly, if a drug can induce a metabolic ab-

normality, check for baseline presence of this metabolic defect.

- Baseline liver function tests and hepatitis viral serology—methotrexate hepatotoxicity (methotrexate "target" organ).
- Baseline renal function assessment; at least creatinine, possibly creatinine clearance—methotrexate hepatotoxicity or pancytopenia (site of methotrexate excretion).
- Baseline eye examination for presence of cataracts—psoralen plus ultraviolet A (PUVA) therapy (PUVA "target" organ).
- Baseline testing for hyperglycemia or hyperlipidemia—prednisone therapy (metabolic abnormalities aggravated by prednisone).

PRINCIPLE

Utilize the most optimal available tests that predict which patients are at increased risk for a specific adverse effect. Typically such tests are ordered only at baseline. (Ideally many more of these predictive tests will be available in the future.)

- Baseline glucose-6-phosphate dehydrogenase (G6PD) level—predicts magnitude of risk for dapsone hemolysis. (This test does not predict dapsone agranulocytosis or hypersensitivity syndrome risk.)
- Baseline thiopurine methyltransferase level—predicts risk for azathioprine hematologic complications, as well as helping to optimize drug dosing. (This test does not predict azathioprine hepatotoxicity or hypersensitivity syndrome reactions.)

There are a few select tests for which a baseline determination is not required. Near the end of long-term high-dose prednisone therapy, an A.M. cortisol determination may be of value in assessing HPA axis function; a baseline determination is virtually never indicated. Some tests may require a delayed baseline determination. A "delayed baseline" ultrasound-guided liver biopsy can be used for methotrexate patients after 6 to 9 months of therapy, once it is clear that the patient tolerates the drug, benefits from the drug, and requires long-term methotrexate therapy. Still the general rule holds—if planning on following a specific test during therapy with a given systemic drug, it is prudent to determine the baseline status of that test.

Concomitant Drug Therapy— Drug Interactions

Chapter 44 is devoted entirely to the subject of drug interactions of importance to the dermatologist and other physicians using similar medications. Still a few principles must be addressed in this setting. The vast majority of drug interactions can be anticipated and thus prevented. Truly life-threatening drug interactions are quite uncommon, and virtually always have been well publicized. The next principles deal with three categories of drug interactions of central importance to maximizing the safety of systemic drug therapy.

PRINCIPLE

Avoid drug combinations that have overlapping sites/target organs of potential toxicity.

- Tetracycline or minocycline plus isotretinoin—pseudotumor cerebri.
- Hydroxychloroquine plus chloroquine—antimalarial retinopathy. (It is acceptable practice to combine quinacrine with either of these two drugs—quinacrine alone does not induce a retinopathy.)
- Methotrexate and a second-generation retinoid (previously etretinate, now acitretin)—probably an increased risk for hepatotoxicity.

PRINCIPLE

Anticipate and avoid interactions involving drugs that alter the same metabolic pathway.

- Methotrexate and trimethoprim/sulfamethoxazole—increased risk for pancytopenia, given that all three drugs affect folate metabolism.
- Azathioprine and allopurinol—increased risk for hematologic complications because these drugs affect parallel purine metabolic pathways.

PRINCIPLE

Anticipate and avoid drug combinations that are metabolized by the same cytochrome P-450

(CYP) pathway, particularly if there is a narrow therapeutic index for one of the drugs involved.

- Rifampin (CYP-enzyme inducer) plus oral contraceptives—loss of efficacy of the contraceptive with potential for unintentional pregnancy.
- Ketoconazole or erythromycin (CYP-enzyme inhibitors) plus cyclosporine—increased risk for toxicity due to increased cyclosporine blood levels.

This area of medicine is very complicated, and it is difficult to stay current (see Chapter 44). Recently released drugs at times have important, potentially life-threatening interactions, which are only discovered several years after the release of the medication. The potential for torsades de pointes with life-threatening dysrhythmias from terfenadine, astemizole, or cisapride (elucidated several years after the drugs' release) in the presence of certain CYP-enzyme inhibitors illustrates this point. The physician should stay current and liberally utilize the numerous electronic resources for information on drug interactions. Frequent utilization of the physician's hospital's drug information pharmacists to deal with this challenging area of medicine is recommended.

Evolving Guidelines—Risk Factors

Typically, with the passage of time, the magnitude of risk for various systemic drugs becomes clarified. The level of concern can go in either of two directions—either increased concern or decreased concern with the availability of new data. Furthermore, specific new risk factors can be elucidated as new scientific information is reported.

PRINCIPLE

Certain risks or risk factors for systemic therapies may be discovered many years after a specific drug is released. It is imperative to be aware of changing standards of care.

- PUVA therapy presents an increased risk for squamous cell carcinoma of the male genitalia (specific risk factor—male gender, without clothing protection of the groin region during PUVA treatments).
- PUVA-induced melanoma—probably an in-

creased risk in patients receiving more than 250 to 350 treatments over a lifetime (specific risk factor—very large number of PUVA treatments).

- Minocycline hypersensitivity syndrome or minocycline-induced lupus erythematosus—the magnitude of risk for these complications was not clarified until over a decade after the drug's release.
- Ketoconazole hepatotoxicity—magnitude of risk overall and potential for fatal outcomes were not clarified until several years after the drug's release.

PRINCIPLE
In contrast, the magnitude of risk for a particular adverse effect may decrease over time as new scientific evidence accumulates.

- Antimalarial retinopathy—markedly lower risk than originally perceived, largely due to more careful antimalarial dosing schemes, and perhaps also due to greater use of hydroxychloroquine over chloroquine.
- PUVA cataracts—primarily a risk in patients who fail to comply with current regimens regarding ultraviolet A (UVA) protective wraparound sunglasses.
- Prednisone bursts and osteonecrosis risk—although this issue is still cloudy in the legal system, the scientific evidence "rules against" there being a true risk of this bone complication with short courses ("bursts") of systemic corticosteroids.

As challenging as it may be, physicians are obligated to stay informed of the latest information on the magnitude of risk from the drugs utilized. Truly important "new risks" tend to be widely and repeatedly disseminated to physicians, with the "Dear Doctor" letters from the FDA being a common vehicle for such dissemination of information.

PREVENTION
Patient Measures
PRINCIPLE
Our patients should utilize all reasonable protective measures to prevent important adverse effects.

- Prevention of squamous cell carcinoma of male genitalia due to PUVA therapy—wearing a "jock strap" or underwear during a PUVA treatment (newer recommended precaution).
- Prevention of cataracts in PUVA therapy—wearing opaque goggles during the PUVA treatment and wearing wrap-around UVA protective sunglasses when exposed to outdoor light at least until sundown the day of the treatment (long-standing requirement).

Therapeutic Interventions to Minimize Drug Risk
There are many occasions in which the patient would benefit from a specific systemic drug, yet there are worrisome risk factors for a given adverse effect. If the drug regimen is essential for the patient, concomitant medical therapy to reduce the risk of the adverse effect is logical and appropriate in most cases.

PRINCIPLE
Physicians should utilize all reasonable adjunctive therapeutic measures to minimize the risk of various adverse effects.

- Daily folic acid therapy in patients receiving methotrexate—prevention of gastrointestinal (GI) adverse effects and to minimize pancytopenia risk. (Ideally, folic acid should be used in all methotrexate patients.)
- Calcium, vitamin D, and possibly estrogens, bisphosphonates, or nasal calcitonin in patients receiving long-term systemic corticosteroid therapy above physiologic doses. (Utilize a greater number of these options in higher risk patients.)

Timing of Risk and Medication Errors
The steps for prevention of many adverse effects require either heightened awareness with more frequent monitoring (drugs with a specific timing of greatest risk) or careful patient education (for potentially serious medication errors). In either setting, a proactive style is preferred to maximize safety.

PRINCIPLE
For the most potentially serious adverse effects from systemic drugs, physicians should learn

the timing of greatest risk for the drug-induced complication and monitor the patient most carefully during this time period.

- Dapsone agranulocytosis or hypersensitivity syndrome—both primarily an issue between weeks 3 and 12 of therapy. (Minocycline hypersensitivity syndrome is a risk in the same interval, leaning towards the first 2 months of therapy.)
- Methotrexate or azathioprine pancytopenia—the risk is greatest primarily in the first 4 to 6 weeks of therapy, unless a drug interaction is a precipitating factor later in the course of therapy.
- Prednisone osteonecrosis—the risk begins to increase substantially by months 2 to 3 of pharmacologic dose corticosteroid therapy. (This risk tends to parallel the overall development of cushingoid changes in the patient.)

PRINCIPLE

Medication errors are largely preventable with careful patient education and, if necessary, cross-checks on potentially unreliable patients. These medication errors can be due to either dose omissions or dose duplications.

- Methotrexate weekly dosing scheme—the literature has many reports of pancytopenia due to inadvertent daily dosing of methotrexate. If necessary, another caregiver or family member should place the drug in the slot for just one specified day in weekly pill containers, particularly for older patients.
- Oral contraceptives and isotretinoin or thalidomide—pregnancy prevention is critical in women of childbearing potential. Omissions of oral contraceptives for even a day can be hazardous in women using these potent teratogens.

DIAGNOSIS
Evolving Guidelines for Monitoring

As previously discussed, newer scientific evidence leads to new or revised guidelines regarding standards of care. As before, the level of concern can increase or decrease when this new scientific information is released.

PRINCIPLE

Physicians should be aware of new guidelines for diagnosing important complications of systemic drug therapy at an early, reversible stage.

- Methotrexate: chest x-rays for pneumonitis—pneumonitis from methotrexate is a significant risk in rheumatoid arthritis patients. In contrast, the negligible risk for this complication in psoriasis patients led to elimination of this yearly requirement for chest x-rays in more recent guidelines.
- Systemic corticosteroids: baseline chest x-ray with a tuberculin skin test—the recent resurgence in incidence of tuberculosis has led many authors to suggest that baseline screening for tuberculosis be performed before long-term, pharmacologic dose prednisone therapy.

A Teamwork Approach to Maximizing the Safety of Drug Therapy

In spite of recent trends of managed care to fragment care and limit access to various medical specialties in the name of cost savings, a teamwork approach for risk reduction is imperative. A "team" consisting of the prescribing physician, the patient, and, in many circumstances, the patient's primary physician or another specialist is of central importance. Each member of the team has an important role in maximizing the safety of systemic drug therapy.

PRINCIPLE

In addition to the importance of the patient's awareness to report symptoms suggesting the early phases of selected complications, the patient often has a role in home monitoring for selected complications.

- Cyclosporine or corticosteroids and hypertension—with a growing number of patients utilizing home blood pressure cuffs or electronic blood pressure monitoring devices, this is a relatively easy area of home surveillance for adverse effects. The patient merely needs to be told what levels of blood pressure elevation should be reported to the prescribing physician.
- Corticosteroids and blood sugar monitoring—even though the history of diabetes

mellitus should lead to careful consideration regarding the necessity of systemic corticosteroids, there are many circumstances in which prednisone therapy is essential. Home glucose monitoring provides easy surveillance and follow-up.

- Corticosteroids and weight gain—the simple bathroom scale can provide useful information on the progression of cushingoid changes or on signs of increasing fluid overload in patients with previously well compensated congestive heart failure.

PRINCIPLE

The prescribing physician's examination is essential for detection or verification of important early signs for various drug complications.

- Full skin examination for PUVA therapy—detection of melanoma, squamous cell carcinoma, and basal cell carcinoma (and precursors thereof).
- Neurologic examination (screening style) for dapsone motor neuropathy or thalidomide sensory neuropathy—screening done by the prescribing physician, possibly verified by a consultant.
- Morbilliform eruption and related hypersensitivity syndrome findings due to dapsone, minocycline, or azathioprine—reported by the patient, but verified by the prescribing physician.

PRINCIPLE

Co-management with another consultant is commonly an essential part of this teamwork approach to maximizing the safety of systemic drug therapy.

- Renal consultation—important for long-term cyclosporine therapy (ideally for cyclosporine therapy over 6 to 12 months duration) to follow more precise tests of glomerular filtration rate and assist with dosing decisions.
- Interventional radiologist—for ultrasound-guided liver biopsies with long-term methotrexate therapy.
- Ophthalmologist—integral part of monitor-

ing guidelines for PUVA and antimalarial therapy.
- Primary physician—for management decisions regarding elevated blood sugar or blood pressure with corticosteroid therapy or for management of hyperlipidemia in patients on long-term systemic retinoid therapy.

Utilizing the Most Optimal Diagnostic Tests
PRINCIPLE

Physicians should be aware of the most optimal diagnostic tests that improve sensitivity and precision for early diagnosis of important adverse effects at a reversible stage.

- Corticosteroid osteonecrosis diagnosis—magnetic resonance imaging is superior to standard x-rays for early diagnosis, which can allow timely performance of core decompression to salvage the affected joint.
- Corticosteroid osteoporosis diagnosis—single and dual photon absorptiometry (Dexascans) have much better sensitivity compared with standard x-rays for early recognition of bone density loss.
- Methotrexate hepatotoxicity diagnosis—ultrasound-guided liver biopsies provide much greater technical precision for avoiding large vessels and bile ducts, thus providing greater safety for liver biopsies.

PRINCIPLE

Physicians should realize that many diagnostic tests provide complementary information.

- Transaminase values and liver histology for methotrexate hepatotoxicity—one set of tests (transaminases) assesses hepatocellular toxicity, whereas the other (liver biopsy/histology) assesses the potential for slow progression from fatty liver to fibrosis to cirrhosis; both tests are essential.
- Ordering both transaminases (SGOT/AST and SGPT/AST) for dapsone, azathioprine, and methotrexate hepatotoxicity—improved sensitivity and specificity when ordering both tests; furthermore, tests for hepatobiliary obstruction (bilirubin, alkaline phosphatase,

γ-glutamyl-transferase [GGT]) can be useful adjuncts if significant transaminase elevation has occurred.

Higher Risk Scenarios

As discussed earlier, all patients are not created equal when it comes to risk factors for adverse effects from systemic drug therapy. The more the physician knows about high-risk scenarios (with corresponding increased surveillance for adverse effects in these settings), the more the physician can maximize the safety of the drug therapy in that particular patient.

PRINCIPLE

Laboratory monitoring and related diagnostic tests should be performed more frequently (1) with higher risk patients, (2) with abnormal test results, and (3) at high-risk periods of time—typically early in therapy.

PRINCIPLE

Become familiar with *thresholds of concern* (levels at which to consider dose reduction and/or more frequent monitoring) and *critical values* (levels at which therapy should be stopped, possibly indefinitely) for various laboratory tests and related monitoring procedures (Table 2-1).

Clinicians should realize that these are merely rough guidelines. The rapidity of change and the overall trend of the laboratory values are of at least equal importance to recognize. Regardless of the actual laboratory test abnormality or the rapidity of change, the clinician should be mindful of the following four possible options (depending on the clinical circumstances in an individual patient): (1) discontinue the drug therapy temporarily or indefinitely, (2) reduce the drug dose, (3) increase the frequency of monitoring, and (4) treat the adverse effect while carefully continuing the therapy with frequent monitoring. These are not mutually exclusive options; generally several of the above steps are instituted simultaneously. Again, the key is to know which circumstances constitute a high-risk clinical scenario and proceed more carefully in these settings.

Efficient Record Keeping

It is quite difficult keeping track of scientific advancements related to dermatologic therapeutics. It is at least an equal challenge to keep track of several aspects of medical record keeping for the four general steps of maximizing safety presented in this chapter. Some of the issues here include: (1) documenting informed consent discussions, (2) the changing frequency of laboratory tests any given patient should have, depending on the stage of therapy and the dose of the drug, (3) keeping track of which patients did not get laboratory tests performed when scheduled, (4) notifying patients about laboratory test results, particularly abnormal results, and the resultant algorithm regarding how to respond to these abnormal re-

---

■ **Table 2-1**   Thresholds of Concern and Critical Value for Selected Diagnostic Tests

	Threshold of Concern	Critical Value
WBC count	<3500/mm^3	<2500-3000/mm^3
Hemoglobin	10-11 g/dl	<10 g/dl
Platelet count	<100,000/mm^3	<50,000/mm^3
Triglycerides	>400-500 mg/dl	>700-800 mg/dl
Creatinine	30% increase from baseline value	>40% to 50% increase from the baseline value
SGOT/SGPT	1.5-2.0 times increase above the upper-normal value	>2.5-3.0 increase above the upper normal value
Dexascan	T-score: −1.0 to −2.5	T-score: −2.5 or less

sults, and (5) how to efficiently document steps (2) through (4) above.

Fortunately the electronic/information era has provided some solutions. Many practitioners previously kept written test result flow sheets on patients. Now, most laboratories can print computer-generated flow sheets of test results. If a clinician can readily find the last 2 to 3 sets of test results, most decision making proceeds without much difficulty. There should be a cross-check system regarding missed appointments and missed laboratory tests for patients on systemic therapy. In general it is helpful to have a patient call about test results (in a specified time frame) if not previously notified by mail or phone calls from the physician's office about the test results. A less time consuming step is a policy that normal test results do not require notification of the patient. The reality is that even with normal test results, commonly the physician (or physician's staff) must contact the patient regarding drug dose increases and thus the need to document and to communicate this decision.

The following principles need to be listed, although some overlap with other chapters (such as Chapter 47).

PRINCIPLE

An important medicolegal dictum states that "if it was not written, it was not done." An individual physician needs to find a balance of thoroughness and efficiency. Dictated chart notes allow this optimal balance—voice recognition software could make thorough documentation in an efficient manner even more achievable.

PRINCIPLE

When possible, with relatively high-risk medications, create backup systems in case the patient, the physician, the office staff, or the laboratory personnel have (hopefully rare) understandable oversights.

PRINCIPLE

Utilize any electronic means available to keep track of important information needed to maximize the safety of systemic drug therapy.

MANAGEMENT
What to Do if Problems Arise
RELATIVELY MINOR COMPLICATIONS.   The vast majority of complications from systemic drug therapy are relatively minor and are fixable. If communication channels are kept open, the physician remains nondefensive and if a solutions-based approach is utilized, keeping the patient's best interests in mind, serious medical complications and adverse medicolegal outcomes are most unlikely. This section addresses a general approach to managing adverse effects if the "anticipation" and "prevention" steps are not fully successful. Parenthetically, these same principles apply to any complication of topical or intralesional therapy as well.

PRINCIPLE

When in doubt, have the patient *stop* the *drug* in question if a potentially serious adverse effect has occurred. The physician generally has at least a few days (having discontinued the drug) to consider the management options and to communicate with consultants. Factors in this decision making include:

- The severity of the disease being treated.
- The magnitude of risk from the adverse effect the patient experienced, particularly if the complication can have a precipitous progression with continuation of the responsible drug.
- Whether the drug in question is uniquely effective for the disease being treated.
- Whether there is a significant risk due to abrupt discontinuation of the responsible drug—most notably the risk of abrupt cessation of high-dose, long-term systemic corticosteroid therapy and the potential for an addisonian crisis.

PRINCIPLE

With less serious medical complications in the setting of a systemic drug that is essential for the patient, specific medical therapy directed at this complication is quite acceptable.

- Retinoid or corticosteroid hyperlipidemia—concomitant treatment with HMG-CoA reductase inhibitors, fenofibrate, or gemfibrozil.

- Corticosteroid or cyclosporine hypertension—any of a wide variety of medical options for blood pressure control. The physician should be mindful of the need to have the therapeutic choice for cyclosporine-induced hypertension preserve renal blood flow as well.

POTENTIALLY SERIOUS COMPLICATIONS
PRINCIPLE
More serious complications generally have a specific remedy, although frequently these management steps come at significant cost or present a life-long risk to the patient. Avoidance of these complications remains the top priority.

- Corticosteroid osteonecrosis—core decompression (if diagnosed relatively early) or joint replacement surgery (if there is more advanced osteonecrosis).
- Methotrexate pancytopenia—if recognized early, leucovorin "rescue" will be quite effective, as is routinely done for high-dose methotrexate therapy in oncology settings.
- Methotrexate, ketoconazole, dapsone liver failure—worst-case scenario may require a liver transplantation.
- Corticosteroid or PUVA cataracts—this outcome is far less catastrophic than even a decade ago, given the availability of safe and predictable lens implants after cataract extraction.

PRINCIPLE
A few complications cannot be fixed and should be *avoided* at all costs.

- Retinoid or thalidomide teratogenesis—absolute and complete prevention is essential.
- Antimalarial retinopathy—although scientific evidence from therapeutic approaches used in the current era downplays the likelihood of this complication.

SUMMARY

Optimally, physicians reading this chapter should use these principles and *never* have a major com-plication from systemic drug therapy in their respective careers. However, this is not likely. The mindset that is more realistic goes as follows:

1. The physician should thoroughly learn the measures necessary to *anticipate* risk factors and *prevent* important complications of systemic drug therapy.
2. The important adverse effects, which infrequently still occur in spite of these steps, should be *diagnosed* at an early and reversible stage through the principles discussed here.
3. Once diagnosed, these complications of therapy should be vigorously *managed* in a proactive fashion, utilizing any consultants necessary and keeping the patients best interests in mind.
4. The more serious and less reversible the complication is, the greater the efforts should be to make sure that this complication *never occurs* (with retinoid or thalidomide teratogenesis as the prototypes).
5. With a proactive mindset for the thorough prevention of and monitoring for adverse effects and a true therapeutic partnership with the patient, the risk for medicolegal consequences of drug therapy becomes quite negligible.
6. Should a serious complication occur (and it almost inevitably will eventually in any physician's career) the most *functional* and *professional approach* has three parts:
   - "Stand by" and work with the patient, regardless of the circumstances.
   - In all ways possible, learn anything possible from the undesirable therapeutic outcome.
   - Focus on the multitudes of patients who have benefited from (and will benefit from) the same drug or therapeutic approach throughout the physician's career.

The gratification that patients and physicians receive from successful outcomes of carefully planned and monitored systemic drug therapy is immense. Physicians should utilize these principles, which are reinforced by further supporting details provided throughout this book.

Bibliography*

Wolverton SE: Major adverse effects from systemic drugs: defining the risks. *Curr Probl Dermatol* 7:1-40, 1995.

Wolverton SE: Monitoring for adverse effects from systemic drugs. In Wolverton SE, Wilkin JK, editors: *Systemic drugs for skin diseases*, Philadelphia, 1991, WB Saunders, pp 385-399.

Wolverton SE: Monitoring for adverse effects from systemic drugs used in dermatology (CME article). *J Am Acad Dermatol* 26:661-679, 1992.

Wolverton SE: Systemic drugs for psoriasis. The most critical issues. *Arch Dermatol* 127:565-568, 1991.

*In addition, the reader is encouraged to consult the various American Academy of Dermatology Guidelines of Care that have been published.

PART II

Systemic Drugs for Infectious Diseases

CHAPTER 3

Neil S. Sadick

Systemic Antibacterial Agents

Antimicrobial agents play an important role in dermatologic practice. When selecting an antimicrobial agent, the dermatologist needs to consider multiple factors, including the host (e.g., pregnancy, underlying disease, age, allergy), the causative pathogen (resistance profile, virulence), and the specific drug (route of administration, dosing, toxicity, plasma and tissue levels, cost, and interaction with other medications). The ever-changing spectrum of newer systemic antimicrobial agents, as well as ever-changing resistance patterns, makes knowledge of these factors very important. The dermatologist must be aware of the adverse effects of antimicrobial agents, as well as various drug interactions that may influence the choice of a drug and specific dosage schedules. In addition, the dermatologist also must be aware that adverse reactions may be more common and severe in immunocompromised patients. More appropriate utilization of these antibacterial agents is possible with a better understanding of the antimicrobial agents presently available.

PENICILLINS

Penicillins inhibit bacterial cell wall synthesis, which leads to unbalanced growth or activation of autolytic enzymes, with resultant bacterial death.[1] Cephalosporins have a similar mechanism of action. Various penicillin-binding proteins and enzymes involved in cell wall metabolism may be affected in different ways by the various antibiotics in this group. In most cases the specific bacterial events are not known.[2]

The first advance over penicillin G for oral therapy was the development of penicillin V (phenoxymethyl penicillin). Penicillin V is more resistant to gastric acid and better absorbed from the gastrointestinal tract than penicillin G (Figure 3-1).

Dicloxacillin is unsurpassed as an oral β-lactamase-resistant penicillin. Oxacillin, cloxacillin, and floxacillin are the other orally effective isoxazolyl penicillins[3] (Table 3-1). The aminopenicillins, amoxicillin and ampicillin, are also of central importance to dermatology.

Antimicrobial Activity

Penicillin V shares the spectrum of penicillin G, although it is less active against some gram-negative organisms, particularly the *Neisseria* species.[4] Ampicillin and amoxicillin are hydrolyzed by β-lactamases, and thus these drugs are not effective against *Staphylococcus aureus* or the many *Enterobacteriaceae* species that make β-lactamases. Of these two antibiotics, amoxicillin is the superior drug with better absorption, less diarrhea, and comparable efficacy. Third- and fourth-generation penicillins, the so-called extended-spectrum penicillins, are

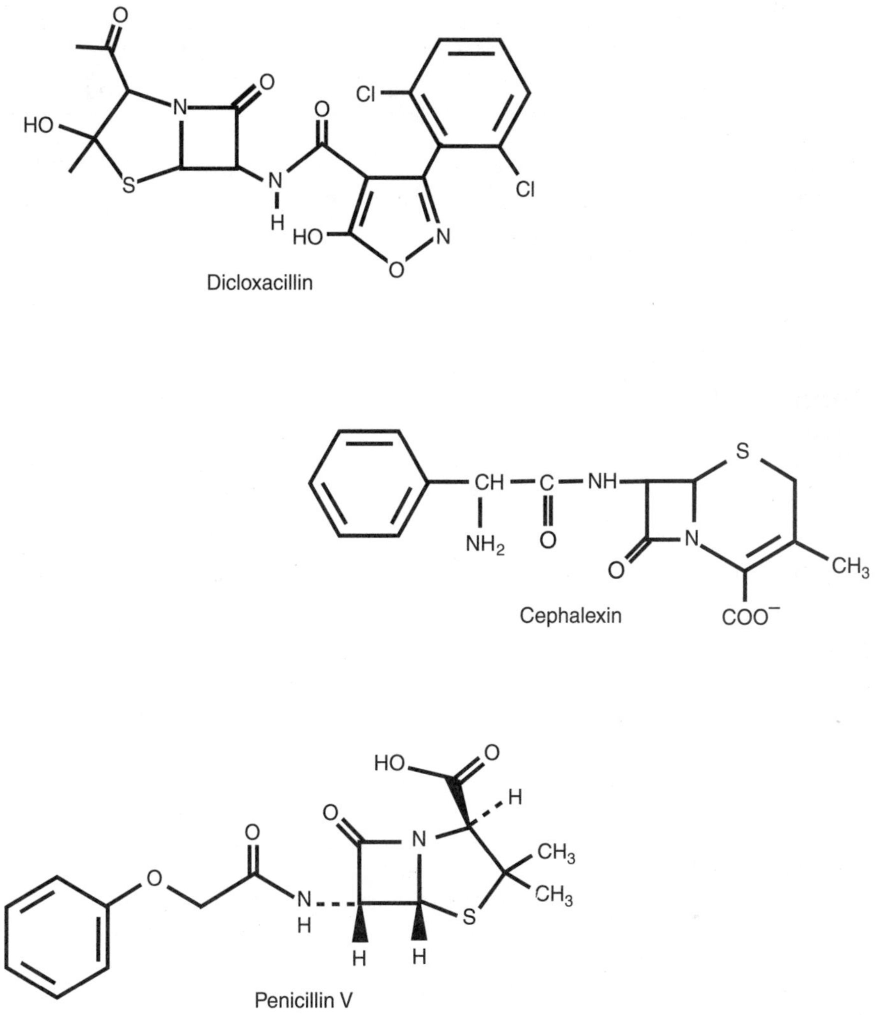

Dicloxacillin

Cephalexin

Penicillin V

Figure 3-1 Systemic antibacterial agents—β-lactam.

many times more potent than the common penicillins against gram-negative microbes.

Pharmacokinetics

Of the β-lactamase–resistant penicillins available for oral use, dicloxacillin is considered to have the best pharmacologic properties. It can be given in doses exceeding 4 g daily. Very high doses can be achieved particularly with concurrent probenecid administration. It is best taken on an empty stomach. A dosage of 2 g daily is adequate for the majority of staphylococcal pyodermas.

Dermatologic Indications

Pyodermas are commonly treated by this class of drugs. Isoxazolyl penicillin shows good cov-

erage for *Streptococcus pyogenes* and *S. aureus*. Either ampicillin or amoxicillin can be a first-line drug for treatment of gonorrhea, *Haemophilus influenzae* infections, and occasionally for other gram-negative infections. For gonorrhea, one of the aminopenicillins may be given as a single-dose treatment (3.5 g for ampicillin and 3 g for amoxicillin) along with probenecid. For other gram-negative infections, a daily dose of 2 to 4 g divided in three or four dosages is given with probenecid if high blood levels are required.

Adverse Effects

Hypersensitivity reactions are the most common adverse effects with the use of penicillins.

◼ **Table 3-1** Currently Available Antibacterial Agents—Penicillins

Generic Name	Trade Name(s)	Routes
NATURAL PENICILLINS		
Penicillin G	None	PO, IM, IV
Penicillin V	PenVee K, V-cillin K	PO
AMINOPENICILLINS		
Ampicillin	Principen	PO, IM, IV
Amoxicillin	Amoxil, Polymax, Larotid	PO
PENICILLINASE-RESISTANT PENICILLINS (ISOXAZOLYL PENICILLINS)		
Dicloxacillin	Dynapen	PO
Cloxacillin	Tegopen	PO, IM, IV
Oxacillin	Bactocill	PO
Nafcillin	Unipen	IM, IV
EXTENDED-SPECTRUM PENICILLINS (CARBOXYPENICILLINS)		
Carbenicillin	Geocillin	PO
Ticarcillin	Ticar	IM, IV
EXTENDED-SPECTRUM PENICILLINS (UREIDOPENICILLINS)		
Azlocillin	Azlin	IV
Mezlocillin	Mezlin	IM, IV
Piperacillin	Pipracil, Pipral	IM, IV
COMBINATION WITH β-LACTAMASE INHIBITORS		
Amoxacillin/clavulanate	Augmentin	PO
Ticarcillin/clavulanate	Timentin	IV
Ampicillin/sulbactam	Unasyn	IV
Piperacillin/tazobactam	Zosyn	IV

◼ **Table 3-2** Commonly Used Oral Penicillins*—Dosage Guidelines

Generic Name	Tab/Caps Sizes	Adult Dosage	Price Index
Penicillin V	250, 500 mg	250-500 mg qid	$ ($)
Ampicillin	250, 500 mg	250-500 mg qid	—
Amoxicillin	250, 500 mg	250-500 mg bid†	$ ($)
Dicloxacillin	250, 500 mg	125-500 mg qid	$/$$ ($)
Cloxacillin	250, 500 mg	250-500 mg qid	—
Oxacillin	250, 500 mg	500-1000 mg q4-6h	—
Amoxicillin/clavulanate	250, 500, 875 mg	500-875 mg bid†	$$$

$, <1.00; $$, 1.01-2.00; $$$, 2.01-5.00; $$$$, 5.01-10.00; $$$$$, >10.00; ( ), generic price; /, two different price ranges from lower dose to higher dose examples of this drug; —, no price listed for this drug.
*All of the drugs in this table have either liquid or suspension formulations available.
†Note: This drug can also be dosed 250-500 mg tid.

The severity of these reactions may range from fatal anaphylaxis through urticaria to morbilliform eruptions.[5,6]

For practical purposes it should be assumed that all of the penicillins cross-react and that if a patient has an allergic reaction to one form of penicillin, he or she will react to all penicillins and possibly to cephalosporins.[7] The aminopenicillins have a higher incidence of allergic reactions than do other penicillins.[8] Intradermal testing with benzyl penicillin G and penicilloyl polylysine (Pre-pen) may be helpful. If an immediate cutaneous reaction does not occur, it is highly unlikely that an immediate or accelerated reaction will occur on administration of the penicillin.

Except for gastrointestinal disturbances, other untoward reactions to penicillin are unusual, especially with oral forms of the medication. Hemolytic anemia, seizures, and electrolyte disturbances are seen only with very large doses of a parenteral drug.[9] Hepatitis and intestinal nephritis are seen rarely with the semisynthetic penicillins.

Dosage

Table 3-2 contains dosage guidelines for commonly used oral penicillins.

CEPHALOSPORINS

The structure of the cephalosporins resembles penicillin. The cephalosporins consist of a 4-membered β-lactam ring attached to a 6-membered dihydrothiazine ring (Figure 3-1). This gives the structure inherent resistance to β-lactamase.[10] As with penicillins, the cephalosporins inhibit a series of enzymes, known as penicillin-binding proteins, that catalyze important steps in the formation of the bacterial cell wall. These enzymes vary from species to species.[11]

Antimicrobial Activity

The cephalosporins have been grouped into "generations" based on their general antimicrobial activity[12] (Table 3-3). *First-generation* cephalosporins are the most active of all the cephalosporins against staphylococci and nonenterococcal streptococci. Methicillin-resistant *S. aureus* (MRSA) and penicillin-resistant *Streptococcus pneumoniae* are usually resistant to these agents. These drugs have less reliable activity

against gram-negative organisms including *H. influenzae* and enterococci.[13] They are active against many of the oral anaerobes but the *Bacteroides fragilis* group are resistant. The in vitro activity of these first-generation agents is almost identical.

Second-generation cephalosporins have increased gram-negative activity but decreased gram-positive activity. Individual agents vary greatly in their spectrum of activity. These agents are often classified into two groups—the true cephalosporins and the cephamycins (cefoxitin, cefotetan). The true cephalosporins have increased activity against *H. influenzae*, *Moraxella catarrhalis*, *Neisseria meningitidis*, *Neisseria gonorrhoeae*, and some *Enterobacteriaceae* organisms. The cephamycins have inferior activity against staphylococci and streptococci. All cephamycins have moderate activity against strains of *B. fragilis*.[14]

Third-generation cephalosporins demonstrate less consistent activity against gram-positive organisms and an increased spectrum of gram-negative activity. This is because of greater β-lactamase stability.[15] Agents such as ceftazidime, cefepime, and cefoperazone have increased antipseudomonal coverage. Ceftazidime has the greatest activity against *Pseudomonas aeruginosa*.

Pharmacokinetics

Absorption properties of the currently available cephalosporins vary greatly. The highest peak serum concentrations depend on their administration in relationship to intake of food. Cefaclor, cefadroxil, cephalexin, and cephradine are best absorbed from an empty stomach. Cefuroxime axetil's bioavailability is increased when taken with food.[16] First- and second-generation cephalosporins are excreted primarily by the kidney; thus dosage adjustments are required for patients with renal insufficiency. Cefixime has significant hepatic elimination. The half-life of most parenterally administered cephalosporins varies between 0.5 and 2 hours. Only ceftriaxone has both renal and hepatic excretion, so dosing does not need to be adjusted for renal insufficiency.[17]

Dermatologic Indications

Cephalosporins are used primarily in dermatologic practice in treating soft tissue infections

■ **Table 3-3**   Currently Available Antibacterial Agents—Cephalosporins

Generic Name	Trade Name(s)	Route
FIRST GENERATION		
Cephalexin	Keflex, Keftab, Biocef	PO
Cephradrine	Velocef, Anspor	PO, IM, IV
Cefadroxil	Duracef, Ultracef	PO
Cephalothin	Keflin	IV
Cefazolin	Ancef, Kefzol	IM, IV
Cephaprin	Cefadyl	IM, IV
SECOND GENERATION		
Cefaclor	Ceclor	PO
Loracarbef	Lorabid	PO
Cefprozil	Cefzil	PO
Cefuroxime axetil	Ceftin	PO
Cefamandole	Mandol	IM, IV
Cefonicid	Monocid	IM, IV
THIRD GENERATION		
Cefpodoxime proxetil	Vantin	PO
Ceftibuten	Cedax	PO
Cefixime	Suprax	PO
Cefotaxime	Claforan	IM, IV
Ceftizoxime	Cefizox	IM, IV
Ceftriaxone	Rocephin	IM, IV
Cefoperozone	Cefobid	IM, IV
Ceftazidime	Fortaz, Tazidime	IM, IV
Cefepime	Maxipime	IM, IV
CEPHAMYCINS		
Cefoxitin	Mefoxin	IM, IV
Cefotetan	Cefotan	IM, IV

such as impetigo, folliculitis, furuncles, carbuncles, cellulitis, ecthyma, erysipelas, postoperative wound infections, and necrotizing fasciitis.[17-19] Table 3-4 contains commonly used cephalosporins as well as dosage guidelines.

Second-generation agents have been efficacious in treating gram-negative cellulitis caused by *H. influenzae* or *Enterobacteriaceae* organisms. Cefuroxime axetil can be used to treat selective cases of Lyme borreliosis.[20] Third-generation agents have also been used in the treatment of soft tissue abscesses and diabetic foot ulcers.[21]

Ceftazidime has been effective in the treatment of *Pseudomonas aeruginosa* infections including ecthyma gangrenosum, diabetic ulcers, diabetic foot ulcers, and infections in burn patients.[22]

Drug Interactions

Certain cephalosporins (cefamandole, cefotetan, and cefoperazone) contain an *N*-methyl-thiotetrazole (NMTT) ring and may induce disulfiram reactions with alcohol ingestion.[23] This same NMTT ring can also prolong prothrombin times, which is a consideration in patients on anticoagulation therapy.[24]

Adverse Effects

Gastrointestinal (GI) toxicity includes nausea, vomiting, diarrhea, and pseudomembranous colitis. Mild elevation of liver enzymes and an association between biliary tract sludge formation and the use of ceftriaxone have been reported.[25]

Hypersensitivity eruptions including urticaria, maculopapular eruptions, and pruritus

■ Table 3-4   Commonly Used Oral Cephalosporins*—Dosage Guidelines

Generic Name	Tab/Caps Sizes	Adult Dosage	Price Index
Cephalexin	250, 500 mg	250-500 mg qid	$$/$$$ ($/$$)
Cephradrine	250, 500 mg	250-500 mg qid	$/$$ ($/$$)
Cefadroxil	500, 1000 mg	1-2 g/d (qd or bid)	$$$/$$$$ ($$$)
Cefaclor	250, 375,† 500 mg	250-500 mg tid	$$/$$$ ($$$)
Loracarbef	200, 400 mg	200-400 mg bid	$$$
Cefprozil	250, 500 mg	250-500 mg/d (qd or bid)	$$$/$$$$
Cefuroxime axetil	125, 250, 500 mg	250-500 mg bid	$$$$
Cefpodoxime proxetil	100, 200 mg	100-400 mg bid	$$$
Ceftibuten	400 mg	400 mg qd	$$$$
Cefixime	200, 400 mg	200 mg bid or 400 mg qd	$$$/$$$$

$, <1.00; $$, 1.01-2.00; $$$, 2.01-5.00; $$$$, 5.01-10.00; $$$$$, >10.00; ( ), generic price; /, two different price ranges from lower dose to higher dose examples of this drug; —, no price listed for this drug.
*All of the drugs listed in this table have either liquid or suspension formulations available.
†Extended-release formulation.

have been reported in 1% to 3% of treated individuals. Approximately 5% to 10% of patients allergic to penicillin will also be allergic to cephalosporins.[26] It is recommended that patients with a history of immediate or accelerated reaction to penicillin (type 1-IgE mediated or severe type IV delayed hypersensitivity reactions) not be treated with cephalosporins.[27] An increased incidence of serum sickness in children receiving cefaclor has been noted.[28]

Local reactions such as thrombophlebitis or pain at injection sites have been described in 1% to 5% of cephalosporin-treated patients.[29]

Hematologic reactions including Coombs' antibody positivity have been reported in cephalosporin-treated patients although hemolytic anemia is rare.[30,31] Eosinophilia and neutropenia have been reported sporadically.[32]

Dosage
Table 3-4 lists dosage guidelines for cephalosporins.

NEWER β-LACTAM ANTIBIOTIC/ β-LACTAMASE INHIBITOR COMBINATIONS

β-Lactamase irreversibly hydrolyzes the amide bond of the β-lactam ring, rendering β-lactam antibiotics inactive. The production of β-lactamases is controlled by either chromosomal or plasmid genes and is readily transferable.[33,34] The introduction of β-lactamase inhibitors, when combined with β-lactam antibiotics, acts synergistically by inhibiting plasma-mediated β-lactamases of the *Enterobacteriaceae* organisms, *S. aureus*, and gram-negative anaerobes.[35] In the United States, clavulanate, sulbactam, and tazobactam are the only inhibitors approved for clinical use.

Available formulations include the following:

1. Amoxicillin-clavulanate (Augmentin)
2. Ampicillin-sulbactam (Unasyn)
3. Ticarcillin-clavulanate (Timentin)
4. Piperacillin-tazobactam (Zosyn)

Antibacterial Activity
None of the β-lactamase inhibitors alone possess clinically useful antibacterial activity; however, when combined with a β-lactam antibiotic, it acts as an irreversible inhibitor of various β-lactamases, thereby restoring and extending the spectrum of activity of the β-lactam.[36] Significant activity for methicillin-sensitive *S. aureus*, *Haemophilus* species, *Klebsiella* species, *Escherichia coli*, *Proteus* species, and *B. fragilis* is noted.

Pharmacokinetics
When clavulanate is given orally with amoxicillin (amox/ca), it is rapidly absorbed.[37] Peak concentrations are reached 40 to 60 minutes af-

ter ingestion, and bioavailability is unaffected by food.[38] Ampicillin/sulbactam (amp/sulb), ticarcillin/clavulanate (tic/ca), and piperacillin/tazobactam (pip/tazo) are administered intravenously. Amp/sulb can also be administered intramuscularly.

Dermatologic Indications
The wide antimicrobial spectrum of amox/ca, amp/sulb, tic/ca, and pip/tazo makes these agents useful for treatment of infections caused by polymicrobial organisms.

Amox/ca is the recommended oral agent for treatment of animal or human bites infected by combined aerobic and anaerobic pathogens. Tic/ca and pip/tazo have an even broader antibacterial spectrum and are thus effective in treating more severe skin and soft tissue infections such as diabetic foot ulcers, infected decubiti, and burn wounds.[39]

Drug Interactions
When administered concomitantly with the β-lactam/β-lactamase inhibitors, oral probenecid slows the rate of the renal tubular secretion of the β-lactam (amoxicillin, ticarcillin, ampicillin, and piperacillin), sulbactam, and tazobactam and produces elevated serum concentrations.[40,41] Allopurinol increases the risk of ampicillin-induced cutaneous hypersensitivity eruptions.[42]

Adverse Effects
Adverse effects most often associated with pip/tazo and amox/ca administration are GI complaints, commonly diarrhea.[35] Diarrhea is more likely to occur in children receiving amox/ca but occurs less commonly when taken with food.[42] Hypersensitivity reactions from the β-lactam/β-lactamase inhibitors are similar to those from the β-lactams alone. Ticarcillin and piperacillin can elongate bleeding times and cause platelet aggregation dysfunction.[44] Hypernatremia has been reported with both ticarcillin and piperacillin administration.[35] Transient elevation of transaminases, positive Coombs' test, thrombocytopenia, neutropenia, and eosinophilia have also been reported with these agents.[45] Sulbactam has been associated with pain at the intramuscular injection sites.[46]

Dosage
Amox/ca is administered orally. Adult dosage is 250 to 500 mg every 8 hours. The tablets and suspension contain either a 2:1 or 4:1 ratio of the drugs. Table 3-2 contains dosage guidelines for oral penicillins. Dosing for the injectable formulations is beyond the scope of this chapter.

CARBAPENEMS AND MONOBACTAMS

There is limited applicability of the carbapenem and monobactam categories of antibacterial agents in dermatology due to the availability only in parenteral forms. A brief discussion is given to the carbapenems and aztreonam.

Carbapenems
The carbapenems differ from other β-lactam antibiotics by the addition of a double bond to the 5-membered ring of the penicillin nucleus and the substitution of a sulfur atom by a carbon atom. The first class of these drugs available in the United States is imipenem (available in combination with cilastatin). Cilastatin is a natural inhibitor of renal dihydropeptidase enzyme, which is the enzyme responsible for the metabolism of imipenem. A cilastatin addition to the imipenem molecule protects the kidney against the drug's potential nephrotoxic effect. Meropenem is a new carbapenem recently approved in the United States.[47]

Carbapenems have the broadest spectrum of activity of any available antibiotics. They are active against most aerobic and anaerobic gram-positive and gram-negative bacteria including most *P. aeruginosa* strains and anaerobic organisms including the *B. fragilis* group.[48,49]

Imipenem is not commonly used by the dermatologist because less expensive, less broad-spectrum agents are usually more appropriate. However, because of its broad spectrum, imipenem is useful in treating infections of mixed flora, such as decubitus and diabetic foot ulcers that would otherwise require the use of multiple agents.[50] It is also useful in treating skin and soft tissue infections caused by pathogens resistant to older agents.

Skin test studies have shown a high degree of cross reactivity between imipenem and penicillins. Thus patients with hypersensitivity responses to one or more of the penicillin determinants should be given imipenem only under close observation with the same precautions as in patients about to receive penicillin.[51]

Aztreonam

Aztreonam has a spectrum of activity limited to aerobic gram-negative organisms.[52,53] Aztreonam has been safely administered to patients with allergies to penicillin and cephalosporins.[54]

Because of its predominant gram-negative spectrum, aztreonam has a limited role in treating skin and soft tissue infections. However, it has been employed as a sole agent in treating gram-negative cutaneous infections, including postoperative wounds, ulcers, burns, and ecthyma gangrenosum, and in conjunction with other drugs that inhibit gram-positive or anaerobic flora.[55]

Aztreonam also has an adverse effect profile similar to other β-lactam antibiotics. Pruritus, purpura, erythema multiforme, toxic epidermal necrolysis, urticaria, exfoliative dermatitis, and petechiae have been reported in less than 1% of patients.[56] Patients who are allergic to penicillin can be safely given aztreonam.

MACROLIDES

Erythromycin is the prototype macrolide. However, it suffers from several drawbacks including nausea and diarrhea, erratic oral bioavailability, short half-life requiring frequent administration, and limited activity against common gram-negative pathogens.[57]

Three new macrolides are available—clarithromycin (Biaxin), azithromycin (Zithromax), and dirithromycin (Dynabac) (Table 3-5 and Figure 3-2).

These new macrolides are similar to erythromycin and act by penetrating cell walls of susceptible bacteria and reversibly binding to the 50S subunit of the ribosome, inhibiting RNA-dependent protein synthesis.[58-60]

Antimicrobial Activity

Both clarithromycin and azithromycin offer enhanced antimicrobial activity. Dirithromycin has antimicrobial activity similar to eryth-

romycin. Clarithromycin is twofold to fourfold more potent than erythromycin against gram-positive organisms.[61] Azithromycin's activity against gram-positive organisms such as staphylococci and streptococci is twofold to fourfold less active than erythromycin. The anaerobic activity of the new macrolides is similar to erythromycin.[62] Clarithromycin and azithromycin possess increased activity against several gram-negative pathogens. Clarithromycin has enhanced activity against *H. influenzae*.[63] Clarithromycin activity against *N. gonorrhoeae* is similar to erythromycin.[64] Azithromycin has enhanced activity against gram-negative pathogens. Azithromycin also has more potent activity against *H. influenzae* than erythromycin.[65] Azithromycin has activity against *E. coli, N. gonorrhoeae, H. ducreyi, Ureaplasma urealyticum*, and *Chlamydia trachomatis*. Azithromycin also has activity against organisms contracted via animal bites including *Pasteurella multocida* and human mouth bites such as *Eikenella corrodens*.[66] Both clarithromycin and azithromycin are effective against atypical mycobacterium such as *Mycobacterium avium intracellulare, M. leprae*, and *M. chelonei*.[67-69] Clarithromycin is the most active macrolide against *M. leprae*. Clarithromycin and azithromycin are also active against *Toxo-*

■ Table 3-5   Currently Available Antibacterial Agents— Macrolides

Generic Name	Trade Name	Route
Azithromycin	Zithromax	PO
Clarithromycin	Biaxin	PO
Dirithromycin	Dynabac	PO
Erythromycin base	ERYC, E-MYCIN, PCE	PO
Erythromycin estolate	Ilosone	PO
Erythromycin ethyl succinate	EES, Pediazole*	PO
Erythromycin lactobionate	None	IV
Troleandomycin	TAO	PO

*Pediazole is a combination of erythromycin ethyl succinate and sulfisoxazole—only available in a liquid formulation.

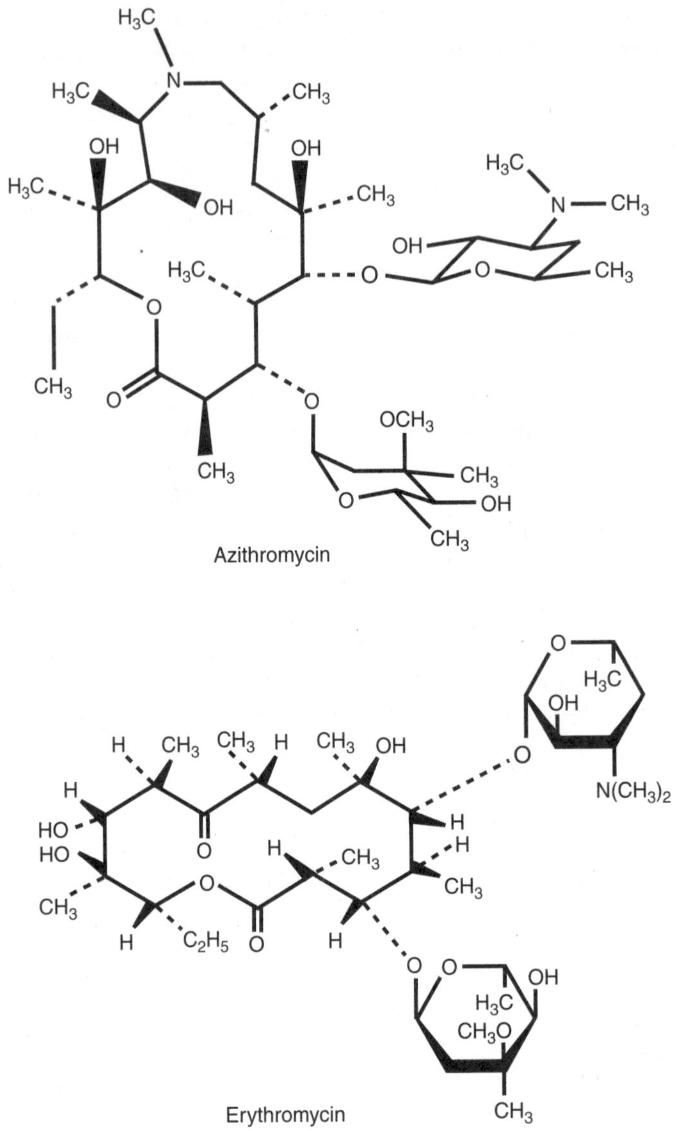

Figure 3-2   Systemic antibacterial agents—macrolides.

plasma gondii, Treponema pallidum, and *Borrelia burgdorferi.*[70-72]

Pharmacokinetics

The new macrolides have excellent bioavailability: clarithromycin is well absorbed with or without food. Azithromycin absorption is decreased with food and should thus be taken 1 to 2 hours before a meal. Clarithromycin is metabolized by the kidney. Thus renal impairment requires dosage adjustments. In contradistinction, azithro-

mycin metabolism is primarily hepatic. Dirithromycin is converted during absorption to an active metabolite, erythromycylamine, which is enhanced by the presence of food. Both dirithromycin and erythromycylamine are predominantly eliminated in the bile and feces.

Dermatologic Indications

The new macrolides are effective in the treatment of skin and soft tissue infection despite the fact that azithromycin's in vitro activity against

■ Table 3-6   Drug Interactions—Macrolides*

Interacting Drug Group	Examples and Comments
CERTAIN MACROLIDES INCREASE THE RISK OF TORSADES DE POINTES DUE TO CYP 3A4 INHIBITION	
Azole antifungal agents	Terfenadine, astemizole (both *off* the market in the United States)
Fluoroquinolone antibacterials	Grepafloxacin,† sparfloxacin
Prokinetic gastrointestinal agents	Cisapride (*off* the market in the United States)
CERTAIN MACROLIDES INCREASE THE SERUM LEVELS (AND POTENTIAL TOXICITY) OF THESE DRUGS—CYP 3A4 INHIBITION	
Anticoagulants	Warfarin anticoagulant effect may be increased
Anticonvulsants	Carbamazepine (other anticonvulsants metabolized by other CYP isoforms)
Antidepressants	Buspirone
Benzodiazepines	Alprazolam, diazepam, midazolam, triazolam
Corticosteroids	Macrolides have the greatest effect on the metabolism of methylprednisolone
HMG CoA reductase inhibitors	Entire drug class—increased risk of myopathy, rhabdomyolysis, hepatotoxicity
Sex steroids	Oral contraceptives—may increase the risk of intrahepatic cholestasis
Signal transduction inhibitors	Cyclosporine, tacrolimus—risk for nephrotoxicity, neurotoxicity increased
Other drugs	Increased levels of disopyramide, felodipine, and ergot alkaloids may occur
CERTAIN MACROLIDES INCREASE THE SERUM LEVELS (AND POTENTIAL TOXICITY) OF THESE DRUGS—CYP 1A2 INHIBITION	
Bronchodilators	Theophylline—risk of CNS toxicity particularly important
Proton pump inhibitors	Omeprazole
OTHER POTENTIALLY IMPORTANT INTERACTIONS	
Digoxin	Drug levels may be elevated due to altered gut flora that metabolize digoxin
Fluconazole	Coadministration may increase clarithromycin levels

Adapted from *CliniSphere 20 CD Rom*, St. Louis, June 2000, Facts & Comparisons.
*Risk for interactions involving CYP 3A4 greatest with erythromycin, moderate with clarithromycin, and negligible risk with azithromycin and dirithromycin; CYP 1A2 inhibition primarily by erythromycin.
†Grepafloxacin is off the market in the United States.

gram-positive organisms is twofold to fourfold lower than that of erythromycin. These newer agents have excellent efficacy in the treatment of pyoderma, abscesses, infected wounds, ulcers, and erysipelas.[73-75]

Skin infections with *M. chelonei, M. simiae, M. avium complex* (MAC), *M. kansasii,* and *M. intracellulare* have been effectively treated with clarithromycin alone.[76]

Drug Interactions

Erythromycin interacts with drugs by inhibiting the hepatic cytochrome P-450 system leading to decreased metabolic decrease of carbamazepine, theophylline, phenytoin, digoxin, warfarin, terfenadine, and methylprednisolone (Table 3-6). Clarithromycin by cytochrome P-450 inhibition can also increase the serum concentrations of carbamazepine and theophylline.

■ **Table 3-7**   Commonly Used Oral Macrolides—Dosage Guidelines

Generic Name	Tab/Caps Sizes	Adult Dosage	Price Index
Azithromycin*	250, 500 mg	500 mg day 1, then 250 mg qd × 4	$$$$/$$$$$
Clarithromycin*	250, 500 mg	250-500 mg bid	$$$
Dirithromycin	250 mg	500 mg qd	—
Erythromycin base†	250, 333, 500 mg	250-500 mg qid‡	$ ($)
Erythromycin estolate*	250 mg	(Not used in adults)	$ ($)
Erythromycin ethyl succinate*	400 mg	400 mg qid	$ ($)

$, <1.00; $$, 1.01-2.00; $$$, 2.01-5.00; $$$$, 5.01-10.00; $$$$$, >10.00; ( ), generic price; /, two different price ranges from lower dose to higher dose examples of this drug; —, no price listed for this drug.
*These drugs are available in either suspension or liquid formulations.
†Enteric-coated formulations are available.
‡Other acceptable regimens include 333 mg tid and 500 mg bid.

Unlike clarithromycin, azithromycin and dirithromycin do not affect the cytochrome P-450 system.[77,78] Clarithromycin may alter the metabolism of nonsedating antihistamines, i.e., terfenadine (Seldane), which may eventuate in ventricular tachycardia. Thus terfenadine is contraindicated in patients receiving clarithromycin or erythromycin.[79,80] Clarithromycin may reduce the absorption of zidovudine (AZT) by 20%.[81] It may also decrease the serum levels of didanosine (ddI).[82]

Adverse Effects
Azithromycin and clarithromycin cause fewer adverse GI effects than erythromycin.[83,84] Dirithromycin appears to have a similar incidence of GI adverse effects. Nausea, abdominal pain, and diarrhea are the most commonly reported effects. Headaches, dizziness, and liver enzyme elevations occur less frequently.[85,86]

Dosage
The adult dosage of clarithromycin is 250 to 500 mg q 12 hours. Clarithromycin is administered in a dosage of 7.5 mg/kg every 12 hours. For azithromycin the adult dosage is 500 mg given as a single dose on day 1 of therapy followed by 250 mg once a day for 4 additional days. For the treatment of uncomplicated chlamydial infections azithromycin is administered 1 gram as a single dose. The adult dose of dirithromycin is 500 mg once daily. Table 3-7 lists dosage guidelines for commonly used oral macrolides.

FLUOROQUINOLONES

There are currently multiple fluoroquinolones available in the United States; these include norfloxacin, ciprofloxacin, ofloxacin, lomefloxacin, enoxacin, levofloxacin, and trovafloxacin (Table 3-8 and Figure 3-3). These agents are more potent than older quinolones (such as nalidixic acid), having a longer serum half-life that allows twice daily administration in most instances. Other advantages of these agents include a low incidence of resistance, high oral bioavailability, and extensive tissue penetration into human cells resulting in antimicrobial activity against intracellular pathogens.[87] These agents are bactericidal, acting via inhibition of DNA gyrase (bacterial topoisomerase II), an enzyme that introduces negative super coiling into bacterial DNA, which results in the interference of DNA replication.[88,89]

Antimicrobial Activity
New fluoroquinolones are effective against most gram-negative organisms, particularly the *Enterobacteriaceae* organisms. Ciprofloxacin is most active against *P. aeruginosa*.[90] This group of agents shows variable efficacy against gram-positive organisms. The fluoroquinolones show minimal

■ Table 3-8 Currently Available Antibacterial Agents— Fluoroquinolones

Generic Name	Trade Name	Route
Ciprofloxacin	Cipro	PO, IV
Enoxacin	Pentrex	PO
Gatifloxacin	Tequin	PO, IV
Levofloxacin	Levaquin	PO
Lomefloxacin	Maxaquin	PO
Moxefloxacin	Avelox	PO
Norfloxacin	Noroxin	PO
Ofloxacin	Floxin	PO, IV
Sparfloxacin	Zagam	PO

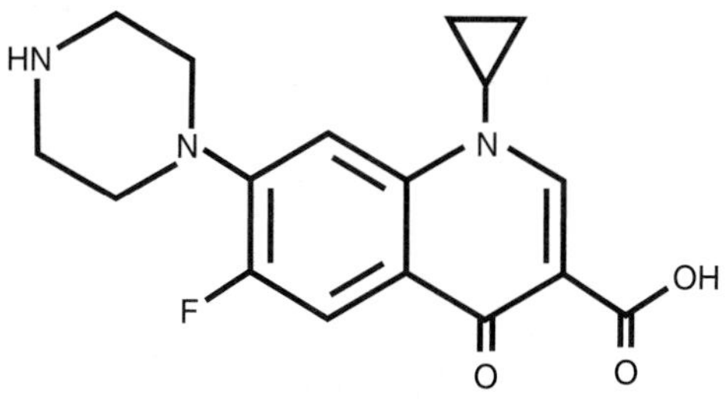

Ciprofloxacin

Figure 3-3 Systemic antibacterial agents— fluoroquinolones.

anaerobic activity. Ciprofloxacin, ofloxacin, and levofloxacin are active against *Mycobacterium* species including *M. tuberculosis*, *M. fortuitum*, and *M. kansasii*.[91-94] *P. aeruginosa* and *S. aureus* commonly develop resistance to these drugs.[95-97]

Pharmacokinetics

The bioavailability of the fluoroquinolones after oral administration is excellent except for norfloxacin.[98,99] These agents are mainly excreted renally and thus require adjustment of dosage in patients with impaired renal function.[100]

Dermatologic Indications

Because of excellent drug levels in the skin and its appendages, the fluoroquinolones are excellent agents for treating cutaneous infections

caused by multiresistant gram-negative bacteria including abscesses, cellulitis, ulcers, and wound infections.[101-104] These agents are also useful in treating external otitis media, gram-negative interdigital web space infections, diabetic foot ulcers, and puncture wounds.

Drug Interactions

All fluoroquinolones show decreased bioavailability when administered with aluminum-, magnesium-, and alum-containing antacids.[105] Antacids should be taken at least 2 hours after the administration of the fluoroquinolone. A similar decreased absorption has been noted with coadministration of iron- or zinc-containing products. Liver metabolism of theophylline is inhibited by enoxacin and to a lesser extent by ciprofloxacin and norfloxacin, resulting in potential theophylline toxicity.[106] Fluoroquinolones are also associated with a decreased seizure threshold. Drug interactions that show a decrease in warfarin and cyclosporine metabolism have also been documented.[107,108] Table 3-9 lists the drug interactions for fluoroquinolones.

Adverse Effects

The most common adverse reactions are nausea, vomiting, diarrhea, headaches, dizziness, agitation, and sleep disturbances.[109] In animals, fluoroquinolones impair cartilage formation and therefore these agents are contraindicated during pregnancy and early childhood.[110]

Hypersensitivity reactions and photosensitivity have also been reported. A decreasing photosensitivity potential of these agents is fleroxacin > lomefloxacin > perfloxacin > ciprofloxacin > enoxacin > norfloxacin > ofloxacin.[111,112] Evening dosing of these agents may minimize phototoxic potential.[113] Blue-black pigmentation of the legs similar to minocycline dyschromia but revealing iron particles within the cytoplasm of dermal macrophages with perfloxacin therapy has been reported.[114]

Dosage

The only fluoroquinolones available for parenteral therapy are ciprofloxacin, levofloxacin, and ofloxacin. Parenteral therapy has no advantage over oral routes and should only be administered to those who are unable to toler-

■ **Table 3-9** Drug Interactions—Fluoroquinolones

Interacting Drug	Mechanism and Comments
DRUGS THAT MAY REDUCE FLUOROQUINOLONE LEVELS*	
Antacids—calcium, aluminum, magnesium	Chelation of fluoroquinolones to divalent (calcium, magnesium) and trivalent (aluminum) cations
Sucralfate	Chelation to sucralfate, which is an aluminum salt of sulfated sucrose
Iron and zinc salts	Chelation of fluoroquinolones to iron and zinc salts
FLUOROQUINOLONES INCREASE SERUM LEVELS (AND POTENTIAL TOXICITY) OF THESE DRUGS	
Theophylline	Increased serum theophylline levels (levels may triple) due to CYP 1A2 inhibition
Aminophylline	Similar to theophylline
Warfarin	Increased protime/INR—uncertain mechanism (CYP 1A2 inhibition may be a factor)
OTHER INTERACTIONS	
Cyclosporine	May increase creatinine levels in transplant patients—can use with careful monitoring

Adapted from *CliniSphere 2.0 CD ROM*, St. Louis, June 2000, Facts & Comparisons.
*Allow at least 2 hours between administration of the fluoroquinolones and these chelating drugs.

■ **Table 3-10** Commonly Used Oral Fluoroquinolones—Dosage Guidelines

Generic Name	Tab/Caps Sizes	Adult Dosage	Price Index
Ciprofloxacin	100, 250, 500, 750 mg	250-750 mg bid	$$$
Levofloxacin	250, 500 mg	250-500 mg qd	$$$$
Sparfloxacin	200 mg	400 mg day 1, then 200 mg qd	$$$$

$, <1.00; $$, 1.01-2.00; $$$, 2.01-5.00; $$$$, 5.01-10.00; $$$$$, >10.00; ( ), generic price; /, two different price ranges from lower dose to higher dose examples of this drug; —, no price listed for this drug.

ate the latter. The preferred dosages for commonly used oral fluoroquinolones are listed in Table 3-10.

TETRACYCLINES

Tetracyclines act via inhibition of protein synthesis by binding to the 30S ribosomal subunit. The tetracyclines exhibit activity against many gram-positive and gram-negative bacteria, as well as mycoplasmas, *Chlamydia* organisms, *Rickettsia* organisms, spirochetes, and some par-

asites. In general they possess greater gram-positive than gram-negative activity. Minocycline and doxycycline are more active against *S. aureus* than is tetracycline (Figure 3-4). Many strains of Group A streptococci are now resistant to tetracycline.[115]

Pharmacokinetics

Tetracycline drugs are better absorbed in the fasting state except for doxycycline and minocycline, which are well absorbed daily in the presence or absence of food. Absorption of tetracycline is impaired by concomitant ingestion of dairy pro-

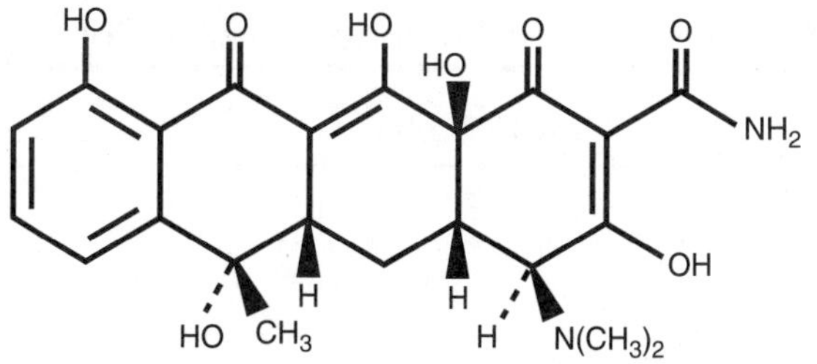

Tetracyclines

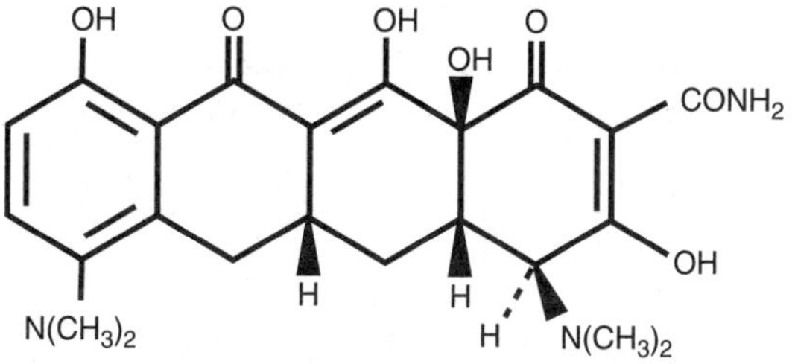

Minocycline

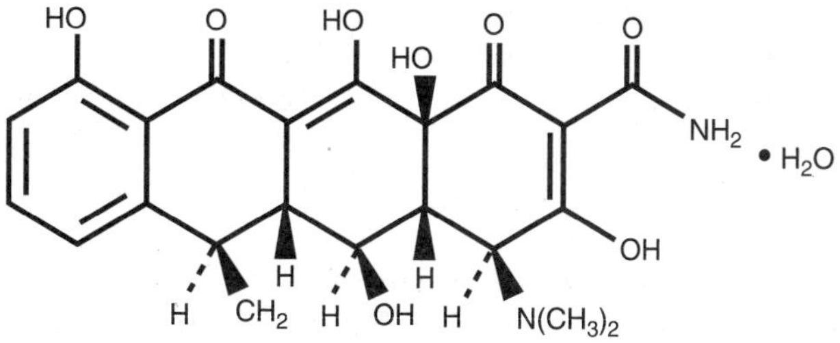

Doxycycline

Figure 3-4   Systemic antibacterial agents—tetracyclines.

ducts, aluminum hydroxide, calcium, iron or zinc salts, and bismuth subsalicylate.[116,117] The tetracyclines are divided into short-acting agents tetracycline (half-life 8.5 hours); intermediate-acting demeclocycline; or long-acting drugs, doxycycline (half-life 14 to 22 hours) and minocycline (half-life 11 to 13 hours) (Table 3-11).

Renal failure prolongs the half-life of most tetracyclines except doxycycline. Unlike other tetracyclines, doxycycline is excreted primarily by the GI tract. The only tetracycline accept-

able for usage in patients with renal failure is doxycycline. Potential hepatotoxicity makes these agents relatively contraindicated in patients with severe liver disease.[118]

Dermatologic Indications

Inhibition of propionibacteria has made treatment of acne rosacea and perioral dermatitis the major usage of this class of drugs.

Other less conventional usages include the combination of tetracycline and nicotinamide in

■ **Table 3-11**   Currently Available Antibacterial Agents—Tetracyclines

Generic Name	Trade Name	Route
SHORT ACTING		
Oxytetracycline	Terramycin	PO, IM
Tetracycline	Sumycin, Achromycin V	PO (IV)
INTERMEDIATE ACTING		
Methacycline	Rondomycin	PO
Demeclocycline	Declomycin	PO
LONG ACTING		
Doxycycline*	Monodox, Vibratabs	PO, IV
Minocycline	Minocin, Dynacin	PO, IV

*Monodox is doxycycline monohydrate; Vibratabs and generic doxycycline formulations are doxycycline hyclate.

the treatment of bullous pemphigoid,[119] dermatitis herpetiformis,[120] and linear IgA bullous dermatosis.[121]

Tetracyclines are also effective in treating rickettsial infections including Rocky Mountain spotted fever, rickettsial pox, and erythema migrans/Lyme disease.[122] Because of activity against *Vibrio vulnificus* and *M. marinum*, tetracyclines have been successfully used to treat infected aquatic injuries.[123,124]

Drug Interactions

Tetracyclines potentiate the effects of oral anticoagulants and lithium by impairing utilization of prothrombin or by decreasing vitamin D production by bacteria. Table 3-12 contains the drug interactions for tetracyclines.

Barbiturates, phenytoin, and carbamazepine decrease the serum concentration of doxycycline but do not affect the concentrations of demeclocycline, oxytetracycline, and tetracycline.[125]

Adverse Effects

GI effects including epigastric burning, abdominal discomfort, nausea, and vomiting are most frequently described. Esophagitis and pancreatitis are less commonly reported sequelae. GI distress may be reduced by administering the drugs with food (nondairy products).[126,127]

The drugs are occasionally hepatotoxic, particularly in large dosages and in pregnant women. Demeclocycline and doxycycline are the most phototoxic of this class of drugs. Phototoxicity may be accompanied by onycholysis. Tetracyclines may cause progression of uremia in patients with renal disease.[128] Demeclocycline has been used in the treatment of diabetes insipidus.[129]

Children receiving tetracycline may develop brown discoloration of teeth and delayed bone growth and thus tetracyclines are not recommended for children younger than 9 years of age. Vestibular toxicity has been described predominantly in women.

Hypersensitivity reactions including exanthems, Stevens-Johnson syndrome, pneumonitis,[130] drug-induced lupus,[131] and serum sickness type reactions have been reported.[132] Sweet's syndrome has been reported with minocycline usage.[133]

Blue-black pigmentation of the nails, skin, scars, and sclerae have also been manifest.[134] Finally, gynecomastia and black tongue[135] have been described.[136] Other less common adverse effects include leukocytosis with atypical lymphocytes, toxic granulation of granulocytes, and thrombocytopenia purpura. Less commonly, pseudotumor cerebri and parenteral administration-related phlebitis have been reported.

Dosing

Table 3-13 contains dosage guidelines for commonly used oral tetracyclines.

■ **Table 3-12**   Drug Interactions—Tetracyclines

Interacting Drug(s)	Mechanism and Comments
DRUGS THAT MAY REDUCE THE GASTROINTESTINAL ABSORPTION OF TETRACYCLINES	
Antacids—calcium, magnesium, aluminum	Chelation of tetracyclines to divalent (calcium, magnesium) and trivalent (aluminum) cations
Other cations—iron, zinc, and bismuth salts	Similarly, chelation with other divalent and trivalent cations may reduce absorption of tetracyclines
Cimetidine	May induce a pH-dependent inhibition of drug dissolution
Sodium bicarbonate	Probably on a similar basis to the inhibition due to cimetidine
TETRACYCLINES MAY INCREASE SERUM LEVELS (AND POTENTIAL TOXICITY) OF THESE DRUGS	
Digoxin	May increase levels in a small portion (<10%) of patients, may persist for months
Lithium	Uncertain mechanism (may also decrease levels of lithium); monitor carefully
Warfarin	Mechanism probably due to tetracycline-induced changes in gut flora affecting enterohepatic recirculation of warfarin
TETRACYCLINES MAY DECREASE SERUM LEVELS OF THESE DRUGS	
Oral contraceptives	Highly *controversial*—theoretically inhibit enterohepatic recirculation of estrogens
OTHER POTENTIALLY IMPORTANT INTERACTIONS	
Anticonvulsants	Phenytoin, phenobarbital, and carbamazepine may induce doxycycline metabolism and thus lower drug levels
Penicillins	Bacteriostatic drugs such as tetracyclines may interfere with bactericidal activity of penicillins
Insulin	Tetracyclines may reduce insulin requirements

Adapted from *CliniSphere 2.0 CD ROM*, St. Louis, June 2000, Facts & Comparisons.

■ **Table 3-13**   Commonly Used Oral Tetracyclines*—Dosage Guidelines

Generic Name	Tab/Caps Sizes	Adult Dosage	Price Index
Tetracycline	250, 500 mg	250-1500 mg/d bid	$ ($)
Doxycycline	20, 50, 100 mg	50-200 mg/d bid	$$$ ($$$)
Minocycline	50, 75, 100 mg	50-200 mg/d bid	$$$ ($$)

$, <1.00; $$, 1.01-2.00; $$$, 2.01-5.00; $$$$, 5.01-10.00; $$$$$, >10.00; ( ), generic price; /, two different price ranges from lower dose to higher dose examples of this drug; —, no price listed for this drug.
*All of the drugs listed in this table have either liquid or suspension formulations available.

RIFAMYCINS

The rifamycins are bactericidal for both intracellular and extracellular organisms. Rifamycin inhibits RNA synthesis by inhibiting DNA-dependent RNA polymerase. Rifampin and rifabutin are the two antibiotic agents commonly employed (Table 3-14).

Antimicrobial Activity

Rifampin has a broad spectrum of activity that includes staphylococci (beta coagulase negative and positive), *Rhodococcus equi*, *N. meningitidis*, *N. gonorrhoeae*, and *H. influenzae*. Poor gram-negative coverage is noted. Sensitivity to *M. tuberculosis* and atypical mycobacteria is also characteristic (especially *M. kansasii* and *M. marinum*).

Rifabutin has a similar spectrum of activity with particular sensitivity to MAC and is commonly used to treat MAC prophylaxis in patients with advanced HIV disease.[137-140]

Pharmacokinetics

Rifampin is available for oral or intravenous infusion. Absorption is impaired if the drug is taken during or right after a meal.[141]

Rifampin is metabolized hepatically in that dosage adjustment is not necessary for renal insufficiency. Placental diffusion contraindicates its usage during pregnancy.[141]

Dermatologic Indications

Cutaneous tuberculosis is a major indication for rifampin therapy.[142] Rifampin is the only drug bactericidal to *M. leprae*.[143] Because of its lack of effect after 6 months, concomitant dapsone therapy is employed.

Rifampin is bactericidal to gram-positive cocci and is thus excellent in treating pyodermas. Cost factors and resistance considerations in antituberculous therapy make its role limited in the treatment of pyodermas caused by staphylococci resistant to other antibiotics.[144] In addition, rapid emergence of resistance has been observed when monotherapy is employed. Thus rifampin should only be used in conjunction with another gram-positive agent.

Cutaneous leishmaniasis and rhinoscleroma also respond well to rifampin because it easily penetrates the cell membrane and attacks intracellular pathogens.[145,146]

■ **Table 3-14**   Other Antibacterial Agents

Generic Name	Trade Name	Route
RIFAMYCINS		
Rifampin	Rifadin, Rimactane	PO, IV
Rifabutin	Mycobutin	PO
FOLATE INHIBITORS		
TMP/SMX*	Septra DS, Bactrim DS	PO, IV
LINCOSAMIDES		
Clindamycin	Cleocin	PO, IV

*DS for this combination of antibacterial agents represents double strength formulation (single strength rarely used).

Rifampin may also play a role in psoriasis by prevention of the carriage state of *S. aureus* and streptococci that produce superantigens, which modulate T-cell function.[147-151]

Rifampin has also been used to reduce staphylococcal nasal colonization and for the pruritus associated with primary biliary cirrhosis by enhancing hepatic microsomal degradation of pruritogenic bile salt metabolites.[152,153]

Drug Interactions

Rifampin is a potent inducer of intestinal and hepatic microsomal enzymes leading to reduced bioavailability and decreased serum half-life of a number of compounds including decreased effect of oral contraceptives, decreased prothrombin time for patients on warfarin therapy, and addisonian crises in patients on steroids.[154] Table 3-15 lists the drug interactions of rifampin.

Adverse Effects

Orange-red discoloration of urine and permanent staining of soft contact lenses are most frequently noted. A hypersensitivity syndrome consisting of flulike symptoms with fever, chills, headache, dizziness, and bone pain, as well as pruritus, urticaria, acneiform eruptions, bullous pemphigoid–like lesions, mucositis, exfoliative dermatitis, and exudative conjunctivitis associated with eosinophilia has been reported with high-dose intermittent therapy.[155] Other reported as-

Table 3-15 Drug Interactions—Rifampin

Interacting Drug Category	Examples and Comments
DRUG LEVELS DECREASED DUE TO CYP 3A4 ENZYME INDUCTION	
Antidysrhythmic agents	Digitoxin, disopyramide, mexiletine, quinidine, tocainide
Antibacterial agents	Chloramphenicol
Anticoagulants	Warfarin (decreased R-warfarin; this enantiomer is less active than S-warfarin)
Anticonvulsants	Phenobarbital, phenytoin
Azole antifungal agents	Concomitant use with ketoconazole may lead to treatment failure of either agent
Bronchodilators	Theophyllines
Cardiovascular agents (other)	β-Blockers, verapamil
Immunosuppressive agents	Cyclosporine, corticosteroids
Miscellaneous drugs/groups	Acetaminophen, benzodiazepines, clofibrate, methadone
Sex steroids	Estrogens (rifampin definitely decreases oral contraceptive effectiveness)
Sulfonamide-related drugs	Dapsone, sulfonylurea, oral hypoglycemic agents
OTHER POTENTIALLY IMPORTANT INTERACTIONS	
Isoniazid	Concomitant use increases the risk of hepatotoxicity from rifampin
Enalapril	Use with rifampin may lead to a significant increase in blood pressure

Adapted from *CliniSphere 2.0 CD ROM*, St. Louis, June 2000, Facts & Comparisons.

 Table 3-16 Other Commonly Used Oral Antibacterial Agents—Dosage Guidelines

Generic Name	Tablet Sizes	Adult Dosage	Price Index
Rifampin	150, 300 mg	300-600 mg/d	$$ ($$/$$$)
TMP/SMX (DS)	160/800 mg*	DS capsule bid	$$ ($)
Clindamycin	75, 150, 300 mg	150-300 mg bid	$$/$$$ ($)

$, <1.00; $$, 1.01-2.00; $$$, 2.01-5.00; $$$$, 5.01-10.00; $$$$$, >10.00; ( ), generic price; /, two different price ranges from lower dose to higher dose examples of this drug; —, no price listed for this drug.
*Fixed combination in this dosage ratio also known generically as cotrimoxazole.

pects of this hypersensitivity syndrome are related to the GI system (anorexia, nausea, diarrhea, abdominal pain, increased hepatic transaminases), possibly accompanied by acute renal failure.[155]

CNS symptoms of headache, drowsiness, ataxia, dizziness, and fatigue have been described. Thrombocytopenia, leukopenia, and hemolytic anemia are rare occurrences.

Dosage

The recommended dosage for treatment of cutaneous infections is usually 10 to 20 mg/kg (600 mg maximum) in a single daily dosage (Table 3-16). The elimination of staphylococcal carriage may require higher dosages as indicated.

TRIMETHOPRIM-SULFAMETHOXAZOLE

This popular antimicrobial agent is a fixed dose ratio of one part trimethoprim (TMP) to five parts sulfamethoxazole (SMX) (Table 3-16 and Figure 3-5).

The two components of this drug inhibit enzymes involved in the bacterial synthesis of

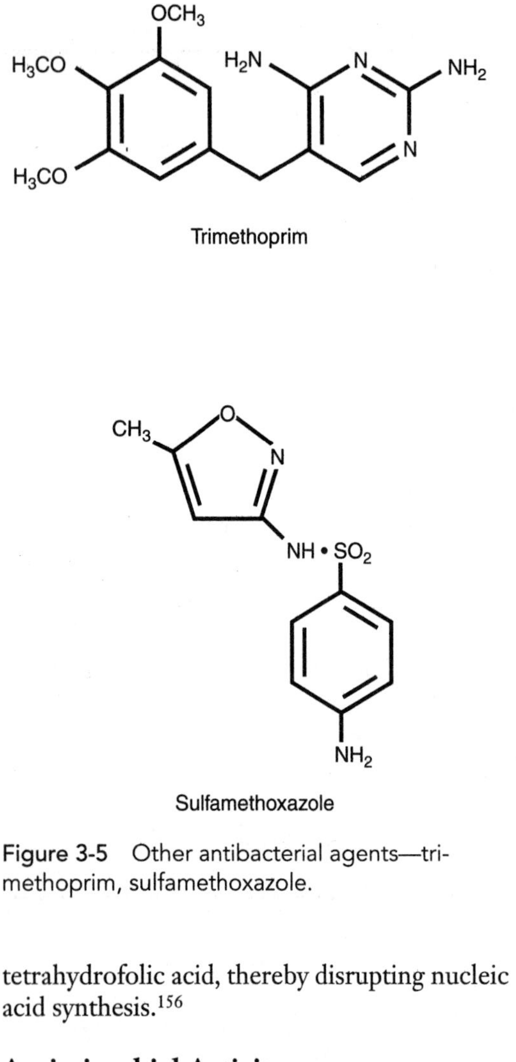

Figure 3-5   Other antibacterial agents—trimethoprim, sulfamethoxazole.

tetrahydrofolic acid, thereby disrupting nucleic acid synthesis.[156]

Antimicrobial Activity

Many gram-positive aerobic cocci including *S. aureus*, *S. pyogenes*, and *S. viridans* are inhibited. Many *Enterobacteriaceae* organisms are also sensitive. *H. influenzae*, *Brucella* species, and *Yersinia* species are also sensitive. *P. aeruginosa* is resistant although other *Pseudomonas* species are often sensitive.[157] Other organisms sensitive to this agent of interest to the dermatologist include *Nocardia asteroides*[158] and atypical mycobacteria.[159] Poor anaerobic activity is present.

Pharmacokinetics

Both TMP and SMX are well absorbed orally with half-lives of 11 and 9 hours, respectively.

Dermatologic Indications

Specific dermatologic indications for TMP-SMX are few, but it may be used as a second or third line agent. TMP-SMX has been used to treat cutaneous *Nocardia* species[160] and *Aeromonas* species infections.[161] TMP-SMX is a treatment option for cat scratch disease,[162] granuloma inguinale,[163] melioidosis,[163] and mycetomas. It may be used as an alternative drug for treatment of pyodermas, chancroid, and lymphogranuloma venereum. TMP-SMX has been used to treat acne vulgaris in tetracycline- and erythromycin-resistant patients.[164]

Drug Interactions

TMP-SMX may prolong the prothrombin time of patients receiving warfarin. It should be avoided in patients receiving methotrexate because it can interfere with folic acid metabolism.[165]

Adverse Effects

Most commonly noted reactions are GI and cutaneous hypersensitivity reactions. Maculopapular eruptions are particularly common in AIDS patients,[165] and pustular eruptions,[166] Sweet's syndrome,[167] Stevens-Johnson syndrome, and toxic epidermal necrolysis have been reported.[168] Aplastic anemia, neutropenia, agranulocytosis, and thrombocytopenia have also been described.[169] CNS effects include headache, fatigue, and tremor.[158] Less common effects include drug fever, cholestatic hepatitis, crystalluria, nephrolithiasis, and interstitial nephritis.

Dosage

A single-strength tablet contains 80 mg TMP and 400 mg SMX. A double-strength tablet contains 160 mg TMP and 800 mg SMX and is given at 12-hour intervals. Dosage adjustment is indicated in patients with renal insufficiency. See Table 3-16 for dosage guidelines for other commonly used oral antibacterial agents.

CLINDAMYCIN

Clindamycin is a 7-chloro, 7-deoxy derivative of lincomycin that has an increased antibacterial potency and is better absorbed than its parent drug.[170]

It binds to the 50S portion of the ribosome and inhibits protein synthesis by blocking transpeptidation. Clindamycin is active against

■ **Table 3-17**   Additional Antibacterial Agents

Aminoglycosides	β-Lactams	Sulfonamides	Other Antibiotics
Amikacin	*Carbapenems*	Sulfadiazine	Chloramphenicol
Gentamicin	Imipenem/Cilastatin	Sulfadoxin	Metronidazole
Kanamycin	Meropenem	Sulfamethoxazole	Nitrofurantoin
Neomycin		Sulfamethizole	Trimethoprim
Netilmicin	*Monobactams*	Sulfapyridine*	Vancomycin
Spectinomycin	Aztreonam	Sulfasalazine	
Streptomycin		Sulfisoxazole	
Tobramycin			

*Sulfapyridine has limited availability in the United States.

most anaerobic organisms, most gram-positive cocci, and certain protozoa. *S. aureus, S. pneumoniae, S. pyogenes,* and *S. viridans* are particularly sensitive. Good anaerobic activity for peptococci, peptostreptococci, propionibacteria, *Clostridium perfringens,* and fusobacteria is noted. Some protozoa including *Toxoplasma gondii* are inhibited.[170] Poor gram-negative activity is characteristic.

Pharmacokinetics

Clindamycin is mainly metabolized in the liver, which necessitates dose adjustment for patients with liver failure.

Dermatologic Indications

Clindamycin is an efficacious agent for treatment of cellulitis, folliculitis, furunculosis, carbuncles, impetigo, ecthyma, and hidradenitis suppurativa.[171] Deep tissue infections including streptococcal myositis, necrotizing fasciitis, and *Clostridium perfringens* infection may better be treated with this agent.

Clindamycin is effective at low doses in preventing recurrent staphylococcal skin infections.[172] It is often used as part of a combination regimen to treat diabetic foot ulcers. The theoretic risk of pseudomembranous colitis has limited its oral usage in the treatment of acne. The actual incidence of this syndrome with clindamycin is actually much lower than originally perceived in the 1970s and 1980s.

Drug Interactions

Clindamycin has been shown to have neuromuscular blocking properties that may enhance other neuromuscular agents such as tubocurare

and pancuronium.[173] Antagonism has been observed between erythromycin and clindamycin in vitro.

Adverse Effects

Pseudomembranous colitis associated with *Clostridium difficile* toxin has been reported in 0.1% to 10% of treated patients.[174]

Other GI adverse effects include nausea, vomiting, diarrhea, and elevated hepatocellular enzymes. Neuromuscular blockage has also been reported.

Cutaneous adverse effects include maculopapular eruptions, urticaria, anaphylaxis, erythema multiforme, and a Stevens-Johnson–type syndrome associated with polyarthritis.[175]

Dosage

The usual adult oral dosage of clindamycin in dermatology is 150 to 300 mg PO q12h. Parenteral dosages vary from 600 to 2700 mg/day in three or four equal doses. See Table 3-16 for dosage guidelines of other commonly used oral antibacterial agents.

SUMMARY

An understanding of the systemic antimicrobial agents available for use by the dermatologist and their associated adverse effects and drug interactions allows the clinician to deliver the most optimal care in the management of cutaneous infectious diseases. This chapter emphasizes the oral formulations of antibacterial agents for skin and soft tissue infections; other antibacterial agents are found in Table 3-17.

Bibliography

General Dermatologic Reviews of Antibacterial Agents

Epstein ME, Amodio-Groton MA, Sadick NA: Antimicrobial agents for the dermatologist. I. β-lactam antibiotics and related compounds. *J Am Acad Dermatol* 37:149-165, 1997.

Epstein ME, Amodio-Groton MA, Sadick NA: Antimicrobial agents for the dermatologist. II. Macrolides, fluoroquinolones, rifamycins, tetracyclines, trimethoprim-sulfamethoxazole and clindamycin. *J Am Acad Dermatol* 37:365-381, 1997.

Reviews of Specific Antibacterial Drug Groups

Alvarez-Elcoro S, Enzler MJ: The macrolides: erythromycin, clarithromycin, and azithromycin. *Mayo Clin Proc* 74:613-634, 1999.

Humbert P, Treffel P, Champuis JF, et al: The tetracyclines in dermatology. *J Am Acad Dermatol* 25:691-697, 1991.

Karchmer AW: Fluoroquinolone treatment of skin and skin structure infections. *Drugs* 58(suppl 2):82-84, 1999.

Klein NC, Cunha BA: Tetracyclines. *Med Clin North Am* 79:789-801, 1995.

Marshall WF, Blair JE: The cephalosporins. *Mayo Clin Proc* 74:187-195, 1999.

Specific Topics in Antimicrobial Therapy

Bisno AL, Stevens DL: Streptococcal infections of skin and soft tissues. *N Engl J Med* 334:240-245, 1996.

Darmstadt GL: Antibiotics in the management of pediatric skin disease. *Dermatol Clin* 16:509-525, 1998.

Haas AF, Grekin RC: Antibiotic prophylaxis in dermatologic surgery. *J Am Acad Dermatol* 32:155-176, 1995.

Leyden JJ: Therapy for acne vulgaris. *N Engl J Med* 336:1156-1162, 1997.

References

Penicillins

1. Tomasz A: Susceptibility to β-lactam antibiotics: from inhibited target proteins to inhibited target cells. In Bearn AG, editor: *Antibiotics in the management of infections: outlook for the 1980's,* New York, 1982, Raven Press, pp 13-28.

2. Feingold D, Wagner R Jr, Boston MA: Antibacterial therapy. *J Am Acad Derm* 14:535-548, 1986.

3. McCarthy CG, Finland M: Absorption and excretion of four penicillins: penicillin G, penicillin V, phenethicillin and phenylmercaptomethyl penicillin. *N Engl J Med* 263:315-326, 1960.

4. Neu HC: Penicillins: microbiology, pharmacology, and clinical usage. In Kagan BM, editor: *Antimicrobial therapy,* Philadelphia, 1980, WB Saunders, p 31.

5. Romano A, Blanca M, Mayorga C, et al: Immediate hypersensitivity to penicillins. Studies on Italian subjects. *Allergy* 52:89-93, 1997.

6. Ponvert C, Le Clainche L, de Blic K, et al: Allergy to beta-lactam antibiotics in children. *Pediatrics* 104:45, 1999.

7. Assem ES, Vickers MR: Test for penicillin allergy in man. II. The immunologic cross-reaction between penicillins and cephalosporins. *Immunology* 27:255-269, 1974.

8. Herman R, Jick H: Cutaneous reaction rates to penicillins: oral versus parenteral. *Cutis* 24:232-234, 1979.

9. Alanis A, Weinstein AJ: Adverse reactions associated with the use of oral penicillins and cephalosporins. *Med Clin North Am* 67:113-129, 1983.

Cephalosporins

10. Neu HC: The new beta-lactamase-stable cephalosporins. *Ann Intern Med* 97:408-419, 1982.

11. Goldberg MD: The cephalosporins. *Med Clin North Am* 71:1113-1133, 1987.

12. Donowitz GR, Mandell GL: Beta-lactam antibiotics (second of two parts). *N Engl J Med* 318:490-500, 1988.

13. Moellering RC Jr, Swartz MN: The new cephalosporins. *N Engl J Med* 294:24-28, 1976.

14. Cuchural GH Jr, Tally FP, Jacobus NV, et al: Comparative activities of newer beta-lactam agents against members of the *Bacteroides fragilis* group. *Antimicrob Agents Chemother* 34:479-480, 1990.

15. Epstein ME, Amodio-Groton MA, Sadick NA: Antimicrobial agents for the dermatologist. I. β-lactam antibiotics and related compounds. *J Am Acad Dermatol* 37:149-165, 1997.

16. Fassberder M, Lode H, Schaberg T, et al: Pharmacokinetics of new oral cephalosporins, including a new carbacephem. *Clin Infect Dis* 16:646-653, 1993.

17. Gustaferro CA, Steckelberg JM: Cephalosporin antimicrobial agents and related compounds. *Mayo Clin Proc* 66:1064-1073, 1991.

18. Johnson JD: The cephalosporins in dermatologic practice. *Int J Dermatol* 25:427-430, 1986.

19. Parish LC, Witkowski JA: Cephalosporin therapy in dermatologic practice. *Clin Dermatol* 9:459-469, 1992.

20. Nadelman RB, Luger SW, Frank E, et al: Comparison of cefuroxime axetil and doxycycline in the treatment of early Lyme disease. *Ann Intern Med* 117:273-280, 1992.

21. Gordin FM, Wofsy CB, Mills J: Once-daily ceftriaxone for skin and soft tissue infections. *Antimicrob Agents Chemother* 27:648-649, 1985.

22. Parish LC, Jungkind DL: Systemic antimicrobial therapy for skin and skin structure infections. Comparison of fleroxacin and ceftazidime. *Am J Med* 94(Suppl 3A):166-173, 1993.

23. Buening MK, Wold JS, Israel KS, et al: Disulfiram-like reactions to beta-lactams (letter). *JAMA* 245:2027, 1981.

24. Quinn EL, Pohlod D, Madhavan T, et al: Clinical experience with cefazolin and other cephalosporins in bacterial endocarditis. *J Infect Dis* 128(Suppl):386-391, 1983.

25. Lopez AJ, O'Keefe P, Mornssey M, et al: Ceftriaxone-induced cholelithiasis. *Ann Intern Med* 115:712-714, 1991.

26. Levine BB: Antigenicity and cross reactivity of penicillins and cephalosporins. *J Infect Dis* 128:364-366, 1973.

27. Saxon A, Beall GN, Rohr AS, et al: Immediate hypersensitivity reactions to beta-lactam antibiotics. *Ann Intern Med* 107:204-215, 1987.

28. Reynolds RD, Grammer LC, Kelsey DK: Cefaclor and serum sickness-like reactions. *JAMA* 276:950-951, 1996.

29. Norrby SR: Side effects of cephalosporins. *Drugs* 34:105-120, 1987.

30. Galnick HR, McGinnis M, Elton W, et al: Hemolytic anemia associated with cephalothin. *JAMA* 217:1193-1197, 1971.

31. Sang N, Kammer RB: Hematologic complications associated with beta-lactam antibiotics. *Rev Infect Dis* 5:380-393, 1983.

32. Fass RJ, Perkins RL, Saslaw S: Cephalexin—a new oral cephalosporin: clinical evaluation in sixty-three patients. *Am J Med Sci* 259:187, 1970.

β-Lactamase Inhibitor/β-Lactam Combination Antibiotics

33. Lindberg F, Normark S: Contribution of chromosomal beta-lactamase to beta-lactam resistance in Enterobacteria. *Rev Infect Dis* 8(Suppl 3):292-304, 1986.

34. Neu HC: Contribution of beta-lactamases to bacterial resistance and mechanisms to inhibit beta-lactamases. *Am J Med* 79 (Suppl 5B):2-12, 1985.

35. Sensakovic JW, Smith LG: Beta-lactamase inhibitor combinations. *Med Clin North Am* 79:695-704, 1995.

36. Maddux MS: Effects of beta-lactamase-mediated antimicrobial resistance: the role of beta-lactamase inhibitors. *Pharmacotherapy* 11:40S-50S, 1991.

37. Stein GE, Gurwith MJ: Amoxicillin-potassium clavulanate, a beta-lactamase-resistant antibiotic combination. *Clin Pharm* 3:591-599, 1984.

38. Staniforth DH, Lilystone KJ, Jackson D: Effect of food on the bioavailability and tolerance of clavulanic acid/amoxicillin combination. *J Antimicrob Chemother* 10:131-139, 1982.

39. Goldstein EJC, Reinhart JF, Murray PM, et al: Outpatient therapy of bite wounds: demographic data, bacteriology and a prospective, randomized trial of amoxicillin-clavulanic acid versus penicillin ± dicloxacillin. *Int J Dermatol* 26:123-131, 1987.

40. Staniforth DH, Jackson D, Clarke HL, et al: Amoxicillin/clavulanic acid: the effect of probenecid. *J Antimicrob Chemother* 12:273, 1983.

41. Ganes D, Batra V, Faulkner K, et al: Effect of probenecid on the pharmacokinetics of piperacillin and tazobactam in healthy volunteers. Proceedings of the Sixth Annual Meeting and Exposition, American Associated of Pharmaceutical Scientists, Washington, DC 1991; Abstract PPDM8293. Pharmaceutical Research 8, S299.

42. Jick D, Porter JB: Potentiation of ampicillin skin reactions by allopurinol or hyperuricemia. *J Clin Pharmacol* 21:456-458, 1981.

43. Ball AP, Mehtar S, Watson A: Clinical efficacy and tolerance of Augmentin in soft tissue infection. *J Antimicrob Chemother* 10:67-74, 1982.

44. Brown CH, Natelson EA, Bradshaw MW, et al: Study of the effects of ticarcillin on blood coagulation and platelet function. *Antimicrob Agents Chemother* 7:652-657, 1975.

45. Bryson HM: Brogden RN: Piperacillin/tazobactam. A review of its antibacterial activity, pharmacokinetic properties and therapeutic potential. *Drugs* 47:506-535, 1994.

46. Itokazu GS, Danziger LH: Ampicillin-sulbactam and ticarcillin-clavulanic acid: a comparison of their in vitro activity and review of their clinical efficacy. *Pharmacotherapy* 11:382-414, 1991.

Carbapenems and Monobactams

47. Hellinger WC, Brewer NS: Imipenem. *Mayo Clin Proc* 66:1074-1081, 1991.

48. Jones RN: Review of the in vitro spectrum of activity of imipenem. *Am J Med* 78:22-32, 1985.

49. Norrby SR: Carbapenems. *Med Clin North Am* 79:745-759, 1995.

50. Fass RJ, Freimer EH, McCloskey RV: Treatment of skin and soft tissue infections with imipenem/cilastatin. *Am J Med* 78:110-112, 1985.

51. Saxon A, Beall GN, Rohr AS, et al: Immediate hypersensitivity reactions to beta-lactam antibiotics. UCLA Conference. *Ann Intern Med* 107:204-215, 1987.

52. Brewer NS, Hellinger WC: The monobactams. *Mayo Clin Proc* 66:1152-1157, 1991.

53. Neu HC: Aztreonam: the first monobactam. *Med Clin North Am* 72:555-566, 1988.

54. Buesing MA, Jorgersen JH: In vitro activity of aztreonam in combination with newer B-lactams and amikacin against multiply resistant bacilli. *Antimicrob Agents Chemother* 25:283-285, 1984.

55. Scully BE, Henry SA: Clinical experience with aztreonam in the treatment of gram-negative bacteremia. *Rev Infect Dis* 7(Suppl 4):789-793, 1985.

56. Anonymous: Aztreonam. AHFS Drug Information 95. American Society of Health System Pharmacists 170-178, 1995.

Macrolides

57. Piscitelli SC, Danziger LH, Rodvold KA: Clarithromycin and azithromycin: new macrolide antibiotics. *Clin Pharmacy* 11:137-152, 1992.

58. Bahal N, Nahata MC: The new macrolide antibiotics: azithromycin, clarithromycin, dirithromycin and roxithromycin. *Ann Pharmacother* 26:46-55, 1992.

59. Brogden RN, Peters DH: Dirithromycin: a review of its antimicrobial activity, pharmacokinetic properties and therapeutic efficacy. *Drugs* 48:599-616, 1994.

60. Schlossberg D: Azithromycin and clarithromycin. *Med Clin North Am* 79:803-815, 1995.

61. Sturgill MG, Rapp RP: Clarithromycin: a review of a new macrolide antibiotic with improved microbiologic spectrum and favorable pharmacokinetic and adverse effect profiles. *Ann Pharmacother* 26:1099-1108, 1992.

62. Retsema J, Girard A, Schelkly W, et al: Spectrum and mode of action of azithromycin (CP-662,993), a new 15-membered-ring macrolide with improved potency against gram-negative organisms. *Antimicrob Agents Chemother* 31:1939-1947, 1987.

63. Hardy DJ, Swanson RN, Rode RA, et al: Enhancement of the in vitro and in vivo activities of clarithromycin against *Haemophilus influenzae* by 14-hydroxy-clarithromycin, its major metabolite in humans. *Antimicrob Agents Chemother* 34:1407-1413, 1990.

64. Bowie WR, Shaw CE, Chan GW, et al: In vitro activity of RO 15-8074, RO 19-5247, A56268, and roxithromycin (RU 28965) against *Neisseria gonorrhoeae* and *Chlamydia trachomatis*. *Antimicrob Agents Chemother* 31:470-472, 1987.

65. Dunkin KT, Jones S, Howard AJ: The in vitro activity of CP-62,993 against *Haemophilus influenzae, Branhamaella catarrhalis, Staphylococci,* and *Streptococci. J Antimicrob Chemother* 21:405-411, 1988.

66. Kitzis MD, Goldstein FW, Miegi M, et al: In vitro activity of azithromycin against various gram-negative bacilli and anaerobic bacteria. *J Antimicrob Chemother* 25(Suppl A):15-18, 1990.

67. Gelber RH, Sui P, Tsang M, et al: Activities of various macrolide antibiotics against *Mycobacterium leprae* infection in mice. *Antimicrob Agents Chemother* 35:760-763, 1991.

68. Perronne C, Gikas A, Truffot-Pernot C, et al: Activities of sparfloxacin, azithromycin, temafloxacin and rifapentine compared with that of clarithromycin against multiplication of *Mycobacterium avium complex* within human macrophages. *Antimicrob Agents Chemother* 35:1356-1359, 1991.

69. Benson CA, Ellner JJ: *Mycobacterium avium complex* infection and AIDS: advances in theory and practice. *Clin Infect Dis* 17:7-20, 1993.

70. Fernandez-Martin J, Leport C, Moriat P, et al: Pyrimethamine-clarithromycin combination for therapy of acute toxoplasma encephalitis in patients with AIDS. *Antimicrob Agents Chemother* 35:2049-2052, 1991.

71. Wynn RF, Leen CLS, Brettle RP: Azithromycin for cerebral toxoplasmosis in AIDS (letter). *Lancet* 341:243-244, 1993.

72. Peterson WL, Graham DY, Marshall B, et al: Clarithromycin as monotherapy for eradication of *Helicobacter pylori:* a randomized, double-blind trial. *Am J Gastroenterol* 88:1860-1864, 1993.

73. Lassus A: Comparative studies of azithromycin in skin and soft tissue infections and sexually transmitted infections by *Neisseria* and *Chlamydia* species. *J Antimicrob Chemother* 25(Suppl A):115-21, 1990.

74. Northcutt VJ, Craft JC, Pichotta P: Safety and efficacy of clarithromycin (C) compared to erythromycin (E) in the treatment (tx) of bacterial skin or skin structure infections (SSSIs) (abstract 1339). In Program and abstracts of the 30th Interscience Conference on Antimicrob Agents and Chemother, Atlanta 1990.

75. Parish LC and the Clarithromycin Study Group: Clarithromycin in the treatment of skin and skin structure infections: two multicenter clinical studies. *Int J Dermatol* 32:528-532, 1993.

76. Franck N, Cabie A, Villette B, et al: Treatment of *Mycobacterium chelonae* induced skin infection with clarithromycin. *J Am Acad Dermatol* 28:1019-1020, 1993.

77. Amacher DE, Schomaker SJ, Retsema JA: Comparison of the effects of the new azalide antibiotic azithromycin, and erythromycin estolate on rat liver cytochrome P-450. *Antimicrob Agents Chemother* 35:1186-1190, 1991.

78. Lindstrom T, Hanssen B, Wrighton S: Cytochrome P450 complex formation by dirithromycin and other macrolides in rat and human livers. *Antimicrob Agents Chemother* 37:265-269, 1993.

79. Product information: Biaxin (R), clarithromycin. Abbott Laboratories, North Chicago, IL 1995.

80. Harris S, Hilligoss D, Colandelo P, et al: Azithromycin and terfenadine: lack of drug interaction. *Clin Pharmacol Ther* 58:310-315, 1995.

81. Peters DH, Clissold SP: Clarithromycin, a review of its antimicrobial activity, pharmacokinetic properties and therapeutic potential. *Drugs* 44:117-164, 1992.

82. Petty B, Polis M, Haneiwick S, et al: Pharmacokinetic assessment of clarithromycin plus zidovudine in HIV patients (abstract). Presented at the 32nd Interscience Conference on Antimicrob Agents Chemother, Anaheim, CA, 1992.

83. Luft BJ, Dattwyler RJ, Johnson RC: Azithromycin compared with amoxicillin in the treatment of erythema migrans. A double-blind, randomized controlled trial. *Ann Intern Med* 124:785-791, 1996.

84. Stein GE, Havlichek DH: The new macrolide antibiotics: azithromycin and clarithromycin. *Postgrad Med* 92:269-280, 1992.

85. Sides GD, Conforti PM: Safety profile of dirithromycin. *J Antimicrob Chemother* 31:(suppl C):175-185, 1992.

86. Jacobson K: Clinical efficacy of dirithromycin in pneumonia. *J Antimicrob Chemother* 31(Suppl C):121-129, 1993.

Fluoroquinolones

87. Suh B, Lorber B: Quinolones. *Med Clin North Am* 29:869-894, 1995.

88. Hooper DC, Wolfson JS: Fluoroquinolone antimicrobial agents. *N Engl J Med* 324:384-394, 1991.

89. Wolfson JS, Hooper DC: Fluoroquinolone antimicrobial agents. *Clin Microbiol Rev* 2:378-424, 1989.

90. Crowe HM, Quintilliani R: Antibiotic formulary section. *Med Clin North Am* 79:476, 1995.

91. Fitton A: The quinolones. An overview of their pharmacology. *Clin Pharmacokinet* 22:1-11, 1992.
92. Chin N-X, Neu HC: Ciprofloxacin, a quinolone carboxylic acid compound active against aerobic and anaerobic bacteria. *Antimicrob Agents Chemother* 25:319-326, 1984.
93. Collins CH, Uttley AHC: In vitro susceptibility of mycobacteria to ciprofloxacin. *J Antimicrob Chemother* 16:575, 1985.
94. Hooton TM, Tartaglione TA: The role of fluoroquinolones in sexually transmitted diseases. *Pharmacotherapy* 13:189-201, 1993.
95. Husain RA: Disturbing susceptibility pattern for ciprofloxacin (letter). *Am J Hosp Pharm* 48:1892, 1991.
96. Jensen T, Pederson SS, Hielson CH, et al: The efficacy and safety of ciprofloxacin and ofloxacin in chronic *Pseudomonas aeruginosa* infection in cystic fibrosis. *J Antimicrob Chemother* 20:585-594, 1987.
97. Bayer AS, Hirano L, Yih J: Development of B-lactam resistance and increased quinolone MICs during therapy of experimental *Pseudomonas aeruginosa* endocarditis. *Antimicrob Agents Chemother* 32:231-235, 1988.
98. Neuman M: Clinical pharmacokinetics of the newer antimicrobial 4-quinolones. *Clin Pharmacokinet* 14:96-121, 1988.
99. Adhami S, Wise R, Wiston D, et al: The pharmacokinetics and tissue penetration of norfloxacin. *J Antimicrob Chemother* 13:87-92, 1984.
100. Fillastre JP, Leroy A, Moulin B, et al: Pharmacokinetics of quinolones in renal insufficiency. *J Antimicrob Chemother* 26(Suppl B):51-60, 1990.
101. Parish LC, Witkowski JA: The quinolones and dermatologic practice. *Int J Dermatol* 2:351-356, 1987.
102. Sanders WE: Oral ofloxacin: a critical review of the new drug application. *Clin Infect Dis* 14:539-554, 1992.
103. Powers RD: Open trial of oral fleroxacin vs amoxicillin/clavulanate in the treatment of infections of skin and soft tissue. *Am J Med* 94:1555-1585, 1993.
104. Smith JW, Nichols RL: Comparison of oral fleroxacin with oral amoxicillin/clavulanate for treatment of skin and soft tissue infections. *Am J Med* 94:1505-1545, 1993.
105. Stein GE: Drug interactions with fluoroquinolones. *Am J Med* 91(Suppl 6A):81S-86S, 1991.
106. Wijnands WJA, Vree TB, Van Herwaarden CLA: The influence of quinolone derivatives on theophylline clearance. *Br J Clin Pharmacol* 22:677-683, 1986.
107. Kamada AK: Possible interaction between ciprofloxacin and warfarin. *Drug Intell Clin Pharm* 24:27-28, 1990.
108. Jolson HM, Tanner A, Green A, et al: Adverse reaction reporting of interactions between warfarin and fluoroquinolones. *Arch Intern Med* 151:1003-1004, 1991.
109. Smith CR: The adverse effects of fluoroquinolones. *J Antimicrob Chemother* 19:709-712, 1987.
110. Poh-Fitzpatrick MB: Lomefloxacin photosensitivity (letter). *Arch Dermatol* 130:261, 1994.
111. Scheife RT, Cramer WR, Decker EL: Photosensitizing potential of ofloxacin. *Int J Dermatol* 32:413-416, 1993.
112. Horio T, Miyauchi H, Asada Y, et al: Phototoxicity and photoallergenicity of quinolones in guinea pigs. *J Dermatol Sci* 7:130-135, 1994.
113. Lowe NJ, Fakouhi TD, Stern RS, et al: Photoreactions with a fluoroquinolone antimicrobial: evening vs morning dosing. *Clin Pharmacol Ther* 56:587-591, 1994.
114. LeCleach L, Chosidu O, Berry JP, et al: Blue-black pigmentation of the legs associated with perfloxacin therapy. *Arch Dermatol* 131:856-857, 1995.

Tetracyclines
115. Klein NC, Cunha BA: Tetracyclines. *Med Clin North Am* 79:789-801, 1995.
116. Neuvonen PJ, Gothoni G, Hackman R, et al: Interference of iron with the absorption of tetracyclines in man. *BMJ* 4:532, 1970.
117. Ericsson CD, Feldman S, Pickering LK, et al: Influence of subsalicylate bismuth on absorption of doxycycline. *JAMA* 247:2266-2267, 1982.
118. Standiford HC: Tetracyclines and chloramphenicol. In Mandell GL, Douglas RG Jr, Bennett JE, editors: *Principles and practice of infectious disease*, ed 4, New York, 1995, Churchill Livingstone, pp 306-317.
119. Berk MA, Lornicz AL: The treatment of bullous pemphigoid with tetracycline and nicotinamide: a preliminary report. *Arch Dermatol* 122:670-674, 1986.
120. Zemtsov A, Neldner KH: Successful treatment of dermatitis herpetiformis with tetracycline and nicotinamide in a patient unable to tolerate dapsone. *J Am Acad Dermatol* 28:505-506, 1993.

121. Chaffins MI, Collinson D, Fivenson DP: Treatment of pemphigus and linear IgA dermatosis with nicotinamide and tetracycline: a review of 13 cases. *J Am Acad Dermatol* 28:998-1000, 1993.

122. Steere AC, Hutchinson GJ, Rahn DW, et al: Treatment of the early manifestations of Lyme disease. *Ann Intern Med* 99:22-26, 1983.

123. Wallace RJ Jr, Wiss K: Susceptibility of *Mycobacterium marinum* to tetracyclines and aminoglycosides. *Antimicrob Agents Chemother* 20:610-612, 1981.

124. Reboli AC, Del Bene VF: Oral antibiotics therapy of dermatologic conditions. *Dermatol Clin* 6:497-520, 1988.

125. Anonymous: Tetracycline. American Hospital Formulary Service. Drug Information 1995. American Society of Health System Pharmacists 95:338-355.

126. Amendda MA, Spera TD: Doxycycline induced esophagitis. *JAMA* 253:1009-1111, 1985.

127. Elmore MF, Rogge JD: Tetracycline induced pancreatitis. *Gastroenterology* 81:1134-1136, 1981.

128. Shils ME: Renal disease and the metabolic effects of tetracycline. *Ann Intern Med* 58:389-408, 1963.

129. Forrest JN Jr, Cox M, Hong C, et al: Superiority of demeclocycline over lithium in the treatment of chronic syndrome of inappropriate secretion of antidiuretic hormone. *N Engl J Med* 298:173-177, 1978.

130. Guillon JM, Joly P, Autran B, et al: Minocycline induced cells mediated hypersensitivity pneumonitis. *Ann Intern Med* 117:476-481, 1992.

131. Matsuura T, Shimizu Y, Fugimoto H, et al: Minocycline-related lupus. *Lancet* 340:1553, 1992.

132. Knowles SR, Shapiro L, Shear NH: Serious adverse reactions induced by minocycline. Report of 13 patients and review of the literature. *Arch Dermatol* 132:934-939, 1996.

133. Thibault MJ, Billick RG, Strolovitz H: Minocycline induced Sweet's syndrome. *J Am Acad Dermatol* 27:801-804, 1992.

134. Angeloni VL, Salashe SJ, Ortiz R: Nail and scleral pigmentation induced by minocycline. *Cutis* 40:229, 1987.

135. Davies JP, Price-Thomas JM: Gynecomastia in association with minocycline (letter). *Br J Clin Pract* 49:179, 1995.

136. Katz J, Barak S, Shemer J, et al: Black tongue associated with minocycline therapy (letter). *Arch Dermatol* 131:620, 1995.

Rifamycins

137. Thornsberry C, Hill BC, Swenson JM, et al: Rifampin: spectrum of antibacterial activity. *Rev Infect Dis* 5(suppl 3):412-417, 1983.

138. Prescott JF: *Rhodococcus equi:* an animal and human pathogen. *Clin Microbiol Rev* 4:20-34, 1991.

139. O'Brien RJ, Lyle MA, Snider DE: Rifabutin (Ansamycin LM427): a new rifamycin-S derivative for the treatment of mycobacterial diseases. *Rev Infect Dis* 9:519-530, 1987.

140. Brogden RN, Fitton A: Rifabutin. A review of its antimicrobial activity, pharmacokinetic properties and therapeutic efficacy. *Drugs* 47:983-1009, 1994.

141. Purohit SD, Supta ML, Gupia PR: Dietary constituents and rifampicin absorption. *Tuberculosis* 68:151, 1987.

142. Tsankov NK, Kamarashev JA: Rifampin in dermatology. *Int J Dermatol* 32:401-406, 1993.

143. Ramesh V, Misra RS, Saxena V, et al: A comparative of efficacy of drug regimens in skin tuberculosis. *Clin Exp Dermatol* 16:106-109, 1991.

144. Bonate JL: Antibiotiques en pathologie cutanee. *Rev Med Toullouse* 19:29-37, 1983.

145. Hoss DM, Feder HM: Addition of rifampicin to conventional therapy for recurrent furunculosis. *Arch Dermatol* 131:647-648, 1995.

146. Gamea AM, El-Tatawi FA: The effect of rifampicin on rhinoscleroma: an electron microscopic study. *J Laryngol Otol* 104:772-777, 1990.

147. Tsankov N, Krasteva M: Rifampin therapy in severe forms of psoriasis. *J Dermatol Treat* 3:69-71, 1992.

148. Johnson TM, Duvic M, Rapini RP: AIDS exacerbation psoriasis (letter). *N Engl J Med* 313:1415, 1985.

149. Green MS, Prystowsky JH, Cohen SR, et al: Infectious complications of erythrodermic psoriasis. *J Am Acad Dermatol* 34:911-914, 1996.

150. Leung DYM, Travers JB, Giorno R, et al: Evidence for streptococcal superantigen driven process in acute guttate psoriasis. *J Clin Invest* 96:2006-2012, 1995.

151. Vincent F, Ross JB, Dalton M, et al: A therapeutic trial of the use of penicillin V or erythromycin with or without rifampin in treatment of psoriasis. *J Am Acad Dermatol* 26:458-461, 1992.

152. Wheat LJ, Kohler RB, White AL, et al: Effect of rifampin on nasal carrier of coagulase-positive staphylococci. *J Infect Dis* 144:177, 1981.

153. Bachs L, Pares A, Elena M, et al: Effects of long-term rifampin administration on primary biliary cirrhosis. *Gastroenterology* 102:2007-2080, 1992.

154. Borcherding SM, Baciewicz AM, Self TH: Update on rifampin drug interactions. *Arch Intern Med* 152:711-716, 1992.

155. Grosset J, Leventis S: Adverse effects of rifampin. *Rev Infect Dis* 5(Suppl 3)S440-446, 1983.

Trimethoprim-Sulfamethoxazole

156. Rubin RH, Schwartz MN: Trimethoprim-sulfamethoxazole. *N Engl J Med* 303:426, 1980.

157. Cockerill FR, Edson RS: Trimethoprim-sulfamethoxazole. *Mayo Clin Proc* 66:1260-1269, 1991.

158. Smego RA Jr, Moeller MB, Gallis HA: Trimethoprim-sulfamethoxazole therapy for nocardia infections. *Arch Intern Med* 143:711-718, 1983.

159. Spitzer PG, Hammer SM, Karchmer AW: Treatment of *Listeria monocytogenes* infection with trimethoprim-sulfamethoxazole. Case report and review of the literature. *Rev Infect Dis* 8:427-430, 1986.

160. Goodgame RW: Understanding intestinal spore-forming protozoa: *Cryptosporidia, Microsporidia, Isospora,* and *Cyclospora*. *Ann Intern Med* 124:429-441, 1996.

161. Gold WI, Salit IE: *Aeromonas hydrophilia* infections of skin and soft tissue: report of 11 cases and review. *Clin Infect Dis* 16:69-74, 1993.

162. Margileth AM: Antibiotic therapy for cat-scratch disease: clinical study of the therapeutic outcome in 268 patients and a review of the literature. *Pediatr Infect Dis J* 11:477-478, 1992.

163. Sookprance M, Boonma P, Susaengrat W, et al: Multicenter positive randomized trial comparing ceftazidime plus cotrimoxazole with chloramphenicol plus doxycycline and cotrimoxazole for treatment of severe melioidosis. *Antimicrob Agents Chemother* 36:158-162, 1992.

164. Magana M, Magana-Garcia M: Mycetoma. *Dermatol Clin* 7:203-217, 1989.

165. Epstein ME, Amodio-Groton MA, Sadick NA: Antimicrobial agents for the dermatologist. II. Macrolides, fluoroquinolones, rifamycins, tetracyclines, trimethoprim-sulfamethoxazole and clindamycin. *J Am Acad Dermatol* 37:365-381, 1997.

166. Bissonnette R, Tousignant J, Allaire G: Drug induced toxic pustuloderma. *Int J Dermatol* 31:172-174, 1992.

167. Walker DC, Cohen PR: Trimethoprim-sulfamethoxazole associated acute febrile neutrophilic dermatosis. Case report and review of drug induced Sweet's syndrome. *J Am Acad Dermatol* 34:918-923, 1996.

168. Jick H: Adverse reactions to trimethoprim-sulfamethoxazole in hospitalized patients. *Rev Infect Dis* 4:426-428, 1982.

169. McGehee RF Jr, Smith CB, Wilcox C, et al: Comparative studies of antibacterial activity in vitro and absorption and excretion of lincomycin and clindamycin. *Am J Med Sci* 256:279-292, 1968.

Clindamycin

170. McGehee RF Jr, Smith CB, Wilcox C, et al: Comparative studies of antibacterial activity in vitro and absorption and excretion of lincomycin and clindamycin. *Am J Med Sci* 256:279-292, 1968.

171. Falagas ME, Gorbach SL: Clindamycin and metronidazole. *Med Clin North Am* 79:845-867, 1995.

172. Klempner MS, Styrt B: Prevention of recurrent staphylococcal skin infections with low dose oral clindamycin therapy. *JAMA* 260:2682, 1988.

173. Anonymous: Clindamycin. American Hospital Formulary Service. Drug Information 1995. American Society of Health System Pharmacists. 1995:357-361.

174. Bartlett JG: Antimicrobial agents implicated in *Clostridium difficile* toxin associated diarrhea or colitis. *Johns Hopkins Med J* 149:6-9, 1981.

175. Dhawan VK, Thadepalli H: Clindamycin: a review of fifteen years of experience. *Rev Infect Dis* 4:1133-1153, 1982.

CHAPTER 4

Aditya K. Gupta

Systemic Antifungal Agents

The systemic antifungal agents used most commonly to treat onychomycosis and other dermatomycoses are the new generation of oral antimycotics: terbinafine, itraconazole, and fluconazole. The older systemic oral antifungal agents are griseofulvin and ketoconazole. This chapter focuses on the new oral antifungals because the traditional agents, griseofulvin and ketoconazole, now have limited use in the management of onychomycosis and other dermatomycoses (Table 4-1). The chapter does not discuss topical therapies for onychomycosis. Ciclopirox nail lacquer has just been approved in the United States for mild-to-moderate dermatophyte toe onychomycosis that does not involve the lunula.

TERBINAFINE

Terbinafine is an allylamine that was discovered in 1974.[1] Oral terbinafine was first approved for use in the United Kingdom in February 1991, in Canada in May 1993, and in the United States in May 1996.[2] Topical terbinafine was approved in the United States in December 1992. The first allylamine to be approved for use in humans was naftifine; however, it is effective only topically.[2] It is estimated that 7.3 million treatment courses of oral terbinafine have been given worldwide as of August 1997.

Pharmacology

Table 4-2 lists key pharmacologic concepts for systemic antifungal agents.

STRUCTURE. Terbinafine hydrochloride has the empirical formula $C_{21}H_{26}ClN$. The molecular weight is 327.9[3] (Figure 4-1).

ABSORPTION AND DISTRIBUTION. When terbinafine is administered orally, 70% to 80% of the dose is absorbed, with the bioavailability not being significantly affected by food intake.[4] The bioavailability of terbinafine as a result of first-pass metabolism is approximately 40%. After a single terbinafine dose of 250 or 500 mg, maximal plasma concentrations are achieved within 2 hours.[5] A maximal plasma concentration of 1.3 mg/mL has been observed in volunteers after repeated administration of 250 mg.[6] Steady-state levels are reached after 10 to 14 days.[6]

Terbinafine is extremely lipophilic and extensively distributed.[5] The allylamine binds strongly (>99%) and nonspecifically to plasma proteins, with binding evenly distributed between all plasma protein fractions.[5] High concentrations of terbinafine are found in the stratum corneum, sebum, and hair.[7-9] The absorption and distribution half-lives of terbinafine are approximately 0.8 hour and 4.6 hours, respectively.[9]

■ **Table 4-1**   Systemic Antifungal Agents

Generic Name	Trade Name	Generic Available	Manu-facturer	Tablet/Capsule Sizes	Special Formu-lations	Price Index
Terbinafine	Lamisil	No	Novartis	250 mg	—	$$$$
Itraconazole	Sporanox	No	Janssen	100 mg	Liquid 10 mg/ml	$$$$
Fluconazole	Diflucan	No	Pfizer	50, 100, 150, 200 mg	Suspension 50 mg/5 ml, 200 mg/5 ml*	$$$$$
Griseofulvin	Gris-PEG†	Yes	Allergan	125, 250 mg	—	$/$$ ($)
	Fulvicin P/G†	Yes	Schering	165, 330 mg	—	$/$$ ($)
	Grifulvin V	Yes	Ortho	250, 500 mg	Suspension 125 mg/5 ml	$$ ($)
Ketoconazole	Nizoral	No	Janssen	200 mg	—	$$$ ($$$)

$, <1.00; $$, 1.01-2.00; $$$, 2.01-5.00; $$$$, 5.01-10.00; $$$$$, >10.00; ( ), generic price; /, two different price ranges from lower dose to higher dose examples of this drug; —, no price listed for this drug.
*Fluconazole also has several injectable formulations available.
†These formulations of griseofulvin are "ultramicrosize" products; Grifulvin V is "microsize."

PHARMACOKINETIC PROFILES IN VARIOUS CUTANEOUS STRUCTURES

Pharmacokinetics in Skin.   When terbinafine is administered orally, the drug has been detected in the stratum corneum as early as 24 hours after commencing therapy.[8] Terbinafine is first detected in the deeper layers of the stratum corneum and probably reaches this site by epidermal diffusion.[8] After a few days of therapy the concentration gradient is lost. Movement of terbinafine through the stratum corneum probably occurs both by diffusion and by incorporation of drug into the corneocytes that are moving outwards.[8] Within 2 days of administering terbinafine 250 mg/day the drug achieves a high level in the sebum but at a slower rate than by diffusion.[7] High concentrations of drug (well above the minimum inhibitory concentration [MIC]) are reached in the stratum corneum within hours of starting therapy.[7] Terbinafine has not been detected in the eccrine sweat.[10] The elimination half-life of terbinafine from the stratum corneum and sebum is 3 to 5 days.[7] After administration of terbinafine 250 mg/day for 12 days, drug concentrations above the MIC for most dermatophytes may be present for 2 to 3 weeks after oral therapy is discontinued.[7]

Pharmacokinetics in Nails.   In patients given terbinafine 250 mg/day, the drug may be detected in the distal nail in the majority of patients within 1 week of starting therapy.[10-12] In peripheral nail clippings, levels of terbinafine were 0.43 μg/g after 7 days of therapy, or 10 to 100 times the MIC for most dermatophytes. The data indicate that terbinafine diffuses into the nail plate via both the nail matrix and the nailbed. When terbinafine 250 mg/day is administered for 6 or 12 weeks to treat onychomycosis, maximum nail levels are detectable after 18 weeks of therapy.[11] After completion of 6 and 12 weeks of therapy, terbinafine is detected in the nail for 30 weeks and 36 weeks, respectively.[11]

Pharmacokinetics in Hair.   Terbinafine has been detected in hair within 1 week of starting therapy.[10] The early detection in hair may be due to delivery of drug to hair via the sebum. The drug may become incorporated into hair by hair matrix cells. When terbinafine 250 mg/day is administered for 14 days, the drug has been detected in hair for at least 50 days.[12] It should be noted that terbinafine may be more effective against tinea capitis caused by endothrix organisms (e.g., *Trichophyton tonsurans*) compared with ectothrix infections (e.g., *Microsporum canis*).[13,14]

METABOLISM AND EXCRETION.   Terbinafine is extensively metabolized in the liver; 15 metabolites have been identified.[2] The metabolites are less lipophilic and lack significant antifungal activity. The main metabolites are the

▋ Table 4-2 Key Pharmacologic Concepts—Systemic Antifungal Agents

Drug	Category	Absorption and Bioavailability			Half-life	Elimination	
		Peak Levels	Bioavail-able (%)	Protein Binding		Metabolism	Excretion
Terbinafine	Allylamine	2 hrs	40%*	99%	22 hrs	Significant first-pass hepatic metabolism; 15 inactive metabolites	Renal 80%, fecal 20% for various metabolites
Itraconazole†	Triazole	4 hrs	55%	99%	56 hrs	Extensive metabolism in liver; has over 30 metabolites; of these one is active—hydroxyitraconazole	Renal 35%, fecal 54%, mostly as inactive metabolites
Fluconazole	Triazole	1-2 hrs	>90%	11%‡	30.2-37.3 hrs	Little first-pass hepatic metabolism, much of dose is excreted as unchanged parent drug	Renal 80% of parent drug, 11% as metabolites, 2% feces
Griseofulvin	Other	4 hrs	99%	??	24 hrs	Hepatic, major metabolites are 6-methyl-griseofulvin and its glucuronide conjugate	Renal, 1% excreted unchanged in urine, 36% in feces

*Initial absorption of terbinafine is in range of 70% to 80% of an oral dose—significant first-pass hepatic metabolism reduces bioavailability to this percentage.
†Itraconazole is highly lipophilic with highest bioavailability when taken with a full meal; extensive storage in fatty tissues including in subcutaneous fat.
‡Fluconazole is much less lipophilic, thus more hydrophilic than other azoles including itraconazole; this accounts for low protein binding.

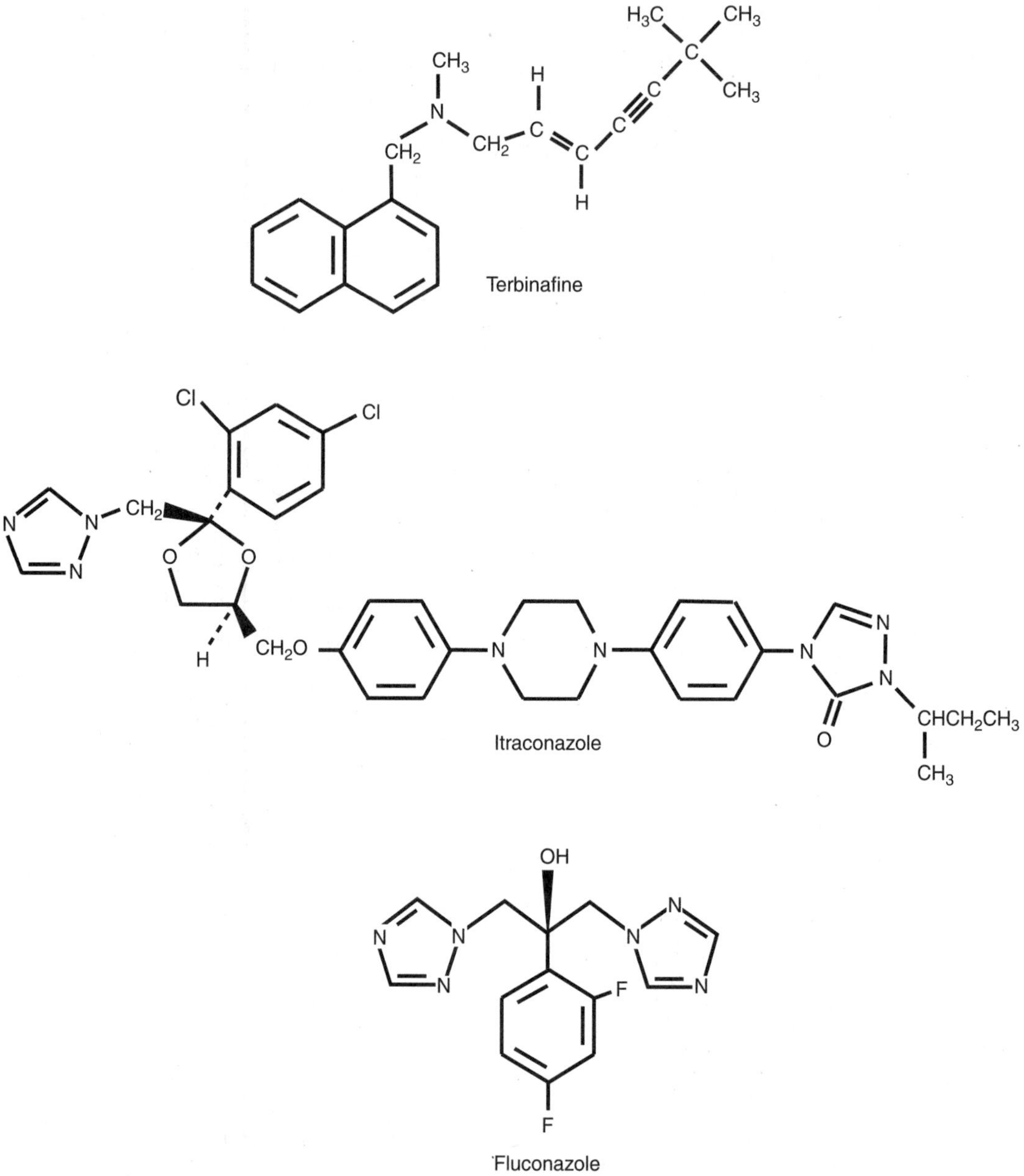

Figure 4-1 Systemic antifungal agents.

N-demethyl and the 2-carboxy metabolites. The elimination of terbinafine in plasma is triphasic, with half-lives of approximately 1.5, 22, and 90 hours.[4] Approximately 80% of the oral dose is excreted in the urine in metabolized form with the remaining 20% being eliminated via the feces.[4,5] About 85% of the terbinafine is recovered within 72 hours.[4] The mean elimination half-life of the parent drug in plasma is 22 days and is in the same range as the metabolites. When therapy is stopped, terbinafine is initially rapidly cleared from plasma; subsequently, the slow half-life probably reflects the gradual release from adipose tissues.

In patients with renal insufficiency, the elimination of terbinafine is reduced with an increase in elimination half-life.[9] It is suggested that the oral terbinafine dosage should be approximately halved when serum creatinine is >300 μmol/L (or creatinine clearance <50 ml/min, that is, 0.83 ml/sec).[9] This may be due to reduced excretion of the *N*-demethyl and carboxylic acid metabolites (the 2 major plasma metabolites of terbinafine) that can compete with the unchanged drug for metabolizing enzymes.[4,5] As a result the metabolic clearance of terbinafine is reduced.[4]

In patients with liver dysfunction, the maximal plasma concentration (Cmax), the time taken to reach Cmax (Tmax), and the absorption half-life of terbinafine may be similar to healthy volunteers.[4] In one study, the elimination of terbinafine was 30% slower in patients with hepatic dysfunction compared with normals as a result of decreased biotransformation.[4]

After a single 500 mg dose, no differences in the pharmacokinetics of terbinafine were observed in elderly subjects, 67 to 73 years of age, compared with young volunteers.[4] Normally, dose adjustments of terbinafine in elderly subjects should not be necessary.[4] However, elderly subjects with age-related renal function impairment may require an adjustment of terbinafine dosage.[9]

MECHANISM OF ACTION. Ergosterol and cholesterol are essential constituents of fungal and mammalian cell membranes, respectively. Allylamines (e.g., naftifine and terbinafine) inhibit squalene epoxidase.[15] Terbinafine does not appear to affect other enzymes of the ergosterol pathway; it may not have a direct effect on nucleic acid, protein, cell wall synthesis, or cell membrane activity. Inhibition of squalene epoxidase may result in both a deficiency of ergosterol and an accumulation of squalene.[15] The fungistatic action in vitro and in vivo may be the result of ergosterol efficiency that interferes with membrane function cell growth leading to an arrest in growth.[15] On the other hand, an accumulation of squalene may be associated with fungicidal action in vitro, possibly by deposition of lipid vesicles with disruption of cellular membranes.[15] Terbinafine is much more selective in its inhibition of fungal rather than human squalene epoxidase by 3 to 4 orders of magnitude.

Terbinafine has been reported to inhibit cytochrome P-450 2D6 in vitro.[16,17] Clinicians should be very cautious regarding concomitant administration of terbinafine with 2D6 substrates such as tricyclic antidepressants.

Clinical Use
Table 4-3 lists indications and contraindications for terbinafine.

APPROVED INDICATIONS
Onychomycosis—Caused by Dermatophytes. Terbinafine is approved for the treatment of onychomycosis of the toenails and fingernails (tinea unguium) caused by dermatophytes. The recommended dosage is 250 mg/day for 6 and 12 weeks for fingernail and toenail onychomycosis, respectively. An analysis of studies where terbinafine 250 mg/day has been administered for 12 to 16 weeks to treat dermatophyte onychomycosis of the toenails demonstrates a metaaverage ± standard error (SE) of 78.7% ± 3.8% (95% CI: 71.2% to 86.2%) (17 trials, n = 1122 patients).[20-36] In one study, approximately 11% of terbinafine responders demonstrated evidence of relapse 18 to 21 months after cessation of treatment.[37] For dermatophyte fingernail onychomycosis, when terbinafine 250 mg/day is given for 6 weeks, the mycologic cure rate, metaaverage ± SE, is 80.9% ± 4.5% (95% CI: 72.0% to 89.9%) (3 trials, n = 74 patients).[27-29] Terbinafine pulse therapy (250 mg twice daily for 1 week a month for 3 to 4 months, with 1 week on and 3 weeks off) has been reported uncommonly.[20,35] This pulse regimen has not received Food and Drug Administration (FDA) approval for the treatment of onychomycosis.

OFF-LABEL USES
Onychomycosis Caused by **Candida** *Species and Nondermatophyte Molds.* In comparison with its efficacy against dermatophytes, terbinafine is less effective when the causative agent of the onychomycosis is *Candida* species, in particular *C. albicans*.[38-40] There are limited data regarding the use of terbinafine to treat nondermatophyte molds, compared with dermatophytes.[39,41,42]

Onychomycosis in Children. Terbinafine is effective and safe when used to treat onychomycosis in children.[43-47] The duration of therapy is similar to that in adults—fingernail and toenail onychomycosis for 6 and 12 weeks, respectively. A dosage schedule is: >40 kg (250 mg/day), 20-40 kg (125 mg/day), and <20 kg (62.5 mg/day).

Tinea Corporis, Tinea Cruris, and Tinea Pedis. In the countries where terbinafine is approved for the treatment of tinea corporis or tinea cruris, the regimen generally is 250 mg/day for 2 to 4 weeks; for tinea pedis the duration is 2 to 6 weeks.[48-54] In some instances, shorter durations of therapy have been reported,

Table 4-3	Terbinafine Indications and Contraindications

FDA-APPROVED INDICATIONS
Onychomycosis—Due to Dermatophytes[18-37]
Tinea unguium fingernails
Tinea unguium toenails

OFF-LABEL USES

Onychomycosis—Other Categories
Candida species[38-40]
Nondermatophyte molds[39,41,42]
Children[43-47]

Other Dermatophyte Infections
Majocchi's granuloma[64]
Tinea imbricata[65]

Dermatophyte Cutaneous Infections[48-54]
Tinea corporis
Tinea cruris
Tinea pedis

Miscellaneous Fungal Infections
Sporotrichosis—cutaneous[66]
Black piedra[67]
Aspergillosis[68]
Chromoblastomycosis[69]

Dermatophyte Hair Infections
Tinea capitis[13,14,55-63]

CONTRAINDICATIONS

Absolute
Hypersensitivity to terbinafine or any
　component of the product

Relative
Preexisting liver disease
Preexisting renal disease (creatinine clearance
　<50 ml/min)

PREGNANCY PRESCRIBING STATUS—CATEGORY B

■ **Table 4-4**　Capsule Dosing of Various Drugs for Tinea Capitis in Children of Various Weights[75,76]

			Weight (kg)				
	Dosage/kg	Duration	10-19	20-29	30-39	40-49	>50
Terbinafine Continuous	5 mg/kg/d	2-4 weeks	62.5 mg qd	125 mg qd	125 mg qd	250 mg qd	250 mg qd
Itraconazole Continuous	5 mg/kg/d	2-4 weeks	100 mg qd	100 mg qd	100 mg qd/ bid alt	200 mg qd	200 mg bid
Itraconazole Pulse*	5 mg/kg/d*	1 to 3 pulses	100 mg qd	100 mg qd	100 mg qd/ bid alt	200 mg qd	200 mg bid

Note: With *Microsporum* species, a longer duration of therapy may be required.
*Itraconazole pulses are 1 week "on" and 3 weeks "off" with the doses listed above; these doses are for capsule formulation; with liquid formulation, the optimal dose is 3 mg/kg/day.

with tinea pedis and tinea corporis requiring 2 and 1 weeks, respectively.

　Tinea Capitis.　There have been a significant number of studies regarding the use of terbinafine for this indication.[56-63] The dosage schedule of terbinafine often used is outlined in Tables

4-4 and 4-5. The duration of therapy is generally 4 weeks, with shorter durations being recently reported to be effective as well.[60] The length of therapy may in part depend on the causative organism, for example, with *M. canis* the duration of therapy may be 6 weeks or longer.[13,14]

■ **Table 4-5**   Suspension Dosing of Various Drugs for Tinea Capitis in Children[75,76]

	Dosage/kg	Duration
SUSPENSION DOSING		
Fluconazole Continuous	6 mg/kg/d	20 days
Fluconazole Pulse*	6 mg/kg/dose q wk	8-12 weeks
Griseofulvin Continuous	15-25 mg/kg/d†	6-12 weeks

*Fluconazole pulses are 1 day "on" and 6 days "off" with the doses listed above.
†Griseofulvin dose based on Grifulvin V suspension 125 mg/5 ml.

■ **Table 4-6**   Adverse Effects Associated With Terbinafine Therapy[70-74]

Gastrointestinal	*Common:* diarrhea, dyspepsia, flatulence, abdominal pain, nausea
	Uncommon: feeling of fullness, gastritis, asymptomatic liver enzyme abnormalities, taste disturbance, symptomatic idiosyncratic hepatobiliary dysfunction (hepatitis)
Cutaneous	*Common:* morbilliform or maculopapular rash
	Uncommon: pruritus, urticaria, eczema, serious skin reaction (e.g., Stevens-Johnson syndrome and toxic epidermal necrolysis), alopecia
Central nervous system	*Common:* headache
	Uncommon: change in concentration, visual disturbance (changes in ocular lens and retina)
Hematologic	*Uncommon:* neutropenia, transient decreases in absolute lymphocyte count
Miscellaneous	*Uncommon:* tiredness, fatigue, allergic reaction, hypersensitivity syndrome

Other Uses.   There have been isolated reports detailing use of terbinafine in patients with Majocchi's granuloma,[64] tinea imbricata,[65] cutaneous sporotrichosis,[66] black piedra,[67] aspergillosis,[68] and chromoblastomycosis.[69]

ADVERSE EFFECTS.[70-74]   Table 4-6 lists adverse effects associated with terbinafine therapy. The more common adverse effects are headache, gastrointestinal symptoms, and dermatologic manifestations.[28,48] The estimated incidence of terbinafine inducing clinically significant symptoms and signs of hepatobiliary function for which no other cause was apparent is 1:45,000 to 1:120,000.[48,73] In postmarketing surveillance studies reported from the United Kingdom and Europe, terbinafine has been found to be safe, with no significant new risks being reported.[70,71]

In the United States, the monitoring requirements include liver function tests (especially transaminase values), which should be performed in patients receiving terbinafine for longer than 6 weeks.[28] If hepatic dysfunction or cholestatic hepatitis develops, treatment should be discontinued.[75] The United States package insert indicates physicians should considering performing complete blood counts in patients with known or suspected immunodeficiency who are administered oral terbinafine for longer than 6 weeks.[28]

USE IN PREGNANCY AND NURSING.   Terbinafine is in the FDA pregnancy category B. There are no adequate and well-controlled studies in pregnant women.[75] It is recommended that terbinafine should not be initiated during pregnancy because treatment for onychomycosis can be postponed until the completion of pregnancy.[75] Terbinafine is excreted in breast milk.[48]

DRUG INTERACTIONS.   The potential drug interactions associated with terbinafine are listed in Table 4-7. Terbinafine has relatively few drug

Table 4-7 Drug Interactions with Terbinafine[16,17,28,77,78]

Interacting Drug	Mechanism and Comments
THESE DRUGS MAY INCREASE THE SERUM LEVELS (AND POTENTIAL TOXICITY) OF TERBINAFINE	
Terfenadine	Decreases terbinafine clearance by 16% (terfenadine a CYP 3A4 substrate)
Cimetidine	Decreases terbinafine clearance by 33% (cimetidine a weak CYP 3A4 inhibitor)
THIS DRUG MAY DECREASE THE SERUM LEVELS OF TERBINAFINE	
Rifampin	Increases terbinafine clearance by 100% (rifampin a CYP 3A4 inducer)
TERBINAFINE MAY INCREASE THE DRUG LEVELS (AND POTENTIAL TOXICITY) OF THESE DRUGS	
Theophylline	Oral clearance of theophylline decreased by 14% and half-life increased by 24%
Nortriptyline	Single case report of nortriptyline intoxication in a patient on terbinafine; rechallenge was positive
Caffeine	Terbinafine decreases intravenously administered caffeine clearance by 19%
TERBINAFINE MAY DECREASE THE DRUG LEVELS OF THIS DRUG	
Cyclosporine	Terbinafine increases cyclosporine clearance by 15%
OTHER POTENTIALLY IMPORTANT DRUG INTERACTIONS	
CYP 2D6 substrates	Recent report of significant CYP 2D6 inhibition by terbinafine in an in vivo pharmacokinetic model; would affect metabolism of 2D6 substrates (e.g., tricyclic antidepressants and narcotics)
Warfarin	Most studies show no significant interaction between the two drugs.[93,94,134] A few case reports show decreased anticoagulant effect of warfarin[135,136]

interactions compared with the azoles and is not contraindicated with any drug.[28,77,78]

ITRACONAZOLE

Itraconazole is a triazole that was synthesized in 1980.[79] It first obtained international registration in 1987. Itraconazole was approved in the United States for the treatment of systemic mycoses in September 1992 and as continuous therapy for onychomycosis of fingernails and toenails in October 1995. Itraconazole pulse therapy has been approved in the United States for the treatment of fingernail onychomycosis since January 1997. It is estimated that itraconazole has been given about 40 million times worldwide, the majority for cases of onychomycosis and other superficial dermatomycoses, rather than for systemic mycoses.[80,81]

Pharmacology
See Table 4-2 for key pharmacologic concepts of itraconazole.

STRUCTURE. Itraconazole is a 1:1:1:1 racemic mixture of four diastereomers (two enantiomeric pairs), each possessing three chiral centers.[3] The molecular formula of itraconazole is $C_{35}H_{38}Cl_2N_8O_4$ with a molecular weight of 705.64[81] (see Figure 4-1).

ABSORPTION AND DISTRIBUTION. Itraconazole is highly lipophilic, a weak base (pKa = 3.7), virtually insoluble in water (<1 mg/L), and ionized only at a low pH.[76] The oral bioavailability of itraconazole is highest when it is taken with a full meal.[82,83] Considerable interpatient variation in absorption may be observed. Absorption of itraconazole in a fasting state, or in individuals with relative or absolute achlorhydria (e.g., those on H_2 inhibitors, antacids, or proton pump inhibitors), may be increased when the itraconazole is administered with at least 8 ounces of a cola beverage.[84] Itraconazole is well absorbed, reaching peak plasma concentrations in approximately 4 hours.[9] When oral solution is administered the absolute oral bioavailability of itraconazole is 55%.[85]

Itraconazole has dose-dependent pharmacokinetics for single and multiple dosing.[86] After oral doses of 50 to 400 mg/day, steady-state concentrations are achieved within 15 days.[81]

Itraconazole binds strongly to plasma proteins (>99%) and is extensively distributed into lipophilic tissues. The concentration of drug in fatty tissues, omentum, liver, kidney, and skin may be 2 to 20 times the corresponding plasma concentration.[85] Aqueous fluids, such as the cerebrospinal fluid and saliva, contain negligible amounts of drug.[85]

PHARMACOKINETIC PROFILE IN VARIOUS CUTANEOUS STRUCTURES

Pharmacokinetics in Skin. Itraconazole is delivered to the skin mainly as a result of passive diffusion from the plasma to the keratinocytes with strong drug adherence to keratin.[80] Itraconazole becomes detectable in the sweat within 24 hours after the initial intake of drug. Despite the early detection in the sweat, the excretion of itraconazole by this route is minimal, in contrast to griseofulvin, ketoconazole, and fluconazole.[83,86] There is extensive excretion of itraconazole into sebum.[80] A negligible amount of itraconazole redistributes back from the skin and appendages to the plasma; therefore itraconazole is eliminated as the stratum corneum renews itself, and the hair and nails grow out.[80,86] Itraconazole may persist in the stratum corneum for 3 to 4 weeks after discontinuation of therapy.[80] In an ex vivo model, the therapeutic effect of itraconazole in the stratum corneum remained for 2 to 3 weeks after stopping therapy.[87]

Pharmacokinetics in Nails. Itraconazole has been detected in the distal end of the fingernail and toenail within 1 and 2 weeks of starting therapy, respectively.[88,89] This is consistent with itraconazole reaching the free end of the nail plate via both the nail matrix and the nailbed. Furthermore, after receiving itraconazole 200 mg/day for 10 days, the concentration of itraconazole in the subungual nail material is more than double the corresponding level in the distal nail clippings. In patients treated with pulse therapy 200 mg twice daily for 1 week, the drug levels exceed the MIC in the fingernail at this time point.[86] After itraconazole intermittent therapy (200 mg twice daily for 1 week a month; active therapy for 1 week and 3 weeks off drug)

for 2 pulses in fingernail onychomycosis the drug is undetectable by 9 months from the initiation of therapy.[86] When toenail onychomycosis is treated with 3 pulses of itraconazole, drug levels have been detected in the nail for 11 months.[86] The faster decline of drug from fingernails compared with toenails is probably because of the faster outgrowth of the former.[89-91] In contrast, plasma levels decrease to very low or negligible levels within 7 to 14 days of stopping itraconazole therapy.

Pharmacokinetics in Hair. Itraconazole may be delivered to the hair primarily by two routes. The faster route is incorporation of the drug in hair via the sebum, and the slower method is incorporation of drug into the hair follicle.[55,92] When itraconazole 100 mg/day is administered as continuous therapy for 4 weeks, drug is detectable in hair after 1 week of therapy.[80] When patients with Majocchi's granuloma have been treated with itraconazole pulse therapy, the drug was detected in the hair after 1 week of therapy.[93] The concentration of itraconazole was 2.6-fold and 3.4-fold higher, respectively, after the second and third pulses compared with the level of drug in hair at the end of the first pulse. After discontinuation of therapy, drug was detectable in hair for up to 9 months, suggesting that the pulse therapy regimen with itraconazole may be a feasible option for the treatment of tinea capitis.

METABOLISM AND EXCRETION. Itraconazole is extensively metabolized in the liver. More than 30 metabolites have been identified and the majority are inactive, having been produced after the azole ring has been cleaved.[94] In contrast with the other azoles, itraconazole undergoes side-chain hydroxylation, which produces hydroxyitraconazole. This is a major metabolite of itraconazole and this metabolite demonstrates antifungal activity. The in vitro antifungal activity of itraconazole is similar to that of hydroxyitraconazole.[86] When itraconazole 200 mg twice daily is administered for 15 days at steady state pharmacokinetics, the area under the curve (AUC) (ng/hr/ml) for itraconazole and hydroxyitraconazole is 22,569 and 38,572, respectively.[75] The corresponding half-lives are 64 and 56 hours, respectively. Itraconazole is excreted in the urine (35%) and in the feces (54%), mostly in the form of inactive metabolites.[90] Fecal and

renal excretion of the parent drug are 3% to 18% and <0.03% of the dose, respectively. The clearance of itraconazole decreases at higher doses, suggesting that the mechanism of clearance may be saturable.[81]

In mild-to-severe renal insufficiency, the plasma concentrations of itraconazole are comparable with those of healthy subjects.[81] When hepatic insufficiency is present, its effect on the plasma concentrations is not known. Thus individuals with hepatic impairment should be carefully monitored.[81]

MECHANISM OF ACTION. The mechanism of action of itraconazole is similar to that of the other azoles.[94] Itraconazole inhibits the cytochrome P-450 enzyme lanosterol 14-α demethlyase, with resultant inhibition in the conversion of lanosterol to ergosterol. Ergosterol is the primary sterol and an essential component of fungal cell membranes. When ergosterol is depleted, there is damage to the fungal cell membrane with an alteration in the permeability and functioning of the fungal cell membrane. Itraconazole has a preferential effect on ergosterol compared with cholesterol, the latter being the major sterol of mammalian cells. When the azoles are used to treat *C. albicans*, they may inhibit the transformation of blastospores into the invasive mycelial form.[9] Like other azoles, itraconazole is primarily fungistatic in vitro.

Clinical Use

Table 4-8 lists indications and contraindications for itraconazole.

APPROVED INDICATIONS

Onychomycosis—Caused by Dermatophytes. Itraconazole is FDA approved for the treatment of the following conditions in nonimmunocompromised patients: dermatophyte onychomycosis of the toenail, with or without fingernail disease, or dermatophyte onychomycosis of fingernails. Continuous itraconazole is approved for toenail onychomycosis, and continuous and pulse regimens are approved for fingernail disease.

Deep Fungal Infections. Itraconazole capsules are also indicated for the treatment of the following fungal infections in immunocompromised and nonimmunocompromised patients:

blastomycosis (pulmonary and extrapulmonary), histoplasmosis (including chronic cavitary, pulmonary, and disseminated, nonmeningeal disease), and aspergillosis (pulmonary and extrapulmonary in patients who are intolerant of or refractory to amphotericin B therapy).

Onychomycosis—Continuous Regimen. When itraconazole 200 mg/day is used as a continuous regimen to treat dermatophyte onychomycosis, the duration of therapy for fingernails and toenails is 6 weeks and 12 weeks, respectively. An analysis of studies where the itraconazole (continuous) regimen has been used for 3 to 4 months to treat toenail dermatophyte onychomycosis indicates that the mycologic cure rate, metaaverage ± SE, is 67.0% ± 5.3% (95% confidence interval, CI: 56.6% to 77.5%) (11 trials, n = 921 patients).* For fingernail dermatophyte onychomycosis, itraconazole (continuous) therapy 200 mg/day for 6 weeks results in a mycologic cure rate, metaaverage ± SE, of 79% ± 1% (95% CI: 78% to 80%)[81,100] (2 trials, n = 58 patients).

Onychomycosis of Fingernails—Pulse Regimen. Itraconazole (pulse) therapy for 2 pulses (each pulse is 200 mg twice daily for 1 week per month, with 1 week on and 3 weeks off between successive pulses) has been used to treat dermatophyte fingernail onychomycosis with a mycologic cure rate, metaaverage ± SE, of 76.9% ± 6.8% (95% CI: 63.5% to 90.2%) (2 trials, n = 38 patients).[101,102]

OFF-LABEL USES

Onychomycosis of Toenails—Pulse Regimen. Itraconazole (pulse) therapy is used widely to treat dermatophyte toenail onychomycosis. The mycologic cure rate when 3 to 4 pulses are used for tinea unguium of the toenails, metaaverage ± SE, is 72.5% ± 6.2% (95% CI: 60.4% to 80.6%) (12 trials, n = 1670 patients).†

Onychomycosis—Candida Species and Nondermatophyte Molds. Itraconazole continuous and pulse regimens are also effective in treating onychomycosis caused by *Candida* species.[100,110,111] The experience with nondermatophyte molds is more limited.[41,42,112,113] The nondermatophytes for which itraconazole may

---

*References 18, 19, 21-23, 36, 81, 89, 95-99.
†References 31, 32, 35, 86, 88, 102-109.

Table 4-8	Itraconazole Indications and Contraindications

FDA-APPROVED INDICATIONS
Onychomycosis—Due to Dermatophytes
Tinea unguium fingernails
Tinea unguium toenails
(*continuous* therapy—either site)*
(*pulse* therapy—fingernails)[101,102]

Systemic Mycoses (Certain Subsets of These Infections)
Blastomycosis
Histoplasmosis
Aspergillosis

OFF-LABEL USES
Onychomycosis—Other Categories
Dermatophyte infections toenails[31,32,35,88,102-109]
Candida species[100,110,111]
Nondermatophyte molds[41,42,112,113]
Children[43,44,46,114]

Pityrosporum Infections
Pityrosporum folliculitis[127,128]
Pityriasis (tinea) versicolor (pulse therapy)[115,129,130]
Seborrheic dermatitis[115]

Dermatophyte Cutaneous Infections
Tinea pedis/manuum (pulse therapy)[52,115,116]
Tinea pedis/manuum (continuous)[115,117]
Tinea corporis/cruris (pulse therapy)[54,115,118]
Tinea corporis/cruris (continuous)[115,118]

Other Dermatophyte Infections
Majocchi's granuloma[93]
Tinea imbricata[65]

Other Yeast Infections
Chronic mucocutaneous candidiasis[110,131]
Vaginal candidiasis[132]

Dermatophyte Hair Infections
Tinea capitis[119-126]

Miscellaneous
HIV-associated eosinophilic folliculitis[127]
Other systemic mycoses[81,132]

CONTRAINDICATIONS
Absolute
Hypersensitivity to the drug or its excipients
Pregnancy

Relative
Uncertain potential for cross-reaction with other azole antifungal agents—use with caution

PREGNANCY PRESCRIBING STATUS—CATEGORY C

*References 18, 19, 21-23, 36, 81, 89, 95-99.

have some efficacy include the *Aspergillus* species.

Onychomycosis in Children.   Itraconazole is effective and safe in the treatment of onychomycosis in children.[43,44,46] A suggested regimen using itraconazole capsules is 2 and 3 pulses for fingernails and toenails, respectively. Each pulse is 5 mg/kg/day lasting for 1 week. Itraconazole oral solution given as pulse therapy may be another option.[114]

Tinea Pedis/Tinea Manuum and Tinea Corporis/Tinea Cruris.   The preferred regimen for treating dermatomycoses is pulse therapy.[115] For tinea pedis/tinea manuum, one pulse of itraconazole 200 mg twice daily for 1 week

should be sufficient.[52,115,116] With continuous therapy for tinea pedis/manuum the regimen is 100 mg/day for 4 weeks or 200 mg/day for 2 weeks.[115,117] When itraconazole pulse therapy is used to treat tinea corporis/tinea cruris the dosage is 200 mg/day for 1 week.[54,115,118] Using continuous therapy for tinea corporis/cruris the regimen is 100 mg/day for 2 weeks.[115,118]

Tinea Capitis.   Itraconazole continuous and pulse therapies have been used to treat tinea capitis effectively. These regimens also appear to be safe and well tolerated[119-126] (see Tables 4-4 and 4-5). A pulse regimen using the oral solution to treat tinea capitis has also been reported.[126]

Pityrosporum *Infections.*   Itraconazole (pulse) therapy 200 mg/day given for 7 days is effective in pityriasis (tinea) versicolor.[115,129-130] Also, seborrheic dermatitis may be effectively treated with itraconazole 200 mg/day given for 1 week.[115]

Other Uses.   Itraconazole may also be effective in the treatment of Majocchi's granuloma,[93] human immunodeficiency virus–associated eosinophilic folliculitis,[127] tinea imbricata,[65] vaginal candidiasis, chronic mucocutaneous candidiasis,[110,131] and other *C. albicans* infections.[132] Off-label uses for itraconazole also include other systemic mycoses.[81,132]

ADVERSE EFFECTS.[74,81,132,133]   Table 4-9 lists adverse effects associated with itraconazole. The more common adverse effects of itraconazole are headache, gastrointestinal disorders, and cutaneous disorders. When itraconazole is given as the pulse regimen for the treatment of onychomycosis, it may be associated with an improved adverse effects profile compared with the continuous regimen using this triazole.[91] The estimated incidence of itraconazole inducing clinically significant symptoms and signs of hepatobiliary dysfunction, for which no other cause was apparent, is 1:500,000.[73] In a prescription-event monitoring postmarketing surveillance of itraconazole carried out in the United Kingdom, Inman and associates[133] found that itraconazole was almost free from clinically important adverse events.

Liver function tests (especially transaminase values) should be monitored periodically when itraconazole is given as continuous therapy for more than 1 month.[81] In general, monitoring should also be carried out in any individual with preexisting hepatic function abnormalities or at any time a patient develops symptoms or signs suggestive of hepatic dysfunction.[81] There are no monitoring requirements in the United States when itraconazole pulse therapy is used to treat dermatophyte fingernail onychomycosis.[81] In the Canadian[106] and international[134] package inserts for itraconazole, there are also no monitoring requirements when the drug is used as pulse therapy to treat onychomycosis.

USE IN PREGNANCY AND WHILE NURSING.   Itraconazole is in FDA pregnancy category C. Itraconazole has been shown to produce teratogenic effects when administered at high doses (40 mg/kg/day or higher) to pregnant rats and to pregnant mice (80 mg/kg/day or higher).[106] There are no studies available on the use of itraconazole in pregnant women.[106] The drug should be used in pregnancy only if the benefit clearly outweighs the potential risk.[106] Itraconazole should not be used for the treatment of onychomycosis or other dermatomycoses in pregnant patients or in women contemplating pregnancy.[106] In a prescription-event monitoring study, 56 individuals took itraconazole during pregnancy, although its use in pregnancy is contraindicated.[133] There was no evidence of fetal damage in this group.[133] Itraconazole is excreted in human milk and the patient should be advised to discontinue nursing while taking itraconazole.[106]

DRUG INTERACTIONS.   In general, before prescribing a new drug, it is important to obtain a complete history of all drugs the patient is cur-

■ **Table 4-9   Adverse Effects Associated With Itraconazole**[74-76,81,106,132]

Gastrointestinal	*Common:* diarrhea, dyspepsia, flatulence, abdominal pain, nausea
	Uncommon: constipation, gastritis, asymptomatic liver enzyme abnormalities, symptomatic hepatobiliary dysfunction (hepatitis)
Cutaneous	*Common:* rash (morbilliform or maculopapular)
	Uncommon: pruritus, urticaria, serious skin reaction (e.g., Stevens-Johnson syndrome)
Central nervous system	*Common:* headache
	Uncommon: dizziness, tremor, somnolence, vertigo, peripheral neuropathy
Hematologic	*Uncommon:* neutropenia
Miscellaneous	*Uncommon:* hypertension, hypertriglyceridemia, fever, edema, menstrual disorder, hypokalemia, allergic reaction

rently taking, both prescription and nonprescription.[18] The inquiry should extend to herbal and recreational agents. In most cases drug interactions are predictable.* The drug interactions associated with itraconazole are listed in Table 4-10.†

---

*References 3, 9, 18, 19, 75, 76.
†References 3, 9, 18, 19, 74-77, 81, 85, 106, 132, 134-136.

FLUCONAZOLE

Fluconazole was initially approved in France and the United Kingdom in 1988 and in the United States in January 1990 for use in humans. Fluconazole is approved for the treatment of onychomycosis in 19 countries. In September 1993, Finland and China were the first countries to receive approval for fluconazole treatment of onychomycosis. In the United

■ Table 4-10   Drug Interactions With Itraconazole*

Interacting Drug Group	Examples and Comments
THESE DRUGS MAY DECREASE THE SERUM LEVELS OF ITRACONAZOLE—CYP ENZYME INDUCERS	
Anticonvulsants	Phenytoin, phenobarbital, carbamazepine—enhance both first-pass metabolism plus CYP 3A4 enzyme induction
Antituberculosis agents	Rifampin, rifabutin, isoniazid—CYP enzyme inducers that decrease drug levels
Nonnucleoside reverse transcriptase inhibitors	Revirapine
THESE DRUGS MAY DECREASE THE SERUM LEVELS OF ITRACONAZOLE DUE TO INCREASED GI pH	
H₂ antihistamines	Cimetidine, azatidine, ranitidine, nizatidine—increased GI pH may decrease itraconazole absorption (administer 1-2 hours before antacid [see below])†
Proton pump inhibitors	Omeprazole, lansoprazole—increased GI pH may decrease itraconazole absorption (administer 1-2 hours before antacid [see below])†
Didanosine	Buffer in product may decrease itraconazole absorption†
ITRACONAZOLE MAY INCREASE THE DRUG LEVELS (AND POTENTIAL TOXICITY) OF THESE DRUGS	
H₁ antihistamines‡	Terfenadine,§ astemizole§—potential for serious tachydysrhythmias associated with torsade de pointes
GI motility agent‡	Cisapride§—likewise a risk for torsades de pointes
HMG CoA reductase inhibitors	Especially simvastatin,§ lovastatin;§ also atorvastatin, cerivastatin—increased levels may increase risk of rhabdomyolysis (and possibly hepatotoxicity)
Benzodiazepines	Triazolam,§ midazolam,§ alprazolam—elevated levels with excessive sedative effects possible
Oral hypoglycemic agents	Particularly with tolbutamide, glyburide, glipizide—hypoglycemia may occur, should monitor blood glucose closely
Ilmmunosuppressants	Cyclosporine, tacrolimus—increased risk for nephrotoxicity, hypertension, neurotoxicity
HIV-1 protease inhibitors	Ritonavir, indinavir in particular at risk

*References 3, 9, 18, 19, 74-77, 81, 85, 106, 132, 134-136.
†Alternative method of decreasing GI pH to more optimal level is to take itraconazole with a full meal or take drug with at least 8 ounces of a cola beverage.
‡These drugs have been withdrawn from the U.S. market due to the risk of life-threatening cardiac dysrhythmias.
§Contraindicated drugs; must avoid concomitant use with itraconazole.   *Continued*

Table 4-10　Drug Interactions With Itraconazole—cont'd

Interacting Drug Group	Examples and Comments
ITRACONAZOLE MAY INCREASE THE DRUG LEVELS (AND POTENTIAL TOXICITY) OF THESE DRUGS—cont'd	
Anticoagulants	Warfarin—drug levels and anticoagulant effect both may be increased
Other drugs	Digoxin, pimozide,§ buspirone, quinidine, vincristine, sildenafil (Viagra)
OTHER POTENTIALLY IMPORTANT DRUG INTERACTIONS	
Oral contraceptives	Isolated case report of possible contraceptive failure—in general drugs that reduce estrogen/progestin levels are due to CYP inducers (not CYP inhibitors)
Calcium channel blockers	Dihydropyridines (amlodipine, felodipine, nicardipine, nifedipine)—edema

States, fluconazole is not approved for the treatment of onychomycosis or other dermatomycoses. It is estimated that fluconazole has been used approximately 50 million times worldwide for all indications.

Pharmacology

See Table 4-2 for key pharmacologic concepts of fluconazole.

STRUCTURE.　Fluconazole is a bis-triazole antifungal agent.[85,137-139] The empirical formula is $C_{13}H_{12}F_2N_6O$ and the molecular weight 306.3 (see Figure 4-1).

ABSORPTION AND DISTRIBUTION.　Fluconazole is very well absorbed when given orally. The bioavailability is over 90% compared with intravenous administration.[137] The high bioavailability may be the result of the relatively low molecular weight and the drug's more hydrophilic nature compared with the other azoles. The absorption of fluconazole is essentially unaffected by alterations in gastric pH. This may be related to its relatively low pKa of 1.76. The absorption of fluconazole is not significantly affected by the presence of food or the administration of antacids. Peak plasma levels are reached within 1 to 2 hours of oral administration.[137] Fluconazole is not highly lipophilic and exhibits a protein binding of 11% to 12%. This is in contrast to ketoconazole and itraconazole, which are approximately 99% protein bound. After continuous administration, the peak plasma concentration is 2.5-fold higher than after a single dose. When fluconazole 50 to 400 mg is given once daily, steady state concentrations are achieved within 5 to 10 days. However, a steady state can be attained more rapidly by doubling the dose on the first day.[137] The volume of distribution of fluconazole is approximately that of total body water, which is consistent with the drug's ability to not extensively bind to protein, fat, or tissue. Fluconazole, in contrast with ketoconazole and itraconazole, has excellent penetration into the cerebrospinal fluid (CSF). The concentration of fluconazole in the CSF compared with plasma is 0.5 to 0.9.

PHARMACOKINETIC PROFILE IN VARIOUS CUTANEOUS STRUCTURES

Pharmacokinetics in Skin.　When fluconazole 150 mg once a week is administered for two doses, the drug accumulates in the stratum corneum through sweat and by direct diffusion through the dermis and epidermis.[140] Excretion in the sebum may be more limited. After discontinuation of therapy, there may be rediffusion of fluconazole from the skin into the systemic circulation but at a rate that is lower than elimination from the plasma.[86] Wildfeuer and associates[141] measured the concentration of fluconazole in plasma and stratum corneum of healthy subjects after daily administration of one 200 mg capsule daily for 5 days. Seven hours after the first administration of a 200 mg capsule, the concentration in the plasma and stratum corneum was 3 µg/ml and 98 µg/g, respectively. The elimination of fluconazole from the stratum corneum occurred with a half-life of approximately 60 to 90 hours. This stratum corneum elimination was 2 to 3 times slower than the elimination from plasma. The pharmacokinetic data suggest that fluconazole 150 mg given once weekly for 2 or more weeks should be effective in the treatment of cutaneous fungal infections.

Pharmacokinetics in Nails. Hay[142] demonstrated that fluconazole can be detected at the distal end of the nail plate within 1 day of starting treatment with 50 mg/day. This suggests that diffusion of fluconazole from the nailbed to the nail plate is an important route of drug delivery.

Faergemann and Laufen[140] reported that fluconazole could be detected in the nail plate for at least 6 months after the discontinuation of therapy. These investigators measured the concentration of fluconazole in fungal toenails of 36 patients treated using a regimen of 150 mg once weekly for 12 months, with discontinuation of therapy earlier if clinically cured.[140] During treatment there was no statistically significant difference in drug levels between healthy and diseased nails. However, the concentration of fluconazole in nails was significantly higher than in serum. After 1 and 6 months of therapy, the mean concentration of fluconazole in healthy nails was 3.09 µg/g and 8.54 µg/g, respectively. In contrast, the serum concentration of fluconazole remained more or less stable at 0.45 to 1.36 µg/ml during therapy. Six months after discontinuation of the drug, fluconazole concentrations in healthy and diseased toenails were 1.4 µg/g and 1.9 µg/g, respectively (n = 3 patients). Both values are higher than the maximal serum levels. These data suggest that there is the potential for ongoing improvement in the onychomycosis even after discontinuation of active drug therapy.

The pharmacokinetics of fluconazole in onychomycosis have also been studied by Rich and co-workers[143] in a dose-finding, placebo-controlled study in which fluconazole (150 mg, 300 mg, 450 mg, or matching placebo) was administered once weekly for the treatment of onychomycosis of the toenails. The investiga-

tors detected fluconazole in both healthy and affected nails within 2 weeks of starting therapy in nearly all patients studied (n = 151). This confirmed the earlier reports of rapid uptake of fluconazole into the nail plate by Hay,[142] as well as Faergemann and Laufen.[140] In the study by Rich,[143] the median time to reach steady-state concentrations of fluconazole in the healthy-appearing nails in each of the 150 mg, 300 mg, and 450 mg groups was 4 to 5 months. It took longer for fluconazole to reach a steady-state concentration in abnormal-appearing (diseased) nails, the median duration being 6 to 7 months. In the three groups treated with active drug, 8 months after starting therapy, the ratio of fluconazole in the nails to plasma concentration ranged from 1.31 to 1.5. These results, where higher concentrations of fluconazole are present in the nail compared with plasma, are similar to the data reported by Faergemann and Laufen.[140] Rich[143] also found that after fluconazole therapy was stopped the concentrations of active drug in toenails decreased gradually with elimination half-lives in the 150 mg, 300 mg, and 450 mg groups being 2.5, 2.4, and 3.7 months, respectively. In fact, in most subjects fluconazole could still be detected in the nail plate 6 months after therapy was discontinued.

Pharmacokinetics in Hair. Relatively little has been published about the pharmacokinetics of fluconazole in hair. Wildfeuer and associates[141] administered 100 mg daily for 5 days to healthy volunteers. Fluconazole was still detectable in scalp hair even 4 to 5 months after completion of therapy.

METABOLISM AND EXCRETION. Unlike the other azoles, fluconazole does not undergo significant first-pass hepatic metabolism. Fluconazole is cleared primarily by renal excretion. Approximately 80% of the dose appears in the urine unchanged and about 11% as metabolites.[137] Two percent of the drug is recovered unchanged in the feces; the fate of the remaining 7% is not known. In healthy volunteers and in women with vaginal candidiasis who have normal renal function the plasma elimination half-life varied from 30.2 to 37.3 hours. This long half-life permits once daily dosing. Because of the long half-life there is an accumulation of drug with multiple dosing. Complete elimination of fluconazole from the systemic circulation takes about 1 week.[86]

In patients with impaired renal function, who are to receive only single-dose therapy for vaginal candidiasis, there is no need to adjust the dosage.[75] However, when a patient with impaired renal function is to receive multiple doses, it is suggested to administer an initial loading dose of 50 to 400 mg.[75] A guideline for subsequent daily doses is when creatinine clearance >50 ml/min, give the entire dosage; however, if creatinine clearance is 11 to 50 mL/min, then 50% of the recommended dose may be sufficient.[75] These are guidelines only, with adjustment depending on factors such as the overall clinical condition.

MECHANISM OF ACTION.   The mechanism of action for fluconazole is similar to that of the other azoles. Like the other azoles, fluconazole exhibits fungistatic activity in vitro. As seen with itraconazole, fluconazole inhibits fungal lanosterol 14-α demethylase to a much greater extent than the corresponding mammalian enzyme.[137] In fact, fluconazole demonstrates a 10,000-fold selectivity for the fungal enzyme.

Clinical Use
Table 4-11 lists indications and contraindications for fluconazole.

INDICATIONS.   In the United States, fluconazole is not officially indicated for the treatment of onychomycosis or other dermatomycoses.[138] Fluconazole is indicated for the treatment of (1) vaginal candidiasis (vaginal yeast infections due to *Candida* species), (2) oropharyngeal and esophageal candidiasis, and (3) cryptococcal meningitis.[138] With regard to prophylaxis, fluconazole is also indicated for use in decreasing the incidence of candidiasis in patients undergoing bone marrow transplantation

---

Table 4-11	Fluconazole Indications and Contraindications

FDA-APPROVED INDICATIONS	
Dermatologic Indications	Nondermatologic[138]
Vaginal candidiasis[138]	Candidiasis—oral or esophageal
	Prophylaxis of candidiasis in immunosuppressed patients
	Cryptococcal meningitis
OFF-LABEL USES	
Onychomycosis—Due to Dermatophytes	Pityrosporum and Candida Infections
Tinea unguium toenails[33,144,148,150]	Pityriasis (tinea) versicolor[163]
Tinea unguium fingernails[149,150]	Cutaneous candidiasis[153,156]
	Chronic mucocutaneous candidiasis[165]
Dermatophyte Cutaneous Infections	
Tinea corporis/cruris[151-156]	Deep Fungal Infections
Tinea pedis[154-158]	Lymphocutaneous sporotrichosis[166]
	Visceral sporotrichosis[166]
Dermatophyte Hair Infections	
Tinea capitis[159-162]	
CONTRAINDICATIONS	
Absolute	Relative
Hypersensitivity to fluconazole or its excipients	Use with caution in patients sensitive to other azoles
Pregnancy	Severe liver disease

PREGNANCY PRESCRIBING STATUS—CATEGORY C

who receive cytotoxic chemotherapy or radiation therapy. Further details on the use of fluconazole to treat systemic mycoses are outside the scope of this chapter.

OFF-LABEL USES

Onychomycosis. In countries where fluconazole is approved for the treatment of onychomycosis, the most frequently used schedule is fluconazole 150 mg once weekly given until the abnormal-appearing nail has grown out. This may occur in 3 to 6 months and 9 to 12 months for dermatophyte fingernail and toenail onychomycosis, respectively. Fluconazole is effective for the treatment of dermatophyte onychomycosis. In six studies (n = 277) the mycologic cure rate in toenail onychomycosis, metaaverage ± SE, is 67.7% ± 8.4 %.[33,144-148] Fluconazole is also effective in the treatment of fingernail onychomycosis, with the mycologic cure rate of 89% after administration of 150 mg once weekly for 9 months.[149]

The experience with fluconazole for the treatment of onychomycosis caused by *Candida* species and other nondermatophyte molds is limited.[150]

Tinea Corporis/Tinea Cruris. The dose of fluconazole for treating tinea corporis/tinea cruris is generally 150 mg once weekly administered for 2 to 4 weeks. Some clinicians may nudge the dose up to 200 mg once weekly for the same duration. The mycologic cure rate (6 trials, n = 583) is metaaverage ± SE, 88.9% ± 1.7%.[151-156]

Tinea Pedis. The dose of fluconazole for treating tinea pedis is usually 150 mg once weekly given for 2 to 6 weeks. The mycologic cure rate (4 trials, n = 327) at follow-up, metaaverage ± SE, is 86.8% ± 3.2%.[154-158]

Tinea Capitis. Short-duration therapy with fluconazole 6 mg/kg/day lasting 2 to 3 weeks may be effective.[159,160] Once weekly therapy with fluconazole for tinea capitis has also been found to be effective.[161,162]

Pityriasis (Tinea) Versicolor. In an open, comparative trial the efficacy of three regimens for the treatment of tinea versicolor was investigated.[163] The most effective regimen was a single dose of fluconazole 300 g repeated 2 weeks later depending on the response to the first dose. The treatment was well tolerated, with only 15 (3.5%) of 603 patients reporting mild-to-moderate adverse events that did not require interruption of therapy.

Cutaneous Candidiasis. Fluconazole is effective in the treatment of cutaneous candidiasis. The dose of fluconazole may be 150 mg once weekly given for 2 to 4 weeks.[153,164]

Mucocutaneous Candidiasis. Fluconazole has been found to be suitable for the management of chronic mucocutaneous candidiasis (CMCC).[165] Eight patients with mycologically confirmed oral candidosis of the tongue and oral mucosa were treated with fluconazole; none had received antifungal therapy for at least 6 weeks before treatment with fluconazole. Each patient received 50 mg fluconazole daily for up to 4 weeks and was assessed clinically and mycologically each week by both microscopy and culture. Clinical and mycologic remissions were induced in all eight patients in a mean period of 10 days (range 7 to 21 days). Three patients relapsed within 4 months (mean 56 days), but all responded to a further short course of oral fluconazole, 50 mg daily for 3 days. The frequency of relapse, however, was less than before and all four patients who were no longer responding to ketoconazole cleared on fluconazole. No patient reported any adverse reactions to the drug and no abnormality of biochemical values was detected during treatment.

Lymphocutaneous and Visceral Sporotrichosis. Thirty patients with documented sporotrichosis were treated with 200 to 800 mg of fluconazole daily.[166] Fourteen patients had lymphocutaneous infection; only five (36%) of these patients had any underlying illnesses. Sixteen patients had osteoarticular or visceral sporotrichosis; 12 (75%) of these patients had relapsed after prior antifungal therapy. Most patients were treated with 400 mg of fluconazole; however, four patients received 200 mg of fluconazole daily for the entire course, and four received 800 mg of fluconazole daily for a portion of their entire course of therapy. Fluconazole therapy cured 10 (71%) of 14 patients with lymphocutaneous sporotrichosis. However, only five (31%) of 16 patients with osteoarticular or visceral sporotrichosis responded to therapy; the conditions of only two of these five improved, and there was no documented cure of their infections. With the exception of alopecia in five patients, toxic effects were minimal.

ADVERSE EFFECTS.[3,138,139,147] Both at the doses used in dermatology, and at higher doses,[167-169] fluconazole has been observed to have a favorable adverse effects profile. The adverse effects that have been reported in patients receiving a single dose for vaginal candidiasis or multiple doses for systemic mycoses may not be applicable to the situation encountered when treating onychomycosis and other dermatomycoses.[3,138,147] In a dose-finding study in which once weekly fluconazole 150 mg, 300 mg, 450 mg, or placebo was given for onychomycosis, the rate of potentially treatment-related adverse effects in the fluconazole and placebo groups was 43% and 29%, respectively (attributable risk [AR] to fluconazole 14%).[147] The incidence of treatment-related adverse effects in the 150 mg groups (n = 89), 300 mg groups (n = 88), and 450 mg groups (n = 92) was 44% (AR to fluconazole 15%), 42% (AR 13%), and 42% (AR 13%), respectively. The number of patients discontinuing the drug in the 150 mg, 300 mg, 450 mg, and placebo groups was 3%, 8%, 4%, and 5%, respectively.[147] The attributable risk to fluconazole in the 150 mg, 300 mg, and 450 mg groups was 2%, 3%, and 1%, respectively.

Most of the adverse events were mild-to-moderate in severity, the most common being (fluconazole versus placebo groups) headache (6% versus 2%), abdominal pain (4% versus 3%), respiratory disorders (4% versus 3%), diarrhea (3% versus 2%), and nausea (2% versus 3%).[147] Fluconazole was discontinued due to a laboratory abnormality in the following proportion of patients: 150 mg group (1%, AR to fluconazole 0%), 300 mg group (2%, AR 1%), 450 mg group (1%, AR 0%) and placebo (1%).[147] The changes in the median laboratory values in the fluconazole and placebo groups were similar; none of the changes in laboratory parameters in the active drug group were clinically significant. Five patients (fluconazole group 4 and placebo group 1) discontinued the study due to liver function test (LFT) abnormalities. The changes in the LFTs were considered to be drug-related in the following instances: 150 mg group (1 patient), 300 mg group (1 patient), and placebo group (1 patient).

Fluconazole has also been reported to be safe at doses higher than those conventionally used in dermatology.[167-169] Stevens and associates[168] detailed the possible adverse effects of chronic, high-dose fluconazole therapy for invasive mycosis (n = 98 patients). Forty-eight patients received 6 months therapy, and 20 received fluconazole for 1 year. Fifty-eight patients received 300 mg/day, and 7 received 600 mg/day. One patient received 1997 g over 86 months. Overall, 27% experienced adverse effects that resulted in two patients discontinuing therapy. In addition, 42% had asymptomatic laboratory abnormalities, none of which were progressive. Headache, hair loss, and anorexia were the most common symptoms experienced (each by 3% of patients). Eosinophilia and aspartate aminotransferase (AST) increases were the most common laboratory findings (12% and 10%, respectively). Fluconazole appears to be well tolerated and safe at these doses and durations.

USE IN PREGNANCY AND NURSING. Fluconazole is in the FDA pregnancy category C. There are no adequate and well-controlled studies in pregnant women. Fluconazole should be used in pregnancy only if the potential benefit clearly justifies the possible risk to the fetus. In women exposed to low-dose fluconazole (median total dose of 150 to 200 mg during the first 12 weeks of gestation), an increased prevalence of congenital anomalies after exposure to fluconazole was not reported.[170-172] However, there have been cases where women received high doses of fluconazole (400 to 800 mg/day) for at least the first 4 months of their pregnancies.[173-175] In one report a patient was given 600 mg/day for 21 days starting in the 14th week of pregnancy (between the first and second trimester) without the development of malformation or abnormality in the child.[175] It is possible that the teratogenic effect of fluconazole is dose-dependent.[175,176]

Fluconazole is distributed in breast milk at a concentration similar to that of plasma.[9] In one report the calculated half-lives of fluconazole in the plasma and breast milk were approximately 35 and 30 hours, respectively.[177] After 3 half-lives (approximately 90 to 105 hours), 87.5% of the drug in the breast milk should be eliminated. It is of note that with impaired renal function there may be a reduced rate of elimination of fluconazole.[178]

■ **Table 4-12**   Drug Interactions With Fluconazole*

Interacting Drug Group	Examples and Comments
THESE DRUGS MAY INCREASE THE SERUM LEVELS (AND POTENTIAL TOXICITY) OF FLUCONAZOLE	
Thiazide diuretics	Primarily with hydrochlorothiazide—reduced renal clearance of fluconazole
H₂ antihistamines	Cimetidine may reduce fluconazole levels—uncertain mechanism
THIS DRUG MAY DECREASE THE SERUM LEVELS OF FLUCONAZOLE	
Antituberculosis agents	Rifampin, rifabutin—reduce drug levels; are potent CYP 3A4 enzyme inducers
FLUCONAZOLE MAY INCREASE THE DRUG LEVELS (AND POTENTIAL TOXICITY) OF THESE DRUGS†	
H₁ antihistamines‡	Terfenadine,§ astemizole—risk of torsades de pointes
GI motility agents‡	Cisapride§—reports of torsades de pointes with concomitant use
Immunosuppressants	Cyclosporine, tacrolimus—increased risk for nephrotoxicity, hypertension, neurotoxicity
Xanthine bronchodilators	Theophylline—increased half-life and decreased clearance
Anticonvulsants	Primarily phenytoin due to CYP 2C9 metabolism of this anticonvulsant
Anticoagulants	Warfarin—levels and anticoagulant effect both may be increased; S-warfarin (which is more potent than R-warfarin) metabolized by CYP 2C9
Oral hypoglycemic agents	Particularly with tolbutamide, glyburide, glipizide—risk of hypoglycemia
HIV nucleoside analogs	Zidovudine—increased drug levels and potential toxicity
OTHER POTENTIALLY IMPORTANT DRUG INTERACTIONS	
Oral contraceptives	Effect unpredictable—both increased and decreased levels of various progestins reported

*References 3, 9, 18, 19, 74-78, 85, 135-139.
†Fluconazole is a CYP 3A4 inhibitor at doses of at least 400 mg per day especially on a continuous basis (less risk with pulse therapy)—many of the other interactions above are due to fluconazole CYP 2C9 inhibition.
‡All three of these drugs are now off the U.S. market due to serious risk associated with torsades de pointes.
§Contraindicated with fluconazole doses of at least 400 mg daily.

DRUG INTERACTIONS.   Potential drug interactions associated with fluconazole are listed in Table 4-12.[77,78,135-139] Coadministration of terfenadine is contraindicated in patients receiving fluconazole at multiple doses of 400 mg or higher.[138]

GRISEOFULVIN

Griseofulvin was isolated from the mold *Penicillium griseofulvum* Dierckx by Oxford in 1939.[179] In the late 1950s and early 1960s griseo-fulvin was found to be effective in the treatment of superficial fungal infections in humans. It was the first significant oral antifungal agent available to manage dermatomycoses. Over the years the use of griseofulvin has decreased; however, it is still widely used for the treatment of tinea capitis. The interested reader can pursue further information on the pharmacology and mechanism of action for griseofulvin.*

---

*References 3, 9, 18, 19, 75, 179.

Clinical Use

INDICATIONS. Griseofulvin is indicated in the United States for the treatment of tinea infections of the skin, hair, and nails. Specific clinical scenarios include tinea capitis, tinea barbae, tinea corporis, tinea cruris, tinea pedis, and tinea unguium associated with *T. rubrum, T. tonsurans, T. mentagrophytes, T. interdigitale, T. verrucosum, T. megninii, T. gallinae, T. schoenleinii, M. audouinii, M. canis, M. gypseum,* and *Epidermophyton floccosum.*[9]

As with other oral antifungal agents, the use of griseofulvin is not justified for the treatment of tinea infections that would be expected to respond satisfactorily to topical antifungals. Griseofulvin is not effective in the treatment of bacterial infections, candidiasis (moniliasis), histoplasmosis, actinomycosis, sporotrichosis, chromoblastomycosis, coccidioidomycosis, North American blastomycosis, cryptococcosis, tinea versicolor, or nocardiosis.

Tinea Capitis. Griseofulvin has an excellent track record in treating tinea capitis.[55,56,61,180-189] In North America, the most common cause of tinea capitis is *T. tonsurans.* This is a shift away from *M. canis* and *M. audouinii,* which were the predominant organisms in the earlier part of the twentieth century in the United States. Griseofulvin is often adminis-tered at a dose of 10 to 15 mg/kg/day, although some children may require the higher dose of 20 to 25 mg/kg/day. When the ultramicrosize formulation is used, the dosage of 10 to 15 mg/kg/day has been successful. The duration of therapy is usually 6 to 8 weeks. Griseofulvin absorption is improved if it is administered with or after a fatty meal. Treatment needs to be continued until there is clinical and mycologic cure. Some patients may require treatment for 12 to 16 weeks, or even longer. Infection with *M. canis* may need to be treated for a longer duration compared to *T. tonsurans.* In some countries including the United States, griseofulvin oral suspension (microsize), 125 mg per 5 ml, is available. Alternatively, the tablets can be pulverized and administered with food.

Griseofulvin has been used as continuous therapy to treat tinea capitis (Table 4-13, and see Tables 4-4 and 4-5)[182-187] with mycologic cure rates generally being in the range of 80% to 95%. Although single-dose and intermittent regimens using griseofulvin are not in regular use in North America, these have been found to be effective in some studies.[188] In these studies the most common organism causing tinea capitis was not *T. tonsurans.*

Use of Adjunctive Therapies for Tinea Capitis. Topical therapies play an important

▪ Table 4-13   Griseofulvin for the Treatment of Tinea Capitis

Lead Author	Dosage Schedule	Organisms	Mycologic Cure
Tanz[182]	250 to 500 mg/d for 6 weeks	Not reported	4/7 (57.1%)
Tanz[183]	10 to 20 mg/kg/d for 12 weeks	*T. tonsurans* 74% *Microsporum* species 13%	23/24 (95.8%)
Gan[184]	15 mg/kg/d for 26 weeks	*T. tonsurans* 74% *M. canis* 13.5% *T. mentagrophytes* 2.7%	28/28 (100%)
Matínez-Roig[185]	350 mg/d for 6 weeks	*T. mentagrophytes* 65% *M. canis* 30%	4/5 (80%)
Lopez-Gomez[186]	500 mg/d (ultramicrosize) for 6 weeks	*M. canis* 94% *T. violaceum* 6%	16/17 (94.1%)
Haroon[187]	125 mg, 250 mg, or 500 mg/d for 8 weeks	*T. violaceum* *T. verrucosum* *T. tonsurans* *T. rubrum* *M. audouinii*	39/49 (79.6%)

role as adjunctive therapy in the management of tinea capitis. This includes the use of ketoconazole shampoo,[189] selenium sulfide,[190,191] and povidone-iodine.[192] These treatments may help reduce the shedding of fungal organisms (spores) and thereby decrease the risk of infection to other individuals.[189,190] Ketoconazole or selenium sulfide shampoo should be applied three times a week and the lather left in the scalp for at least 5 minutes.[189] The topical therapy should be continued until there is a complete cure.[189]

Fomites and symptom-free carriers may play a role in the management of tinea capitis,[193-199] especially when *M. audouini* is the predominant organism implicated in causing tinea capitis.[199] Children should be counseled about not sharing objects that may help spread tinea capitis to other contacts, including items such as caps, combs, and toys. It is also possible that symptom-free adult carriers living at home may act as a reservoir for the infection.[195,199] Furthermore, the contacts and environment at home may be a greater source of infection than contacts in school.[199] When a zoophilic organism such as *M. canis* is the causative organism for the tinea capitis, the possibility of an animal source such as a cat or dog should be investigated.

KETOCONAZOLE

Ketoconazole was the first significant oral imidazole to become available for the treatment of mycotic infections. The drug was released in the United States in 1981. Previous therapies for systemic mycoses or severe dermatomycoses required intravenous administration (e.g., amphotericin B or miconazole), or had a limited spectrum of action (e.g., griseofulvin for dermatophytes or nystatin for *C. albicans*). The interested reader can pursue further information on the pharmacology and mechanism of action for ketoconazole.*

---

*References 3, 9, 18, 19, 75, 179.

Clinical Use
APPROVED INDICATIONS

Dermatophyte Infections.   Ketoconazole tablets are FDA approved for the treatment of patients with severe recalcitrant cutaneous dermatophyte infections who have not responded to topical therapy or oral griseofulvin, or who are unable to take griseofulvin.[85] This could include recalcitrant or very severe disfiguring or disabling pityriasis versicolor, tinea corporis, tinea cruris, and tinea pedis infections unresponsive to griseofulvin, or in patients allergic to or unable to tolerate griseofulvin.[9]

Deep Fungal Infections.   Ketoconazole is also indicated for the treatment of the following systemic fungal infections: candidiasis, chronic mucocutaneous candidiasis, oral thrush, candiduria, blastomycosis, coccidioidomycosis, histoplasmosis, chromomycosis, and paracoccidioidomycosis.[75]

OFF-LABEL USES

Various Fungal and Yeast Infections.   Ketoconazole has been used to treat onychomycosis (etiology: *Trichophyton* and *Candida* species),[179] pityriasis (tinea) versicolor, tinea pedis, and tinea corporis (dosage: 200 to 400 mg/day), tinea capitis (3.3 to 6.6 mg/kg/day), pityrosporum folliculitis (200 mg/day for 28 days), seborrheic dermatitis (200 mg/day for 28 days), cutaneous lesions of Reiter's syndrome, and vaginal candidiasis. Ketoconazole is no longer recommended for the treatment of onychomycosis, which requires long-term therapy.

Pityriasis (Tinea) Versicolor.   The majority of cases of pityriasis versicolor are treated with topical therapy. When ketoconazole tablets have been used, several dosage regimens exist, including 200 mg/day for 5 days, 200 mg/day for 3 to 5 weeks, and 400 mg on one or two occasions 1 week apart.[188,200-204] Because a significant amount of ketoconazole is excreted in eccrine sweat, ingestion of the tablets followed by exercise that produces sweat may enhance the efficacy of therapy. Regimens for prophylaxis include 400 mg once a month or 200 mg administered for 3 consecutive days each month.[204]

Bibliography

Antifungal Drug Therapy Overviews

Gupta AK, Sauder DN, Shear NH: Antifungal agents: an overview. Part I. *J Am Acad Dermatol* 30:677-698, 1994.

Gupta AK, Sauder DN, Shear NH: Antifungal agents: an overview. Part II. *J Am Acad Dermatol* 30:911-933, 1994.

Reviews of Individual Drugs and Specific Fungal Infections

Elewski BE: Tinea capitis: a current perspective. *J Am Acad Dermatol* 42:1-20, 2000.

Grant SM, Clissold SP: Fluconazole: a review of its pharmacodynamic and pharmacokinetic properties, and therapeutic potential in superficial and systemic mycoses. *Drugs* 39:877-917, 1990.

Gupta AK, Shear NH: Terbinafine: an update. *J Am Acad Dermatol* 37:979-988, 1997.

Gupta AK, Shear NH: The new oral antifungal agents for onychomycosis of the toenails. *J Eur Acad Dermatol Venereol* 13:1-13, 1999.

Haria M, Bryson HM, Goa KL: Itraconazole. A reappraisal of its pharmacological properties and therapeutic use in the management of superficial fungal infections. *Drugs* 51:585-620, 1996.

Jones TC: Overview of the use of terbinafine (Lamisil) in children. *Br J Dermatol* 132:683-689. (#45), 1995.

Adverse Effects and Drug Interactions

Gupta AK, Katz, I, Shear NH: Drug interactions with itraconazole, fluconazole, and terbinafine and their management. *J Am Acad Dermatol* 41:237-248, 1999.

Gupta AK, Shear NH: A risk-benefit assessment of the newer oral antifungal agents used to treat onychomycosis. *Drug Safety* 22:33-52, 2000.

Hall M, Monka C, Krupp P, et al: Safety of oral terbinafine: results of a postmarketing surveillance study in 25,884 patients. *Arch Dermatol* 133:1213-1219, 1997.

Hay RJ: Risk/benefit ratio of modern antifungal therapy: focus on hepatic reactions. *J Am Acad Dermatol* 29:S50-S54, 1993.

References

Terbinafine—Pharmacology

1. Berney D, Schuh K: Heterocyclic spironaphthalenones. Part 1: synthesis and reactions of some spiro [(1 H-naphthalenome)]-1,3,-piperidines. *Helv Chir Acta* 61:1262-1273, 1978.

2. Gupta AK, Shear NH: Terbinafine: an update. *J Am Acad Dermatol* 37:979-988, 1997.

3. *Physicians' desk reference*, ed 51, Montvale NJ, 1997, Medical Economics, pp 1345-1348.

4. Jensen JC: Clinical pharmacokinetics of terbinafine (Lamisil). *Clin Exp Dermatol* 14:110-113, 1989.

5. Balfour JA, Faulds D: Terbinafine. A review of its pharmacodynamic and pharmacokinetic properties, and therapeutic potential in superficial mycoses. *Drugs* 43:259-284, 1992.

6. Faergemann J, Zehender H, Jones T, et al: Terbinafine levels in serum, stratum corneum, dermis-epidermis (without stratum corneum), hair, sebum, and eccrine sweat. *Acta Derm Venereol* 71:322-326, 1990.

7. Lever LR, Dykes PJ, Thomas R, et al: How orally administered terbinafine reaches the stratum corneum. *J Dermatol Treat* 1:23-25, 1990.

8. Faergemann J, Zehender H, Jones T, et al: Terbinafine levels in serum, stratum corneum, dermis-epidermis (without stratum corneum), hair, sebum, and eccrine sweat during and after 250 mg terbinafine orally once per day in men. *J Invest Dermatol* 24:523, 1994.

9. Drug Information for the Health Care Professional, USP DI, The United States Pharmacopeial Convention, Inc., ed 17, Taunton MA, 1997, Rand McNally, pp 296-308.

10. Faergemann J, Zehender H, Denouël J, et al: Levels of terbinafine in plasma, stratum corneum, dermis-epidermis (without stratum corneum), sebum, hair and nails during and after 250 mg terbinafine orally once per day for four weeks. *Acta Derm Venereol* 73:305-309, 1993.

11. Schatz F, Bräutigam M, Dobrowolski E, et al: Nail incorporation kinetics of terbinafine in onychomycosis patients. *Clin Exp Dermatol* 20:377-383, 1995.

12. Faergemann J, Zehender H, Millerioux L: Levels of terbinafine in plasma, stratum corneum, dermis-epidermis (without stratum corneum), sebum, hair and nails during and after 250 mg terbinafine orally once daily for 7 and 14 days. *Clin Exp Dermatol* 19:121-126, 1994.

13. Baudraz-Rosselet F, Monod M, Jaccoud S, et al: Efficacy of terbinafine treatment of tinea capitis in children varies according to the dermatophyte species. *Br J Dermatol* 135:1011-1012, 1996.

14. Dragoš V, Lunder M: Lack of efficacy of 6-week treatment with oral terbinafine for tinea capitis due to *Microsporum canis* in children. *Pediatr Dermatol* 14:46-48, 1997.

15. Ryder NS: Terbinafine: mode of action and properties of the squalene epoxidase inhibition. *Br J Dermatol* 126:2-7, 1992.

16. Abdel-Rahman SM, Gotschall RR, Kaufmann RE, et al: Investigation of terbinafine as a CYP 2D6 inhibitor in vivo. *Clin Pharmacol Ther* 65:465-472, 1999.

17. Abdel-Rahman SM, Marcucci K, Boge T, et al: Potent inhibition of cytochrome P-450 2D6-mediated dextromethorphan O-demethylation by terbinafine. *Drug Metab Dispos* 27:770-775, 1999.

18. Gupta AK, Shear NH: A risk-benefit assessment of the newer oral antifungal agents used to treat onychomycosis. *Drug Saf* 22:33-52, 2000.

Terbinafine—Clinical Use

19. Gupta AK, Shear NH: The new oral antifungal agents for onychomycosis of the toenails. *J Eur Acad Dermatol Venereol* 13:1-13, 1999.

20. Alpsoy E, Yilmaz E, Basaran E: Intermittent therapy with terbinafine for dermatophyte toe-onychomycosis: a new approach. *J Dermatol* 34:595-600, 1996.

21. Arenas R, Dominguez-Cherit J, Fernández LM: Open randomized comparison of itraconazole versus terbinafine in onychomycosis. *Int J Dermatol* 34:138-143, 1993.

22. Bräutigam M, Nolting S, Schopf RE, et al: Randomized double blind comparison of terbinafine and itraconazole for treatment of toenail tinea infection. *BMJ* 311:919-922, 1995.

23. De Backer M, De Keyser P, De Vroey C, et al: A 12-week treatment for dermatophyte toe onychomycosis: terbinafine 250 mg/day vs. itraconazole 200 mg/day—a double-blind comparative trial. *Br J Dermatol* 134(Suppl 46):16-17, 1996.

24. Galimberti R, Kowalczuk A, Flores V, et al: Onychomycosis treated with a short course of oral terbinafine. *Int J Dermatol* 35:374-375, 1996.

25. Goodfield MJD, Andrew L, Evans EGV: Short term treatment of dermatophyte onychomycosis with terbinafine. *BMJ* 304:1151-1154, 1992.

26. Svejgaard EL, Brandrup F, Kragballe K, et al: Oral terbinafine in toenail dermatophytosis. *Acta Derm Venereol* 77:66-69, 1997.

27. Taush I, Bräutigam M, Weidinger G, et al: Evaluation of 6 weeks treatment of terbinafine in tinea unguium in a double-blind trial comparing 6 and 12 weeks therapy. *Br J Dermatol* 136:737-742, 1997.

28. Terbinafine package insert (United States): East Hanover NJ, Novartis, 1996.

29. van der Schroeff JG, Cirkel PKS, Crijns MB, et al: A randomized treatment duration-finding study of terbinafine in onychomycosis. *Br J Dermatol* 126:36-39, 1992.

30. Watson A, Marley J, Ellis D, et al: Terbinafine in onychomycosis of the toenail: a novel treatment protocol. *J Am Acad Dermatol* 33:775-779, 1995.

31. Evans EGV, Sigurgeirsson B, Billstein S: Double blind, randomised study of continuous terbinafine compared with intermittent itraconazole in treatment of toenail onychomycosis. The L.I.O.N. Study Group. *BMJ* 17:1031-1035, 1999.

32. Svejgaard E, et al; In De Doncker P, Van Custem J, PiJrard G, et al: Itraconazole compared to terbinafine in superficial fungal infections: from petri dish to patient. Poster P 206. Presented at The Fifty-sixth Annual American Academy of Dermatology Meeting, Orlando, Florida, February 27-March 4, 1998.

33. Havu V, Heikkilä H, Stubb S, et al: A study to compare the efficacy of Lamisil® (terbinafine) and Diflucan® (fluconazole) in patients with onychomycosis. Poster 132. *J Eur Acad Dermatol Venereol* 7(Suppl 2):S154, 1996.

34. Török I, Simon G, Dobozy A, et al: Long-term post-treatment follow-up of onychomycosis treated with terbinafine: a multicenter trial. *Mycoses* 41:63-65, 1998.

35. Tosti A, Piraccini BM, Stinchi C, et al: Treatment of dermatophyte nail infections: an open randomized study comparing intermittent terbinafine therapy with continuous terbinafine treatment and intermittent itraconazole therapy. *J Am Acad Dermatol* 34:595-600, 1996.

36. Honeyman JF, Talarico FS, Arruda LHF, et al: Itraconazole versus terbinafine (Lamisil®): which is better for the treatment of onychomycosis? *J Eur Acad Dermatol* 9:215-221, 1997.

37. Drake LA, Shear NH, Arlette JP, et al: Oral terbinafine in the treatment of toenail onychomycosis: North American multicenter trial. *J Am Acad Dermatol* 37:740-745, 1997.

38. Roberts DT, Richardson MD, Dwyer PK, et al: Terbinafine in chronic paronychia and *Candida* onychomycosis. *J Dermatol Treat* 2(Suppl 1):39-42, 1992.

39. Nolting S, Bräutigam M, Weidinger G: Terbinafine in onychomycosis with involvement by non-dermatophytic fungi. *Br J Dermatol* 30(Suppl 43):16-21, 1994.

40. Segal R, Kitzman A, Cividalli L, et al: Treatment of *Candida* nail infection with terbinafine. *J Am Acad Dermatol* 35:958-961, 1996.

41. Tosti A, Piraccini BM, Stinchi C, et al: Onychomycosis due to *Scopulariopsis brevicaulis:* clinical features and response to systemic antifungals. *Br J Dermatol* 135:799-802, 1996.

42. Tosti A, Piraccini BM, Lorenzi S: Onychomycosis caused by non-dermatophyte molds: clinical features and response to treatment of 59 cases. *J Am Acad Dermatol* 42:217-224, 2000.

43. Gupta AK, Sibbald RG, Lynde CW, et al: The prevalence of onychomycosis in children and treatment strategies. *J Am Acad Dermatol* 36:395-402, 1997.

44. Gupta AK, Chang P, Del Rosso JQ, et al: Onychomycosis in children: prevalence and management. *Pediatr Dermatol* 15:464-471, 1998.

45. Jones TC: Overview of the use of terbinafine (Lamisil) in children. *Br J Dermatol* 132:683-689, 1995.

46. Gupta AK, Del Rosso JQ: Management of onychomycosis in children. *Postgrad Med* (Suppl 38):29-35, 1999.

47. Goulden V, Goodfield MJD: Treatment of childhood dermatophyte infections with oral terbinafine. *Pediatr Dermatol* 12:53-54, 1995.

48. Terbinafine product monograph: Canada. Dorval, Quebec, Sandoz Canada, 1-33, 1995.

49. Savin RC: Oral terbinafine versus griseofulvin in the treatment of moccasin-type tinea pedis. *J Am Acad Dermatol* 23:807-809, 1990.

50. Hay RJ, Logan RA, Moore MK: A comparative study of terbinafine versus griseofulvin in "dry type" dermatophyte infections. *J Am Acad Dermatol* 24:243-246, 1991.

51. De Keyser P, De Backer M, Massart DL, et al: Two-week oral treatment of tinea pedis, comparing terbinafine (250 mg/day) with itraconazole (100 mg/day): a double-blind, multicentre study. *Br J Dermatol* 130:22-25, 1994.

52. Tausch I, Decroix J, Gwiedzdzinski Z, et al: Short-term itraconazole versus terbinafine in the treatment of tinea pedis or manus. *Int J Dermatol* 37:128-144, 1998.

53. Cole GW, Sticklin G: A comparison of a new oral antifungal, terbinafine, with griseofulvin as therapy for tinea corporis. *Arch Dermatol* 125:1537-1539, 1989.

54. Decroix J, Fritsch P, Picoto A, et al: Short-term itraconazole versus terbinafine in the treatment of superficial dermatomycoses of the glabrous skin (tinea corporis or cruris). *Eur J Dermatol* 7:353-357, 1997.

55. Gupta AK, Hofstader SLR, Adam P, et al: Tinea capitis: an overview with an emphasis on management. *Pediatr Dermatol* 16:171-189, 1999.

56. Gupta AK, Summerbell RC: Tinea capitis. *Medical Mycology* 38:255-287, 2000.

57. Nejjam JF, Zatula M, Cabiac MD, et al: Pilot study of terbinafine in children suffering from tinea capitis: evaluation of efficacy, safety and pharmacokinetics. *Br J Dermatol* 132:98-105, 1995.

58. Gruseck E, Splanemann V, Bleck O, et al: Oral terbinafine in tinea capitis in children. *Mycoses* 39:237-240, 1996.

59. Kullavanijaya P, Reangchainam S, Ungpakorn R: Randomized single-blind study of efficacy and tolerability of terbinafine in the treatment of tinea capitis. *J Am Acad Dermatol* 37:272-273, 1997.

60. Haroon TS, Hussain I, Aman S, et al: A randomized double-blind comparative study of terbinafine for 1, 2 and 4 weeks in tinea capitis. *Br J Dermatol* 135:86-88, 1996.
61. Elewski BE: Tinea capitis: a current perspective. *J Am Acad Dermatol* 42:1-20, 2000.
62. Gupta AK, Adam P: Terbinafine pulse therapy is effective in tinea capitis. *Pediatr Dermatol* 15:56-58, 1998.
63. Abdel-Rahman SM, Nahata MC: Treatment of tinea capitis. *Ann Pharmacother* 31:338-348, 1997.
64. Gupta AK, Prussick R, Sibbald RG, et al: Terbinafine in the treatment of Majocchi's granuloma. *Int J Dermatol* 34:489, 1995.
65. Budimulja U, Kuswadji K, Bramono S, et al: A double-blind, randomized, stratified controlled study of the treatment of tinea imbricata with oral terbinafine or itraconazole. *Br J Dermatol* 130:29-31, 1994.
66. Hull PR, Vismer HF: Treatment of cutaneous sporotrichosis with terbinafine. *Br J Dermatol* 126:51-55, 1992.
67. Gip L: Black piedra: the first case treated with terbinafine (Lamisil). *Br J Dermatol* 130:26-28, 1994.
68. Schiraldi GF, Circero SL, Colombo MD, et al: Refractory pulmonary aspergillosis: compassionate trial with terbinafine. *Br J Dermatol* 134(Suppl 46):25-29, 1996.
69. Esterre P, Inzan CK, Ratsioharana M, et al: A multicenter trial of terbinafine in patients with chromoblastomycosis: effect on clinical and biological criteria. *J Dermatol Treat* 9(Suppl 1):S29-S34, 1998.

Terbinafine—Adverse Effects and Drug Interactions

70. Hall M, Monka C, Krupp P, et al: Safety of oral terbinafine: results of a postmarketing surveillance study in 25,884 patients. *Arch Dermatol* 133:1213-1219, 1997.
71. O'Sullivan DP, Needham CA, Bangs A, et al: Postmarketing surveillance of oral terbinafine in the UK: report of a large cohort study. *Br J Clin Pharmacol* 41:1-7, 1996.
72. Stricker BHC, Van Riemsdijk MM, Sturkenboom MCJM, et al: Taste loss to terbinafine: a case-control study of potential risk factors. *Pharmacoepidemiol Drug Safety* 4:S22, 1995.
73. Hay RJ: Risk/benefit ratio of modern antifungal therapy: focus on hepatic reactions. *J Am Acad Dermatol* 29:S50-S54, 1993.
74. Gupta AK, Shear NH: Safety review of the new oral antifungal agents to treat superficial mycoses. *Int J Dermatol* 38(Suppl 2):40-52, 1999.
75. *Drugs facts and comparisons,* St. Louis, 1998, A Wolters Kluwer, pp 358-358(b).
76. Gupta AK, Sauder DN, Shear NH: Antifungal agents: an overview. Part II. *J Am Acad Dermatol* 30:911-933, 1994.
77. Gupta AK, Katz, I, Shear NH: Drug interactions with itraconazole, fluconazole, and terbinafine and their management. *J Am Acad Dermatol* 41:237-248, 1999.
78. Katz HI, Gupta AK: Oral antifungal drug interactions. *Dermatol Clin* 15:535-544, 1997.

Itraconazole—Pharmacology

79. Heeres J, Backx LJ, Van Custem J, et al: Antimycotic azoles. 7. Synthesis and antifungal properties of a series of novel triazol-3-ones. *J Med Chem* 27:894-900, 1984.
80. Cauwenbergh G, Degreef H, Heykants J, et al: Pharmacokinetic profile of orally administered itraconazole in human skin. *J Am Acad Dermatol* 18:263-268, 1988.
81. Itraconazole package insert (USA): Titusville NJ, Janssen, 1996.
82. Van Peer A, Woestenborghs R, Heykants J, et al: The effects of food and dose on the oral systemic availability of itraconazole in healthy subjects. *Eur J Clin Pharmacol* 36:423-426, 1989.
83. Grant SM, Clissold SP: Itraconazole: a review of its pharmacodynamic and pharmacokinetic properties, and therapeutic use in superficial and systemic mycoses. *Drugs* 37:310-344, 1989.
84. Jaruratanasirikul S, Kleepkaew A: Influence of an acidic beverage (Coca-Cola) on the absorption of itraconazole. *Eur J Clin Pharmacol* 52:235-237, 1997.
85. *Mosby's complete drug reference physicians GenRx,* St. Louis, Mosby-Year Book, 1997, II-1017 to II-1020.
86. De Doncker P: Pharmacokinetics of oral antifungal agents. *Dermatol Ther* 3:46-57, 1997.
87. Piérard G, Arrese J, De Doncker P: Antifungal activity of itraconazole and terbinafine in human stratum corneum: a comparative study. *J Am Acad Dermatol* 32:429-435, 1995.

88. De Doncker P, Decroix J, Piérard GE, et al: Itraconazole pulse therapy is effective in the treatment of onychomycosis: a pharmacokinetic/pharmacodynamic and clinical evaluation. *Arch Dermatol* 132:34-41, 1996.

89. Willemsen M, De Doncker P, Willems J, et al: Post-treatment itraconazole levels in the nail. New implications for treatment in onychomycosis. *J Am Acad Dermatol* 26:731-735, 1992.

90. De Doncker P: Effects of itraconazole in relation to drug distribution and penetration in the nail. PhD thesis. Antwerp: Universiteit Antwerpen, 1995.

91. Gupta AK, De Doncker P, Scher RK, et al: Itraconazole for the treatment of onychomycosis: an overview. *Int J Dermatol* 37:303-308, 1998.

92. Van Cutsem J: Therapeutic oral treatment with itraconazole solution of experimental microsporosis in cats. Efficacy and hair antifungal levels. Preclinical research report on itraconazole (R51211/85), December 1991, Janssen Research Foundation, Belgium.

93. Gupta AK, Groen K, De Doncker P: Itraconazole is effective in the treatment of Majocchi's granuloma: a clinical and pharmacokinetic evaluation. II. Implications for the effectiveness of itraconazole pulse therapy in tinea capitis. *Clin Exp Dermatol* 23:103-108, 1998.

94. Haria M, Bryson HM, Goa KL: Itraconazole. A reappraisal of its pharmacological properties and therapeutic use in the management of superficial fungal infections. *Drugs* 51:585-620, 1996.

Itraconazole—Clinical Use

95. Elewski BE, Scher RK, Aly R, et al: Double-blind, randomized comparison of itraconazole capsules vs. placebo in the treatment of toenail onychomycosis. *Cutis* 59:217-220, 1997.

96. Jones HE, Zaias N: Double-blind, randomized comparison of itraconazole capsules and placebo in onychomycosis of toenail. *Int J Dermatol* 35:589-590, 1996.

97. Haneke E, Delescluse J, Plinck EPB, et al: The use of itraconazole in onychomycosis. *Eur J Dermatol* 6:7-10, 1996.

98. Odom R, Daniel R, Aly R: A double-blind, randomized comparison of itraconazole capsules and placebo in the treatment of onychomycosis of the toenail. *J Am Acad Dermatol* 35:110-111, 1996.

99. Havu V, Brandt H, Heikkilä H, et al: A double-blind, randomized study comparing itraconazole pulse therapy with continuous dosing for the treatment of toe-nail onychomycosis. *Br J Dermatol* 136:230-234, 1997.

100. Kim JA, Ahn KJ, Kim JM, et al: Efficacy and tolerability of itraconazole in patients with fingernail onychomycosis: a 6-week pilot study. *Curr Ther Res* 56:1066-1075, 1995.

101. Odom RB, Aly R, Scher R, et al: A multicenter, placebo-controlled, double-blind study of intermittent therapy with itraconazole for the treatment of onychomycosis of the fingernail. *J Am Acad Dermatol* 36:231-235, 1997.

102. Wu J, Wen H, Liao W: Small-dose itraconazole pulse therapy in the treatment of onychomycosis. *Mycoses* 40:397-400, 1997.

103. Havu V, Brandt H, Heikkilä H, et al: A double-blind, randomized study comparing itraconazole pulse therapy with continuous dosing for the treatment of toe-nail onychomycosis. *Br J Dermatol* 136:230-234, 1997.

104. De Doncker P, Van Lint J, Dockx P, et al: Pulse therapy with one-week itraconazole monthly for three or four months in the treatment of onychomycosis. *Cutis* 56:180-183, 1995.

105. Bonifaz A, Carrasco-Gerard E, Saúl A: Itraconazole in onychomycosis: intermittent dose schedule. *Int J Dermatol* 36:70-72, 1997.

106. Itraconazole package insert (Canada): Janssen Canada, 1997.

107. Haneke E, Abeck D, Ring J: The safety and efficacy of intermittent therapy with itraconazole for finger and toenail onychomycosis: a multicenter trial. *Zeitschriftfuer Hautkrankheiten* 10:737-740, 1997.

108. Ginter G, De Doncker P: An intermittent 1-week dosing regimen for the treatment of toenail onychomycosis in dermatological patients. *Mycoses* 41:235-238, 1998.

109. Wang DP, Wang AP, Li RY, Wang R: Treatment efficacy and safety of 1-week intermittent therapy with itraconazole for onychomycosis in a Chinese patient population. *Dermatology* 199:47-49, 1999.

110. Tosti A, Piraccini DM, Vincenzi C, et al: Itraconazole in the treatment of two young brothers with chronic mucocutaneous candidiasis. *Pediatr Dermatol* 14:146-148, 1997.

111. Hay RJ, Clayton YM, Moore MK, et al: An evaluation of itraconazole in the management of onychomycosis. *Br J Dermatol* 119:359-366, 1988.

112. Scher RK, Barnett JM: Successful treatment of *Aspergillus flavus* onychomycosis with oral itraconazole. *J Am Acad Dermatol* 23:749-750, 1990.

113. De Doncker PRG, Scher RK, Baran RL, et al: Itraconazole therapy is effective for pedal onychomycosis caused by some nondermatophyte molds and in mixed infection with dermatophytes and molds: a multicenter study with 36 patients. *J Am Acad Dermatol* 36:173-177, 1997.

114. Gupta AK, Adam P, Hofstader SLR: Itraconazole oral solution for the treatment of onychomycosis. *Pediatr Dermatol* 15:472-474, 1998.

115. De Doncker P, Gupta AK, Marynissen G, et al: Itraconazole pulse therapy for onychomycosis and dermatomycoses: an overview. *J Am Acad Dermatol* 37:969-974, 1997.

116. Gupta AK, De Doncker P, Heremans A, et al: Itraconazole for the treatment of tinea pedis: a dose of 400 mg/day given for 1 week is similar in efficacy to 100 or 200 mg/day given for 2 to 4 weeks. *J Am Acad Dermatol* 36:789-792, 1997.

117. Lachapelle JM, De Doncker P, Tennstedt D, et al: Itraconazole compared with griseofulvin in the treatment of tinea corporis/cruris and tinea pedis/manus: an interpretation of the clinical results of all completed double-blind studies with respect to the pharmacokinetic profile. *Dermatology* 184:45-50, 1992.

118. Parent D, Decroix J, Heenen M: Clinical experience with short schedules of itraconazole in the treatment of tinea corporis and/or tinea cruris. *Dermatology* 189:378-381, 1994.

119. Gupta AK, Nolting S, Prost Y, et al: The use of itraconazole to treat superficial fungal infections in children. *Dermatology* 199:248-252, 1999.

120. Gupta AK, Alexis ME, Raboobee N, et al: Itraconazole pulse therapy is effective in the treatment of tinea capitis in children: an open multicentre study. *Br J Dermatol* 137:251-254, 1997.

121. Elewski BE: Treatment of tinea capitis with itraconazole. *Int J Dermatol* 36:537-541, 1997.

122. Gupta AK, Hofstader SLR, Summerbell RC, et al: Itraconazole pulse therapy for the treatment of tinea capitis. *J Am Acad Dermatol* 39:216-219, 1998.

123. Gupta AK, Adam P, De Doncker P: Itraconazole pulse therapy for tinea capitis: a novel treatment schedule. *Pediatr Dermatol* 15:225-228, 1998.

124. Ginter G: *Microsporum canis* infections in children: results of a new oral antifungal therapy with itraconazole. Third meeting of the European Confederation of Medical Mycology, Lisbon, Portugal, May 9-11, 1996.

125. Abdel-Rahaman SM, Powell DA, Nahata MC: Efficacy of itraconazole in children with *Trichophyton tonsurans* tinea capitis. *J Am Acad Dermatol* 38:443-446, 1998.

126. Gupta AK, Solomon RS, Adam P: Itraconazole oral solution for the treatment of tinea capitis. *Br J Dermatol* 139:104-106, 1998.

127. Berger TG, Heon V, King C, et al: Itraconazole therapy for human immunodeficiency virus-associated eosinophilic folliculitis. *Arch Dermatol* 31:358-360, 1995.

128. Kavanagh GM, Leeming JP, Marshman GM, et al: Folliculitis in Down's syndrome. *Br J Dermatol* 129:696-699, 1993.

129. Delescluse J: Itraconazole in tinea versicolor: a review. *J Am Acad Dermatol* 23:551-554, 1990.

130. Faergemann J: Treatment of pityriasis versicolor with itraconazole: a double-blind placebo controlled study. *Mycoses* 31:377-379, 1988.

131. Burke WA: Use of itraconazole in a patient with chronic mucocutaneous candidiasis. *J Am Acad Dermatol* 21:1309-1310, 1989.

132. Itraconazole oral solution product monograph: Titusville NJ, Janssen, 1997.

Itraconazole—Adverse Effects and Drug Interactions

133. Inman W, Kubota K, Pierce G, et al: PEM report number 7. Itraconazole. *Pharmacoepidemiol Drug Safety* 2:423-443, 1993.

134. Itraconazole International Product Monograph: Breese, Belgium, 1996, 1-7.

135. Tatro DS, editor: *Drug interaction facts. Facts and comparisons*, St. Louis, 1998, A Wolters Kluwer.

136. Stockley IH: *Drug interactions*, ed 4, London, 1996, The Pharmaceutic Press.

Fluconazole—Pharmacology

137. Grant SM, Clissold SP: Fluconazole: a review of its pharmacodynamic and pharmacokinetic properties, and therapeutic potential in superficial and systemic mycoses. *Drugs* 39:877-917, 1990.

138. Fluconazole package insert: New York, Pfizer Roerig, 1997.

139. Fluconazole package insert: Pfizer Canada.

140. Faergemann J, Laufen H: Levels of fluconazole in serum, stratum corneum, epidermis-dermis (without stratum corneum) and eccrine sweat. *Clin Exp Dermatol* 18:102-106, 1993.

141. Wildfeuer A, Faergemann J, Laufen H, et al: Bioavailability of fluconazole in the skin after oral medication. *Mycoses* 37:127-130, 1994.

142. Hay RJ: Pharmacokinetic evaluation of fluconazole in skin and nails. *Int J Dermatol* 1(Suppl 2):6-7, 1992.

143. Rich P, Scher R, Brenneman D, et al: Pharmacokinetics of three doses of once-weekly fluconazole (150, 300, and 400 mg) in the management of distal subungual onychomycosis of the toenail. *J Am Acad Dermatol* 38:S103-S109, 1998.

Fluconazole—Clinical Use

144. Fräki J, Heikkilä H, Kero M, et al: An open-label, non-comparative, multicenter evaluation of fluconazole with or without urea nail pedicure for treatment of onychomycosis. *Curr Ther Res* 58:481-491, 1997.

145. Kuokkanen K, Alava S: Fluconazole in the treatment of onychomycosis caused by dermatophytes. *J Derm Treat* 3:115-117, 1992.

146. Montero Gei F, Robles-Soto ME, Schlager H: Fluconazole in the treatment of severe onychomycosis. *Int J Dermatol* 35:587-588, 1996.

147. Scher RK, Brenneman D, Rich P, et al: A placebo-controlled, randomized, double-blind trial of once-weekly fluconazole (150 mg, 300 mg, or 450 mg) in the treatment of distal subungual onychomycosis of the toenail. *J Am Acad Dermatol* 38:S77-S86, 1998.

148. Sadeque Z, Rahmatullah H, Latif Khan A: A comparison of the efficacy of oral griseofulvin, fluconazole and terbinafine in the treatment of onychomycosis. *Bangladesh J Dermatol* 13:29-32, 1996.

149. Drake L, Babel D, Stewart DM, et al: Once-weekly fluconazole (150, 300 or 450 mg) in the treatment of distal subungual onychomycosis of the fingernail. *J Am Acad Dermatol* 38:S87-S94, 1998.

150. Smith SW, Sealy DP, Schneider E, et al: An evaluation of the safety and efficacy at fluconazole in the treatment of onychomycosis. *South Med J* 88:1217-1220, 1995.

151. Faergemann J, Mork NJ, Haglund A, et al: A multicentre (double-blind) comparative study to assess the safety and efficacy of fluconazole and griseofulvin in the treatment of tinea corporis and tinea cruris. *Br J Dermatol* 136:575-577, 1997.

152. Stary A, Sarnow E: Fluconazole in the treatment of tinea corporis and tinea cruris. *Dermatology* 196:237-241, 1998.

153. Suchil P, Montero Gei F, Robles M, et al: Once-weekly oral doses of fluconazole 150 mg in the treatment of tinea corporis/cruris and cutaneous candidiasis. *Clin Exp Dermatol* 17:397-401, 1992.

154. Haroon TS, Asghar HA, Aman S, et al: An open, non-comparative study for the evaluation of oral fluconazole in the treatment of tinea corporis. *Specialist* 13:417-423, 1997.

155. Papini M, Difonzo EM, Cilli P, et al: Itraconazole versus fluconazole, a double-blind comparison in tinea corporis. *J Mycologie Medicale* 7:77-80, 1997.

156. Kotogyan A, Harmanyeri Y, Tahsin Gunes A, et al: Efficacy and safety of oral fluconazole in the treatment of patients with tinea corporis, cruris or pedis or cutaneous candidiasis. A multicentre, open, non-comparative study. *Clin Drug Invest* 12:59-66, 1996.

157. Gomez M, Arenas R, Salazar JJ, et al: Tinea pedis. A multicentre trial to evaluate the efficacy and tolerance of a weekly dose of fluconazole. *Dermatologia Revista Mexicana* 40:251-255, 1996.

158. Del Aguila R, Montero Gei F, Robles M, et al: Once-weekly oral doses of fluconazole 150 mg in the treatment of tinea pedis. *Clin Exp Dermatol* 17:402-406, 1992.

159. Solomon BA, Collins R, Sharma R, et al: Fluconazole for the treatment of tinea capitis in children. *J Am Acad Dermatol* 37:274-275, 1997.

160. Gupta AK, Adam P, Hofstader SL, et al: Intermittent short duration therapy with fluconazole is effective for tinea capitis. *Br J Dermatol* 41:304-306, 1999.

161. Montero Gei F: Fluconazole in the treatment of tinea capitis. *Int J Dermatol* 37:870-871, 1998.

162. Gupta AK, Dlova N, Taborda P, et al: Once weekly fluconazole is effective in the treatment of tinea capitis: a prospective, multicentre study. *Br J Dermatol* 142:965-968, 2000.

163. Amer MA: Fluconazole in the treatment of tinea versicolor. *Int J Dermatol* 36:940-942, 1997.

164. Stengel F, Robbo-Soto N, Galinberti R, Suchil P: Fluconazole versus ketoconazole in the treatment of dermatophytoses and cutaneous candidiasis. *Int J Dermatol* 33:726-729, 1994.

165. Hay RJ, Clayton YM: Fluconazole in the management of patients with chronic mucocutaneous candidosis. *Br J Dermatol* 119:683-684, 1988.

166. Kauffman CA, Pappas PG, McKinsey DS, et al: Treatment of lymphocutaneous and visceral sporotrichosis with fluconazole. *Clin Infect Dis* 22:46-50, 1996.

167. Anaissie EJ, Kontoyiannis DP, Huls C, et al: Safety, plasma concentrations, and efficacy of high-dose fluconazole in invasive mold infections. *J Infect Dis* 172:599-602, 1995.

Fluconazole—Adverse Effects and Drug Interactions

168. Stevens DA, Diaz M, Negroni R, et al: Safety evaluation of chronic fluconazole therapy. *Chemotherapy* 43:371-377, 1997.

169. Duswald KH, Penk A, Pittrow L: High-dose therapy with fluconazole greater than or equal to 800 mg per day. *Mycoses* 40:267-277, 1997.

170. Mastroiacovo P, Mazzone T, Botto LD, et al: Prospective assessment of pregnancy outcomes after first-trimester exposure to fluconazole. *Am J Obstet Gynecol* 175:1645-1650, 1996.

171. Inman W, Pearce G, Wilton L: Safety of fluconazole in the treatment of vaginal candidiasis. *Eur J Clin Pharmacol* 46:115-118, 1994.

172. Rubin PC, Wilton LV, Inman WHW: Fluconazole and pregnancy: results of a prescription event-monitoring study. *Int J Gynecol Obstet* 37:25-27, 1992.

173. Lee BE, Feinberg M, Abraham JJ, et al: Congenital malformations in an infant born to a woman treated with fluconazole. *Pediatr Infect Dis J* 11:1062-1064, 1992.

174. Pursley TJ, Blomquist IK, Abraham J, et al: Fluconazole-induced congenital anomalies in three infants. *Clin Infect Dis* 22:336-340, 1996.

175. Krcmery V, Huttova M, Masar O: Teratogenicity of fluconazole. *Pediatr Infect Dis J* 15:841, 1996.

176. Inman W, Pearce G, Wilton L: Safety of fluconazole in the treatment of vaginal candidiasis. A prescription-event monitoring study, with special reference to the outcome of pregnancy. *Eur J Clin Pharmacol* 46:115-118, 1994.

177. Force RW: Fluconazole concentrations in breast milk. *Pediatr Infect Dis J* 14:235-236, 1995.

178. Debruyne D, Ryckeelynck JP, Moulin M, et al: Pharmacokinetics of fluconazole in patients undergoing continuous ambulatory peritoneal dialysis. *Clin Pharmacokinet* 18:491-498, 1990.

Griseofulvin

179. Gupta AK, Sauder DN, Shear NH: Antifungal agents: an overview. Part I. *J Am Acad Dermatol* 30:677-698, 1994.

180. Schwartz RA, Janniger CK: Tinea capitis. *Cutis* 55:29-33, 1995.

181. Abdel-Rahman SM, Nahata MC, Powell DA: Response to initial griseofulvin therapy in pediatric patients with tinea capitis. *Ann Pharmacother* 31:406-410, 1997.

182. Tanz RR, Stagl S, Esterly NB: Comparison of ketoconazole and griseofulvin for the treatment of tinea capitis in childhood: a preliminary study. *Pediatr Emerg Care* 1:16-18, 1985.

183. Tanz RR, Herbert AA, Esterly NB: Treating tinea capitis: should ketoconazole replace griseofulvin? *J Pediatr* 112:987-991, 1988.

184. Gan VN, Petruska M, Ginsburg CM: Epidemiology and treatment of tinea capitis: ketoconazole vs. griseofulvin. *Pediatr Infect Dis J* 6:46-49, 1987.

185. Martinez-Roig A, Torres-Rodriguez JM, Bartlett-Coma A: Double-blind study of ketoconazole and griseofulvin in dermatophytoses. *Pediatr Infect Dis J* 7:37-40, 1988.

186. Lopez-Gomez S, Del Palacio A, Van Custem J, et al: Itraconazole versus griseofulvin in the treatment of tinea capitis: a double-blind randomized study in children. *Int J Dermatol* 33:743-747, 1994.

187. Haroon TS, Hussain I, Aman S, et al: A randomized double-blind comparative study of terbinafine and griseofulvin in tinea capitis. *J Dermatol Treat* 6:167-169, 1995.

188. Gupta AK, Del Rosso JQ: An evaluation of intermittent therapies used to treat onychomycosis and other dermatomycoses with the oral antifungal agents. *Int J Dermatol* 39:401-411, 2000.

189. Elewski B: Tinea capitis. *Dermatol Clin* 14:23-31, 1996.

190. Allen HB, Honig PJ, Leyden JJ, et al: Selenium sulfide: adjunctive therapy for tinea capitis. *Pediatrics* 69:81-83, 1982.

191. Givens TG, Murray MM, Baker RC: Comparison of 1% and 2.5% selenium sulfide in the treatment of tinea capitis. *Arch Pediatr Adolesc Med* 149:808-811, 1995.

192. Neil G, Hanslo D, Buccimazza S: Control of the carrier state of scalp dermatophytes. *Pediatr Infect Dis J* 14:2-8, 1990.

193. Abdel-Rahaman SM, Nahata MC: Treatment of tinea capitis. *Ann Pharmacother* 31:338-348, 1997.

194. Williams JV, Honig PJ, McGinley KJ, et al: Semiquantitative study of tinea capitis and the asymptomatic carrier state in inner-city school children. *Pediatrics* 96:265-267, 1995.

195. Babel DE, Baughmann SA: Evaluation of the adult carrier state in juvenile tinea capitis caused by *Trichophyton tonsurans*. *J Am Acad Dermatol* 21:1209-1212, 1989.

196. Herbert AA, Head ES, MacDonald EM: Tinea capitis caused by *Trichophyton tonsurans*. *Pediatr Dermatol* 2:219-223, 1985.

197. MacKenzie DWR, Burrows D, Walby AL: *Trichophyton sulphureum* in a residential school. *BMJ* 2:1055-1058, 1960.

198. Arnow PM, Houchins SG, Pugliese G: An outbreak of tinea corporis in hospital personnel caused by a patient with *Trichophyton tonsurans* infection. *Pediatr Infect Dis J* 10:355-359, 1991.

199. Greer DL: Treatment of symptom-free carriers in the management of tinea capitis. *Lancet* 348:350-351, 1996.

Ketoconazole

200. Gupta AK, Einarson TR, Summerbell RC, et al: An overview of topical antifungal therapy in dermatomycoses: a North American perspective. *Drugs* 55:645-674, 1998.

201. Zaias N: Pityriasis versicolor with ketoconazole (letter). *J Am Acad Dermatol* 20:703-704, 1989.

202. Faergemann J, Djäru L: Tinea versicolor: treatment and prophylaxis with ketoconazole. *Cutis* 30:542-545, 1982.

203. Rausch LJ, Jacobs PH: Tinea versicolor: treatment and prophylaxis with monthly administration of ketoconazole. *Cutis* 34:470-471, 1984.

204. Jones HE: Pityriasis versicolor with ketoconazole (letter reply). *J Am Acad Dermatol* 20:704-705, 1989.

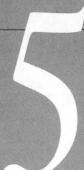

CHAPTER 5

Tanya Y. Evans
Melody R. Vander Straten
Daniel A. Carrasco
Soni Carlton
Stephen K. Tyring

Systemic Antiviral Agents

Viral diseases in dermatology can be very frustrating to treat. Exposure controls, such as vaccines, sanitation, vector controls, blood testing, condom use/abstinence, and education, remain extremely important methods in managing viral spread. Once viruses, such as human herpesvirus (HHV), human papillomavirus, and human immunodeficiency virus (HIV), are acquired, antivirals are important methods of treatment. A large number of antiviral agents received approval from the U.S. Food and Drug Administration (FDA) over the past decade. New antiviral agents and new vaccines are continuously being researched for more effective control of viral diseases.

To date there are 17 FDA-approved systemic antiviral drugs for treatment of infections due to HHV and HIV. This chapter deals with the current use of systemic antiviral agents in dermatology, as well as new agents that are currently under investigation.

The first section of this chapter focuses on drugs for HHV infections. The second major section focuses on drugs for HIV-1. Because these drugs for HIV-1 are prescribed by only a small percentage of practicing dermatologists, relatively little text is devoted to each of these drugs.

DRUGS FOR HUMAN HERPESVIRUS INFECTIONS

Infection with any of the double-stranded linear DNA viruses may cause a variety of different clinical manifestations. The HHV family includes herpes simplex virus (HSV) type 1 and type 2, commonly causing herpes labialis (cold sores) and genital lesions, respectively; however, both types of lesions can be caused by either virus (Table 5-1). HSV type 1 and type 2 (HSV-1 and HSV-2) have also been shown to cause gingivostomatitis, herpes gladiatorum, eczema herpeticum, herpetic whitlow, neonatal herpes, lumbosacral herpes, herpetic keratoconjunctivitis, herpes encephalitis, and cervicitis and are also a leading cause of erythema multiforme.[1] Varicella zoster virus (VZV) is HHV type 3, more commonly known as chickenpox in its primary form and herpes zoster or shingles in a recurrent form. The remaining members of the HHV family and resulting conditions are listed in Table 5-1.[1,2]

Drugs that have at least some degree of efficacy against the spectrum of HHV infections include acyclovir, valacyclovir (the prodrug of acyclovir), and famciclovir. These three

■ **Table 5-1** Human Herpes Virus (HHV) Nomenclature

HHV Number	Older Nomenclature	Resultant Diseases
HHV 1	Herpes simplex virus type 1 (HSV-1)	Herpes labialis, a variety of others
HHV 2	Herpes simplex virus type 2 (HSV-2)	Genital herpes, a variety of others
HHV 3	Varicella-zoster virus (VZV)	Chicken pox, herpes zoster
HHV 4	Epstein-Barr virus (EBV)	Mononucleosis, Burkitt's lymphoma
HHV 5	Cytomegalovirus (CMV)	CMV retinitis in HIV patients
HHV 6	No prior viral name	Roseola infantum, others
HHV 7	No prior viral name	Pityriasis rosea,* others
HHV 8	Kaposi's sarcoma herpes virus (KSHV)	Kaposi's sarcoma (classic and epidemic)

*The causal role of HHV 7 in pityriasis rosea has not been fully established.

■ **Table 5-2** Systemic Antiviral Agents (Used to Treat Human Herpes Virus Infections)

Generic Name	Trade Name	Generic Available	Manu- facturer	Tablet/ Capsule Sizes	Special Formula- tions	Standard Dosage Range	Price Index
Acyclovir	Zovirax	Yes	Glaxo- Wellcome, various others	200, 400, 800 mg	Oral suspension 200 mg/ 5 ml	See Table 5-8	$$$/$$$$ ($/$$$)
Valacyclovir	Valtrex	No	Glaxo- Wellcome	500 mg	No	See Table 5-8	$$$
Famciclovir	Famvir	No	SmithKline Beecham	125, 250, 500 mg	No	See Table 5-8	$$$/$$$$

$, <1.00; $$, 1.01-2.00; $$$, 2.01-5.00; $$$$, 5.01-10.00; $$$$$, >10.00; ( ) , generic price; /, two different price ranges from lower dose to higher dose examples of this drug; —, no price listed for this drug.

drugs receive the greatest focus in this chapter (Table 5-2).

Acyclovir

PHARMACOLOGY.   The most well known and widely used antiviral drug in the world is acyclovir (9-2-hydroxyethoxymethyl guanine or acycloguanosine) (ACV)[1,3] (Figure 5-1). This drug's activation requires a thymidine kinase (TK) specifically for the herpesvirus; herpesvirus infected cells produce TK 100 times faster than uninfected cells. This high rate of TK production results in a monophosphory-lated form of ACV that must then be biphos-phorylated and triphosphorylated by cellular enzymes. The triphosphorylated form of ACV inhibits viral DNA polymerase greater than human DNA polymerase, which results in chain termination (i.e., complete and irreversible inhibition of further viral DNA synthesis).[1,4]

Table 5-3 contains the key pharmacologic concepts for ACV.

CLINICAL USE.   Indications and contraindications for ACV are found in Table 5-4.

   FDA-Approved Indications
   Herpes Simplex Virus Infections.   There are several modalities of administration of ACV. The most widely used form of administration is the oral form. Oral ACV is used for several types

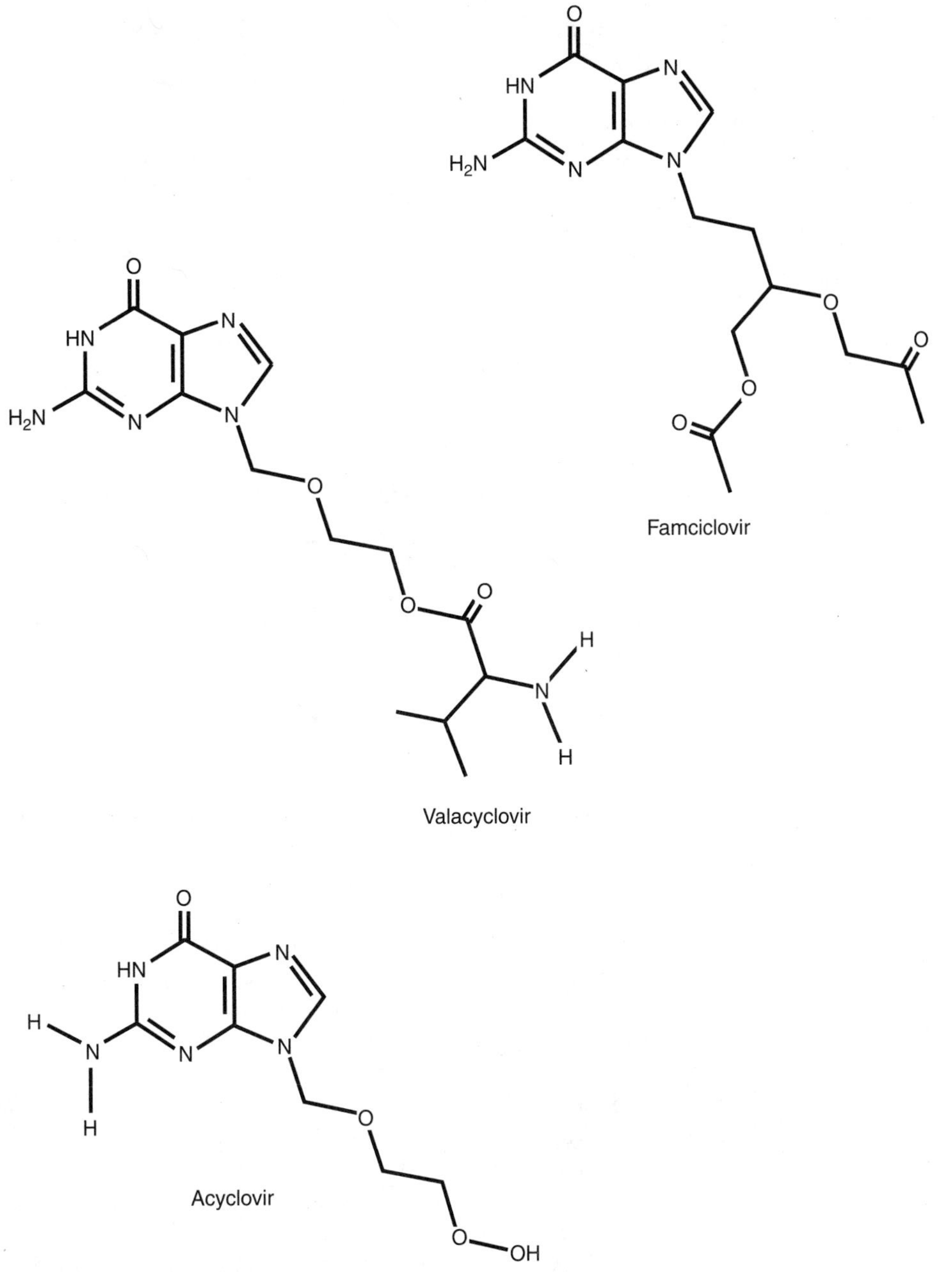

Figure 5-1 Systemic antiviral agents.

of HSV infections. The usual dose of ACV for first-episode genital herpes is 200 mg five times per day for 10 days, and the same dose can be used for 5 days for recurrent episodes of genital herpes.[1,4] Alternatively, ACV can be used as 400 mg three times per day for recurrences, leading to greater convenience and increased compli-ance. Even though ACV has a greater effect when used for first-episode genital herpes, it may show significant benefit in recurrent dis-ease if therapy is initiated during the prodrome phase.[1,4] ACV can also be taken at a dose of 400 mg twice daily on a continuous basis as sup-pressive therapy. This continuous suppressive

■ Table 5-3　Key Pharmacologic Concepts—Acyclovir, Valacyclovir, and Famciclovir

Drug Name	Absorption and Bioavailability			Elimination		
	Peak Levels	Bioavail-able (%)	Protein Binding	Half-life	Metabolism	Excretion
Acyclovir	1.5-2.0 hrs	15%-30%	9%-33%	1.3-1.5 hrs	No hepatic microsomal metabolism	Roughly equal urine and fecal—mostly unchanged free drug (acyclovir)
Valacyclovir	Uncertain	54.5%	13.5%-17.9%	2.5-3.3 hrs	No hepatic microsomal metabolism; rapid conversion to acyclovir	(Same as acyclovir)
Famciclovir	0.9 hr	77%	<20%	2.3-3.0 hrs	No hepatic microsomal metabolism; rapid conversion to penciclovir	73% urine, 27% fecal; mostly penci-clovir, also 6-deoxypenciclovir

Adapted from *CliniSphere 2.0 CD ROM,* St. Louis, June 2000, Facts & Comparisons.

therapy can reduce recurrences of genital herpes by 80% to 90% and reduce asymptomatic viral shedding of HSV-2 by 95%.[1,5] The twice daily suppressive dose can also reduce the frequency of herpes labialis recurrences by 50% to 78%.[1,6,7]

Chickenpox. ACV can also be used at an oral dose of 20 mg/kg four times daily (up to a maximum of 800 mg per dose) for chickenpox, but the usual adult dose is 800 mg five times daily.[1,8] In order for treatment of chickenpox to be effective, ACV needs to be initiated early in the disease process. Studies evaluating therapy for chickenpox initiated therapy in the first 24 hours after appearance of the characteristic skin eruption. ACV use in chickenpox does not adversely affect immunity to the virus because therapy would begin with the appearance of the first vesicle. This would be approximately 2 weeks after viral replication began, which is more than sufficient time to mount an adequate immune response. ACV treatment of chickenpox, even in otherwise healthy children, is con-

sidered cost effective because it allows the child to return to school at least 2 days earlier, thus enabling the parent to return to work at least 2 days earlier.

Herpes Zoster. ACV can also be used for recurrences of VZV in adulthood known as herpes zoster.[1] Acute herpes zoster requires 800 mg of ACV to be taken five times per day for 7 to 10 days. Therapy ideally should begin within 1 to 2 days of the initial symptoms and signs of herpes zoster. Although there is much controversy regarding the effects of ACV on herpes zoster, this dose has been shown to reduce the mean duration of postherpetic neuralgia (PHN) from 62 days for patients treated with placebo to 20 days for patients treated with ACV.[1,9]

Immunocompromised Patients. Due to the 15% to 30% bioavailability of oral ACV, the intravenous preparation is used in severely ill patients, including immunocompromised patients with HSV or VZV, especially with disseminated disease, as well as in immunocompe-

Table 5-4	Acyclovir Indications and Contraindications

FDA-APPROVED INDICATIONS
Herpes Simplex Infections[1,4-8]
Primary episode
Recurrent episodes
Suppressive therapy

Varicella-Zoster Infections
Chicken pox[1,8]
Herpes zoster[1,9]

Herpes Simplex or Varicella-Zoster Infections
Immunocompromised patients (such as HIV infections)[1,10-14]

OFF-LABEL USES
Recurrent erythema multiforme (presumed/proven due to HSV)[15-18]
Other subsets of herpes simplex infections (see text)

CONTRAINDICATIONS
Hypersensitivity to acyclovir
Hypersensitivity to any component of the formulation

PREGNANCY PRESCRIBING STATUS—CATEGORY C*

*With doses at least 60 times human doses, acyclovir causes some fetal abnormalities in laboratory animals.

tent persons with severe trigeminal nerve distribution herpes zoster (especially cases involving the ophthalmic branch).[1] In a recent metaanalysis of randomized individual patient data looking at clinical efficacy of high-dose ACV in patients with HIV infection, ACV offered a modest survival benefit to patients infected with HIV.[10] Although ACV has no antiretroviral activity, reduction in the incidence of HSV and VZV infections suggests that the suppression of the bursts of HIV replication occurring during active herpesvirus infections is one possible explanation for prolonged survival.[10-14] Topical preparations of ACV continue to be available for HSV regardless of the low efficacy of ACV in that form.[1,4] (See the Therapeutic Guidelines—Drugs

for HHV Infections section for a summary of the use of ACV in patients with HSV and VZV.)

Off-Label Uses
Recurrent Erythema Multiforme.   Over the past 15 years there have been a variety of studies and case series evaluating intermittent or suppressive ACV therapy for recurrent erythema multiforme proven or presumed to be due to HSV.[16-19] One of studies evaluated the response of children, with a dosage range of 20 to 25 mg/kg/day.[16] The majority of patients in these studies had oral mucosal involvement. Overall, about 55% of patients had a favorable response. When suppressive therapy was utilized, ACV 400 mg twice daily was given. ACV is a reasonable therapeutic option for frequent, painful recurrences of erythema multiforme that are likely due to preceding HSV infections.

Other Herpes Simplex Infections.   A variety of subsets of HSV can be treated with ACV in a similar fashion to the regimens outlined for oral and genital herpes simplex infections that have FDA approval. These subsets include primary gingivostomatitis, recurrent herpes labialis, herpes gladiatorum, eczema herpeticum, herpetic whitlow, and herpetic keratoconjunctivitis. Empiric dosages can be identical to those utilized for primary infections, recurrences, and suppressive regimens outlined in the Therapeutic Guidelines—Drugs for HHV Infections section.

Adverse Effects.   ACV is generally well tolerated regardless of the route of administration. Infrequent adverse effects with oral and intravenous treatment include nausea, vomiting, diarrhea, and headache. Intravenous infusions are associated with phlebitis and infusion-site inflammation in addition to reversible renal impairment due to a crystalline nephropathy.

Drug Interactions.   Since ACV is not metabolized by hepatic microsomal enzymes, there is a relative paucity of important drug interactions. A few minor interactions are detailed in Table 5-5.

Valacyclovir
PHARMACOLOGY.   Two additional antiherpes agents were approved for easier dosing and increased bioavailability. These two agents include valacyclovir (VACV) and famciclovir (FCV). VACV is a 1-valyl ester of ACV with a bioavailability about 3 to 5 times that of

■ **Table 5-5**   Acyclovir, Valacyclovir, and Famciclovir Drug Interactions

Precipitant Drug	Target Drug	Mechanism
DRUGS THAT INCREASE ANTIVIRAL DRUG LEVELS		
Probenecid	Acyclovir, famciclovir	↑ bioavailability, ↓ renal clearance due to ↓ renal tubular secretion
Zidovudine	Acyclovir	Uncertain mechanism—severe drowsiness and lethargy can occur
Cimetidine	Famciclovir	Small ↑ penciclovir levels—no clinical importance
Theophylline	Famciclovir	Small ↓ penciclovir renal clearance—no clinical importance
DRUG LEVELS INCREASED BY ANTIVIRAL AGENTS		
Famciclovir	Digoxin	Uncertain mechanism—levels ↑ 19%
DECREASED RATE OF CONVERSION VALACYCLOVIR TO ACYCLOVIR		
Cimetidine	Valacyclovir	↓ rate but not extent of conversion to acyclovir
Probenecid	Valacyclovir	Same as above

Adapted from *CliniSphere 2.0 CD ROM*, St. Louis, June 2000, Facts & Comparisons.

oral ACV, making it nearly as potent (in the oral form of VACV) as intravenous ACV when comparing blood levels of the two drugs[1] (see Figure 5-1). VACV is a prodrug, with the active metabolite being acyclovir. Aside from the differences in bioavailability between the two drugs, one would expect that the mechanism, clinical spectrum, and adverse effects would be similar overall (see Pharmacology section and Table 5-3).

CLINICAL USE.   Indications and contraindications for VACV are found in Table 5-6.

FDA-Approved Indications

Herpes Simplex Infections. VACV is FDA-approved for the episodic treatment of recurrent genital herpes at a dose of 500 mg orally twice a day for 5 days. First-episode genital herpes is treated with 1000 mg of VACV twice daily for 10 days.[1] Ten-day courses of both ACV five times daily and VACV twice daily are equally effective in accelerating the resolution of first-episode genital herpes.[15] The twice-daily regimen is also more convenient for patients to take, which leads to potentially greater patient compliance. Continuous therapy with 500 mg of VACV taken daily for suppression of recurrent genital herpes is approved for persons with nine or fewer episodes/year; persons with 10 or more

episodes/year may need 1 g/day. A current study in persons who are HIV seronegative will determine if once daily use of VACV can prevent HSV transmission via decreasing HSV recurrences and decreasing asymptomatic HSV shedding.

A recent study presented at the International Congress on Infectious Diseases compared 3 days versus 5 days of VACV in 800 patients with recurrent genital herpes and showed similar results in terms of reduced time to lesion healing, duration of pain, and length of episode, and an increased proportion of patients whose outbreaks stopped after treatment began.[20] A 3-day course offers a more cost-effective method of treating recurrent genital herpes.

VACV has also been tested for recurrent genital herpes in patients who are HIV positive. In a recent double-blind controlled trial, 1062 patients infected with HIV with a history of recurrent anogenital herpes were randomized to receive VACV 500 mg twice daily, VACV 1000 mg daily, or ACV 400 mg twice daily for 1 year.[21] There was no significant difference between VACV 1000 mg daily versus ACV 400 mg twice daily; however, a significant improvement was noted with 500 mg of VACV given twice daily in terms of protection against recurrent genital herpes in patients who are HIV positive.[21]

Table 5-6	Valacyclovir Indications and Contraindications

FDA-APPROVED INDICATIONS
Herpes Simplex Infections[1,19-21]
Primary episode
Recurrent episodes
Suppressive therapy

Varicella-Zoster Infections
Herpes zoster[22,23]

Herpes Simplex or Varicella-Zoster Infections
Immunocompromised patients (such as HIV infections)

OFF-LABEL USES
Recurrent erythema multiforme (presumed/proven due to HSV)[24]
Other subsets of herpes simplex infections (see text)

CONTRAINDICATIONS
Hypersensitivity to valacyclovir or acyclovir
Hypersensitivity to any component of the formulation

PREGNANCY PRESCRIBING STATUS—CATEGORY B

Herpes Zoster.   VACV also has an FDA indication for use in herpes zoster. The usual treatment of herpes zoster with VACV requires 1000 mg three times per day for 7 days. This treatment with VACV has been shown to be as effective as ACV in its effect on the appearance of new lesions, time to crusting, and time to 50% healing.[22] VACV does have an advantage over ACV when evaluating pain associated with PHN. VACV patients had a median duration of 40 days of pain after lesion resolution compared to 60 days of pain after lesion resolution for ACV recipients.[22] In terms of zoster-related discomfort overall, it was estimated that VACV provided a 25% benefit over ACV.[22,23] The more convenient dosing schedule, as well as quicker cessation of pain, makes VACV more efficacious than ACV in treating acute herpes zoster. Current clinical trials are exploring the use of 1.5 g of ACV twice daily for acute herpes zoster in immunocompetent patients. The use of VACV for immunocompromised patients with herpes zoster has not been reported, but current trials are investigating the use of 1 g versus 2 g three times per day for 7 days for herpes zoster in this population. (See the Therapeutic Guidelines—Drugs for HHV Infections section for a summary regarding the use of VACV for HSV and VZV infections.)

Other Dermatologic Uses
Recurrent Erythema Multiforme.   There is just one brief report in the English language literature on suppressive VACV therapy for recurrent erythema multiforme due to HSV infection.[24] Given the reasonable level of success with ACV for this condition and the significantly greater bioavailability of VACV, further evaluation of this potential indication for VACV is in order.

Other Herpes Simplex Infections.   A variety of subsets of HSV can be treated with VACV in a similar fashion to the regimens outlined for oral and genital HSV infections that have FDA approval. These subsets include primary gingivostomatitis, recurrent herpes labialis, herpes gladiatorum, eczema herpeticum, herpetic whitlow, and herpetic keratoconjunctivitis. Empiric dosages can be identical to those utilized for primary infection, recurrences, and suppressive regimens outlined in the Therapeutic Guidelines—Drugs for HHV Infections section.

Adverse Effects.   The reported adverse effects of VACV include nausea and headaches (as in ACV), with incidences usually not significantly different from placebo. As with ACV, VACV is a strikingly safe drug with excellent patient tolerance.

Drug Interactions.   Given that VACV and its active form ACV are not metabolized by hepatic microsomal enzymes, there is a relative paucity of important drug interactions. A few minor interactions are detailed in Table 5-5.

Famciclovir

PHARMACOLOGY.   FCV is the oral prodrug form of penciclovir (PCV), an acyclic nucleoside (see Figure 5-1). Like ACV, PCV must be phosphorylated to PCV triphosphate to be pharmacologically active. PCV triphosphate has a much longer intracellular half-life (10 to 20 hours in HSV-infected cells and 7 hours in VZV-infected cells) compared with ACV triphosphate (less than 1 hour in either HSV- or VZV-infected cells).[1,4] Oral FCV has a 77% bioavailability compared with 15% to 30% bioavailability of oral ACV and 55% for oral VACV.[1,4,25-31] Pharmacologic key concepts of FCV can be found in Table 5-3.

CLINICAL USE.   Indications and contraindications for FCV are found in Table 5-7.

FDA-Approved Indications

Herpes Simplex Infections.   FCV is FDA-approved at a dose of 125 mg twice daily for 5 days for the treatment of recurrent genital herpes. It has been shown that FCV causes a significant reduction in pain, burning, tenderness, and tingling in patients with recurrent genital herpes.[1,32] FCV has also been recently licensed for suppression of recurrent genital herpes. A metaanalysis from multiple 2-year, multicenter, placebo-controlled trials, which compared FCV 250 mg twice daily versus placebo in male and female patients over 18 years of age with a history of recurrent genital herpes, demonstrated that FCV-treated patients had approximately 80% fewer recurrences per year compared with placebo recipients.[33] FCV was well tolerated for suppression with a safety profile similar to that seen with placebo.[33] No significant difference was seen when comparing ACV with FCV in the treatment of first-episode genital herpes in terms of decreasing viral shedding, time for complete healing, and loss of all symptoms.[1,33]

FCV has also proven to be effective for the treatment of HSV-1 and HSV-2 in immunocompromised patients. It has been approved recently by the FDA at a dose of 500 mg twice daily for 7 days for treatment of recurrent genital herpes in people who have HIV infection and is the first oral drug approved for this purpose.[20] HSV is one of the most common viral infections complicating HIV infection.[34] Up to 95% of patients who are HIV positive are seropositive for either HSV-1, HSV-2, or both.[34-41] In a recent study conducted on 12 men with HIV infection with a history of symptomatic HSV-2 infection, HIV-1 virions were consistently detected (via polymerase chain reaction) in genital ulcers caused by HSV-2.

Table 5-7	Famciclovir Indications and Contraindications

FDA-APPROVED INDICATIONS
Herpes Simplex Infections[1,32,33]
Primary episode
Recurrent episodes
Suppressive therapy
Immunocompromised patients (such as HIV infections)[20,34-43]

Varicella-Zoster Infections
Herpes zoster[27,44-46]

OFF-LABEL USES
Other subsets of herpes simplex infections (see text)
Primary varicella

CONTRAINDICATIONS
Hypersensitivity to famciclovir
Hypersensitivity to any component of the formulation

PREGNANCY PRESCRIBING STATUS—CATEGORY B

This suggests that genital herpes infection probably increases the efficiency of the sexual transmission of HIV-1.[42] A recent double-blind, placebo-controlled trial to test FCV for the suppression of symptomatic and asymptomatic HSV reactivation in persons with HIV infection was conducted on 48 patients. It was noted that the time to first HSV reactivation was delayed in the FCV group versus the placebo group.[34] FCV resulted in a marked decrease in total, symptomatic, and asymptomatic HSV shedding. Daily therapy with FCV reduced total HSV-2 shedding by 87%, and the frequency of genital signs and symptoms was reduced by 65%.[34] The percentage of days with genital lesions was reduced from 13.8% to 4.9% in the FCV-treated population. In another blinded trial conducted on 293 patients who were HIV positive with recurrent genital herpes, 500 mg of FCV taken twice daily for 7 days was equivalent in efficacy to high-dose ACV 400 mg five times daily for 7 days.[43] In another double-blind, placebo-controlled, cross-over study conducted on patients who are seropositive for HIV and HSV, 500 mg FCV taken twice daily for 8 weeks was shown to suppress HSV-2 reactivation in 83% of patients compared with 36% of placebo-treated patients. HSV-2–associated lesions were reduced from 9.7% of days in the placebo group to 1.3% of days in the FCV-treated group, and asymptomatic shedding was also reduced from 5.1% of days on placebo to only 1.2% of days in the FCV-treated group.[43]

Herpes Zoster. Famciclovir has been shown to be highly effective in the treatment of herpes zoster.[27,44] The FDA-recommended FCV dose for zoster in immunocompetent patients is 500 mg taken orally three times per day for 7 days. At this dose, FCV has been shown to decrease the time of healing of cutaneous manifestations of zoster, as well as reduce the duration of PHN.[1,45] Postherpetic neuralgia resolved twice as fast in patients who received FCV for acute herpes zoster compared with patients who received a placebo.[46] Patients at least 50 years of age are at increased risk for developing PHN with a longer duration of pain. In these patients, FCV was shown to cause resolution of pain 2.6 times faster, which resulted in a 3½-month reduction in the median duration of PHN.[46]

In immunocompromised patients, such as bone marrow and organ transplant recipients, cancer patients receiving chemotherapy and irradiation, and patients who are HIV positive, VZV infection can be particularly severe with significant morbidity and mortality. Intravenous ACV has been the mainstay of therapy for the immunocompromised patient with VZV, requiring hospitalization or home intravenous care. Oral FCV compared favorably with oral ACV in the treatment of herpes zoster in immunocompromised patients.[46] The recommended dose of FCV in immunocompromised patients is 500 mg three times daily for 10 days. This dosing regimen provides more convenient and effective dosing for immunocompromised patients with herpes zoster. There were also minimal adverse effects in the use of FCV for acute herpes zoster, including nausea, headache, and vomiting at a rate similar to that of oral ACV.[46] In an open-label study conducted on 25 patients who are HIV positive receiving 500 mg FCV three times daily for 10 days, times to full crusting and healing compared favorably with historical data reported for ACV therapy of immunocompromised patients with herpes zoster.[43] See Tables 5-8 and 5-9 regarding the use of FCV for HSV and VZV infections.

Other Dermatologic Uses
Other Herpesvirus Infections. A variety of subsets of HSV can be treated with FCV in a similar fashion to the regimens outlined for oral and genital herpes simplex infections that have FDA approval. These subsets include primary gingivostomatitis, recurrent herpes labialis, herpes gladiatorum, eczema herpeticum, herpetic whitlow, and herpetic keratoconjunctivitis. Empiric dosages can be identical to those used for primary infections, recurrences, and suppressive regimens outlined in the Therapeutic Guidelines—Drugs for HHV Infections section later. FCV may also be utilized for primary varicella infections, although this indication needs further clinical evaluation.

Adverse Effects. FCV, like ACV, can rarely cause such adverse effects as headache, nausea, or diarrhea. FCV shares with ACV and VACV an excellent safety profile and patient tolerance.

Drug Interactions. Given that FCV and its active form PCV are not metabolized by hepatic microsomal enzymes, there is a relative paucity of important drug interactions. A few minor interactions are detailed in Table 5-5.

Therapeutic Guidelines—Drugs for HHV Infections

In general, ACV, VACV, and FCV are equivalent in their safety and efficacy. The primary exception to this rule is the finding that VACV was somewhat more effective in reducing the duration of zoster-associated pain than was ACV. If cost and availability are not major factors, either VACV or FCV is generally preferred over ACV due to greater dosing frequency required with ACV (secondary to the drug's relatively low bioavailability). Although there are no published studies to document the assumption, VACV and FCV are considered equivalent for therapy of HSV or VZV infections (despite pharmacologic differences). Table 5-8 outlines clinical regimens for the immunocompetent patient with an HHV infection. Table 5-9 outlines the clinical

■ **Table 5-8**　Clinical Regimens for Human Herpes Virus Infections
　　　　　　　　in *Immunocompetent* Patients

Clinical Scenario	Acyclovir	Valacyclovir	Famciclovir
Herpes simplex—primary	200 mg 5 × day for 10 days	1000 mg bid for 10 days	250 mg tid for 10 days
Herpes simplex—recurrences	400 mg tid for 5 days	500 mg bid for 5 days	125 mg bid for 5 days
Herpes simplex—suppression	400 mg bid	500 mg qd*	250 mg bid
Herpes zoster—acute treatment	800 mg 5 × day for 7-10 days	1000 mg tid for 7-10 days	500 mg tid for 7 days
Primary varicella—children	20 mg/kg qid up to 800 mg/dose for 5-7 days	Not well evaluated yet	Not well evaluated yet

Note: All oral regimens.
*Recommend VACV 1000 mg daily suppressive dose (single dose) if 10 or more HSV recurrences each year.

■ **Table 5-9**　Clinical Regimens for Human Herpes Virus Infections
　　　　　　　　in *Immunocompromised* Patients

Clinical Scenario	Acyclovir	Valacyclovir	Famciclovir
Herpes simplex—primary	200-400 mg 5 × day for 10 days *or* 5 mg/kg IV q8h for 7-10 days	Studies in progress	No studies reported
Herpes simplex—recurrences	No studies reported	Studies in progress	500 mg bid for 7 days
Herpes simplex—suppression	At least 400 mg bid	Studies in progress	500 mg bid
Herpes zoster—acute treatment	10 mg/kg IV q8h for 7-10 days	Studies in progress	500 mg tid for 10 days
Primary varicella—children	10 mg/kg IV q8h for 7-10 days	Studies in progress	No studies reported

Note: All oral regimens unless otherwise noted.

regimens for the immunocompromised patient with an HHV infection. Both tables include various clinical scenarios of HSV, herpes zoster, and primary varicella.

Any one of these drugs can be used to suppress recurrent genital herpes or herpes labialis, although few data are available for the latter entity. Reasons to offer suppression versus episodic therapy include (1) frequency of outbreaks (e.g., six or greater per year), (2) severity of outbreaks (physical and/or emotional), (3) lack of a sufficient prodrome (such that episodic therapy would have little benefit, and (4) having a sexual partner who is seronegative via western blotting for HSV (particularly HSV-2), thus reducing outbreaks and asymptomatic viral shedding with the possibility of reducing transmission.

Immunocompromised patients include those with HIV, patients with organ transplants, persons taking systemic immunosuppressive drugs, and patients with internal malignances. A spectrum in the degree of immunosuppression, from mild to severe, exists within each of these conditions. Oral preparations of these three drugs have been used to treat HSV and VZV infections, as well as suppress HSV infections in immunocompromised persons, but relatively few data exist on the individual drugs. Even less information is available comparing the relative safety and efficacy of these agents in immunocompromised persons.

Therefore there is little basis to recommend one oral drug over another, except for the greater convenience of VACV and FCV (relative to ACV) and the greater volume of published studies on FCV in immunocompromised patients. Reasons for recommending intravenous ACV over the oral drugs include the following: (1) severe immunosuppression, (2) inability to swallow oral medication, (3) impaired memory and/or mental capacity, and (4) long distance or lack of transportation to medical care in case of complications with oral therapy.

Investigational Drugs

Sorivudine, a thymidine analog, is an investigational antiviral drug with extremely potent (2000 to 5000 times as potent as ACV) in vitro activity against VZV.[47] Sorivudine, like ACV, must be monophosphorylated by a virally encoded thymidine kinase; however, unlike ACV, diphosphorylation is also dependent on viral enzymes.[47] The triphosphate form blocks viral DNA replication by inhibiting DNA polymerase activity, but it does not become incorporated into elongating viral DNA.[47-49] In a randomized placebo-controlled study comparing sorivudine versus ACV for treatment of dermatomal herpes zoster in patients with HIV infection, patients were given 40 mg daily of sorivudine versus 800 mg five times daily of ACV.[50,51] At this dose, sorivudine was found to be superior to ACV in terms of cessation of new lesion formation, less time to complete crusting, reduced duration of positive viral cultures, and decreased incidence of recurrent disease.[50,51] One of the metabolites of sorivudine is bromovinyluracil (BVU), a potent metabolite of dihydropyrimidine dehydrogenase (DPD).[47] DPD is involved in the metabolism of 5-fluorouracil (5-FU), a cancer chemotherapeutic agent.[47,52] The concomitant use of BVU with 5-FU results in sustained activity of 5-FU due to inhibition of DPD, leading to severe bone marrow suppression.[47] Due to this significant drug reaction, sorivudine is not FDA-approved for treatment of herpes zoster.

Netivudine (882C87, 1-(beta-D-arabinofuranosyl)-5-propynyluracil) is a potent agent with selective inhibitory activity against VZV.[53,54] This drug shares several characteristics with sorivudine including structure, the specific mode of activation to the triphosphate form, the propensity for a drug interaction with 5-FU, and a high degree of protein binding.[53] In vitro studies showed that this drug is 10 times more potent against VZV than is ACV.[53,55] However, like sorivudine, further development of netivudine has been terminated after the results of carcinogenicity studies in animals.[53]

Lobucavir (LBV) is a guanine nucleoside analog synthesized from 2'-deoxy-guanosine, with replacement of the sugar by a cyclobutyl ring. In tissue culture models, it has been shown to have a broad spectrum of antiviral activity against DNA and RNA viruses. In a recent study, 1917 patients were enrolled to receive 100 mg twice daily or 200 mg daily or 200 mg twice daily of LBV versus placebo to treat recurrent genital herpes. All doses of LBV shortened the median time to healing by 0.5 day and the median time to resolution by up to 1 day.[56] Subset analysis showed a decrease in time to healing by 1.43 days in subjects self initiating treatment and up to 1.37 days in subjects with classic lesions.[56] The adverse events that were noted with LBV were comparable with the ones noted with placebo and were minimal. LBV development, however, has been discontinued secondary to the results of carcinogenicity studies in animals.

Vaccines for HHV Infections

The first available vaccine for prevention of herpesvirus infection is a live attenuated vaccine given for the prophylaxis of primary varicella. About 4 million Americans are infected annually with chickenpox, resulting in over 100 deaths and more than 9000 hospitalizations, which leads to an annual cost of hundreds of million dollars in medical bills and lost productivity.[4] Varicella is the leading cause of vaccine-preventable death in children in the United States. Studies have shown that the varicella vaccine is 70% to 90% effective in completely preventing varicella and results in milder disease in the remaining recipients.[4] This vaccine may be administered along with the measles-mumps-rubella (MMR) vaccine at approximately 1 year of age. For children under the age of 12 who have not yet had chickenpox, a single dose of this vaccine is advised. For ages 13 and older, two injections 4 to 8 weeks apart are suggested. Herpes zoster appears less commonly in persons given the vaccine to prevent primary VZV, but it is not clear if the vaccine can prevent herpes zoster if given after natural chickenpox. Studies are currently being conducted to answer that question.

There are also ongoing investigations with vaccines for the prophylaxis of HSV infections in persons who are seronegative for HSV. The first documentation of the use of a herpes simplex vaccine for treatment of HSV was published in 1994[4,57]; patients with recurrent genital herpes received a recombinant glycoprotein D (gD2) vaccine of HSV-2. These patients experienced a one-third reduction in recurrences compared with placebo recipients during the subsequent year.[4] Since then, multiple large phase III trials using recombinant vaccines containing glycoprotein B (gB2) and/or gD2 have been conducted for patients who are at risk of acquiring genital herpes but who are seronegative for HSV-2 (and for HSV-1 in some studies). Some of these studies are still ongoing and results are therefore pending.

The development of a disabled infectious single cycle (DISC) HSV-2 vaccine candidate (designated DISC HSV) for the prophylaxis and therapy of genital herpes is currently under investigation. The DISC HSV vaccine mimics HSV-2 with the deletion of the gene encoding glycoprotein H (gH), an essential gene for cell infection by HSV.[58] After inoculation, DISC HSV undergoes one cycle of replication resulting in noninfectious progeny. DISC HSV has the immunogenicity of a live virus vaccine, while maintaining the safety of an inactivated one. The first human trial of DISC HSV has been completed. In this phase I trial the safety of three doses of DISC HSV (2×10^3, 3×10^4, and 3×10^5 pfu/dose) was compared with placebo. Six subjects with different sero-status (HSV-1 positive and HSV-2 negative or both HSV-1 and HSV-2 negative) were randomized to each group, who received their first two immunizations 8 weeks apart. The vaccine was safe and well tolerated at all doses. This vaccine induced a lymphoproliferative response and in vitro in-

terferon gamma production in a dose-related manner in HSV-seronegative subjects. Subjects immunized with 3×10^5 pfu/dose had a lymphoproliferative response that was maintained 6 months after immunization. Neither cell-mediated nor humoral responses increased significantly in HSV-seropositive subjects.[58] Higher doses of this vaccine are currently being studied with the hope of effectively preventing the transmission of HSV.

DRUGS FOR HUMAN IMMUNODEFICIENCY VIRUS INFECTIONS

Cutaneous manifestations of HIV often lead to its diagnosis. Most commonly, the clinical manifestations of the disease include a papulosquamous exanthem that is similar to a variety of other viral diseases.[1] Early in the disease process the exanthem lasts about 2 weeks and then spontaneously regresses. However, as the disease progresses to AIDS, 90% of patients develop mucocutaneous manifestations secondary to infections, neoplasms, or other causes.[1,59,60] Herpesviruses, poxviruses, and papillomaviruses are the most common opportunistic viral infections that lead to cutaneous manifestations in individuals who are HIV positive.[1]

The search for a cure for this deadly virus has lead to extensive study of different modalities of therapy. Currently, there are 14 FDA-approved antiretroviral drugs falling into three categories: nucleoside analogs (zidovudine, lamivudine, didanosine, zalcitabine, stavudine, abacavir), nonnucleoside analogs (nevirapine, delavirdine, efavirenz), and protease inhibitors (saquinavir, indinavir, ritonavir, nelfinavir, amprenavir) (Table 5-10).

Nucleoside Analogs

ZIDOVUDINE. Nucleoside analogs exert their effect by incorporating into the DNA and interfering with HIV reverse transcriptase, thus inhibiting replication of HIV RNA. Zidovudine (azidothymidine [AZT]) was the first FDA-approved drug for therapy of HIV infections. Zidovudine must be phosphorylated to zidovudine triphosphate, the active form that inhibits HIV reverse transcriptase (RT), thus

Table 5-10 FDA-Approved Antiretroviral Agents for HIV Infections

Generic Name	Trade Name	Adult Daily Dosing
NUCLEOSIDE ANALOGS		
Zidovudine	Retrovir	200 mg tid (capsules) 300 mg bid (tablets)
Didanosine	Videx	200 mg bid
Zalcitabine	Hivid	0.75 mg bid
Stavudine	Zerit	40 mg bid
Lamivudine	Epivir	150 mg bid
Lamivudine/ Zidovudine	Combivir	150/300 mg bid
Abacavir	Ziagen	300 mg bid
NONNUCLEOSIDE REVERSE TRANSCRIPTASE INHIBITORS		
Nelvirapine	Viramune	200 mg bid
Delavirdine	Rescriptor	400 mg tid
Efavirenz	Sustiva	600 mg qhs
HIV-1 PROTEASE INHIBITORS		
Saquinavir (hard gel)	Invirase	600 mg tid
Saquinavir (soft gel)	Fortovase	1200 mg tid
Ritonavir	Norvir	600 mg bid
Indinavir	Crixivan	800 mg q8h
Nelfinavir	Viracept	750 mg tid
Amprenavir	Agenerase	1200 mg bid

blocking the infectivity and cytopathic effects of HIV at concentrations that do not interfere with normal T cell functions.[1,61] Initially, AZT was the most commonly prescribed drug for HIV.[1,62] This drug is no longer used as monotherapy due to minor effects on increasing survival and reduction in frequency and severity of opportunistic infections.[1,63] There are also reports of resistance to AZT in some individuals. The adverse effect profile of AZT includes headache, insomnia, nausea, gastrointestinal pain, anorexia, diarrhea, myalgia, and rash. The most serious adverse effect is bone marrow suppression causing anemia and granulocytopenia.[1]

Zidovudine gained approval in 1996 for treatment of HIV infections in pregnant females during their third trimester to reduce the risk of perinatal transmission.[1] This drug has been shown to reduce the transmission of HIV from a mother infected with HIV to her newborn by 66% when administered during the antepartum and intrapartum periods and to the newborn during the first 6 weeks of life.[50,64] It is usually given orally between weeks 14 and 34 of gestation, and then the intravenous route is employed during labor.[1]

DIDANOSINE. The second FDA-approved nucleoside analog was didanosine (ddI, ideoxyinosine), a pyrimidine nucleoside analog. To inhibit the function of reverse transcriptase, ddI needs to be phosphorylated to its active form, dideoxyadenosine triphosphate (ddATP). This drug is used in patients who are not able to tolerate or who are resistant to AZT. It is common for patients with HIV infections that are resistant to AZT to also be resistant to ddI. Didanosine has been shown to cause a decrease in serum p24 antigen and an increase in the CD4 count. However, after 1 year of use, studies show ddI to be less effective than AZT in increasing CD4 levels or on disease progression, as well as mortality rates.[1,63] Pancreatitis is the major toxicity seen with ddI. Other less common adverse events include oral and esophageal ulcers, cardiomyopathy, peripheral neuropathy, rash, fever, and malaise.

AZT and ddI are absorbed more readily in a basic environment; hence they should be taken on an empty stomach to avoid a highly acidic postprandial environment. The concomitant use of certain antifungals (ketoconazole and itraconazole) and the quinolone antibiotics with ddI is contraindicated because these latter drugs require an acidic environment for absorption.

ZALCITABINE. The third drug to be FDA-approved for treatment of HIV was zalcitabine (ddC, dideoxycytidine). Zalcitabine is a pyrimidine nucleoside analog that is primarily used for patients with advanced HIV disease who are intolerant of or have disease progression while on alternate therapeutic regimens.[1] This medication needs to be converted to dideoxycitadine 5'-triphosphate to inhibit viral replication. Zalcitabine has minimal benefits when used alone; however, its greatest effects are seen when used in combination with AZT. The adverse effect profile of ddC includes oral and esophageal ulcers, pancreatitis, hepatic toxicity, and peripheral neuropathy.[1]

STAVUDINE.   Stavudine (d4T) is the fourth FDA-approved nucleoside analog. This drug is used for patients who are intolerant of the other nucleoside analogs or who have significant clinical or immunologic deterioration while taking other antiretroviral drugs.[1] In a randomized double-blind trial conducted for 12 weeks comparing AZT with d4T, there was an increase in the CD4 cell count with d4T, while AZT was associated with a decrease in the CD4 count.[1,66] Peripheral neuropathy is the major clinical toxicity, seen in 20% of patients who use d4T.[1]

LAMIVUDINE.   The fifth nucleoside reverse transcriptase inhibitor approved by the FDA was lamivudine (3TC, 3' thiacytidine). Initial results of a phase I/II single-dose pharmacokinetic study indicated that lamivudine treatment sustained the reduction of virologic markers of infection despite the development of a high level of drug resistance.[1,67] The major limitation to the use of 3TC as monotherapy is the rapid development of resistance within 4 weeks of initiating therapy.[1,68] The adverse effects profile of 3TC includes insomnia, headache, diarrhea, abdominal pain, pruritus, peripheral neuropathy, and pancreatitis.[1] High doses of lamivudine (over 20 mg/kg/day) can cause significant neutropenia.

Reports of combination therapy of lamivudine with zidovudine have shown long-lasting positive effects on surrogate markers like CD4 cell count and viral load.[1,69] As a result of commonly combining zidovudine with lamivudine, a new drug combining these two medications, has recently been FDA-approved (see Table 5-10).

ABACAVIR.   Abacavir is a second-generation nucleoside reverse transcriptase inhibitor recently given accelerated FDA approval for use in multidrug treatment of HIV infection.[70,71] It is a synthetic carboxycyclic nucleoside with a 6-cyclopropylamino modification. Abacavir is the most powerful nucleoside analog and one of the most powerful antiretroviral drugs currently available. Its use results in reduction in viral loads and increases in CD4 counts that are unparalleled by any other nucleoside analog and are similar to most potent protease inhibitors. Resistance to zidovudine and lamivudine gives cross-resistance to abacavir. In patients who have previously been heavily treated with other nucleoside analogs, the addition of abacavir would be ineffective.

Adverse effects seen with abacavir include fatigue, nausea, vomiting, headache, diarrhea, loss of appetite, malaise, fever, and rash. Approximately 5% of treated patients experience a hypersensitivity reaction with a rash in addition to fever, nausea/vomiting, malaise, or body aches.[70,72] The rash typically is morbilliform or urticarial, but the clinical presentation may vary. The hypersensitivity reaction usually resolves with cessation of the drug; however, a rechallenge of abacavir after this hypersensitivity reaction resolves can be life-threatening.

INVESTIGATIONAL DRUGS.   Phase III clinical trials to test the efficacy of Bis-pom PMEA (adefovir dipivoxil, a nucleotide analog inhibitor of reverse transcriptase) are currently under way for treatment of individuals with HIV infections. Studies are also ongoing with integrase inhibitors as well as fusion inhibitors.

Nonnucleoside Analogs

NEVIRAPINE.   Nonnucleoside reverse transcriptase inhibitors (NNRTI) work at the same stage of replication as the nucleoside reverse transcriptase inhibitors; however, this family of drugs utilizes a different mechanism of action. Nevirapine was the first FDA-approved NNRTI for HIV. This drug exerts its action by binding directly onto the reverse transcriptase enzyme, altering its structure and inhibiting its function. Nevirapine has higher potency and lower toxicity than AZT; however, the rapid development of resistance (as quickly as 1 week) has limited its use to combination therapy.[1,73] Nevirapine is used in combination with nucleoside analogs in patients who have clinical and/or immunologic deterioration while on an initial therapeutic regimen.[1] Due to the high rate of resistance, this medication should be discontinued if no benefit is seen shortly after its addition. The adverse effect profile of nevirapine includes rash, diarrhea, and drug fever.

DELAVIRDINE. Delavirdine was the second NNRTI to be FDA-approved for use in combination therapy to treat HIV. The efficacy profile of this medication in combination therapy is currently under investigation.

EFAVIRENZ. Efavirenz is the most recent FDA-approved NNRTI.[74] It is a potent drug that is well tolerated and can be given once daily. Like all NNRTIs, resistant viruses emerge rapidly when efavirenz is used as monotherapy. Thus it cannot be used as a single agent to treat HIV or added on as a sole agent to a failing regimen. It must be administered with a protease inhibitor and/or a nucleoside reverse transcriptase inhibitor. In clinical trials, 52% of patients receiving efavirenz reported central nervous system or psychiatric symptoms. Most of these adverse effects were mild in severity.

INVESTIGATIONAL DRUGS. New NNRTIs that are currently undergoing clinical efficacy and safety trials include loviride, MKC-442, and DMP-266.

HIV-1 Protease Inhibitors

HIV-1 protease inhibitors (PI) have offered a new dimension to the treatment of HIV. These drugs block the protease enzyme involved in the final processing of viral proteins, resulting in decreased assembly of new progeny viruses from newly infected and chronically infected cells. This offers a greater advantage over the RT inhibitors, which only inhibit replication in newly infected cells.[1,75] Five currently approved PIs are used in combination with RT inhibitors or NNRTIs. This combination can produce at least a 2-log decrease in viral load in most patients, but RT inhibitors used in monotherapy usually only produce a 0.5 log decrease.

SAQUINAVIR. Saquinavir was the first PI to be FDA-approved for patients with HIV. Saquinavir has an oral bioavailability of only 4% due to first pass hepatic metabolism.[1,75] Taking this medication 2 hours after eating does increase the bioavailability but not to a significant extent. A soft gel formulation of saquinavir with increased bioavailability has been formulated and was recently FDA-approved for treatment in patients with HIV infection. The soft gel formulation taken with two nucleoside analogs showed a significantly greater viral load reduction than saquinavir taken with two nucleoside analogs.[50] The adverse effect profile of the new soft gel formulation when used in combination therapy with other antiviral agents includes diarrhea, nausea, abdominal discomfort, and dyspepsia. Current studies are investigating the possible use of the gel formulation in the pediatric population.

RITONAVIR. The second FDA-approved PI for the treatment of HIV was ritonavir. This drug has excellent oral bioavailability. It has a unique mechanism of action in that it reduces metabolism of other drugs, leading to higher serum levels of other protease inhibitors as well as other agents.[1] Studies on HIV-negative volunteers have shown a fiftyfold to 100-fold increase in the plasma saquinavir level when combined with ritonavir; the safety of this combination is still being investigated.[1,75,76] Due to the unique metabolic effects of ritonavir, caution should be taken with concomitant use of drugs like rifabutin and the hepatically metabolized benzodiazepines because of increased levels of these agents.[1,75] Concomitant use of ritonavir with terfenadine, astemizole, and cisapride may lead to fatal dysrhythmias due to decreased metabolism of these agents. The cytochrome 3A4 inhibition potential of ritonavir is central to the potentially serious interactions due to markedly increased drug levels of 3A4 targets (substrates) such as terfenadine, astemizole, and cisapride. A similar mechanism explains the drug interactions of nelfinavir as well.

The adverse effect profile of ritonavir is varied. The most common adverse effects include gastrointestinal disturbances such as nausea, vomiting, and diarrhea. Taking ritonavir with a large meal can reduce the severity of these symptoms. Less common adverse effects include altered taste sensation and circumoral and peripheral paresthesias.[1,75] After initiation of ritonavir therapy, toxicity may occur due to high plasma trough levels leading to fatigue. Reversible elevation in hepatic aminotransferase and serum triglyceride levels without clinical consequences may occur in patients taking ritonavir. It is recommended that ritonavir be initiated at a less than maximal dose and then be increased gradually to the maximum dose to prevent the occurrence of resistance.[1,75] Once resistance develops, cross-resistance to other protease inhibitors can occur, rendering them ineffective in treating patients with HIV.

INDINAVIR. The third PI approved by the FDA for treatment in patients with HIV was indinavir. This PI can significantly reduce the amount of viremia in HIV-infected patients. Combination of indinavir with AZT and 3TC has been shown to reduce the viral load to an undetectable level after 16 weeks of therapy in approximately 90% of patients.[50,77] Indinavir is well absorbed orally when taken on an empty stomach. Absorption is drastically impaired when it is coadministered with high amounts of protein or fatty foods.[1,75]

The adverse effect profile of indinavir includes reversible elevation in bilirubin levels and the potential to cause nephrolithiasis due to crystallization of indinavir into the urine.[1,75] Other reported adverse effects include insomnia, dry skin, a mild rash, and pharyngitis in addition to abnormal fat deposits known as a "buffalo hump" and "protease pouch."[1,75] These latter conditions also have been reported with other protease inhibitors. As with ritonavir, resistance with indinavir causes cross-resistance with the other protease inhibitors.

NELFINAVIR. Nelfinavir was the fourth FDA-approved PI for treatment in patients with HIV. This drug has excellent bioavailability, especially when administered with food.[1] The most common toxic adverse effect that has been reported with nelfinavir includes a mild-to-moderate diarrhea that occurs in about 20% of patients.[1,78] This problem can be controlled with over the counter antimotility agents. Other adverse effects that have been reported include asthenia, decreased concentration, and moderate hypertension.[1,79,80]

Concomitant administration of nelfinavir with terfenadine, astemizole, or cisapride can cause life-threatening dysrhythmias.[50] Nelfinavir,

in combination with either triazolam or midazolam, may cause prolonged sedation. As with indinavir and ritonavir, nelfinavir results in potent and durable suppression of viral replication when used in combination with two nucleoside analogs in minimally pretreated patients.[50,81]

AMPRENAVIR. Amprenavir is the newest protease inhibitor to receive FDA approval and is indicated for use in combination regimens with other antiretroviral agents.[82] Interestingly, amprenavir has been shown to lower virus levels in semen as well as in plasma. Amprenavir has a long half-life that permits twice-daily dosing. The chief adverse effects of amprenavir are usually mild to moderate in intensity, and include perioral paresthesias, diarrhea, nausea, vomiting, and headache. A morbilliform rash develops in 28% of patients, with or without pruritus. Severe skin reactions, such as Stevens-Johnson syndrome, occur in 1% of treated patients.[82] Like other protease inhibitors, amprenavir has been associated with diabetes mellitus, hyperglycemia, and acute hemolytic anemia.

Investigational Drugs
A new PI, 141W94, is currently in phase III clinical trials. A potent PI, ABT378, is also currently undergoing clinical evaluation. There are novel PIs with unique mechanisms of action that are currently in the preclinical stages of development.[50,83]

Therapeutic Guidelines—Drugs for HIV Infections
Monotherapy is no longer considered the mainstay of treatment for HIV infection.[1,84,85] The International AIDS Society-USA panel continues to recommend antiretroviral therapy for any patient with established HIV infection and a confirmed plasma HIV-1 RNA level greater than 5000 to 10,000 copies/mL.[86] For asymptomatic patients with low plasma HIV RNA levels (<5000 to 10,000 copies/mL) and high CD4 cell count (>350 to 500/uL), treatment may be deferred with close follow-up to avoid the risk of adverse effects and consequences of recurrence.[86] For patients with low HIV RNA levels (<5000 to 10,000 copies/mL) and low CD4 cell count (<500 and particularly <350/uL), initiation of therapy is recommended.[86,89] Current recommendations in-

clude the combined use of two nucleoside RT inhibitors and one PI. There are no specific guidelines on which PI to use, and several different combinations of RT inhibitors have been tried.[86] Ritonavir, indinavir, and nelfinavir are all equally effective when administered in combination with RT inhibitors.[1,75] Possible RT inhibitor combinations include zidovudine plus didanosine, zalcitabine, lamivudine, or didanosine plus stavudine.[1,75] Drug failure is usually due to resistance, especially in patients on monotherapy, or to noncompliance with complicated multidrug regimens. Patients on chronic therapy with RT inhibitors should be switched to new ones if no clinical benefit is seen to avoid resistance. As with RT inhibitors, PI also should be switched if no clinical benefit is seen with their use. If resistance to indinavir or ritonavir develops, then salvage therapy with PI-containing regimens is difficult due to cross-resistance; however, if resistance to saquinavir or nelfinavir emerges, then preliminary data have shown that salvage therapy may be possible, but further studies are needed to confirm this.

Summary

Although great progress has been made in the study and treatment of HIV, a great deal of work still remains to find a cure. New protease inhibitors, nucleoside reverse transcriptase inhibitors, and nucleoside and nonnucleoside reverse transcriptase inhibitors continue to be tested daily in multicenter trials.[1,90] Agents with different mechanisms of action are also being developed for future use. These agents under development include drugs that focus on various targets such as virion-cell-membrane fusion, HIV-1 integrase, nucleocapsid formation, and HIV-chemokine-receptor interactions. The most effective method of reducing transmission is through education on safe sex and abstinence, testing of blood products, the use of sterile needles, and proper handling of body fluids potentially containing HIV.

HIV Vaccine Development

The greatest hope for the future of HIV control is to minimize transmission by using a prophylactic vaccine. Different types of vaccines are currently being investigated including subunit vaccines, recombinant vector vaccines, vaccine combinations (recombinant vector vaccine followed by subunit vaccine booster), peptide vaccines, virus-like particle vaccines, antiidiotype vaccines, whole-inactivated virus vaccines, and a live-attenuated virus vaccine.[50,91] Clinical trials with a new prophylactic candidate vaccine made from a protein called gp120, which is part of the HIV outer coat, have begun. The clinical potential of a vaccine to prevent infection with a rapidly mutating virus has been questioned, but the vaccine currently under study is derived from the constant (i.e., nonmutating) region of the gp120 molecule. This new "bivalent" vaccine has a new, additional molecular component that may contribute to a broader range of protection against subtypes of HIV found in North America, Europe, Australia, Central America, and South America.[92] A different molecular component has been added to this vaccine to target antigens of HIV subtypes found among injection drug users in Thailand and other Asian countries.[92] In tests conducted on 1200 volunteers beginning in early 1992, this vaccine elicited neutralizing antibodies against HIV in more than 99% of the vaccinated participants.[92] New trials with this vaccine are intended to determine the effectiveness in protecting people with high-risk behavior such as risky sexual practices or needle sharing in injection drug users.

Bibliography

Erlich KS: Management of herpes simplex and varicella-zoster virus infections. *West J Med* 166:211-215, 1997.

Evans T, Tyring SK: Advances in antiviral therapy in dermatology. *Dermatol Clin* 16:409-420, 1998.

Perry CM, Faulds D: Valaciclovir: a review of its antiviral activity, pharmacokinetic properties and therapeutic efficacy in herpesvirus infections. *Drugs* 52:754-772, 1996.

Severson JL, Tyring SK: Viral disease update. *Curr Probl Dermatol* 11:37-72, 1999.

Trizna Z, Tyring SK: Antiviral treatment of diseases in pediatric dermatology. *Dermatol Clin* 16:539-552, 1998.

References

Antiviral Agents for Human Herpes Virus Infections

1. Evans TY, Tyring SK: Advances in antiviral therapy in dermatology. *Dermatol Ther* 16:409-420, 1998.
2. Whitley RJ: The biology of B viruses (cercopithecine virus). In Roizman B, Whitley RJ, Lopez C, editors: *The human herpesviruses*, New York, 1993, Raven Press, p 317.

Acyclovir

3. Wagstaff AJ, Faulds D, Goak L: Acyclovir, a reappraisal of its antiviral activity, pharmacokinetic properties and therapeutic efficacy. *Drugs* 47:153-205, 1994.
4. Herne K, Cirelli R, Lee P, et al: Advances in antiviral therapy. *Curr Opin Dermatol* 3:195-201, 1996.
5. Wald A, Zeh J, Barnum G, et al: Suppression of subclinical shedding of herpes simplex virus type 2 with acyclovir. *Ann Intern Med* 124:8-15, 1996.
6. Goldberg LH, Kaufman R, Kurtz TO, et al: The acyclovir study group. Long-term suppression of recurrent genital herpes with acyclovir: a 5-year benchmark. *Arch Dermatol* 129:582-587, 1993.
7. Spruance SL: Prophylactic chemotherapy with acyclovir for recurrent herpes simplex labialis. *J Med Virol* 1(Suppl):27-32, 1993.
8. Thandi A, Tyring SK: Newer aspects of herpesvirus infections. In Dahl MV, editor: *Current opinions in dermatology*, Philadelphia, 1997, Rapid Science Publishers, p 42-50.
9. Huff JC, Drucker JL, Clemmer A, et al: Effects of oral acyclovir on pain resolution in herpes zoster. A reanalysis. *J Med Virol* 1(Suppl):93-96, 1993.
10. Ioannidis JPA, Collier AC, Cooper DA, et al: Clinical efficacy of high-dose acyclovir in patients with human immunodeficiency virus infection: a meta-analysis of randomized individual patient data. *J Infect Dis* 178:349-359, 1998.
11. Golden MP, Kim S, Hammer SM, et al: Activation of human immunodeficiency virus by herpes simplex virus. *J Infect Dis* 166:494-499, 1992.
12. Griffiths PD: Studies to define viral cofactors for human immunodeficiency virus. *Infect Agents Dis* 1:237-244, 1992.
13. Heng MC, Heng SY, Allen SG: Co-infection and synergy of human immunodeficiency virus-1 and herpes simplex virus-1. *Lancet* 343:255-258, 1994.
14. Mole L, Ripich S, Margolis D, et al: The impact of active herpes simplex virus infection on human immunodeficiency virus load. *J Infect Dis* 176:766-770, 1997.
15. Weston WL, Morelli JG: Herpes simplex virus-associated erythema multiforme in prepubertal children. *Arch Pediatr Adoles Med* 151:1014-1016, 1997.
16. Lemak MA, Duvic M, Bean SF: Oral acyclovir for the prevention of herpes-associated erythema multiforme. *J Am Acad Dermatol* 15:50-54, 1986.
17. Schofield JK, Tatnall FM, Leigh IM: Recurrent erythema multiforme: clinical features and treatment in a large series of patients. *Br J Dermatol* 128:542-545, 1993.
18. Tatnall FM, Schofield JK, Leigh IM: A double-blind, placebo-controlled trial of continuous acyclovir therapy in recurrent erythema multiforme. *Br J Dermatol* 132:267-270, 1995.

Valacyclovir

19. Fife KH, Barbarash RA, Rudolph T, et al: Valaciclovir versus acyclovir in the treatment of first-episode genital herpes infection: results of an international, multicenter, double-blind, randomized clinical trial. *Sex Trans Dis* 24:481-486, 1997.
20. Leone PA, Trottier S, Miller JM, and the International Valaciclovir Study Group: A comparison of oral valaciclovir 500 mg twice daily for three or five days in the treatment of recurrent genital herpes. ICID, 15-18 May 1998, Boston, USA.
21. Lawrence AG, Bell AR, International Valaciclovir HSV Study Group: Valaciclovir for prevention of recurrent herpes simplex virus infection in HIV-infected individuals–a double-blind controlled trial. 8th ECCMID, 1997.

22. Herne K, Cirelli R, Lee P, et al: Antiviral therapy of acute herpes zoster in older patients. *Drugs Aging* 8:97-112, 1996.
23. Beutner K: Antivirals in the treatment of pain. *J Geriatr Dermatol* 2:23A-28A, 1994.
24. Kerob D, Assier-Bonnet H, Esnault-Gelly P, et al: Recurrent erythema multiforme unresponsive to acyclovir prophylaxis and responsive to valacyclovir continuous therapy (letter). *Arch Dermatol* 134:876-877, 1998.

Famciclovir

25. Tyring SK: Advances in the treatment of herpesvirus infections: the role of famciclovir. *Clin Ther* 20:661-670, 1998.
26. Pratt SK, Fairless AJ, Pue MA, et al: The absolute bioavailability of the antiviral compound, penciclovir, following a single oral administration of 500 mg famciclovir. Presented at the 3rd Congress of the European Academy of Dermatology and Venereology, Copenhagen, Denmark, 1993 (poster).
27. Pue MA, Benet LZ: Pharmacokinetics of famciclovir in man. *Antiviral Chem Chemother* 4:47-55, 1993.
28. Valtrex. *Physicians' desk reference* ed 51, Montvale, NJ, 1997, Medical Economics Data, pp 1167-1169.
29. Weller S, Blum MR, Doucette M, et al: Pharmacokinetics of the acyclovir pro-drug valaciclovir after escalating single and multiple-dose administration to normal volunteers. *Clin Pharmacol Ther* 54:595-605, 1993.
30. Pue MA, Pratt SK, Fairless AJ, et al: Linear pharmacokinetics of penciclovir following administration of single oral doses of famciclovir 125, 250, 500 and 750 mg to healthy volunteers. *J Antimicrob Chemother* 33:119-127, 1994.
31. Miranda P, Blum MR: Pharmacokinetics of acyclovir after intravenous and oral administration. *J Antimicrob Chemother* 12(Suppl B):29-37, 1983.
32. Sacks SL, Aoki F, Diaz-Mitoma F, et al: Patient-initiated, twice daily oral famciclovir for early recurrent genital herpes. *JAMA* 276:44-49, 1996.
33. Loveless M, Harris W, Sacks S: Treatment of first episode genital herpes with famciclovir (abstract H12). American Society for Microbiology, 35th ICAAC meeting. San Francisco, California, September, 1995.

34. Schacker T, Hu H, Koelle DM, et al: Famciclovir for the suppression of symptomatic and asymptomatic herpes simplex virus reactivation in HIV-infected persons: a double-blind, placebo-controlled trial. *Ann Intern Med* 128:21-28, 1998.
35. Enzensberger R, Braun W, July C, et al: Prevalence of antibodies to human herpesviruses and hepatitis B virus in patients at different stages of human immunodeficiency virus (HIV) infection. *Infection* 3:140-145, 1991.
36. Mann SL, Meyers JD, Holmes KL, et al: Prevalence and incidence of herpesvirus infections among homosexually active men. *J Infect Dis* 149:1026-1027, 1984.
37. Siegel D, Golden E, Washington AE, et al: Prevalence and correlates of herpes simplex infections. The population-based AIDS in Multiethnic Neighborhoods Study. *JAMA* 268:1702-1708, 1992.
38. Quinn TC, Piot P, McCormick JB, et al: Serologic and immunologic studies in patients with AIDS in North America and Africa. The potential role of infectious agents as cofactors in human immunodeficiency virus infection. *JAMA* 257:2617-2621, 1987.
39. Mertz GJ: Genital herpes simplex virus infections. *Med Clin North Am* 74:1433-1454, 1990.
40. Nahmias A, Lee F, Beckman-Nahmias S: Sero-epidemiological and sociological patterns of herpes simplex virus infection in the world. *Scand J Infect Dis* 69(Suppl):19-36, 1990.
41. Safrin S, Arvin A, Mills J, et al: Comparison of the Western immunoblot assay and a glycoprotein G enzyme immunoassay for detection of serum antibodies to herpes simplex virus type 2 patients with AIDS. *J Clin Microbiol* 30:1312-1314, 1992.
42. Schacker T, Ryncarz AJ, Goddard J, et al: Frequent recovery of HIV-1 from genital herpes simplex virus lesions in HIV-1-infected men. *JAMA* 280:61-66, 1998.
43. Schacker T, Romanowski B, Tyring S, et al: Famciclovir for the management of herpes virus infections in HIV-infected patients. 4th International Congress on Drug Therapy in HIV Infection, Glasgow, Nov 8-12, 1998.
44. Friedman-Kien AE: The pathogenesis and treatment of varicella zoster infection in the immunocompromised host. *J Geriatr Dermatol* 2(Suppl A):11A-16A, 1994.

45. Tyring S, Barbarash RA, Nahlik J, et al: Famciclovir for the treatment of acute herpes zoster: Effects on acute disease and postherpetic neuralgia. *Ann Intern Med* 123:89-96, 1995.

46. Tyring S, Belanger R, Bezwoda W, et al: Famciclovir treatment of herpes zoster in immunocompromised patients: a multicenter, double-blind, randomized, acyclovir-controlled trial. 56th Annual Meeting of the AAD. 27 Feb-3 Mar, 1998, Orlando, Florida, Poster 243.

Investigational Drugs and Vaccines for HHV Infections

47. Gnann JW Jr, Crumpacker CS, Lalezari JP, et al: Sorivudine versus acyclovir for treatment of dermatomal herpes zoster in human immunodeficiency virus-infected patients: results from a randomized, controlled clinical trial. *Antimicrob Agents Chemo* 42:1139-1145, 1998.

48. Descamps J, Sehgal RK, DeClereq E, et al: Inhibitory effects of E-5-(bromovinyl)-1-β-D-arabinofuranosyluracil on herpes simplex virus replication and DNA synthesis. *J Virol* 43:332-336, 1982.

49. Yokata T, Kono K, Mori S, et al: Mechanism of selective inhibition of varicella-zoster virus replication by 1-beta-D-arabinofuranosyl-E-5-(2-bromovinyl)uracil. *Mol Pharmacol* 36:312-316, 1989.

50. Carlton S, Evans T, Tyring SK: New antiviral agents for dermatologic disease. *Semin Cutan Med Surg* 17:243-255, 1998.

51. Bodsworth N, Boag F, Burdge D, et al: Evaluation of sorivudine (BV-araU) versus acyclovir in the treatment of acute localized herpes zoster in human immunodeficiency virus-infected adults. *J Infect Dis* 176:103-111, 1997.

52. Desgranges C, Razaka G, DeClerq E, et al: Effects of E-5-(2-bromovinyl)uracil on the catabolism and antitumor activity of 5-fluorouracil in rats and leukemic mice. *Cancer Res* 46:1094-1101, 1986.

53. Soltz-Szots J, Tyring S, Andersen PL, et al: A randomized controlled trial of acyclovir versus netivudine for treatment of herpes zoster. *J Antimicrob Chemother* 41:549-556, 1998.

54. Rahim SG, Trevidi N, Selway J, et al: 5-Alkynyl pyrimidine nucleosides as potent selective inhibitors of varicella zoster virus. *Antiviral Chem Chemother* 3:293-297, 1992.

55. Purifoy DJM, Beauchamp LM, de Miranda P, et al: Review of research leading to new antiherpesvirus agents in clinical development: valaciclovir hydrochloride (256U, the L-valyl ester of acyclovir) and 882C, a specific agent for varicella zoster virus. *J Med Virol* 41(Suppl 1):139-145, 1993.

56. Wilber R, Buffington D, Tyring S, et al: Efficacy and safety of oral lobucavir (LBV) in patients with recurrent genital herpes. Presented at ICAAC, San Diego, CA, Sept, 1998.

57. Straus SE, Corey L, Burke RL, et al: Placebo controlled trial of vaccination with recombinant glycoprotein D of herpes simplex type 2 for immunotherapy of genital herpes. *Lancet* 343:1460-1463, 1994.

58. Hickling JK, Chisholm SE, Duncan IA, et al: Immunogenicity of a disabled infectious single cycle (DISC) HSV-2 vaccine in phase 1 clinical trials. Presented at ICID, Boston, USA, May 15-18, 1998.

Antivirals Used for Human Immunodeficiency Virus Infections—Overview

59. Kaplan MH, Sadick N, McNutt NS, et al: Dermatologic findings and manifestations of acquired immunodeficiency syndrome (AIDS). *J Am Acad Dermatol* 16:485, 1987.

60. Zalla MJ, Su WP, Fransway AF: Dermatologic manifestations of human immunodeficiency virus infection. *Mayo Clin Proc* 67:1089, 1992.

Nucleoside Analogs

61. Mitsuya H, Weinhold KJ, Furman PA, et al: Double-blind, placebo-controlled trial comparing long-term suppression with short term oral acyclovir therapy for management of recurrent genital herpes. *Am J Med* 85(Suppl 2A):20-25, 1988.

62. Goldshmidt RH, Moy A: Antiretroviral drug treatment for HIV/AIDS. *Am Fam Phys* 54:574-580, 1996.

63. Volberding PA, Lagakos SW, Koch MA, et al: Zidovudine in asymptomatic human immunodeficiency virus infection: A controlled trial in persons with fewer than 500 CD4-positive cells per cubic millimeter. *N Engl J Med* 322:941-949, 1990.

64. Connor EM, Sperling RS, Gelber R, et al: Reduction of maternal-infant transmission of human immunodeficiency virus type 1 with zidovudine treatment. *N Engl J Med* 331:1173-1180, 1994.

65. Torres RA, Barr MR, McIntyre KI, et al: A comparison of zidovudine, didanosine, zalcitabine and no antiretroviral therapy in patients with advanced HIV disease. *Int J STD AIDS* 6:19-26, 1995.

66. Dunkle LM: Stavudine (d4t) vs zidovudine (ZDV) for the treatment of HIV infected patients with CD4 counts of 50-500 cells/mm^3 following at least 6 months of zidovudine. Presented at the American Society for Microbiology 34th ICAAC. Orlando, Florida, October 1994.

67. Cammack N: Lamivudine in the therapy of HIV infection. *Int Antiviral News* 4:127-128, 1996.

68. Shuurman R, Nijhuis M, van Leeuwen R, et al: Rapid changes in human immune deficiency virus type 1 RNA load and appearance of drug-resistant virus populations in persons treated with lamivudine. *J Infect Disease* 171:1431, 1995.

69. Katlama C: Second International Congress on Drug Therapy of HIV Infection (abstract 2831). Glasgow, Scotland, November 1994.

70. Staszewski S: Coming therapies: abacavir. *Int J Clin Pract* 103(Suppl):35-38, 1999.

71. Foster RH, Faulds D: Abacavir. *Drugs* 55:729-738, 1998.

72. Clay PG, Rathbun RC, Slater LN: Management protocol for abacavir-related hypersensitivity reaction. *Ann Pharmacother* 34:247-249, 2000.

Nonnucleoside Analogs

73. Wynn P: Class of AIDS drugs boost combination therapy approach. *Dermatol Times* 17:33, 1996.

74. Ruiz N: Clinical history of efavirenz. *Int J Clin Pract* 103(Suppl):3-7, 1999.

Protease Inhibitors

75. McDonald CK, Kurtzkes DR: Human immunodeficiency virus type 1 protease inhibitors. *Arch Intern Med* 157:951-959, 1997.

76. Cameron W, Sun E, Markowitz M, et al: Combination use of ritonavir and saquinavir in HIV-infected patients: Preliminary safety and activity data. In Program and Abstracts of the 11th International Conference on AIDS (abstract Th.B 934). Vancouver, British Columbia, July 1996.

77. Martinez LJ: Approval of new protease inhibitors. *Res Initiative Treat Action* 2:1-3, 1996.

78. Wynn P: Class of AIDS drugs boost combination therapy approach. *Dermatol Times* 17:33, 1996.

79. Gathe J, Burkhardt B, Hawley P, et al: A randomized phase II study of Viracept, a novel HIV protease inhibitor, used in combination with stavudine vs stavudine alone (abstract M.B 413). In Program and Abstracts of the XI International Conference on AIDS. Vancouver, British Columbia, July 1996.

80. Moyle GJ, Youle M, Higgs C, et al: Extended follow-up and safety and activity of Agouron's HIV proteinase inhibitor from the UK phase I/II dose finding study (abstract M.B. 173). In Program and Abstracts of the 11th International Conference on AIDS. Vancouver, British Columbia, July 1996.

81. Saag M, Knowles M, Chang Y, et al: Durable effects of VIRACEPT (nelfinavir mesylate, NFV) in triple combination therapy. Programs and abstracts of the 37th International Conference on Antimicrobial Agents and Chemotherapy. Toronto, Canada, 1997.

82. Adkins JC, Faulds D: Amprenavir. *Drugs* 55:837-844, 1998.

83. Deeks S, Loftus R, Cohen P, et al: Incidence and predictors of virologic failure to indinavir or/and ritonavir in an urban health clinic. Programs and abstracts of the 37th International Conference on Antimicrobial Agents and Chemotherapy. Toronto, Canada ,1997.

84. Jacobsen H, Yasargil IC, Winslow DL, et al: Characterization of human immunodeficiency virus type 1 mutants with decreased sensitivity to proteinase inhibitor Ro 31-8959. *Virology* 206:527-534, 1995.

85. Richman E: HIV infection and AIDS update: advances in clinical care. *Int Med World Rep* 11:3, 5-7, 1996.

86. Carpenter CCJ, Fischl MA, Hammer SM, et al: Antiretroviral therapy for HIV infection in 1998: updated recommendations of the International AIDS Society-USA Panel. *JAMA* 280:78-86, 1998.

87. Mellors JW, Munoz AM, Giorgi JV, et al: Plasma viral load and CD4$^+$ lymphocytes as prognostic markers of HIV-1 infection. *Ann Intern Med* 126:946-954, 1997.

88. Delta Coordinating Committee: Delta: a randomised double-blind controlled trial comparing combinations of zidovudine plus didanosine or zalcitabine with zidovudine alone in HIV-infected individuals. *Lancet* 348:283-291, 1996.

89. Hammer SM, Katzenstein DA, Hughes MD, et al: A trial comparing therapy in HIV-infected adults with CD4$^+$ cell counts from 200-500 per cubic millimeter. *N Engl J Med* 335:1081-1090, 1996.

90. Chopra KF, Tyring SK: Current antiviral therapy in the treatment of human immunodeficiency virus infections. *Semin Cutan Med Surg* 16:224-234, 1997.

91. Shelton DL: Vaccines now being tested around the world. *Am Med News* January 20, 1997.

92. AIDS vaccine moves into phase 3 trials (Medical News & Perspectives). *JAMA* 280:7-8, 1998.

PART III

Systemic Immunomodulatory and Antiproliferative Agents

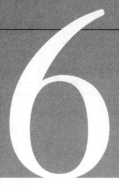

CHAPTER 6

Stephen E. Wolverton

Systemic Corticosteroids

Kendall[1] described compound E (cortisone) in 1935. A Mayo clinic group first described the use of cortisone and adrenocorticotropic hormone (ACTH) in patients with rheumatoid arthritis in 1948.[1] In 1950 Hench and colleagues[2] presented the first report on the basic effects and toxicities of corticosteroids (CS).

Sulzberger and colleagues' 1951 report[3] described the use of cortisone and ACTH in a variety of inflammatory dermatoses. This report on CS radically changed the therapeutic approach of dermatologists. As the list of steroid-responsive dermatoses grew, so did the list of potential adverse effects. In 1961 Reichling and Kligman[4] suggested alternate-day CS use. This was an important step toward decreasing adverse effects and yet maintaining antiinflammatory effect over the 48-hour period between doses.

Two major advances in CS therapy occurred during the 1970s and 1980s. Adjunctive therapy with immunosuppressive drugs, such as azathioprine and cyclophosphamide, has been used increasingly for "steroid-sparing" effect. These drugs allow lower CS doses to be used, which lessens the risk of serious adverse effects while maintaining an adequate immunosuppressive effect. High-dose pulse intravenous methylprednisolone therapy was increasingly utilized through the 1980s. Quicker remission with lower risk from therapy is the goal of this method of CS administration.

This chapter deals with the pharmacology and clinical use of systemic CS. Particular attention is given to the risks of systemic CS, especially focusing on measures to minimize the risk of these important complications. The physician who is thoroughly familiar with these measures can more comfortably and intelligently use systemic CS to the benefit of many grateful patients.

Included in this chapter are special sections covering the following topics: normal hypothalamic-pituitary-adrenal (HPA) axis function, intramuscular CS administration, pulse intravenous CS administration, HPA axis suppression, and therapeutic guidelines.

PHARMACOLOGY

Table 6-1 lists key pharmacologic concepts for systemic corticosteroids.

Structure

The basic structure of all CS consists of three hexane rings and one pentane ring.[1,5] The combined ring structure is known as the cyclopentenoperhydrophenanthrene nucleus. The rings are designated by letters A, B, C, and D, and each carbon is assigned a number from 1 to 21 (Figure 6-1). The designations alpha (α, away from the CS receptor) and beta (β, toward the CS receptor) refer to the position of any added molecules in reference to the stereochemical plane.

Cortisone and hydrocortisone both possess a 4,5 double bond and a ketone (carbonyl) group

■ **Table 6-1** Key Pharmacologic Concepts—Systemic Corticosteroids[5-8]

Drug	Equivalent Dose (mg)	Gluco-corticoid Potency*	Mineralo-corticoid Potency	Plasma Half-life (min)	Biologic Half-life (hrs)
SHORT-ACTING					
Cortisone	25	0.8	2+	30-90	8-12
Hydrocortisone	20	1	2+	60-120	8-12
INTERMEDIATE-ACTING					
Prednisone	5	4	1+	60	24-36
Prednisolone	5	4	1+	115-212	24-36
Methylprednisolone	4	5	0	180	24-36
Triamcinolone	4	5	0	78-188	24-36
LONG-ACTING					
Dexamethasone	0.75	20-30	0	100-300	36-54
Betamethasone	0.6-0.75	20-30	0	100-300	36-54

*Glucocorticoid potency is expressed in a relative scale without specific units of measure; this relative potency number is inversely related to the equivalent dose in the first column.

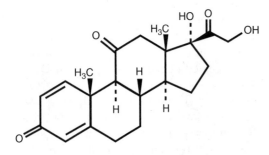

Hydrocortisone (Cortisol)

Prednisone

Figure 6-1 Systemic corticosteroids.

at the 3 position.[5,9] Cortisone, which is an inactive form, has a ketone at the 11 position. The active form, hydrocortisone (cortisol), is formed through hepatic conversion of the 11-ketone to an 11-hydroxyl group. The addition of a 1,2 double bond results in increased glucocorticoid activity and a decreased rate of degradation. This results in prednisone (with an 11-ketone group), and through 11-hydroxylation the active analog, prednisolone, is formed. Methylprednisolone is formed through the addition of a 6-methyl group to prednisolone, which leads to slightly increased glucocorticoid potency.

The addition of fluorine to hydrocortisone at the 9α position leads to increased glucocorticoid, but excessive mineralocorticoid (MC) activity.[5,9] The resulting compound is 9α-fluorohydrocortisone (fludrocortisone, Florinef). This compound is the basic structure of most fluorinated topical steroids. In general, the MC effect is decreased in topical steroids by the masking of the 16- or 17-hydroxyl group with various esters (e.g., acetonide, valerate, or propionate).

With systemic CS, 9α fluorohydrocortisone with an added 1,2 double bond is also modified further.[5,9] By adding a 16α-hydroxyl group (triamcinolone), a 16α-methyl group (dexamethasone), or a 16β-methyl group (betamethasone), one can form three compounds with high glucocorticoid and low MC effects. Because all have an 11-hydroxyl group, these three compounds are in biologically active forms. All CS have a hydroxyl group at the 17 position (17-hydroxycorticosteroids). Androgenic steroid compounds have a 17-ketone group and a 19-carbon basic ring structure (17-ketosteroids).

Absorption/Distribution

Exogenous CS are absorbed in the upper jejunum.[1] More than 50% of prednisone is absorbed. Food delays but does not decrease the amount absorbed. Peak plasma levels are reached 30 to 100 minutes after the drug is taken.

The primary endogenous carrier protein is cortisol-binding globulin (CBG, transcortin).[5] Overall, 80% to 90% of endogenous cortisol is bound; the free fraction represents the active form. CBG is a low-capacity, high-affinity binding system. Albumin (corticosteroid-binding albumin) represents a low-affinity, high-capacity binding reserve. The avidity with which synthetic CS bind to these carrier proteins is less than the avidity with endogenous cortisol. Thus for synthetic CS a greater free fraction is available. Prednisolone is reported to bind to carrier proteins with greater affinity than other synthetic forms, with resultant displacement of endogenous cortisol from the protein-binding sites.

CBG is decreased by hypothyroidism, liver disease, renal disease, and obesity, all of which may result in increased amount of the free CS fraction.[10] CBG is increased by estrogen therapy, pregnancy, and hyperthyroidism, all of which may decrease the free fraction of endogenous and synthetic CS. High-dose therapy results in a greater proportion of free CS in the body. Likewise, prolonged CS treatment typically increases the free fraction.

Overall, CS are widely distributed to most body tissues. All endogenous and synthetic CS are well distributed into fetal tissue with the exception of prednisone.[5]

Metabolism/Excretion

All the biologically active CS and their synthetic congeners have a double bond in the 4,5 position and a ketone group at the 3 position.[5,9] Reduction at the 4,5 double bond can occur at both hepatic and extrahepatic sites, yielding an inactive substance. Reduction of the 3-ketone substituent to a 3-hydroxyl group to form tetrahydrocortisol has been demonstrated only in the liver. Most of the aforementioned metabolites are conjugated at the 3-hydroxyl site with sulfate or glucuronic acid to form water-soluble metabolites, which are excreted by the kidney.

Of importance is that the action of 11β-hydroxydehydrogenase in the liver is necessary to convert cortisone to hydrocortisone and to convert prednisone to prednisolone.[5] Of these four CS, only hydrocortisone and prednisolone are biologically active. Severe liver disease may impair this conversion. Thus the administration of prednisolone rather than prednisone to patients with advanced liver disease would be appropriate. In addition, liver disease may result in decreased albumin, which would increase the free fraction of CS.

The plasma half-lives of the various synthetic CS do not correlate well with the duration of biologic activity[1] (see Table 6-1). A much more important measure of duration of activity is the duration of ACTH suppression after the administration of a single dose of a given CS. This duration of activity correlates well with glucocorticoid and antiinflammatory effects.[7,8] There is an inverse correlation between the duration of action and the MC effect.

Mechanism of Action

The most important immunosuppressive and antiinflammatory effects of systemic CS are listed in Table 6-2. In addition, the mechanisms responsible for 15 of the most important CS adverse effects are listed in Table 6-3. The interested reader should spend adequate time to thoroughly understand the information in these two tables to have a broad comprehension of the overall benefits and risks of systemic CS. A concise discussion on normal HPA axis function, glucocorticoid effects, and MC effects follows, concluding with relatively new information on glucocorticoid receptors, corticosteroid resistance, and tachyphylaxis, apoptosis, and transcription factors.

NORMAL HPA AXIS FUNCTION. It is important to understand the normal function of

■ **Table 6-2**   Immunosuppressive and Antiinflammatory Effects
of Corticosteroids[11-13]

Corticosteroid Action	Mechanism and Biologic Result
EFFECTS ON GLUCOCORTICOID RECEPTOR (GCR)	
Normal response	On ligand (CS) binding, the GCR is activated and translocates to the nucleus, binding to glucocorticoid-response elements of multiple genes. CS can function as an agonist or antagonist for these genes; GCR is ubiquitous throughout body.
Resistance	Generally a dynamic, temporary, relative resistance, with mechanisms not fully known; usually no evidence of GCR mutations or polymorphisms
TRANSCRIPTION FACTOR EFFECTS	
NFκB inhibition	Increased IκB production, direct NFκB binding; net result ↓ production of multiple cytokines such as IL-1, TNF-α, adhesion molecules, growth factors, etc.
AP-1 inhibition	Decreased production of multiple cytokines; cytokine spectrum similar to NFκB
APOPTOSIS INDUCTION	
Lymphocyte apoptosis	Apoptosis of autoreactive T cells (in autoimmune disorders) and neoplastic T cells (in various lymphomas); AP-1 and caspase cascade probably involved in process
Eosinophil apoptosis	Apoptosis of eosinophils with potential implications for various allergic disorders
SIGNAL TRANSDUCTION	
Phospholipase A_2 inhibition	CS effect probably mediated indirectly via ↑ lipocortin-1 (now called "annexins")
↓ "downstream" eicosanoids	As a result of phospholipase A_2 inhibition, ↓ production of various prostaglandins, leukotrienes, 12-HETE, and 15-HETE inflammatory mediators
COX-2	↓ eicosanoid production generated by this inducible (with inflammation) enzyme; CS effect on COX-2 >> COX-1

GCR, Glucocorticoid receptor; *NFκB*, nuclear factor κB; *IκB*, inhibitor κB; *AP-1*, activating protein-1; *HETE*, hydroxyeicosatetraenoic (acid); *COX-2*, cyclo-oxygenase 2 inhibition; *COX-1*, cyclo-oxygenase 1 inhibition; *WBC*, white blood cell; *NK*, natural killer; *PMN*, polymorphonuclear neutrophil leukocyte.

the HPA axis to better understand the potential for HPA axis suppression by synthetic CS. For further background information, several reviews are particularly helpful.[10,14,19-21]

The primary stimulus for release of endogenous cortisol originates in the hypothalamus. The tropic hormone is known as corticotropin-releasing factor (CRF). ACTH is subsequently released by the anterior pitui-

tary. ACTH is produced from the prohormone pro-ACTH/endorphin. There are approximately 10 bursts of ACTH released throughout the day. The greatest frequency of these bursts occurs in the early morning hours during a normal sleep cycle. The zona fasciculata of the adrenal cortex is then stimulated to produce and release cortisol. ACTH also stimulates adrenal androgen synthesis. However, ACTH is not sig-

Table 6-2   Immunosuppressive and Antiinflammatory Effects of Corticosteroids[11-13]—cont'd

Corticosteroid Action	Mechanism and Biologic Result
EFFECTS ON VARIOUS WBC SUBSETS AND OTHER IMMUNOLOGIC CELLS	
B cells	With higher CS doses significant B-cell effect, reduced immunoglobulin production
T cells	Greater effect on T cells (CD4 > CD8 effect) at lower doses compared to above B-cell effect; net result ↓ IL-2 production and resultant ↓ amplification effect
Other lymphocyte subsets	↓ NK cell activity, ↓ antibody-dependent cellular cytotoxicity mediated by K cells
PMNs	↓ PMN marginization, ↓ chemotaxis, small effect on microbicidal respiratory burst; also ↓ apoptosis of PMNs (in contrast with ↑ apoptosis of T cells and eosinophils)
Mast cells	Inhibit degranulation, with resultant ↓ release of histamine, kinins, other mediators
Monocytes, macrophages	↓ monocyte maturation; ↓ access to inflammatory sites, ↓ IL-1 and IFN-γ release
Langerhans' cells	↓ characteristic surface markers, impaired antigen processing and presentation
Eosinophils, basophils	Reduced numbers and function both cell types, ↓ recruitment to inflammatory sites
Fibroblasts	↓ production of collagen, ground substance, fibronectin, and collagenase
Membrane stabilization	Both lysosomal and cell membrane stabilization; probable role in mast cell, PMN, other inflammatory cell effects
Bottom line *generalizations*	CS overall effects—cell trafficking > cellular function; cellular immunity > humoral immunity; major portion of effects mediated via above cytokine alterations
VASCULAR EFFECTS	
Angiogenesis	↓ angiogenesis in wound healing and with proliferative lesions (hemangiomas)
Vasoconstriction	Net result of vasocortin and vasoregulin, potentiate response to catecholamines
Decreased permeability	Decreased vascular smooth muscle response to histamine and bradykinin

nificantly involved in the release of the MC aldosterone.

The three main controls of endogenous cortisol production are discussed in Box 6-1.

GLUCOCORTICOID EFFECTS. Table 6-4 lists physiologic glucocorticoid and MC effects. CS play an important teleologic role in maintaining adequate blood glucose levels for brain function.[5] Gluconeogenesis generates glucose at the expense of amino acids derived from en-dogenous proteins. CS also produce peripheral insulin resistance, which impedes glucose absorption by various body tissues. In addition, glycogen storage in the liver is enhanced. Lipid stores are stimulated to undergo lipolysis, generating increased amounts of triglycerides from which to derive energy.

The net effect is a catabolic state that produces carbohydrates at the expense of protein and fat stores.[5] Through gluconeogenesis, proteins from muscle, trabecular bone (especially

■ Table 6-3   Mechanisms Responsible for Selected Corticosteroid Adverse Effects[11,12,14-18]

Adverse Effect	Proposed Mechanisms
HPA AXIS EFFECTS	
Adrenal crisis	Reduced GC and MC reserves—normally there are adequate compensatory mechanisms for GC and MC effects such that major complications very rare
METABOLIC EFFECTS	
Hyperglycemia	GC effects—↑ hepatic glucose/glycogen production, ↑ gluconeogenesis via protein catabolism, induce insulin resistance producing ↓ glucose entry into cells
Hypertension	MC effects—sodium retention; also in part due GC-induced vasoconstriction
Congestive heart failure	MC effects—↑ sodium retention, resultant fluid overload in predisposed individuals
Hyperlipidemia	GC effects—overall result of catabolic state, in part initiated by ↑ lipoprotein lipase
Cushingoid changes	Altered fat distribution, uncertain mechanism; result of overall fat catabolism
BONE EFFECTS	
Growth impairment	Due to ↓ growth hormone and IGF-1 production; net result delayed skeletal maturation
Osteoporosis*	↑ osteoclast activity, ↓ osteoblast activity, ↓ GI absorption of calcium, ↑ renal excretion of calcium; resultant secondary hyperparathyroidism and bone resorption
Osteonecrosis	↑ marrow fat deposition, compression of interosseous vessels; hypercoagulability due to endogenous disorders or exogenous factors such as smoking, alcohol, trauma
GASTROINTESTINAL EFFECTS	
Bowel perforation	GC catabolic effects producing ↓ wound healing after recent bowel anastomosis
Peptic ulcer disease	↓ mucus production, ↑ acid production; CS not a direct gastric irritant
OTHER ADVERSE EFFECTS	
Cataracts	Altered lens proteins, with uncertain mechanism (typically posterior subcapsular location)
Agitation/psychosis	Possibly due to electrolyte shifts, altered nerve excitability, ? mild cerebral edema
Opportunistic infections	Impaired immunologic responses (see Table 6-2)
Myopathy	↓ glucose and amino acid uptake by muscles, leading to muscle atrophy/wasting

GC, Glucocorticoid; MC, mineralocorticoid; GI, gastrointestinal.
*Greatest CS effect on bone resorption at sites of high trabecular bone content such as ribs, vertebral bodies, and flat bones of pelvis, correspond to sites with greatest risk of fractures.

vertebral and hip), dermal connective tissue, and vascular proteins are metabolized. Lipolysis results in triglyceride release with additional fat redistribution to areas that are characteristic of Cushing's syndrome.

MINERALOCORTICOID EFFECTS. Aldosterone is the primary endogenous MC hormone. The primary aldosterone effect is sodium reabsorption and resultant water reabsorption at the proximal tubule site in the kidneys.

Box 6-1

HPA Axis in a Nutshell[10,14,19-21]

COMPONENTS OF HPA AXIS AND HORMONE PRODUCED Hypothalamus—CRF Pituitary (anterior)—ACTH Adrenal—cortisol (same as hydrocortisone) **BASAL AND STRESS LEVELS OF CS PRODUCTION** Basal production of *cortisol*—20 to 30 mg daily Basal production in *prednisone equivalents*—5 to 7.5 mg daily Maximal stress production of *cortisol*—300 mg daily Maximal stress production in *prednisone equivalents*—75 mg daily Minor stress production of cortisol—probably 2 to 3 times basal production **RESPONSE OF VARIOUS COMPONENTS TO EXOGENOUS CS AND SUBSEQUENT STRESS** Hypothalamus—first to be suppressed, first to recover full function, most critical component for adequate stress responsiveness Adrenal—slower to be suppressed, much slower to recover full function	**REGULATORY MECHANISMS AND SOURCES OF VARIABILITY** Circadian variations—CRF (and thus ACTH) have innate diurnal variations tied to sleep cycle (highest production mid-sleep, lowest late afternoon) Negative feedback—increased cortisol levels reduce CRF and ACTH production Stress response—increased CRF release and subsequently increased ACTH release **BACKUP MECHANISMS FOR CS PRODUCTION IN SETTING OF ADRENAL INSUFFICIENCY** CRF alternate sites of production—cerebral cortex and limbic system, which can be released by acetylcholine and serotonin Alternative inducers of ACTH release—catecholamines, vasopressin All the above means serve to maintain glucose homeostasis

Note: ACTH has no role in endogenous MC production.
CRF, Corticotropin-releasing factor; *ACTH,* adrenocorticotropic hormone; *MC,* mineralocorticoid.

Table 6-4   Physiologic Glucocorticoid and Mineralocorticoid Effects[5,11,12,22]

Glucocorticoid Effects*	Mineralocorticoid Effects†
GLUCOSE METABOLISM Gluconeogenesis at expense of protein catabolism Peripheral insulin resistance—reduced glucose into cells Glycogen storage in liver	**ALDOSTERONE EFFECTS— ENDOGENOUS** Major effect is sodium and water retention This effect is primarily at proximal tubule in kidney Potassium is excreted in exchange sodium at this site
LIPID METABOLISM Lipolysis releasing triglycerides as source of energy Fat redistribution to central locations	**CORTICOSTEROID EFFECTS— EXOGENOUS** Endogenous/exogenous cortisol significant MC effects See Table 6-1 for MC effect of various CS
REGULATION OF ABOVE PROCESSES ACTH (pituitary) induces release of cortisol (adrenal) Negative feedback loop to hypothalamus (site of CRF)	**REGULATION OF ENDOGENOUS ALDOSTERONE** ACTH has no role in aldosterone production Regulation primarily by renin-angiotensin, potassium

MC, Mineralocorticoid; *ACTH,* adrenocorticotropic hormone; *CRF,* corticotropin-releasing factor.
*Conceptually all the glucocorticoid effects are prioritized to maintain brain glucose homeostasis.
†Major priority for MC is to maintain sodium and fluid homeostasis.

Sodium is exchanged for potassium, which leads to hypokalemia when there is excessive MC effect. ACTH has no direct control on MC production. The primary MC control mechanisms are through the renin-angiotensin system and serum potassium levels.[10,19] CS with significant MC effect, such as hydrocortisone, have a similar effect on sodium, potassium, and fluid balance as aldosterone. Long-acting CS, such as dexamethasone and betamethasone, have essentially no MC effect (see Table 6-2).

GLUCOCORTICOID RECEPTOR AND CORTICOSTEROID RESISTANCE.   There is only one glucocorticoid receptor (GCR), accounting for endogenous glucocorticoid effects, as well as the pharmacologic effects of synthetic CS (both beneficial and adverse effects).[11,12] This cytosolic receptor can function directly as a transcription factor, which on translocation to the nucleus binds directly to various glucocorticoid responsive elements of multiple genes in DNA. In addition, the ligand-GCR complex can activate other transcription factors as detailed in the next section.

There are rare cases of hereditary glucocorticoid resistance in which there are mutations in the GCR gene and GCR protein.[23] In clinical practice, GCR sensitivity is much more dynamic than previously appreciated. Furthermore, relative resistance at the GCR in otherwise healthy individuals is much more common than previously recognized. These cases of relative resistance lack mutations or polymorphisms in the GCR gene.[24] In addition, relative resistance is not due to altered bioavailability, altered ligand binding to GCR, or altered translocation of the activated GCR complex to the nucleus.[25] Conceptually, this resistance could represent a negative feedback system of sorts, with down regulation of GCR after prolonged or high-dose CS therapy. The transcription factor activating protein-1 (AP-1) is thought to play a role in this process as well.[25]

CORTICOSTEROIDS AND TRANSCRIPTION FACTORS.   The two well-described transcription factors with a central role in amplification of the inflammatory response are nuclear factor κB (NFκB) and AP-1. NFκB is biologically inactive as long as it is bound to inhibitor κB (IκB).[26,27] NFκB is activated when any of a wide variety of stimuli degrade IκB, thus freeing the

transcription factor. Free NFκB translocates to the nucleus where it induces transcription of numerous genes, such as "immunoawakening" cytokines (IL-1β, TNF-α); "immunomodulatory" cytokines (IL-2, IL-8); growth factors (G-CSF, GM-CSF); adhesion molecules (ICAM-1, E-selectin); receptors (IL-2 receptor); and inflammatory enzymes (COX-2, phospholipase A_2), to name just some of the list.[26]

CS reduce the effects of NFκB in two ways.[26,27] The CS-GCR complex leads to increased IκB formation and subsequent NFκB binding by this inhibitory protein. The CS-GCR complex can also directly bind to NFκB. By either means, there can be a dramatic reduction of a wide variety of components of the inflammatory response.

AP-1 is actually a collective term for dimeric transcription factors composed of Jun, Fos, or activating transcription factor (ATF), all of which bind to a common DNA site, the AP-1 binding site.[28] There is tremendous overlap with the inflammatory response genes induced by AP-1 and NFκB.[29] The CS inhibition of AP-1 activation and DNA binding serves to further augment the biologic effects of NFκB inhibition by CS. It is unknown whether sustained inhibition of NFκB and AP-1 gene transcription may be responsible for important CS adverse effects.

CORTICOSTEROID-INDUCED APOPTOSIS. Apoptosis is an orderly process of programmed cell death. The process is a biologically active, noninflammatory sequence of cellular changes that occur with an intact plasma membrane in spite of nuclear fragmentation. CS can directly induce apoptosis in lymphocytes and eosinophils.[30] CS can induce apoptosis at least in part through down regulation of the CD3 molecule of T cells; this molecule plays an important role in T cell activation.[31] There can also be an indirect effect on lymphocytes and eosinophils through CS-induced suppression of cytokines essential to cellular survival.[30]

The logical application of these facts is an underlying explanation for CS effects in autoimmune disorders (apoptosis of autoreactive T cells), allergic disorders (apoptosis of eosinophils), and certain neoplastic disorders (apoptosis of malignant T cells). It is doubtful that the ability of CS to induce apoptosis is limited to these white blood cell subsets.

CLINICAL USE
Indications

A number of the dermatoses listed in Table 6-5 are discussed selectively to illustrate various principles of CS therapy. Conditions in which dermatologists play a central role in CS management are discussed in significant detail. Al-

ternative and adjunctive systemic therapies are briefly described as well.

Overall, well-controlled studies of CS use in dermatoses are quite uncommon. When available, controlled studies sometimes produced results contrary to traditional beliefs on CS indications (see later section on postherpetic

Table 6-5   Systemic Corticosteroid Indications and Contraindications

DERMATOLOGIC USES

Bullous Dermatoses
Pemphigus vulgaris/superficial forms*[32-46]
Bullous pemphigoid*[47-52]
Cicatricial pemphigoid[47,53-57]
Herpes gestationis[47,58,59]
Epidermolysis bullosa acquisita[60]
Linear IgA bullous dermatosis[61,62]
SJS/TEN*[63-73]
Erythema multiforme minor*[74]

Autoimmune Connective Tissue Diseases
Lupus erythematosus[75,76] (systemic*)
Dermatomyositis*[77-80]

Vasculitis
Cutaneous[81-85,88]
Systemic[86,87]

Neutrophilic Dermatoses
Pyoderma gangrenosum[89-94]
Behçet's disease/aphthous ulcers[95-97]
Sweet's syndrome[98,99]

Dermatitis/Papulosquamous Dermatoses
Contact dermatitis[100]
Atopic dermatitis[101,102]
Exfoliative erythroderma[103]
Lichen planus[104-108]

Other Dermatoses
Sarcoidosis[109-111]
Sunburn[112]
Urticaria (severe*)[113]
Androgen excess (acne/hirsutism)[114,115]
Postherpetic neuralgia prevention[116-123]

Intramuscular CS[124,125]

Pulse IV Methylprednisolone (*Experimental*)
Pyoderma gangrenosum[89,90,131,132]
Pemphigus vulgaris[36,37,133]
Bullous pemphigoid[134]
Sweet's syndrome[135]
Urticarial vasculitis[136]
Alopecia areata[137,138]

CONTRAINDICATIONS

Absolute
Systemic fungal infections
Herpes simplex keratitis
Hypersensitivity (primarily occurs with ACTH, occasionally noted with IV preparations)

Relative†
Cardiovascular: hypertension, CHF
Central nervous system: prior psychosis, severe depression
Gastrointestinal: active PUD, recent anastomosis
Infections: active TB, positive tuberculin skin test
Metabolic: diabetes mellitus
Musculoskeletal: osteoporosis
Ocular: cataracts, glaucoma
Pregnancy

PREGNANCY PRESCRIBING STATUS—CATEGORY C

SJS, Stevens-Johnson syndrome; *TEN*, toxic epidermal necrolysis; *ACTH*, adrenocorticotropic hormone; *IV*, intravenous; *CHF*, congestive heart failure; *PUD*, peptic ulcer disease; *TB*, tuberculosis.
*FDA-approved indications.
†The severity of the disease to be treated and the anticipated dose and duration of CS therapy determine whether relative contraindications prohibit CS therapy.

neuralgia [PHN]). In clinical practice, it is actually quite easy in most cases to have a high level of certainty about the benefits of CS in an individual patient. Recent studies and reviews are given priority here. Definitions of importance are listed in Table 6-6.

PEMPHIGUS VULGARIS.   The best-studied purely dermatologic indication for systemic CS therapy is pemphigus vulgaris. The emphasis here is high-dose CS therapy with use of adjunctive immunosuppressive therapy. CS are appropriate at the start of therapy for any significant case of pemphigus vulgaris that has no absolute contraindications to CS use. Adjunctive therapy is generally used with a choice of azathioprine, cyclophosphamide, cyclosporine, methotrexate, gold, or plasmapheresis.[32-34] More recently, antiinflammatory antibiotics, such as the tetracyclines, have been utilized for milder cases of pemphigus vulgaris and for pemphigus foliaceus.[35] Pulse methylpred-

nisolone may be indicated to attain rapid disease control in more severe cases of pemphigus vulgaris.[36,37]

Early reports on oral CS therapy for pemphigus vulgaris describe doses of 120 to 140 mg/day of prednisone (up to more than twice that dose).[38-40] Disease- and treatment-related deaths occurred in up to 44% of patients. This death rate still was a significant improvement from the reported 90% disease fatality rate before the availability of CS therapy in the 1950s. In the early 1970s there was further reduction of disease- and treatment-related fatalities to as low as 9.5% from treatment-induced mortality and 24% from combined treatment- and disease-induced mortality.[39,40] Current series report much lower death rates.[32-34,41,42] Earlier diagnosis, lower doses of CS therapy, improved treatment of secondary infections, and adjunctive azathioprine, cyclophosphamide, cyclosporine, or methotrexate therapy are probably responsible for the improved survival statistics.

■ Table 6-6   Some Pharmacologic Definitions

DOSING LEVEL DEFINITIONS

Decrement	Amount of reduction in CS dose, either a fixed percentage or fixed interval decrease
Increment	Amount of increase in CS dose, guided by the urgency to attain disease control
Induction	Initial CS dose focused on quickly attaining disease control
Maintenance	Relatively constant dose of CS to maintain disease control attained by induction dose
Minimal effective dose	The lowest dose of CS just adequate to almost completely control the disease process
Pharmacologic	Generally considered to be any dose above physiologic levels (see text)
Physiologic	Dose of exogenous CS that is similar to the quantity of endogenous CS produced
Replacement	Synonym of physiologic dose, term also used to refer to endogenous MC levels
Supraphysiologic	Synonym of pharmacologic dose
Tapering	Any effort to reduce the CS dose, given that reasonable disease control is attained

DOSING FREQUENCY OR DURATION DEFINITIONS

Alternate-day	CS doses given every other day, result is an "on" day and an "off" day
Burst	Short course of CS (generally 2-3 weeks or less) to control self-limited disease
Consolidation	Change from a divided dose to a single daily dose without changing the daily dose; necessary step before tapering
Divided	Any dosing frequency that is more frequent than daily dosing; usually bid or qid
"Off" day	With alternate-day therapy, day in which CS is omitted (or lower dose is given)
"On" day	With alternate-day therapy, day in which CS is administered (or higher dose is given)
Pulse	Usually represents a very brief course (5-7 days) of very high dose (10-15 mg/kg/day) of IV methylprednisolone (see text for other usage of this term)

MC, Mineralocorticoid; *IV,* intravenous.

Current management includes prednisone doses no greater than 2 mg/kg/day in divided doses. In general, it is reasonable to start prednisone at 1 mg/kg/day, increasing to the above dosage range as indicated for more severe cases of pemphigus. Disease control is usually attained in 4 to 6 weeks. At this time, the divided dose should be consolidated into a single daily dose and tapered rapidly to the 40 mg/day range. Azathioprine or related immunosuppressive drugs can be added at the time of prednisone tapering in many cases. For more severe cases, it is wise to add the steroid-sparing agent at the start of therapy. Management of oral involvement needs to be reasonably aggressive, both to limit progression to more serious cutaneous involvement and to maintain adequate fluid and nutrition intake.[43] Juvenile pemphigus vulgaris is similar to that just described, with CS doses appropriate for body weight.[44,45] The challenge of managing paraneoplastic pemphigus has been reviewed by Anhalt.[46]

BULLOUS PEMPHIGOID.   In patients with bullous pemphigoid, moderate doses of CS up to 1 mg/kg/day are used.[47] In addition, the CS course is typically given for a defined duration of time (generally 6 to 12 months). Nonsteroidal immunosuppressants should be the mainstay of therapy if the disease persists beyond this time period. The heterogeneous nature of the disease dictates that the dosage level should be individualized for generalized bullous pemphigoid cases. Dapsone for children and tetracycline and related drugs for adults are alternative therapies. About half of patients require concomitant immunosuppressive therapy with drugs such as azathioprine or methotrexate.[48,49] Plasma exchange has given inconsistent results in treating bullous pemphigoid.[49,50]

In general, 60 to 80 mg/day (1 mg/kg/day) of prednisone in divided doses is successful in eliminating new blister formation within several weeks. Should the patient not respond to this dose or require a high maintenance dose, adjunctive immunosuppressive therapy can be added. In the absence of new blisters over 5 to 7 days' time, the prednisone dose can be gradually tapered. Contrary to prior reports, Schmidt and colleagues[51] reported that disease activity can be monitored by determining bullous pemphigoid antigen 180 (BPA 180) titers.

Deaths still occasionally occur in older patients with more extensive involvement; more conservative management utilizing alternatives to CS may help lessen the risk of sepsis in this population.[52]

CICATRICIAL PEMPHIGOID.   In contrast, cicatricial pemphigoid is less responsive to CS than is bullous pemphigoid.[47,53-55] Consultation with an ophthalmologist is necessary in every case with ocular involvement. The course of the disease is variable; early institution of treatment leads to better results. Azathioprine, cyclophosphamide, or cyclosporine is usually needed as adjunctive therapy when there is significant ocular involvement.[53,56] Dapsone therapy for initial management is often successful for milder ocular involvement and for oral involvement.

In general, 1 to 1.5 mg/kg/day of prednisone is required for controlling moderate-to-severe cases. Aggressive management is important in ocular cases because of the significant potential for blindness. Early diagnosis, moderately aggressive therapy, and subsequent mucous membrane grafting by an experienced oculoplastic surgeon are key elements for management. The immunosuppression should be carried out at least 3 months before the grafting; otherwise, there may be deleterious results.[57]

STEVENS-JOHNSON SYNDROME AND TOXIC EPIDERMAL NECROLYSIS.   There is still significant controversy regarding the use of systemic CS for the spectrum of Stevens-Johnson syndrome (SJS) and toxic epidermal necrolysis (TEN). Recent trends towards the use of cyclosporine or intravenous (IV) immunoglobulin for these patients have taken some of the heat off the debate. A number of studies support routine CS therapy.[63-65] A majority of studies, however, present data that support routine utilization of burn unit care in the absence of systemic CS therapy.[66-69] These studies report a higher fatality rate, particularly from sepsis, in CS-treated patients, compared with patients managed in a burn unit without CS therapy. In one burn unit study, systemic CS were not associated with higher morbidity or mortality.[70] Still others promote careful nursing care in a well-staffed floor or an intensive care unit, in the absence of systemic CS.[71]

Proponents of routine systemic CS use suggest that for patients who have SJS and TEN, systemic CS treatment early in the disease course (before significant sloughing of skin) followed by rapid tapering of CS may be beneficial and even life-saving. After widespread sloughing occurs, the risk of infection clearly outweighs the potential CS benefits. Of importance is that drug and infectious precipitators be sought and eliminated if possible. Should CS therapy be indicated, doses up to 2 to 2.5 mg/kg/day of IV methylprednisolone in divided doses are generally used.

In the late 1990s, there were two somewhat puzzling, if not counterintuitive, studies on this subject. One study reported that CS therapy for other indications before the onset of SJS or TEN did not decrease the risk of these disorders.[72] Another study noted an increased risk of SJS or TEN in patients previously on systemic CS.[73] Further investigation in these areas would be of value.

A more common indication for moderate CS doses is recurrent oral erythema multiforme minor.[74] Painful oral erosions respond promptly to prednisone in doses up to 1 mg/kg/day, rapidly tapered over 2 to 3 weeks. For recurrent cases, one should also consider acyclovir, valacyclovir, or famciclovir on a long-term daily basis, particularly if herpes simplex virus is proved or strongly suspected to be the etiology.

LUPUS ERYTHEMATOSUS.   The lupus erythematosus (LE) spectrum represents a setting in which CS therapy is generally indicated only for systemic disease manifestations. Vasculitis and bullous LE, as well as widespread disfiguring discoid LE, are the primary cutaneous indications.[75,76] With vasculitis and bullous findings, there is generally underlying systemic disease. Numerous alternatives to CS are available. Antimalarial agents, dapsone, retinoids, thalidomide, and oral gold all are reasonable options for many of the cutaneous findings. Most cutaneous LE cases can be managed with sunscreens, topical or intralesional CS, or antimalarial therapy. Should systemic CS be indicated, doses of 20 mg every other day up to 60 mg/day of prednisone may be required. The dose should be individualized; low-to-moderate doses are favored.

DERMATOMYOSITIS.   Comanagement with either a rheumatologist or a neurologist is appropriate when there is significant muscle disease. In contrast, a number of patients present with purely cutaneous features.[77,78] When indicated, systemic CS therapy is often successful as monotherapy.[78,79] Dermatomyositis is a condition in which very slow tapering of systemic CS over at least 6 to 12 months is in order. Although their efficacy has not been established in controlled trials, systemic CS are generally accepted as the treatment of choice. About 90% of patients respond to a prednisone dose of 1 to 1.5 mg/kg/day. The dose is adjusted on the basis of examination of muscle strength and muscle enzyme levels. Frequently azathioprine or methotrexate is needed as adjunctive therapy for control of muscle involvement. Juvenile dermatomyositis management has been reviewed by Shehata and associates.[80]

Antimalarial agents may improve cutaneous findings as an adjunctive measure. High-potency topical CS and sunscreens are essential components of the cutaneous disease management.

VASCULITIS.   Vasculitis may be the cutaneous manifestation of a large variety of conditions. Palpable purpura from leukocytoclastic vasculitis and persistent urticarial lesions associated with urticarial vasculitis are the most common presentations.[81,82] In both settings, drugs such as colchicine, dapsone, indomethacin, and perhaps antihistamines will frequently control the cutaneous findings. Gastrointestinal, renal, and joint involvement may indicate systemic CS therapy.[83,84] Patients with chronic cutaneous leukocytoclastic vasculitis with ulcers, infarction, or persistent painful lesions may require doses up to 1 mg/kg/day of prednisone. Rapid tapering to alternate-day dosing is suggested; prednisone 20 mg (or less) on alternate days is often successful in maintaining the improvement attained by daily doses. Callen and Ekenstam[85] reported a more than 90% response to relatively low-dose CS therapy in a tertiary care setting. Colchicine is a predictably effective alternative to CS therapy in most cases of chronic cutaneous leukocytoclastic vasculitis.

Patients with more serious types of systemic vasculitis, such as Wegener's granulomatosis and allergic granulomatosis, generally require a multidisciplinary approach.[86,87] Although periarteritis nodosa (PAN) traditionally requires a similar aggressive therapeutic approach, the subset benign cutaneous PAN may respond to relatively low doses of prednisone.[88]

PYODERMA GANGRENOSUM. Although pulse IV methylprednisolone is used for severe cases,[89,90] "bursts" of moderate-dose oral prednisone may initiate improvement in less severe cases.[91,92] Alternatively, dapsone is often successful for mild cases of pyoderma gangrenosum (PG). Azathioprine and related immunosuppressive drugs may be required in refractory cases.[91,92] In general, 40 to 60 mg/day of prednisone, tapered over 1 month to low-dose alternate-day therapy, is successful as initial therapy. Gradual tapering of doses below 20 to 30 mg on alternate days is in order. Periostomal PG following bowel excision for inflammatory bowel disease can be a particularly challenging management problem.[93] Prednisone is frequently used for children with various subsets of PG.[94]

Prednisone therapy initiated at 1 mg/kg/day is useful in quickly attaining disease control in patients for whom dapsone will be used for long-term maintenance therapy. Both drugs are started simultaneously, with prednisone tapered after 1 to 3 months, depending on the rate of disease response. Intralesional CS may be a useful adjunct to the above two systemic drugs.

ACUTE DERMATITIS. Severe acute contact dermatitis due to poison ivy/poison oak is a classic situation in which a 2 to 3 week burst of systemic CS therapy is usually successful at minimal risk.[100] Potential rebound of disease activity due to prednisone courses of less than 10 to 14 days is important to consider. Cases with widespread cutaneous involvement or significant facial involvement treated early in their course typically respond rapidly. Doses up to 1 mg/kg/day (generally 40 to 60 mg/day of prednisone) tapered over 2 to 3 weeks yield adequate improvement with minimal risk of rebound flare after cessation of therapy. A simple approach that is easy for patients to follow uses just 20 mg prednisone tablets. The patient receives 5 days each of 60 mg, 40 mg, and 20 mg. Various "dose packs" of prednisone and methylprednisolone typically do not provide an adequate dose (to quickly attain disease control) for an adequate duration (to avoid a rebound flare).

Acute flares of *chronic* atopic, nummular, or contact dermatitis can be managed in a similar fashion.[101,102] Maintenance CS therapy is best avoided in these settings.

Exfoliative erythroderma management uncommonly requires systemic CS therapy.[103] Given that psoriasis has been excluded, exfoliative erythroderma refractory to aggressive topical management or to phototherapy may respond to prednisone up to 1 mg/kg/day. This dose is tapered rapidly to low-dose alternate-day therapy.

LICHEN PLANUS. A relatively long burst of systemic CS may be indicated at times to minimize the disfiguring hyperpigmentation possible from lichen planus. Prednisone given at 40 to 60 mg/day and tapered over 4 to 6 weeks consistently eradicates or reduces the intensity of generalized lichen planus. Ideally the regimen should reach a physiologic dose range by the end of a month. This use is potentially important for darkly pigmented races in whom pigment incontinence is most notable. Acitretin and psoralen plus ultraviolet A (PUVA) photochemotherapy provide several alternatives to systemic CS use.[104]

Severe oral erosive lichen planus may require judicious low-to-moderate–dose CS therapy.[105-107] Because of the chronicity of therapy required, lower doses of systemic CS are indicated for severe oral erosive lichen planus. Alternatives such as high-potency topical CS gels, intralesional CS therapy, systemic retinoids, and cyclosporine ("swish and spit") all should be considered for patients with oral erosive lichen planus. Lichen planus presenting as desquamative vaginitis is an appropriate indication for even briefer bursts of CS therapy.[108]

SARCOIDOSIS. Cutaneous findings of sarcoidosis alone rarely justify systemic CS therapy. However, these cutaneous lesions predictably respond to such therapy if there is a systemic indication for CS therapy.[109] Ulcerative sarcoidosis or aggressive facial involvement, such as that seen with lupus pernio, may indicate judicious systemic CS therapy.[110] Alternatives to CS include antimalarial agents, low-dose methotrexate, and intralesional CS. Children with cutaneous features of sarcoidosis in addition to systemic findings predictably respond to CS therapy.[111]

ANDROGEN EXCESS SYNDROMES.

For hirsutism and recalcitrant acne vulgaris due to elevated adrenal androgens (most commonly mild DHEA-S elevations), a unique CS approach is often indicated. In these patients, nighttime suppressive therapy with low-dose dexamethasone (below physiologic replacement levels) therapy is predictably successful. Most cases can be controlled with 0.125 to 0.375 mg of dexamethasone at bedtime.[114,115] This timing is important to suppress the early morning peak of ACTH, which stimulates adrenal androgen production. A reasonable approach is to start with dexamethasone 0.125 mg nightly and repeat the laboratory test in 6 to 8 weeks. If the test result has not normalized, dose increases of 0.125 mg up to a maximum of 0.375 mg may be utilized, with follow-up testing 6 to 8 weeks after the dose increment. For a more complete discussion on androgen excess syndromes, see Chapter 19.

POSTHERPETIC NEURALGIA.

Another controversial area of systemic CS therapy is prevention of PHN pain. An early study by Eaglstein[116] suggested that moderate-dose CS could minimize the risk of PHN. A variety of systematic reviews[117-119] and a metaanalysis[120] evaluated various studies that allow several conclusions. The overall incidence of PHN is not reduced by acute therapy with 2 to 3 weeks of prednisone with an initial dose of 40 to 60 mg daily, although acute pain and quality of life measures will commonly improve to a moderate degree. Subsequently, a case-control study[121] and two well-controlled prospective studies[122,123] reached similar conclusions. The latter studies both evaluated acyclovir therapy (with and without CS therapy) versus placebo.[122,123] Similar studies evaluating moderate-dose CS along with valacyclovir or famciclovir would be of tremendous interest, given the much higher drug levels attained by these antiviral drugs.

It is reasonable to treat patients with facial involvement, patients with severe acute pain during the cutaneous eruption, and patients over 60 years of age with combined antiviral and CS therapy, ideally quite early in the disease course. Although disseminated herpes zoster from CS therapy is a theoretic concern, this is a distinctly uncommon complication in patients with normal baseline immunity.

INTRAMUSCULAR CORTICOSTEROID ADMINISTRATION.

Dermatologists have long held widely divergent viewpoints regarding the pros and cons of intramuscular CS therapy. Table 6-7 attempts to summarize both sides of the argument. In addition, the relatively unique complications of intramuscular CS are listed in Box 6-2.

A pivotal point of debate is the effect of intramuscular CS on the HPA axis. Kusama and associates[127] detected suppression up to 3 to 4 weeks after each injection of triamcinolone acetonide as measured by plasma cortisol and urine 17-hydroxycorticosteroids. Mikhail and colleagues[128] studied patients receiving intramuscular triamcinolone acetonide every 6 weeks for 1.5 to 5 years. Roughly half the patients had impaired responses to the insulin hypoglycemia test. Mikhail and coauthors[128] noted that the interval between doses is a more important factor in HPA axis suppression than is the dose. Low-dose intramuscular CS at 2- to 4-week intervals produced greater suppression than did higher doses at 6-week intervals. Using the metyrapone test, Carson and associates[129] found evidence of HPA axis suppression up to 10 months after treatment. Droszcz and colleagues[130] detected abnormal ACTH stimulation in 6 of 48 patients (13%) receiving doses of intramuscular triamcinolone acetonide in 2- to 6-week intervals. In the previously mentioned study, Carson and associates[129] evaluated triamcinolone acetonide, 40 mg given every 3 weeks for four doses. This resulted in anovulatory menstrual cycles in women because of decreased gonadotropin levels.

After these arguments and data are presented, a reasonably balanced viewpoint follows. Serious adverse effects are rare with either a single intramuscular CS injection or a burst of oral prednisone. Rarely do oral bursts, single injections, or long-term use of either form result in adrenal insufficiency of clinical importance. Neither route of administration has an advantage in withdrawal from chronic CS use. It is

◼ **Table 6-7**   Comparison of Oral Versus Intramuscular Corticosteroid Administration[124,125]

Issue	Oral Administration	Intramuscular Administration
Absorption	Reasonably predictable	Highly variable from patient to patient
Compliance	Variable based on patient reliability	Guaranteed that dose is administered
Duration of therapy	Any duration possible	Must utilize short-, intermediate-, and long-acting IM versions
Patient illness affecting dosing	Requires "cooperative" GI tract	Can be given with nausea/vomiting
Patient participation in dosing	Requires active patient participation	Patient in a passive role
Physician level of control	Can vary the doses based on disease and adverse effects	Can be certain the patient received the medication
Reproduces diurnal variation	With AM dosing reproduces somewhat	Constant levels without diurnal variance
Tapering	Precise tapering possible	Gradual tapering as drug metabolized

MC, Mineralocorticoid; *GI,* gastrointestinal.

Box 6-2

Complications Relatively Unique to Intramuscular Corticosteroids[18,124-126]

> **INJECTION SITE COMPLICATIONS**
> Cold abscess
> Subcutaneous fat atrophy
> Crystal deposition
>
> **OTHER ADVERSE EFFECTS**
> Menstrual irregularities
> Purpura (incidence appears to be increased)

important to focus on altering disease precipitators and providing adequately aggressive topical therapy when either oral or intramuscular CS are given. Should repeated intramuscular CS therapy be desired, one should use short-to-intermediate–acting products such as Celestone and Aristocort. When a long-acting form such as Kenalog is used, a reasonable limit would be 3 to 4 injections per year. Each clinician has to make up his or her own mind concerning the relative advantages and disadvantages of intramuscular versus oral CS therapy. As is often the case, the correct answer depends on the clinical situation; neither form has a clear-cut advantage over the other method of administration. The author favors the precision of dosing and the active patient participation that oral CS regimens require for most dermatoses.

PULSE INTRAVENOUS CORTICOSTEROID ADMINISTRATION. Pulse CS therapy has been proposed as a means to rapidly control life-threatening or serious conditions with minimal toxicity, allowing for less aggressive long-term maintenance CS therapy. Typically, 500 to 1000 mg of methylprednisolone (~10 to 15 mg/kg/day) is given intravenously over at least 60 minutes. This dose is repeated on a daily basis for 5 consecutive days. Pulse methylprednisolone is typically administered in an inpatient setting with cardiac monitoring highly recommended. Alternate-day CS or a nonsteroidal immunosuppressive drug is used to maintain the improvement from the pulse IV CS.

Systemic vasculitis and systemic LE are indications for pulse IV CS therapy that are of peripheral interest to the dermatologist. The initial dermatologic use was in the treatment of PG by Johnson and Lazarus in 1982.[89] In a follow-up report, Prystowsky and colleagues[90] described a total of eight patients with PG treated by pulse IV methylprednisolone; six patients responded favorably. Subsequently, several more reports were published documenting favorable response of PG in small case series.[131,132] The most extensive evaluation of pulse IV CS therapy has been for pemphigus vulgaris.[36,37,133] After evaluating six different studies regarding pulse IV CS for pemphigus vulgaris, Roujeau[133] concluded that this modality had comparable results to traditional therapy with 1 to 2 mg/kg/day prednisone as a starting dose, with or without adjunctive immunosuppressive therapy.

The only other significant series of cases for a serious dermatologic indication for pulse IV CS has been for bullous pemphigoid.[134] Eight patients were treated with pulse methylprednisolone therapy, followed by more moderate-dose CS therapy. In seven of the eight patients, blistering decreased within 24 hours. In addition, this therapeutic approach has been used for Sweet's syndrome,[135] urticarial vasculitis,[136] and refractory alopecia areata.[137,138] The results of this aggressive therapy for refractory alopecia areata have been interestingly promising.[137,138] The two key questions regarding use of pulse IV CS for alopecia areata are (1) would the benefits be sustained and (2) would the potential risk be justified for the potential cosmetic and psychosocial benefits to these patients? Further evaluation of these issues is in order before widespread use could be recommended.

Sudden death of presumed cardiac origin is a notable complication of pulse IV CS therapy.[139,140] Atrial fibrillation has been reported as well.[141] Furthermore, anaphylaxis due to pulse IV CS is a potentially life-threatening complication.[142] Acute electrolyte shifts have been postulated to explain the rare cases of sudden cardiac death.[139,140] It is interesting that careful potassium infusions may minimize the risk of these potentially serious cardiac adverse effects.[143] Given that the vast majority of cardiac complications occurred outside of dermatologic settings, some authors question the need for hospitalization and cardiac monitoring for dermatologic purposes.[144] This issue needs very careful study before outpatient administration of pulse IV methylprednisolone or dexametha-

sone can be recommended. Additional adverse effects apparently unique to this mode of CS administration include seizures and acute electrolyte abnormalities.

The suppression of various lymphocyte subsets is greater with pulse CS therapy than with standard doses of oral CS therapy.[18] CS-induced apoptosis likely plays a key role in this effect. In addition, there appears to be a persistent decrease in natural killer (NK) cell activity. Other immunologic effects are qualitatively similar to those of oral administration.

Interest in pulse CS therapy with IV methylprednisolone appears to have leveled off over the past decade. This modality should be used only when the severity of the patient's condition and lack of response to alternative modes of therapy indicate its appropriateness. Pulse IV methylprednisolone therapy should be considered experimental and used very selectively in an individualized fashion.

Adverse Effects

Box 6-3 lists potential adverse effects from the use of systemic CS. Brief bursts of CS for 2 to 3 weeks are surprisingly safe and very useful in self-limiting dermatoses. Box 6-4 lists common adverse effects with prednisone bursts. Lower-dose, long-term regimens at or near replacement (physiologic) levels of CS also are reasonably safe. With supraphysiologic doses longer than 3 to 4 weeks, there is an increased risk for more serious complications. The most serious adverse effects come from chronic use at doses well above replacement (physiologic) levels. Patients with bullous dermatoses, autoimmune connective tissue diseases, vasculitis, and neutrophilic dermatoses all frequently need such chronic, pharmacologic-level doses of CS. Cutaneous adverse effects and proposed underlying mechanisms are listed in Table 6-8.

GENERAL POINTS REGARDING ADVERSE EFFECTS.   Understanding risk factors for corticosteroid adverse effects (Table 6-9) and measures for prevention, diagnosis, and management of important adverse effects (Table 6-10) are essential to maximize safety when prescribing systemic CS. The tables are not intended to be comprehensive; instead the focus is on central issues for the most important CS adverse ef-

Box 6-3

Important Adverse Effects of Systemic Corticosteroids by Category[14-18,145]

HPA AXIS
Steroid withdrawal syndrome
Addisonian crisis

METABOLIC
Glucocorticoid Effects
Hyperglycemia
Increased appetite (and weight)

Mineralocorticoid Effects (Due to Sodium Retention, Potassium Loss)
Hypertension
Congestive heart failure
Excessive weight gain
Hypokalemia

Lipid Effects (↑ Lipolysis and Altered Deposition)
Hypertriglyceridemia
Cushingoid changes

Other Metabolic Effects
Menstrual irregularity (with IM CS)
Hypocalcemia

BONE
Osteoporosis
Osteonecrosis

GASTROINTESTINAL
Peptic ulcer disease
Bowel perforation
Fatty liver changes
Esophageal reflux
Nausea, vomiting

OCULAR
Cataracts
Glaucoma

OCULAR—cont'd
Infections-especially staphylococcal
Refraction changes (from CS-induced hyperglycemia)

PSYCHIATRIC
Psychosis
Agitation or personality change
Depression

NEUROLOGIC
Pseudotumor cerebri
Epidural lipomatosis
Peripheral neuropathy

INFECTIOUS
Tuberculosis reactivation
Opportunistic, deep fungi, others
Prolonged herpesvirus infections

MUSCULAR
Myopathy (with muscle atrophy)

PEDIATRIC
Growth impairment

CUTANEOUS
See Table 6-8

PULSE THERAPY
Electrolyte shifts
Cardiac dysrhythmias
Seizures

OTHER
"Opportunistic" malignancies (see Table 6-11)
Teratogenicity—doubtful

IM, Intramuscular.

Box 6-4

Common Adverse Effects With Prednisone Bursts in Absence of Relative Contraindications

METABOLIC
Increased appetite with weight gain
Fluid retention with edema and possible weight gain

PSYCHIATRIC
Occasional patient may become "wired" or "weird"

PSYCHIATRIC—cont'd
Some patients may become depressed during tapering phase

GASTROINTESTINAL
Mild gastroenteritis symptoms

■ **Table 6-8**   Cutaneous Adverse Effects from Systemic Corticosteroids[14-18,145]

Category	Mechanism	Adverse Effects
Wound healing and related changes	↓ collagen, ground substance; ↓ reepithelialization, angiogenesis	Nonhealing wounds, ulcers, striae, atrophy, telangiectasias
Pilosebaceous	Pityrosporum ovale, androgenicity	"Steroid acne," "steroid rosacea"
Vascular	Catabolic effects on vascular smooth muscle (see above)	Purpura, including actinic purpura
Cutaneous infections	See Table 6-2	Staphylococcal, herpesvirus infections in particular
Hair effects	Uncertain for telogen effluvium	Telogen effluvium, hirsutism
Injectable CS	Lipolysis of subcutaneous fat	Fat atrophy; crystallization of injectable material
Other skin effects	↓ CS immunosuppression (while tapering)	Pustular psoriasis flare, rebound of poison ivy/oak
	Insulin resistance	Acanthosis nigricans

fects from a standpoint of magnitude of risk and frequency of occurrence.

POTENTIALLY FATAL COMPLICATIONS.   It is most unusual to have a fatal outcome when CS are prescribed for dermatologic indications. Drug-induced fatalities in older studies of CS (and other immunosuppressive agents) for pemphigus vulgaris are a noteworthy exception of historical significance. Table 6-11 provides relevant references for the complications of systemic CS that have even a remote potential for a fatal outcome.

PREGNANCY RISK.   Several older studies demonstrated increased teratogenesis in laboratory animals that is due to CS therapy. Cleft lip and cleft palate are the most common specific malformations. Multiple studies in humans of patients with CS-dependent systemic conditions during pregnancy demonstrated no increased risk of congenital malformations.[169] In general, these studies have evaluated the use of CS for conditions for which there is a risk of major maternal complications if systemic CS are withheld during pregnancy. These studies that demonstrated no increased risk of teratogenicity include patients with systemic LE and related connective tissue diseases,[170,171] severe asthma,[172-174] and organ transplantation.[175] As with any drug in pregnancy, CS should be used only when the drug is clearly indicated and the potential ben-

efits far exceed the potential risk to the mother and fetus.

Fetal HPA axis suppression is important to consider, particularly when CS therapy is used near the time of delivery. There may be an increased risk of stillbirth and spontaneous abortion.[18]

OTHER CONDITIONS WITH THE POTENTIAL FOR SERIOUS MORBIDITY.   A number of potentially serious complications of systemic CS (as well as adrenal crisis and immunosuppression carcinogenesis, which were previously discussed) have been reviewed.[14] This monograph included thorough reviews of the following important potential CS complications:

• Osteonecrosis (avascular necrosis, aseptic necrosis)—brief bursts of systemic CS simply do not create a risk for osteonecrosis. The medicolegal implications of this statement are very important. The vast majority of cases in the literature are with pharmacologic doses of prednisone (or comparable doses of other systemic CS) for at least 2 to 3 months for life-threatening conditions.

• Osteoporosis—preventive measures to retard the expected CS-induced bone calcium depletion for any patient receiving pharmacologic doses of CS for at least 1 month are imperative. The hierarchy of options includes calcium (1000 to 1500 mg daily), vitamin D,

■ **Table 6-9**   Risk Factors for Selected Corticosteroid Adverse Effects[14-18,145]

Adverse Effect	Corticosteroid Therapy Factors	Additional Risk Factors
HPA AXIS EFFECTS		
Adrenal crisis	Abrupt cessation of CS (in addition to major stressors)	Major surgery, trauma, or illness; severe gastroenteritis with fluid and electrolyte loss
METABOLIC EFFECTS		
Hyperglycemia	Especially with high CS dose	Family or personal history of DM, obesity; rarely *de novo* DM development (is generally reversible)
Hypertension	CS with high MC effect, therapy over 1 yr, pulse CS	Prior hypertension, elderly patients; rarely occurs with bursts of CS
Congestive heart failure	CS with high MC effect	Prior well- or partially-compensated CHF
Hyperlipidemia	Especially with high CS dose	Caloric/saturated fat excesses, personal or family history of hyperlipidemia, DM, hypothyroidism
Cushingoid changes	CS for at least 2-3 mos	Excessive caloric intake due to increased appetite
BONE EFFECTS		
Growth impairment	Chronic pharmacologic dose CS therapy, ↓↓ with qod	Transplantation or autoimmune condition in children requiring indefinite corticosteroid therapy
Osteoporosis	No decrease with qod CS	Female gender, increased age, thin, inactive patients at highest risk; no doubt men at risk as well
Osteonecrosis	Continuous, pharmacologic CS for at least 2-3 mos	Significant trauma, smoking, alcohol abuse, hypercoagulable conditions, hyperlipidemia
GASTROINTESTINAL EFFECTS		
Bowel perforation	Dose, duration of CS not a key determinant of risk	Recent bowel anastomosis, active diverticulitis
Peptic ulcer disease	Total CS dose of 1 g	Concomitant ASA, NSAID therapy, history of PUD, or autoimmune connective tissue disease
OTHER ADVERSE EFFECTS		
Cataracts	No decrease with qod CS	Baseline lens opacities, older patients, children
Agitation/psychosis	CS at least 40 mg/d; doses above 80 mg/d high risk	Family history of psychosis, baseline high anxiety, female gender (especially day 15-30 of CS course)
Opportunistic infections	Prolonged high CS dose; ↓↓ risk with qod CS	Multidrug immunosuppressive therapy, transplantation patients with foreign antigen present long-term
Myopathy	Possibly from fluorinated CS, rapid CS taper	Lack of exercise

DM, Diabetes mellitus; *MC,* mineralocorticoid; *CHF,* congestive heart failure; *ASA,* acetylsalicylic acid (aspirin); *NSAID,* nonsteroidal antiinflammatory drug; *PUD,* peptic ulcer disease.

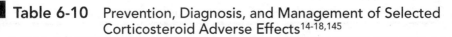 **Table 6-10**   Prevention, Diagnosis, and Management of Selected Corticosteroid Adverse Effects[14-18,145]

Adverse Effect	Prevention*	Diagnosis	Management
HPA AXIS EFFECTS			
CS withdrawal syndrome	Appropriate CS tapering	History (see text)	Raise CS dose, then taper much more slowly
METABOLIC EFFECTS			
Hyperglycemia	Dietary measures	Fasting glucose levels	ADA diet, insulin, OHGA, insulin sensitizers
Hypertension	Sodium restriction, choose CS with low MC effect	Monitor blood pressure; usually mild elevation	Initially sodium restriction, thiazide diuretic
Hyperlipidemia	Low-calorie, low-saturated-fat diet	Triglycerides† (milder cholesterol elevations)	Gemfibrozil, "statins"
Cushingoid changes	Dietary measures, exercise	Examination, weights	Low-calorie diet, exercise
BONE EFFECTS			
Growth impairment	Low single AM dose of CS; qod also helpful	Plotting height and weight on growth chart in kids	If possible taper CS; possibly growth hormone
Osteoporosis	Calcium and vitamin D, physical activity	Serial Dexascans; consider "baseline" by 1-2 mos	Bisphosphonates, nasal calcitonin, estrogens
Osteonecrosis	Avoidance trauma, alcohol excess, smoking	Focal pain in hip, shoulder, or knee; MRI scan is the definitive test	Prompt referral, core decompression, joint replacement
GASTROINTESTINAL EFFECTS			
Bowel perforation	Caution with CS after bowel surgery	CS may mask signs and symptoms of perforation	Prompt surgical referral
Peptic ulcer disease	H_2 antihistamines in higher risk patients	History; upper GI endoscopy	H_2 antihistamines, proton pump inhibitors
OTHER ADVERSE EFFECTS			
Cataracts	Sunglasses may help	Slit-lamp examination every 6-12 mos	If advanced, cataract removal and lens implant
Agitation/psychosis	Careful patient selection if prior psychiatric disorder	History; depression may occur during tapering	Doxepin (if agitation); may need antipsychotics
Myopathy	Exercise, caution with CS tapering after high-dose therapy	Proximal muscle weakness, may have pain; muscle enzymes often normal	Gradual taper of CS dose; exercise especially if muscle atrophy/wasting

OHGA, Oral hypoglycemic agents; *MC*, mineralocorticoid; *MRI*, magnetic resonance imaging; GI, gastrointestinal.
*In each of the above adverse effects, careful dosing is important for prevention; anticipate high-risk patients.
†Particular caution should be exercised with triglyceride levels over 400-500 mg/dl; risk of pancreatitis is very high with levels above 800 mg/dl.

▪ Table 6-11   Corticosteroid Complications That May Rarely Be Fatal

Complication	Comments
Adrenal crisis[7,146-148]	Distinctly uncommon currently perhaps due to heightened awareness, aggressive emergency room or postoperative preventive and therapeutic measures
Bowel perforation[149-152]	Best strategy is prevention; can have catastrophic outcome if late diagnosis
Perforated PUD[153-155]	Typically factors such as NSAIDs, known history of PUD present; gastric ulcer perforation more common than duodenal ulcer perforation
Pancreatitis[156-159]	Primarily a result of triglyceride elevations > 800 mg/dl; possible role of increased viscosity of pancreatic secretions leading to obstruction
Severe hyperglycemia[160,161]	Risk primarily if diabetic ketoacidosis or hyperosmolar nonketotic coma results; overall these complications are rare, perhaps in part due to home glucose monitoring
Opportunistic infections*[162-167]	Strikingly uncommon in dermatologic therapy; greater risk with multidrug immunosuppressive regimens common with organ transplantation
"Opportunistic" malignancies†[14,168]	Primarily with CS in multidrug immunosuppression regimens in transplantation settings; Kaposi's sarcoma may be an exception with CS use alone

PUD, Peptic ulcer disease; *NSAIDs*, nonsteroidal antiinflammatory drugs.
*Opportunistic infections occasionally present in patients receiving CS for inflammatory or autoimmune conditions; include infections due to candidiasis (unusual locations), cryptococcosis, aspergillosis, listeriosis, herpesvirus (widespread), cytomegalovirus, *Pneumocystis carinii*, and strongyloidiasis.
†"Opportunistic" in this case refers to predominantly virus-induced malignancies that are markedly increased with multidrug immunosuppressive regimens most commonly used in transplantation setting, especially non-Hodgkin's lymphomas, Kaposi's sarcoma, and cutaneous/female genitourinary tract squamous cell carcinomas.

bisphosphonates, estrogens, and nasal calcitonin. Bone density assessment with Dexascans revolutionized the surveillance for this important complication.

- Growth impairment in children—rarely an issue for dermatologic indications. Even with CS use in transplantation settings and for serious systemic autoimmune conditions in children, catch-up growth is possible as CS doses reach physiologic levels or below.

HPA Axis Suppression

ADRENAL INSUFFICIENCY DEFINITIONS.
It is important to have a clear set of definitions for the various types of adrenal insufficiency. The three types of adrenal insufficiency are listed in Table 6-12.[12,17] In order for the patient to present with Addison-like symptoms, more than 90% of the cortisol-producing zona fasciculata must be destroyed, reflecting the inherent reserve capacity of the adrenal gland. Note that significant MC reduction (risk for fluid and electrolyte abnormalities) and increased ACTH production (with hyperpigmentation) are noted

only in primary adrenal insufficiency. Furthermore, only in secondary endogenous adrenal insufficiency is there reduction of other tropic hormones such as the gonadotropins (luteinizing hormone, follicle-stimulating hormone), growth hormone, and thyroid-stimulating hormone.

The most important type of adrenal insufficiency for dermatologists to understand is the secondary exogenous type, typically due to systemic CS therapy.[10,19] There is striking individual variability in susceptibility to secondary exogenous adrenal insufficiency. There are no significant MC abnormalities, no increased ACTH production, and no pituitary tropic hormone abnormalities.

HPA AXIS SUPPRESSION OVERVIEW.
It is important to consider the HPA axis as a unit, rather than to simply focus on the adrenal gland.[14] This is because of the importance of the entire HPA axis in stress responses. The hypothalamus is not only the site most susceptible to drug-induced suppression but is also the quickest to recover after cessation of therapy. This re-

■ **Table 6-12**   Major Categories of Adrenal Insufficiency[10,19]

Category	Etiologies	Mineralo-corticoid Levels	ACTH Levels	Pituitary Findings
Primary	Addison's disease	Reduced*	Increased†	No other pituitary findings
Secondary–endogenous	Usually neoplasms of pituitary gland	Normal	Normal	Other pituitary tropic hormones also reduced
Secondary–exogenous	Prolonged, high-dose CS therapy	Normal	Normal	No other pituitary findings

ACTH, Adrenocorticotropic hormone.
*When MC levels are reduced, the patient is at risk for severe hypotension and electrolyte abnormalities; if the levels are normal, fluid/electrolyte abnormalities are not a key component of this type of adrenal insufficiency.
†When ACTH levels are increased, there is a stimulatory effect on melanocytes resulting in hyperpigmentation characteristic of Addison's disease.

covery occurs in most clinical scenarios within 14 to 30 days after cessation of CS therapy. The adrenal gland is more resistant to suppression and, likewise, is slower to recover once CS therapy is stopped. Overall, the hypothalamus is the most important part of the axis in terms of stress responsiveness.

The susceptibility to HPA axis suppression is a function of both dose and duration of CS therapy.[14] Doses significantly exceeding physiologic levels for at least 1 month produce significant laboratory-detectable HPA axis suppression. Divided-dose regimens and single-dose therapy given at a time other than morning increase the risk of suppression. Finally, the longer-acting CS preparations are more likely to produce HPA axis suppression than are short- and intermediate-duration CS.

Minor laboratory-detectable suppression may occur within days of moderate-to-high–dose therapy.[14] This suppression is short-lived and of little clinical importance. Significant HPA axis suppression with physiologic (replacement) doses of CS for a prolonged duration is distinctly uncommon. With long-term, high-dose CS therapy, morning cortisol levels may generally require 6 to 9 months or more to return to normal limits. Some authors report a period of up to 12 to 16 months of increased vulnerability to stress, which is based on impaired ACTH stimulation test production of cortisol.

There is only slight blunting of HPA axis function with off-day testing during prolonged alternate-day therapy. Even though alternate-day therapy lessens the risk of HPA axis suppression, it does not speed the recovery once this suppression occurs. Pulsatile administration of CRF has been shown to speed the rate of recovery from HPA axis suppression.

ALTERNATIVE MEANS OF STRESS RESPONSIVENESS. The direct CS effect in producing elevated blood glucose is much slower than the catecholamine response. Both ACTH and cortisol can indirectly induce rapid glucose elevation through release of epinephrine[14,19] (see Box 6-1).

The MC aldosterone does not play a significant role in the HPA axis stress response. Secondary exogenous adrenal insufficiency from CS therapy typically leaves MC production intact. Thus the risk of hypotension and electrolyte abnormalities is quite low. In addition, through direct and indirect catecholamine, acetylcholine, vasopressin, and serotonin effects, blood glucose responses remain intact. Finally, the hypothalamus' response to stress is typically reversible over 2 to 4 weeks, which makes prolonged supplementation with "stress doses" of CS overall unnecessary.

HPA AXIS TESTS.   Table 6-13 lists primary tests used to evaluate adrenal insufficiency. These tests are uncommonly utilized in derma-

■ **Table 6-13**   Primary Tests Used to Evaluate Adrenal Insufficiency[20,176-178]

Test Name	Basal Versus Stress	Part of HPA Axis Tested	How Test Is Performed	Comments
AM cortisol	Basal	Adrenal gland	Check 8 AM serum cortisol level	Ideally omit CS dose that day
24-hour urine-free cortisol	Basal	Adrenal gland	Simple 24 urine collection, check free cortisol levels	More expensive, more precise test of basal status
ACTH stimulation	Stress	Adrenal gland	Check basal, 30′, and 60′ cortisol levels after ACTH* injection	Most commonly utilized provocative test
Insulin hypoglycemia†	Stress	Entire HPA axis	Levels of cortisol checked after insulin injection	Must have normal ACTH after stimulation test first
Metyrapone†	Stress	Entire HPA axis	11-Deoxycortisol levels measured after metyrapone injection	Must have normal ACTH after stimulation test first
Corticotropin-releasing factor (CRF)†	Stress	Entire HPA axis	Level of cortisol checked after CRF injection	Very expensive; perhaps best test of entire axis

ACTH, Adrenocorticotropic hormone.
*The ACTH form injected cosyntropin (IM or IV) utilizing a 250 μg dose after baseline cortisol determination.
†These tests are cumbersome, have some inherent risk, and require endocrine consultation; the counterpoint is that these are the only tests that evaluate function of the entire HPA axis under stressful conditions.

tologic practice. Nevertheless, clinicians in all fields should be familiar with the various tests, including the strengths and limitations of each test. In particular, one should know whether a given test reflects function of the entire axis or only one particular organ such as the adrenal gland. In addition, it is important whether the test performed examines basal function versus stress responsiveness.

The primary test of basal HPA axis function is that of the morning cortisol level.[20,176-178] The normal peak cortisol value occurs around 8:00 AM, and the trough value occurs in the late afternoon. Current radioimmunoassay techniques are minimally altered by exogenous prednisone, prednisolone, and dexamethasone therapy. Nevertheless, it is generally recommended to omit the morning CS dose on the day that the cortisol level is checked. Cortisol levels generally range from 5 to 30 μg/dl, with levels up to 60 μg/dl with stress. With prolonged therapy,

AM cortisol levels below 10 μg/dl suggest impaired basal HPA axis function.

The reader is referred to several reviews of HPA axis testing for further details for tests listed in Table 6-13. In general, endocrine consultation is required for tests other than basal testing of AM cortisol levels. It is important to reiterate here that the commonly used ACTH stimulation test does not reflect the entire HPA axis. Many physicians, in spite of a normal ACTH stimulation test, still supplement the patients with stress doses of CS. This practice limits the value of the ACTH test, and the morning cortisol alone may be sufficient to at least ascertain adequate basal HPA axis function.

ADRENAL CRISIS AND STEROID WITHDRAWAL SYNDROME.   Given the millions of patients who have received systemic CS therapy since the 1950s, there is a striking paucity of well-documented cases of deaths that were due to acute addisonian crisis.[7,146-148] Such patients exhibit characteristic symptoms of adrenal insufficiency, hypotension, and markedly decreased cortisol levels with no alternative explanations for these findings (Table 6-14). In general, momentous stressors are required to produce vascular collapse due to secondary exogenous adrenal insufficiency. The paucity of serious outcomes is largely explained by the preservation of MC function in (drug-induced) secondary exogenous adrenal insufficiency. Alternative nonsteroidal mechanisms of stress response discussed previously also help sustain sodium and glucose homeostasis in these settings.

Given its much greater incidence, dermatologists should be familiar with a condition known as steroid withdrawal syndrome (SWS).[20,181] In such patients there is no significant change in the serum cortisol level. However, it is postulated that there may be a sudden decrease of CS available at the cellular level. More recent evidence suggests that IL-6 (and to a lesser extent IL-1β and TNF-α) is responsible for much of the symptomatology associated with SWS.[182]

The condition is precipitated by abrupt CS tapering with intermediate- and chronic-duration therapy. At pharmacologic doses beyond 2 to 3 weeks, it is possible to develop SWS. Presenting signs and symptoms include arthralgias and myalgias, mood swings and headache, fatigue and lethargy, and in severe cases, anorexia, nausea, and vomiting. The return to higher CS doses with more gradual tapering will eliminate these symptoms.

STRESS CORTICOSTEROID DOSES. The question of stress CS doses arises primarily with surgery performed on patients who received prolonged pharmacologic levels of CS therapy. Through the effects of anesthesia, surgical trauma, or both, most major surgical procedures stimulate a rise in endogenous cortisol production.[19,20] The regimens are based on the rise of basal cortisol production of about 30 mg/day to a maximum of 300 mg/day with major physical stressors. Typically, the IV form of hydrocortisone (Solu-Cortef) is administered at a dose of 100 mg the night before surgery, perioperatively, and every 8 hours the day of surgery. The dose is decreased by 50% daily until the previous CS dose is reached. Although the risk associated with these stress

---

■ **Table 6-14**   Comparison of Steroid Withdrawal Syndrome Versus Adrenal Crisis Clinical Findings[19,179-181]

Stage and Category	Clinical Findings
STEROID WITHDRAWAL SYNDROME—MILD-TO-MODERATE SEVERITY	
General findings	Fatigue, lethargy
Neuropsychiatric findings	Depression, mood swings, headache
Musculoskeletal findings	Myalgias, arthralgias, flulike symptoms
STEROID WITHDRAWAL SYNDROME—MORE SEVERE	
Gastrointestinal findings	Anorexia, nausea, vomiting, weight loss
ADRENAL (ADDISONIAN) CRISIS (ABOVE FINDINGS PLUS THE FOLLOWING)	
Glucocorticoid deficiency*	Hypoglycemia, although glucose values may be normal
MC deficiency†	Hypotension (including postural), shock, hypokalemia, sodium depletion (may have normal serum sodium levels in spite of total body sodium depletion)

MC, Mineralocorticoid.
*See text for comments on multiple compensatory mechanisms the body utilizes to preserve serum glucose levels.
†Aldosterone production is intact with CS-induced secondary exogenous adrenal insufficiency; there is some MC effect reduction with ↓ endogenous cortisol levels or with abrupt tapering of exogenous CS (typically prednisone).

doses is low, supplementing patients during major surgery beyond 1 to 2 months after cessation of CS therapy is probably unnecessary. Major infections, trauma, and myocardial infarction may require stress doses, as previously outlined.

Minor physical stresses, such as febrile illnesses, can be supplemented at a dose level 2 to 3 times the basal production of endogenous CS. This amount is rapidly tapered back to the dose the patient was taking before the stressful event. This minor stress supplementation is required only for patients taking less than 15 to 20 mg of prednisone per day.

These more traditional approaches have recently been challenged by a wide variety of authors.[183-186] These authors cite data suggesting that replacement doses of systemic CS may suffice with surgical stress and for other nonsurgical physiologic stressors. The final verdict is not in yet; pending a widespread consensus to the contrary, brief courses using stress doses listed previously are safe and prudent.

Drug Interactions

Table 6-15 lists the clinically relevant drug interactions involving systemic CS. There are a relatively small number of potentially serious drug interactions, with very few involving prednisone or prednisolone.

■ **Table 6-15**   Corticosteroid Drug Interactions of Importance[6]

Interacting Drug or Group	Examples and Comments
THESE DRUGS MAY INCREASE THE SERUM LEVELS (AND POTENTIAL TOXICITY) OF VARIOUS CORTICOSTEROIDS	
Azole antifungal agents	Ketoconazole increases levels of various CS, potent CYP 3A4 inhibitor
Macrolide antibacterial agents	Erythromycin > clarithromycin effect on CS levels, CYP 3A4 inhibitors
Sex steroids	Estrogens and oral contraceptives may increase half-life and decrease CS clearance
THESE DRUGS MAY DECREASE THE SERUM LEVELS OR ACTIVITY OF VARIOUS CORTICOSTEROIDS	
Aminoglutethimide	Possible loss of *dexamethasone*-induced adrenal suppression
Anticonvulsants	Phenytoin, phenobarbital, decreased levels of multiple CS, CYP 3A4 inducers
Antituberculous therapy	Rifampin decreases levels of multiple CS, CYP 3A4 inducers
Cholestyramine	May decrease levels of *hydrocortisone*
Ephedrine	May decrease the half-life and increase the clearance of *dexamethasone*
CORTICOSTEROIDS MAY INCREASE THE DRUG LEVELS (AND POTENTIAL TOXICITY) OF THESE DRUGS	
Diuretics—potassium depleting	Hypokalemia potential of the diuretics may be aggravated by CS potassium loss
Immunosuppressants	Cyclosporine in combination with CS is standard in transplantation and for autoimmune disorders; increased toxicity of cyclosporine may occur at times
Inotropic agents	Digitali glycoside risk may be increased by CS-induced hypokalemia
CORTICOSTEROIDS MAY DECREASE THE DRUG LEVELS OR ACTIVITY OF THESE DRUGS	
Antituberculous therapy	Isoniazid levels may be decreased by various CS

Continued

Table 6-15   Corticosteroid Drug Interactions of Importance[6]—cont'd

Interacting Drug or Group	Examples and Comments
CORTICOSTEROIDS MAY DECREASE THE DRUG LEVELS OR ACTIVITY OF THESE DRUGS—cont'd	
Insulin	CS induce state of relative insulin resistance; result is increased blood glucose
Salicylates	Serum levels and efficacy may be decreased
OTHER POTENTIALLY IMPORTANT DRUG INTERACTIONS	
Anticoagulants	CS may increase or decrease warfarin anticoagulant activity; is unpredictable
Xanthine bronchodilators	Alterations in either theophylline or CS activity may occur

Monitoring Guidelines

Table 6-16 lists adverse effects of corticosteroids in which home monitoring by the patient is possible.

Therapeutic Guidelines

INDIVIDUALIZED RISK/BENEFIT ANALYSIS. Any decision to use CS can always be simplified to a risk/benefit ratio. The risks in the equation are specifically the risks of CS for that particular patient. This includes any contraindications present or risk factors that put the patient at increased risk for a specific adverse effect. The anticipated dose and duration of CS therapy are very important in determining these risks.

The benefits of CS therapy are through the reduction or eradication of the potential risk of the disease to be treated. The inherent severity and natural history of the disease, as well as the ability of CS to alter this natural history, are central to the risk/benefit decision. CS therapy is optimal (benefits >> risk) when the disease can be suppressed quickly with minimal toxicity.

In brief, the decision resolves around whether the CS therapy can be given soon enough, at high enough doses, and for a long enough duration to obtain the desired benefits. This is balanced by whether the therapy can be administered at a low enough dose and for a short enough duration to minimize the risks. Box 6-5 contains important principles to maximize the safety of systemic CS.

■ **Table 6-16**   Corticosteroid Adverse Effects That Can Be Home Monitored by Patient

Adverse Effect	Home Monitoring Measure
Hyperglycemia	Home glucose monitoring devices
Hypertension	Home blood pressure cuffs/electronic devices
Fluid overload	Weighing self on bathroom scale
Weight gain	Weighing self on bathroom scale

ACUTE DOSAGE OPTIONS.   Most CS therapy is given as a single oral daily dose in the morning with an intermediate-duration CS such as prednisone. This method most closely approximates the body's own diurnal variation of cortisol production. Divided doses, typically given twice daily, are reserved for acute therapy for severe, life-threatening illnesses such as pemphigus vulgaris. Administration four times daily is generally used with IV methylprednisolone in high-dose therapy (up to 2 to 2.5 mg/kg/day; but not at doses used in pulse therapy) for selected patients with early SJS. When a

Corticosteroid Monitoring Guidelines[14,22]

BASELINE (WHEN ANTICIPATING LONG-TERM CS THERAPY)

Examination

- Blood pressure, weight
- Height and weight plotted on a growth curve (in children)
- Ophthalmoscopic examination for cataracts

Laboratory

- TB screening (strongly consider)—tuberculin skin test, chest x-ray
- Fasting glucose and triglycerides; potassium level

FOLLOW-UP (WITH LONG-TERM CS THERAPY ABOVE PHYSIOLOGIC DOSE LEVELS)

Examination

At 1 month, then at least every 2 to 3 months:

- Blood pressure, weight
- Height and weight plotted on a growth curve (in children)
- Thorough history each visit for adverse effects*

At least every 6 months initially; at least every 12 months long-term

- Ophthalmologic examination for cataracts and glaucoma

Laboratory

At 1 month, then at least every 3 to 4 months while on pharmacologic dose CS

- Potassium levels
- Glucose levels (fasting)
- Triglycerides (fasting)

Near time of cessation of long-term pharmacologic dose CS therapy (optional)

- AM cortisol level (or another suitable test of adrenal function or the entire HPA axis)

PULSE INTRAVENOUS METHYLPREDNISOLONE THERAPY

- Cardiac monitoring
- Daily electrolyte and glucose levels

Note: More frequent surveillance is needed if laboratory values are abnormal or with high-risk patients.

*Many potentially serious musculoskeletal, gastrointestinal, central nervous system, infectious, and ocular adverse effects are detected only by careful attention to patients' symptoms, by examination findings, and by well-directed laboratory or radiologic testing.

Box 6-5

Important Principles to Maximize the Safety of Systemic Corticosteroids in General*

First and foremost, prescribe systemic CS only for *appropriate*, well-documented *indications*.

Thoroughly understand (and use all possible measures to avoid) the most *serious* potential CS *complications*.

Stress thorough *patient education* reinforced by a patient handout, striving to form a true therapeutic partnership.

Match the aggression of CS therapy with *risk* of the *disease* being treated.

Find the *lowest* possible *effective* CS *dose* as soon as possible.

Use a *nonperfectionistic mindset* regarding the completeness of disease control.

Attack (quickly control the disease process), then reasonably quickly *retreat* (taper CS) philosophy.

Seek to attain physiologic or alternate-day doses within 1 to 2 months; if this is not possible (or unlikely to be possible) utilize steroid-sparing therapy.

Steroid-sparing therapy in a broad sense includes *any* topical or systemic *adjunctive therapy* that may allow a reduced CS dose.

Proactively deal with *precipitators* for the disease being treated.

In the presence of a relative contraindication to CS therapy, *medical management* of this contraindication may allow careful CS therapy.

Laboratory *monitoring* particularly for metabolic changes in potassium, glucose, and triglycerides (likewise follow the blood pressure closely).

In general, the proactive, careful clinician will do the following:

Anticipate (risk factors and relative contraindications)

Prevent (be proactive regarding measures to prevent adverse effects)

Diagnose early (monitor labs, home monitoring, and patient awareness)

Manage (should a significant adverse effect occur) potential adverse effects from CS therapy

*See also Chapter 2.

constant total daily dose is given, divided-dose regimens have greater therapeutic benefits than equivalent daily-dose regimens.

The briefer the duration for which CS therapy exceeds physiologic doses, the lower the risk of significant adverse effects. *Brief bursts* (2 to 3 weeks or less), *intermediate duration* (over 3 to 4 weeks up to perhaps 3 to 4 months at most), and *chronic therapy* (indefinite) are the key options regarding therapeutic duration.

Physiologic (replacement) CS therapy is 5 to 7.5 mg/day of prednisone or its equivalent. Pharmacologic dosage ranges at the initiation of therapy include *high dose* (greater than 60 mg/day), *moderate dose* (40 to 60 mg/day), and *low dose* (less than 40 mg/day). Aside from potentially life-threatening dermatoses, such as pemphigus vulgaris and bullous pemphigoid, most dermatologic conditions can be controlled by moderate-to-low–dosage regimens. It is important to determine initially how the disease activity will be followed. Once a desired outcome is achieved, the patient will conclude the acute phase of therapy, and the tapering principles described later in this section should be followed.

PEDIATRIC DOSAGE RANGE. Pediatric patients uncommonly require CS therapy for dermatologic conditions.[188,189] Conditions, such as severe rhus dermatitis, occasionally require a 2- to 3-week burst of CS. Typically, 1 mg/kg/day is initially given; the dose is halved every 4 to 7 days. This approach has no significant effect on growth and is safe for the pediatric patient who has no significant relative contraindications.

CORTICOSTEROID FORMULATION CHOICE. Prednisone is generally the CS of choice for most dermatoses. Prednisone is inexpensive and comes in multiple-dosage options, which allow easy titration of the dose to obtain maximal therapeutic efficacy. The prednisone dosage ranges are reasonably well standardized for most conditions treated. In addition, the prednisone duration of action is optimal for allowing daily or alternate-day therapy. In Europe, prednisolone is commonly used instead of prednisone. Prednisolone requires no metabolic conversion to be active, has a quicker onset of action, and has a greater cortisol-binding globulin affinity compared with prednisone. Drawbacks to prednisolone use include its greater cost and smaller number of dosage options (only 5 mg tablets available).

Overall, MC effect and duration of action are much more important factors in the choice of CS therapy than is the antiinflammatory potency of the product. There is equivalent antiinflammatory efficacy of various preparations at therapeutically equivalent doses. Prednisone and prednisolone share a reasonable profile of MC effect and duration of action in comparison with other alternatives. Lower-potency, short-acting CS, such as hydrocortisone, may not allow for steady day-long control of the disease activity. The MC effect of hydrocortisone is excessive, should fluid retention be deleterious to a specific patient.

TAPERING PRINCIPLES. Box 6-6 contains general principles for successfully and safely tapering systemic corticosteroids. Tapering based on the disease activity is performed to avoid undesirable flare-ups of a previously controlled dermatologic condition. Excessively rapid tapering occasionally allows a marked rebound of disease activity, such as that seen at times with brief (less than 10 to 14 days) courses of CS, therapy of severe poison ivy/poison oak (rhus dermatitis). Identification at the onset of key historic, examination, and laboratory parameters of disease activity is important to guide tapering of therapy.

At pharmacologic doses, it is important to periodically attempt CS tapering to determine the minimal effective dose that a given patient requires. A rough guideline for tapering intermediate-to-chronic–duration CS therapy (greater than 1 month) would be to decrease the dose by 20% to 30% every 1 to 2 weeks as disease activity allows. More serious conditions, such as pemphigus vulgaris, commonly require more gradual tapering at intervals of 3 to 4 weeks or more.

The prednisone dose should be increased to the last effective dose level if a significant disease flare-up occurs during the tapering process. When the daily dose exceeds physiologic levels for more than 1 month, the physician should consider attempting alternate-day therapy.

Nearing the end of long-term high-dose CS therapy, basal HPA function can be determined through an AM cortisol level. A cortisol value above 10 µg/dl ensures adequate basal HPA

Box 6-6

General Principles for Successfully and Safely Tapering Systemic Corticosteroids

TWO MAIN REASONS TO TAPER CS AT ANY TIME

Disease control is a reason to taper CS from beginning of therapy.

Potential for HPA axis suppression becomes important in tapering decisions after 3 to 4 weeks of therapy.

DETERMINATION OF THE MINIMAL EFFECTIVE CS DOSE

Must periodically decrease dose with maintenance therapy until a very mild flare occurs.

At this point, level off dose (ideally) or increase the dose slightly.

DECREMENTS UTILIZED IN TAPERING WITH LONG-TERM, HIGH-DOSE CS THERAPY (roughly 20% to 30% decrements, more gradual decrements with more serious dermatoses)

With high-dose therapy, consolidate to a daily dose first:

100 mg down to 60 mg—20 mg decrements

60 mg down to 20 to 30 mg—10 mg decrements*

20-30 mg down to 10 mg—5 mg decrements

10 mg until off therapy—2.5 mg decrements (consider 1 mg decrements if serious disease, after long-term CS therapy)

RATE OF TAPERING IN GENERAL

Above physiologic CS levels, in general taper more rapidly.

Below physiologic CS levels, in general taper more gradually.

THREE MAIN GOALS OF TAPERING FOR RELATIVELY SHORT-TERM THERAPY

First priority is to be *off* therapy by 2 to 3 weeks.

Otherwise, attempt to reach physiologic CS doses by 3 to 4 weeks.

If the above goals are not reached, change to alternate-day therapy as soon as possible, add steroid-sparing measures, or both.

VARIABLES OF DISEASE BEING TREATED THAT INFLUENCE TAPERING

Serious (potentially life-threatening) disease, taper CS more slowly (longer intervals) and more gradually (smaller decrements)

Self-limited disorders (poison ivy) taper over 2 to 3 weeks.

Various rates of tapering between these two extremes.

*Conversion from 10 to 5 mg decrements reasonable anywhere in range of 20 to 30 mg of prednisone or its equivalent.

function, although stress doses of CS may still be required. Most clinical scenarios do not require this AM cortisol testing.

ALTERNATE-DAY CORTICOSTEROID THERAPY. The conceptual basis for alternate-day therapy is that the antiinflammatory benefits of CS therapy persist longer than HPA axis suppression when intermediate-duration CS therapy, such as prednisone, is used.[4,190,191] During the off day, cell-mediated immunity, white blood cells subset levels, and potassium excretion are all normalized.

Alternate-day CS therapy should be used to maintain disease activity suppression once adequate disease control has been obtained with daily CS therapy. Patients should be aware that

complete suppression of disease activity on the off day may not be possible. However, either small prednisone doses or other nonsteroidal therapeutic measures can be used for minor symptoms during the off day.

Various options for conversion from daily to alternate-day CS therapy are listed in Box 6-7. The risk of cataracts, osteoporosis, and possibly osteonecrosis is not decreased by alternate-day CS therapy. The HPA axis advantages of alternate-day therapy no longer exist once the dose reaches physiologic levels (10 to 15 mg of prednisone on alternate days). If tapering is proceeding quickly, it is reasonable to finish the tapering schedule with alternate-day doses. Otherwise, consider converting back to daily prednisone therapy at 5 mg daily (or less) and

Box 6-7

General Principles for Successful Conversion to Alternate-Day Corticosteroid Therapy

PREREQUISITES BEFORE CONVERSION TO ALTERNATE-DAY THERAPY

Complete or nearly complete disease control has been attained.

Conversion to alternate-day therapy is most likely to succeed when prednisone dose is down to 20 to 30 mg daily (or less).

Conversion only from daily AM doses (not from divided doses).

Intermediate-duration CS, such as prednisone, is essential for alternate-day therapy to succeed.

OPTIONS FOR CONVERSION TO ALTERNATE-DAY THERAPY*

1. Double the prior daily dose for _on_ day, and drop dose for _off_ day (if mild flare occurs or for more serious conditions, consider 2.5 times prior daily dose for _on_ day dose).

OPTIONS FOR CONVERSION TO ALTERNATE-DAY THERAPY—cont'd

2. Gradually increase dose for _on_ day, while decreasing by a similar amount for _off_ day.

3. Keep a constant dose for _on_ day, while gradually decreasing dose for _off_ day.

EXAMPLES FOR THE ABOVE THREE CONVERSION OPTIONS IN MG BY DAY*

1. 20-20-40-0-40-0 (serious dermatoses consider 20-20-50-0)
2. 20-20-25-15-30-10-35-5-40-0†
3. 20-20-20-15-20-10-20-5-20-0†

**Note:* Only options 1 and 2 keep the 2-day total CS dose at least at prior levels before initiating conversion to alternate-day therapy; in general this constant cumulative dose decreases the likelihood of a disease flare.
†For options 2 and 3, the clinician may continue each dosing level for two or more cycles, depending on the severity of the disease treated.

proceeding slowly with subsequent tapering. Some clinicians suggest conversion to the shorter-acting hydrocortisone at this point with unusually long courses of CS.

PATIENT INVOLVEMENT.   Involvement of the patient and the patient's family is important for long-term CS therapy. These individuals should be educated about important adverse effects to report, follow-up visits required, and laboratory tests or special examinations necessary to monitor CS therapy. The patient (and family) should be informed about clinical scenarios that require stress doses of CS. Measures to decrease adverse effects, such as calcium and vitamin D supplements for prevention of osteoporosis, should be discussed. Medic Alert bracelets or an identification card in the wallet should be carried to notify medical personnel of the patient's long-term, pharmacologic dose of CS therapy. Because of the numerous potential adverse effects of CS therapy, the active participation of the patient and the patient's family is of tremendous importance.

Bibliography

Book Chapters

Schimmer BP, Parker KL: Adrenocortical steroids and their synthetic analogs. In Hardman JG, Limbird LE, Molinoff PB, et al: editors: *Goodman and Gilman's the pharmacological basis of therapeutics*, ed 9, New York, 1996, McGraw-Hill, pp 1459-1486.

Wolverton SE: Glucocorticosteroids. In Wolverton SE, Wilkin JK, editors: *Systemic drugs for skin diseases*, Philadelphia, 1991, WB Saunders, pp 86-124.

Adverse Effects Overviews

Baxter JD: Minimizing the side effects of gluco-corticoid therapy. *Adv Intern Med* 35:173-194, 1990.

Gallant C, Kenny P: Oral glucocorticoids and their complications: a review. *J Am Acad Dermatol* 14:161-177, 1986.

Lester RS, Knowles SR, Shear NH: The risks of systemic corticosteroid use. *Dermatol Clin* 16:277-288, 1998.

Nesbitt LT: Minimizing complications from systemic glucocorticosteroid use. *Dermatol Clin* 13:925-937, 1995.

Wolverton SE: Major adverse effects from systemic drugs: defining the risks. *Curr Probl Dermatol* 7:1-40, 1995.

Mechanisms of Action

Boumpas DT, Chrousos GP, Wilder RL, et al: Glu-cocorticoid therapy for immune-mediated diseases: basic and clinical correlates. *Ann Intern Med* 119:1198-1208, 1993.

Feldman SR: The biology and clinical application of systemic glucocorticosteroids. *Curr Probl Dermatol* 4:211-234, 1992.

Pediatric Dermatology Use of Corticosteroids

Lucky AW: Principles of the use of glucocortico-steroids in the growing child. *Pediatr Dermatol* 1:226-235, 1984.

Melo-Gomes JA: Problems related to systemic glucocorticoid therapy in children. *J Rheumatol* 20(suppl 37):35-39, 1993.

References

Introduction and Pharmacology

1. Lester RS: Corticosteroids. *Clin Dermatol* 7 (3):80-97, 1989.

2. Hench PS, Kendall EC, Slocumb CH, et al: Effects of cortisone acetate and pituitary ACTH on rheumatoid arthritis, rheumatic fever, and certain other conditions; study in clinical physiology. *Arch Intern Med* 85:545-556, 1950.

3. Sulzberger MB, Witten VH, Yaffe SN: Cortisone acetate administered orally in dermatologic therapy. *Arch Dermatol Syphilol* 64:573-578, 1951.

4. Reichling GH, Kligman AM: Alternate-day corticosteroid therapy. *Arch Dermatol* 83:980-983, 1961.

5. Schimmer BP, Parker KL: Adrenocortical steroids and their synthetic analogs. In Hardman JG, Limbird LE, Molinoff PB, et al: editors: *Goodman and Gilman's the pharmacological basis of therapeutics,* ed 9, New York, 1996, McGraw-Hill, pp 1459-1486.

6. *CliniSphere 2.0 CD ROM,* St. Louis, June 2000, Facts & Comparisons.

7. Axelrod L: Glucocorticoid therapy. *Medicine* 55:39-65, 1976.

8. Fauci AS, Dale DC, Balow JE: Glucocorti-coid therapy: mechanism of action and clinical considerations. *Ann Intern Med* 84:304-315, 1976.

9. Ziment I: Steroids. *Clin Chest Med* 7:341-354, 1986.

10. Wand GS, Ney RL: Disorders of the hypothalamic-pituitary-adrenal axis. *Clin Endocrinol Metab* 14:33-53, 1985.

Mechanisms of Action

11. Feldman SR: The biology and clinical application of systemic glucocorticosteroids. *Curr Probl Dermatol* 4:211-234, 1992.

12. Boumpas DT, Chrousos GP, Wilder RL, et al: Glucocorticoid therapy for immune-mediated diseases: basic and clinical correlates. *Ann Intern Med* 119:1198-1208, 1993.

13. Barnes PJ: Anti-inflammatory actions of glucocorticoids: molecular mechanisms. *Clin Sci* 94:557-572, 1998.

14. Wolverton SE: Major adverse effects from systemic drugs: defining the risks. *Curr Probl Dermatol* 7:1-40, 1995.

15. Nesbitt LT: Minimizing complications from systemic glucocorticosteroid use. *Dermatol Clin* 13:925-937, 1995.

16. Lester RS, Knowles SR, Shear NH: The risks of systemic corticosteroid use. *Dermatol Clin* 16:277-288, 1998.

17. Baxter JD: Minimizing the side effects of glucocorticoid therapy. *Adv Intern Med* 35:173-194, 1990.

18. Gallant C, Kenny P: Oral glucocorticoids and their complications: a review. *J Am Acad Dermatol* 14:161-177, 1986.

19. Glick M: Glucocorticosteroid replacement therapy: a literature review and suggested replacement therapy. *Oral Surg Oral Med Oral Pathol* 67:614-620, 1989.

20. Krasner AS: Glucocorticoid-induced adrenal insufficiency. *JAMA* 282:671-676, 1999.

21. Werbel SS, Ober KP: Acute adrenal insufficiency. *Endocrinol Metab Clin North Am* 22:303-328, 1993.

22. Wolverton SE: Glucocorticosteroids. In Wolverton SE, Wilkin JK, editors: *Systemic drugs for skin diseases,* Philadelphia, 1991, WB Saunders, pp 86-124.

23. DeRijk R, Sternberg EM: Corticosteroid resistance and disease. *Ann Med* 29:79-82, 1997.

24. Koper JW, Stolk RP, deLange P, et al: Lack of association between five polymorphisms in the human glucocorticoid receptor gene and glucocorticoid resistance. *Hum Genet* 99:663-668, 1997.

25. Lane SJ, Lee TH: Mechanisms of corticosteroid resistance in asthmatic patients. *Int Arch Allergy Immunol* 113:193-195, 1997.

26. Barnes PJ, Karin M: Nuclear factor-kappa B: a pivotal transcription factor in chronic inflammatory diseases. *N Engl J Med* 336:1066-1171, 1997.

27. Scheinman RI, Cogswell PC, Lofquist AK, et al: Role of transcriptional activation of I kappa B alpha in mediation of immunosuppression by glucocorticoids. *Science* 270:283-286, 1995.

28. Karin M, Liu ZG, Zandi E: AP-1 function and regulation. *Curr Opin Cell Biol* 9:240-246, 1997.

29. Foletta VC, Segal DH, Cohen DR: Transcriptional regulation in the immune system: all roads lead to AP-1. *J Leukocyte Biol* 63:139-152, 1998.

30. Ohta K, Yamashita N: Apoptosis of eosinophils and lymphocytes in allergic inflammation. *J Allergy Clin Immunol* 104:14-21, 1999.

31. Scudeletti M, Lanza L, Monaco E, et al: Immune regulatory properties of corticosteroids: prednisone induces apoptosis of human T lymphocytes following the CD3 down-regulation. *Ann N Y Acad Sci* 876:164-179, 1999.

Clinical Use—Pemphigus Spectrum

32. Mourellou O, Chaidemenos GC, Koussidou T, et al: The treatment of pemphigus vulgaris. Experience with 48 patients seen over an 11-year period. *Br J Dermatol* 133:83-87, 1995.

33. Lapidoth M, David M, Ben-Amatai D, et al: The efficacy of combined treatment with prednisone and cyclosporine in patients with pemphigus: preliminary study. *J Am Acad Dermatol* 30:752-757, 1994.

34. Carson PJ, Hameed A, Ahmed AR: Influence of treatment on the clinical course of pemphigus vulgaris. *J Am Acad Dermatol* 34:645-652, 1996.

35. Calebotta A, Saenz AM, Gonzalez F, et al: Pemphigus vulgaris: benefits of tetracycline as adjuvant therapy in a series of 13 patients. *Int J Dermatol* 38:217-221, 1999.

36. Chryssomallis F, Dimitriades A, Chaidemenos GC, et al: Steroid-pulse therapy in pemphigus vulgaris long term follow-up. *Int J Dermatol* 34:438-442, 1995.

37. Werth VP: Treatment of pemphigus vulgaris with brief, high-dose intravenous glucocorticoids. *Arch Dermatol* 132:1435-1439, 1996.

38. Lever WF, White H: Treatment of pemphigus with corticosteroids: results obtained in 46 patients over a period of 11 years. *Arch Dermatol* 87:52-66, 1963.

39. Lever WF, Schaumberg-Lever G: Immunosuppressants and prednisone in pemphigus vulgaris: therapeutic results obtained in 63 patients between 1961 and 1975. *Arch Dermatol* 113:1236-1241, 1977.

40. Rosenburg FR, Sander S, Nelson CT: Pemphigus: a 20-year review of 107 patients treated with corticosteroids. *Arch Dermatol* 112:962-970, 1976.

41. Alsaleh QA, Nanda A, Al-Baghli NM, et al: Pemphigus in Kuwait. *Int J Dermatol* 38:351-356, 1999.

42. Kanwar AJ, Dhar S: Factors responsible for death in patients with pemphigus. *J Dermatol* 21:655-659, 1994.

43. Scully C, Paes De Almeida O, Porter SR, et al: Pemphigus vulgaris: the manifestations and long-term management of 55 patients with oral lesions. *Br J Dermatol* 140:84-89, 1999.

44. David M, Zaidenbaum M, Sandbank M: Juvenile pemphigus vulgaris: a 4- to 19-year follow-up of 4 patients. *Dermatologica* 177:165-169, 1988.

45. Bjarnason B, Flosadottir E: Childhood, neonatal, and stillborn pemphigus vulgaris. *Int J Dermatol* 38:680-688, 1999.

46. Anhalt GJ: Paraneoplastic pemphigus. *Adv Dermatol* 12:77-97, 1997.

Clinical Use—Pemphigoid Spectrum

47. Anhalt GJ, Morrison LH: Pemphigoid: bullous, gestational, and cicatricial. *Curr Probl Dermatol* 1:128-156, 1989.

48. Paul MA, Jorizzo JL, Fleischer AB Jr, et al: Low-dose methotrexate treatment in elderly patients with bullous pemphigoid. *J Am Acad Dermatol* 31:620-625, 1994.

49. Guilamme JC, Vaillant L, Bernard P, et al: Controlled trial of azathioprine and plasma exchange in addition to prednisolone in the treatment of bullous pemphigoid. *Arch Dermatol* 129:49-53, 1993.

50. Roujeau JC, Morel P, Dalle E, et al: Plasma exchange in bullous pemphigoid. *Lancet* 2:468-469, 1984.

51. Schmidt E, Obe K, Brocker EB, et al: Serum levels of autoantibodies to BP180 correlate with disease activity in patients with bullous pemphigoid. *Arch Dermatol* 136:174-178, 2000.

52. Roujeau JC, Lok C, Bastuji-Garin S, et al: High risk of death in elderly patients with extensive bullous pemphigoid. *Arch Dermatol* 134:465-469, 1998.

53. Ahmed AR, Kurgis BS, Rogers RS III: Cicatricial pemphigoid. *J Am Acad Dermatol* 24:987-1001, 1991.

54. Mondino BJ, Brown SI: Immunosuppressive therapy in ocular cicatricial pemphigoid. *Am J Ophthalmol* 96:453-459, 1983.

55. Vincent SD, Lilly GE, Baker KA: Clinical, historic, and therapeutic features of cicatricial pemphigoid. A literature review and open therapeutic trial with corticosteroids. *Oral Surg Oral Med Oral Pathol* 76:453-459, 1993.

56. Elder MJ, Lightman S, Dart JK: Role of cyclophosphamide and high dose steroid in ocular cicatricial pemphigoid. *Br J Ophthalmol* 79:264-266, 1995.

57. Heiligenhaus A, Shore JW, Rubin PA, et al: Long-term results of mucous membrane grafting in ocular cicatricial pemphigoid. Implications for patient selection and surgical considerations. *Ophthalmology* 100:1283-1288, 1993.

58. Lawley TJ, Stingl G, Katz SI: Fetal and maternal risk factors in herpes gestationis. *Arch Dermatol* 114:552-555, 1978.

59. Morrison LH, Anhalt GJ: Herpes gestationis. *J Autoimmun* 4:37-45, 1991.

Clinical Use—Other Autoimmune Bullous Dermatoses

60. Callot-Mellot C, Bodemer C, Caux F, et al: Epidermolysis bullosa acquisita in childhood. *Arch Dermatol* 133:1122-1126, 1997.

61. Mobacken H, Kastrup W, Ljunghall K, et al: Linear IgA dermatosis: a study of ten adult patients. *Acta Derm Venereol* 63:123-128, 1983.

62. Jablonska S: The therapies for linear IgA bullous dermatosis of childhood. *Pediatr Dermatol* 16:415, 1999.

Clinical Use—Stevens-Johnson Syndrome and Toxic Epidermal Necrolysis

63. Rasmussen JE: Toxic epidermal necrolysis: a review of 75 cases in children. *Arch Dermatol* 111:1135-1139, 1975.

64. Kakourou T, Klontza D, Soteropoulou F, et al: Corticosteroid treatment of erythema multiforme major (Stevens-Johnson syndrome) in children. *Eur J Pediatr* 156:90-93, 1997.

65. Cheriyan S, Patterson R, Greenberger PA, et al: The outcome of Stevens-Johnson syndrome treated with corticosteroids. *Allergy Proc* 16:151-155, 1995.

66. Halebian PH, Madden MR, Findlestein JL, et al: Improved burn center survival of patients with toxic epidermal necrolysis managed with corticosteroids. *Ann Surg* 204:504-512, 1986.

67. Kelemen JJ III, Cioffi WG, McManus WF, et al: Burn center care for patients with toxic epidermal necrolysis. *J Am Coll Surg* 180:273-278, 1995.

68. Sheridan RL, Weber JM, Schulz JT, et al: Management of severe toxic epidermal necrolysis in children. *J Burn Care Rehab* 20:497-500, 1999.

69. Murphy JT, Purdue GF, Hunt JL: Toxic epidermal necrolysis. *J Burn Care Rehab* 18:417-420, 1997.

70. Engelhardt SL, Schurr MJ, Helgerson RB: Toxic epidermal necrolysis: an analysis of referral patterns and steroid usage. *J Burn Care Rehab* 18:520-524, 1997.

71. Prendiville JS, Hebert AA, Greenwald MJ, et al: Management of Stevens-Johnson syndrome and toxic epidermal necrolysis in children. *J Pediatr* 115:881-887, 1989.

72. Guibal F, Bastuji-Garin S, Chosidow O, et al: Characteristics of toxic epidermal necrolysis in patients undergoing long-term glucocorticoid therapy. *Arch Dermatol* 131:669-672, 1995.

73. Roujeau JC, Kelly JP, Naldi L, et al: Medication use and the risk of Stevens-Johnson syndrome or toxic epidermal necrolysis. *N Engl J Med* 333:1600-1607, 1995.

74. Bean SF: Diagnosis and management of chronic oral mucosal bullous diseases. *Dermatol Clin* 5:751-760, 1987.

Clinical Use—Connective Tissue Diseases

75. Lee LA, David KM: Cutaneous lupus erythematosus. *Curr Probl Dermatol* 1:165-200, 1989.

76. Callen JP, Klein J: Subacute cutaneous lupus erythematosus. *Arthritis Rheum* 31:1007-1013, 1988.

77. Krain LS: Dermatomyositis in six patients without initial muscle involvement. *Arch Dermatol* 111:241-245, 1975.

78. Callen JP: Dermatomyositis. *Lancet* 355:53-57, 2000.

79. Dawkins MA, Jorizzo JL, Walker FO, et al: Dermatomyositis: a dermatology-based case series. *J Am Acad Dermatol* 38:397-404, 1998.

80. Shehata R, al-Mayouf S, al-Dalaan A, et al: Juvenile dermatomyositis: clinical profile and disease course in 25 patients. *Clin Exp Rheumatol* 17:115-118, 1999.

Clinical Use—Vasculitis and Neutrophilic Dermatoses

81. Chua SH, Lim JT, Ang CB: Cutaneous vasculitis seen at a skin referral center in Singapore. *Singapore Med J* 40:147-150, 1999.

82. Lotti T, Ghersetich I, Comacchi C, et al: Cutaneous small-vessel vasculitis. *J Am Acad Dermatol* 39:667-690, 1998.

83. Saulsbury FT: Henoch-Schonlein purpura in children. Report of 100 patients and review of the literature. *Medicine* 78:395-409, 1999.

84. Martinez-Taboada VM, Blanco R, et al: Clinical features and outcome of 95 patients with hypersensitivity vasculitis. *Am J Med* 102:186-191, 1997.

85. Callen JP, Ekanstam EA: Cutaneous leukocytoclastic vasculitis: clinical experience in 44 patients. *South Med J* 80:848-851, 1987.

86. Fauci AS: Wegener's granulomatosis: prospective clinical and therapeutic experience with 85 patients for 21 years. *Ann Intern Med* 98:76-85, 1983.

87. Guillevin L, Cohen P, Sayraud M, et al: Churg-Strauss syndrome. Clinical study and long-term follow-up of 96 patients. *Medicine* 78:26-37, 1999.

88. Khoo BP, Ng SK: Cutaneous polyarteritis nodosa: a case report and literature review. *Ann Acad Med Singapore* 27:868-872, 1998.

89. Johnson RB, Lazarus GS: Pulse therapy: therapeutic efficacy in the treatment of pyoderma gangrenosum. *Arch Dermatol* 118:76-84, 1982.

90. Prystowski JH, Kahn SN, Lazarus GS: Present status of pyoderma gangrenosum. *Arch Dermatol* 125:57-74, 1989.

91. Chow RK, Ho VC: Treatment of pyoderma gangrenosum. *J Am Acad Dermatol* 34:1047-1060, 1996.

92. Bennett ML, Jackson JM, Jorizzo JL, et al: Pyoderma gangrenosum. A comparison of typical and atypical forms with an emphasis on time of remission. Case review of 86 patients from 2 institutions. *Medicine* 79:37-46, 2000.

93. Cairns BA, Herbst CA, Sartor BR, et al: Periostomal pyoderma gangrenosum and inflammatory bowel disease. *Arch Surg* 129:769-772, 1994.

94. Graham JA, Hansen KK, Rabinowitz LG, et al: Pyoderma gangrenosum in infants and children. *Pediatr Dermatol* 11:10-17, 1994.

95. Jorizzo JL: Behçet's disease: an update based on the 1985 international conference in London. *Arch Dermatol* 122:556-558, 1986.

96. Kaklamani VG, Vaiopoulos G, Kaklamanis PG: Behçet's disease. *Semin Arthritis Rheum* 27:197-217, 1998.

97. MacPhail L: Topical and systemic therapy for recurrent aphthous stomatitis. *Semin Cutan Med Surg* 16:301-307, 1997.

98. Fett DL, Gibson LE, Su WP: Sweet's syndrome: systemic signs and symptoms and associated disorders. *Mayo Clin Proc* 70:234-240, 1995.

99. von den Driesch P: Sweet's syndrome (acute febrile neutrophilic dermatosis). *J Am Acad Dermatol* 31:535-556, 1994.

Clinical Use—Dermatitis and Papulosquamous Dermatoses

100. Baer RL: Poison ivy dermatitis. *Cutis* 46:34-36, 1990.

101. Raimer SS: Managing pediatric atopic dermatitis. *Clin Pediatr* 39:1-14, 2000.

102. Tay YK, Khoo BP, Goh CL: The profile of atopic dermatitis in a tertiary dermatology outpatient clinic in Singapore. *Int J Dermatol* 38:689-692, 1999.

103. Mogavero HS: Exfoliative erythroderma. In Provost TT, Farmer ER, editors: *Current therapy in dermatology-2,* Toronto, 1988, Decker, pp 20-21.

104. Cribier B, Frances C, Chosidow O: Treatment of lichen planus. An evidence-based medicine analysis of efficacy. *Arch Dermatol* 134:1521-1530, 1998.

105. Lozada-Nur F, Miranda C: Oral lichen planus: topical and systemic therapy. *Semin Cutan Med Surg* 16:295-300, 1997.

106. Silverman S Jr, Bahl S: Oral lichen planus update: clinical characteristics, treatment responses, and malignant transformation. *Am J Dent* 10:259-263, 1997.

107. Thorn JJ, Holmstrup P, Rindum J, et al: Course of various clinical forms of oral lichen planus. A prospective study of 611 patients. *J Oral Pathol* 17:213-218, 1988.

108. Edwards L, Friedrich EG: Desquamative vaginitis: lichen planus in disguise. *Obstet Gynecol* 71:832-836, 1988.

Clinical Use—Other Dermatoses

109. Muthiah MM, Macfarlane JT: Current concepts in the management of sarcoidosis. *Drugs* 40:231-237, 1990.

110. Albertini JG, Tyler W, Miller OF III: Ulcerative sarcoidosis. Case report and review of the literature. *Arch Dermatol* 133:215-219, 1997.

111. Milman N, Hoffman AL, Byg KE: Sarcoidosis in children. Epidemiology in Danes, clinical features, diagnosis, treatment and prognosis. *Acta Paediatr* 87:871-878, 1998.

112. Stone JJ, Elpern DJ: Sunburn. In Provost TT, Farmer ER, editors: *Current therapy in dermatology-2,* Toronto, 1988, Decker, p 164.

113. Negro-Alvarez JM, Carreno-Rojo A, Funes-Vera E, et al: Pharmacologic therapy for urticaria. *Allergol Immunopathol* 25:36-51, 1997.

114. Redmond GP, Gidwani GP, Gupta MK, et al: Treatment of androgenic disorders with dexamethasone: dose-response relationship for suppression of dehydroepiandrosterone sulfate. *J Am Acad Dermatol* 22:91-93, 1990.

115. Lucky AW: Hormonal correlates of acne and hirsutism. *Am J Med* 98(1A):89S-94S, 1995.

116. Eaglstein WH, Katz R, Brown JA: The effects of early corticosteroid therapy on the skin eruption and pain of herpes zoster. *JAMA* 211:1681-1683, 1970.

117. Post BT, Philbrick JT: Do corticosteroids prevent post-herpetic neuralgia? *J Am Acad Dermatol* 18:605-610, 1988.

118. Watson CPN: Post-herpetic neuralgia. *Neurol Clin* 7:231-248, 1989.

119. Ernst ME, Santee JA, Klepser TB: Oral corticosteroids for pain associated with herpes zoster. *Ann Pharmacother* 32:1099-1103, 1998.

120. Lycka BA: Postherpetic neuralgia and systemic corticosteroid therapy. Efficacy and safety. *Int J Dermatol* 29:523-527, 1990.

121. Choo PW, Galil K, Donahue JG, et al: Risk factors for postherpetic neuralgia. *Arch Intern Med* 157:1217-1224, 1997.

122. Whitley RJ, Weiss H, Gnann JW Jr, et al: Acyclovir with and without prednisone for the treatment of herpes zoster. A randomized, placebo-controlled trial. *Ann Intern Med* 125:376-383, 1996.

123. Wood MJ, Johnson RW, McKendrick MW, et al: A randomized trial of acyclovir for 7 days or 21 days with and without prednisolone for treatment of acute herpes zoster. *N Engl J Med* 330:896-900, 1994.

Clinical Use—Intramuscular and Intravenous Corticosteroids

124. Storrs FJ: Intramuscular corticosteroids: a second point of view. *J Am Acad Dermatol* 5:600-602, 1981. (Replies by Rees RB, Arnold HL, Mikhail GR, pp 602-606.)

125. Arnold HL: Oral prednisone—an illogical therapy. *Int J Dermatol* 26:286-288, 1987.

126. Olson RK, Woorhees RE, Eitzen HE, et al: Cluster of postinjection abscesses related to corticosteroid injections and use of benzalkonium chloride. *West J Med* 10:143-147, 1999.

127. Kusama M, Sakauchi N, Kumaoka S: Studies of plasma levels and urinary excretion after intramuscular injection of triamcinolone acetonide. *Metabolism* 20:590-596, 1971.

128. Mikhail GR, Sweet LC, Mellinger RC: Parenteral long-acting corticosteroids: effect on hypothalamic-pituitary-adrenal function. *Ann Allergy* 31:337-342, 1973.

129. Carson TE, Daane TA, Lee PA, et al: Effect of intramuscular triamcinolone acetonide on the human ovulatory cycle. *Cutis* 19:633-637, 1977.

130. Droszcz W, Malunowicz E, Lech B, et al: Assessment of adrenocortical function in asthmatic patients on long-term triamcinolone acetonide treatment. *Ann Allergy* 42:41-43, 1979.

131. Pinto GM, Cabecas MA, Riscado M, et al: Pyoderma gangrenosum associated with systemic lupus erythematosus: response to pulse steroid therapy. *J Am Acad Dermatol* 24:818-821, 1991.

132. Resnik BI, Rendon M, Kerdel FA: Successful treatment of aggressive pyoderma gangrenosum with pulse steroids and chlorambucil. *J Am Acad Dermatol* 27:635-636, 1992.

133. Roujeau JC: Pulse glucocorticoid therapy. The "big shot" revisited. *Arch Dermatol* 132:1499-1502, 1996.

134. Siegel J, Eaglstein WH: High-dose methylprednisolone in the treatment of bullous pemphigoid. *Arch Dermatol* 120:1157-1165, 1984.

135. Case JD, Smith SZ, Callen JP: The use of pulse methylprednisolone and chlorambucil in the treatment of Sweet's syndrome. *Cutis* 44:125-129, 1989.

136. Asherson RA, D'Cruz D, Stephens CJ, et al: Urticarial vasculitis in a connective tissue disease clinic: patterns, presentations, and treatment. *Semin Arthritis Rheum* 20:285-296, 1991.

137. Fridli A, Labarthe MP, Engelhardt E, et al: Pulse methylprednisolone therapy for severe alopecia areata: an open prospective study of 45 patients. *J Am Acad Dermatol* 39:597-602, 1998.

138. Kiesch N, Stene JJ, Goens J, et al: Pulse steroid therapy for children's severe alopecia areata? *Dermatology* 194:395-397, 1997.

139. Bocanegra TS, Castaneda MD, Espinoza LR, et al: Sudden death after methylprednisolone pulse therapy. *Ann Intern Med* 95:122, 1981.

140. Baethge BA, Lidsky MD, Goldber JW: A study of adverse effects of high-dose intravenous (pulse) methylprednisolone therapy in patients with rheumatic disease. *Ann Pharmacother* 26:316-320, 1992.

141. McLuckie AE, Savage RW: Atrial fibrillation following pulse methylprednisolone therapy in an adult. *Chest* 104:622-623, 1993.

142. Freedman MD, Shocket AI, Chapel N, et al: Anaphylaxis after intravenous methylprednisolone administration. *JAMA* 245:607-608, 1981.

143. Bonnotte B, Chauffer B, Martin F, et al: Side-effects of high-dose intravenous (pulse) methylprednisolone therapy cured by potassium infusion. *Br J Rheumatol* 37:109, 1998.

144. White KP, Driscoll MS, Rothe MJ, et al: Severe adverse cardiovascular effects of pulse steroid therapy: is continuous cardiac monitoring necessary? *J Am Acad Dermatol* 30:768-773, 1994.

Adverse Effects

145. David DS, Grieco H, Cushman P Jr: Adrenal glucocorticoids after twenty years—A review of their clinically relevant consequences. *J Chron Dis* 22:637-711, 1970.

146. Allanby KD: Deaths associated with steroid-hormone therapy. *Lancet* 1:1104-1110, 1957.

147. Kehlet H, Binder C: Adrenal-cortical function and clinical course during and after surgery in unsupplemented glucocorticoid-treated patients. *Br J Anaesth* 45:1043-1048, 1973.

148. Christy N: Clinical significance of pituitary-adrenal suppression by exogenous corticosteroids. *J Chronic Dis* 26:261-264, 1973.

149. Lauber JS, Abrams HL, Ray MC: Silent bowel perforation occurring during corticosteroid treatment for pemphigus vulgaris. *Cutis* 43:27-28, 1989.

150. Webb PK, Conant MA, Maibach HI: Perforation of the colon in high-dose corticosteroid therapy of pemphigus. *J Am Acad Dermatol* 6:1040-1041, 1982.

151. Myllykangas-Luosujarvi R, Aho K, Isomaki H: Death attributed to antirheumatic medication in a nationwide series of 1666 patients with rheumatoid arthritis who have died. *J Rheumatol* 22:2214-2217, 1995.

152. Weiner HL, Rezai AR, Cooper PR: Sigmoid diverticular perforation in neurosurgical patients receiving high-dose corticosteroids. *Neurosurgery* 33:40-43, 1993.

153. Saag KG, Koehnke R, Caldwell JR, et al: Low dose long-term corticosteroid therapy in rheumatoid arthritis: an analysis of serious adverse events. *Am J Med* 96:115-123, 1994.

154. Dayton MT, Kleckner SC, Brown DK: Peptic ulcer perforation associated with steroid use. *Arch Surg* 122:376-380, 1987.

155. Henry DA, Johnston A, Dobson A, et al: Fatal peptic ulcer complications and the use of non-steroidal anti-inflammatory drugs, aspirin, and corticosteroids. *BMJ* 295:1227-1229, 1987.

156. Hamed I, Lindeman RD, Czerwinski AW: Case report: acute pancreatitis following corticosteroid and azathioprine therapy. *Am J Med Sci* 276:211-219, 1978.

157. Yoshizawa Y, Ogasa S, Izaki S, et al: Corticosteroid-induced pancreatitis in patients with autoimmune bullous disease: case report and prospective study. *Dermatology* 198:304-306, 1999.

158. Guillevin L, Le Thi Huong D, Godeau P, et al: Clinical findings and prognosis of polyarteritis nodosa and Churg-Strauss angiitis: a study in 165 patients. *Br J Rheumatol* 27:258-264, 1988.

159. Keefe M, Munro F: Acute pancreatitis: a fatal complication of treatment of bullous pemphigoid with systemic corticosteroids. *Dermatologica* 179:73-75, 1989.

160. Waer M, Vanrenterghem Y, Roels L, et al: Immunological and clinical observations in diabetic kidney graft recipients pretreated with total-lymphoid irradiation. *Transplantation* 43:371-379, 1987.

161. Yang JY, Cui XL, He XJ: Non-ketotic hyperosmolar coma complicating steroid treatment in childhood nephrosis. *Pediatr Nephrol* 9:621-622, 1995.

162. Wiest PM, Flanigan T, Salata RA, et al: Serious infectious complications of corticosteroid therapy for COPD. *Chest* 95:1180-1184, 1989.

163. Hellmann DB, Petri M, Whiting-O'Keefe Q: Fatal infections in systemic lupus erythematosus: the role of opportunistic organisms. *Medicine* 66:341-348, 1987.

164. Le Thi Huong D, Wechsler B, Piette JC, et al: Pregnancy and its outcome in systemic lupus erythematosus. *QJM* 87:721-729, 1994.

165. Kraus A, Cabral AR, Sifuentes-Osornio J, et al: Listeriosis in patients with connective tissue disease. *J Rheumatol* 21:635-638, 1994.

166. Katz A, Ehrenfeld M, Livneh A, et al: Aspergillosis in systemic lupus erythematosus. *Semin Arthritis Rheum* 26:635-640, 1996.

167. Takeshita T: Bilateral herpes simplex virus keratitis in a patient with pemphigus vulgaris. *Clin Exp Dermatol* 21:291-292, 1996.

168. Qian XC, Huang YZ, Huang RK: Kaposi's sarcoma after steroid therapy for pemphigus foliaceus. *Chinese Med J* 102:647-649, 1989.

169. Fraser FC, Sajoo A: Teratogenic potential of corticosteroids in humans. *Teratology* 51:45-46, 1995.

170. Rayburn WF: Glucocorticoid therapy for rheumatic disease: maternal, fetal, and breast-feeding considerations. *Am J Reprod Immunol* 28:138-140, 1992.

171. Buchanan NM, Khamashta MA, Morton KE, et al: A study of 100 high-risk lupus pregnancies. *Am J Reprod Immunol* 28:192-194, 1992.

172. Stenius-Aarniala B, Piirila P, Teramo KA: Asthma and pregnancy: a prospective study of 198 pregnancies. *Thorax* 43:12-18, 1988.

173. Stenius-Aarniala B, Hedman J, Teramo KA: Acute asthma during pregnancy. *Thorax* 51:411-414, 1996.

174. Schatz M, Zeiger RS, Harden K, et al: The safety of asthma and allergy medications during pregnancy. *J Allergy Clin Immunol* 100:301-306, 1997.

175. Wong KM, Bailey RR, Lynn KL, et al: Pregnancy in renal transplant recipients: the Christchurch experience. *N Z Med J* 108:190-192, 1995.

HPA Axis Suppression

176. Snow K, Jiang NS, Kao PC, et al: Biochemical evaluation of adrenal dysfunction: the laboratory perspective. *Mayo Clin Proc* 67:1055-1065, 1992.

177. Hasinski S: Assessment of adrenal glucocorticoid function. Which tests are appropriate for screening? *Postgrad Med* 104:61-64, 69-72, 1998.

178. Grinspoon SK, Biller BM: Clinical review 62; laboratory assessment adrenal insufficiency. *J Clin Endocrinol Metab* 79:923-931, 1994.

179. Weiss AH: Adrenal suppression after corticosteroid injection of periocular hemangiomas. *Am J Ophthalmol* 107:518-522, 1989.

180. Jacobs TP, Whitlock RT, Edsall J, et al: Addisonian crisis while taking high-dose glucocorticoids. An unusual presentation of primary adrenal failure in two patients with underlying inflammatory diseases. *JAMA* 260:2082-2084, 1988.

181. Kahl L, Medsger TA Jr: Severe arthralgias after wide fluctuations in corticosteroid dosage. *J Rheumatol* 13:1063-1065, 1986.

182. Papanicolaou DA, Tsigos C, Oldfield EH, et al: Acute glucocorticoid deficiency is associated with plasma elevations of interleukin-6; does the latter participate in the symptomatology of the steroid withdrawal syndrome and adrenal insufficiency? *J Clin Endocrinol Metab* 81:2303-2306, 1996.

183. Fabrega AJ, Corwin C, Martin M: Adrenal insufficiency (letter, comment). *N Engl J Med* 336:1105-1107, 1997.

184. Levy A: Perioperative steroid cover (letter). *Lancet* 347:846-847, 1996.

185. Friedman RJ, Schiff CF, Bromberg JS: Use of supplemental steroids in patients having orthopaedic operations. *J Bone Joint Surg Am* 77:1801-1806, 1995.

186. Salem M, Tainsh RE Jr, Bromberg J, et al: Perioperative glucocorticoid coverage. A reassessment 42 years after emergence of a problem. *Ann Surg* 219:416-425, 1994.

Therapeutic Guidelines

187. Lucky AW: Principles of the use of glucocorticosteroids in the growing child. *Pediatr Dermatol* 1:226-235, 1984.

188. Melo-Gomes JA: Problems related to systemic glucocorticoid therapy in children. *J Rheumatol* 20(suppl 37):35-39, 1993.

189. Fauci AS: Alternate-day corticosteroid therapy. *Am J Med* 64:729-731, 1978.

190. Dale DC, Fauci AS, Wolff SM: Alternate-day prednisone: leukocyte kinetics and susceptibility to infection. *N Engl J Med* 291:1154-1158, 1974.

Jeffrey P. Callen
Carol L. Kulp-Shorten
Stephen E. Wolverton

Methotrexate

In 1951, Gubner and colleagues recognized that the folic acid antagonist aminopterin was effective for the treatment of psoriasis.[1] Shortly after this observation, it was recognized that methotrexate (amethopterin), another folic acid antagonist, was also an excellent therapeutic agent for the control of psoriasis. Despite this discovery, it took nearly 20 years for the US Food and Drug Administration (FDA) to approve methotrexate for use in psoriasis, a nonmalignant condition.[2] Only in the late 1980s was rheumatoid arthritis approved as another indication for the use of methotrexate.[3] Despite large numbers of patients who have been treated with methotrexate, there remain many areas of controversy and confusion regarding the indications for and the safety of this chemotherapeutic and immunosuppressive agent. Included among these controversies are the criteria for selection of the psoriatic patient to receive methotrexate, the method of laboratory evaluation, and the role of liver biopsies in surveillance. In this chapter we review the existing data on the pharmacology of, the indications for, and the toxicity of methotrexate.

PHARMACOLOGY
Structure
Methotrexate (4-amino-N^{10}methyl pteroglyglutamic acid) is a potent inhibitor of the enzyme dihydrofolate reductase. It is structurally similar to folic acid, the natural substrate for this enzyme, differing from folic acid in only two areas. The amino group in the 4-carbon position takes the place of a hydroxyl group, and a methyl group at the N^{10} position substitutes for the hydrogen atom (Figure 7-1).

Absorption and Distribution
Methotrexate can be administered orally, intravenously, or intramuscularly. It is rapidly absorbed through the gastrointestinal tract, although peak levels occur more slowly (1 hour after ingestion) through this route than through the other two routes of administration. Although absorption of oral methotrexate may be incomplete and variable with higher doses, this route of administration provides more reliable blood levels than parenteral administration.[4] Concurrent food intake, especially milk-based meals, may decrease bioavailability in children.[5] However, in adults, the drug is unaffected by food.[6] In addition, nonabsorbable antibiotics such as neomycin may reduce the absorption of methotrexate significantly. The drug is well distributed throughout the body except in the brain, penetrating the blood-brain barrier poorly.

Metabolism and Excretion
Once absorbed, the level of methotrexate in the plasma has a triphasic reduction. The first phase occurs rapidly ($\frac{3}{4}$ of an hour) and reflects dis-

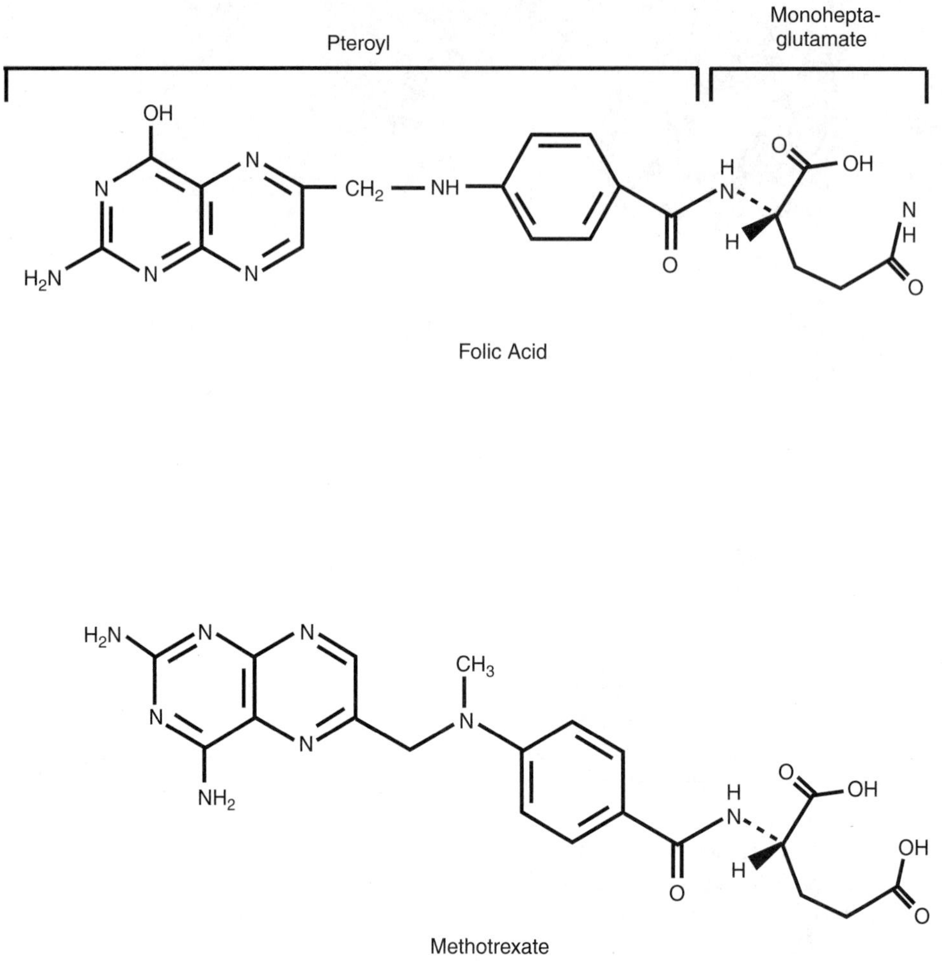

Figure 7-1 Methotrexate and folic acid.

tribution of the drug throughout the body. The second phase of the reduction is represented by renal excretion and occurs over 2 to 4 hours. Methotrexate is a weak organic acid that is excreted predominantly through the kidneys. Therefore glomerular filtration and active tubular secretion are susceptible to drug interactions with other weak acids, such as salicylates, probenecid, and sulfonamides. The third phase represents the terminal half-life and varies between 10 and 27 hours. This phase is thought to reflect a slow release of methotrexate, primarily bound to dihydrofolate reductase, from the tissues.

Approximately 50% of methotrexate is bound to plasma proteins, and the active portion of the drug is the free fraction (unbound) in the plasma. Thus any drug that may increase the unbound portion (e.g., sulfonamides, salicylates, tetracycline, chloramphenicol, sulfonylureas, retinoids, barbiturates, probenecid, and phenytoin) may play a role in the beneficial tissue effects, as well as in the potential for toxicity. Methotrexate is transported into cells actively, rather than entering by diffusion. It was previously thought that methotrexate is not substantially metabolized; however, evidence suggests that the drug is metabolized intracellularly, including by the liver, to polyglutamated forms.[7,8] These metabolites, also potent inhibitors of dihydrofolate reductase, are postulated to play a key role in methotrexate toxicity.

Mechanism of Action
Methotrexate competitively and irreversibly binds to dihydrofolate reductase within 1 hour

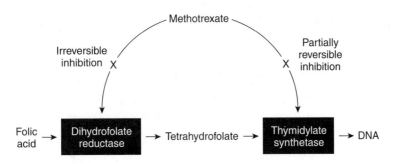

Figure 7-2   Methotrexate mechanism of action diagram.

with a greater affinity than folic acid. This prevents the conversion of dihydrofolate to tetrahydrofolate. Tetrahydrofolate is a necessary cofactor in the production of 1-carbon units, which are critical for the synthesis of thymidylate and purine nucleotides needed for DNA and RNA synthesis. A less rapid, but partially reversible, competitive inhibition of thymidylate synthetase also occurs within 24 hours after administration of methotrexate (Figure 7-2).

Thus the overall effect of methotrexate is inhibition of cell division, being specific for the S phase (DNA synthesis) of the normal cell cycle. The inhibition of dihydrofolate reductase can be bypassed by leucovorin (N^5-formyl-tetrahydrofolate: folinic acid, citrovorum factor) or thymidine. Leucovorin, a fully reduced, functional folate coenzyme, bypasses the reaction catalyzed by dihydrofolate reductase. Thymidine, converted to thymidylate by thymidine kinase, bypasses the reaction catalyzed by thymidylate synthetase. Thus acute hematologic toxicity secondary to methotrexate can be reversed by high doses of folinic acid (leucovorin).

The mechanism of action of methotrexate in psoriasis was originally thought to be due to the suppression of hyperproliferation of keratinocytes. However, Jeffes and colleagues[9] demonstrated that the effect of methotrexate on lymphoid cells is 1000 times more than its effect on human keratinocytes in an in vitro experiment. Thus at concentrations reached in vivo, it is most likely that methotrexate acts via an immunosuppressant mechanism rather than as an antiproliferative agent directed against the keratinocyte.

Methotrexate has activity as an immunosuppressive agent. The effect probably occurs because of inhibition of DNA synthesis in immunologically competent cells. The drug can suppress primary and secondary antibody responses.[10,11] There is no significant effect on delayed type hypersensitivity.

Recent work by Cronstein[12] has shed new light on the apparent paradox that folic acid can inhibit methotrexate-induced gastrointestinal adverse effects and reduce the risk of pancytopenia, without impairing the efficacy of methotrexate. First, methotrexate inhibits AICAR (*aminoimidocarboxyamido-ribonucleotide*) transformylase, a pivotal enzyme in DNA synthesis. The net result of this inhibition is increased local tissue adenosine concentration; adenosine is a potent antiinflammatory mediator. Secondly, methotrexate also inhibits methionine synthetase. This enzyme leads to an increased production of S-adenyl methionine (SAM), a proinflammatory mediator. Reduction of SAM production has a net antiinflammatory effect. Through increased adenosine and decreased SAM, methotrexate has at least two mechanisms for antiinflammatory effects, which are totally independent of the folate metabolic pathway. It is almost certain that further mechanisms for the beneficial effect of methotrexate on various autoimmune and inflammatory dermatoses will be discovered in the foreseeable future.

CLINICAL USE
Indications
Methotrexate is available as a 2.5-mg tablet. Methotrexate is also available in vials of sterile injectable solution, which may be used for intramuscular or intravenous administration (2-ml vials with 2.5 mg/ml and 25 mg/ml available). This agent is approved for use by patients with malignancies, including mycosis fungoides,

along with approval for psoriasis vulgaris[13] and rheumatoid arthritis. However, it is widely used in dermatology practices for other conditions, including bullous disorders, selected collagen vascular disorders, proliferative conditions such as pityriasis rubra pilaris (PRP) and pityriasis lichenoides et varioliformis acuta (PLEVA), and miscellaneous unrelated diseases. It has also been reported to be effective for inflammatory bowel disease[15,16] and asthma.[17,18] See Table 7-1 for indications and contraindications for methotrexate.

FDA-Approved Dermatologic Indication
PSORIASIS.   The major clinical use of methotrexate in dermatologic practice is in the therapy of psoriasis.[13] The selection of the patient for

Table 7-1	Methotrexate Indications and Contraindications

FDA-APPROVED INDICATIONS
Psoriasis[13]
Sézary syndrome[14]

OFF-LABEL USES

Proliferative Dermatoses	**Vasculitis—Neutrophilic Dermatoses**
Pityriasis rubra pilaris[19-21]	Leukocytoclastic vasculitis[33]
Pityriasis lichenoides et varioliformis acuta[22]	Cutaneous polyarteritis nodosa[34]
Reiter's disease[23]	Behçet's disease[34]
	Pyoderma gangrenosum[35,36]
Immunobullous Dermatoses	
Pemphigus vulgaris[24,25]	**Dermatitis**
Bullous pemphigoid[25,26]	Atopic dermatitis[37]
Autoimmune Connective Tissue Diseases	**Other Dermatoses**
Dermatomyositis[28-30]	Sarcoidosis[38-40]
Systemic lupus erythematosus[31]	Keloids[41]
Scleroderma[32]	Lymphomatoid papulosis[42]
	Keratoacanthomas[43]
	Mycosis fungoides[44,45]
	Psoriatic arthritis[46]

CONTRAINDICATIONS[12]	
Absolute	**Relative**
Pregnancy	Unreliable patient—including excessive alcohol
Lactation	intake
	Decreased renal function (dosage must be reduced)
	Metabolic: diabetes mellitus or obesity
	Hepatic disease: abnormal liver function tests, active hepatitis; history of liver disease, cirrhosis
	Severe hematologic abnormalities
	Man or woman contemplating conception (3 months off drug for men, off one ovulatory cycle for women)
	Active infectious disease or history of potentially serious infection that could reactivate (such as tuberculosis)
	Immunodeficiency syndrome: hereditary or acquired

PREGNANCY PRESCRIBING STATUS—CATEGORY X

the initiation of methotrexate therapy should be carefully considered. The benefits and risks of therapy, as well as available alternative therapies, should be discussed fully before its initiation. In general, the patient who is considered to be a methotrexate candidate should have debilitating disease that either is uncontrolled by conventional methods or is not amenable to more conservative therapies. Physicians should consider each patient on an individual basis, taking into account not only the characteristics of the disease, but also the socioeconomic aspects of the individual. For example, it may be impractical for the patient to receive Goeckerman therapy or psoralens plus ultraviolet A (PUVA) therapy because of job-related needs or because the patient may not reside near a phototherapy facility. Similarly, retinoid therapy may be inappropriate because of hyperlipidemia or because the patient may be a woman with childbearing potential. Patients in our practices with recalcitrant psoriasis are presented with the risks and benefits of each of these treatment modalities and participate in the selection of the best therapeutic option for them. Roenigk and colleagues summarized the indications for the use of methotrexate in psoriasis[13] (Box 7-1).

The selection of the patient is made after the relative and absolute contraindications to the drug's use are considered. The only absolute contraindications are pregnancy and lactation (see Table 7-1). The relative contraindications can be waived when the probable benefits of the therapy outweigh the potential risks. In general,

Box 7-1

Indications for Methotrexate Therapy of Psoriasis

- Erythrodermic psoriasis
- Psoriatic arthritis: not responsive to conventional therapy
- Pustular psoriasis: generalized or debilitating localized disease
- Psoriasis that adversely affects ability to maintain employment
- Extensive, severe plaque psoriasis: not responsive to conventional therapy (usually >20% surface involvement)
- Lack of response to phototherapy (PUVA or UVB) or systemic retinoids

75% to 80% of psoriatics treated with methotrexate respond, typically demonstrating an initial response within 1 to 4 weeks. Complete response usually occurs by 2 to 3 months. Specifics regarding dosing and follow-up of the psoriatic patient are addressed in the Monitoring Guidelines and Therapeutic Guidelines sections of this chapter.

Off-Label Uses

OTHER PROLIFERATIVE DISORDERS. Methotrexate has been reported to be useful for several other conditions. Patients with other presumed epidermal proliferative diseases, such as PRP,[19-21] PLEVA,[22] and Reiter's disease,[23] responded favorably to methotrexate. PRP seems to respond less well to methotrexate than does psoriasis. In general, the doses necessary to control PRP are 1.5 to 2 times higher than those necessary for control of psoriasis with a similar amount of involved body surface area. Furthermore, anecdotal reports suggested that for patients with PRP, the drug should be administered on a daily low-dose regimen rather than a weekly basis. An important disadvantage of this daily-dosage regimen in comparison with the same total weekly given over 24 hours is an increased incidence of adverse effects. Methotrexate has only a secondary role in the treatment of this disease with the availability and efficacy of retinoids for PRP (see Chapter 13). Exquisitely small doses of methotrexate (as little as 2.5 to 5 mg weekly) often can be used to control the disease process in patients with PLEVA.[13] Reiter's disease can at times be controlled with methotrexate. For this disease, the doses necessary are slightly higher than the doses for psoriasis, and the drug can be beneficial for both the rheumatologic and the cutaneous aspects.[21] Methotrexate therapy can also improve psoriatic arthritis.

IMMUNOBULLOUS DERMATOSES. Diseases of presumed immunologic origin may also respond to methotrexate. Specifically, bullous diseases, such as pempigus,[24,25] bullous pemphigoid (BP),[25,26] and epidermolysis bullosa acquisita, may respond.[27] Paul and associates[25] have described their experience in elderly patients with BP. These patients are treated cautiously because of the decreased renal function that may be present.

AUTOIMMUNE CONNECTIVE TISSUE DISEASES.   Patients with collagen vascular diseases (autoimmune connective tissue diseases), such as dermatomyositis,[28-30] lupus erythematosus,[31] and scleroderma,[32] can respond well to methotrexate. Methotrexate has been extremely useful to patients with dermatomyositis or polymyositis who either do not respond to corticosteroids or develop corticosteroid-related side effects. The drug is very effective in the control of the muscle disease. In patients with cutaneous dermatomyositis, doses higher than those for psoriasis or rheumatoid arthritis are generally needed. Often, up to 30 to 35 mg per week has been utilized for dermatomyositis patients; however, the average weekly dose we use is 25 mg per week. In dermatomyositis the disease may be quantified. Thus one can objectively measure a response by following the muscle strength or the levels of muscle enzymes. The drug is initiated at an empiric weekly dose while the same dose of corticosteroids is maintained. The onset of noticeable improvement is generally within 4 to 8 weeks. Of the patients treated with methotrexate for dermatomyositis/polymyositis, three fourths will respond, and the dose of systemic corticosteroids can be significantly reduced.

VASCULITIS AND NEUTROPHILIC DERMATOSES.   Systemic vasculitis[33] and cutaneous polyarteritis nodosa[34] have been successfully treated with methotrexate. Neutrophilic dermatoses, such as Behçet's disease,[34] pyoderma gangrenosum,[35,36] and Sweet's syndrome, may benefit from methotrexate therapy. The drug is most often used for these diseases as a means of sparing the patient from chronic high doses of corticosteroids.

OTHER DERMATOSES.   Significant personal experience and some literature experience with methotrexate therapy for recalcitrant atopic dermatitis in adults suggest that this drug is a reasonable backup option for difficult cases.[37] Anecdotal reports suggest that methotrexate is beneficial for patients with cutaneous sarcoidosis,[38-40] keloids,[41] lymphomatoid papulosis,[42] keratoacanthomas,[43] mycosis fungoides,[44,45] Sézary syndrome,[14,45] and psoriatic arthritis.[46] Methotrexate is uncommonly used in children

for various dermatoses.[47] Great caution should be exercised for use in this age group.

SUMMARY.   The use of methotrexate for "off-label" indications (with the exception of dermatomyositis and the neutrophilic dermatoses) has been less rewarding than the use of other immunosuppressive/cytotoxic agents (e.g., azathioprine, cyclophosphamide, cyclosporine, or chlorambucil). In general for dermatomyositis and neutrophilic dermatoses, methotrexate must be used in weekly doses ranging from 25 to 35 mg to achieve control of these diseases.

Adverse Effects

HEPATOTOXICITY.   Hepatotoxicity resulting from long-term use of methotrexate is the most frequent significant problem that must be considered.[13,48] Hepatotoxicity differs in the two large populations in which this drug is used on a long-term basis: patients with psoriasis and patients with rheumatoid arthritis. Perhaps there are differences between the populations that may relate to a hereditary predisposition to liver disease, the rate of alcoholism, or some other factor as yet unidentified. However, over time it has become evident that among patients with rheumatoid arthritis, methotrexate-related liver damage is possible.[49] Although liver function tests may be abnormal in the presence of liver toxicity, they are frequently normal.[50,51] Therefore it is essential to examine the histologic appearance of the liver during long-term therapy. The data on the risk of methotrexate-induced cirrhosis have varied widely, with reported frequencies from 0% to 25%.[13,48] It appears that the risk of liver damage is low for patients whose cumulative dosage is below 1.5 g.[13] Although methotrexate cumulative doses at or above 4.0 g have been traditionally considered particularly risky for liver fibrosis and cirrhosis, recent studies with more careful patient selection to avoid important risk factors (renal insufficiency, diabetes mellitus, obesity, and excessive alcohol intake) demonstrated a much lower incidence of this important complication.[52-54]

The clinical course of the cirrhosis induced by methotrexate is often nonaggressive. In fact, many of the Scandinavian patients in one study continued therapy without a deterioration of their liver histopathology.[55] The patient who has an abnormal liver biopsy may with time experience a reversal of the findings while off therapy.[50,55] Thus it may be possible for that patient to resume methotrexate therapy after a significant period of time off the drug.

A noninvasive test to diagnose methotrexate-induced hepatotoxicity would be ideal. Although hepatic ultrasound may be useful according to one study,[56] other studies reported the inability of ultrasound to discriminate fat from fibrosis.[57,58] Radionuclide scans and the aminopyrine breath test are inadequate to screen for hepatotoxicity that is due to methotrexate.[57,59] The amino-terminus of type III procollagen peptide (PIIINP) is a serum test that may be of value in assessing ongoing hepatic fibrosis.[60,61] The key limitation of PIIINP assessments is the lack of site specificity regarding identifying which organ is undergoing fibrosis; this test is not reliable in patients with significant psoriatic arthritis. Based on these various noninvasive tests, Zachariae made a strong plea to consider using tests such as ultrasound, dynamic radionuclide scans, and the PIIINP assay to at least *reduce* (not eliminate) the number of liver biopsies required for patients on methotrexate therapy.[61]

The liver biopsy remains the gold standard diagnostic test for most accurate diagnosis of methotrexate-induced hepatic fibrosis and cirrhosis. Zachariae's viewpoint is definitely worth investigating further (see section on Monitoring Guidelines and Table 7-4).

PULMONARY TOXICITY.   In rare instances, pulmonary toxicity, such as acute pneumonitis, can occur.[62-67] This pulmonary toxicity is idiosyncratic, can occur with extremely small doses of methotrexate, and can be life-threatening if the methotrexate is not stopped. In addition, some patients develop a more gradual pulmonary toxicity that is manifest by pulmonary fibrosis on chest x-ray. Routine chest x-ray studies and pulmonary function testing are not useful in the detection or prevention of pulmonary toxicity.[64] The great majority of the pulmonary toxicity reports has occurred in patients with rheumatoid arthritis. The prevalence of pulmonary toxicity in up to 5% of these patients has been reported. Methotrexate-induced pneumonitis has infrequently been reported in psoriasis patients.[65] A chest x-ray should be done only if the patient develops symptoms suggesting pneumonitis.

HEMATOLOGIC EFFECTS.   Hematologic toxicity, such as pancytopenia, presents the greatest potential for loss of life due to methotrexate. By far, the greatest amount of data on pancytopenia due to methotrexate is found in the rheumatology literature.[68-72] There are a number of definable risk factors for pancytopenia in these patients that are all essentially avoidable (Table 7-2). There are far fewer reports of pancytopenia in dermatologic patients.[73-75] It is not clear if the risk for pancytopenia in psoriasis is less than the risk for rheumatoid arthritis patients or if the dermatology has been less systematic in collating and reporting this complication. Either way, all clinicians routinely should (1) be vigilant about potential drug interactions with methotrexate, particularly those involving trimethoprim/sulfamethoxazole combinations[76,77] or NSAIDs[78] in combination with methotrexate and (2) supplement methotrexate patients with 1 to 5 mg/day of folic acid (folate), regardless of whether the patient is experiencing nausea or other gastrointestinal (GI) adverse effects.[79,80]

Frequent blood counts are important monitors for bone marrow toxicity.[13] Should significant myelosuppression develop, the patient can be treated with leucovorin (folinic acid), which can bypass the enzyme dihydrofolate reductase and allow normal cell division to resume. This procedure is commonly used for cancer patients treated with much higher methotrexate doses. Macrocytic indices without anemia are common with dermatologic dosage levels.

MALIGNANCY INDUCTION.   With the wider use of methotrexate in collagen vascular diseases, a number of patients with lymphoma have been reported.[81-84] This occurrence has only rarely been reported in patients with psoriasis.[85] Many of the patients have been found to have Epstein-Barr virus within the lymphomas, and many, but not all, demonstrated regression of their lymphoma with cessation of immunosuppressive therapy.[81]

There is no evidence that methotrexate increases the risk of developing a subsequent malignancy in patients with psoriasis.[86,87]

■ **Table 7-2**   Risk Factors for Methotrexate Pancytopenia[68-72]

Risk Factor	Comments
MORE COMMON RISK FACTORS FOR METHOTREXATE PANCYTOPENIA	
Drug interactions	Can occur at any time of methotrexate therapy; especially TMP/SMX and NSAIDs
Renal disease	Even slight increase in creatinine to 1.5-2.0 range an important risk factor
Elderly patients	Vast majority of cases in patients >65-70; largely due to reduced renal function
No folate supplementation	In studies cited, pancytopenia virtually never occurred in patients receiving folate supplementation
LESS COMMON RISK FACTORS FOR METHOTREXATE PANCYTOPENIA	
Daily methotrexate dosing	In current era, primarily inadvertent given unique once weekly normal dosing scheme
First 4-6 wks of therapy	In absence of drug interactions or recent major illness, most cases occur early in therapy
Albumin <3.0 g/dl	Reduced methotrexate protein binding capacity, results in increased free drug levels
Major illnesses	Antecedent infections, major surgery, bleeding episodes a factor in some cases

TMP/SMX, Trimethoprim/sulfamethoxazole; *NSAIDs,* nonsteroidal antiinflammatory drugs.

GASTROINTESTINAL EFFECTS. Nausea and anorexia are adverse reactions to methotrexate that are commonly encountered. Diarrhea, vomiting, and ulcerative stomatitis are less frequently observed. The presence of ulcerative stomatitis or severe diarrhea requires cessation of the methotrexate therapy. Cautious reinstitution after these problems resolve may be considered. Studies in both psoriatic and rheumatoid patients demonstrated that folic acid reduces GI toxicity without compromising the efficacy.[79,80,88] It is intriguing that doses of folic acid up to 50 mg/day have been given to rheumatoid arthritis patients without impairing the efficacy of methotrexate.[80]

REPRODUCTIVE EFFECTS. Methotrexate has long been considered a potent teratogen and abortifacient, but it has far less long-term mutagenic and carcinogenic potential than do the alkylating agents.[13] Recently, however, one systematic review of the literature found the teratogenicity risk to be very small.[89] It remains prudent to be very cautious regarding the complete avoidance of fetal exposure to methotrexate.

Women of childbearing potential who take methotrexate should use reliable birth control. Previously treated patients do not have an increased risk of fetal abnormalities in subsequent pregnancies. Men should be counseled with regard to possible reversible oligospermia and should avoid impregnating a woman while on methotrexate.[90]

RENAL EFFECTS. High-dose therapy (i.e., 50 to 250 mg/m^2 intravenously; dosages used only in chemotherapy for malignant disease) may lead to renal toxicity secondary to precipitation of methotrexate in the renal tubules. This toxicity is not likely to be encountered with low-dose therapy for psoriasis.

OTHER ADVERSE EFFECTS. Other reported adverse reactions to methotrexate include mild alopecia, headaches, fatigue, and dizziness. If these reactions occur, the dose can be lowered or the drug can be stopped. Methotrexate is also thought to be potentially phototoxic.[91,92] It may cause an unusual reaction in which either a recent sunburn is "recalled" or previously irradiated skin develops a toxic reaction with the administration of the drug. Other rare reactions are anaphylaxis,[93] acral erythema,[94] epidermal necrosis,[95] vasculitis,[96] and osteopathy.[97] Recently Morgan and colleagues[98] suggested that increased levels of homocysteine complicate long-term, low-dose methotrexate and can be lowered by concomitant use of folic

■ **Table 7-3**   Methotrexate Drug Interactions[13,99]

Interacting Drug	Mechanism/Comments
DRUGS THAT INCREASE METHOTREXATE DRUG LEVELS AND TOXICITY	
Salicylates	Decreased renal excretion; displacement from plasma proteins
NSAIDs	Decreased renal excretion; displacement from plasma proteins
Sulfonamides (see below)	Decreased renal function; displacement from plasma proteins
Dipyridamole	Increased intracellular accumulation of methotrexate
Probenecid	Increased intracellular accumulation of methotrexate; decreased renal tubular function
Chloramphenicol	Displacement from plasma proteins
Phenothiazines	Displacement from plasma proteins
Phenytoin	Displacement from plasma proteins
Tetracyclines	Displacement from plasma proteins
DRUGS THAT SIMULTANEOUSLY INHIBIT FOLATE METABOLIC PATHWAY— INCREASE HEMATOLOGIC TOXICITY	
Trimethoprim*	Inhibition of dihydrofolate reductase
Sulfonamides*	Inhibition of dihydropteroate synthetase
Dapsone	Inhibition of dihydropteroate synthetase
DRUGS THAT MAY SYNERGISTICALLY INCREASE HEPATOTOXICITY—COMMON TARGET ORGAN	
Systemic retinoids	Common target organ for toxicity—liver
Alcohol	Common target organ for toxicity—liver

NSAIDs, Nonsteroidal antiinflammatory drugs.
*Trimethoprim and sulfamethoxazole in combination (Bactrim, Septra) markedly increase the risk of hematologic toxicity when used with methotrexate due to more complete inhibition of two-step folate metabolic pathway.

acid. Higher levels of homocysteine in the serum have been associated with increased potential for cardiovascular disease.

DRUG INTERACTIONS

Table 7-3 lists drug interactions for methotrexate. It is important to be fully aware of the many well-documented drug interactions involving methotrexate. The patient should be reminded to notify other physicians that he or she is taking methotrexate when a physician is considering adding new medications.

MONITORING GUIDELINES

Before the first dose, a thorough evaluation of the patient should be completed. The pre-

methotrexate evaluation begins with a thorough history and physical examination. This evaluation assists the physician in the identification of patients at increased risk for toxicity. The minimal laboratory evaluation should consist of a complete blood count (CBC) and a platelet count, tests of renal function, liver enzyme determinations, and serologic tests for hepatitis A, B, and C. For patients at risk for acquired immunodeficiency syndrome (AIDS), a human immunodeficiency virus (HIV) antibody determination should be part of the screening.

The type of renal function testing is a critical issue in elderly patients. Methotrexate is excreted by the kidneys, and even subtle abnormalities in the clearance can result in a markedly prolonged half-life of the drug and eventuate in methotrexate toxicity.[100] Thus in patients over 50 years of age, the serum determinations of the blood urea nitrogen and creatinine may not be

Methotrexate Monitoring Guidelines[13]

BASELINE

Examination
- Careful history and physical examination
- Identification of patients at increased risk for toxicity
- Recording concomitant medications that may interact with methotrexate

Laboratory
- CBC and platelet count*
- Liver function tests (especially transaminases)*
- Serologic tests for hepatitis A, B, C antibodies
- Renal function tests: blood urea nitrogen, creatinine†
- HIV testing in patients at risk for AIDS

Liver Biopsy
- Delayed baseline after 3-6 months in most patients—once it is certain that methotrexate is effective, is well tolerated, and will be necessary for long-term therapy

Liver Biopsy—cont'd
- Consider true baseline liver biopsy in higher risk patients (probably best to avoid methotrexate altogether in these higher risk patients)

FOLLOW-UP

Laboratory
- CBC, platelet count and liver function tests*
  Weekly for 2-4 weeks
  5-6 days after dose escalations
  Gradually decrease frequency of tests to every 3-4 months long-term
- Renal function tests (once or twice yearly)†

Liver Biopsy
- After every 1.5-2.0 g total dose for low-risk patients
- After every 1.0 g total dose for higher risk patients
- Every 6 months for patients with grade IIIA liver biopsy changes

Note: More frequent surveillance is needed if laboratory values are abnormal or with high-risk patients.
*Most optimal timing for laboratory tests is 5-6 days after the preceding methotrexate dose.
†Methotrexate is not nephrotoxic at standard dermatologic doses; the risk of other toxicities markedly increases with a reduction of renal function due to any etiology.

sufficient. Reliable measurement of creatinine clearance is often difficult. Therefore Farris and co-workers[101] suggested a means of estimating creatinine clearance based on serum creatinine, weight, age, and gender. The drug should be used much more cautiously in patients with creatinine clearance less than 50 ml/minute.

Liver Biopsy

The need for routine liver biopsy before the initiation of therapy has been questioned. In the largest study to date, in which more than 68,000 consecutive liver biopsies (performed for the full spectrum of liver biopsy indications) were evaluated, six deaths occurred.[102] Of importance is that all six patients who died had advanced cirrhosis or hepatic malignancies. The five largest biopsy series, each for blind percutaneous liver biopsy technique[102-106] and ultrasound-guided liver biopsy technique,[107-111] are analyzed in Table 7-4. As with the Piccinino study, others have documented that the extremely rare fatalities with either technique had a major risk fac-

tor present (portal hypertension, hepatic malignancy, coagulation defects, or acute hepatitis) that is not relevant to patients with psoriasis who are carefully monitored while on methotrexate. A single fatal outcome in these 10 large studies (over 110,000 patients for all biopsy indications) occurred with a premethotrexate liver biopsy using the blind technique.[105] Overall, patients strongly prefer the greater physical comfort and the psychologic reassurance with the ultrasound-guided technique.

On the other hand, deaths due to methotrexate-induced cirrhosis in patients with psoriasis occurred. These deaths may be avoidable with proper surveillance.[112] In addition, a case series was published regarding patients who developed severe cirrhosis and subsequently underwent a liver transplantation after receiving long-term methotrexate in the absence of liver biopsy surveillance.[113]

There are many situations in which pretreatment liver biopsy may not be necessary. Not all patients with psoriasis improve with methotrex-

■ **Table 7-4**   Major Liver Biopsy Studies: Fatal Complications—Blind versus Ultrasound-Guided Liver Biopsies*

Author	Study Year	Biopsy #	Deaths	Deaths-Baseline MTX Biopsy	Deaths (A)	Deaths (B)	Deaths (C)	Deaths (D)	Deaths (E)
BLIND LIVER BIOPSIES									
Piccicino[102]	1986	68,276	6	None	3	3	—	—	—
Wildhirt[103]	1981	19,563	0	None	—	—	—	—	—
Van Thiel[104]	1993	12,695	0	None	—	—	—	—	—
McGill[105]	1990	9212	10	1	1	6	—	—	2
Sherlock[106]	1985	6379	2	None	—	—	—	1	1
ULTRASOUND-GUIDED LIVER BIOPSIES									
Lang[107]	1999	3670	0	None	—	—	—	—	—
Buscarini[108]	1990	2091	0	None	—	—	—	—	—
Drinkovic[109]	1996	1750	2	None	—	1	1	—	—
Columbo[110]	1988	1192	0	None	—	—	—	—	—
Bret[111]	1988	1060	1	None	—	—	1	—	—

A, Biopsy deaths attributed to cirrhosis and portal hypertension; B, biopsy deaths attributed to liver metastases; C, biopsy deaths attributed to primary hepatic carcinoma; D, biopsy deaths attributed to a coagulation defect; E, biopsy deaths attributed to acute hepatitis.
*Five largest studies evaluating each liver biopsy technique.

ate. Furthermore, some patients cannot tolerate the drug even in small doses. In these instances, performing a pretreatment liver biopsy has placed the patient at risk without any foreseeable benefit. Therefore many physicians are postponing the initial biopsy until the third to sixth month of therapy for patients with potential liver disease, or to a cumulative dose of 1500 mg in otherwise healthy patients with psoriasis with normal liver function testing. It is still imperative that a full discussion with the patient takes place so that the patient understands that a biopsy will be needed at some time in the near future. An advantage of a premethotrexate liver biopsy is that it impresses on patients the serious nature of the agent with which they are about to be treated.

There are several other instances in which a premethotrexate liver biopsy is necessary. For patients with a personal or familial history of liver disease, a liver biopsy before therapy is helpful. Similarly, for those patients with a history of exposure to known hepatotoxins, including alcohol or intravenous drugs, liver histology is important. Patients with diabetes or obesity are presumed to be at greater risk for liver toxicity, and pretreatment biopsies are deemed necessary. Finally, in patients with abnormal baseline liver function tests or serologic tests for hepatitis, a liver biopsy before receiving the first dose of methotrexate is usually recommended. It is quite reasonable to strongly consider avoiding methotrexate therapy altogether in the patients mentioned here, given the significantly increased risk of hepatotoxicity in these patient populations.

Current dermatology guidelines offer the option of waiting until 1 to 1.5 g cumulative methotrexate dose before performing a "baseline" liver biopsy.[13] From references cited in these current guidelines, a substantial portion of all psoriasis patients who developed cirrhosis had full-blown cirrhosis present at the 1.5 g cumulative dose (frequently with completely normal "liver function tests"). We still believe that the delayed "baseline" liver biopsy, performed routinely 3 to 6 months into the methotrexate course for lower risk patients, is a prudent standard of care.

The need for repeated liver biopsies is based on the total dose taken by the patient.[13]

■ **Table 7-5**   Classification of Liver Biopsy Findings

Biopsy Grade	Liver Histopathologic Findings
I	Normal; fatty infiltration—mild; portal inflammation—mild
II	Fatty infiltration—moderate-to-severe; portal inflammation—moderate-to-severe
IIIA	Fibrosis—mild
IIIB	Fibrosis—moderate-to-severe
IV	Cirrhosis

Adapted from Roenigk HH Jr, Auerbach R, Maibach HI, et al: *J Am Acad Dermatol* 19:145-156, 1988.

The cumulative dose should be periodically calculated and recorded in the patient's medical record to more effectively deal with the discussion of the need for a liver biopsy. In general, a liver biopsy is repeated after every 1 to 1.5 g total dose. The time needed to reach this level of intake varies, depending on the weekly dose. Continuation or discontinuation of methotrexate is based on liver biopsy findings (Table 7-5). The following recommendations have been proposed by Roenigk and colleagues[13]:

1. Patients with grade I or II changes may continue to receive methotrexate therapy.
2. Patients with grade IIIA changes may continue to receive methotrexate therapy but should have another liver biopsy after approximately 6 months of continuous therapy.
3. Patients with grades IIIB and IV should not be given further methotrexate except under exceptional circumstances with careful follow-up of liver biopsies.

The discrimination of grade IIIA versus grade IIIB changes is somewhat subjective, despite the impact on the decision-making process. Equally important is the trend of histologic changes when previous liver biopsies are compared.

Laboratory Monitoring

The patient should be monitored closely with frequent CBCs, liver function panels, and serum creatinine measurements during the initial phase of therapy, regardless of the disease for which methotrexate is being used. If the white blood cell count (WBC) is less than 3500/mm^3, the platelet count is less than 100,000/mm^3, or there is an increase over twice the upper normal value for liver transaminase levels, discontinue or reduce the dosage of methotrexate. The drug may be restarted at a lower dose after a 2- to 3-week rest period, if the laboratory abnormality has resolved. After the first month of therapy, this laboratory monitoring can be gradually reduced in frequency to a range of every 3 to 4 months.

More frequent monitoring is necessary if the dose is being escalated, if there is an intercurrent illness, or if additional systemic therapy with other drugs is begun. This is particularly important if the additional drug (such as acitretin) has an inherent potential for liver toxicity.

Published guidelines recommend hematologic laboratory follow-up every month.[13] In practice, it is rare to develop an abnormal WBC or platelet count after the first few months of therapy on a constant or tapering methotrexate dose. An exception is the potential risk for pancytopenia to occur at any stage of therapy, when potential drug interactions are not recognized. The potential risk is greatest with the addition of either trimethoprim-sulfamethoxazole or a nonsteroidal antiinflammatory drug to a patient already receiving a full dose of methotrexate.[76-78] Furthermore, late hematologic complications occasionally occur due to patient errors, in which methotrexate is inadvertently taken on a daily basis.[104]

THERAPEUTIC GUIDELINES

Once the decision has been made to administer methotrexate, the next step is to decide on the dosage and the route of administration. For patients with psoriasis, oral weekly doses are usually effective and reasonably well tolerated. An occasional patient who is poorly compliant may be treated with weekly intramuscular methotrexate, as may the patient who develops nausea from oral but not parenteral administration. There are two methods of weekly administration of oral methotrexate: a single weekly dose and three divided doses over a 24-hour period each week. The divided-dose regimen consists of taking the medication on a schedule such as 8 AM and 8 PM on the first day and 8 AM on the second day; with the development of the dose pack, sold under the trade name Rheumatrex (three of the 2.5 mg tablets per dose pack), this schedule may be easier to explain. The rationale behind this schedule relates to the presumed cell cycle kinetics in psoriasis. However, the two methods of administration are equally effective and have similar toxicity. Given the simplicity of a single weekly dose, with all other issues equal, this would be the most logical dosing scheme. Either way, the patient should always be reminded to carefully adhere to the unique weekly schedule of methotrexate administration (whether the physician is utilizing a single-dose or three-dose regimen). Major hematologic complications of inadvertent daily methotrexate dosing are almost inevitable.[114]

The initial dose should be fairly conservative to prevent myelosuppression. In general, a test dose of 5 to 10 mg is given, and a CBC and liver function tests are taken 7 days later. The dose is gradually escalated (2.5 to 5 mg/week) to a level that provides reasonable benefit without noticeable toxicity. Patients receiving intramuscular or intravenous methotrexate are able to tolerate higher doses because of more rapid renal clearance. One can measure the response to the drug by quantifying the area of surface involvement or by evaluating the characteristics of an individual lesion such as a scale, erythema, or elevation. In general, patients with psoriasis are able to achieve benefits at 10 to 15 mg/week. The total weekly dose rarely exceeds 30 mg. When maximal benefit is reached, the methotrexate may be tapered by 2.5 mg/week to determine the lowest possible dosage that provides disease control. For patients treated with intramuscular methotrexate, it may be more convenient to taper by increasing the interval between doses to 2 weeks or more. The dosage and the schedule of administration for other disorders may differ from those recommended for psoriasis. These differences have been discussed previously.

Bibliography

Pharmacology

Cronstein BN: The mechanism of action of methotrexate. *Rheum Dis Clin North Am* 23:739-755, 1997.

Olson EA: The pharmacology of methotrexate. *J Am Acad Dermatol* 25:300-318, 1993.

Dermatology Guidelines

Roenigk HH Jr, Auerbach R, Maibach HI, et al: Methotrexate in psoriasis: consensus conference. *J Am Acad Dermatol* 38:478-485, 1998.

Zachariae H: Liver biopsies and methotrexate: a time for reconsideration. *J Am Acad Dermatol* 42:531-534, 2000.

Adverse Effects Overviews

Ahern MJ, Smith MD, Roberts-Thomson PJ: Methotrexate hepatotoxicity: what is the evidence? *Inflam Res* 47:148-151, 1998.

Cleach LL, Bocquet, Roujeau JC: Reactions and interactions of some commonly used systemic drugs in dermatology. *Dermatol Clin* 16:421-429, 1998.

van Ede AE, Laan, RFJM, Blom H, et al: Methotrexate in rheumatoid arthritis: an update with focus on mechanisms involved in toxicity. *Semin Arthritis Rheum* 27:277-292, 1998.

Wolverton SE: Major adverse effects from systemic drugs: defining the risks. *Curr Prob Dermatol* 7:1-40, 1995.

Rheumatology Viewpoint

Anonymous: Guideline for methotrexate drug therapy in rheumatoid arthritis. *Arthritis Rheum* 39:723-731, 1996.

Special Patient Groups—Children and Pregnant Women

Kallen B: The teratogenicity of antirheumatic drugs—what is the evidence? *Scand J Rheumatol* 107:119-124, 1998.

Paller AS: Dermatologic use of methotrexate in children. *Pediatr Dermatol* 2:238-243, 1985.

References

Introduction and Pharmacology

1. Gubner R, August S, Ginsberg V: Therapeutic suppression of tissue reactivity: effect of aminopterin in rheumatoid arthritis and psoriasis. *Am J Med Sci* 221:176-182, 1951.
2. Weinstein GD: Methotrexate. *Ann Intern Med* 86:199-204, 1977.
3. Healy LA: The current status of methotrexate use in rheumatoid disease. *Bull Rheum Dis* 35:1-10, 1986.
4. Balis FM, Savitch JL, Bleyer WA: Pharmacokinetics of oral methotrexate in children. *Cancer Res* 43:2242-2245, 1983.
5. Dupuis LL, Koren G, Silverman ED, et al: Influence of food on the bioavailability of oral methotrexate in children. *J Rheumatol* 22:1570-1573, 1995.
6. Hamilton RA, Kremer JM: The effects of food on methotrexate absorption. *J Rheumatol* 22:630-632, 1995.
7. Galivan J, Pupons A, Rhee M: Hepatic parenchymal cell glutamylation of methotrexate studied in monolayer culture. *Cancer Res* 46:670-675, 1986.
8. Kamen BA, Nylen PA, Camitta DM, et al: Methotrexate accumulation in cells as a possible mechanism of chronic toxicity to the drug. *Br J Haematol* 49:355-360, 1981.
9. Jeffes EWB III, McCullough JL, Pittelkow MR, et al: Methotrexate therapy of psoriasis. Differential sensitivity of proliferating lymphoid and epithelial cells to the cytotoxic and growth-inhibitory effects of methotrexate. *J Invest Dermatol* 104:183-188, 1995.
10. Hersh EM, Carbone PP, Wond VG, et al: Inhibition of primary immune response in man by antimetabolites. *Cancer Res* 25:1997-2001, 1965.
11. Mitchells MS, Wade ME, DeCenti RC, et al: Immune suppressive effects of cytosine arabinoside and methotrexate in man. *Ann Intern Med* 70:535-547, 1969.
12. Cronstein BN: The mechanism of action of methotrexate. *Rheum Dis Clin North Am* 23:739-755, 1997.

Clinical Use—Approved Indications

13. Roenigk HH, Auerbach R, Maibach HI, et al: Methotrexate in psoriasis: revised guidelines. *J Am Acad Dermatol* 38:478-485, 1998.

14. Zackheim HS, Epstein EH Jr: Low-dose methotrexate for the Sézary syndrome. *J Am Acad Dermatol* 21:757-762, 1989.

Indications—Medical Indications

15. Feagan BFG, Rochon J, Fedorak RN, et al: Methotrexate for the treatment of Crohn's disease. *N Engl J Med* 332:292-297, 1995.
16. Kozarek RA, Patterson DJ, Gelfand MD, et al: Methotrexate induced clinical and histologic remission in patients with refractory inflammatory bowel disease. *Ann Intern Med* 110:353-356, 1989.
17. Shiner RJ, Numm AJ, Chung KF, et al: Randomized, double-blind, placebo-controlled trial of methotrexate in steroid-dependent asthma. *Lancet* 336:137-140, 1990.
18. Mullarkey MF, Lammert JK, Blumenstein BA: Long-term methotrexate treatment in corticosteroid-dependent asthma. *Ann Intern Med* 112:577-581, 1990.

Indications—Proliferative Dermatoses

19. Borrie P: Pityriasis rubra pilaris treated with methotrexate. *Arch Dermatol* 79:115-116, 1967.
20. Knowles WR, Chernosky ME: Pityriasis rubra pilaris: prolonged treatment with methotrexate. *Arch Dermatol* 102:603-612, 1970.
21. Hanke CW, Steck WD: Childhood-onset pityriasis rubra pilaris treated with methotrexate administered intravenously. *Cleve Clin Quart* 50:201-203, 1983.
22. Cornelison RL, Knox JM, Everett MA: Methotrexate for the treatment of Mucha-Habermann disease. *Arch Dermatol* 106:507-508, 1972.
23. Lally EV, Ho G Jr: A review of methotrexate therapy in Reiter syndrome. *Semin Arthritis Rheum* 15:139-145, 1985.

Indications—Bullous Dermatoses

24. Lever WF, Schaumburg-Lever G: Immunosuppressants and prednisone in pemphigus vulgaris. *Arch Dermatol* 13:1236-1241, 1977.
25. Levene GM: The treatment of pemphigus and pemphigoid. *Clin Exp Dermatol* 7:643-652, 1982.
26. Paul MA, Jorizzo JL, Fleischer AB Jr, et al: Low-dose methotrexate treatment in elderly patients with bullous pemphigoid. *J Am Acad Dermatol* 31:620-625, 1994.

27. Gammon WR, Briggaman RA, Wheeler CE Jr: Epidermolysis bullosa acquisita presenting as an inflammatory bullous disease. *J Am Acad Dermatol* 7:382-387, 1982.

Indications—Autoimmune Connective Tissue Diseases

28. Metzer AL, Bohan A, Goldberg LS, et al: Polymyositis and dermatomyositis: combined methotrexate and corticosteroid therapy. *Ann Intern Med* 81:182-189, 1974.
29. Giannini M, Callen JP: Treatment of dermatomyositis with methotrexate and prednisone. *Arch Dermatol* 115:1251-1252, 1979.
30. Kasteler JS, Callen JP: Low-dose methotrexate administered weekly is an effective corticosteroid-sparing agent for the treatment of cutaneous manifestations of dermatomyositis. *J Am Acad Dermatol* 36:67-71, 1997.
31. Rothenberg FJ, Graziano FM, Grandone JT, et al: The use of methotrexate in steroid-resistant systemic lupus erythematosus. *Arthritis Rheum* 31:612-615, 1988.
32. Wallace CA: The use of methotrexate in childhood rheumatic diseases. *Arthritis Rheum* 41:381-391, 1998.

Vasculitis and Neutrophilic Dermatoses

33. Langford CA, Sneller MC, Hoffman GS: Methotrexate use in systemic vasculitis. *Rheum Dis Clin North Am* 23:841-853, 1997.
34. Jorizzo JL, White WL, Wise CM, et al: Low-dose weekly methotrexate for unusual neutrophilic vascular reactions: cutaneous polyarteritis nodosa and Behçet's disease. *J Am Acad Dermatol* 42:973-978, 1991.
35. Phan JC, Hargadon AP, Salpeter SR: Association between pyoderma gangrenosum and psoriasis (letterl). *Lancet* 348:547, 1996.
36. Teitel AD: Treatment of pyoderma gangrenosum with methotrexate. *Cutis* 57:326-328, 1996.

Other Indications

37. Cooper KD: New therapeutic approaches in atopic dermatitis. *Clin Rev Allergy* 11:543-559, 1993.
38. Laeher MJ: Spontaneous remission or response to methotrexate in sarcoidosis. *Ann Intern Med* 69:1247-1248, 1968.
39. Veien NK, Brodthagen H: Cutaneous sarcoidosis treated with methotrexate. *Br J Dermatol* 97:213-216, 1977.
40. Gedalia A, Molina JF, Ellis GS Jr, et al: Low-dose methotrexate therapy for childhood sarcoidosis. *J Pediatr* 130:25-29, 1997.
41. Onwukwe MF: Treating keloids by surgery and methotrexate. *Arch Dermatol* 116:158, 1980.
42. Wantzin GL, Thomsen K: Methotrexate in lymphomatoid papulosis. *Br J Dermatol* 111:93-95, 1984.
43. Melton JL, Nelson BR, Stough DB, et al: Treatment of keratoacanthoma with intralesional methotrexate. *J Am Acad Dermatol* 25:1017-1023, 1991.
44. Zackheim HS: Treatment of cutaneous T-cell lymphoma. *Semin Dermatol* 13:207-215, 1994.
45. Schappell DL, Alper JC, McDonald CJ: Treatment of advanced mycosis fungoides and Sézary syndrome with continuous infusions of methotrexate followed by fluorouracil and leucovorin rescue. *Arch Dermatol* 131:307-313, 1995.
46. Kragballe K, Zachariae E, Zachariae H: Methotrexate in psoriatic arthritis. A retrospective study. *Acta Derm Venereol* 63:165-167, 1983.
47. Paller AS: Dermatologic use of methotrexate in children. *Pediatr Dermatol* 2:238-243, 1985.

Hepatotoxicity

48. Robinson JK, Baughman RD, Auerbach R, et al: Methotrexate hepatotoxicity in psoriasis. Consideration of liver biopsies at regular intervals. *Arch Dermatol* 116:413-415, 1980. (In Fitzpatrick TB, editor: Methotrexate therapy for psoriasis II: a liver biopsy is indicated in patients who have received more than 2000 mg of methotrexate. *Dermatol Capsule & Comment* 2:61-63, 1980.)
49. Weinblatt ML, Raimer JM: Methotrexate in rheumatoid arthritis. *J Am Acad Dermatol* 19:126-128, 1988.
50. Newman M, Auerbach R, Feiner H, et al: The role of liver biopsies in psoriatic patients receiving long-term methotrexate: improvement of liver abnormalities after cessation of treatment. *Arch Dermatol* 125:1218-1224, 1989.
51. O'Connor GT, Olmstead EM, Zug K, et al: Detection of hepatotoxicity associated with methotrexate therapy for psoriasis. *Arch Dermatol* 125:1209-1217, 1989.

52. Boffa MJ, Chalmers RJ, Haboubi HY, et al: Sequential liver biopsies during long-term methotrexate treatment for psoriasis: a reappraisal. *Br J Dermatol* 133:774-778, 1995.

53. Van Dooren-Greebe RJ, Kuijpers AL, Mulder J, et al: Methotrexate revisited: effects of long-term treatment in psoriasis. *Br J Dermatol* 130:204-210, 1994.

54. Malatjalian D, Ross J, Colwell S, et al: Methotrexate hepatotoxicity in psoriatic patients submitted to long-term therapy. *Can J Gastroenterol* 10:369-375, 1996.

55. Zachariae H, Sogaard H: Methotrexate-induced liver cirrhosis. A follow-up. *Dermatologica* 175:178-182, 1987.

56. Miller JA, Dodd H, Rustin MHA, et al: Ultrasound as a screening procedure for methotrexate-induced hepatic damage in severe psoriasis. *Br J Dermatol* 113:699-705, 1985.

57. Mitchell D, Johnson RD, Testa HJ, et al: Ultrasound and radionuclide scans—poor indicators of liver damage in patients treated with methotrexate. *Clin Exp Dermatol* 12:243-245, 1987.

58. Coulson HH, McKenzie J, Neild VS, et al: A comparison of liver ultrasound with liver biopsy histology in psoriatics receiving long-term methotrexate therapy. *Br J Dermatol* 116:491-495, 1987.

59. Williams CN, McNauley D, Malatjalian DA, et al: The aminopyrine breath test, an inadequate early indicator of methotrexate-induced liver disease in patients with psoriasis. *Clin Invest Med* 10:54-58, 1987.

60. Zachariae H, Aslam HM, Bjerring P, et al: Serum aminoterminal propeptide of type III procollagen in psoriasis and psoriatic arthritis: relation to liver fibrosis and arthritis. *J Am Acad Dermatol* 25:50-53, 1991.

61. Zachariae H: Liver biopsies and methotrexate: a time for reconsideration. *J Am Acad Dermatol* 42:531-534, 2000.

Pulmonary Toxicity

62. Sostman HD, Matthay RA, Putman CE, et al: Methotrexate-induced pneumonitis. *Medicine* 55:371-388, 1976.

63. Searles G, McKenry RJR: Methotrexate pneumonitis in rheumatoid arthritis: potential risk factors. Four case reports and a review of the literature. *J Rheumatol* 14:1164-1171, 1987.

64. Cottin V, Tébib J, Massonnet B, et al: Pulmonary function in patients receiving long-term low-dose methotrexate. *Chest* 109:933-938, 1996.

65. Phillips TJ, Jones DH, Baker H: Pulmonary complications following methotrexate therapy. *J Am Acad Dermatol* 16:373-375, 1987.

66. Verdich J, Christensen AL: Pulmonary disease complicating intermittent methotrexate therapy of psoriasis. *Acta Derm Venereol* 59:471-473, 1979.

67. Kaplan RL, Waite DH: Progressive interstitial lung disease from prolonged methotrexate therapy. *Arch Dermatol* 114:1800-1802, 1978.

Hematologic Toxicity

68. Gutierrez-Urena S, Molina JF, Garcia CO, et al: Pancytopenia secondary to methotrexate therapy in rheumatoid arthritis. *Arthritis Rheum* 39:272-276, 1996.

69. Nygaard H: Pancytopenia secondary to methotrexate therapy in rheumatoid arthritis: comment on the article by Gutierrez-Urena (letter). *Arthritis Rheum* 40:194-196, 1997.

70. Berthelot JM: Pancytopenia secondary to methotrexate therapy in rheumatoid arthritis: comment on the article by Gutierrez-Urena (letter). *Arthritis Rheum* 40:193-196, 1997.

71. Kassai A, Rautenstrauch H: Incidence of pancytopenia with methotrexate treatment of rheumatoid arthritis in Germany: comment on the article by Gutierrez-Urena (letter). *Arthritis Rheum* 40:195-196, 1997.

72. Ohosone Y, Okano Y, Kameda H, et al: Clinical characteristics related to methotrexate-induced pancytopenia (letter). *Clin Rheumatol* 16:321-323, 1997.

73. Shupack JL, Webster GF: Pancytopenia following low-dose oral methotrexate therapy for psoriasis. *JAMA* 259:3594-3596, 1988.

74. Mayall B, Poggi G, Parkin JD: Neutropenia due to low-dose methotrexate therapy for psoriasis and rheumatoid arthritis may be fatal. *Med J Austral* 155:480-484, 1991.

75. Abel EA, Farber EM: Pancytopenia following low-dose methotrexate therapy. *JAMA* 259:3612, 1988.

76. Groenendal H, Rampen FHJ: Methotrexate and trimethoprim-sulphamethoxazole—a potentially hazardous combination. *Clin Exp Dermatol* 15:358-360, 1990.

77. Thomas DR, Dover JS, Camp RD: Pancytopenia induced by the interaction between methotrexate and trimethoprim-sulfamethoxazole. *J Am Acad Dermatol* 17:1055-1056, 1987.

78. Frenia ML, Long KS: Methotrexate and non-steroidal antiinflammatory drug interactions. *Ann Pharmacother* 26:234-237, 1992.

79. Duhra P: Treatment of gastrointestinal symptoms associated with methotrexate therapy for psoriasis. *J Am Acad Dermatol* 28:466-469, 1993.

80. Morgan SL, Alarcon SG, Krumdieck CL: Folic acid supplementation during methotrexate therapy: it makes sense. *J Rheumatol* 20:929-930, 1993.

Malignancy Induction

81. Kamel OW, van de Rijn M, Weiss LM, et al: Reversible lymphomas associated with Epstein-Barr virus occurring during methotrexate therapy for rheumatoid arthritis and dermatomyositis. *N Engl J Med* 328:1317-1321, 1993.

82. Moder KG, Tefferi A, Cohen MD, et al: Hematologic malignancy and the use of methotrexate in rheumatoid arthritis. A retrospective study. *Am J Med* 99:276-281, 1995.

83. Bleyer WA: Methotrexate induced lymphoma? *J Rheumatol* 25:404-408, 1998.

84. Kamel OW: Lymphomas during long-term methotrexate therapy. *Arch Dermatol* 133:907-908, 1997.

85. Paul C, Tourneau AL, Cayuela JM, et al: Epstein-Barr virus-associated lymphoproliferative disease during methotrexate therapy for psoriasis. *Arch Dermatol* 133:867-871, 1997.

86. Bailin TL, Tindall JP, Roenigk HH, et al: Is methotrexate therapy for psoriasis carcinogenic? A modified retrospective-prospective analysis. *JAMA* 232:359-362, 1975.

87. Nyfors A, Jensen H: Frequency of malignant neoplasms in 248 long-term methotrexate-treated psoriatics: a preliminary study. *Dermatologica* 167:260-261, 1983.

Other Adverse Effects

88. Ortiz Z, Shea B, Suarez-Almazor ME, et al: The efficacy of folic acid and folinic acid in reducing methotrexate gastrointestinal toxicity in rheumatoid arthritis: a meta-analysis of randomized controlled trials. *J Rheumatol* 25:36-43, 1998.

89. Kallen B: The teratogenicity of antirheumatic drugs—what is the evidence? *Scand J Rheumatol* 107(suppl):119-124, 1998.

90. Morris LE, Harrod MJ, Menter A, et al: Methotrexate and reproduction in men: case report and recommendations. *J Am Acad Dermatol* 29:913-916, 1993.

91. Armstrong RB, Poh-Fitzpatrick MB: Methotrexate and ultraviolet radiation. *Arch Dermatol* 118:177-178, 1982.

92. Guzzo C, Kaidby K: Recurrent recall of sunburn by methotrexate. *Photodermatol Photoimmunol Photomed* 11:55-56, 1995.

93. Adkins SA, Byrd JC, Morgan SK, et al: Anaphylactoid reactions to methotrexate. *Cancer* 77:2123-2126, 1996.

94. Hellier I, Bessis D, Sotho A, et al: High dose methotrexate induced bullous variant of acral erythema. *Arch Dermatol* 132:590-591, 1996.

95. Harrison PV: Methotrexate-induced epidermal necrosis. *Br J Dermatol* 116:867-869, 1987.

96. Halevy S, Giryes H, Avinoach I, et al: Leukocytoclastic vasculitis induced by low-dose methotrexate: in vitro evidence for an immunologic mechanism. *J Eur Acad Dermatol Venereol* 10:81-85, 1998.

97. Maenaut K, Westhovens R, Dequeker J: Methotrexate osteopathy, does it exist? *J Rheumatol* 23:2156-2159, 1996.

98. Morgan SL, Baggott JE, Lee JY, et al: Folic acid supplementation prevents deficient blood folate levels and hyperhomocysteinemia during long-term low dose methotrexate therapy for rheumatologic arthritis. Implications for cardiovascular disease prevention. *J Rheumatol* 25:441-446, 1998.

Monitoring and Therapeutic Guidelines

99. Evans WE, Christensen ML: Interactions with methotrexate. *J Rheumatol* 12(suppl 12):15-20, 1985.

100. Ostergard K, Weismann K, Huttes L: Renal function and the rate of disappearance of methotrexate from serum. *Eur J Clin Pharmacol* 8:439-444, 1975.

101. Fairris GM, Dewhurst AG, White JE, et al: Methotrexate dosage in patients over aged 50 with psoriasis. *BMJ* 298:801-802, 1989.

102. Piccinino F, Sagnelli E, Pasquale G, et al: Complications following percutaneous liver biopsy: A multicenter retrospective study of 68,276 biopsies. *J Hepatol* 2:165-173, 1986.

103. Wildhirt E, Moller E: Experience with nearly 20,000 blind liver punctures. *Medizinische Klinik* 76:254-255, 1981.

104. Van Thiel DH, Gavaler JS, Wright H, et al: Liver biopsy. Its safety and complications as seen at a liver transplant center. *Transplantation* 55:1087-1090, 1993.

105. McGill DB, Rakela J, Zinsmeister AR, et al: A 21-year experience with major hemorrhage after percutaneous liver biopsy. *Gastroenterology* 99:1396-1400, 1990.

106. Sherlock S, Dick R, van Leeuwen DJ: Liver biopsy today. The Royal Free Hospital experience. *J Hepatol* 1:75-85, 1985.

107. Lang M, Neumann UP, Muller AR, et al: Complications of percutaneous liver biopsy in patients after liver transplantation. *Zeitschrift fur Gastroenterologie* 37:205-208, 1999.

108. Buscarini L, Fornari F, Bolondi L, et al: Ultrasound-guided fine-needle biopsy of focal liver lesions: techniques, diagnostic accuracy and complications. A retrospective study on 2091 biopsies. *J Hepatol* 11:344-348, 1990.

109. Drinkovic I, Brkljacic B: Two cases of lethal complications following ultrasound-guided percutaneous fine-needle biopsy of the liver. *Cardiovasc Intervent Radiol* 19:360-363, 1996.

110. Columbo M, Del Ninno E, de Franshis R, et al: Ultrasound-assisted percutaneous liver biopsy: superiority of the Tru-Cut over the Menghini needle for diagnosis of cirrhosis. *Gastroenterology* 95:487-489, 1988.

111. Bret PM, Labadie M, Bretagnolle M, et al: Hepatocellular carcinoma: diagnosis by percutaneous fine needle biopsy. *Gastrointest Radiol* 13:253-255, 1988.

112. Wolverton SE: Major adverse effects from systemic drugs: defining the risks. *Curr Prob Dermatol* 7:1-40, 1995.

113. Gilbert SC, Klintmalm G, Menter A, et al: Methotrexate-induced cirrhosis requiring liver transplantation in three patients with psoriasis. A word of caution in light of the expanding use of this "steroid sparing" agent. *Arch Intern Med* 150:889-891, 1990.

114. Brown AM, Corrigan AB: Pancytopenia after accidental overdose of methotrexate: a complication of low-dose therapy for rheumatoid arthritis. *Med J Austral* 155:493-494, 1991.

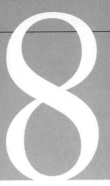

Stephanie Badalamenti
Francisco A. Kerdel

Azathioprine

Azathioprine (Imuran) was synthesized in 1959 from its parent drug 6-mercaptopurine (6-MP).[1] Clinical research showed that azathioprine was less toxic than 6-MP for an equivalent degree of immunosuppression, and hence azathioprine has eclipsed 6-MP as an immunosuppressant.[2] The parent drug, 6-MP, is now used exclusively as a cytotoxic agent in the treatment of acute lymphoblastic leukemia. Azathioprine made its clinical debut in 1961 as an immunosuppressant for renal transplantation.[2] Its usefulness in this setting resulted in azathioprine becoming the drug of choice for organ transplantation during the 1960s and 1970s. During this time it became apparent that azathioprine had not only immunosuppressant but also antiinflammatory qualities and was therefore sought by physicians treating a number of diverse immunologic disorders. In particular, rheumatologists, gastroenterologists, neurologists, and dermatologists began using azathioprine for a wide variety of inflammatory diseases, many of which occur on an autoimmune basis. The drug delivery, dose, and cost are shown in Table 8-1.

Dermatologists accumulated more than 30 years of experience using this drug in at least 40 dermatologic diseases.[1,3] Historically, empiric dosing has generally been 100 mg/day.[3] Subsequently, the manufacturer of the drug (Faro Pharmaceutical) and a number authors suggested that the dose be adjusted according to body weight.[3-5] More recently, advances in knowledge of the genetics of azathioprine metabolism led many dermatologists to adjust doses of azathioprine relative to enzyme activity of thiopurine methyltransferase (TPMT), a critical enzyme in the catabolism of azathioprine.[6]

PHARMACOLOGY

Key pharmacologic concepts of azathioprine can be found in Table 8-2.

Absorption and Distribution

Azathioprine (Figure 8-1) is usually prescribed in its oral form. After oral administration, greater than 88% of the drug is absorbed through the gastrointestinal tract.[2] The peak plasma levels occur in under 2 hours. The drug is rapidly metabolized to numerous products and distributed throughout the body. The transformed metabolites slowly accumulate and eventually provide maximal clinical immunosuppression by 8 to 12 weeks using traditional dosage schemes. This conservative dosing scheme reflects empiric experience given a population with variability in the activity of thiopurine methyltransferase. However, with the recent dissection of azathioprine metabolism and an awareness that 89% of patients are homozygous for the high TPMT activity, it is likely that more aggressive azathioprine dosing may lead to a more rapid clinical effect. In spite of the considerable research and

■ Table 8-1   Azathioprine

Generic name	Azathioprine
Trade name	Imuran
Date released	1959
Drug formulation	50 mg scored tablet
	100 mg vials
Drug dosing—empiric	Up to 2-2.5 mg/kg/d
Drug dosing by TPMT level	
High TPMT >19 U	Up to 2.5 mg/kg/d
Medium TPMT 13.7-19 U	Up to 1.5 mg/kg/d
Low TPMT 5-13.7 U	Up to 0.5 mg/kg/d
Price index	$$($$)

$, <1.00; $$, 1.01-2.00; $$$, 2.01-5.00; $$$$, 5.01-10.00; $$$$$, >10.00; ( ), generic price; /, two different price ranges from lower dose to higher dose examples of this size; —, no price listed for this drug.

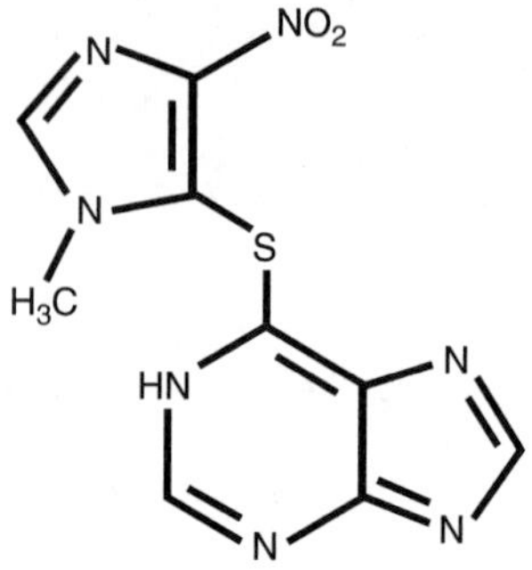

Figure 8-1   Azathioprine.

■ Table 8-2   Key Pharmacologic Concepts—Azathioprine

	Absorption and Bioavailability			Elimination		
	Peak Level	Bioavailable (%)	Protein Binding	Half-life	Metabolism	Excretion
Azathioprine	1 to 2 hrs	88%	30%	5 hrs	Thiopurine methyltransferase Xanthine oxidase HGPRT (active 6-thioguanine metabolites)	Negligible azathioprine is excreted; virtually completely metabolized

■ Table 8-3   Three Metabolic Pathways of Azathioprine

Enzyme Pathway	End Product	Inhibition of Pathway
Thiopurine methyltransferase (TPMT)	Inactive metabolites	Genetic predisposition
Xanthine oxidase (XO)	Inactive metabolites	Allopurinol
Hypoxanthine guanine phospho-ribosyltransferase (HGPRT)	Active purine analogs—especially 6-thioguanine	Lesch-Nyhan syndrome

clinical experience, the pharmacokinetics of azathioprine are not entirely understood.

Metabolism and Excretion

There are three pathways by which azathioprine's first metabolite (6-MP) is metabolized.[7] The clinical importance of each of these pathways is detailed below and is summarized in Table 8-3.

Azathioprine is rapidly converted to 6-MP on absorption. This conversion occurs mainly in erythrocytes. The fate of 6-MP is determined by one of the following three competing pathways: (1) anabolized to its active form, a purine analog, by the enzyme hypoxanthine-guanine phosphoribosyltransferase (HGPRT), (2) catabolized by TPMT to inactive metabolites, or (3) catabolized by xanthine oxidase (XO) to inactive metabolites. The anabolic pathway eventually leads to purine analogs such as thioguanine monophosphate (and other 6-thioguanine metabolites), which interfere with DNA and RNA synthesis and repair. Both catabolic pathways lead to inactive, nontoxic metabolites. Reduced activity (either genetically or by drug interaction) of either of the catabolic pathways will, however, have a potentially dramatic effect clinically. Such reduced activity will shift more of the 6-MP into the HGPRT anabolic or active pathway, potentially leading to excessive immunosuppression clinically with an increased risk of pancytopenia or bone marrow failure.[7]

Pharmacologically reduced (XO) or genetically reduced (TPMT) activity of these catabolic pathways has been demonstrated. The reduced activity of TPMT results from polymorphisms at this allele.[8] Enzyme function testing and enzyme allele sequencing are now possible. The enzyme function test involves measuring the activity of TPMT in red blood cells and has been shown to correlate with systemic TPMT activity. Through this functional assay system, three groups of patients (in a largely Caucasian population) were identified.[9] The large majority of patients (89%) show high levels of TPMT activity. Intermediate levels of TPMT activity were identified in 11% of patients, and very low levels of TPMT were identified in 1 of 300 patients.[8] Patients with low TPMT activity have markedly increased accumulation of 6-thioguanine metabolites, which increases the risk of pancytopenia. Those with high levels of this enzyme may be therapeutically underdosed.[10,11] This variation in enzyme activity can now be explained on a genetic level. The TPMT gene has been cloned.[12,13] It is 34 kB in length and consists of 10 exons and 9 introns and maps to chromosome band 6p22.3. TPMT activity is inherited as an autosomal codominant trait. Patients with high levels of TPMT are homozygotes for the high activity allele. Those with intermediate activity are heterozygous for the high activity allele and one of the over seven known low activity alleles.[13-18] Finally, those with low activity are homozygous for one of the low activity alleles or are compound heterozygotes for two different low activity alleles.

The question of ethnic variation at the TPMT locus resulted in part from an observation that different ethnicities have different success responding to thioguanine. Research into this ethnic diversity has yielded interesting and sometimes conflicting data with respect to overall activity of TPMT in various populations. Data suggest that Chinese persons may have higher activity relative to white Americans who in turn may have higher activity than black Americans.[19] The clinical relevance of this finding is unclear. It is clear, however, that the frequency of low activity alleles appears constant among white Americans, black Americans, Norwegians, Europeans, and Ghanaians. However, the exact mutations accounting for the low activity alleles are different among these ethnicities. Certain mutations are shared among different ethnicities and others are unique to a given ethnic group.[13-18]

The diversity of mutations among different races makes it difficult to create a genetic test to identify low activity alleles. This is compounded by the fact that TPMT mutations have been found in the promoter region, exons, and within introns, allowing for the possibility of new mutations anywhere within the genomic DNA. Unfortunately, the functional enzyme assay is not a simple solution to identify patients with mutant alleles or low TPMT activity phenotype. The functional enzyme test has recently been shown to have variability between testing sites. Furthermore, the functional enzyme test has inherent variability because different test kits may contain varying amounts of enzyme inhibitor.[20] It is for these reasons that these authors do not test TPMT activity before prescribing azathioprine. The awareness of these three TPMT phenotypes allows the physician to monitor for pancytopenia while at the same time increasing the dose of azathioprine in patients who tolerate azathioprine well but are not showing an adequate clinical response (presumed homozygotes for the high activity allele).

XO is another enzyme that catabolizes azathioprine. Decreased activity of this enzyme has been identified and is a result of drug interactions and not genetic variability. Specifically, the XO pathway can be inhibited by allopurinol. Allopurinol is commonly used in the treatment of gout because it decreases uric acid accumulation by inhibiting the enzyme XO. In patients concurrently taking allopurinol and azathioprine, the allopurinol shunts more 6-MP from the XO catabolic pathway to the HGPRT anabolic pathway, creating an excess of purine analogs. This in turn may lead to excessive immunosuppression and risk for pancytopenia as well.[21] In patients receiving allopurinol who require azathioprine therapy, the dose of azathioprine should be reduced by 75%. Unlike TPMT, there is little genetic variation in individual XO activity, and hence there is no need for assessment of this enzyme activity with respect to azathioprine dosing.[7]

Reduced activity of the anabolic pathway has no known adverse effects. However, one would expect less immunosuppression if azathioprine could not be transformed to its active molecule. The absence of adverse effects is a consequence of shunting from the anabolic pathway toward both catabolic pathways, resulting in an accumulation of nontoxic, inactive metabolites. Patients with Lesch-Nyhan syndrome have a genetic absence of HGPRT. Patients with Lesch-Nyhan syndrome taking azathioprine will experience no immunosuppression and no adverse effects.[2] This confirms the importance of HGPRT in metabolizing the 6-MP into its active 6-thioguanine metabolites and further confirms that the XO and TPMT metabolic pathways produce both nontoxic and clinically inactive metabolites.

To summarize, pharmacologic inhibition or genetically reduced activity of either catabolic pathway (XO or TPMT) will result in excessive HGPRT conversion of azathioprine (via 6-MP), with resultant clinically enhanced immunosuppression and risk of bone marrow toxicity.

Mechanism of Action

Azathioprine with its immunosuppressive and antiinflammatory effects has been used to treat autoimmune diseases of the skin. This most notably includes autoimmune bullous disorders, such as pemphigus vulgaris and bullous pemphigoid, as well as a multitude of other cutaneous inflammatory diseases.[4] The mechanism of action is not well understood.

Azathioprine's active metabolite is a purine analog, which inhibits DNA/RNA synthesis and repair and possesses immunosuppressive activity. The active metabolite of azathioprine (6-thioguanine) is structurally similar to the endogenous purines adenine and guanine. In contrast to endogenous purines, which have an amino group or hydroxyl group, 6-thioguanine contains a thiol group. This structural similarity allows 6-thioguanine to be incorporated into DNA and RNA, subsequently inhibiting purine metabolism and cell division.[22,23] However, the mechanism of activity of azathioprine goes beyond simple incorporation and subsequent inhibition of DNA and RNA synthesis because it actually affects the function of T and B cells.[1] In the T cell, cell-mediated function is depressed, and antibody production is diminished in the B cell.[1] Azathioprine also decreases the number of Langerhans' cells and other antigen-presenting cells in the skin, as well as decreasing the ability of these cells to present antigens, further enhancing the drug's immunosuppressive effects.[24]

CLINICAL USE

Table 8-4 contains indications and contraindications for azathioprine.

Indications

Azathioprine is approved by the US Food and Drug Administration (FDA) only for use in certain organ transplantations and in severe rheumatoid arthritis patients. However, the moderately potent immunosuppressive and antiinflammatory effects, a reasonable risk/benefit profile, and low cost have resulted in a

Table 8-4	Azathioprine Indications and Contraindications

FDA-APPROVED INDICATIONS (NONE SPECIFIC TO DERMATOLOGY)
Organ transplantation
Severe rheumatoid arthritis

OFF-LABEL USES

Immunobullous Dermatoses
Bullous pemphigoid[27,28]
Pemphigus vulgaris[29-33]
Cicatricial pemphigoid[34-36]

Vasculitis
Leukocytoclastic vasculitis[37,38]
Wegener's granulomatosis[39,40]
Polyarteritis nodosa[41]

Neutrophilic Dermatoses
Behçet's disease[42-44]
Pyoderma gangrenosum[45,46]

Autoimmune Connective Tissue Diseases
Systemic lupus erythematosus[38,47-54]
Dermatomyositis[55-58]
Sjögren's syndrome[59]
Scleroderma[60,61]
Relapsing polychondritis[62]

Dermatitis and Papulosquamous Dermatoses
Psoriasis[63-66]
Atopic dermatitis[26,67,70,71]
Contact dermatitis[68,69]
Lichen planus[72,73]

Photodermatoses
Chronic actinic dermatitis[74,75]
Polymorphous light eruption[76]
Persistent light reaction[77]

Other Dermatoses
Sarcoidosis (especially pulmonary features)[78,79]
Erythema multiforme[80]
Weber-Christian disease[81]
Chronic graft-versus-host disease[82]

CONTRAINDICATIONS

Absolute
Pregnancy
Hypersensitivity to azathioprine
Active clinically significant infections

Relative
Allopurinol use—can prescribe azathioprine
  cautiously with significantly reduced dose
Prior use of alkylating agents

PREGNANCY PRESCRIBING STATUS—CATEGORY D

variety of "off-label" uses. Physicians from various disciplines most frequently employed azathioprine in diseases responding to corticosteroids as a corticosteroid-sparing agent. Azathioprine is commonly used in the treatment of inflammatory bowel disease and multiple sclerosis.

Dermatologists should follow the guidelines in Box 8-1 to determine the appropriateness of azathioprine use.

IMMUNOBULLOUS DERMATOSES. Dermatologists have gained over 30 years of experience using azathioprine for the treatment of immunobullous diseases, including pemphigus vulgaris, bullous pemphigoid, and cicatricial pem-

Box 8-1

General Guidelines for Use of Azathioprine in Dermatology

- Disease should be serious or life threatening.
- Disease should be reversible or controllable.
- Disease is unresponsive to less potentially risky therapies.
- Disease should have measurable clinical or laboratory measures of improvement.
- Risks and adverse effects should be carefully discussed with the patient.
- Alternative therapies should be discussed with patient.
- Patient should be compliant with various laboratory monitoring tests.

phigoid. In fact, dermatologists are most likely to prescribe azathioprine for the management of this category of diseases.[3] Several excellent reviews on the use of azathioprine in the management of these diseases have been published.[1,4,5,26] As early as 1978, controlled trials of azathioprine plus prednisone versus prednisone alone suggested the corticosteroid-sparing effects of this drug in the management of bullous pemphigoid.[27] However, a subsequent controlled trial comparing azathioprine and prednisone versus plasma exchange and prednisone vs. prednisone alone revealed no benefit of adjuvant therapy to corticosteroids alone during a 6-month period.[28] The authors of this study acknowledged the low statistic power of the study, limited follow-up, and wide confidence intervals among the treatment groups.

Similarly, prospective and retrospective studies on the use of azathioprine in treatment of pemphigus vulgaris also suggested a corticosteroid-sparing effect.[29-32] This observation was also challenged by authors who reviewed the literature and concluded there was no benefit of adjuvant treatment (such as azathioprine) to corticosteroids in the treatment of pemphigus vulgaris.[33] Again the strength of this argument is based on a review of the literature and not on a clinical trial. Despite the conflicting data, dermatologists frequently prescribe azathioprine for pemphigus vulgaris and bullous pemphigoid.[4,25] More than 30 years of clinical experience combined with the data appears to tip the balance of the argument towards using azathioprine as a corticosteroid-sparing agent.

Azathioprine has been used in the treatment of cicatricial pemphigoid, particularly to treat corticosteroid-refractory eye involvement.[34-36]

VASCULITIS.   Giant cell arteritis, polyarteritis nodosa, Wegener's granulomatosis, retinal vasculitis, and leukocytoclastic vasculitis have all been successfully treated with azathioprine. Particularly impressive results have been reported with the use of azathioprine for leukocytoclastic vasculitis (LCV). A review of rheumatoid arthritis–related LCV suggested that azathioprine plus prednisone, compared with continuation of conventional rheumatic drugs, had lower incidence of vasculitis relapse, fewer serious complications, and relatively low mortality.[37] In another study evaluating patients with idiopathic LCV refrac-

tory to corticosteroids, azathioprine therapy resulted in five of six patients improving, with complete disease control in two of six.[38]

Azathioprine has been used by pulmonologists, otolaryngologists, and dermatologists alike for the treatment of Wegener's granulomatosis. Both renal and lung disease showed improvement with the combination of corticosteroids and azathioprine.[39,40] Renal disease in polyarteritis also showed improvement with the use of azathioprine.[41]

NEUTROPHILIC DERMATOSES.   Azathioprine has been used extensively in the treatment of Behçet's disease and to a lesser extent in managing pyoderma gangrenosum. Two placebo-controlled, double-blind trials of azathioprine used in Behçet's disease showed decreased eye problems including hypopyon and emergent blindness.[42,43] Furthermore, both studies revealed decreased extraocular complications including fewer oral ulcers, genital ulcers, and arthritis.[42,43] Dermatologists have also used azathioprine to treat Behçet's disease skin involvement.[44] Occasionally, azathioprine has been used to treat pyoderma gangrenosum with variable success.[45,46]

AUTOIMMUNE CONNECTIVE TISSUE DISEASES.   Azathioprine is commonly used in the treatment of systemic lupus erythematosus, particularly in the treatment of lupus nephritis. Three retrospective studies and one prospective study showed that azathioprine in combination with prednisone and/or cyclophosphamide helps preserve renal function and reduce disease flares.[47-50] A more recent study showed azathioprine to be successful in treating lupus-associated cardiomyopathy.[51] Azathioprine has occasionally been documented to treat cutaneous features of lupus, discoid lupus erythematosus, subacute cutaneous lupus erythematosus, and systemic lupus erythematosus have all responded in selected patients. Azathioprine appears particularly useful in extensive discoid lesions with palmoplantar involvement.[52-54]

Polymyositis and dermatomyositis have also been successfully treated with azathioprine.[55-58] The respiratory and muscle symptoms may respond to azathioprine, but the successful resolution of skin lesions has not been consistently demonstrated.[55,56]

Azathioprine has been used in other connective tissue diseases including Sjögren's syndrome,[59] scleroderma,[60,61] and relapsing polychondritis.[62] The drug appears particularly useful in treating the eye involvement in relapsing polychondritis.[62]

DERMATITIS AND PAPULOSQUAMOUS DERMATOSES. In the 1960s and 1970s several articles were published documenting the treatment of psoriasis with azathioprine.[63-65] A more recent review published in 1992 describes azathioprine as a forgotten alternative in the treatment of psoriasis.[66] Yet azathioprine remains a rare drug choice in the treatment of psoriasis. Perhaps with the addition of cyclosporine and systemic retinoids, in addition to the widespread accessibility of ultraviolet light treatment, the utility of azathioprine for psoriasis therapy has diminished.

Atopic dermatitis and contact dermatitis have both been treated with azathioprine.[67-71] Usually these dermatoses can be controlled with topical corticosteroids, but in severe cases oral corticosteroids or cytotoxic agents are required. It was recently shown that severe atopic eczema responds well to azathioprine and provides a less expensive alternative to cyclosporine.[67] This conclusion was supported in a retrospective study of azathioprine therapy in atopic dermatitis.[26] In this retrospective study, patients receiving azathioprine required fewer antibiotic courses, fewer courses of high potency corticosteroids, and less hospitalization, and had fewer outpatient visits. These authors also commented on the safety and simple monitoring of azathioprine compared with cyclosporine.

Lichen planus (both erosive and generalized disease) responded to azathioprine as monotherapy.[72] In another case report, azathioprine was successfully used as a corticosteroid-sparing agent in lichen planus.[73]

PHOTODERMATOSES. Azathioprine has been used in the treatment of photodermatoses, including chronic actinic dermatitis and polymorphous light eruption. A double-blind placebo-controlled trial of azathioprine therapy for chronic actinic dermatitis demonstrated that azathioprine was so successful and well tolerated that statistical significance was quickly reached

and the trial was terminated early.[74] In another study, azathioprine improvement of chronic actinic dermatitis appeared to be permanent after a mean duration of 11.5 months of treatment.[75]

Two case reports show the success of azathioprine in the treatment of severe polymorphous light eruption and persistent light reactors,[76,77] but the authors remarked that azathioprine was used to treat only the most severe cases.

OTHER DERMATOSES. Azathioprine has been used in a number of other skin disorders. The lung disease of sarcoidosis has been shown to respond to azathioprine, with less predictable improvement of the cutaneous features of sarcoidosis.[78,79] The spectrum of diseases successfully treated with azathioprine has also included erythema multiforme,[80] Weber-Christian panniculitis,[81] and chronic graft-versus-host disease.[82]

Adverse Effects

IMMUNOSUPPRESSION CARCINOGENESIS. Azathioprine's immunosuppressive effects may be associated with malignancy in selected patient populations.[84-86] The most common malignancies associated with azathioprine include lymphoproliferative malignancies (especially non-Hodgkin's B-cell lymphomas) and squamous cell carcinomas of the skin.[85] The likelihood of developing these cancers is influenced by factors including ethnicity, duration of treatment, depth of immunosuppression, and underlying disease state.[83-89]

Depth of immunosuppression is related to the dose of the immunosuppressant and the number of immunosuppressants required to achieve the desired therapeutic result. Renal transplantation patients require a much greater depth of immunosuppression to prevent organ rejection than do liver transplantation patients. This intense suppression of immunity needed to prevent organ rejection may interfere with the immune system's ability to provide routine cancer surveillance functions. This theory is supported by the fact that renal transplantation patients taking either cyclosporine or azathioprine are at greater risk for malignancy than comparable liver transplantation patients.[8]

The underlying medical condition requiring immunosuppressive therapy also plays a role in malignancies related to azathioprine use.

Patients with rheumatoid arthritis have a three-fold to eightfold incidence of lymphoproliferative malignancy (independent of drug therapy) when compared with the normal population.[83,90] This increased incidence is related to the underlying immunopathogenesis of rheumatoid arthritis. Patients with this predisposition to malignancy induced by immunosuppressive agents (such as azathioprine) have an increased risk for lymphoproliferative malignancies.[83,89] Studies of immunosuppressants other than azathioprine have likewise demonstrated an increased risk of lymphoproliferative malignancies in rheumatoid arthritis patients.[83,92] Therefore malignancy is likely a phenomenon related to immunosuppression in rheumatoid arthritis patients in general, rather than the use of azathioprine specifically.

Patients with Crohn's disease and ulcerative colitis do not have an innate predisposition to malignancy and interestingly do not appear to be at greater risk for malignancy while on azathioprine.[90] Not only do these patients lack a predisposition to malignancy, they do not require the great depth of immunosuppression or indefinite immunosuppressive therapy required in renal transplantation recipients.

There are no significant studies evaluating the incidence of lymphoproliferative malignancies or squamous cell carcinomas in patients taking azathioprine for dermatologic disease. Likewise, there are no case reports of lymphoproliferative malignancies in patients receiving azathioprine for dermatologic disease. There are, however, three case reports of aggressive squamous cell carcinomas presenting in patients on azathioprine for eczema, atopic dermatitis, and chronic actinic dermatitis.[92] These aggressive squamous cell carcinomas were found on the head and neck in fair-skinned patients, with two of three patients reporting excessive sun exposure.[92] One patient developed an invasive squamous cell carcinoma that metastasized to local lymph nodes after 4 years on azathioprine. The second patient developed a recurrent squamous cell carcinoma on the face requiring enucleation of the eye after 6 years on azathioprine. The third patient developed a rapidly growing squamous cell carcinoma on the ear requiring wide excision after 4 years on azathioprine therapy.

Dermatologists prescribing azathioprine should be aware of the increased risk of lymphoproliferative malignancies and cutaneous squamous cell carcinomas in selected patients receiving azathioprine. Although the increased incidence of these malignancies has not been convincingly demonstrated in dermatology patients, regular physical examinations with attention to these issues for patients on long-term azathioprine are important.

PANCYTOPENIA. Pancytopenia (bone marrow failure) is a rare adverse event resulting from excessive immunosuppression by azathioprine. Pancytopenia occurs in a specific subset of patients with the low TPMT phenotype discussed earlier.[8] These patients have low TPMT activity leading to a massive accumulation of 6-thioguanine metabolites, overwhelmingly interfering with DNA/RNA synthesis in cells with a high turnover rate, such as hematologic precursor cells.[1,7] Cessation of the drug therapy if significantly reduced blood counts occur (WBC <4000 to 4500/mm^3, hemoglobin <10 g/dl, platelets <100,000/mm^3) should allow recovery of the bone marrow (see Chapter 42). To prevent catastrophic bone marrow failure, physicians should perform regular complete blood count (CBC) monitoring as outlined in the Monitoring Guidelines section to identify patients who are evolving towards pancytopenia.

OPPORTUNISTIC INFECTIONS. In addition, patients on azathioprine are at higher risk of infection secondary to their immunosuppressive state.[94] This increased infection rate is typically seen in patients on higher doses of azathioprine or patients who are on multiple immunosuppressive agents, such as organ transplant recipients. However, any patient on azathioprine must be considered at a potentially increased risk for infection.[25,94] These infections include herpes virus infections, scabies infections, and human papillomavirus infections.[95]

USE IN PREGNANCY. Azathioprine is contraindicated in pregnancy and is a category D drug.[94] Azathioprine readily crosses the placenta. Furthermore, in animal studies, azathioprine caused fetal abnormalities at doses similar to those given to humans. These abnormalities include skeletal malformations and visceral anomalies.[95] Despite azathioprine's contraindication during pregnancy, a summary of data in over 440 pregnant women who were concurrently taking azathioprine failed to demonstrate an increased risk of fetal anomalies.[96] There are, however, case reports of bone marrow suppression in some of these pregnancies and two case reports of fetal cytomegalovirus (CMV) infection.[97,98] Two other case reports describe congenital abnormalities in two children born from mothers receiving azathioprine during pregnancy.[99,100] These abnormalities include preaxial polydactyly in one child and myelomeningocele, bilateral hip dislocation, and bilateral talipes equinovarus in the other child.

HYPERSENSITIVITY SYNDROME. A rare side effect of azathioprine is the potential for a drug-induced hypersensitivity syndrome. The diversity of associated symptoms includes cardiovascular collapse, cutaneous eruptions, fever, leukocytosis, gastrointestinal discomfort ranging from nausea to hepatotoxicity and pancreatitis, arthralgias and myalgias, rhabdomyolysis, headaches, renal insufficiency, and respiratory involvement ranging from cough to pneumonitis.[101-103] The specific cutaneous eruption is diverse and includes macular erythema or maculopapular eruptions, macular eruptions with vesicles or pustules within it, and purpuric or petechial lesions. Other describe erythema multiforme, urticaria, angioedema, or erythema nodosum due to azathioprine hypersensitivity.[101] Hypersensitivity reactions typically develop between 1 and 4 weeks of starting therapy.[104] This reaction appears more commonly in patients who are simultaneously receiving cyclosporine and methotrexate therapy.[104] Rechallenge of these patients with the drug is contraindicated because this rechallenge may cause a life-threatening reaction.[101,105]

GASTROINTESTINAL EFFECTS. The most common adverse effects of azathioprine are gastrointestinal including nausea, vomiting, and diarrhea. The gastrointestinal symptoms often present between the first and tenth days of therapy. The mechanism for this effect is unknown; however, decreasing the dose, dividing the dose, and taking azathioprine with food often alleviates these symptoms.[4,11]

DRUG INTERACTIONS

There are relatively few drug interactions with azathioprine. The most important drug interaction occurs between azathioprine and allopurinol. As discussed in the pharmacology section, allopurinol inhibits XO, one of two metabolic pathways involved in the detoxification of azathioprine to inactive metabolites. This inhibition leads to an excess of the active purine analog, leading to an increased risk of pancytopenia.[1] Three other drugs can potentially interact with azathioprine: captopril, warfarin, and pancuronium. Captopril use may increase the risk of leukopenia.[106] An increase in warfarin dose may be required in patients on azathioprine therapy.[107] Patients on pancuronium may require an increased dose of this paralytic agent for appropriate control.

MONITORING GUIDELINES

A review of the literature regarding the recommended guidelines for monitoring azathioprine treatment is compiled for the Monitoring Guidelines. These guidelines are drawn from a variety of articles published in the late 1990s.[3-6,11,25] Authors have a variety of dosing preferences in the treatment of bullous pemphigoid and pemphigus vulgaris. These various approaches are discussed clearly in the individual articles cited for these immunobullous dermatoses.

SUMMARY

Azathioprine was developed almost four decades ago. During this time, azathioprine has been used successfully in a number of inflammatory and autoimmune diseases. The major contraindications and adverse effects are clearly identified, allowing dermatologists to inform patients reasonably well regarding the pros and cons of therapy in a given clinical situation. Although there are no FDA-approved indications for azathioprine in dermatology, there is ample evidence to support azathioprine therapy in a variety of autoimmune and inflammatory dermatoses. The most well-studied use of this drug in dermatology is the for treatment of immunobullous diseases.

Azathioprine Monitoring Guidelines[3-6,11,25]

BASELINE

Clinical Evaluation
- Discuss the risk/benefit profile and adverse effects with each patient.
- Discuss alternative treatments and the requirement for multiple blood tests.
- Discuss sun avoidance and birth control/abstinence in women of childbearing age.
- Elicit history of prior alkylating agents or current use of allopurinol.
- Perform careful physical examination with focus on skin and lymphoreticular system.

Laboratory
- Pregnancy test (for women of childbearing potential)
- CBC with platelet count
- Serum chemistry profile
- Urine analysis
- Tuberculin skin test (at least strongly consider performing, depending on clinical situation)

Special Tests
- If using the TPMT assay dose according to the enzyme activity*
  TPMT < 5.0 U = no treatment with azathioprine

Special Tests—cont'd
  TPMT between 5.0 U and 13.7 U = 0.5 mg/kg maximum azathioprine dose
  TPMT between 13.7 U and 19.0 U = 1.5 mg/kg maximum azathioprine dose
  TPMT > 19.0 U = 2.5 mg/kg maximum azathioprine dose

FOLLOW-UP

Clinical Evaluation
- Biannual physical examination with particular attention to possible lymphoreticular and squamous cell malignancy.

Laboratory
(Monthly for the first 3 months,† every 2 months thereafter)
- CBC with differential WBC count (consider a 2-week determination with more aggressive dosing)
- Liver function tests focusing on the transaminases (AST and ALT)

Special Tests
- *Do not* need to repeat the TPMT assay subsequent to baseline determination

*If GFR <10 ml/min decrease AZA dose by 50%; if GFR 10 to 50 ml/min decrease AZA dose by 25%.
†Laboratory testing frequency based on performance of baseline TPMT determination; if this test is not obtained at baseline, the clinician should monitor hematologic parameters more closely.

Bibliography

Pharmacology

Canafax DM, Johnson CA: The therapeutic use of azathioprine in renal transplantation. *Pharmacotherapy* 7:165-177, 1987.

Lennard L: The clinical pharmacology of 6-mercaptopurine. *Eur J Clin Pharmacol* 43:329-339, 1992.

Clinical Use and Practice Guidelines

Callen JP: Immunosuppressive and cytotoxic drugs in dermatology: a practical overview and personal perspective. *J Cut Med Surg* 1:58-64, 1996.

Korman NJ: Update on the use of azathioprine in the management of pemphigus and bullous pemphigoid. *Med Surg Dermatol* 3:209-213, 1996.

Tan BB, Lear JT, Gawakrodger DJ, et al: Azathioprine in dermatology: a survey of current practices in the U.K. *Br J Dermatol* 136:351-355, 1997.

Wolverton SE: Major adverse effects from systemic drugs: defining the risks. *Curr Prob Dermatol* 7:1-40, 1995.

Younger IR, Harris DWS, Clover GB: Azathioprine in dermatology. *J Am Acad Dermatol* 25:281-288, 1991.

References

1. Younger IR, Harris DWS, Clover GB: Aza-thioprine in dermatology. *J Am Acad Dermatol* 25:281-288, 1991.
2. Chan GLC, Canafax DM, Johnson CA: The therapeutic use of azathioprine in renal transplantation. *Pharmacotherapy* 7:165-177, 1987.
3. Tan BB, Lear JT, Gawkrodger DJ, et al: Aza-thioprine in dermatology: a survey of current practice in the U.K. *Br J Dermatol* 136:351-355, 1997.
4. Korman NJ: Update on the use of azathio-prine in the management of pemphigus and bullous pemphigoid. *Med Surg Dermatol* 3:209-213, 1996.
5. Wolverton SE: Major adverse effects from systemic drugs: defining the risk. *Curr Prob Dermatol* 7:1-40, 1995.
6. Jackson AP, Hall AG, McLelland J: Thio-purine methyltransferase levels should be measured before commencing patients on azathioprine. *Br J Dermatol* 136:132-148, 1997.

Pharmacology

7. Lennard L: The clinical pharmacology of 6-mercaptopurine. *Eur J Clin Pharmacol* 43:329-339, 1992.
8. Weinshilboum RM, Sladek SL: Mercapto-purine pharmacogenetics: monogeneic in-heritance of erythrocyte thiopurine methyl-transferase activity. *Am J Human Gen* 32:651-662, 1980.
9. Bergan S, Rugstad HE, Kelmetdal B, et al: Possibilities for therapeutic drug monitoring of azathioprine: 6-thioguanine nucleotide concentrations and thiopurine methyltrans-ferase activity in red blood cells. *Ther Drug Monitor* 19:318-326, 1997.
10. Snow JL, Gibson LE: The role of genetic variation in thiopurine methyltransferase ac-tivity and the efficacy and/or side effects of azathioprine therapy in dermatologic pa-tients. *Arch Dermatol* 131:193-197, 1995.
11. Snow JL, Gibson LE: A pharmacogenetic basis for the safe and effective use of aza-thioprine and other thiopurine drugs in der-matologic patients. *J Am Acad Dermatol* 32:114-116, 1995.
12. Honchel R, Aksoy I, Szumlanski C, et al: Thiopurine methyltransferase: molecular cloning and expression of T84 colon carci-noma cell cDNA. *Mol Pharmacol* 43:878-887, 1993.
13. Szumlanski C, Otterness D, Her C, et al: Thiopurine methyltransferase pharmacoge-netics: human gene cloning and characteri-zation of a common polymorphism. *DNA Cell Biol* 1:17-30, 1996.
14. Otterness DM, Szumlanski CL, Wood TC, et al: Human thiopurine methyltransferase pharmacogenetics. *J Clin Invest* 101:1036-1044, 1998.
15. Spire-Vayron de la Moureyre C, Debuysere H, Mastain B, et al: Genotypic and pheno-typic analysis of the polymorphic thiopurine S-methyltransferase gene (TPMT) in a Euro-pean population. *Br J Pharmacol* 125:879-887, 1998.
16. Ameyaw MM, Collie-Duguid ESR, Powrie RH, et al: Thiopurine methyltransferase al-leles in British and Ghanaian populations. *Hum Mol Genet* 8:367-370, 1999.
17. Hon YY, Fessing MY, Pui CH, et al: Polymor-phisms of the thiopurine S-methyltrans-ferase gene in African-Americans. *Hum Mol Genet* 8:371-376, 1999.
18. McLeod HL, Pritchard SC, Githang J, et al: Ethnic differences in thiopurine methyl-transferase pharmacogenetics: evidence for allele specificity in Caucasian and Kenyan individuals. *Pharmacogenetics* 9:773-776, 1999.
19. McLeod HL, Lin JS, Scott EP, et al: Thio-purine methyltransferase activity in Ameri-can white subjects and black subjects. *Clin Pharmacol Ther* 55:15-20, 1994.
20. Kroplin T, Fisher C, Iven H: Inhibition of thiopurine S-methyltransferase activity by impurities in commercially available sub-strates: a factor for different results of TPMT measurements. *Eur J Clin Pharmacol* 55:285-291, 1999.
21. Kennedy DT, Hayney MS, Lake KD: Azathio-prine and allopurinol: the price of an avoid-able drug interaction. *Ann Pharmacother* 30:951-954, 1996.
22. Loo TL, Luce JK, Sullivan MP, et al: Clinical pharmacologic observations of 6-mercap-topurine and 6-methythipurine ribonucleo-side. *Clin Pharmacol Ther* 9:180-194, 1968.
23. Elion GB: Biochemistry and pharmacology of purine analogs. *Fed Proc* 26:898-904, 1967.

24. Liu H, Wong C: In vitro immunosuppressive effects of methotrexate and azathioprine on Langerhans cells. *Arch Dermatol Res* 289:94-97, 1997.

Clinical Use—Immunobullous Dermatoses

25. Callen JP: Immunosuppressive and cytotoxic drugs in dermatology: a practical overview and personal perspective. *J Cut Med Surg* 1:58-64, 1996.
26. Lear JT, English JSC, Jones P, et al: Retrospective review of the use of azathioprine in severe atopic dermatitis. *J Am Acad Dermatol* 35:642-643, 1996.
27. Burton JL, Harman RR, Peachey RD, et al: Azathioprine plus prednisone in treatment of pemphigoid. *BMJ* 2:1190-1201, 1978.
28. Guillaume JC, Vaillant L, Bernard P, et al: Controlled trial of azathioprine and plasma exchange in addition to prednisolone in the treatment of bullous pemphigoid. *Arch Dermatol* 129:49-53, 1993.
29. Carson PJ, Hameed A, Ahmed AR: Influence of treatment on the clinical course of pemphigus vulgaris. *J Am Acad Dermatol* 34:645-652, 1996.
30. Fine JD, Appell ML, Green LK, et al: Pemphigus vulgaris. Combined treatment with intravenous corticosteroid pulse therapy, plasmapheresis, and azathioprine. *Arch Dermatol* 124:236-239, 1988.
31. Aberer W, Wolff-Schreiner EC, Stingl G, et al: Azathioprine in the treatment of pemphigus vulgaris. A long-term follow-up. *J Am Acad Dermatol* 16:527-533, 1987.
32. Mourellou O, Chaidemenos GC, Koussidou T, et al: The treatment of pemphigus vulgaris: experience with 48 patients seen over an 11-year period. *Br J Dermatol* 133:83-87, 1995.
33. Bystryn J, Steinman NM: The adjuvant therapy of pemphigus. *Arch Dermatol* 132:203-212, 1996.
34. Warren SD, Lesher JL Jr: Cicatricial pemphigoid. *South Med J* 86:461-464, 1993.
35. Tauber J, Sainz de la Maza M, Foster CS: Systemic chemotherapy for ocular cicatricial pemphigoid. *Cornea* 10:185-195, 1991.
36. Dave VK, Vickers CF: Azathioprine in the treatment of mucocutaneous pemphigoid. *Br J Dermatol* 90:183-186, 1974.

Vasculitis

37. Heurkens AH, Westedt ML, Breedveld FC: Prednisone plus azathioprine treatment in patients with rheumatoid arthritis complicated by vasculitis. *Arch Int Med* 151:2249-2254, 1991.
38. Callen JP, Spencer LV, Burruss JB, et al: Azathioprine. An effective, corticosteroid-sparing therapy for patients with recalcitrant cutaneous lupus erythematosus or with recalcitrant cutaneous leukocytoclastic vasculitis. *Arch Dermatol* 127:515-522, 1991.
39. Thorkelsen H, Berdal P: Wegener's granulomatosis immunosuppressive therapy. *Acta Otolaryngol* 82:208-211, 1976.
40. Wishart JM: Wegener's granulomatosis—controlled by azathioprine and corticosteroids. *Br J Dermatol* 92:471-477, 1975.
41. Brock PG, Richard P: Reversal of rapidly progressive renal failure associated with polyarteritis. *Proc Roy Soc Med* 66:656-657, 1973.

Neutrophilic Dermatoses

42. Hamuryudan V, Ozyazgan Y, Hizli N, et al: Azathioprine in Behcet's syndrome: effects on long-term prognosis. *Arthritis Rheum* 40:769-774, 1997.
43. Yazici H, Pazarli H, Barnes CG, et al: A control trial of azathioprine in Behcet's syndrome. *N Engl J Med* 322:281-285, 1990.
44. Nethercott J, Lester RS: Azathioprine therapy in complete Behçet's syndrome. *Arch Dermatol* 110:432-434, 1974.
45. Duffill MB: Cyclosporine, azathioprine and local therapy for pyoderma gangrenosum. *Austral J Dermatol* 35:15-18, 1994.
46. Breathnach SM, Wells GC, Valdimarsson H: Idiopathic pyoderma gangrenosum and impaired lymphocyte function: failure of azathioprine and corticosteroids. *Br J Dermatol* 104:567-577, 1981.

Autoimmune Connective Tissue Diseases

47. D'Cruz D, Cuadroado MJ, Mujic F, et al: Immunosuppressive therapy in lupus nephritis. *Clin Exp Rheumatol* 15:275-282, 1997.
48. Oelzner P, Abendroth K, Hein G, et al: Predictors of flares and long-term outcome of systemic lupus erythematosus during combined treatment with azathioprine and low-dose prednisolone. *Rheumatol Int* 16:133-139, 1996.

49. Chan TM, Li EK, Wong RW, et al: Sequential therapy for diffuse proliferative and membranous lupus nephritis: cyclophosphamide and prednisolone followed by azathioprine and prednisolone. *Nephron* 71:321-327, 1995.

50. Swaak AJ, Statius van Eps LW, Aarden LA, et al: Azathioprine in the treatment of systemic lupus erythematosus. A three-year prospective study. *Clin Rheumatol* 3:285-291, 1984.

51. Naarendorp M, Kerr LD, Kahn AS, et al: Dramatic improvement of left ventricular function after cytotoxic therapy in lupus patients with acute cardiomyopathy: report of 6 cases. *J Rheumatol* 26:2257-2260, 1999.

52. Ashinoff R, Werth VP, Franks AG Jr: Resistant discoid lupus erythematosus of palms and soles: successful treatment with azathioprine. *J Am Acad Dermatol* 19:961-965, 1988.

53. Shehade S: Successful treatment of generalized discoid skin lesions with azathioprine. *Arch Dermatol* 122:376-377, 1986.

54. Tsokos GC, Caughman SW, Klippel JH: Successful treatment of generalized discoid skin lesions with azathioprine. Its use in a patient with systemic lupus erythematosus. *Arch Dermatol* 121:1323-1325, 1985.

55. Rowen AJ, Reichel J: Dermatomyositis with lung involvement, successfully treated with azathioprine. *Respiration* 44:143-146, 1983.

56. Brunch TW: Prednisone and azathioprine for polymyositis: long-term follow-up. *Arthritis Rheum* 21:45-48, 1981.

57. Jacobs JC Jr: Treatment of dermatomyositis. *Arthritis Rheum* 20:208-211, 1977.

58. Lever WF: Dermatomyositis. *Arch Dermatol* 105:771-772, 1972.

59. Deheinzelin D, Capelozzi VL, Kairalla RA, et al: Interstitial lung disease in primary Sjogren's syndrome. Clinical-pathological evaluation and response to treatment. *Am J Resp Crit Care Med* 154:794-799, 1996.

60. Nachbar F, Stolz W, Volkenandt M, et al: Squamous cell carcinoma in localized scleroderma following immunosuppressive therapy with azathioprine. *Acta Derm Venereol* 73:217-219, 1993.

61. Jansen GT, Barraza DF, Ballard JL, et al: Generalized scleroderma. Treatment with an immunosuppressive agent. *Arch Dermatol* 97:690-698, 1968.

62. Hoang-Xaun T, Foster CS, Rice BA: Scleritis in relapsing polychondritis. Response to therapy. *Ophthalmology* 97:892-898, 1990.

Dermatitis and Papulosquamous Dermatoses

63. Munro DD: Azathioprine in psoriasis. *Proc Roy Soc Med* 66:747-748, 1973.

64. Dawber RP: The effect of methotrexate, corticosteroids and azathioprine on fingernail growth in psoriasis. *Br J Dermatol* 83:315-323, 1970.

65. Greaves MW, Dawber RP: Azathioprine in psoriasis. *BMJ* 703:237-238, 1970.

66. Hacker SM, Ramos-Caro FA, Ford MJ, et al: Azathioprine: a forgotten alternative for treatment of severe psoriasis. *Int J Dermatol* 31:873-874, 1992.

67. Buckley DA. Baldwin P, Rogers S: The use of azathioprine in severe adult atopic eczema. *J Eur Acad Dermatol Venereol* 11:137-140, 1998.

68. Lear JT, English JSC: Severe and chronic allergic contact dermatitis responding to azathioprine therapy. *J Dermatol Treat* 7:109-110, 1996.

69. Roed-Petersen J, Thomsen K: Azathioprine in the treatment of airborne contact dermatitis form compositae oleoresins and sensitivity to UVA. *Acta Derm Venereol* 60:275-277, 1980.

70. Morrison JG, Schulz EJ: Treatment of eczema with cyclophosphamide and azathioprine. *Br J Dermatol* 98:203-207, 1978.

71. Gunnar S, Johansson O, Juhlin L: Immunoglobulin E in "healed" atopic dermatitis and after treatment with corticosteroids and azathioprine. *Br J Dermatol* 82:10-13, 1970.

72. Lear JT, English JS: Erosive and generalized lichen planus responsive to azathioprine. *Clin Exp Dermatol* 21:56-57, 1996.

73. Klien LR, Callen JP: Azathioprine: effective steroid-sparing therapy for generalized lichen planus. *South Med J* 82:198-201, 1992.

Photodermatoses

74. Murphy GM, Maurice PD, Norris PG, et al: Azathioprine treatment in chronic actinic dermatitis: a double-blind controlled trial with monitoring of exposure to ultraviolet radiation. *Br J Dermatol* 121:639-646, 1989.

75. Leigh IM, Hawk JL: Treatment of chronic actinic dermatitis with azathioprine. *Br J Dermatol* 110:691-695, 1984.

76. Norris PG, Hawk JL: Successful treatment of severe polymorphous light eruption with azathioprine. *Arch Dermatol* 125:1377-1379, 1989.

77. De Castro JL, Pereira MA, Nunes FP, et al: Successful treatment of a musk ambrette-sensitive persistent light reactor with azathioprine. *Photodermatology* 3:241-242, 1986.

Other Dermatoses

78. Lewis SJ, Ainslie GM, Bateman ED: Efficacy of azathioprine as second-line treatment in pulmonary sarcoidosis. *Sarcoid Vasc Diff Lung Dis* 16:87-92, 1999.
79. Pacheco Y, Marechal C, Marchal F, et al: Azathioprine treatment of chronic pulmonary sarcoidosis. *Sarcoidosis* 2:107-113, 1985.
80. Jones RR: Azathioprine therapy in the management of persistent erythema multiforme. *Br J Dermatol* 105:465-467, 1981.
81. Hotta T, Wakamatsu Y, Matsumura N, et al: Azathioprine-induced remission in Weber-Christian disease. *South Med J* 74:234-237, 1981.
82. Sullivan KM, Shulman HM, Storb R, et al: Chronic graft-versus-host disease in 52 patients: adverse natural course and successful treatment with combination immunosuppression. *Blood* 57:267-276, 1981.

Adverse Effects—Carcinogenesis

83. Kinlen JL: Incidence of cancer in rheumatoid arthritis and other disorders after immunosuppressive treatment. *Am J Med* 78:44-49, 1985.
84. Kinlen LJ, Sheil AGR, Peto J, et al: Collaborative United Kingdom-Australian study of cancer in patients treated with immunosuppressive drugs. *BMJ* 2:1461-1466, 1979.
85. Gruber SA, Skjei KL, Sothern RM, et al: Cancer development in renal allograft recipients treated with conventional and cyclosporine immunosuppression. *Transplant Proc* 23:1101-1103, 1991.
86. Tennis P, Andrews E, Bombardier C, et al: Record linkage to conduct an epidemiologic study on the association of rheumatoid arthritis and lymphoma in the province of Saskatchewan, Canada. *J Clin Epidemiol* 46:685-695, 1993.
87. Cockburn I: Assessment of the risks of malignancy and lymphoma developing in patients using Sandimmune. *Transplant Proc* 19:1804-1807, 1987.
88. Penn I: Cancers in cyclosporine-treated vs azathioprine-treated patients. *Transplant Proc* 28:876-878, 1996.

89. Silman AJ, Petrie J, Hazelman B, et al: Lymphoproliferative cancer and other malignancy in patients with rheumatoid arthritis treated with Imuran: a 20 year follow up study. *Ann Rheumatol Dis* 47:988-992, 1988.
90. Kinlen LJ: Malignancy in autoimmune disease. *J Autoimmun* 5:363-371, 1992.
91. Connell WR, Kamm MA, Dickson M, et al: Long term neoplasia risk after azathioprine treatment in inflammatory bowel disease. *Lancet* 343:1249-1252, 1994.
92. Baker GL, Kahl LE, Zee BC, et al: Malignancy following treatment of rheumatoid arthritis with cyclophosphamide. *Am J Med* 83:1-9, 1987.
93. Bottomley WW, Ford G, Cunliffe WJ, et al: Aggressive squamous cell carcinoma developing in patients receiving long-term azathioprine. *Br J Dermatol* 133:460-462, 1995.

Adverse Effects—Other

94. Faro Pharmaceutical: Azathioprine medication profile. Drug insert information.
95. Whisnant JK, Perlkey J: Rheumatoid arthritis: treatment with azathioprine: clinical side effects and laboratory abnormalities. *Ann Rheum Dis* 41:44-47, 1982.
96. Tagatz GE, Simmons RL: Pregnancy after renal transplantation. *Ann Intern Med* 82:113-114, 1975.
97. Cote CJ, Meuwissen HJ, Pickering RJ: Effects on the neonate of prednisone and azathioprine administered to the mother during pregnancy. *J Pediatr* 85:324-328, 1974.
98. DeWitte DB, Buick MK, Stephen EC, et al: Neonatal pancytopenia and severe combined immunodeficiency associated with antenatal administration of azathioprine and prednisone. *J Pediatr* 105:625-628, 1984.
99. Williamson RA, Karp LE: Azathioprine teratogenicity: review of the literature and case report. *Obstet Gynecol* 58:247-250, 1981.
100. Ostensen M: Treatment with immunosuppressive and disease modifying drugs during pregnancy and lactation. *Am J Reproduct Immunol* 28:148-152, 1992.
101. Knowles SR, Gupta AK, Shear NH, et al: Azathioprine hypersensitivity-like reactions—a case report and a review of the literature. *Clin Exp Dermatol* 20:353-356, 1995.

102. Compton MR, Crosby DL: Rhabdomyolysis associated with azathioprine hypersensitivity syndrome. *Arch Dermatol* 132:1254-1255, 1996.

103. Jones JJ, Ashworth J: Azathioprine-induced shock in dermatology patients. *J Am Acad Dermatol* 29:795-796, 1993.

104. Blanco R, Martinez-Taboada VM, Gonzalez-Gay MA, et al: Acute febrile toxic reaction in patients with refractory rheumatoid arthritis who are receiving combined therapy with methotrexate and azathioprine. *Arthritis Rheum* 39:1016-1020, 1996.

105. Pandhi RK, Gupta LK, Girdhar M: Azathioprine-induced drug fever. *Int J Dermatol* 33:198, 1994.

Interactions and Monitoring

106. Gossmann J, Kachel HG, Schoeppe W, et al: Anemia in renal transplant recipients caused by concomitant therapy with azathioprine and angiotensin-converting enzyme. *Transplantation* 56:585-589, 1993.

107. River G, Khamashta MA, Hughes GR: Warfarin and azathioprine: a drug interaction does exist. *Am J Med* 95:342, 1993.

Teddy D. Pan
Charles J. McDonald

Cytotoxic Agents

The treatment of skin diseases with cytotoxic drugs is an important aspect of dermatologic practice. When used properly, cytotoxic drugs can substantially improve the quality of life and in some cases save lives. However, these drugs have significant adverse effects (such as carcinogenicity, bone marrow suppression, and teratogenicity) that the dermatologist must be aware of before their use. These adverse effects preclude their widespread use in many benign skin diseases and restrict their application to selected severe skin diseases, such as mycosis fungoides, recalcitrant psoriasis, bullous dermatoses, and connective tissue diseases.[1,2] When cytotoxic agents are indicated, the physician should be familiar with their application, toxicities, and proper monitoring. In addition, patients must understand the risks and benefits of these medications so that they can make an informed decision regarding their use.[3-6] Systemic cytotoxic agents commonly used in dermatology include the antimetabolites (methotrexate and azathioprine) and the alkylating agents (chlorambucil, cyclophosphamide, and hydroxyurea). The focus in this chapter will be on chlorambucil, cyclophosphamide, hydroxyurea, and mycophenolate mofetil (Table 9-1). Melphalan and 5-fluorouracil will also be discussed but in lesser detail.

The clinician should be aware that myelosuppression is a potentially serious and unnecessary adverse reaction from these medications. Cytotoxic agents can produce a substantial immunosuppressive effect without myelosuppression.[1]

In general, cytotoxic drugs exert their effects by interfering with protein and nucleic acid synthesis, thereby affecting cell replication, which may ultimately result in cell death. The individual cell cycle for cellular replication is composed of five phases. The G_1 phase involves preparation for DNA synthesis. The cell primarily synthesizes DNA in the S phase. After DNA synthesis is complete, the cell prepares for mitosis in the G_2 phase. If the cell undergoes mitosis, the cell enters the M phase. Alternatively, the cell can enter into a resting phase, G_0 (from either G_1 or G_2), and remain in this phase until the proper stimulus to undergo cell division is received.[1] Through their effect on protein synthesis, cytotoxic drugs also interfere with the production of cytokines, growth factors, adhesion molecules, and other substances associated with cell growth and differentiation. It is these various actions by cytotoxic agents that make them useful for the treatment of benign and malignant skin diseases.

Antimetabolites can be incorporated as analogs to natural molecules in DNA and result in cell death by chain scission or missense mutations. As a result, their actions are cell-cycle specific to the S phase. Similarly, adverse effects are most evident in tissues with high mitotic indices such as the gastrointestinal tract and the bone marrow. Alkylating agents primarily exert their effects by altering the chemical properties of DNA,

■ **Table 9-1** Cytotoxic Agents

Generic Name	Trade Name	Generic Available	Manufacturer	Formula- tions	Special Formulations	Standard Dosage Range	Price Index
Cyclophosphamide	Cytoxan, Neosar	No	Bristol-Myers Squibb	25 mg, 50 mg	IV 100, 200, 300 mg vials	(PO) 1-3 mg/kg/d (IV) 0.5-1 g/m^2	$$$
Chlorambucil	Leukeran	No	Glaxo Wellcome	2 mg		(initial) 0.05-0.2 mg/ kg/d typically 4-10 mg/d (maint.) 2-4 mg/d	$$
Hydroxyurea	Hydrea	Yes	Bristol-Myers Squibb	500 mg		1.0-1.5 g/d	$$ ($$)
Mycophenolate mofetil	CellCept	No	Roche	250 mg, 500 mg		1.25-2.0 g/d	$$$
Fluorouracil	Adrucil	Yes	Pharmacia/ Upjohn, Roche	None	IV 50 mg/ml	3-12 mg/kg/d (max 800 mg/d)	—
Melphalan	Alkeran	No	Glaxo Wellcome	2 mg		(initial) 2-6 mg (maint.) 0.05-0.1 mg/ kg/d	—

$, <1.00; $$, 1.01-2.00; $$$, 2.01-5.00; $$$$, 5.01-10.00; $$$$$, >10.00; ( ), generic price; /, two different price ranges from lower dose to higher dose examples of this size; —, no price listed for this drug.

regardless of cell cycle. They are considered cell-cycle nonspecific, although their biochemical effects are more significant in proliferating cells. Their adverse effects, correspondingly, are not limited to sites with a high proliferation index. As a result, these drugs are often mutagenic.[1]

Patient education is an important aspect of prescribing cytotoxic therapy. Patients should be made aware of the common potential adverse effects such as fever, chills, diaphoresis, cough, dyspnea, or headache when infection is imminent. The physician should assess patient compliance with proper monitoring and overall safety measures.

CYCLOPHOSPHAMIDE

Cyclophosphamide was first synthesized in the late 1950s as a derivative of nitrogen mustard (mechlorethamine). It is classified as an oxazaphosphorine that is inactive until metabolized in the body.[7]

Pharmacology
Cyclophosphamide (Figure 9-1) is 2-bis [(2-chloroethyl)amino] tetrahydro-2H-1,3,2-oxazaphosphorine 2-oxide monohydrate. Like other bifunctional alkylating agents, cyclophosphamide contains two highly reactive electrophilic sites

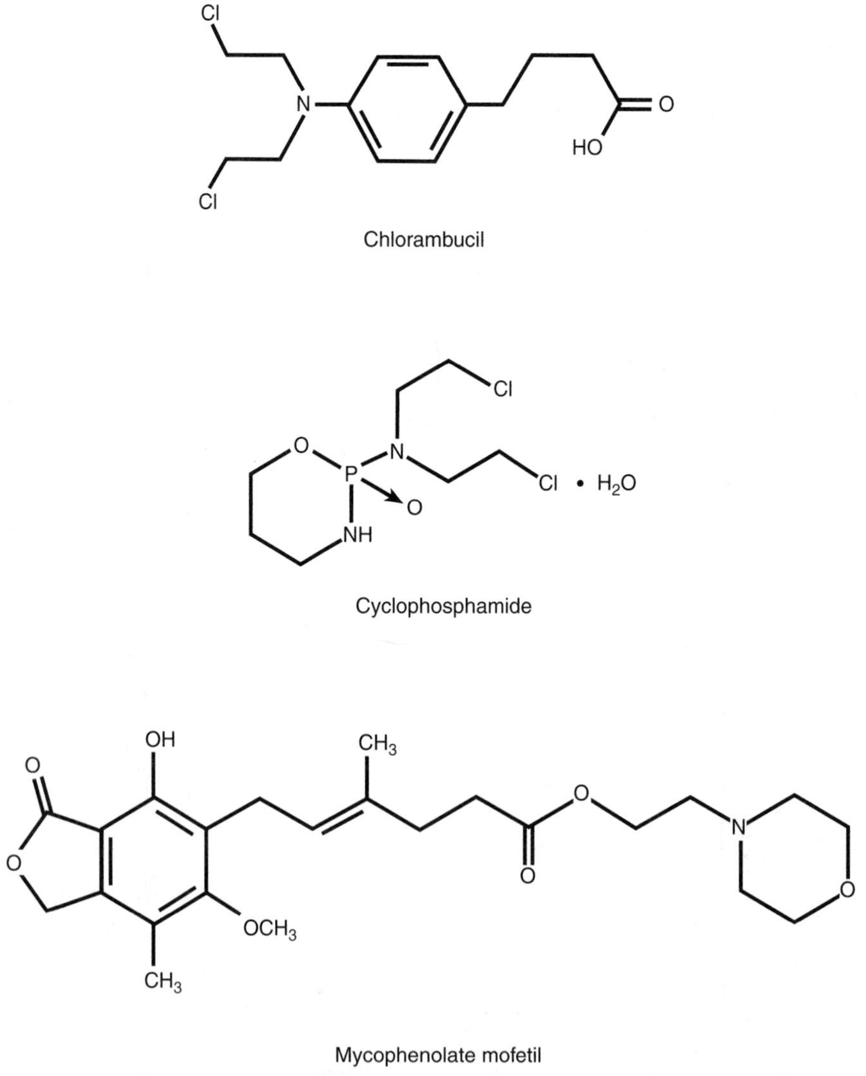

Chlorambucil

Cyclophosphamide

Mycophenolate mofetil

Figure 9-1 Cytotoxic agents.

that give this drug the ability to bind with nucleophilic, electron-rich regions of nucleic acids and proteins. Base pairing with substances on guanine in DNA can lead to miscodings and depurination and ultimately damage the DNA molecule. Table 9-2 contains key pharmacologic concepts for cytotoxic agents.

The oral bioavailability of cyclophosphamide is 74% with peak plasma levels occurring at 1 hour. Cyclophosphamide is widely distributed throughout the body, including the cerebrospinal fluid. The half-life of the drug ranges from 2 to 10 hours. Plasma half-life is increased in cirrhosis, but is decreased in children. The drug is only 13% protein-bound, but its metabolites are approximately 50% protein-bound in plasma.

Cyclophosphamide is primarily metabolized by the liver. The kidneys account for 10% to 20% of the excretion of the unchanged drug. Unusual for alkylating agents, cyclophosphamide requires modification by the cytochrome P-450 (2B, 2C) system to become biologically active. Cyclophosphamide is first converted by the cytochrome P-450 system to the metabolite 4-hydroxycyclophosphamide. This molecule exists in equilibrium with aldophosphamide. Aldophosphamide is nonenzymatically cleaved to phosphoramide mustard and acrolein, of which only phosphoramide

mustard is active. Aldophosphamide can alternatively be converted into an inactive metabolite carboxyphosphamide by aldehyde dehydrogenase. 4-Hydroxycyclophosphamide can alternatively be enzymatically cleaved into its inactive metabolite 4-ketocyclophosphamide. Acrolein, a pharmacologically inactive metabolite, is believed to be the cause of bladder toxicity. Unlike the excretion of the unchanged drug, the kidneys account for 50% of the excretion of the metabolites. The half-life of phosphoramide mustard and nornitrogen mustard is 9 hours and 3.3 hours, respectively. Of the cyclophosphamide metabolites, only phosphoramide mustard and 4-hydroxycyclophosphamide are biologically active.[8-12]

MECHANISM OF ACTION. Cyclophosphamide is a cell-cycle nonspecific drug. It depresses B cell function more so than T cell function. The effect on T cell activity is variable, with greater activity when the drug is given before antigen presentation and diminished activity when the drug is given after antigen presentation. In addition, suppressor T cells appear to be more affected than helper T cells.[13,15] Table 9-3 lists mechanisms of action of cytotoxic drugs.

The alkylating functions of cyclophosphamide are a result of the highly reactive bis-

Table 9-2   Key Pharmacologic Concepts—Cytotoxic Agents

| Drug Name | Absorption and Bioavailability | | | Elimination | | |
	Peak Levels	Bioavailable (%)	Protein Binding	Half-life	Metabolism	Excretion
Cyclophosphamide[1,8-12*]	2 hrs	74%	13%	2-3 hrs (up to 10 hrs)	Hepatic†	Mostly hepatic Renal 10%-20% 50% metabolites in urine
Chlorambucil[1,9,12]	1 hr	87%	99%	1.3 hrs	Hepatic	Hepatic (renal <1%)
Hydroxyurea[1,9*]	1-2 hrs	100%	(minimal)	5.5 hrs	(unclear)	Renal 80%
Mycophenolate mofetil	6-12 hrs	94%	(minimal)	17.9 hrs	Hepatic	Renal 93% (metabolites)

*Cyclophosphamide and hydroxyurea also penetrate the cerebrospinal fluid.
†Cyclophosphamide has two active metabolites: phosphoramide mustard and nornitrogen mustard.

■ **Table 9-3**   Mechanisms of Action of Cytotoxic Drugs

Drug Name	Mechanism	Resultant Clinical Effect(s)
Cyclophosphamide[9,13]	Cell-cycle nonspecific Suppresses B cells > T cells Affects T suppressor cells more than T helper cells Forms DNA cross-linkages	Immunosuppression, cell death Bone marrow suppression, carcinogenicity
Chlorambucil[9,14]	Cell-cycle nonspecific Forms DNA cross-linkage	Immunosuppression, cell death Bone marrow suppression, carcinogenicity
Hydroxyurea[9]	S phase specific Inhibits ribonucleotide reductase preventing DNA synthesis and repair Hypomethylation of genes	Immunosuppression, radiation sensitization, cell death Normalization of psoriatic skin Bone marrow suppression, megaloblastic changes, carcinogenicity
Mycophenolate mofetil[15]	Noncompetitive inhibitor of inosine monophosphate dehydrogenase	Immunosuppression, bone marrow suppression

(2-chloroethyl) grouping. With the release of chlorides, a very reactive ethyleniminium intermediate is formed that can covalently bind with nucleophilic centers within DNA. Nucleophilic moieties include phosphate, amino, sulfhydryl, hydroxyl, carboxyl, and imidazole groups. The most susceptible part of the DNA molecule is the 7-nitrogen atom of guanine. Other susceptible areas include the 1- or 3-nitrogens of adenine, the 3-nitrogen of cytosine, the 6-oxygen of guanine, the phosphate atoms of the DNA backbone, and the various proteins associated with DNA. Four effects result from alkylation. DNA may cross-link with another nucleophilic residue such as a separate DNA strand or protein. An abnormal base pair with thymine may be formed, which can result in the eventual substitution of a C-G pair with an A-T pair. Depurination may occur with resultant chain scission. The imidazole ring on the base residue may be cleaved, resulting in depurination and chain scission. If these mutations overwhelm the DNA repair system, the result is either cell death or mutagenesis and carcinogenesis.[9,14]

Resistance to cyclophosphamide and other alkylating agents can occur. The mechanisms include the following: decreased penetration of the drugs into cells, increased production of competing nucleophilic substances, increased activity of the DNA repair system, or increased metabolism to inactive metabolites.[9,14]

Clinical Use
INDICATIONS.   Cyclophosphamide is indicated for use in a variety of benign and malignant diseases (Table 9-4). In benign skin diseases it is most often used as a corticosteroid-sparing agent. Thus cyclophosphamide is often combined with prednisone to induce disease remission. In such instances cyclophosphamide may be continued as the single agent for maintenance of a response after the prednisone is tapered. Certain laboratory criteria should be met before a patient is started on cyclophosphamide therapy for benign diseases. The white blood cell count should be greater than 5000/mm³. The granulocyte count should be greater than 2000/mm³. The leukocyte count nadir occurs 8 to 12 days after cyclophosphamide therapy is initiated.[12]

Dosage Guidelines.   Cyclophosphamide comes as 25 and 50 mg tablets labeled Cytoxan. Dosages range from 1 to 5 mg/kg/day. This is usually given as 50 to 200 mg/day in equally divided doses or as a single morning dose. For nonmalignant disease, doses rarely need to exceed 2 to 3 mg/kg/day. Doses above 200 mg/day

Table 9-4   Cyclophosphamide Indications and Contraindications

FDA-APPROVED INDICATIONS
Mycosis fungoides (advanced)[2,17]

OFF-LABEL USES

Vasculitis
Wegener's granulomatosis[17-20]
Lymphomatoid granulomatosis[21]
Polyarteritis nodosa[17,22]
Leukocytoclastic vasculitis[23,24]
Other forms of necrotizing vasculitis[17,18,25]
Cryoglobulinemia[17,26]
Rheumatoid vasculitits[17]

Bullous Dermatoses
Pemphigoid[17,27]
Pemphigus[17,28-31]

Neutrophilic Dermatoses
Pyoderma gangrenosum[32,33]
Behçet's disease[17,34,35]
Erythema elevatum diutinum[36]

Connective Tissue Diseases
Dermatomyositis[37-40]
Lupus erythematosus[14,15,17,41-44]
Scleroderma[17,45,46]
Relapsing polychondritis[47]

Malignancies
Histiocytosis X[3,48]

Infiltrative Diseases
Lichen myxedematosus[49]
Scleromyxedema[50]

Miscellaneous
Psoriatic arthritis[51]
Severe eczematous dermatitis[52]
Severe nonresponsive bullous erythema
    multiforme[53]
Multicentric reticulohistiocytosis[54,55]
Cytophagic histiocytic panniculitis[56,57]
Ichthyosis linearis circumflexa[58]

CONTRAINDICATIONS

Absolute
Pregnancy (teratogenic)
Lactation (found in breast milk)
Hypersensitivity to cyclophosphamide
    (may cross-react with chlorambucil or
    mechlorethamine)[59,60]
Depressed bone marrow function

Relative
Infections (depends on severity)
Impaired hepatic function
Impaired renal function

PREGNANCY PRESCRIBING STATUS—CATEGORY D

almost invariably cause myelosuppression. It should be reemphasized that it is not necessary to induce myelosuppression to produce an immunosuppressive effect. Patients should be advised to drink plenty of fluids throughout the day to decrease the risk of hemorrhagic cystitis. In patients with impaired hepatic or renal function, the dose should be reduced.[1,2]

Cyclophosphamide can also be given parenterally although it is rarely used this way by dermatologists. It has been shown that daily IV boluses of cyclophosphamide (5 to 9 mg/kg/day) given over 7 to 15 days may be effective in the treatment of proteinuric lupus nephropathy and severe lupus vasculitis. A monthly IV pulse regimen of 0.5 to 1.0 g/m^2 of cyclophosphamide followed by vigorous hydration may also be used.[41-44]

Cytotoxic Drug Choice. The use of cyclophosphamide is not without risks and drawbacks. If one excludes cyclosporine, tacrolimus, and some of the newer immunosuppressive agents, cyclophosphamide is the most potent immunosuppressive drug available for general use. Although it may require more than 6 weeks of cyclophosphamide therapy to determine if there has been an adequate disease response, its onset of action is equivalent to that of newer immunosuppressive drugs and more rapid than that of azathioprine. Cyclophosphamide is reasonably easy to use and to monitor its associated adverse effects. Patients need to be made aware of these potential adverse effects before initiating therapy.

Life-Threatening Dermatoses.   Cyclophosphamide may be used alone or in conjunction with other drugs in the treatment of advanced mycosis fungoides, although other modalities are probably more effective.[17] In patients with pemphigus or pemphigoid, cyclophosphamide may be used as a first line agent to induce early disease control, or it may be used as a second line agent in combination with pred-

nisone when azathioprine or prednisone alone has failed.[27-31] In Wegener's granulomatosis and lymphomatoid granulomatosis, cyclophosphamide is the drug of choice.[18-21]

ADVERSE EFFECTS.   Box 9-1 lists the adverse effects of cyclophosphamide.

Carcinogenicity.   Cyclophosphamide has a well-established increased risk of malignancy in transplant patients for whom prolonged high dosages are frequently used. Reported malignancies associated with cyclophosphamide include non-Hodgkin's lymphoma, leukemia, bladder carcinoma, and squamous cell carcinomas. There is a slightly increased risk of non-Hodgkin's B-cell lymphoma reported in rheumatologic use.[23,62,66] There is also an 8 to 10 times greater risk of transitional cell carcinoma of the bladder.[62-65] This is thought to follow chronic, untreated episodes of hemorrhagic cystitis. Acute leukemia, especially acute myelogenous leu-

---

Box 9-1

Adverse Effects of Cyclophosphamide[1,11,12,61]

CARCINOGENICITY
- Increased risk of transitional cell bladder carcinoma (eightfold to tenfold increased relative risk)[62-65]
- Leukemia (AML), non-Hodgkin's lymphoma, squamous cell carcinoma[23,62,66-70]

HEMATOLOGIC
- Leukopenia (common, dose-limiting)
- Thrombocytopenia (usually at higher doses)
- Anemia (less common)
- Aplastic anemia (rare, reversible)

BLADDER[8,65]
- Dysuria, urgency, microscopic hematuria
- Hemorrhagic cystitis (5% to 40%)—dose-related; probably caused by acrolein metabolite; increases risk of bladder carcinoma
- Bladder fibrosis, necrosis, contracture, vesicoureteral reflux

DERMATOLOGIC[71,72]
- Anagen effluvium (5% to 30%, can be irreversible), pigmented band on teeth (irreversible)

DERMATOLOGIC[71,72]**—cont'd**
- Diffuse hyperpigmentation of skin, transverse ridging of nails, acral erythema, Stevens-Johnson syndrome[73]
- Rarely, urticaria and mucosal ulcerations

GASTROINTESTINAL
- Nausea, vomiting, diarrhea (most common; seen in up to 70% of patients)
- Anorexia, stomatitis, hepatotoxicity (high doses), hemorrhagic colitis

REPRODUCTIVE
- Amenorrhea, azoospermia (after prolonged therapy and may be irreversible)

OTHER RARE ADVERSE EFFECTS
- Cardiomyopathy (high doses), pneumonitis, interstitial pulmonary fibrosis, SIADH,[74] CNS effects (convulsions, progressive muscular paralysis, cholinergic effects), fever, anaphylaxis
- Opportunistic infections

SIADH, Syndrome of inappropriate antidiuretic hormone; *CNS,* central nervous system.

kemia,[67] is increased when cyclophosphamide has been used as adjuvant chemotherapy. The risk of malignancy (lymphoma, leukemia, and squamous cell carcinoma) in dermatologic patients receiving cyclophosphamide is probably much lower than the risk in transplant patients. Careful screening for hematuria can help to prevent the development of bladder carcinoma.

Bladder Toxicity.   The major difficulty with this drug is hemorrhagic cystitis, which occurs in 5% to 40% of patients. This issue requires careful monitoring, as hemorrhagic cystitis can be fatal and can increase the future risk of transitional cell carcinoma. Cyclophosphamide should be discontinued once hematuria is noted. It is recommended that patients drink plenty of fluids and void frequently to decrease the risk of hemorrhagic cystitis. This toxicity is probably due to the acrolein metabolite of cyclophosphamide. Mesna (sodium 2-mercaptoethanesulfonate) has been used to reduce this adverse effect when cyclophosphamide has been given in large doses.[8,68]

DRUG INTERACTIONS.   The major drug interactions involving cyclophosphamide are listed in Table 9-5.

CHLORAMBUCIL

Chlorambucil was first synthesized in the 1950s. It is a bifunctional alkylating agent like cyclophosphamide that is also derived from nitrogen mustard.

Pharmacology

Chlorambucil (see Figure 9-1) is 4-bis ([cholethyl] amino)-benzenebutanoic acid. Its oral bioavailability is 87% with peak plasma levels occurring 1 hour after administration. Like cyclophosphamide, chlorambucil is widely distributed after absorption. The plasma half-life is 1.3 hours. The drug is 99% protein-bound in plasma. Less than 1% of the total drug dose is excreted by the kidneys. The majority of the drug metabolism is performed in the liver. Chlorambucil does not require hepatic metabolism

 Table 9-5   Cyclophosphamide Drug Interactions[13]

Interacting Drug	Mechanism/Clinical Result
DRUGS THAT INCREASE CYCLOPHOSPHAMIDE DRUG LEVELS AND TOXICITY	
Allopurinol	Inhibits metabolism, increases leukopenic effects
Cimetidine	Inhibits CYP enzymes, increases leukopenic effects
Chloramphenicol	Inhibits metabolism, increases leukopenic effects
CYCLOPHOSPHAMIDE ENHANCES THE THERAPEUTIC EFFECTS OF THIS DRUG[75]	
Succinylcholine	Inhibits metabolism of succinylcholine, prolonging its effects
OTHER DRUG INTERACTIONS INVOLVING CYCLOPHOSPHAMIDE	
Halothane	Unclear/concomitant exposure results in unpredictable effects and may result in increased morbidity or mortality
Nitrous oxide	Unclear/concomitant exposure results in unpredictable effects and may result in increased morbidity or mortality
Barbiturates	Induce CYP enzymes, reduce cyclophosphamide drug levels
Doxorubicin	Increases the myocardial toxicity of doxorubicin
Digoxin[76]	Decreases oral absorption of digoxin
Viral vaccines	May reduce the effectiveness of viral vaccines because of cyclophosphamide immunosuppression
Immunosuppressive drugs	In combination may have additive immunosuppressive and carcinogenic effects

Cyclophosphamide Monitoring Guidelines[2]

BASELINE
Examination
- Complete physical examination

Laboratory
- CBC with differential and platelet count
- Serum chemistry profile
- Urinalysis

FOLLOW-UP
Examination (at least every 6 months)
- Complete physical examination
- Special emphasis on lymph node screen and cutaneous examination for malignancies
- Pap smear (for women) and stool guaiac

Laboratory
Weekly (frequency may be reduced to biweekly if results are unremarkable after 2 to 3 months of therapy)
- CBC with differential and platelet count

Laboratory—cont'd
- Urinalysis (stop treatment if red blood cells appear in urine)
Monthly (after 3 to 6 months, frequency of these tests may be reduced to every 3 months if stable)
- Serum chemistry profile with emphasis on liver function test values
Periodically (at least every 6 months)
- Chest x-ray
- Urine cytology when cumulative dose exceeds 50 g or if patient has had hemorrhagic cystitis

INDICATIONS FOR DISCONTINUING THERAPY (OR AT LEAST REDUCING DOSE)
- WBC < 4000 to 4500 cells/mm³ or platelets < 100,000 cells/mm³*
- Red cells in urine (refer to urologist for persistent hematuria)

Note: More frequent surveillance is needed if laboratory values are abnormal or with high-risk patients.
*A gradual reduction in WBC to 4000 to 4500 range may require closer surveillance or a small dose reduction rather than discontinuation of therapy.

to become biologically active.[9,12] (See Table 9-2 for key pharmacologic concepts of chlorambucil.)

MECHANISM OF ACTION.   Like cyclophosphamide, chlorambucil is an alkylating agent and is therefore not cell-cycle specific. Chlorambucil exerts its effects through DNA cross-linkages. This mechanism is explained in greater detail in the previous section on cyclophosphamide (see Table 9-3). Chlorambucil is also the slowest acting and least toxic nitrogen mustard derivative.[9,14]

Clinical Use
INDICATIONS
Dosage Guidelines.   Table 9-6 lists indications and contraindications for chlorambucil. Chlorambucil is supplied as Leukeran 2 mg tablets. The recommended oral dosage is 0.05 to 0.2 mg/kg/day. Dosages for benign diseases should remain at the lower end of the spectrum. Initial dosages of 4 to 10 mg/day are to induce disease control, followed by maintenance dosages of 2 to 4 mg/day. In comparison with cyclophosphamide, chlorambucil is less effective, although probably less toxic with less frequent gastrointestinal adverse effects. Chlorambucil can be tolerated as a once daily medication. Like cyclophosphamide, chlorambucil is often used in conjunction with prednisone. The therapeutic benefits of chlorambucil begin to appear in 3 to 6 weeks. However, this drug is infrequently used in dermatology. Its short-term and long-term use should be tailored to each individual.

Cytotoxic Drug Choice.   As in most cases with cyclophosphamide, chlorambucil is not the first-line treatment for any of the diseases listed in Table 9-6. Like most cytotoxic agents, it is associated with significant risks of malignancy induction and bone marrow toxicity in transplant patients.[69,70] Therefore the patient and physician should clearly outline the risks and benefits of the drug before initiating therapy. In dermatologic doses, the incidence of malignancy is not clear and likely to be overrepresented by the in-

Table 9-6	Chlorambucil Indications and Contraindications

FDA-APPROVED INDICATIONS
None specific to dermatology

OFF-LABEL USES

Vasculitis
Cryoglobulinemia[26]
Wegener's granulomatosis[19]
Other forms of necrotizing vasculitis[77]

Bullous Dermatoses
Pemphigoid[78]
Epidermolysis Bullosa Acquisita[79]
Pemphigus[31]

Neutrophilic Dermatoses
Pyoderma gangrenosum[80-82]
Behçet's disease[34,83,84]
Sweet's syndrome[85]

Connective Tissue Diseases
Dermatomyositis[37,86]
Lupus erythematosus[16,41]
Relapsing polychondritis[47]
Scleroderma[3,46]

Malignancies
Histiocytosis X[48]
Mycosis fungoides/Sezary syndrome[3,87,88]
Necrobiotic xanthogranuloma with
    paraproteinemia[89]

Infiltrative Diseases
Lichen myxedematosus[49,90]
Scleromyxedema[50]

Miscellaneous
Mastocytosis[3,91]
Sarcoidosis[92,93]
Granuloma annulare[94]
Amyloidosis[95]

CONTRAINDICATIONS

Absolute
Pregnancy (teratogenic)
Lactation (not known if present in breast
    milk but does have effect on
    infant)
Hypersensitivity to chlorambucil (may
    cross-react with cyclophosphamide or
    mechlorethamine)[59,60]

Relative
Infections (depends on severity)
Impaired hepatic function
Children (may have increased risk of seizures)

PREGNANCY PRESCRIBING STATUS—CATEGORY D

cidence in the transplant population. Complicating the decision making process, the FDA-approved package insert for Leukeran states that chlorambucil should not be used for treating nonmalignant diseases.

ADVERSE EFFECTS

Box 9-2 contains the adverse effects of chlorambucil.

Carcinogenicity. Chlorambucil therapy has a well-documented risk of inducing malig-

nancy in transplant patients.[69,70] There is a significantly increased risk of non-Hodgkin's B-cell lymphoma. Acute leukemia, especially acute myelogenous leukemia, is also increased in this population. In addition, there is a significant increase in the incidence of squamous cell carcinomas, principally of the skin.[62,67,69,70]

DRUG INTERACTIONS. The most important drug interactions for chlorambucil are listed in Table 9-7.

Box 9-2

Adverse Effects of Chlorambucil[1,13,61]

CARCINOGENICITY
- Leukemia (AML), lymphoma, squamous cell carcinoma[62,66,67,69,70]

HEMATOLOGIC
- Leukopenia (common, dose-limiting, persists for 10 days after last dose)
- Thrombocytopenia (less common)
- Anemia (less common)
- Aplastic anemia (irreversible, uncommon)

DERMATOLOGIC[71,72]
- Alopecia (rare), morbilliform rash, urticaria (uncommon), mucosal ulcerations (uncommon)

GASTROINTESTINAL (LESS COMMON)
- Nausea, vomiting, diarrhea
- Hepatotoxicity (uncommon)

REPRODUCTIVE
- Amenorrhea, azoospermia

CNS
- Generalized tonic-clonic seizures (especially in children with nephrotic syndrome, adults with seizure history, or high dose therapy)[96,97]
- Peripheral neuropathy (uncommon), myoclonus[98]

OTHER RARE ADVERSE EFFECTS
- Pneumonitis, interstitial pulmonary fibrosis,[99-101] fever, sterile cystitis
- Opportunistic infections

Table 9-7   Chlorambucil Drug Interactions

Interacting Drug	Mechanism/Clinical Result
Viral vaccines	May reduce the effectiveness of viral vaccines because of chlorambucil immunosuppression
Immunosuppressive drugs	In combination may have drug's additive immunosuppressive and carcinogenic effects

Adapted from *CliniSphere 2.0 CD ROM*, St. Louis, June 2000, Facts & Comparisons.

Chlorambucil Monitoring Guidelines[2]

BASELINE
Examination
- Complete physical examination

Laboratory
- CBC with differential and platelet count
- Serum chemistry profile
- Urinalysis

FOLLOW-UP
Examination (At Least Every 6 Months)
- Complete physical examination
- Special emphasis on lymph node screen and cutaneous examination for malignancies
- Pap smear (for women) and stool guaiac

Laboratory
Weekly (frequency may be reduced to biweekly if results are unremarkable after 3 months of therapy)

Examination (At Least Every 6 Months)—cont'd
- CBC with differential and platelet count
Monthly (after 3 to 6 months, frequency of these tests may be reduced to every 3 months if stable)
- Serum chemistry profile
- Urinalysis
Periodically (at least every 6 months)
- Chest x-ray

INDICATIONS FOR DISCONTINUING THERAPY (OR AT LEAST REDUCING DOSAGE)
- WBC < 4000 to 4500 cells/mm^3 or platelets < 100,000 cells/mm^{3*}

Note: More frequent surveillance is needed if laboratory values are abnormal or with high-risk patients.
*A gradual reduction in WBC to 4000 to 4500 range may require closer surveillance or a small dose reduction rather than discontinuation of therapy.

HYDROXYUREA

Hydroxyurea was first synthesized in 1869 by Dressler and Stein.[102] It was later found to induce leukopenia, anemia, and megaloblastic changes in the bone marrow of rabbits by Rosenthal in 1928.[103] Hydroxyurea preferentially affects cells with a high proliferative index. Yarbro in 1969 was the first to report hydroxyurea therapy for psoriasis.[104]

Pharmacology

Hydroxyurea is a small molecule that has the chemical structure of urea with an added hydroxyl group (see Table 9-2). It is well absorbed orally with peak plasma levels occurring at 1 to 2 hours.[9,105] The onset of action is fairly rapid with tissue effects noted by 5 hours, peaked in 8 hours, and persisting for 20 hours.[106] Hydroxyurea is widely distributed throughout body tissues, including the cerebrospinal fluid with peak levels in 3 hours.[1] The half-life of the drug is 5.5 hours. Within 24 hours, negligible levels of the drug remain within the body. Hydroxyurea is not significantly protein bound but does bind with plasma fibrinogen. Overall, 80% of the drug is excreted by the kidneys.[107] The actual metabolism of the drug is unclear, although it may be metabolized to acetohydroxamic acid.[108] In addition, hydroxyurea exists in higher concentrations within leukocytes than in erythrocytes.[105]

MECHANISM OF ACTION.   Hydroxyurea affects DNA synthesis, DNA repair, and gene regulation (see Table 9-3). Withdrawal of the drug results in the rapid reversal of its effects. The primary mechanism of action is through the inhibition of ribonucleotide reductase, a rate-limiting enzyme in DNA synthesis. This enzyme catalyzes the reductive conversion of ribonucleotides to deoxyribonucleotides, which are integral to DNA synthesis.[109,110] Ribonucleotide reductase is composed of two subunits, a regulatory (M_1) protein and a catalytic (M_2) protein.[111] Hydroxyurea inactivates a tyrosyl free radical in the center of the M_2 subunit while leaving the M_1 subunit unaffected. Inhibition of ribonucleotide reductase results in a decrease of intracellular levels of deoxyadenosine, deoxyguanosine, and deoxycytidine, and in an increase in deoxythymidine levels. The imbalance

of these DNA precursors may also contribute to DNA damage. Ultimately, these effects result in DNA strand breakage.[112]

Another important feature of this drug is its action as a radiation sensitizer. This probably occurs because the cells are arrested in the G_1 phase and are therefore unable to repair damage induced by ultraviolet and ionizing radiation.[113,114] Hydroxyurea may also affect gene expression directly. Hydroxyurea causes hypomethylation of the fetal hemoglobin gene, thereby increasing transcription.[115,116] Hypomethylation may play three important roles: fetal hemoglobin induction, normalization of psoriatic skin by the induction of differentiation, and induction of other genes. Epigenetic changes, such as the loss of amplified genes on episomes, have also been induced by hydroxyurea.[117] In the treatment of B16 melanoma cells, hydroxyurea has been shown to increase the activity of cellular glutathione reductase and glutathione peroxidase, which help maintain levels of glutathione.[118]

Resistance to hydroxyurea has been attributed to two mechanisms. Levels of ribonucleotide reductase may be increased through gene amplification. Additionally, the biochemical properties of ribonucleotide reductase may be altered, resulting in a decreased sensitivity to hydroxyurea.[119-121]

Clinical Use
INDICATIONS.   Table 9-8 lists indications and contraindications for hydroxyurea.

Dosage Guidelines.   Hydroxyurea is supplied as Hydrea in 500 mg tablets. Dosages range from 1 to 1.5 g/day taken in divided doses. The usual dosage is 20 to 30 mg/kg/day. Dosages beyond 2 g/day are probably not of greater benefit. The drug may be taken with food. Patients should be advised to take the medication with milk or antacids if complaints of dyspepsia arise.

Cytotoxic Drug Choice.   Hydroxyurea appears to have its greatest benefit in treating patients whose psoriasis has been refractory to topical methods of therapy, or whose medical comorbidities preclude other more potent therapies such as psoralen plus ultraviolet A (PUVA), acitretin, methotrexate, and cyclosporine. Studies have shown its positive efficacy in various forms of psoriasis including erythrodermic,

Table 9-8	Hydroxyurea Indications and Contraindications

FDA-APPROVED INDICATIONS
Squamous cell carcinoma of head and
  neck[122,123]
Metastatic melanoma and gastrointestinal
  melanoma[124-126]

OFF-LABEL USES

Vasculitis
Cryoglobulinemia[26]

Neutrophilic Dermatoses
Pyoderma gangrenosum[127]
Sweet's syndrome[128]

Malignancies
Chronic granulocytic leukemia cutis (who have
  failed radiation and busulfan)[129]

Infiltrative Diseases
Scleromyxedema[130]

Miscellaneous
Psoriasis[131-134]
Polycythemia vera[135]
Hypereosinophilic syndrome[136,137]
Sickle cell anemia[138]

CONTRAINDICATIONS

Absolute
Pregnancy (teratogenic)
Lactation (not known if present in breast milk
  but does have effect on infant)
Drug allergy

Relative
Concomitant administration of ara-C
Blood dyscrasias
Poor patient compliance
Substance abuse
Ongoing infection
Hepatic/renal/cardiopulmonary disease
Psoriatic arthropathy (ineffective)
Unstable/fulminant psoriasis
Renal disease (may need to reduce dose)

PREGNANCY PRESCRIBING STATUS—CATEGORY D

plaque, guttate, and pustular psoriasis. However, experience has shown that hydroxyurea is of little use as a single agent for the induction or maintenance of clearing in psoriasis.[131-134] The authors believe hydroxyurea is most effective when used for maintenance once initial clearance of psoriasis is achieved with other modalities such as ultraviolet B (UVB), PUVA, or retinoids.

Hypereosinophilic syndrome, when unresponsive to steroids, may respond to doses of 0.5 to 1.5 g/day of hydroxyurea.[136,137] Hydroxyurea has been used in the past as treatment for malignant melanoma in combination with other therapies such as dimethylaminotrizenocarboxamide (DTIC) and bischloroethylnitrosourea (BCNU).[124-126]

ADVERSE EFFECTS. Hydroxyurea is generally well tolerated. Layton and associates[134] noted that only 18% of patients receiving 1.5 g/day of hydroxyurea experienced adverse effects significant enough to stop the medication while 57% of patients reported no adverse effects. Older populations, however, are more susceptible to adverse effects.

Carcinogenicity. Hydroxyurea has been rarely associated with the development of acute leukemia. Three cases of acute leukemia were described by Donovan and associates[135] in patients being treated for polycythemia vera. Another case of acute myelogenous leukemia was discovered in a patient receiving hydroxyurea for 7 years.[139] Five cases of cutaneous carcino-

Note: More frequent surveillance is needed if laboratory values are abnormal or with high-risk patients.
*A small decrease of 1 to 2 g/dl in hemoglobin and an increase in MCV should be expected.

mas, including basal cell carcinomas and squamous cell carcinomas, have also been reported by Callot-Mellot and colleagues.[140]

Hematologic Toxicity. The most common adverse effects of hydroxyurea are various hematologic effects. Anemia is the most common finding present in 12% to 34% of cases. Leukopenia is present in 7% of cases. Thrombocytopenia is least common; it is present in only 2% to 3% of cases.[121] Megaloblastic changes are virtually ubiq-

uitous to patients receiving hydroxyurea.[1] This probably results from the selective inhibition of DNA synthesis, whereas RNA synthesis remains unaffected.[141] These effects (other than megaloblastosis) may occur within 48 hours of beginning therapy. They are often the dose-limiting factor in continued treatment. Like the therapeutic effects, these adverse effects resolve rapidly within a few days of withdrawal of the medication.[114]

Gastrointestinal Toxicity. Hepatitis with elevated transaminases and bilirubin has been reported but is reversible and transient.[114] Acute hepatitis is often associated with a "flu-like" syndrome. Other symptoms reported by patients include nausea, vomiting, anorexia, constipation, and stomatitis.

Renal Toxicity. Elevated blood urea nitrogen levels and creatinine levels have been reported in patients. Hematuria, proteinuria, and uricosuria have also been attributed to hydroxyurea. Renal failure is exceedingly rare but also has been reported.[114]

Cutaneous Toxicity. Hydroxyurea produces several rare cutaneous adverse reactions. Poikiloderma, affecting the dorsum of the hands with a bandlike distribution on the fingers and toes, has been seen with hydroxyurea in the treatment of chronic myelogenous leukemia.[142] Diffuse hyperpigmentation was noted in 4.7% of patients by Layton and co-workers.[134] Leg ulcers that reversed on withdrawal of the drug have also been reported.[143,144] Other cutaneous reactions include lichen planus,[145] dermatomyositis-like reactions,[146] vasculitis, fixed drug eruption,[147] focal or diffuse hyperpigmentation, radiation recall,[148] alopecia,[149] photosensitivity, palmar/plantar keratoderma, urticaria, pruritus, erythema multiforme, nail changes,[150,151] acral erythema, xerosis, and atrophy of skin and nails.[152]

Other Toxicity. Patients have also reported arthralgia, depression, diaphoresis, epistaxis, fatigue, fever,[153,154] flulike illnesses, loss of libido, lower leg swelling, and nasal septum ulceration.[155]

MYCOPHENOLIC ACID AND MYCOPHENOLATE MOFETIL

Mycophenolic acid (MPA) was originally used to treat psoriasis successfully in the 1970s.[156] Its use had fallen out of favor until recently when mycophenolate mofetil (MMF), an esterified form with greater bioavailability, was introduced.

Pharmacology

MPA is a weak organic acid that has a good oral bioavailability. On systemic absorption, the drug is inactivated by glucuronidation in the liver and subsequently converted back to its active form by β-glucuronidase within the epidermis and gastrointestinal tract.[1] MMF (see Figure 9-1) is a morpholinoester of MPA that has a greater oral bioavailability. MMF is cleaved to MPA after ingestion.[157,158]

MECHANISM OF ACTION.   MPA acts by inhibiting de novo purine synthesis. It is a noncompetitive inhibitor of inosine monophosphate dehydrogenase. This enzyme is important in the conversion of inosine-5-phosphate and xanthine-5-phosphate to guanosine-5-phosphate. Cells relying on de novo purine synthesis rather than the purine salvage pathway are preferentially affected. Therefore the proliferative responses of T lymphocytes and B lymphocytes, which lack the purine salvage pathway, are blocked.[159,160] MPA also leads to decreased levels of immunoglobulins and delayed-type hypersensitivity responses.[161]

Clinical Use

INDICATIONS.   Table 9-9 lists indications and contraindications of MMF.

Dosage Guidelines.   The usual doses are in the range of 3.0 to 4.8 g/day for MPA and of 1.3 to 2.0 g/day for MMF. The greatest effectiveness of MMF in dermatologic diseases is at doses of at least 1000 mg/day.

Cytotoxic Drug Choice.   MMF is FDA approved for the treatment of renal allograft rejection in combination with cyclosporine

Table 9-9	Mycophenolate Mofetil Indications and Contraindications

FDA-APPROVED INDICATIONS
Renal allograft rejection[162,163]

OFF-LABEL USES	
Neutrophilic Dermatoses	Miscellaneous
Refractory pyoderma gangrenosum[164]	Psoriasis[169-172]
	Dyshidrotic eczema[173]
Bullous Diseases	Metastatic Crohn's disease[170]
Bullous pemphigoid[165,166]	
Pemphigus vulgaris[167,168]	
Pemphigus foliaceus[168]	

CONTRAINDICATIONS	
Absolute	Relative
Pregnancy (teratogenic)	Lactation (may be present in breast milk)
Drug allergy	Peptic ulcer disease
	Hepatic/renal disease
	Azathioprine (concomitant administration has not been studied)
	Drugs that interfere with enterohepatic recirculation (cholestyramine)
	Hepatic/renal/cardiopulmonary disease
	Psoriatic arthropathy (ineffective)
	Unstable/fulminant psoriasis
	Renal disease (may need to reduce dose)

PREGNANCY PRESCRIBING STATUS—CATEGORY C

and corticosteroids.[162,163] In 1993, Goldblum[174] reported clinical improvement in rheumatoid arthritis patients given MMF. MPA and MMF have been reported to be effective for refractory pyoderma gangrenosum,[164] bullous pemphigoid,[165,166] pemphigus vulgaris,[167,168] pemphigus foliaceus,[168] psoriasis,[169-172] dyshidrotic eczema,[173] and metastatic Crohn's disease.[170] It should be noted that in most of the studies, MMF was used in conjunction with another agent, most commonly systemic corticosteroids.

ADVERSE EFFECTS.   MMF is very well tolerated. The most common adverse effects are gastrointestinal (Box 9-3).

Carcinogenicity.   In 1977, Lynch and Roenigk[171] reported the development of neoplasms in three patients receiving MPA for psoriasis. One woman had breast carcinoma. She had been receiving methotrexate for 5 years before beginning MPA. Another patient had a recurrent carcinoma on the scalp. The other patient had a squamous cell carcinoma of the epiglottis after 46 weeks of therapy. Epinette and associates[172] reported no incidence of carcinogenesis in their population of patients being treated with MPA for psoriasis.

Gastrointestinal Toxicity.   This organ system is the most common site of adverse reaction to MPA and MMF. It is dose dependent and includes nausea, diarrhea, soft stools, anorexia, abdominal cramps, frequent stools, vomiting, and anal tenderness.[157,164,170,173]

FLUOROURACIL

Fluorouracil (5-FU, Adrucil) is a fluorinated pyrimidine analog that was first synthesized in 1957. The oral absorption of 5-FU is poor and unpredictable, and therefore the drug is available only in an intravenous form. Most of the drug remains unbound in plasma, with a half-life of 11 hours. Principally, 5-FU is metabolized by the liver. The mechanism of action appears to be through its interaction with DNA, RNA, and protein synthesis as an antimetabolite. This drug covalently binds to thymidylate synthetase, thereby inactivating the enzyme complex and preventing the conversion of deoxyuridine monophosphate (dUMP) to deoxythymidine monophosphate (dTMP), which is required for DNA synthesis. Cell growth is also inhibited because 5-FU incorporates itself into RNA as an abnormal base pair.[9] 5-FU does not have any FDA-approved dermatologic indications; however, there have been reports of clinical use in recalcitrant psoriasis,[175] mycosis fungoides,[176] scleroderma,[177,178] and metastatic melanoma.[179,180] As an intralesional agent, 5-FU has been efficacious for keratoacanthoma, basal cell carcinoma, psoriasis, and squamous cell carcinoma. Its primary use has been as a topical agent for actinic keratosis, superficial basal cell carcinomas, verruca plana, and other benign, premalignant, and malignant lesions. (Topical use of 5-FU is discussed in Chapter 29.) The toxicity of parenteral 5-FU can be severe, with

Box 9-3

Adverse Effects of Mycophenolate Mofetil[168,170]

CARCINOGENICITY
- Controversial (see text)

GASTROINTESTINAL
- Dose-dependent, most common
- Nausea, diarrhea, soft stools, anorexia, abdominal cramps, frequent stools, vomiting, anal tenderness

GENITOURINARY
- Urgency, frequency, dysuria, burning, sterile pyuria (occasionally)

GENITOURINARY—cont'd
- Decrease in frequency after first year
- Does not cause nephrotoxicity

INFECTIOUS
- Increased incidence of herpes zoster
- Increased incidence of viral and bacterial infections (postulated)

NEUROLOGIC
- Weakness, fatigue, headache, tinnitus, insomnia

Mycophenolate Mofetil Monitoring Guidelines[2,168,170]

BASELINE

Examination
- Complete physical examination

Laboratory
- CBC with differential and platelet count
- Serum chemistry profile
- Serum liver function tests

FOLLOW-UP

Examination (At Least Every 6 Months)
- Complete physical examination

Laboratory
Weekly to *biweekly*
- CBC with differential and platelet count weekly for first month

Laboratory—cont'd
- CBC with differential and platelet count bi-weekly for second and third months

Monthly
- CBC with differential for first year (starting fourth month of therapy)
- Serum liver function tests

INDICATIONS FOR DISCONTINUING THERAPY (OR AT LEAST REDUCING DOSE)
- WBC < 4000 to 4500 cells/mm^3

Note: More frequent surveillance is needed if laboratory values are abnormal or with high-risk patients.

adverse effects including severe bone marrow suppression, gastrointestinal effects, and cutaneous reactions. Given its parenteral administration, narrow therapeutic window, and the availability of other equally effective and safer agents, 5-FU is rarely used in dermatology.

MELPHALAN

Melphalan (Alkeran), like cyclophosphamide and chlorambucil, is an alkylating agent and a phenylalanine derivative of nitrogen mustard. Melphalan's oral bioavailability is variable at 71% ± 23%. Approximately 80% to 90% of the drug is protein-bound in plasma. The half-life is 90 minutes, with only 10% to 15% of the drug excreted unchanged in the urine while the remainder is metabolized by the liver.[9] Melphalan has been used for amyloidosis,[181,182] cryoglobulinemia,[63] metastatic melanoma,[183] necrobiotic xanthogranuloma,[184] pyoderma gangrenosum,[185] relapsing polychondritis,[47] and scleromyxedema.[186,187] The usual dose is 6 mg daily to induce disease control, followed by 2 mg daily for maintenance therapy. Like other alkylating agents, its adverse effects are bone marrow suppression, increased risk of malignancies (especially leukemia), gastrointestinal effects, reproductive effects, and cutaneous reactions.[9] Melphalan is uncommonly used by dermatologists.

Bibliography

Ahmed AR, Hombal SM: Cyclophosphamide (Cytoxan): a review on relevant pharmacology and clinical uses. *J Am Acad Dermatol* 11:1115-1126, 1984.

Boyd A, Neldner K: Hydroxyurea therapy. *J Am Acad Dermatol* 16:518-524, 1991.

Calabresi P, Chabner BA: Chemotherapy of neoplastic diseases. In Goodman LS, Gilman AG, Rall TW, et al, editors: *The pharmacological basis of therapeutics,* New York, 1995, Pergamon Press, pp 1232-1287.

Lind MJ, Ardiet C: Pharmacokinetics of alkylating agents. *Cancer Surv* 17:157-188, 1993.

McDonald CJ, editor: *The use of immunomodu-latory and cytotoxic agents in dermatological diseases,* New York, 1997, Marcel Dekker, Inc.

McDonald CJ: Cytotoxic agents for use in dermatology: I. *J Am Acad Dermatol* 12:753-775, 1985.

McDonald CJ: Use of cytotoxic drugs in dermatologic diseases: II. *J Am Acad Dermatol* 12:965-975, 1985.

Nashel DJ: Mechanisms of action and clinical applications of cytotoxic drugs in rheumatic disorders. *Med Clin North Am* 69:817-840, 1985.

Shupack JL, Stiller MJ, Webster GF: Cytotoxic agents and dermatologic therapy. In Fitzpatrick TB, Eisen AZ, Wolff R, et al, editors: *Dermatology in general medicine,* Philadelphia, 1993, JB Lippincott, pp 2872-2883.

References

Overviews

1. McDonald CJ: Cytotoxic agents for use in dermatology. I. *J Am Acad Dermatol* 12:753-775, 1985.
2. McDonald CJ: Use of cytotoxic drugs in dermatologic diseases. II. *J Am Acad Dermatol* 12:965-975, 1985.
3. Dantzig PI: Immunosuppressive and cytotoxic drugs in dermatology. *Arch Dermatol* 110:393-406, 1974.
4. Schwartz RS, Gowans JDC: Guidelines for the use of cytotoxic drugs in rheumatic diseases (letter). *Arthritis Rheum* 14:134, 1971.
5. Steinberg AD, Plotz PH, Wolff SM, et al: Cytotoxic drugs in the treatment of nonmalignant disease. *Ann Intern Med* 76:619-642, 1972.
6. Whitehouse JMA: Cytotoxic drugs for non-neoplastic disease. *BMJ* 287:79-80, 1983.

Cyclophosphamide—Pharmacology

7. Gerschwin ME, Goetzl EJ, Stienberg AD: Cyclophosphamide: use in practice. *Ann Intern Med* 80:531-540, 1974.
8. Colvin M, Hilton J: Pharmacology of cyclophosphamide and metabolites. *Cancer Treat Rep* 65:89-95, 1981.
9. Calabresi P, Chabner BA: Chemotherapy of neoplastic diseases. In Goodman LS, Gilman AG, Rall TW, et al, editors: *The pharmacological basis of therapeutics,* New York, 1990, Pergamon Press, pp 1202-1263.
10. Bagley CM, Bostick FW, DeVita VT: Clinical pharmacology of cyclophosphamide. *Cancer Res* 33:226-223, 1973.

11. Jardine I, Fenselau C, Appler M, et al: Quantification by gas chromatography chemical ionization. Mass spectrometry of cyclophosphamide, phosphoramide mustard, and nor-nitrogen mustard in the plasma and urine of patients receiving cyclophosphamide therapy. *Cancer Res* 38:408-415, 1978.
12. Lind MJ, Ardiet C: Pharmacokinetics of alkylating agents. *Cancer Surv* 17:157-188, 1993.
13. Rapini RP: Cytotoxic drugs in the treatment of skin disease. *Int J Dermatol* 30:313-321, 1991.
14. Hall AG, Tilby MJ: Mechanisms of action of, and modes of resistance to, alkylating agents used in the treatment of haematological malignancies. *Blood Rev* 6:163-173, 1992.
15. Sievers TM, Rossi SJ, Ghobrial RM, et al: Mycophenolate mofetil. *Pharmacotherapy* 17:1178-1197, 1997.
16. Fox DA, McCune WJ: Immunosuppressive drug therapy of systemic lupus erythematosus. *Rheum Dis Clin North Am* 20:265-299, 1994.

Cyclophosphamide—Indications

17. Ahmed AR, Hombal SM: Cyclophosphamide (Cytoxan): A review on relevant pharmacology and clinical uses. *J Am Acad Dermatol* 11:1115-1126, 1984.
18. Novack SN, Pearson CM: Cyclophosphamide therapy in Wegener's granulomatosis. *N Engl J Med* 284:938-942, 1971.
19. Morton CE, Easton DJ: Cytotoxic therapy for Wegener's granulomatosis (letter). *Lancet* 1:1411, 1984.

20. DeRemee RA, McDonald TJ, Weiland LH: Wegener's granulomatosis: observations on treatment with antimicrobial agents. *Mayo Clin Proc* 60:27-32, 1985.

21. Brodell RT, Miller CW, Eisen AZ: Cutaneous lesions of lymphomatoid granulomatosis. *Arch Dermatol* 122:303-306, 1986.

22. Leib ES, Restivo C, Paulus HE: Immunosuppressive and corticosteroid therapy for polyarteritis nodosa. *Am J Med* 67:941-947, 1979.

23. Kinlen LJ: Incidence of cancer in rheumatoid arthritis and other disorders after immunosuppressive treatment. *Am J Med* 78(Suppl 1A):44-49, 1985.

24. Taylow HG, Samanta A: Treatment of vasculitis. *Br J Clin Pharmacol* 35:93-104, 1993.

25. Fauci AS, Katz P, Haynes BF, et al: Cyclophosphamide therapy of severe systemic necrotizing vasculitis. *N Engl J Med* 301:235-238, 1979.

26. Ristow SC, Griner PF, Abraham GN, et al: Reversal of systemic manifestations of cryoglobulinemia: treatment with melphalan and prednisone. *Arch Intern Med* 136:467-470, 1976.

27. Brody HJ, Pirozzi DJ: Benign mucous membrane pemphigoid. Response to therapy with cyclophosphamide. *Arch Dermatol* 113:1598-1599, 1977.

28. Ebringer A, Mackay IR: Pemphigus vulgaris successfully treated with cyclophosphamide. *Ann Intern Med* 71:125-127, 1969.

29. McKelvey EM, Hasegaga J: Cyclophosphamide and pemphigus vulgaris. *Arch Dermatol* 103:198-200, 1971.

30. Fellner MJ, Katz JM, McCabe JB: Successful use of cyclophosphamide and prednisone for initial treatment of pemphigus vulgaris. *Arch Dermatol* 114:889-894, 1978.

31. Piamphongsant T, Ophaswongse S: Treatment of pemphigus. *Int J Dermatol* 30:139-146, 1991.

32. Crawford SE, Sherman R, Farara B: Pyoderma gangrenosum with response to cyclophosphamide therapy. *J Pediatr* 71:255-258, 1967.

33. Newell LM, Malkinson FD: Pyoderma gangrenosum: response to cyclophosphamide therapy. *Arch Dermatol* 119:495-497, 1983.

34. Arbesfeld SJ, Kurban AK: Behçet's disease: new perspectives on an enigmatic syndrome. *J Am Acad Dermatol* 19:767-779, 1988.

35. Buckeley CE III, Gillis JR Jr: Cyclophosphamide therapy of Behçet's disease. *J Allergy Clin Immunol* 43:273-283, 1969.

36. Chow R, Benny W, Coupe RL, et al: Erythema elevatum diutinum associated with IgA paraproteinemia successfully controlled with intermittent plasma exchange. *Arch Dermatol* 132:1360-1364, 1993.

37. Ansell BM: Management of polymyositis and dermatomyositis. *Clin Rheum Dis* 10:205-213, 1984.

38. El Ghobarch A, Balint GD: Dermatomyositis: observation on the use of immunosuppressive therapy and review of literature. *Postgrad Med* 54:516-527, 1978.

39. Yoshioka M, Okuno T, Mikawa H: Prognosis and treatment of polymyositis with particular reference to steroid-resistant patients. *Arch Dis Child* 60:236-244, 1985.

40. Bombardieri S, Hughes GRV, Neri R, et al: Cyclophosphamide in severe polymyositis (letter). *Lancet* 1:1138-1139, 1989.

41. Sabbour MS, Osman LM: Comparison of chlorambucil, azathioprine, or cyclophosphamide combined with corticosteroids in the treatment of lupus nephritis. *Br J Dermatol* 100:113-125, 1979.

42. Dinant HJ, Decker JL, Klippel JH, et al: Alternate modes of cyclophosphamide and azathioprine therapy in lupus nephritis. *Ann Intern Med* 96:728-736, 1982.

43. Hecht B, Siegel N, Adler M, et al: Prognostic indices in lupus nephritis. *Medicine* 55:163-181, 1976.

44. McCune WJ, Golbus J, Zeldes W, et al: Clinical and immunological effects of monthly administration of intravenous cyclophosphamide in severe systemic lupus erythematosus. *N Engl J Med* 318:1423-1431, 1988.

45. Steigerwal JC: Progressive systemic sclerosis. Management: III. Immunosuppressive agents. *Clin Rheum Dis* 5:284-294, 1979.

46. Torres MA, Furst DE: Treatment of generalized systemic sclerosis. *Rheum Dis Clin North Am* 16:217-241, 1990.

47. Cohen PR, Rapini RP: Relapsing polychondritis. *Int J Dermatol* 25:280-285, 1986.

48. Roper SS, Spraker MK: Cutaneous histiocytosis syndromes. *Pediatr Dermatol* 3:19-30, 1985.

49. Jessen RT, Straight M, Becker LE: Lichen myxedematosus: treatment with cyclophosphamide. *Int J Dermatol* 17:833-839, 1978.

50. Gabriel SE, Perry HO, Oleson GB, et al: Scleromyxedema: a scleroderma-like disorder with systemic manifestations. *Medicine* 67:58-65, 1988.

51. Higgins LC Jr, Thompson JG: Psoriasis with arthritis: chemotherapy with cyclophosphamide, nitrogen mustard and 6-mercaptopurine. *South Med J* 59:1191-1193, 1966.

52. Morrison JGL, Schulz EJ: Treatment of eczema with cyclophosphamide and azathioprine. *Br J Dermatol* 98:203-207, 1978.

53. Eastham JH, Segal JL, Gomez MF, et al: Reversal of erythema multiforme major with cyclophosphamide and prednisone. *Ann Pharmacother* 30:606-607, 1996.

54. Liang GC, Granston AS: Complete remission of multicentric reticulohistiocytosis with combination therapy of steroid, cyclophosphamide, and low-dose pulse methotrexate. Case report, review of the literature, and proposal for treatment. *Arthritis Rheum* 39:171-174, 1996.

55. Coupe MO, Whittaker SJ, Thatcher N: Multicentric reticulohistiocytosis. *Br J Dermatol* 116:245-247, 1987.

56. Koizumi K, Sawada K, Nishio M, et al: Effective high-dose chemotherapy followed by autologous peripheral blood stem cell transplantation in a patient with the aggressive form of cytophagic histiocytic panniculitis. *Bone Marrow Transplant* 20:171-173, 1997.

57. Matsue K, Itoh M, Tsukuda K, et al: Successful treatment of cytophagic histiocytic panniculitis with modified CHOP-E. Cyclophosphamide, Adriamycin, vincristine, prednisone, and etoposide. *Am J Clin Oncol* 17:470-474, 1994.

58. Klein E, Hahn GM, Solomon JA, et al: Explorations of antimitotic agents in the treatment of a congenital disease, ichthyosis linearis circumflexa. *J Surg Oncol* 11:85-88, 1979.

59. Weiss RB, Bruno S: Hypersensitivity reactions to cancer chemotherapy agents. *Ann Intern Med* 94:66-72, 1981.

60. Kritharides L, Lawrie K, Varigos GA: Cyclophosphamide hypersensitivity and cross-reactivity with chlorambucil (letter). *Cancer Treat Rep* 71:1323-1324, 1987.

Cyclophosphamide—Adverse Effects

61. Luqmani RA, Palmer RG, Bacon PA: Azathioprine, cyclophosphamide and chlorambucil. *Baillieres Clin Rheumatol* 4:595-619, 1990.

62. Baker GL, Kahl LE, Zee BC: Malignancy following treatment of rheumatoid arthritis with cyclophosphamide. *Am J Med* 83:1-9, 1987.

63. Pedersen-Bjergaard J, Ersboll J, Hansen VL, et al: Carcinoma of the urinary bladder after treatment with cyclophosphamide for non-Hodgkin's lymphoma. *N Engl J Med* 318:1028-1032, 1988.

64. Fairchild WV, Spence CR, Soloman HD, et al: The incidence of bladder cancer after cyclophosphamide therapy. *J Urology* 1222:163-164, 1979.

65. Brock N, Pohl J, Stekar J: Studies on the urotoxicity of oxazaphosphorine cytostatics and its prevention. I. Experimental studies on the urotoxicity of alkylating agents. *Eur J Cancer Clin Oncol* 17:596-607, 1981.

66. Baltus JAM, Boersma JW, Hartman AP, et al: The occurrence of malignancies in patients with rheumatoid arthritis treated with cyclophosphamide: a controlled retrospective follow-up. *Ann Rheum Dis* 42:368-370, 1983.

67. Ellis M, Lishner M: Second malignancies following treatment in non-Hodgkin's lymphoma. *Leuk Lymph* 9:337-342, 1993.

68. Haas JF, Kittelmann B, Mehnert WH, et al: Risk of leukemia in ovarian tumor and breast cancer patients following treatment by cyclophosphamide. *Br J Cancer* 55:213-218, 1987.

69. Palmer RG, Denman AM: Malignancies induced by chlorambucil. *Cancer Treat Rev* 11:121-129, 1984.

70. Berk PP, Goldberg JD, Silverstein MN, et al: Increased incidence of acute leukemia in polycythemia vera associated with chlorambucil therapy. *N Engl J Med* 304:441-447, 1981.

71. DeSpain JD: Dermatologic toxicity of chemotherapy. *Semin Oncol* 19:501-507, 1992.

72. Bronner AK, Hood AF: Cutaneous complications of chemotherapeutic agents. *J Am Acad Dermatol* 9:645-663, 1983.

73. Assier-Bonnet H, Aractingi S, Cadranel J, et al: Stevens-Johnson syndrome induced by cyclophosphamide: report of two cases. *Br J Dermatol* 135:864-866, 1996.

74. DeFronzo RA, Braine H, Colvin OM: Water intoxication in man after cyclophosphamide therapy. Time course and relation to drug activation. *Ann Intern Med* 78:861-869, 1973.

75. Dillman JB: Safe use of succinylcholine during repeated anesthetics in a patient treated with cyclophosphamide. *Anesth Analg* 66:351-353, 1987.

76. Bjornsson TD, Huang AT, Roth P, et al: Effects of high-dose cancer chemotherapy on the absorption of digoxin in two different formulations. *Clin Pharmacol Ther* 39:25-28, 1986.

77. Bradley JD, Brandt KD, Kath BP: Infectious complications of cyclophosphamide treatment for vasculitis. *Arthritis Rheum* 32:45-53, 1989.

Chlorambucil—Indications

78. Milligan A, Hutchinson PE: The use of chlorambucil in the treatment of bullous pemphigoid. *J Am Acad Dermatol* 22:796-801, 1990.

79. Kofler H, Wambacher-Gasser B, Topar G, et al: Intravenous immunoglobulin treatment in therapy-resistant epidermolysis bullosa acquisita. *J Am Acad Dermatol* 36:331-335, 1997.

80. Callen JP, Case JD, Sager D: Chlorambucil—An effective corticosteroid-sparing therapy for pyoderma gangrenosum. *J Am Acad Dermatol* 21:515-519, 1989.

81. Resnik BI, Rendon M, Kerdel FA: Successful treatment of aggressive pyoderma gangrenosum with pulse steroids and chlorambucil. *J Am Acad Dermatol* 27:635-636, 1992.

82. Burruss JB, Farmer ER, Callen JP: Chlorambucil is an effective corticosteroid-sparing agent for recalcitrant pyoderma gangrenosum. *J Am Acad Dermatol* 35:720-724, 1996.

83. Mamo JG, Azzam SA: Treatment of Behçet's disease with chlorambucil. *Arch Ophthalmol* 84:446-450, 1970.

84. Wong RC, Ellis CB, Diz LA: Behçet's disease. *Int J Dermatol* 23:25-32, 1984.

85. Case JD, Smith SZ, Callen JP: The use of pulse methylprednisolone and chlorambucil in the treatment of Sweet's syndrome. *Cutis* 44:125-129, 1989.

86. Sinoway PA, Callen JP: Chlorambucil: an effective corticosteroid-sparing agent for patients with recalcitrant dermatomyositis. *Arthritis Rheum* 36:319-324, 1993.

87. Hamminga L, Hargrink-Groenveld CA, van Vloten WA: Sézary's syndrome: a clinical evaluation of eight patients. *Br J Dermatol* 100:291-296, 1979.

88. McEvoy MT, Zelickson BD, Pineda AA, Winkelmann RK: Intermittent leukapheresis: an adjunct to low-dose chemotherapy for Sézary syndrome. *Acta Derm Venereol* 69:73-76, 1989.

89. Mehregan DA, Winkelmann RK: Necrobiotic xanthogranuloma. *Arch Dermatol* 128:94-100, 1992.

90. Wieder JM, Barton KL, Baron JM, et al: Lichen myxedematosus treated with chlorambucil. *J Dermatol Surg Oncol* 19:475-476, 1993.

91. Moschella SL: Chemotherapy used in dermatology. *Cutis* 19:603-612, 1977.

92. Kataria YP: Chlorambucil in sarcoidosis. *Chest* 78:36-43, 1980.

93. Selroos O: Treatment of sarcoidosis. *Sarcoidosis* 11:80-83, 1994.

94. Winkelmann RK, Stevens JC: Successful treatment response of granuloma annulare and carpal tunnel syndrome to chlorambucil. *Mayo Clin Proc* 69:1163-1165, 1994.

95. Gertz MA, Kyle RA: Amyloidosis: prognosis and treatment. *Semin Arthritis Rheum* 24:124-138, 1994.

Chlorambucil—Adverse Effects

96. Salloum E, Khan KK, Cooper DL: Chlorambucil-induced seizures. *Cancer* 79:1009-1013, 1997.

97. Williams SA, Makker SP, Grupe WE: Seizures: a significant side effect of chlorambucil therapy in children. *J Pediatr* 93:516-518, 1978.

98. Wyllie AR, Bayliff CD, Kovacs MJ: Myoclonus due to chlorambucil in two adults with lymphoma. *Ann Pharmacother* 31:171-174, 1997.

99. Mohr M, Kingreen D, Ruhl H, Huhn D: Interstitial lung disease—an underdiagnosed side effect of chlorambucil? *Ann Hematol* 67:305-307, 1993.

100. Giles FJ, Smith MP, Goldstone AH: Chlorambucil lung toxicity. *Acta Haematol* 83:156-158, 1990.

101. Carr ME Jr: Chlorambucil induced pulmonary fibrosis: report of a case and review. *Va Med* 113:677-680, 1986.

Hydroxyurea—Pharmacology

102. Dressler WF, Stein R: Uber den hydroxylharnstuff. *Justus Liebigs Ann Chem* 150:242-252, 1869.

103. Rosenthal F, Wislicki L, Kollek L: Ueber die beziehungen von schwersten blutgiften zu abbauprodukten des eiweisses: ein beitrag zum entsehungsmechanismus der perniziosen anamie. *Klin Wochenschr* 7:972-977, 1928.

104. Yarbro JW: Hydroxyurea in the treatment of refractory psoriasis. *Lancet* 2:846-847, 1969.

105. Donehower RC: Hydroxyurea. In Chabner BA, Collins JM, editors: *Cancer chemotherapy*, Philadelphia, 1990, JB Lippincott, pp 225-233.

106. McDonald CJ: Uses of systemic chemotherapeutic agents in psoriasis. *Pharmacol Ther* 14:1-24, 1981.

107. Yarbro JW: Mechanism of action of hydroxyurea. *Semin Oncol* 19:1-10, 1992.

108. Fishbein WN, Carbone PP: Hydroxyurea: mechanism of action. *Science* 142:1069-1070, 1963.

109. Krakoff IH, Brown NC, Reichard P: Inhibition of ribonucleoside diphosphate reductase by hydroxyurea. *Cancer Res* 28:1559-1565, 1968.

110. Thelander L, Reichard P: Reduction of ribonucleotides. *Annu Rev Biochem* 48:133-158, 1979.

111. Reichard P, Ehrenberg A: Ribonucleotide reductase: a radical enzyme. *Science* 221:514-519, 1983.

112. Li JC, Kaminskas E: Progressive formation of DNA lesions in cultured Ehrlich ascites tumor cells treated with hydroxyurea. *Cancer Res* 47:2755-2758, 1987.

113. Francis AA, Blevins RD, Carrier WL, et al: Inhibition of DNA repair in ultraviolet-irradiated human cells by hydroxyurea. *Biochem Biophys Acta* 563:385-392, 1979.

114. Donehower RC: An overview of the clinical experience with hydroxyurea. *Semin Oncol* 19:11-19, 1992.

115. Galanello R, Stamatoyannopoulos G, Papyannopoulou T: Mechanism of HbF stimulation by S-stage compounds: in vitro studies with bone marrow cells exposed to 5-azacytidine, ara-C, or hydroxyurea. *J Clin Invest* 81:1209-1216, 1988.

116. Watson JD, Hopkins NH, Roberts JW, et al, editors: *Molecular biology of the gene*, Reading, MA, 1987, Benjamin/Cummings.

117. Christen RD, Shalinsky DR, Howell SB: Enhancement of the loss of multiple drug resistance by hydroxyurea. *Semin Oncol* 19:94-100, 1992.

118. Eskenazi AE, Pinkas, J, Whitin JC, et al: Role of antioxidant enzymes in the induction of increased experimental metastasis by hydroxyurea. *J Natl Cancer Inst* 9:711-721, 1993.

119. Wright JA: Altered mammalian ribonucleoside diphosphate reductase from mutant cell lines. *Int Encycl Pharmacol Ther* 128:89, 1989.

120. Choy BK, McClarty GA, Chan AK, et al: Molecular mechanisms of drug resistance involving ribonucleotide reductase: hydroxyurea resistance in a series of clonally related mouse cell lines selected in the presence of increasing drug concentrations. *Cancer Res* 48:2029-2035, 1988.

121. Hurta RA, Wright JA: Amplification of the genes for both components of ribonucleotide reductase in hydroxyurea resistant mammalian cells. *Biochem Biophys Res Commun* 167:258-264, 1990.

Hydroxyurea—Indications

122. Gandia D, Wibault P, Guillot T, et al: Simultaneous chemoradiotherapy as salvage treatment in locoregional recurrences of squamous head and neck cancer. *Head Neck* 15:8-15, 1993.

123. Vokes EE, Haraf DJ, Panje WR, et al: Hydroxyurea with concomitant radiotherapy for locally advanced head and neck cancer. *Semin Oncol* 19(3 Suppl 9):53-58, 1992.

124. Willbanks OL, Fogelman MJ: Gastrointestinal melanosarcoma. *Am J Surg* 120:602-606, 1970.

125. Gottlieb JA, Frei E III, Luce K: Dose schedule studies with hydroxyurea in malignant melanoma. *Cancer Chemother Rep* 55:277-280, 1971.

126. Costanzi JJ, Vaitkevicius V, Quagliana JM, et al: Combination chemotherapy for disseminated malignant melanoma. *Cancer* 35:342-346, 1975.

127. Schiefke I, Halm U, Paasch U, et al: Pyoderma gangrenosum and portal vein thrombosis in a 33-year-old female patient. *Deutsche Med Wschr* 124:142-145, 1999.

128. Osterwalder B, Schmid L, Jungi WF, et al: Myeloproliferative syndrome and acute febrile neutrophilic dermatosis (Sweet syndrome)—a rare association. *Schweiz Med Wschr* 117:1896-1901, 1987.

129. Friedhoff FW, Atamer MA, Thelmo WL: Chronic granulocytic leukemia cutis treated with hydroxyurea. *Chemotherapy* 24:321-326, 1978.

130. Harris RB, Perry HO, Kyle RA, et al: Treatment of scleromyxedema with melphalan. *Arch Dermatol* 115:295-299, 1979.
131. Leavell UW, Yarbro JW: Hydroxyurea: a new treatment for psoriasis. *Arch Dermatol* 102:144-150, 1970.
132. Stein KM, Shelley WB, Weinberg RA: Hydroxyurea in the treatment of pustular psoriasis. *Br J Dermatol* 85:81-85, 1971.
133. Moschella SL, Greenwald MA: Psoriasis with hydroxyurea: an 18-month study of 60 patients. *Arch Dermatol* 107:363-368, 1973.
134. Layton AM, Sheehan-Dare RA, Goodfield MJD, et al: Hydroxyurea in the management of therapy resistant psoriasis. *Br J Dermatol* 121:647-653, 1989.
135. Donovan PB, Kaplan ME, Goldberg JD, et al: Treatment of polycythemia vera with hydroxyurea. *Am J Hematol* 17:329-334, 1984.
136. Fauci AS: The idiopathic hypereosinophilic syndrome. *Ann Intern Med* 97:78, 1982.
137. Parrillo JE, Fauci AS, Wolff SM: Therapy of the hypereosinophilic syndrome. *Ann Intern Med* 89:167-172, 1978.
138. Goldberg MA, Brugnara C, Dover GJ, et al: Treatment of sickle cell anemia with hydroxyurea and erythropoietin. *N Engl J Med* 323:366-372, 1990.

Hydroxyurea—Adverse Effects

139. van den Anker-Lugtenburg PJ, Sizoo W: Myelodysplastic syndrome and secondary acute leukemia after treatment of essential thrombocythemia with hydroxyurea. *Am J Hematol* 33:152, 1990.
140. Callot-Mellot C, Bodemer C, Chosidow O, et al: Cutaneous carcinoma during long-term hydroxyurea therapy: a report of 5 cases. *Arch Dermatol* 132:1395-1397, 1996.
141. Spier S, Solomon LM, Esterly NB, et al: Hydroxyurea and macrocytosis. *Br J Dermatol* 89:199-205, 1973.
142. Kennedy BJ, Smith LR, Goltz RW: Skin changes secondary to hydroxyurea therapy. *Arch Dermatol* 111:183-187, 1975.
143. Best PJ, Daoud MS, Pittelkow MR, et al: Hydroxyurea-induced leg ulceration in 14 patients. *Ann Intern Med* 128:29-32, 1998.
144. Montefusco E, Alimena G, Gastaldi R, et al: Unusual dermatologic toxicity of long-term therapy with hydroxyurea in chronic myelogenous leukemia. *Tumori* 72:317-321, 1986.
145. Renfro L, Kamino H, Raphael J, et al: Ulcerative lichen planus like dermatitis associated with hydroxyurea. *J Am Acad Dermatol* 24:143-145, 1991.
146. Senet P, Aractingi S, Porneuf M, et al: Hydroxyurea-induced dermatomyositis-like eruption. *Br J Dermatol* 133:455-459, 1995.
147. Moschella SL: Chemotherapy of psoriasis: ten years of experience. *Int J Dermatol* 15:373-378, 1976.
148. Sears ME: Erythema in areas of previous irradiation in patients treated with hydroxyurea (NSC-32065). *Cancer Chemother Rep* 40:31-32, 1964.
149. Ariel IM: Therapeutic effects of hydroxyurea: experience with 118 patients with inoperable solid tumors. *Cancer* 25:705-714, 1970.
150. Richard M, Truchetet F, Friedel J, et al: Skin lesions simulating chronic dermatomyositis during long-term hydroxyurea therapy. *J Am Acad Dermatol* 21:797-799, 1989.
151. Delmas-Marsalet B, Beaulieu P, Teillet-Thiebaud F, et al: Longitudinal melanonychia induced by hydroxyurea: four case reports and review of the literature. *Nouv Rev Fr Hematol* 37:205-210, 1995.
152. Kennedy BJ, Smith LR, Goltz RW: Skin changes secondary to hydroxyurea. *Arch Dermatol* 111:183-187, 1975.
153. Lossos IS, Matzner Y: Hydroxyurea-induced fever: case report and review of the literature. *Ann Pharmacother* 29:132-133, 1995.
154. Van der Klooster JM, Sucec PM, Stiegelis WF, et al: Fever caused by hydroxyurea: a report of three cases and review of the literature. *Neth J Med* 51:114-118, 1997.
155. Boyd A, Neldner K: Hydroxyurea therapy. *J Am Acad Dermatol* 16:518-524, 1991.

Mycophenolic Acid and Mycophenolate Mofetil—Pharmacology

156. Jones EL, Hackney VC, Menendez L, et al: Treatment of psoriasis with oral mycophenolic acid. *J Invest Dermatol* 65:537-542, 1975.
157. Platz KP, Sollinger HW, Hullett DA, et al: RS-61443: a new, potent immunosuppressive agent. *Transplantation* 51:27-31, 1991.
158. Lee WA, Gu L, Miksztal AR, et al: Bioavailability improvement of mycophenolic acid through amino ester derivatization. *Pharm Res* 7:161-166, 1990.
159. Eugui EM, Mirkovitch A, Allison AC: Lymphocyte-selective anti-proliferative and immunosuppressive effects of mycophenolic acid in mice. *Scand J Immunol* 33:175-183, 1991.

160. Eugui EM, Almquist S, Muller CD, et al: Lymphocyte-selective cytostatic and immunosuppressive effects of mycophenolic acid in vitro: role of deoxyguanosine nucleotide depletion. *Scand J Immunol* 33:161-173, 1991.

161. Schiff MH, Goldblum R, Rees MMC: New DMARD. Mycophenolate mofetil (Myco-M) effectively treats refractory rheumatoid arthritis (RA) patients for one year. *Arthritis Rheum* 34:S89, 1991.

Mycophenolic Acid and Mycophenolate Mofetil—Indications

162. European Mycophenolate Mofetil Cooperative Study Group: Placebo-controlled study of mycophenolate mofetil combined with cyclosporine and corticosteroids for prevention of acute rejection. *Lancet* 345:1321-1325, 1995.

163. Solinger HW, US Renal Transplant Mycophenolate Mofetil Study Group: Mycophenolate mofetil for the prevention of acute rejection in cadaveric renal allograft recipients. *Transplantation* 60:225-232, 1995.

164. Hohenleutner U, Mohr VD, Michel S, et al: Mycophenolate mofetil and cyclosporine treatment for recalcitrant pyoderma gangrenosum (letter). *Lancet* 350:1748, 1997.

165. Bohm M, Beissert S, Schwartz T, et al: Bullous pemphigoid treated with mycophenolate mofetil. *Lancet* 349:541, 1997.

166. Nousari HC, Griffin WA, Anhalt GJ: Successful therapy of bullous pemphigoid with mycophenolate mofetil. *J Am Acad Dermatol* 39:497-498, 1998.

167. Enk AH, Knop J: Treatment of pemphigus vulgaris with mycophenolate mofetil (letter). *Lancet* 350:494, 1997.

168. Nousari HC, Sragovich A, Kimyai-Asadi A, et al: Mycophenolate mofetil in autoimmune and inflammatory skin disorders. *J Am Acad Dermatol* 40:265-268, 1999.

169. Haufs MG, Beissert S, Grabbe S, et al: Psoriasis vulgaris treated successfully with mycophenolate mofetil. *Br J Dermatol* 138:179-181, 1998.

170. Kitchin JE, Pomeranz MK, Pak G, et al: Rediscovering mycophenolic acid: a review of its mechanism, side effects, and potential uses. *J Am Acad Dermatol* 37:445-449, 1997.

171. Lynch WS, Roenigk HH Jr: Mycophenolic acid for psoriasis. *Arch Dermatol* 113:1203-1208, 1977.

172. Epinette WW, Parker CM, Jones EL, et al: Mycophenolic acid for psoriasis: a review of pharmacology, long-term efficacy, and safety. *J Am Acad Dermatol* 17:962-971, 1987.

173. Picknacker A, Luger TA, Schwarz T: Dyshidrotic eczema treated with mycophenolate mofetil. *Arch Dermatol* 134:378-379, 1998.

174. Goldblum R: Therapy of rheumatoid arthritis with mycophenolate mofetil. *Clin Exp Rheum* 11:S117-119, 1993.

5-Fluorouracil

175. Alper JC, Wiemann MC, Rueckl FS, et al: Rationally designed combination chemotherapy for the treatment of patients with recalcitrant psoriasis. *J Am Acad Dermatol* 13:567-577, 1985.

176. Schappell DL, Alper JC, McDonald CJ: Treatment of advanced mycosis fungoides and Sézary syndrome with continuous infusions of methotrexate followed by fluorouracil and leucovorin rescue. *Arch Dermatol* 131:307-313, 1995.

177. Casas JA, Subauste CP, Alarcon GS: A new promising treatment in systemic sclerosis: 5-fluorouracil. *Ann Rheum Dis* 46:763-767, 1987.

178. Casas JA, Saway PA, Villarreal I, et al: 5-fluorouracil in the treatment of scleroderma: a randomized, double blind, placebo controlled international collaborative study. *Ann Rheum Dis* 49:926-928, 1990.

179. Klausner JM, Gutman M, Rozin RR, et al: Conventional fractionation radiotherapy combined with 5-fluorouracil for metastatic malignant melanoma. *Am J Clin Oncol* 10:448-450, 1987.

180. Olver IN, Bishop JF, Green M, et al: A phase II study of cisplatinum and continuous infusion 5-fluorouracil for metastatic melanoma. *Am J Clin Oncol* 15:503-505, 1992.

Melphalan

181. Kyle RA, Greipp PR, Garton JP, et al: Primary systemic amyloidosis: comparison of melphalan/prednisone versus colchicine. *Am J Med* 79:708-716, 1985.

182. Benson MD: Treatment of AL amyloidosis with melphalan, prednisone, and colchicine. *Arthritis Rheum* 29:683-687, 1986.

183. Lazarus HM, Herzig RH, Wolff SN, et al: Treatment of metastatic melanoma with intensive melphalan and autologous bone marrow transplantation. *Cancer Treat Rep* 69:473-477, 1985.

184. Finan MC, Winkelmann RK: Necrobiotic xanthogranuloma with paraproteinemia: a review of 22 cases. *Medicine* 65:376-388, 1986.

185. Moeller H, Waldenstroem JG, Zettervall O: Pyoderma gangrenosum (dermatitis ulcerosa) and monoclonal (IgA) globulin healed after melphalan treatment. Case report and review of the literature. *Acta Med Scand* 203:293-296, 1978.

186. Harris RB, Perry HO, Kyle RA, et al: Treatment of scleromyxedema with melphalan. *Arch Dermatol* 115:295-299, 1979.

187. Wright RC, Franco RS, Denton MD, et al: Scleromyxedema. *Arch Dermatol* 112:63-66, 1976.

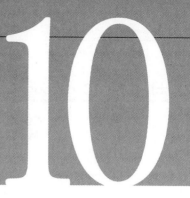

CHAPTER 10

John Y. M. Koo
Chai Sue Lee
Jack E. Maloney

Cyclosporine and Related Drugs

In 1970, Borel at the Sandoz Laboratories in Basel, Switzerland, discovered and isolated cyclosporine from the soil fungus *Tolypocladium inflatum gams* during a search for antifungal agents. Although it was found to have only weak antibiotic activity, cyclosporine, also known as Cyclosporin A (CsA), was identified as a potent immunosuppressive agent in 1976.[1] CsA's therapeutic effects in psoriasis were discovered fortuitously in 1979 by Mueller and Herrmann[2] during a pilot study to investigate CsA efficacy in rheumatoid arthritis. These investigators observed that in patients who had psoriatic arthritis, the psoriasis improved with CsA treatment. Since 1979, more than 60,000 patients worldwide have been treated for psoriasis with CsA.

The original formulation of CsA (Sandimmune) was approved for prophylaxis of organ rejection in the United States in 1983. Neoral, a more bioavailable and more consistently absorbed microemulsion formulation of CsA, was approved for prophylaxis of organ rejection in the United States in 1995. Neoral was approved for the treatment of rheumatoid arthritis and psoriasis in 1997. In comparison with other immunosuppressive drugs that have been used to treat psoriasis, such as methotrexate, hydroxyurea, and

6-thioguanine, CsA is not cytotoxic, does not suppress bone marrow, and is not teratogenic.

Even though CsA has excellent efficacy for psoriasis and has been used worldwide to treat patients with psoriasis for many years, most dermatologists in the United States are not experienced with its use. Moreover, many dermatologists shy away from learning how to use CsA to treat psoriasis because of the misconception that it is associated with severe adverse effects such as renal failure and cancer. Consequently, in this chapter, an emphasis will be placed on communicating a proper perspective regarding the use of CsA in the treatment of psoriasis, in addition to discussing CsA pharmacology and guidelines for safe use of CsA (Table 10-1). There will be relatively minimal information on the related medications tacrolimus and sirolimus (rapamycin) because neither of these medications is yet FDA-approved for any dermatologic indications, and their future in dermatology is still not clear.

PHARMACOLOGY

Table 10-2 contains key pharmacologic concepts for cyclosporine and related drugs.

■ Table 10-1   Cyclosporine and Related Drugs

Generic Name	Trade Name	Generic Available	Manu-facturer	Tablet/Capsule Sizes	Special Formu-lations	Standard Dosage Range	Price Index
Cyclosporine	Sandimmune	No	Novartis	25, 50, 100 mg	IV 50 mg/ml PO soln. 100 mg/ml	2.5-5 mg/kg/d	—
Cyclosporine	Neoral	Yes	Novartis	25, 100 mg	PO soln. 100 mg/ml	2.5-4 mg/kg/d*	$$$/$$$$‡
Tacrolimus	Prograf	No	Fujisawa	1, 5 mg	IV 5 mg/ml	??	$$$/$$$$$
Sirolimus†	Rapamune	No	Wyeth	—	1 mg/ml (1, 2, 5 ml)	??	$$$$/$$$$$

$, <1.00; $$, 1.01-2.00; $$$, 2.01-5.00; $$$$, 5.01-10.00; $$$$$, >10.00; ( ), generic price; /, two different price ranges from lower dose to higher dose examples of this size; —, no price listed for this drug.
*FDA-recommended dosage—see text regarding authors' viewpoint on starting Neoral at 5 mg/kg/d.
†Formerly known as rapamycin.
‡Recently released CsA generic has similar price index to Neoral.

■ Table 10-2   Key Pharmacologic Concepts—Cyclosporine and Related Drugs

Drug Name	Absorption and Bioavailability			Elimination		
	Peak Levels	Bioavail-able (%)	Protein Binding	Half-life	Meta-bolism	Excretion
Cyclosporine (Sandimmune)	2-4 hrs	30%	90%	5-18 hrs	Primarily hepatic	Primarily hepatobiliary (renal 6%)
Cyclosporine (Neoral)	2-4 hrs	(Increased versus Sandimmune)*	90%	5-18 hrs	Primarily hepatic	Primarily hepatobiliary (renal 6%)
Tacrolimus†	0.4-4 hrs	17%-22 %	75%-99%	4-40 hrs	Hepatic >99%	Primarily hepatobiliary

Adapted from *Physicians' desk reference*, ed 53, Montvale, NJ, 1999, Medical Economics Co, Inc.
*Absolute bioavailability not determined; Neoral has more complete and more predictable absorption than Sandimmune.
†Tacrolimus is commonly referred to by its prior designation—FK 506.

Structure

CsA is a neutral cyclic peptide composed of 11 amino acids (Figure 10-1). It is available in original formulation (Sandimmune) or a more consistently bioavailable microemulsion formulation (Neoral). Neoral, the only formulation of CsA approved for treatment of psoriasis, is avail-able as an oral solution or in capsules. The oral solution contains 100 mg/mL and should be diluted preferably with orange juice or apple juice immediately before it is administered to make it more palatable. Grapefruit juice affects metabolism of CsA and should be avoided. The combination of Neoral solution with milk can be un-

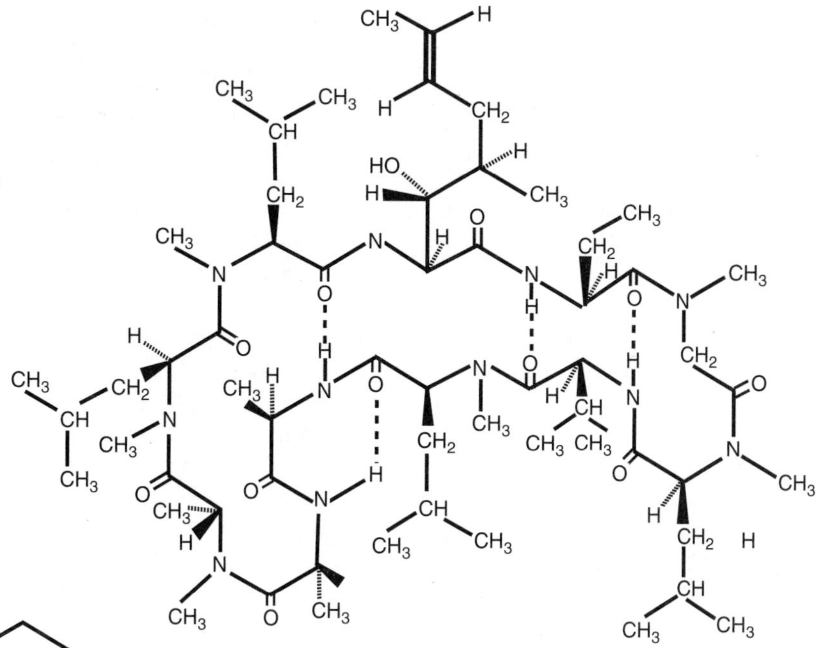

Figure 10-1   Cyclosporine and a related drug.

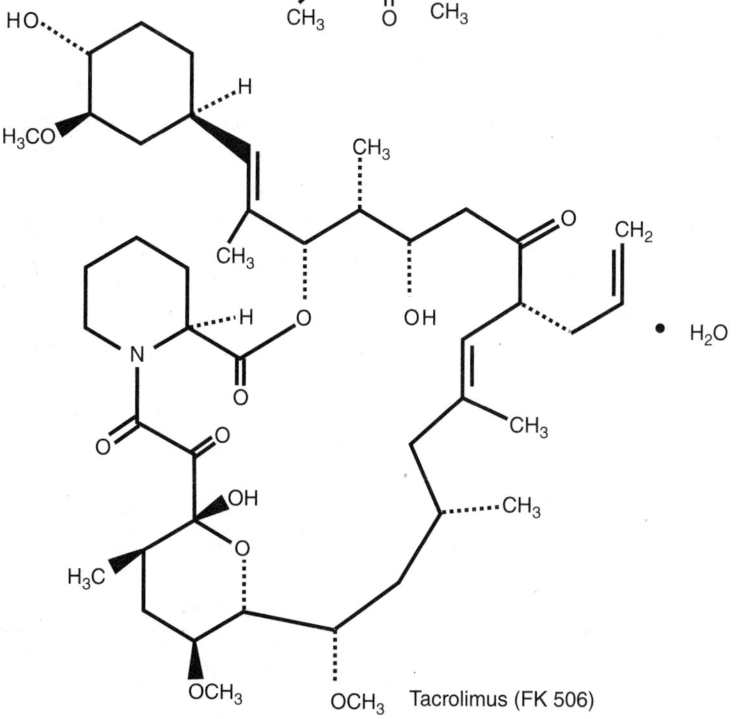

palatable. The soft gelatin capsules are much more convenient and are available in 25 mg and 100 mg strengths.

Absorption and Bioavailability

Neoral is an oral formulation of CsA that immediately forms a microemulsion in an aqueous environment. The absolute bioavailability of CsA administered as Neoral has not been determined; however, it has increased bioavailability compared to Sandimmune. When compared with Sandimmune at the same dose, Neoral shows a 20% to 50% increase in area under the concentration versus time curve (AUC) and a 40% to 106% increase in the peak blood CsA concentration (C_{max}).[3] This mainly results from the fact that Neoral is a "predigested" form of CsA that is less dependent on bile, food, diet, and the gastrointestinal environment for proper absorption. CsA is excreted in human milk, and breast-feeding should be avoided while on CsA.

Metabolism and Excretion

CsA is extensively metabolized by the cytochrome P-450 3A4 (CYP 3A4) enzyme system in the liver and is primarily excreted by way of the bile through feces with only 6% of the dose (parent drug and metabolites) excreted in urine. Neither dialysis nor renal failure significantly alters the drug's clearance.

Mechanisms of Action

The most established role of CsA in psoriasis is its effect on T lymphocytes. CsA inhibits interleukin-2 (IL-2) production by activated CD4+ T cells.[4] This is thought to be accomplished by the inhibition of calcineurin, a calcium- and calmodulin-dependent phosphatase, by a complex formed between CsA and cyclophilin, an intracellular receptor.[5-7] Because IL-2 causes the proliferation of helper T cells (CD4) and cytotoxic T cells (CD8), impaired IL-2 production leads to a decline in the number of activated CD4 and CD8 cells in the epidermis.[8] As CsA inhibits T-cell secretion of cytokines such as interferon-γ (IFN-γ), which promotes release of proinflammatory cytokines by keratinocytes, lymphocyte infiltration and inflammation may also be reduced.[4,9] Also, several in vitro studies have demonstrated that CsA inhibits the growth of keratinocytes at high concentrations,[10-13] although in actual usage the concentration of CsA attained in vivo appears to be too low to exert a direct antiproliferative effect on keratinocytes.[14] CsA also reduces the chemotactic ability of polymorphonuclear neutrophils by inhibiting the production of chemoattractant cytokines by psoriatic monocytes and probably other cells as well.[15] CsA's direct effect may extend to other cells, including antigen-presenting cells (such as Langerhans' cells) and mast cells.[16-20] Table 10-3 lists the mechanisms of action for cyclosporine and tacrolimus.

Certain cytokines such as IFN-γ are known to increase the expression of intercellular adhesion molecule 1 (ICAM-1).[8,21] These molecules are expressed on the surface of various cells such as keratinocytes and dermal capillary endothelium and play a role in the immune process by affect-

■ **Table 10-3**   Cyclosporine and Tacrolimus Mechanisms of Action[14]

Mechanism	Resultant Clinical Effect(s)
Inhibit production of IL-2 by inhibiting calcineurin	Decreased T-cell proliferation on activation
Calcineurin inhibition leads to reduced activity of the transcription factor NFAT-1	Inhibits T-cell proliferation
Inhibits IFN-γ production by T lymphocytes	Reduced HLA DR-positivity; reduced keratinocyte proliferation
Binds to steroid receptor associated heat-shock protein 56	Inhibits transcription of proinflammatory cytokines such as GM-CSF, IL-1, IL-3, IL-4, IL-5, IL-6, IL-8, TNF-α

Adapted from Faulds D, Goa KL, Benfield P: *Drugs* 45:953-1040, 1993; Beals CR, Clipstone NA, Ho SN, et al: *Genes Dev* 11:824-834, 1997; Cristillo AD, Heximer SP, Russell L, et al: *DNA Cell Biol* 16:1449-1458, 1997.

ing "trafficking" of various inflammatory cells. Conceivably, these cytokines could enable the endothelium to attract circulating leukocytes more effectively, and once in the epidermis, inflammatory cells may stay near keratinocytes longer. CsA inhibits the production of IFN-γ[4,19,22] and in turn down-regulates ICAM-1.

CLINICAL USE
Indications

Table 10-4 lists indications and contraindications for cyclosporine. There are a large number of dermatoses for which CsA is helpful. Except for psoriasis, these uses are not FDA-approved in the United States; however, physicians may prescribe CsA "off-label" for any dermatosis for which there is reasonable literature support of efficacy and safety of CsA.

PSORIASIS.   There are at least three types of psoriasis (Box 10-1) that can come under consideration for CsA therapy. CsA is particularly useful in patients who present with widespread, intensely inflammatory, or frankly erythrodermic psoriasis. Instituting CsA usually results in a rapid "cool-down." The second group of patients are those who are unable to tolerate, have contraindications to, or have failed all other treatment modalities. The third group are those with generalized plaque-type psoriasis for whom CsA may be considered as a rotational therapeutic option or as a first-line treatment.

OTHER DERMATOLOGIC USES.   CsA has also been reported to be effective in the treatment of a variety of dermatologic disorders, including atopic dermatitis,[30-35] lichen planus,[36-38] pemphigus,[39-48] pemphigoid,[49-55] epidermolysis bullosa acquisita,[56-64] dermatomyositis,[65-71] lupus erythematosus,[72-78] scleroderma,[79-83] Behçet's disease,[84-87] pyoderma gangrenosum,[88-96] cutaneous T-cell lymphoma,[97-103] contact dermatitis,[104-108] alopecia,[109-116] granuloma annulare,[117,118] sarcoidosis,[119-123] pityriasis rubra pilaris,[124-126] ichthyosis,[127,128] Darier's disease,[129] photodermatoses,[130-134] graft-versus-host disease,[135-144] erythema nodosum leprosum,[145,146] vitiligo,[129] chronic urticaria,[147] hidradenitis suppurativa,[129] and pityriasis lichenoides chronica.[129]

Of all the above off-label indications, prob-ably the best studied and most popular indications are with the use of CsA for atopic dermatitis and pyoderma gangrenosum. A brief overview of these two uses of CsA is presented in the next sections, serving to further illustrate how this important drug works for a variety of immunologic dermatoses.

Atopic Dermatitis.   A number of placebo-controlled, crossover studies evaluating the use of CsA in atopic dermatitis have been reported, with the greatest number of studies from the United Kingdom.[30-33] In addition, two large open trials are discussed here.[34,35] In only one study were children with atopic dermatitis evaluated,[34] with the remaining studies evaluating purely an adult atopic population. In the majority of studies a starting CsA dose of 5 mg/kg/day was utilized. Maintenance doses as low as 2 mg/kg/day were successful.[32] In later studies, starting doses as low as 2.5 mg/kg/day were utilized, with the option to gradually increase or decrease the dose as necessary to maximize disease control.[35]

In general, a greater percentage of patients had significant to marked improvement in the first 1 to 2 months of therapy, with a smaller number of patients clearing completely. This improvement was typically both subjective (reduced pruritus) and objective (decreased disease severity scores). The great majority of patients would relapse within 2 to 4 weeks of discontinuing CsA, albeit a significant number of patients would persist with a relatively mild disease activity subsequent to CsA cessation.[34] Serious adverse effects were rare, with relatively frequent, minor, reversible alterations in renal function reported.[31,33]

Pyoderma Gangrenosum.   In contrast to atopic dermatitis, primarily uncontrolled large[88,89] and small case series[90-92] characterized the literature experience regarding the use of CsA in pyoderma gangrenosum. Several single case reports[93-95] detailing the use of oral CsA and a single report on intralesional CsA in pyoderma gangrenosum[96] are of interest as well. A variety of generalizations can be made as detailed below.

CsA doses of 5 to 7 mg/kg/day are typically used at the outset,[88,89] ideally tapering below 5 mg/kg/day once there is a clear therapeutic response to the drug. Initial doses of CsA at the lower end of this interval would be currently recommended. As a rule, 2 to 3 months of CsA

Table 10-4   Cyclosporine Indications and Contraindications

USA FDA-APPROVED INDICATIONS
Psoriasis[23-29]
Severe psoriasis
Recalcitrant, treatment-resistant psoriasis
Disabling psoriasis (including localized versions
  such as hand and foot psoriasis)

**APPROVED INDICATIONS OTHER
COUNTRIES***
Psoriasis
Atopic dermatitis[30-35]

OFF-LABEL USES
Papulosquamous Dermatoses
Lichen planus[36-38]

Alopecia
Alopecia areata[109-113]
Male pattern alopecia[114-116]

Bullous Dermatoses
Pemphigus[39-48]
Pemphigoid[49-55]
Epidermolysis bullosa acquisita[56-64]

Granulomatous Dermatoses
Granuloma annulare[117,118]
Sarcoidosis[119-123]

Autoimmune Connective Tissue Diseases
Dermatomyositis[65-71]
Lupus erythematosus[72-78]
Scleroderma[79-83]

Disorders of Keratinization
Pityriasis rubra pilaris[124-126]
Ichthyosis[127,128]
Darier's disease[129]

Neutrophilic Dermatoses
Behçet's disease[84-87]
Pyoderma gangrenosum[88-96]

Photosensitivity Dermatoses
Actinic reticuloid[130-132]
Reticular erythematous mucinosis[133,134]

Neoplastic
Sézary's syndrome[97-98]
Mycosis fungoides[99-103]

Other Dermatoses
Graft-versus-host disease[135-144]
Erythema nodosum leprosum[145,146]
Vitiligo[129]

Dermatitis
Atopic dermatitis[30-35]
Contact hypersensitivity[104-108]

Chronic urticaria[147]
Hidradenitis suppurativa[129]
Pityriasis lichenoides chronica[129]

CONTRAINDICATIONS
Absolute
Significantly decreased renal function
Uncontrolled hypertension
Hypersensitivity to CsA or any ingredients in
  formulation
Clinically cured or persistent malignancy
  (except nonmelanoma skin cancers)

Relative
Age <18 years or >64 years
Controlled hypertension
Planning to receive a live attenuated
  vaccination
On medications that interfere with CsA
  metabolism or potentiate renal dysfunction
Active infection or evidence of
  immunodeficiency
Concomitantly receiving phototherapy,
  methotrexate, or other immunosuppressive
  agents
Pregnancy or lactation
Unreliable patients

PREGNANCY PRESCRIBING STATUS—CATEGORY C

*Australia.

Box 10-1

Specific Indications for Cyclosporine Therapy of Psoriasis*

- Patients with severe psoriasis who have *failed to respond* to at least one systemic therapy (such as PUVA, retinoids, or methotrexate)
- Patients with severe psoriasis who *cannot tolerate* or *have contraindications to* other systemic therapies
  - Women of childbearing potential
  - PUVA logistically difficult; inconvenient for patients
  - Methotrexate inappropriate because of significant alcohol use or concerns about liver biopsy
- Patients with severe acute flare-ups

*In each of these indications, cyclosporine therapy should be given for 3 to 6 months ideally, 12 months at most.

Box 10-2

Common Adverse Effects of Cyclosporine

RENAL
Renal dysfunction

CARDIOVASCULAR
Hypertension

NEUROLOGIC
Tremor
Headache
Paresthesia, hyperesthesia

MUCOCUTANEOUS
Hypertrichosis
Gingival hyperplasia

GASTROINTESTINAL
Nausea, abdominal discomfort
Diarrhea

MUSCULOSKELETAL
Myalgia, lethargy
Arthralgia

LABORATORY ABNORMALITIES
Hyperkalemia
Hyperuricemia (occasionally precipitates gout)
Hypomagnesemia
Hyperlipidemia

therapy are required for complete healing of the ulcers. In the two largest studies discussed here, 14 of 18 patients cleared completely.[88,89] Some of the relatively wide variation in time to complete ulcer healing can be explained in the variety of ulcer sizes treated. Initial CsA administration at 3 to 3.5 mg/kg/day successfully healed two patients in 3 and 5 months, respectively, in one report.[90] As with atopic dermatitis, serious adverse effects are distinctly uncommon. Patients who had minor alterations in renal function routinely reverted back to baseline values over a few months off therapy.[89,93]

Contraindications

Contraindications to the use of CsA are largely based on avoiding adverse effects on the kidney and on the ability of the patient's immune system to fight cancer and infection (see Table 10-4).

Adverse Effects

The adverse effects of CsA are listed in Box 10-2. These adverse effects are usually reversible on discontinuation of CsA. The most troublesome adverse effects involve nephrotoxicity and hypertension; the risk increases with increasing dose and duration of therapy. Neurologic effects are the most common adverse effects noted in patients using CsA for 2 months or less because nephrotoxicity and hypertension are rarely encountered from short-term usage in patients who do not have a history of preexisting kidney disease or hypertension.

RENAL EFFECTS.   The most important misconceptions about the use of CsA for treating psoriasis involve the adverse reaction of renal dysfunction and an increased risk of developing malignancies. There is a commonly held belief that the use of CsA puts psoriasis patients at risk for renal failure or serious renal dysfunction. Because most American dermatologists are not familiar with the proper guidelines for use of CsA, many do not realize that some of the published studies that address the risk of adverse effects represent an improper use of CsA and may take the findings at face value.[150,151] For example, in the study involving kidney biopsies by Zachariae and associates,[150] CsA was used in a manner inconsistent with current established guidelines (dosing schedules exceeding the current maximum recommended CsA dosage of 5 mg/kg/day and using the drug continuously for more than 1 year, even when serum creatinine has increased beyond 30% of the baseline value), which unquestionably contributed to the renal toxicity reported.

Many precautions have been built into current guidelines to safeguard against kidney damage. Historically, the threshold for adjusting the CsA dose was if serum creatinine is increased by 50% of the baseline. This was based on recommendations from nephrologists that if a 50% increase in baseline creatinine was not maintained for more than 3 months, elevation of serum creatinine will most likely revert back to normal, and the risk of irreversible damage to the kidneys is unlikely. Over the years, the worldwide consensus conference group determined that if the threshold for changing the dose is decreased from 50% to 30% to reflect greater caution, it will not be necessary to do creatinine clearance testing or kidney biopsies to safeguard the kidneys.[148,149] When Neoral was approved for psoriasis use in the United States, the FDA arbitrarily "shaved off" another 5% from the worldwide guidelines to recommend an adjustment in the CsA dosage when there is a 25% increase from the baseline creatinine value. With these cautious measures, the fact is that despite many years of widespread use worldwide outside of the United States where more than 60,000 psoriasis patients were treated with CsA, there is not a single documented case in the world literature to date of a patient who ended up with renal failure or any *clinically* significant kidney damage from the use of CsA for psoriasis *according to guidelines* (serum creatinine is kept within 30% of the patient's baseline creatinine level). This is not at all surprising because renal failure or significant renal insufficiency, almost by definition, requires a serum creatinine elevation much greater than 30% of the baseline. Furthermore, the creatinine level for all research subjects whose serum creatinine increased above 30% of the baseline either normalized or came back within 5% of the baseline after dose reduction or discontinu-

ation of CsA, as long as they were using CsA continuously for no more than 2 years.[153]

CARCINOGENESIS RISK. Another common misconception regarding the use of CsA for treating psoriasis involves an increased risk of developing lymphoma, other internal malignancies, or skin cancers. In a worldwide study involving more than 1000 research subjects who were exposed to CsA for up to 2 years, the prevalence of internal malignancies, including lymphoma, was not significantly increased in comparison with the general public.[152] Only two cases of lymphoma were found. The first case was a man 59 years of age who was found to have generalized mycosis fungoides within approximately 6 weeks after starting CsA.[153] Because it is extremely unlikely that the patient would develop mycosis fungoides all over his body in only 6 weeks, this patient probably never had psoriasis; he probably had mycosis fungoides to start with. However, because the lymphoma was discovered during the study, the case was listed as a case of lymphoma related to the use of CsA. The second case involved a man 66 years of age who developed lymphoma and died from it.[154] However, this very aggressive lymphoma was discovered more than 6 months after CsA was discontinued. Because CsA has a half-life of only 8 hours and is not stored in the body, and because this B-cell lymphoma was such an aggressive lymphoma that killed the patient within months, it is questionable whether this lymphoma was present more than half a year earlier when CsA was still being used. Nevertheless, once again, because the patient was involved in a CsA study earlier, he is listed as the second case of lymphoma associated with the CsA clinical trial.

There is no question that the risk of cancer is increased among *transplant* patients who are exposed not only to CsA in much higher dosages (7 to 15 mg/kg/day) in a chronic, lifelong fashion but also to many other immunosuppressive agents such as prednisone, azathioprine, and cyclophosphamide. When CsA is used in the relatively low, maximum dermatologic dose of 5 mg/kg/day by psoriatic patients who are not using other systemic immunosuppressants concurrently and who are generally healthy, the increased cancer risk is

Cyclosporine Monitoring Guidelines[148,149,156,157]

BASELINE:
Examination
- Complete history and physical examination (to rule out active infection, tumor)
- At least two baseline blood pressures

Laboratory
- At least two baseline serum creatinine levels
- Other baseline renal evaluation—BUN, urinalysis with microscopic examination
- CBC* and liver function tests (especially SGOT and SGPT)*
- Fasting lipid profile—triglycerides, cholesterol, HDL cholesterol
- Other laboratory tests: magnesium (may decrease†), potassium (may increase), uric acid (mainly relevant for those at risk for gout)

FOLLOW-UP:
Examination
- *Reevaluate the patient every 2 weeks for 1 to 2 months, then monthly while on cyclosporine*
- Blood pressure checked at each visit

Laboratory
- *Laboratory surveillance every 2 weeks for the first 1 to 2 months, then monthly while on cyclosporine*
- Renal function—serum creatinine, BUN, urinalysis
- CBC and liver function tests (especially SGOT and SGPT)*
- Lipids—triglycerides, cholesterol (consider doing only on alternate visits)
- Other laboratory tests—magnesium, potassium, uric acid

Indicated Infrequently on Selected Patients
- Serum CsA level,‡ creatinine clearance (consider if >6 months therapy), kidney biopsy (very rarely)

Note: More frequent surveillance is needed if laboratory values are abnormal or with high-risk patients.
*CBC and liver function tests are very seldom affected by cyclosporine.
†Serum magnesium may not be relevant if CsA usage is ≤4 months in duration.
‡Consider doing trough whole cyclosporine drug levels if inadequate clinical response and for suspected drug interactions.

not evident as long as CsA is used continuously for no more than 2 years at a time.

HYPERTENSION.   In many cases, the development of hypertension during the use of CsA was thought to be due to the direct vasoconstrictive effect of CsA on the vascular smooth muscles in the kidneys.[155] The development of hypertension, however, could also be secondary to renal dysfunction. Hypertension develops in approximately 27% of psoriasis patients on CsA.[3] It is usually mild with low-dose CsA and is generally reversible after dose reduction or discontinuation of CsA. The development of hypertension by itself does not constitute a contraindication to continuing therapy with CsA, as long as the hypertension can be brought under control with appropriate antihypertensive agents. In psoriasis patients treated in U.S. controlled clinical studies within the recommended dose range, CsA was discontinued in 1% of patients because of hypertension.[3]

DRUG INTERACTIONS

Table 10-5 lists drug interactions for cyclosporine. The list of drugs with which CsA interacts is quite long, and the clinical effects of that interaction can be substantial. Because CsA is metabolized by the hepatic cytochrome P-450 3A4 enzyme system, concomitant use of medications that compete for this P-450 isoform or induce cytochrome P-450 3A4 activity may in-

Table 10-5   Cyclosporine Drug Interactions

Interacting Drug or Drug Group	Comments and Examples
DRUGS THAT INCREASE CYCLOSPORINE DRUG LEVELS—CYP 3A4 *INHIBITION*	
Macrolide antibiotics	Erythromycin >> clarithromycin > azithromycin
Fluoroquinolone antibiotics	Norfloxacin (also ciprofloxacin)
Other antibiotics	Cephalosporins, doxycycline
Azole antifungal agents	Ketoconazole >> itraconazole > fluconazole
HIV-1 protease inhibitors	Ritonavir, indinavir >> saquinavir, nelfinavir
Calcium channel blockers	Diltiazem, verapamil, nicardipine > all others
H_2 antihistamines	Cimetidine >> ranitidine, famotidine, azatidine = 0
Corticosteroids	Primarily methylprednisolone (? Dexamethasone)
Diuretics	Thiazides, furosemide
Miscellaneous drugs	Allopurinol, bromocriptine, danazol, amphotericin B, metoclopramide, oral contraceptives, warfarin
(Food items)	Grapefruit, grapefruit juice
DRUGS THAT DECREASE CYCLOSPORINE DRUG LEVELS—CYP 3A4 *INDUCTION*	
Antituberculous drugs	Rifampin, rifabutin
Other antibacterial agents	Nafcillin
Anticonvulsants	Carbamazepine, phenobarbital, phenytoin, valproate
Miscellaneous drugs	Octreotide, ticlopidine
DRUGS USED IN COMBINATION WITH CYCLOSPORINE THAT MAY POTENTIATE RENAL TOXICITY	
Aminoglycosides	Tobramycin, gentamicin
Other antibiotics	Trimethoprim/sulfamethoxazole, vancomycin
Antifungal agents	Amphotericin B
NSAIDs	Indomethacin, naproxen, diclofenac
Immunosuppressants	Tacrolimus, melphalan
OTHER DRUGS THAT OCCASIONALLY INTERACT WITH CYCLOSPORINE	
Digoxin	Cyclosporine reduces renal clearance
Lovastatin	Cyclosporine reduces renal clearance
Prednisolone	Cyclosporine reduces renal clearance
ACE inhibitors	Increased risk of hyperkalemia with concurrent use
Potassium supplements	Increased risk of hyperkalemia with concurrent use
Potassium-sparing diuretics	Increased risk of hyperkalemia with concurrent use

Adapted from *CliniSphere 2.0 CD ROM*, St. Louis, June 2000, Facts & Comparisons.

crease or decrease the serum concentration of CsA, respectively. In addition, the metabolism of the interacting drug may be either raised or lowered with concurrent use of CsA.

MONITORING GUIDELINES

Once CsA therapy is initiated, periodic follow-ups are required for proper monitoring as out-lined later in this section. A serum cyclosporine level is not needed on a routine basis because CsA is known to share significant interpatient variation in blood levels for a given dosage, and there is not a good correlation between serum levels and the efficacy or toxicity of CsA in the treatment of psoriasis.[156] Drug levels are most important if the question of an unexpected drug interaction involving CsA arises.

In the event that hypertension develops,

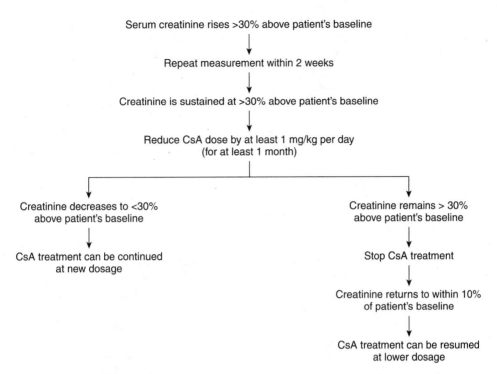

Serum creatinine rises >30% above patient's baseline

↓

Repeat measurement within 2 weeks

↓

Creatinine is sustained at >30% above patient's baseline

↓

Reduce CsA dose by at least 1 mg/kg per day
(for at least 1 month)

Creatinine decreases to <30%
above patient's baseline

↓

CsA treatment can be continued
at new dosage

Creatinine remains > 30%
above patient's baseline

↓

Stop CsA treatment

↓

Creatinine returns to within 10%
of patient's baseline

↓

CsA treatment can be resumed
at lower dosage

Figure 10-2   Steps to follow with rising creatinine. (*Adapted from Berth-Jones J, Voorhees J: Br J Dermatol 135:775-777, 1996.*)

the dose of CsA may be reduced or the hypertension may be treated with calcium antagonists such as nifedipine or isradipine because these two agents do not alter serum CsA levels.[157] Isradipine has one advantage over nifedipine in that it has not been associated with gingival hyperplasia, whereas nifedipine, by itself, has. Diltiazem and verapamil are not recommended because they may alter CsA blood levels. Potassium-sparing diuretics are probably best avoided as CsA tends to raise serum potassium levels.

If the serum creatinine rises to more than 30% above the patient's baseline creatinine level, recheck serum creatinine within 2 weeks. If an elevation of greater than 30% is confirmed, the dose of CsA should be reduced by at least 1 mg/kg/day for at least 2 to 4 weeks. If the creatinine then decreases to less than 30% above the patient's baseline, treatment can be continued; if not, adjust the dose again or discontinue therapy. These guidelines are summarized in the algorithm in Figure 10-2. The U.S. FDA has conservatively recommended decreasing this threshold to 25% of the baseline creatinine for American dermatologists. In practice this distinction seldom translates to a significant clinical difference between the 25% versus 30% guidelines.

THERAPEUTIC GUIDELINES

In evaluating patients for CsA therapy, key issues include patient selection, preliminary work-up, and continued monitoring throughout therapy.

Baseline Assessment

The patient should be carefully instructed regarding the nature and implementation of CsA treatment. Thorough history and physical examination should be conducted to rule out the existence of any active infection or tumor, with careful attention being paid to measurement of blood pressure. Before therapy, laboratory evaluation should be done as outlined in the previous section.

Dosage and Treatment Regimens

There are two schools of thought regarding the proper approach to dosing CsA. One advocates the initial use of a high-dose regimen, with gradual transition to a lower dosage, and the other advocates the initial use of a low dose, with upward adjustment as indicated.

More important than any guidelines or "schools of thought," the initial dosage of CsA for the treatment of psoriasis should depend on the clinical state of the patient being treated. For patients with severe, inflammatory flares of psoriasis or truly recalcitrant cases (psoriasis that has failed to respond to many other treatment modalities), where rapid improvement is critical, the authors recommend starting with the maximum dermatologic dosage of 5 mg/kg/day administered once or twice daily because 3 mg/kg/day is not even adequate as a *maintenance* dose in half of these cases of severe psoriasis. As soon as the patient is no longer in great distress, the dosage of CsA can be decreased in decrements of 1 mg/kg/day every other week until the minimum effective dosage for maintenance therapy is defined for the patient. On the other hand, for patients with generalized but relatively stable plaque-type psoriasis or cases where the severity lies between moderate and severe, it is reasonable to start with a low dose, typically 2.5 mg/kg/day. If improvement in psoriasis has not occurred by 1 month, it is important to remember to increase the CsA dosage in increments of 0.5 to 1.0 mg/kg/day every 2 weeks as necessary but not to exceed the maximum dose of 5 mg/kg/day. Both the rate of clearance and the overall success rate are related to the starting dose. It has been well demonstrated that 5 mg/kg/day dosing on the average is much more efficacious, in terms of both rapidity of the onset of therapeutic effect and the probability of clearing, compared with lower dosages such as 2.5 or 1.25 mg/kg/day (Figures 10-3 and 10-4).[158] If there is insufficient response after 3 months on the maximum dose of 5 mg/kg/day, CsA should be discontinued.

For obese patients, the *ideal* body weight should be used to calculate the daily dosage of CsA. If clinical response is not adequate, then gradually increase the dosage because calculation based on actual body weight is likely to result in an excessive dosage.

The previously mentioned guidelines are consistent with the scientific data available and closely reflect the results of the 1996 and 1998 worldwide consensus conferences on CsA.[148,149] It should be noted, however, that the US FDA has recommended a maximum dermatologic dosage of 4 mg/kg/day to reflect adjustments from Sandimmune to Neoral based on bioavailability data.

Conversion from Sandimmune to Neoral Formulation

When converting patients from the original CsA formulation (Sandimmune) to the microemulsion formulation (Neoral), a 1:1 dose-conversion strategy is recommended. In the majority of patients who absorb the original formulation adequately, the absorption of CsA is unlikely to change postconversion. However, in patients who were relatively poor absorbers of CsA from the original formulation, absorption will increase postconversion. As a result, it may be necessary to make subsequent dose reduction in these patients to ensure that they are receiving the lowest effective dose. Dose adjustments should also be made, as required, to comply with the safety guidelines as stated previously.

Careful safety monitoring is mandatory postconversion. Blood pressure and serum creatinine should be measured before conversion, in addition to 2, 4, and 8 weeks thereafter. Hypertension or a significant increase in serum creatinine should be managed according to the guidelines above.

Sequential Therapy Involving Neoral and Acitretin

According to the US FDA guidelines, CsA can be used continuously for up to 1 year at a time or up to 2 years according to the worldwide consensus guidelines.[148,149] Nevertheless, we feel that the optimal use of CsA is for a period of 3 to 4 months at a time as an acute agent to control a flare of psoriasis or to eliminate or greatly improve generalized psoriasis. The clinician should transition to another therapeutic modality for long-term maintenance by the end of that

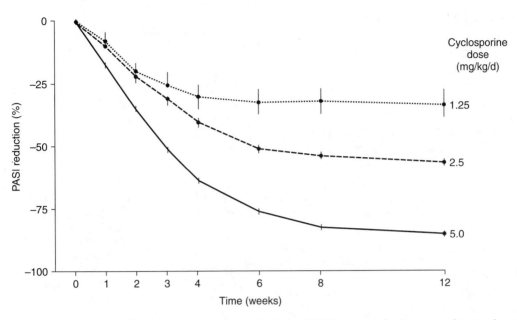

Figure 10-3 Percentage of psoriasis area and severity index (PASI) score reduction according to dose in the first 3 months of treatment with cyclosporine. (*Adapted from Timonen P, Friend D, Abeywickrama K, et al: Br J Dermatol 122:33-39, 1990.*)

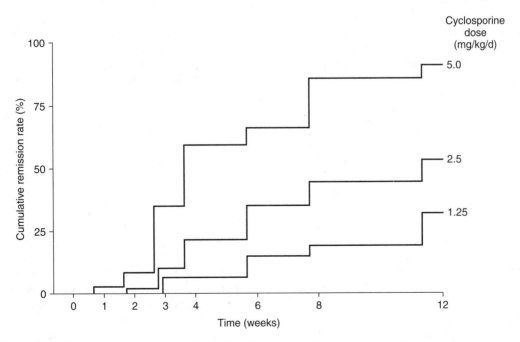

Figure 10-4   Cumulative success rate in the first 3 months of treatment according to cyclosporine dose. (*Adapted from Timonen P, Friend D, Abeywickrama K, et al: Br J Dermatol 122:33-39, 1990.*)

time period. Medications are like people in that they have both strengths and weaknesses. The idea behind this type of therapy (Box 10-3) is that you can use specific medications in a deliberate sequence to optimize each drug's strengths while minimizing each drug's weaknesses. This is in contrast to the usual approach where a psoriasis patient is given one main therapeutic agent with the expectation that if it works well, it will be continued and, if it does not, it will be replaced by something else.

Several issues should be considered in making a transition to another therapeutic agent. First of all, the risk of recurrence is much higher if CsA is discontinued abruptly than if it is gradually tapered. Therefore unless there is an overwhelming and urgent reason, CsA should always be gradually tapered and not stopped "cold turkey." Second, it is important for the practitioner to plan ahead so that another therapeutic agent is in place with decent therapeutic efficacy before the dosage of CsA is tapered and eventually discontinued. The number of studies that show the efficacy of CsA in combination with other agents is very limited. If one were to transition from CsA to phototherapy without risking relapse, one would probably have to overlap the two treatments for several weeks because phototherapy (UVB or PUVA) is not optimally therapeutic from day one. However, there is a theoretic concern about increased risk of skin cancer with concurrent use of CsA and phototherapy (albeit for a brief period of time), at least among fair-skinned Caucasian patients. When transitioning from CsA to methotrexate, the concurrent use of methotrexate and CsA in dermatology patients has not yet been determined to be safe. This is due in part to the fact that CsA and methotrexate can theoretically inhibit each other's metabolism.

It is our experience that the sequential use of CsA and acitretin (Soriatane) appears to be safe with close monitoring, considering their almost mutually exclusive side-effect profiles. For example, acitretin has the potential to affect the liver but virtually never alters kidney function, whereas CsA may alter kidney function with prolonged therapy but almost never has liver toxicity. Acitretin tends to induce hair loss, whereas CsA tends to induce hair growth. CsA

Box 10-3

Rationale for Sequential Therapy for Psoriasis

- Some medications are more ideal for "quick fixes" whereas others are more ideal for maintenance therapy.
- Systemic medications for psoriasis have both strengths and weaknesses for individual patients.
- Maximize the strength and minimize the weakness of each therapeutic agent involved.
- Sequential therapy involves three stages:
  Stage 1—Clearing phase
  Stage 2—Transitional phase
  Stage 3—Maintenance phase
- Sequential therapy with cyclosporine and acitretin can be a useful alternative to methotrexate therapy, although possible sequential therapy options include cyclosporine followed by methotrexate.

may increase potassium and decrease magnesium levels, but acitretin produces neither of these adverse effects. The only overlap in their side-effect profiles involves the fact that both medications can cause increases in cholesterol or triglyceride levels. However, this is generally reversible after dose reduction or discontinuation of CsA.[3] In addition, these two medications are metabolized by different enzymes minimizing the risk of drug interactions. In fact, the concurrent use of CsA and acitretin is not unprecedented; they have been used concurrently in *transplant* patients who are at increased risk for developing skin cancer.[159,160] Figure 10-5 defines a particular sequential use of CsA and acitretin. This sequence makes the best use of the property of Neoral as a "quick fix" agent that works rapidly, is well tolerated at high doses, and induces complete clearing. The most optimal attribute of acitretin is that this drug has the best long-term safety profile of the FDA-approved systemic agents for psoriasis. The major possible cumulative risk to consider with acitretin is the potential effect oral retinoids have on the skeletal system (such as the DISH syndrome). The magnitude of this retinoid skeletal risk is markedly lower than originally believed.[161]

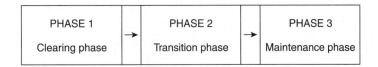

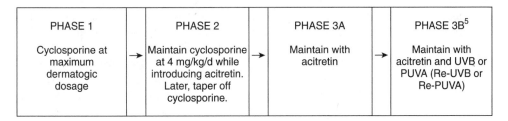

Figure 10-5   An example of oral sequential therapy.

Acitretin appears to be a very good long-term maintenance agent at low doses. In contrast, this drug is not particularly ideal as a clearing agent, has a slow onset of action, and has annoying adverse effects at high doses, such as hair loss and cheilitis. CsA, on the other hand, seems to be a very good clearing agent, but its merit for long-term use as a maintenance agent is questionable due to an increased risk of decreased kidney function and possible development of hypertension with long-term (over 6 to 12 months) use of CsA. Thus with patients with severe psoriasis, it is logical to use CsA first for inducing clearance followed by acitretin for maintenance therapy. Used in combination, CsA and acitretin are very effective in clearing severe psoriasis and in safely maintaining that clearance on a long-term basis.

One of our favorite ways of maximizing the benefits of both Neoral and acitretin is to first clear the psoriasis or greatly improve it with the use of Neoral at the maximum dermatologic dosage of 5 mg/kg/day. After 3 to 4 weeks of CsA therapy to establish the fact that the CsA is well tolerated, acitretin is introduced at 25 mg daily and increased by 10 to 25 mg increments every 2 to 4 weeks. The acitretin dose is increased in this fashion until a maximally tolerated dose for that particular patient is established; the dose of Neoral is maintained at the maximum dermatologic dosage. Once the psoriasis is cleared or greatly improved (which generally takes 3 months or less when CsA is used at the maximal derma-

tologic dosage), the patient is gradually weaned from CsA no faster than 1 mg/kg per month, and the patient is maintained on acitretin alone. After discontinuation of CsA, the acitretin may in certain patients prove inadequate at keeping the psoriasis under control. In that situation, UVB or PUVA phototherapy can be introduced to enhance the therapeutic effects through "Re-UVB" (retinoid *plus* UVB) or "Re-PUVA" (retinoid *plus* PUVA) therapy. These options for "sequential therapy" conform to the recommendation that CsA and phototherapy not be utilized simultaneously or consecutively because of the theoretic risk of increase in skin cancer in fair-skinned Caucasian patients if CsA and phototherapy are used concurrently.

Sequential Therapy—an Alternative to Methotrexate

Methotrexate is a very useful oral agent that has been considered the "gold standard" of oral therapy for the treatment of psoriasis for several decades. Despite its good efficacy and the option of long-term use, there is a definite need for a safe and effective systemic alternative to methotrexate. This is because there are many patients who cannot tolerate methotrexate due to such adverse effects as fatigue, nausea, vomiting, and changes in liver function tests. There are also some rare patients for whom methotrexate is not adequately efficacious. Moreover, the most pressing reason for a need for an alternative to methotrexate is the concern regarding cumulative toxicity of methotrexate, an area where most studies show that the risk of fibrosis or cirrhosis increases with an increase in the cumulative dose of methotrexate. In fact, the classic studies, one by Nyfors[162] and another by Zachariae and associates,[163] documented that once the cumulative dose of methotrexate is increased beyond 4 g, the risk of fibrosis and cirrhosis of the liver is at least 50%, even though there are multiple recent studies that give a much lower incidence of hepatotoxicity from methotrexate.[164-167] The fact that kidney damage from use of CsA can be predictably minimized by a simple blood test such as serum creatinine determination (and subsequent dosing adjustments) is in marked contrast to methotrexate therapy in which fibrosis or cirrhosis of the liver is not reliably predicted by blood tests alone. With CsA, all one has to do is follow serum creatinine and adjust the dose if serum creatinine increases by 30% of the baseline. There are no organ biopsy requirements with the use of CsA. In contrast, according to the latest proposed "more liberal" methotrexate guidelines, a liver biopsy is recommended for those who have no risk factors at 1 to 1.5 g cumulative methotrexate dose, and repeat biopsies are recommended at 3 g and at 4 g.[168]

There are two other ways in which CsA is safer than methotrexate. First, because there are no acute, catastrophic adverse effects such as pancytopenia associated with CsA, no "test dose" is needed before use of CsA at the maximum dermatologic dosage. Given that the patient does not have preexisting kidney disease or hypertension, the most serious adverse effects of CsA (decrease in kidney function or hypertension) do not occur in a precipitous fashion. Therefore unlike methotrexate, which requires a "test dose" and ideally gradually increasing doses, CsA therapy can be initiated at a full dose as soon as the preliminary laboratory evaluations are completed. Lastly, CsA is not known to be a teratogen (although it is listed as FDA category C), whereas methotrexate is a known teratogen.[170] The fact that CsA has no known teratogenicity can be an asset in treating teenagers with severe psoriasis, given the inherent tendency for teenagers to be unreliable with contraceptive measures.

NEWER IMMUNOSUPPRESSIVE DRUGS

Tacrolimus and Sirolimus (Rapamycin)

Tacrolimus (FK 506) and sirolimus are two immunosuppressive agents that have been utilized for organ transplantation purposes (Tables 10-1 and 10-2). These two drugs are now being investigated for use in dermatology to treat inflammatory skin diseases such as psoriasis and atopic dermatitis. Both of these medications have a chemical structure different from CsA; both have the structure of a hydrophobic macrolide antibiotic.[171] Like CsA, tacrolimus inhibits the activation of helper T cells and production of the T-cell growth factor IL-2. As a matter of fact, tacrolimus is known to be 10 to 100 times more potent dose for dose than CsA at inhibiting T-cell activation.[172-175] In addition, tacrolimus inhibits the production of other cytokines, including the inflammatory mediator IL-8, which is known to be elevated in psoriatic lesions.[176,177] IL-8 appears to be involved in the accumulation of neutrophils and T cells in the psoriatic dermis and epidermis.[176,178]

Sirolimus (formerly rapamycin) interferes with both T- and B-cell activation and is a potent inhibitor of T-cell proliferation. In vitro studies show sirolimus to be more potent in suppressing keratinocyte proliferation than either CsA or tacrolimus, and sirolimus does not produce nephrotoxicity.[171,179] However, studies evaluating the use of sirolimus in skin disorders have yet to be done, whereas tacrolimus has been more extensively studied as both a systemic and a topical agent in skin diseases. Kaplan and coworkers[180] reported two patients with psoriasis who developed capillary leak syndrome characterized by clinical signs of vascular leakage with fever and anemia after oral administration of sirolimus, with resolution after stopping treatment with the drug.

TACROLIMUS FOR PSORIASIS.   Jegasothy and coworkers[181] evaluated systemic tacrolimus in seven psoriatic patients undergoing organ transplantation. These patients had a dramatic improvement in their psoriasis with a marked reduction in erythema and scale after just 1 week of use and complete remission by the fourth week of treatment. However, the patients developed changes in their renal function; all had increased serum creatinine and blood urea nitrogen that did not return to baseline after the medication was discontinued. Also, three of the patients developed mild hypertension. Serial skin biopsies of the seven patients revealed a rapid resolution of the inflammatory infiltrate in the dermis but a slower improvement of the epidermal changes, such as the hyperkeratosis and acanthosis seen in psoriatic plaques. Another study evaluating keratinocyte growth showed that tacrolimus, unlike CsA and sirolimus, had no inhibitory effect on cell growth.[171] Therefore its antipsoriasis properties appear to be more closely linked to effects on T lymphocytes rather than on keratinocytes.

In 1996, the European FK 506 Multicentre Psoriasis Study Group published its results from the first double-blind, placebo-controlled study evaluating systemic tacrolimus for psoriasis.[176] This study involved 50 patients with severe and recalcitrant plaque psoriasis. The patients were randomized to receive either oral tacrolimus or placebo over a 9-week treatment period. At the end of the treatment period, there was a significantly greater reduction in the Psoriasis Area and Severity Index (PASI) for those patients who received tacrolimus than for the placebo-treated patients. In this study, the most frequently reported adverse effects in the tacrolimus group were diarrhea, paresthesias, and insomnia. Mild hypertension developed in just one of the 27 patients treated with tacrolimus, and it resolved without an antihypertensive medication or dose reduction. Only two patients treated with tacrolimus showed a change in renal function. However, the study duration of 9 weeks is much shorter than clinical studies involving CsA, most of which are 6 months to 1 year in duration. The results of this study are encouraging; they demonstrate that systemic tacrolimus is effective for psoriasis and that further studies should be done.

TOPICAL TACROLIMUS.   Tacrolimus is effective even when applied topically by affecting local immunosuppression at areas of application. Phase I and II studies evaluating topical tacrolimus for atopic dermatitis in adults and children show that it is safe and effective.[182,183] Thirty-nine patients with atopic dermatitis were evaluated in a phase I study of tacrolimus 0.3%, which was applied to various body regions that ranged from 0.5% to 27% of the body surface area (BSA).[182] Ninety-five percent of patients showed at least good improvement after 8 days of treatment. The most common adverse effect at the application site was burning, which occurred in 15% of patients. All adverse effects were transient. There was no evidence of systemic accumulation of tacrolimus, and no consistent laboratory changes were observed. In a recent phase II study, 213 patients with atopic dermatitis were evaluated over a period of 3 weeks.[183] The patients were randomized to receive one of four treatments: 0.03%, 0.1%, or 0.3% tacrolimus, or vehicle alone. All three groups that received tacrolimus ointment showed significantly greater improvement than the placebo group. Again, the most common adverse effect was a burning sensation at the site of application—44% in those who received tacrolimus and 15% in those treated with vehicle alone. The clinical studies currently being done to further evaluate topical tacrolimus also show promise. See Chapter 30 for a more detailed discussion on topical tacrolimus.

SUMMARY

Because of good efficacy and tolerability, CsA is a great addition to our therapeutic armamentarium in the treatment of psoriasis. Even though fear, lack of knowledge, and misconceptions are prevalent among dermatologists in the United States regarding this agent, once CsA is properly understood by clinicians, its advantages and benefits can be made available to patients, especially for short-term, effective control of severe psoriasis patients. Sequential therapy with CsA and acitretin may offer an alternative for many patients to the use of methotrexate in the treatment of severe psoriasis.

Bibliography

Berth-Jones J, Voorhees JJ: Consensus conference on cyclosporin A microemulsion for psoriasis, June 1996. *Br J Dermatol* 135:775-777, 1996.

Finzi AF, della Casa Alberighi O: The place of cyclosporin in the treatment of severe psoriasis. *Clin Drug Invest* 10(Suppl 1):45-52, 1995.

Gilleaudeau P, McClelland PB: Cyclosporine: a new therapeutic option for severe, recalcitrant psoriasis. *Dermatol Nurs* 6:395-405, 1994.

Koo J, Lee J: Cyclosporine: what clinicians need to know. *Dermatol Clin* 13:897-907, 1995.

Koo J: Sequential therapy of psoriasis. Introducing a new therapeutic paradigm for better clinical results. *J Am Acad Dermatol* 41:S25-28, 1999.

Lebwohl M, Ellis C, Gottlieb A, et al: Cyclosporine consensus conference: with emphasis on the treatment of psoriasis. *J Am Acad Dermatol* 39:464-475, 1998.

Stutz JA, Ellis CN: Dermatological uses of cyclosporine: management of dermatoses other than psoriasis and atopic dermatitis. *Clin Drug Invest* 10(Suppl 1):22-35, 1995.

Wong RL, Winslow CM, Cooper KD: The mechanisms of action of cyclosporin-A in the treatment of psoriasis. *Immunol Today* 114:69-74, 1993.

References

1. Borel JF, Feurer C, Gubler HU: Biological effects of cyclosporin A: a new antilymphocyte agent. *Agents Act* 6:468-475, 1976.
2. Mueller W, Hermann B: Cyclosporin A for psoriasis. *N Engl J Med* 301:555, 1979.

Pharmacology

3. Neoral Prescribing Information, Novartis Pharmaceuticals Corporation.
4. Granelli-Piperno A: The effect of immunosuppressive agents on the induction of nuclear factors that bend to sites on the interleukin-2 promotor. *J Exp Med* 171:533-544, 1990.
5. Flanagan WM, Corthesy B, Bram RJ, et al: Nuclear association of a T-cell transcription factor blocked by FK-506 and cyclosporin. *Nature* 352:803-807, 1991.
6. Liu J, Farmer JD Jr, Lane WS, et al: Calcineurin is a common target of cyclophilin-cyclosporin and FKPP-FK5-6 complexes. *Cell* 66:807-815, 1991.
7. Schreiber SL, Crabtree GR: The mechanism of action of cyclosporin and FK506. *Immunol Today* 13:136-142, 1992.
8. Baker BS, Griffiths CEM, Lambert S, et al: The effects of cyclosporin A on T lymphocyte and dendritic cell sub-populations in psoriasis. *Br J Dermatol* 116:503-510, 1987.
9. Kalman VK, Klimpel GR: Cyclosporin A inhibits the production of gamma interferon (IFN-γ), but does not inhibit production of virus-induced IFN-γ. *Cell Immunol* 78:122-129, 1983.
10. Fisher GJ, Duell EA, Nickoloff BJ, et al: Levels of cyclosporin in epidermis of treated psoriasis patients differentially inhibit growth of keratinocytes cultured in serum free versus serum containing media. *J Invest Dermatol* 91:142-146, 1988.
11. Nickoloff BJ, Fisher GJ, Mitra RS, et al: Additive and synergistic antiproliferative effects of cyclosporin A and gamma interferon on cultured human keratinocytes. *Am J Pathol* 131:12-18, 1988.
12. Sharpe GR, Fisher C: Time-dependent inhibition of growth of human keratinocytes and fibroblasts by cyclosporin A: Effect on keratinocytes at therapeutic blood levels. *Br J Dermatol* 123:207-213, 1990.
13. Won Y, Sauder ON, McKenzie RC: Cyclosporin A inhibits keratinocyte cytokine gene expression. *Br J Dermatol* 130:312-319, 1994.
14. Wong RL, Winslow CM, Cooper KD: The mechanisms of action of cyclosporin A in the treatment of psoriasis. *Immunol Today* 14:69-74, 1993.

15. Mozzanica N, Pigatto PD, Finzi AF: Cyclosporin in psoriasis: pathophysiology and experimental data. *Dermatology* 187(Suppl 1):3-7, 1993.
16. Demidem A, Taylor JR, Grammer SF, et al: T-lymphocyte-activating properties of epidermal antigen-presenting cells from normal and psoriatic skin: evidence that psoriatic epidermal antigen-presenting cells resemble cultured normal Langerhans cells. *J Invest Dermatol* 97:454-460, 1991.
17. Dupuy P, Bagot M, Michel L, et al: Cyclosporin A inhibits the antigen-presenting functions of freshly isolated human Langerhans cells in vitro. *J Invest Dermatol* 96:408-413, 1991.
18. Furue M, Katz SI: The effect of cyclosporin on epidermal cells: cyclosporin inhibits accessory cell functions of epidermal Langerhans cells in vitro. *J Immunol* 140:4139-4143, 1988.
19. Hultsch T, Rodriguez JL, Kaliner MA, et al: Cyclosporin A inhibits degranulation of rat basophilic leukemia cells and human basophils: inhibition of mediator release without affecting PI hydrolysis or Ca^{2+} fluxes. *J Immunol* 144:2659-2664, 1990.
20. Triggiani M, Cirillo R, Lichtenstein LM, et al: Inhibition of histamine and prostaglandin D_2 release from human lung mast cells by cyclosporin A. *Intern Arch Allergy Appl Immunol* 88:253-255, 1989.
21. Baadsgaard O, Tong P, Elder JT, et al: UM4D4+ (CDw60) T cells are compartmentalized into psoriatic skin and release lymphokines that induce a keratinocyte phenotype expressed in psoriatic lesions. *J Invest Dermatol* 95:275-282, 1990.
22. Korstanje MJ, Bilo HJG, Stoof TJ: Sustained renal function loss in psoriasis patients after withdrawal of low-dose cyclosporin therapy. *Br J Dermatol* 127:501-504, 1992.

Clinical Use—Psoriasis

23. Griffiths CEM, Powles AV, McFadden J, et al: Long term cyclosporin for psoriasis. *Br J Dermatol* 120:256-266, 1989.
24. Powles AV, Baker BS, Valdimarsson H, et al: Four years experience with cyclosporin in psoriasis. *Br J Dermatol* 122(Suppl 36):13-19, 1990.
25. Laburte C, Grossman R, Abi-Rached J, et al: Efficacy and safety of oral cyclosporin for long term treatment of chronic severe plaque psoriasis. *Br J Dermatol* 130:366-375, 1994.
26. Levell NJ, Schuster S, Munro CS, et al: Remission of ordinary psoriasis following a short clearance course of cyclosporin. *Acta Derm Venereol (Stockh)* 75:65-69, 1995.
27. Mahrle G, Shultze HJ, Farber L, et al: Low dose short-term cyclosporin versus etretinate in psoriasis. *J Am Acad Dermatol* 32:78-88, 1995.
28. Berth-Jones J, Henderson CA, Munro CS, et al: Treatment of psoriasis with intermittent short course cyclosporin (Neoral®). A multicentre study. *Br J Dermatol* 136:527-530, 1997.
29. Zachariae H, Steen Olsen T: Efficacy of cyclosporin A in psoriasis: an overview of dose/response, indications, contraindications and side effects. *Clin Nephrol* 43:154-158, 1995.

Atopic Dermatitis

30. Wahlgren CF, Scheynius A, Hagermark O: Antipruritic effect of oral cyclosporin in atopic dermatitis. *Acta Derm Venereol (Stockh)* 70:323-329, 1990.
31. Sowden JM, Berth-Jones J, Ross JS, et al: A multicentre, double blind, placebo controlled crossover study to assess the efficacy and safety of cyclosporin in adult patients with severe refractory atopic dermatitis. *Lancet* 338:137-140, 1991.
32. Munro CS, Levell NJ, Shuster S, et al: Maintenance treatment with cyclosporin in atopic eczema. *Br J Dermatol* 130:376-380, 1994.
33. Van Joost TH, Heule F, Korstanje M, et al: Cyclosporin in atopic dermatitis: a multicentre placebo controlled study. *Br J Dermatol* 130:634-640, 1994.
34. Berth-Jones J, Finlay AY, Zaki I, et al: Cyclosporin in severe childhood atopic dermatitis: a multicentre study. *J Am Acad Dermatol* 34:1016-1021, 1996.
35. Berth-Jones J, Graham-Brown RAC, Marks R, et al: Long-term efficacy and safety of cyclosporin in severe adult atopic dermatitis. *Br J Dermatol* 136:76-81, 1997.

Lichen Planus

36. Ho VC, Gupta AK, Ellis CN, et al: Treatment of severe lichen planus with cyclosporine. *J Am Acad Dermatol* 22:64-68, 1990.
37. Fornasa CV, Catalano P: Effect of local applications of ciclosporin in chronic ulcerative lichen planus. *Dermatologica* 182:65, 1991.

38. Jemec GB, Baadsgaard O: Effect of cyclosporine on genital psoriasis and lichen planus. *J Am Acad Dermatol* 29:1048-1049, 1993.

Pemphigus
39. Thivolet J, Barthélémy H, Rigot-Muller G, et al: Effects of cyclosporin on bullous pemphigoid and pemphigus (letter). *Lancet* 1:334-335, 1985.
40. Barthélémy H, Biron F, Caludy A, et al: Cyclosporine: new immunosuppressive agent in bullous pemphigoid and pemphigus. *Transplant Proc* 18:913-914, 1986.
41. Balda BR, Rosenzweig D: Cyclosporin A in the treatment of pemphigus foliaceus and pemphigus erythematosus. *Hautarzt* 37:454-457, 1986.
42. Cunliffe WJ: Pemphigus foliaceous and response to cyclosporin. *Br J Dermatol* 117:114-116, 1987.
43. Barthélémy H, Frappaz A, Cambazard F, et al: Treatment of nine cases of pemphigus vulgaris with cyclosporine. *J Am Acad Dermatol* 18:1262-1266, 1988.
44. Lapidoth M, David M, Ben-Amitai D, et al: The efficacy of combined treatment with prednisone and cyclosporine in patients with pemphigus: preliminary study. *J Am Acad Dermatol* 30:752-757, 1994.
45. Bondesson L, Hammar H: Treatment of pemphigus vulgaris with cyclosporine. *Dermatologica* 181:308-310, 1990.
46. Tappeiner G, Groh V: Treatment of pemphigus with ciclosporin. In Schindler R, editor: *Ciclosporin in autoimmune diseases,* Berlin, 1985, Springer-Verlag, pp 205-208.
47. Ormerod AD, Duncan J, Stankler L: Benign familial pemphigus responsive to cyclosporin, a possible role for cellular immunity in pathogenesis (letter). *Br J Dermatol* 124:299-300, 1991.
48. Jitsukawa K, Ring J, Weyer U, et al: Topical cyclosporine in chronic benign familial pemphigus (Hailey-Hailey disease). *J Am Acad Dermatol* 27:625-626, 1992.

Pemphigoid
49. Barthélémy H, Thivolet J, Cambazard F, et al: Cyclosporin in the treatment of bullous pemphigoid: preliminary study. *Ann Dermatol Venereol* 113:309-313, 1986.
50. Cunliffe WJ: Bullous pemphigoid and response to cyclosporin. *Br J Dermatol* 117(Suppl 32):113-114, 1987.

51. Bianchi L, Gatti S, Nini G: Bullous pemphigoid and severe erythrodermic psoriasis: combined low-dose treatment with cyclosporine and systemic steroids (letter). *J Am Acad Dermatol* 27:278, 1992.
52. Curley RK, Holden CA: Steroid-resistant bullous pemphigoid treated with cyclosporin A. *Clin Exp Dermatol* 16:68-69, 1991.
53. Boixeda JP, Soria C, Medina S, et al: Bullous pemphigoid and psoriasis: treatment with cyclosporine (letter). *J Am Acad Dermatol* 24:52, 1991.
54. Eisen D, Ellis CN: Topical cyclosporine for oral mucosal disorders. *J Am Acad Dermatol* 23:1259-1263, 1990.
55. Azana JM, de Misa RF, Boixeda JP, et al: Topical cyclosporine for cicatricial pemphigoid (letter). *J Am Acad Dermatol* 28:134-135, 1993.

Epidermolysis Bullosa Acquisita
56. Connolly SM, Sander HM: Treatment of epidermolysis bullosa acquisita with cyclosporine (letter). *J Am Acad Dermatol* 16:890, 1987.
57. Zachariae H: Cyclosporine A in epidermolysis bullosa acquisita (letter). *J Am Acad Dermatol* 17:1058-1059, 1987.
58. Crow LL, Finkle JP, Gammon WR, et al: Clearing of epidermolysis bullosa acquisita with cyclosporine. *J Am Acad Dermatol* 19:937-942, 1988.
59. Klein JS, Goldin HM, Keegan C, et al: Clear-cell carcinoma of the lung in a patient treated with cyclosporine for epidermolysis bullosa acquisita. *J Am Acad Dermatol* 24:297, 1991.
60. Mallett RB, Holden CA: Clearing of epidermolysis bullosa acquisita with cyclosporine (letter). *J Am Acad Dermatol* 24:1034-1035, 1991.
61. Crow LL, Woodley DT: Reply: clearing of epidermolysis bullosa acquisita with cyclosporine. *J Am Acad Dermatol* 24:1034, 1991.
62. Clement M, Ratnesar P, Thirumoorthy T, et al: Epidermolysis bullosa acquisita—a case with upper airway obstruction requiring tracheostomy and responding to cyclosporin. *Clin Exp Dermatol* 18:548-551, 1993.
63. Layton AM, Cunliffe WJ: Clearing of epidermolysis bullosa acquisita with cyclosporine (letter). *J Am Acad Dermatol* 22:535-536, 1990.

64. Merle C, Blanc D, Zultak M, et al: Intractable epidermolysis bullosa acquisita: efficacy of cyclosporin A. *Dermatologica* 181:44-47, 1990.

Dermatomyositis

65. Pistoia V, Buoncompagni A, Scribanis R, et al: Cyclosporin A in the treatment of juvenile chronic arthritis and childhood polymyositis-dermatomyositis. Results of a preliminary study. *Clin Exp Rheumatol* 11:203-208, 1993.
66. Dantzig P: Juvenile dermatomyositis treated with cyclosporine. *J Am Acad Dermatol* 22:310-311, 1990.
67. Grau JM, Herrero C, Casadermont J, et al: Cyclosporine A as first choice therapy for dermatomyositis. *J Rheumatol* 21:381-382, 1994.
68. Danko K, Szegedi G: Cyclosporine A treatment of dermatomyositis. *Arthritis Rheum* 34:933-934, 1991.
69. Correia O, Polonia J, Nunes JP, et al: Severe acute form of adult dermatomyositis treated with cyclosporine. *Int J Dermatol* 31:517-519, 1992.
70. Casato M, Bonomo L, Caccavo D, et al: Clinical effects of cyclosporin in dermatomyositis. *Clin Exp Dermatol* 15:121-123, 1990.
71. Mehregan DR, Su WP: Cyclosporine treatment for dermatomyositis/polymyositis. *Cutis* 51:59-61, 1993.

Lupus Erythematosus

72. Feutren G, Querin S, Tron F, et al: The effects of cyclosporine in patients with systemic lupus. *Transplant Proc* 18:643-644, 1986.
73. Miescher PA, Favre H, Mihatsch MJ, et al: The place of cyclosporine A in the treatment of connective tissue diseases. *Transplant Proc* 20(Suppl 4):224-237, 1988.
74. Ter Borg EJ, Tegzess AM, Kallenberg CGM: Unexpected severe reversible cyclosporine A-induced nephrotoxicity in a patient with systemic lupus erythematosus and tubulointerstitial renal disease. *Clin Nephrol* 29:93-95, 1988.
75. Huele F, Van Joost T, Beukers R: Cyclosporine in the treatment of lupus erythematosus. *Arch Dermatol* 122:973-974, 1986.

76. Makover D, Freundlich B, Zurier RB: Relapse of systemic lupus erythematosus in a patient receiving cyclosporine A. *J Rheumatol* 15:117-119, 1988.
77. Deteix P, Lefrancois N, Laville M, et al: Open therapeutic trial of ciclosporin in systemic lupus erythematosus. Preliminary results in 4 patients. In Schindler R, editor: *Ciclosporin in autoimmune diseases,* Berlin, 1985, Springer-Verlag, pp 361-365.
78. Feutren G, Querin S, Noel LH, et al: Effects of cyclosporine in severe systemic lupus erythematosus. *J Pediatr* 111:1063-1068, 1987.

Scleroderma

79. Vayssairat M, Baudot N, Biotard C, et al: Cyclosporine therapy for severe systemic sclerosis associated with the anti-Scl-70 autoantibody. *J Am Acad Dermatol* 22:695-696, 1990.
80. Zachariae H, Halkier-Sorensen L, Heickendorff L, et al: Cyclosporin A treatment of systemic sclerosis. *Br J Dermatol* 122:677-681, 1990.
81. Gisslinger H, Burghuber OC, Stacher G, et al: Efficacy of cyclosporine A in systemic sclerosis. *Clin Exp Rheumatol* 9:383-390, 1991.
82. Clements PJ, Lachenbruch PA, Sterz M, et al: Cyclosporine in systemic sclerosis. Results of a forty-eight-week open safety study in ten patients. *Arthritis Rheum* 36:75-83, 1993.
83. Morle B, Hein R, Krieg T, et al: Ciclosporin in localized and systemic scleroderma—a clinical study. *Dermatologica* 181:215-220, 1990.

Behçet's Disease

84. BenEzra D, Cohen E, Chajek T, et al: Evaluation of conventional therapy versus cyclosporine A in Behçet's disease. *Transplant Proc* 20(Suppl 4):136-143, 1988.
85. Masuda K, Nakajima A, Urayama A, et al: Double-masked trial of cyclosporin versus colchicine and long-term open study of cyclosporin in Behçet's disease. *Lancet* 1:1093-1096, 1989.
86. Pacor ML, Biasi D, Lunardi C, et al: Cyclosporin in Behçet's disease: results in 16 patients after 24 months of therapy. *Clin Rheumatol* 13:224-227, 1994.
87. Suss R, al-Ayoubi M, Ruzicka T: Cyclosporine therapy in Behçet's disease. *J Am Acad Dermatol* 29:101-102, 1993.

Pyoderma Gangrenosum

88. Matis WL, Ellis CN, Griffiths CEM, et al: Treatment of pyoderma gangrenosum with cyclosporine. *Arch Dermatol* 128:1060-1064, 1992.

89. Elgart G, Stover P, Larson K, et al: Treatment of pyoderma gangrenosum with cyclosporine: results in seven patients. *J Am Acad Dermatol* 24:83-86, 1991.

90. Schmitt EC, Pigatto PD, Boneschi V, et al: Pyoderma gangrenosum treated with low-dose cyclosporin (letter). *Br J Dermatol* 128:230-231, 1993.

91. Soria C, Allegue F, Martin M, et al: Treatment of pyoderma gangrenosum with cyclosporin A. *Clin Exp Dermatol* 16:392-394, 1991.

92. Kavanagh GM, Ross JS, Cronin E, et al: Recalcitrant pyoderma gangrenosum—two cases successfully treated with cyclosporin A. *Clin Exp Dermatol* 17:49-52, 1992.

93. O'Donnell B, Powell FC: Cyclosporine treatment of pyoderma gangrenosum (letter). *J Am Acad Dermatol* 24:141-143, 1991.

94. Bijmer-Iest JC, Rompelman-Schiere SI, Van Ginkel CJ: Treatment of pyoderma gangrenosum with cyclosporin (letter). *Br J Dermatol* 125:283, 1991.

95. Fedi MC, Quercetani R, Lotti T: Recalcitrant pyoderma gangrenosum responsive to cyclosporine. *Int J Dermatol* 32:119, 1993.

96. Mrowietz U, Christophers E: Clearing of pyoderma gangrenosum by intralesional cyclosporin A (letter). *Br J Dermatol* 125:499, 1991.

Cutaneous T-cell Lymphoma

97. Catterall MD, Addis BJ, Smith JL, Coode PE: Sézary syndrome: Transformation to a high grade T-cell lymphoma after treatment with cyclosporin A. *Clin Exp Dermatol* 8:159-169, 1983.

98. Street ML, Muller SA, Pittelkow MR: Cyclosporine in the treatment of cutaneous T cell lymphoma. *J Am Acad Dermatol* 23:1084-1089, 1990.

99. Maddox AM, Kahan BD, Tucker S, et al: Remission in skin infiltrate of a patient with mycosis fungoides treated with cyclosporine. *J Am Acad Dermatol* 12:952-956, 1985.

100. Moreland AA, Robertson DB, Heffner LT: Treatment of cutaneous T cell lymphoma with cyclosporin A (letter). *J Am Acad Dermatol* 12:886-887, 1985.

101. Jensen JR, Thestrup-Pedersen K, Zachariae H, et al: Cyclosporin A therapy for mycosis fungoides. *Arch Dermatol* 123:160-163, 1987.

102. Kreis W, Budman DR, Shapiro PE: Cyclosporin A (cyclosporine) in the treatment of cutaneous T cell lymphoma (mycosis fungoides) (letter). *J Am Acad Dermatol* 18:1138-1140, 1988.

103. Cooper DL, Braverman IM, Sarris AH, et al: Cyclosporine treatment of refractory T-cell lymphomas. *Cancer* 71:2335-2341, 1993.

Contact Dermatitis

104. Rullan PP, Barr RJ, Cole GW: Cyclosporine and murine allergic contact dermatitis. *Arch Dermatol* 120:1179-1183, 1984.

105. Kakagawa S, Oka D, Jinno Y, et al: Topical application of cyclosporine on guinea pig allergic contact dermatitis. *Arch Dermatol* 124:907-910, 1988.

106. Lembo G, Balato N, Patruno C, et al: Influence of topical cyclosporin A on patch test reactions. *Contact Dermatitis* 20:155-156, 1989.

107. Cole GW, Shimomaye S, Goodman M: The effect of topical cyclosporin A on the elicitation phase of allergic contact dermatitis. *Contact Dermatitis* 19:129-132, 1988.

108. Aldridge RD, Sewell HF, King G, et al: Topical cyclosporin A in nickel contact hypersensitivity: results of a preliminary clinical and immunohistochemical investigation. *Clin Exp Immunol* 66:582-589, 1986.

Alopecia

109. Parodi A, Rebora A: Topical cyclosporine in alopecia areata (letter). *Arch Dermatol* 123:165-166, 1987.

110. Gupta AK, Ellis CN, Cooper KD, et al: Oral cyclosporine for the treatment of alopecia areata. *J Am Acad Dermatol* 22:242-250, 1990.

111. Teshima H, Urabe A, Irie M, et al: Alopecia universalis treated with oral cyclosporine A and prednisolone: immunologic studies. *Int J Dermatol* 31:513-516, 1992.

112. Mauduit G, Lenvers P, Barthelemy H, et al: Treatment of severe alopecia areata with topical applications of cyclosporin A. *Ann Dermatol Venereol* 114:507-510, 1987.

113. Gilhar A, Pillar T, Etzioni A: Topical cyclosporin A in alopecia areata. *Acta Derm Venereol* 69:252-253, 1989.

114. Picascia DD, Roenigk HH Jr: Effects of oral and topical cyclosporine in male pattern alopecia. *Transplant Proc* 20(Suppl 4):109-111, 1988.

115. Gilhar A, Pillar T, Etzioni A: Topical cyclosporine in male pattern alopecia. *J Am Acad Dermatol* 22:251-253, 1990.

116. Picascia DD, Roenigk HH Jr: Cyclosporine and male-pattern alopecia (letter). *Arch Dermatol* 123:1432, 1987.

Granulomatous Dermatoses

117. Filotico R, Vena GA, Coviello C, et al: Cyclosporine in the treatment of generalized granuloma annulare. *J Am Acad Dermatol* 30:487-488, 1994.

118. Ho V: Cyclosporine in the treatment of generalized granuloma annulare. *J Am Acad Dermatol* 32:298, 1995.

119. Rebuck AS, Stiller CR, Braude AC, et al: Cyclosporin A in the treatment of pulmonary sarcoidosis. *Lancet* 1:1174, 1984.

120. Bain VG, Kneteman N, Brown NE: Sarcoidosis, liver transplantation, and cyclosporine (letter). *Ann Intern Med* 119:1148, 1993.

121. York EL, Paul Man SF, Sproule BJ: Cyclosporine A in a case of refractory systemic and cutaneous sarcoidosis. *Chest* 89(Suppl 89):519, 1986.

122. York EL, Kovithavongs T, Man SF, et al: Cyclosporine and chronic sarcoidosis. *Chest* 98:1026-1029, 1990.

123. Bielory L, Holland C, Gascon P, et al: Uveitis, cutaneous and neurosarcoid: treatment with low-dose cyclosporine A. *Transplant Proc* 20:144-148, 1988.

Disorders of Keratinization

124. Meyer P, van Voorst Vader PC: Lack of effect of cyclosporin A in pityriasis rubra pilaris (letter). *Acta Derm Venereol* 69:272, 1989.

125. Rosenbach A, Lowe NJ: Pityriasis rubra pilaris and cyclosporine (letter). *Arch Dermatol* 129:1346-1348, 1993.

126. Ghazi A, Laso-Dosal F: Cyclosporin A and pityriasis rubra pilaris (letter). *Acta Derm Venereol* 70:181, 1990.

127. Velthius PJ, Jesserun RF: Improvement of ichthyosis by cyclosporin (letter). *Lancet* 1:335, 1985.

128. Ho VC, Gupta AK, Ellis CN, et al: Cyclosporine in lamellar ichthyosis. *Arch Dermatol* 125:511-514, 1989.

129. Gupta AK, Ellis CN, Nickoloff BJ, et al: Oral cyclosporine in the treatment of inflammatory and noninflammatory dermatoses. A clinical and immunopathologic analysis. *Arch Dermatol* 126:339-350, 1990.

Photosensitivity Dermatoses

130. Norris PG, Camp RD, Hawk JL: Actinic reticuloid: response to cyclosporine. *J Am Acad Dermatol* 21:307-309, 1989.

131. Gardeazabal J, Arregui MA, Gil N, et al: Successful treatment of musk ketone-induced chronic actinic dermatitis with cyclosporine and PUVA. *J Am Acad Dermatol* 27:838-842, 1992.

132. Thestrup-Pedersen K, Zachariae C, Kaltoft K, et al: Development of cutaneous pseudolymphoma following ciclosporin therapy of actinic reticuloid. *Dermatologica* 177:376-381, 1988.

133. Duschet P, Schwarz T, Oppolzer G, et al: Persistent light reaction. Successful treatment with cyclosporin. *Acta Derm Venereol (Stockh)* 68:176-178, 1988.

134. Bulengo-Ransby SM, Ellis CN, Griffiths CE, et al: Failure of reticular erythematous mucinosis to respond to cyclosporine. *J Am Acad Dermatol* 27:825-828, 1992.

Other Dermatoses

135. Towpik E, Kupiec-Weglinski JW, Schneider TM, et al: Cyclosporine and experimental skin allografts. *Transplantation* 40:714-718, 1985.

136. Gilhar A, Wojciechowski ZJ, Piepkorn MW, et al: Description of and treatment to inhibit the rejection of human split-thickness skin grafts by congenitally athymic (nude) rats. *Exp Cell Biol* 54:263-274, 1986.

137. Biren CA, Barr RJ, McCullough JL, et al: Prolonged viability of human skin xenografts in rats by cyclosporine. *J Invest Dermatol* 86:611-614, 1986.

138. Achauer BM, Hewitt CW, Black KS, et al: Long-term skin allograft survival after short-term cyclosporin treatment in a patient with massive burns. *Lancet* 1:14-15, 1986.

139. Frame JD: Short-term cyclosporin and meshed allograft in burns. *Lancet* 1:154-155, 1987.

140. Harper JI, Kendra JR, Desai S, et al: Dermatological aspects of the use of cyclosporin A for prophylaxis of graft-versus-host disease. *Br J Dermatol* 110:469-474, 1984.

141. Powles RL, Clink HM, Spence D, et al: Cyclosporine A to prevent graft-versus-host disease in man after allogenic bone-marrow transplantation. *Lancet* 1:327-329, 1980.

142. Powles RL, Barrett AJ, Clink HM, et al: Cyclosporin A for the treatment of graft-versus-host disease in man. *Lancet* 2:1327-1331, 1978.

143. Al Rustom K, Pierard-Franchimont C, Peirard GE: Présentation anatomo-clinique de la maladie du greffon contre l'hôte traitée par cyclosporine A. *Dermatologica* 171:65-71, 1985.

144. Barrett AJ, Kendra JR, Lucas CF, et al: Cyclosporin A as prophylaxis against graft-versus-host disease in 36 patients. *BMJ* 285:162-166, 1982.

145. Miller RA, Shen JY, Rea TH, et al: Treatment of chronic erythema nodosum leprosum with cyclosporine A produces clinical and immunohistologic remission. *Int J Lepr Mycobact Dis* 55:441-449, 1987.

146. Uyemura K, Dixon JF, Wong L, et al: Effect of cyclosporine A in erythema nodosum leprosum. *J Immunol* 137:3620-3623, 1986.

147. Fradin MS, Ellis CN, Goldfarb MT, et al: Oral cyclosporine for severe chronic idiopathic urticaria and angioedema. *J Am Acad Dermatol* 25:1065-1067, 1991.

Adverse Effects

148. Berth-Jones J, Voorhees JJ: Consensus conference on cyclosporin A microemulsion for psoriasis, June 1996. *Br J Dermatol* 135:775-777, 1996.

149. Lebwohl M, Ellis C, Gottlieb A, et al: Cyclosporine consensus conference: with emphasis on the treatment of psoriasis. *J Am Acad Dermatol* 39:464-475, 1998.

150. Zachariae H, Hansen HE, Kragballe K, et al: Morphologic renal changes during cyclosporine treatment of psoriasis. *J Am Acad Dermatol* 26:415-419, 1992.

151. Powles AV, Cook T, Hulme B, et al: Renal function and biopsy findings after 5 years' treatment with low-dose cyclosporin for psoriasis. *Br J Dermatol* 128:159-165, 1993.

152. Data on file with Sandoz Clinical Research Division, East Hanover, NJ.

153. In file with Novartis Pharmaceuticals Corporation.

154. Koo J, Kadonaga JN, Wintroub BV, et al: The development of B-cell lymphoma in a patient with psoriasis treated with cyclosporine. *J Am Acad Dermatol* 26:836-840, 1992.

155. Luke RG: Mechanism of cyclosporine-induced hypertension. *Am J Hypertension* 4:468-471, 1991.

Monitoring and Therapeutic Guidelines

156. Timonen P, Friend D, Abeywickrama K, et al: Efficacy of low-dose cyclosporin A in psoriasis; results of dose-finding studies. *Br J Dermatol* 122(Suppl 36):33-39, 1990.

157. Feutren G, Friend D, Timonen P, et al: Predictive value of cyclosporin A level for efficacy or renal dysfunction in psoriasis. *Br J Dermatol* 122(Suppl 36):85-93, 1990.

158. Mihatsch MJ, Wolff K: Report of a meeting: Consensus conference on cyclosporine A for psoriasis, February 1992. *Br J Dermatol* 126:622, 1992.

159. Bavinck JNB, Tieben LM, Van der Woude FJ, et al: Prevention of skin cancer and reduction of keratotic skin lesions during acitretin therapy in renal transplant recipients: A double-blind, placebo-controlled study. *J Clin Oncol* 13:1933-1938, 1995.

160. Yuan Z, Davis A, Macdonald K, et al: Use of acitretin for the skin complications in renal transplant recipients. *N Z Med J* 108:255-256, 1995.

161. Van Dooren-Greebe RJ, Lemmens JAM, De Boo T, et al: Prolonged treatment with oral retinoids in adults: no influence on the frequency and severity of spinal abnormalities. *Br J Dermatol* 134:71-76, 1996.

162. Nyfors A: Liver biopsies from psoriatics related to methotrexate therapy. Findings in post-methotrexate liver biopsies from 160 patients. *Acta Pathol Microbiol Scand (A)* 85:511-518, 1977.

163. Zachariae H, Kragballe K, Sogaard H: Methotrexate induced liver cirrhosis. Studies including serial liver biopsies during continued treatment. *Br J Dermatol* 102:407-412, 1980.

164. Ahern MJ, Smith MD, Roberts-Thomson PJ: Methotrexate hepatotoxicity: what is the evidence? *Inflammation Research* 47:148-151, 1998.

165. Ashton RE, Millward-Sadler GH, White JE: Complications in methotrexate treatment of psoriasis with particular reference to liver fibrosis. *J Invest Dermatol* 79:229-232, 1992.

166. Themido R, Loureiro M, Pecegueiro M, et al: Methotrexate hepatotoxicity in psoriatic patients submitted to long-term therapy. *Acta Derm Venereol* 72:361-364, 1992.

167. Van Dooren-Greebe RJ, Kuijpers AL, Mulder J, et al: Methotrexate revisited: effects of long-term treatment in psoriasis. *Br J Dermatol* 130:204-210, 1994.

168. Roenigk HH Jr, Auerbach R, Maibach H, et al: Methotrexate in psoriasis: consensus conference. *J Am Acad Dermatol* 38:478-485, 1998.

169. Georgescu L, Quinn GC, Schwartzman S, et al: Lymphoma in patients with rheumatoid arthritis: association with the disease state or methotrexate treatment. *Semin Arthritis Rheum* 26:794-804, 1997.

170. Methotrexate sodium tablets, Methotrexate sodium for injection, Methotrexate LPF sodium (Methotrexate sodium injection) and Methotrexate sodium injection (package insert). Carolina, PR: Lederle Parenterals Inc; Pearl River, NY: Lederle Laboratories Division; Jan 25, 1996.

Tacrolimus and Sirolimus (Rapamycin)

171. Duncan JI: Differential inhibition of cutaneous T-cell-mediated reactions and epidermal cell proliferation by cyclosporin A, FK-506, and rapamycin. *J Invest Dermatol* 102:84-88, 1994.

172. Aoyama H, Tabata N, Tanaka M, et al: Successful treatment of resistant facial lesions of atopic dermatitis with 0.1% FK 506 ointment. *Br J Dermatol* 133:494-496, 1995.

173. Sawada S, Suzuki G, Kawase Y, et al: Novel immunosuppressive agent, FK506. In vitro effects on cloned T cell activation. *J Immunol* 139:1797-1803, 1987.

174. Kino T, Hatanaka H, Hashimoto M, et al: FK506, a novel immunosuppressant isolated from a Streptomyces. I. Fermentation, isolation, and physico-chemical and biological characteristics. *J Antibiot* 40:1249-1255, 1987.

175. Kino T, Hatanaka H, Miyata S, et al: FK506, a novel immunosuppressant isolated from a Streptomyces. II. Immunosuppressive effects of FK506 in vitro. *J Antibiot* 40:1256-1265, 1987.

176. The European FK 506 Multicentre Psoriasis Study Group: Systemic tacrolimus (FK 506) is effective for the treatment of psoriasis in a double-blind, placebo-controlled study. *Arch Dermatol* 132:419-423, 1996.

177. Michel G, Kemény L, Homey B, et al: FK 506 in the treatment of inflammatory skin disease: promises and perspectives. *Immunol Today* 17:106-108, 1996.

178. Schulz BS, Michel G, Wagner S, et al: Increased expression of epidermal IL-8 receptor in psoriasis. *J Immunol* 151:4399-4406, 1993.

179. Groth CG: Immunosuppressive regimens of tomorrow. *Transplantation Proc* 27:2971-2973, 1995.

180. Kaplan MJ, Ellis CN, Bata-Csorgo Z, et al: Systemic toxicity following administration of sirolimus (formerly rapamycin) for psoriasis: association of capillary leak syndrome with apoptosis of lesional lymphocytes. *Arch Dermatol* 135:553-557, 1999.

181. Jegasothy BV, Ackerman CD, Todo S, et al: Tacrolimus (FK 506)—a new therapeutic agent for severe recalcitrant psoriasis. *Arch Dermatol* 128:781-785, 1992.

182. Alaiti S, Kang S, Fiedler VC, et al: Tacrolimus (FK506) ointment for atopic dermatitis: A phase I study in adults and children. *J Am Acad Dermatol* 38:69-76, 1998.

183. Ruzicka T, Bieber T, Schöpf E, et al: A short-term trial of tacrolimus ointment for atopic dermatitis. *N Engl J Med* 337:816-821, 1997.

Russell P. Hall III

Dapsone

In 1947 Costello[1] reported on the successful use of sulfapyridine in the treatment of dermatitis herpetiformis (DH). This observation resulted in the investigation of a number of different sulfonamide-type drugs for the treatment of DH, which culminated in the studies of Kruizinga and Hamminga,[2] who documented the efficacy of a sulfone, 4, 4'-diamino-diphenyl sulfone (DDS) or dapsone, in the treatment of DH. This chapter focuses on the use of dapsone in the treatment of DH and other skin diseases (Table 11-1). Although dapsone has many associated pharmacologic and idiosyncratic adverse effects, a complete understanding of the pharmacology, proposed mechanisms of action, and adverse benefits allows the clinician to use the drug in a manner that maximizes the therapeutic benefit and minimizes any associated adverse effects of the drug.

Sulfonamides were first synthesized for use as dyes (derived from coal tar) for the fabric industry in the early twentieth century. The original use of these drugs in humans focused on the treatment of streptococcal infections. Dapsone was synthesized in 1908, and because of its structural similarity to other sulfonamides, it was tested as an antistreptococcal antibiotic.[3] In 1941 dapsone was shown to be effective in experimental tuberculosis and later in experimental leprosy, leading to its use in human leprosy, for which it remains a mainstay of therapy.[4]

In 1940 Costello[1] reported on the treatment of a patient with DH with sulfapyridine, with excellent results. It was thought that DH represented a reaction to the presence of bacteria somewhere in the body and that the sulfapyridine was functioning as an antibiotic in the treatment of DH. Cornbleet[5] recognized that sulfapyridine did not cure DH; he then treated patients with DH with sulfoxone sodium and found it to be more effective than sulfapyridine. In 1953 Kruizinga and Hamminga[2] introduced the use of the parent drug of sulfoxone, dapsone, for the treatment of DH, and since that time it has remained the mainstay of treatment for DH.

Dapsone (DDS) is available as 25 mg and 100 mg tablets. Other sulfones, such as diasone, are currently not available in the United States. Sulfapyridine, which has also been found to be effective in DH and other skin diseases, is also not currently available in the United States, although clinical trials are underway. Dapsone is inexpensive, with a typical dosage of 100 mg daily costing the pharmacy approximately $0.15 to $0.60 per day. Although sulfasalazine is metabolized in the large intestine to sulfapyridine, the amount of sulfapyridine that is absorbed is highly dependent on gut transit time, gut flora, and other factors, resulting in a less predictable clinical response than sulfapyridine.[6]

PHARMACOLOGY

Table 11-2 contains key pharmacologic concepts for dapsone and related drugs. Figure 11-1 demonstrates the structure of dapsone.

■ Table 11-1   Dapsone and Related Drugs

Generic Name	Trade Name	Generic Available	Manu-facturer	Tablet/ Capsule Sizes	Special Formu-lations	Standard Dosage Range	Price Index
Dapsone	Dapsone	No	Jacobus	25, 100 mg	None	50-200 mg/d	$
Sulfapyridine	Currently unavailable	NA	Jacobus	500 mg (in studies)	NA	1-2 g/d	—
Sulfasalazine	Azulfidine Azulfidine EN	Yes	Pharmacia Upjohn, various others	500 mg	None	1-2 g/d	$ ($)

$, <1.00; $$, 1.01-2.00; $$$, 2.01-5.00; $$$$, 5.01-10.00; $$$$$, >10.00; ( ), generic price; /, two different price ranges from lower dose to higher dose examples of this drug; —, no price listed for this drug.

Absorption and Bioavailability

Dapsone is a lipid-soluble, water-insoluble compound that penetrates well into cells and tissues. Dapsone is well absorbed from the gut with approximately 70% to 80% of a single oral dose absorbed and an absorption half-life of approximately 1 hour.[7-9] The observed increased effectiveness of dapsone compared with other sulfones (e.g., diasone, the prodrug of dapsone; no longer available in the United States) and sulfonamides (e.g., sulfapyridine) is probably related to the superior absorption of dapsone from the gut and its effective penetration into the cell.

Dapsone is able to cross the placenta and is excreted into breast milk.[9] Hemolysis has been known to occur in nursing infants of mothers taking dapsone.[10] No harmful effects of dapsone have been demonstrated on fetal development in utero.[11]

After a single oral dose of 100 mg of dapsone, a maximum serum level of 1.70 mg/L is achieved. In a steady state condition, a 100 mg dose of dapsone results in a mean level at 24 hours of 1.95 mg/L, with a peak dapsone level of approximately 3 mg/L. The elimination half-life of dapsone has been shown to average between 24 and 30 hours (with significant individual variability ranging from 10 to 50 hours), with a peak serum level occurring at 2 to 6 hours after an oral dose. This long elimination half-life results in dapsone remaining in the circulation for as long as 30 days after a single oral dose. The long half-life of dapsone may be a result of a significant enterohepatic recirculation and of the strong protein binding of both dapsone and its major metabolite monoacetyldapsone (MADDS).[9]

Metabolism

Dapsone is primarily metabolized by N-acetylation and N-hydroxylation. Dapsone is acetylated in the liver by N-acetyltransferase and subsequently deacetylated. An equilibrium develops rapidly between acetylation and deacetylation; however, during the early phases of absorption an increased ratio of MADDS/DDS is observed, probably due to the stronger protein binding of MADDS compared with DDS.[9] There is a significant variability in individual acetylation, resulting in some individuals being labeled as slow acetylators; however, this variability is not relevant in the clinical utilization of dapsone.[12,13]

The second major pathway of metabolism of dapsone is hydroxylation. N-hydroxylation of dapsone occurs in the liver and this metabolic product is thought to be responsible for the hematologic adverse effects associated with dapsone including methemoglobinemia and the development of a hemolytic anemia.[14,15] This N-hydroxylation of dapsone can be inhibited in vivo by the use of cimetidine, which has been demonstrated to decrease methemoglobinemia in animal studies and in man, although the clinical relevance has yet to be demonstrated.[16] No significant change in either hemoglobin levels

Table 11-2 Key Pharmacologic Concepts—Dapsone and Related Drugs

| Drug Name | Drug Category | Absorption and Bioavailability | | | Elimination | | |
		Peak Levels	Bioavailable (%)	Protein Binding	Half-life	Metabolism	Excretion
Dapsone	Sulfone	2-6 hrs	70%-80% absorbed	70%-90%	10-50 hrs mean 28 hrs	N-acetylation, N-hydroxylation	Hepatic and renal
Sulfapyridine	Sulfonamide	1.5-4 hrs	>80%	50%-70%	5-14 hrs	N-acetylation, N-hydroxylation	Hepatic and renal
Sulfasalazine	Sulfonamide	10-30 hrs	15%	99%	6-15 hrs	Mostly acetylation; in bowel converted to SP and 5-ASA	Hepatic and renal

SP, Sulfapyridine; 5-ASA, 5-acetylsalicylic acid.

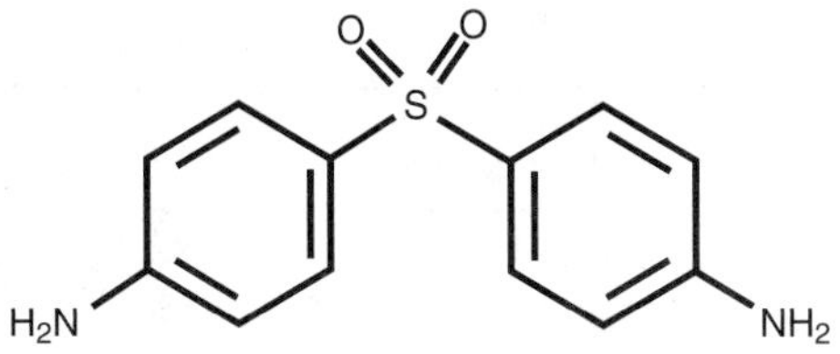

Figure 11-1   Dapsone.

or reticuloctye counts, however, was noted in the human studies.[17]

Excretion

Dapsone and its metabolites are also conjugated in the liver as dapsone glucuronide, which is rapidly excreted via the kidneys because it is more water soluble. These conjugates represent the major metabolites of dapsone found in the urine and are not easily detectable in the circulation, suggesting that they are rapidly cleared. Dapsone has been suggested to have a significant enterohepatic circulation, in part due to the observation that treatment with activated charcoal increases the rate of elimination of dapsone up to 5 times. Dapsone is excreted via the kidneys. The parent drug and N-hydroxy dapsone are the main products detected and are most often conjugated with glucuronide.[9] The observation that treatment with probenicid decreases renal clearance implies renal tubular transport.[9]

The role of liver failure in the clinical use of dapsone has been evaluated in patients with cirrhosis, and although minor changes in the metabolism of dapsone have been documented, no dosage adjustment appears to be needed.[18] The role of renal failure in the clinical use of dapsone has not been thoroughly investigated. No clinically significant difference in the absorption of dapsone has been observed in patients with DH, despite the presence of a gluten-sensitive enteropathy in these patients.[13,19]

In summary, dapsone is well absorbed from the gut and metabolized by N-acetylation and N-hydroxylation. The N-hydroxylated forms of dapsone are important because they play a critical role in the hematologic adverse effects noted with dapsone. Dapsone is excreted via the

kidney with a significant enterohepatic circulation. This results in an effective half-life of approximately 24 to 36 hours, which allows for daily dosing.

Mechanisms of Action

While the mechanism of action of dapsone in the treatment of leprosy has been shown to be a result of inhibition of the folic acid pathway, the mechanism of action of dapsone in inflammatory diseases is not well understood.[7] Clinically it appears that dapsone is most useful in treating diseases with neutrophilic infiltrates in the skin. This has led to suggestions that dapsone may directly affect neutrophil function. Table 11-3 contains a list of dapsone mechanisms and potential clinical effects.

NEUTROPHIL RESPIRATORY BURST.   Initial observations suggested that dapsone might inhibit complement function. Dapsone has not, however, been demonstrated to affect either the presence of complement deposits in the skin of patients with DH or the activation of complement in experimental systems.[20] The frequent presence of neutrophils in the inflammatory infiltrate of many "dapsone responsive" skin diseases also led to the suggestion that dapsone may inhibit lysosomal enzymes[21]; however, this effect has been demonstrated only at concentrations of dapsone up to 20 times that seen in serum after a 300 mg dose of dapsone. If dapsone does exert an effect on lysosomal enzymes, it must be concentrated in the lysosome, which to date has not been demonstrated.[22] Stendahl and co-workers[23] investigated the effect of dapsone on neutrophils and found no evidence of an effect on random movement, chemotaxis, release of lysosomal enzymes, or oxidative metabolism by dapsone at concentrations of 1 to 30 μg/ml. They did however demonstrate that dapsone was able to inhibit the myeloperoxidase-peroxide-halide–mediated cytotoxic system, which likely plays a role in controlling the degree of destruction in lesions.[23] However, these findings do not address the observation that neutrophils do not accumulate in the skin of patients treated with dapsone.

NEUTROPHIL CHEMOTAXIS.   The lack of neutrophils in the skin of patients being treated

Table 11-3 Dapsone Mechanisms

Postulated Mechanisms	Resultant Clinical Effects
Inhibition of neutrophil myeloperoxidase	Inhibition of neutrophil respiratory burst mechanisms with inhibition of neutrophil tissue damage
Inhibition of neutrophil adhesion to vascular endothelium integrins	Impaired neutrophil chemotaxis
Inhibition of chemotaxis in part by inhibition of f-met leu phe-mediated chemotaxis	Impaired neutrophil chemotaxis
Inhibition of LTB_4 binding	Impaired neutrophil chemotaxis
Inhibition of generation of 5-lipogenase products in neutrophils and macrophages	Inhibition of chemotaxis and inflammatory damage to tissue
Inhibition of eosinophil myeloperoxidase	Potential mechanism by which dapsone may affect some eosinophil-mediated dermatoses such as eosinophilic cellulitis

with dapsone suggests that dapsone may affect the chemotaxis of neutrophils. Initial investigation showed no consistent inhibition of chemotaxis by dapsone.[23-25] Harvath and co-workers[26] did demonstrate a selective inhibition of neutrophil chemotaxis in vitro by dapsone. They showed that while neutrophil chemotaxis to either C5a- or leukocyte-derived chemotactic factor was not affected by dapsone, chemotaxis to the chemoattractant *N*-formyl-methionyl-leucyl-phenylalanine (F-met-leu-phe) was inhibited by dapsone.[26] The mechanism of this effect is not known, but dapsone did inhibit the binding of F-met-leu-phe to neutrophils, and this effect was specific for human neutrophils. Other investigations into neutrophil chemotaxis demonstrated that dapsone inhibits the adherence of neutrophils to IgA. Thuong-Nguyen and associates[27] showed that dapsone was able to inhibit the migration and binding of neutrophils to IgA deposits in skin in an in vitro neutrophil adherence assay. Nelson and co-authors investigated the possible role of dapsone in the inhibition of integrin-mediated neutrophil adherence. Their results demonstrated that dapsone can inhibit the CD11b/CD18-mediated binding of neutrophils in vitro and that this is associated with an inhibition of the chemoattractant-induced signal transduction in neutrophils.[28,29] Investigators also demonstrated that some sulfones can inhibit synthesis of chemotactic lipids and interfere with LTB_4-mediated chemotaxis in neutrophils.[30-33]

These studies suggest that although the actual mechanism of dapsone is not clearly known, it does have a specific effect on human neutrophils, probably both by moderating the level of damage by neutrophils at the site of lesions and by decreasing neutrophil migration to lesions.

CLINICAL USE

Table 11-4 lists indications and contraindications for dapsone.

Dermatologic Indications—Consistent Efficacy

Dapsone has been approved by the FDA for the treatment of patients with DH or leprosy. In addition, dapsone has been recognized to be an effective therapy for a variety of skin diseases and for selected infectious diseases (malaria and *Pneumocystis carinii* prophylaxis). Dapsone-responsive dermatoses can be divided into two general categories—those in which a response has been clearly documented and those in which the response has been noted only anecdotally or in a minority of patients treated (Table 11-4). A common element in many of the inflammatory conditions that have been found to be most responsive to dapsone is the predominance of a neutrophilic infiltrate in the skin. Due to the relative toxicity of dapsone and the erratic nature of many inflammatory skin diseases, it is important that clear criteria be es-

Table 11-4	Dapsone Indications and Contraindications

FDA-APPROVED INDICATIONS
Dermatitis herpetiformis
Leprosy

**DERMATOLOGIC INDICATIONS
(CONSISTENT EFFICACY)**
Dermatitis herpetiformis[35-37]
Linear IgA dermatosis (bullous dermatosis of
   childhood)[38-41]
Bullous eruption of systemic lupus
   erythematosus[42]
Leprosy[43]
Erythema elevatum diutinum[44]

**OTHER DERMATOLOGIC USES
(VARIABLE EFFICACY)**

Autoimmune Bullous Dermatoses
Bullous pemphigoid[45,49,50,56]
Cicatricial pemphigoid[52,53,55]
Pemphigus vulgaris/foliaceus[46,48,51,54]
Subcorneal pustular dermatosis (IgA
   pemphigus)[47]

Neutrophilic Dermatoses
Pyoderma gangrenosum[60]
Acute febrile neutrophilic dermatosis (Sweet's
   syndrome)[59]
Behçet syndrome/aphthous stomatitis[61,63]

Vasculitis
Cutaneous vasculitis (leukocytoclastic)[57]
Urticarial vasculitis[58]

Other Dermatoses
Subacute cutaneous lupus erythematosus[64,65]
Relapsing polychondritis[66-68]
Granuloma annulare[69]
Brown recluse spider bites[70,71]

CONTRAINDICATIONS

Absolute
Prior hypersensitivity to dapsone, including
   agranulocytosis and hypersensitivity syndrome

Relative
Allergy to sulfonamide antibiotics
Significant cardiopulmonary disease
G6PD deficiency

PREGNANCY PRESCRIBING STATUS—CATEGORY C

tablished for dapsone responsiveness in diseases in which the efficacy has not been firmly established. Most often if dapsone is going to be effective in the treatment of an inflammatory dermatosis, the patient will experience a relatively rapid response (within 24 to 48 hours) to dapsone therapy, with a relatively rapid recurrence of the disease after withdrawal of the medication. In general, sulfapyridine has a similar, albeit less effective, profile of activity than dapsone. In a similar manner, sulfasalazine (Azulfidine) is less effective for most dermatologic diseases, most

probably because of the poor absorption of sulfapyridine from the large bowel. An important exception may be psoriasis, in which one controlled trial demonstrated a significant benefit of sulfasalazine.[34] It is not clear whether this effect was secondary to the sulfapyridine, the 5-aminosalicylate, or the sulfasalazine itself.

DERMATITIS HERPETIFORMIS. Dapsone is the drug of choice for the treatment of DH.[35-37] Although patients may also be treated with a gluten free diet with good results, the difficulty of following that diet often makes treatment with dapsone the treatment of choice for most patients. Most patients respond within 24 to 36 hours with marked decrease in itching and new blister formation. Similarly, withdrawal of dapsone results in a rapid (within 12 to 48 hours) recurrence of the signs and symptoms of DH. This is a reproducible finding and should be the measure against which all therapy with dapsone is judged. The majority of patients with DH can be maintained on 100 to 200 mg of dapsone per day. There is however, considerable variability in this response, with some patients controlled on 25 mg per day or less while others may have significant skin lesions occurring despite therapy with up to 400 mg per day of dapsone. The majority of patients, however, can be managed on 100 to 200 mg per day of dapsone.[35] If no significant risk factors such as severe cardiac, pulmonary, or hematologic disease exist for the pharmacologic side effects of dapsone (e.g., hemolytic anemia and methemoglobinemia), therapy can begin with 100 mg daily. This results in rapid control of the disease in most patients. Adjustment of the dosage can then be undertaken to achieve the lowest possible dose needed to control the disease. Because toxicity from the pharmacologic adverse effects is directly related to the dose of the drug, patients must be warned against self-medication and self-adjustment of the dosage of dapsone in response to small changes in disease activity. The severity of DH also may vary with time for reasons that are not clear. This oftentimes allows the dapsone dose to be reduced, reducing toxic adverse effects with no change in clinical symptoms.

It is critical that patients be evaluated before institution of therapy for any factors that may place them at high risk from the pharmacologic adverse effects of dapsone and that they be followed-up closely during therapy (see later section on Monitoring Guidelines). Sulfapyridine is also effective in patients with DH although less effective than dapsone.[35] The pharmacologic adverse effects of sulfapyridine are also less prominent than seen with dapsone, making it a useful drug when patients cannot tolerate dapsone. Most patients with DH that can be controlled with sulfapyridine are treated with 1 to 2 g daily. Currently sulfapyridine is not available in the United States, but approval by the FDA is expected in the near future.

LINEAR IGA BULLOUS DERMATOSIS AND CHRONIC BULLOUS DERMATOSIS OF CHILDHOOD. Patients with linear IgA disease generally present with clinical and histologic features that are very similar to those seen in patients with DH.[38-41] These patients for the most part also respond to treatment with dapsone in a similar manner as do patients with DH. Most patients can be controlled with 100 to 200 mg of dapsone daily. Occasionally patients with linear IgA dermatosis cannot be controlled on dapsone alone and may require adjunctive therapy, often with low dose systemic corticosteroids. This seems to be the case more often in some children with linear IgA disease (chronic bullous dermatosis of childhood). However, this response is difficult to predict, and decisions about the addition of systemic corticosteroids should be made on an individual basis.

BULLOUS ERUPTION OF SYSTEMIC LUPUS ERYTHEMATOSUS. Patients with the bullous eruption of systemic lupus erythematosus (SLE) have a vesicular eruption with a histologic picture similar to that seen in patients with DH. These patients often have a dramatic response to dapsone therapy in doses as low as 50 mg daily.[42] The presence of neutrophils in a vesicular eruption in a patient with SLE suggests that dapsone will be effective and may lessen the need for systemic corticosteroids. Because patients with SLE may have other manifestations that could increase the clinical severity of the pharmacologic effects of dapsone, special care should be taken in both pretreatment and posttreatment monitoring (see later section on Monitoring Guidelines).

LEPROSY. The treatment of leprosy is constantly under review, and a discussion of this use of dapsone is beyond the scope of this discussion. The World Health Organization issues frequent guidelines that should be consulted when treating patients with leprosy. It is important to emphasize that monotherapy with dapsone is ineffective in essentially all cases of leprosy.[43]

ERYTHEMA ELEVATUM DIUTINUM. Patients with erythema elevatum diutinum, a distinct type of leukocytoclastic vasculitis, often respond dramatically to dapsone therapy.[44] The dosages used are similar to those for DH and other blistering diseases.

Other Dermatologic Indications— Variable Efficacy

A wide variety of other diseases have been proposed to be responsive to treatment with dapsone; however, the response is often highly variable. In most of these conditions, there are not controlled studies demonstrating the effectiveness of dapsone, and most of the evidence consists of case reports or small uncontrolled series of patients. The diseases with the most consistent response are those with a predominant neutrophilic infiltrate. Evaluating the nature of the histologic infiltrate and using dapsone when neutrophils are found to be the predominant inflammatory cell increase the likelihood of a good therapeutic response to dapsone therapy. Dapsone has proven to be a useful adjunctive agent in the treatment of inflammatory diseases of the skin for which systemic corticosteroids are the treatment of choice.[45,46] Although the response to dapsone therapy is unpredictable in many of these patients, the alternative drugs used as "steroid-sparing agents" often have more long-term toxicity making a trial of dapsone a reasonable clinical consideration. Careful evaluation of both the clinical and the histologic characteristics of the disease with particular concern for the nature of the inflammatory infiltrate will increase the likelihood of therapeutic success when using dapsone.

AUTOIMMUNE BULLOUS DERMATOSES.

Dapsone has been reported to be of some use in the treatment of a variety of autoimmune blistering diseases such as bullous pemphigoid, cicatricial pemphigoid, IgA pemphigus (subcorneal pustular dermatosis), pemphigus vulgaris, pemphigus foliaceus, and epidermolysis bullosa acquisita.[45-56] The response in these diseases is often highly variable. In bullous pemphigoid, the presence of a predominant neutrophilic infiltrate is often associated with a higher likelihood of successful therapy with dapsone.

VASCULITIS.

Dapsone has been used with varying success in the treatment of cutaneous leukocytoclastic vasculitis and in the treatment of urticarial vasculitis.[57,58] The response to ther-

apy is variable; however, dapsone may be useful as a steroid-sparing agent in some patients.

NEUTROPHILIC DERMATOSES.

Successful use of dapsone has been described in individual cases or small series of patients with a variety of neutrophilic dermatoses such as Sweet's syndrome and pyoderma gangrenosum, as well as in cutaneous leukocytoclastic vasculitis and erythema elevatum diutinum.[59,60] Dapsone has also been demonstrated to be useful in the cutaneous and oral mucosal manifestations of Behçet's disease.[61-63] One study demonstrated that dapsone decreased the pathergic response that is often seen in the skin of patients with Behçet's disease.[61]

OTHER DERMATOSES.

Dapsone has been described to be effective in some patients with cutaneous manifestations of lupus erythematosus such as chronic cutaneous and subacute cutaneous lupus.[64,65] Successful therapy of relapsing polychondritis has also been reported using dapsone.[66-68] However, no controlled studies have been performed, and the unpredictable course of this disease makes it difficult to judge the true effectiveness of the use of dapsone in relapsing polychondritis. In a similar manner, granuloma annulare has been reported to respond to dapsone therapy; however, no controlled studies have been performed.[69]

Recently dapsone has been suggested to be of benefit in the management of brown recluse spider bites.[70] Prospective clinical trials comparing immediate surgery with treatment with dapsone followed by delayed surgical excision suggested a benefit for dapsone.[71] Other studies, however, have not indicated a clear benefit.[70,72] Experimental studies have not clearly demonstrated that dapsone provides any benefit in the management of the bite of the brown recluse spider.[73-75] Although clear evidence supporting the use of dapsone in severe brown recluse spider bites is not available, the use of dapsone may be considered in some patients. It should be emphasized that one of the systemic manifestations of brown recluse spider bites is a hemolytic anemia, which is also an adverse effect associated with dapsone therapy.[72]

A number of other dermatologic diseases and conditions such as granuloma faciale, pustular psoriasis, panniculitis, acne rosacea, and nodulocystic acne have been reported to be somewhat responsive to dapsone, but for the most part these reports represent case reports of one or two patients or small uncontrolled series of patients and have not been confirmed by larger series or prospective trials.[76-82] Indeed, in nodulocystic acne a randomized, prospective trial of dapsone compared to 13-cis-retinoic acid demonstrated only marginal benefit with dapsone therapy, clearly inferior to that seen with the use of 13-cis-retinoic acid. One controlled, double blind study has been published suggesting that sulfasalazine improves psoriasis; however, this finding has not been confirmed by other investigators.[34]

Contraindications

Dapsone is contraindicated in patients with documented hypersensitivity to the drug (see Table 11-4). Sulfapyridine is also contraindicated when hypersensitivity to that drug has been documented. It is important to note, however, that cross-sensitivity with sulfapyridine and with other sulfonamide-type drugs is relatively rare.[83,84] A relative contraindication to the use of both drugs is related to the pharmacologic adverse events. Great care should be taken in treatment with dapsone in patients that are at increased risk for the development of the pharmacologic adverse effects due to pulmonary, cardiovascular, or hematologic disease or glucose-6-phosphate dehydrogenase (G6PD) deficiency.

Adverse Effects—Pharmacologic

Box 11-1 lists selected adverse effects of dapsone.

HEMOLYTIC ANEMIA. Dapsone is associated with both pharmacologic and idiosyncratic adverse events. The development of hemolytic anemia or methemoglobinemia has long been recognized as an adverse event associated with dapsone and occurs to some degree in all individuals who take dapsone. However, there is a significant variability as to the extent of the toxicity and in the clinical significance of the hematologic changes observed. This hematotoxicity is dose-related and can occur in individuals receiving a single 100 mg dose of dapsone.[85] The observation that dapsone is not directly toxic when incubated with erythrocytes in vitro led to investigation into what metabolic product(s) of

---

Box 11-1

Selected Adverse Effects of Dapsone

PHARMACOLOGIC
Hemolytic anemia
Methemoglobinemia—symptoms include
    headache, lethargy

IDIOSYNCRATIC
Hematologic
Leukopenia
Agranulocytosis

Hepatic
Hepatitis (predominantly transaminase
    elevations)
Infectious mononucleosis–like syndrome
    (dapsone hypersensitivity syndrome)
Cholestatic jaundice
Hypoalbuminemia

Cutaneous Hypersensitivity Reactions
Morbilliform eruption (including dapsone
    hypersensitivity syndrome)
Exfoliative erythroderma
Toxic epidermal necrolysis (rare)

Gastrointestinal
Gastric irritation
Anorexia

Neurologic
Psychosis
Peripheral neuropathy (motor predominant)

---

dapsone may be responsible for the hematotoxicity. It is now recognized that the major hematotoxicity of dapsone is related to the N-hydroxy metabolites (N-hydroxy-dapsone equals dapsone hydroxylamine and N-hydroxy-monoacetyl dapsone equals monoacetyl dapsone hydroxylamine) of dapsone.[15,85,86] These metabolites are formed in the liver via the cytochrome P-450 (CYP) system and are potent oxidants. The ability of the red blood cell to tolerate oxidative stresses is related to the presence of red blood cell–reduced glutathione and the ability of the hexose monophosphate shunt and red blood cell glycolysis to maintain effective antioxidants. Because red blood cells do not synthesize new protein, the ability of the red blood cell to resist oxidative stress decreases with the age of the red blood cells, making older cells more susceptible to damage and removal from the circulation. This may result in patients having an initial decrease in the hemoglobin followed by a partial correction due to increased production of new red blood cells from the bone marrow.

N-hydroxy metabolites of dapsone are potent oxidants and present to the red blood cell a persistent oxidative stress. They may act directly on the red blood cell, leading to the depletion of red blood cell–reduced glutathione, the formation of protein (including hemoglobin and red blood cell membrane)–glutathione disulfides, structural changes in the red blood cell, Heinz-body formation, and splenic sequestration of the red blood cells.[85] In addition, lipid peroxidation of red blood cell membrane has been documented to occur in vitro, which may also contribute to membrane changes and sequestration in the spleen of the erythrocytes. Significant individual variability in susceptibility to this effect has been described, especially in individuals who are deficient in G6PD. G6PD-deficient individuals are more susceptible to oxidative stresses, including that from dapsone metabolites. It is important to remember that although this enzyme is more frequently absent in African-Americans, those of Middle Eastern ancestry, and Asians, significant variability in G6PD function exists in all populations, which can result in significant hemolysis.[87,88] The degree of hemolysis, however, does not correlate with the acetylator phenotype of the individual.[89]

METHEMOGLOBINEMIA.   The second major hematologic adverse event associated with dapsone is the formation of methemoglobin. The formation of methemoglobin is also related to the *N*-hydroxy metabolites of dapsone. This is also dose-related, and small amounts of methemoglobin can be seen in individuals on low doses of dapsone. The methemoglobin that is formed is acted on by methemoglobin reductase in the red blood cell leading to the regeneration of hemoglobin.[85] This regeneration of oxyhemoglobin is independent of G6PD, and there is not a clear relationship between the hemolytic anemia associated with dapsone and the formation of methemoglobin. The clinical significance of methemoglobin relates to the decreased oxygen-carrying capacity of methemo-

globin and therefore is directly related to the total hemoglobin and the clinical status of the patient's cardiopulmonary system. It is not possible to accurately predict the amount of methemoglobin based on the degree of cyanosis of the patient. In addition, the percent of methemoglobin may not accurately reflect the clinical significance of the methemoglobinemia. For example, a patient with 10% methemoglobin but with a total hemoglobin of 15 g/dl will have a functional hemoglobin of approximately 13.5 g/dl, whereas the same percentage of methemoglobin (10%) in a patient with a total hemoglobin of 10 g/dl will have a functional hemoglobin concentration of 9 g/dl and may develop symptoms. Similarly, patients with significant cardiac or pulmonary disease may be less able to tolerate relatively low levels of methemoglobin.

It is important to remember that both the hemolytic anemia and methemoglobinemia are predictable events in patients taking dapsone and that significant variability in the magnitude of these effects can be seen from patient to patient. Safe use of dapsone relies on the clinician's awareness of these side effects, predicting any possible serious clinical effects on the patient, and managing the dosage of dapsone with all of these factors taken into account. Vitamin E (800 IU/day) has been demonstrated to provide a small amount of protection against the formation of methemoglobin and hemolysis; however, the clinical benefit of this effect has not been documented.[90] Cimetidine (400 mg PO three times daily) has also been demonstrated to decrease methemoglobin formation in man.[17] This effect is thought to be mediated by inhibition of the formation of the *N*-hydroxy metabolites of dapsone, which cause hematotoxicity. In an emergency, oral methylene blue (100 to 300 mg/day) can also be used to acutely decrease methemoglobin levels, although this drug is not effective if the patient is G6PD deficient.[91] Although these drugs may improve the laboratory manifestations of dapsone toxicity, the clinical significance of the changes has not been documented.

Adverse Effects—Idiosyncratic

The mechanisms associated with the idiosyncratic adverse effects of dapsone are not as well understood. These adverse effects range from relatively minor cutaneous manifestations similar to other drug eruptions to severe life threatening complications such as agranulocytosis.

AGRANULOCYTOSIS. Agranulocytosis is one of the most serious idiosyncratic reactions to dapsone.[92,93] The mechanism of the agranulocytosis is not known; however, some data suggest that the *N*-hydroxy metabolites may also play a role in this reaction. Hornsten and coworkers[93] estimated an incidence of agranulocytosis from dapsone of 1 case per every 3000 patient years of exposure to dapsone or in approximately 1 in 240 to 1 in 425 patients with DH who were treated with dapsone. The median duration of therapy with dapsone before the development of agranulocytosis was 7 weeks, with an average dosage of 100 mg daily. It is difficult to accurately determine the earliest onset of this agranulocytosis because uniform timing of monitoring of white blood cell counts is not noted in the literature. However, it is clear that agranulocytosis has occurred as early as 3 weeks after beginning therapy.[92-94] In addition, essentially all cases of agranulocytosis developed within the first 12 weeks of therapy. Evaluation of the bone marrow of these patients most often reveals severe depression of granulopoieses. Patients may present with fever, pharyngitis, and occasionally signs of sepsis. The initial reports suggested a mortality rate of 50% when agranulocytosis is discovered early. Patients for whom dapsone is promptly discontinued recover in 7 to 14 days.[92] Granulocyte colony–stimulating factor has been used successfully to speed the recovery of normal granulocyte numbers.[95] The potential severity of this reaction and the fact that it always occurs gradually within the first 3 months of therapy suggest that frequent early monitoring of complete blood counts be undertaken.[93,94] Patients should be instructed to discontinue the medication if they develop persistent fevers or flulike symptoms.

NEUROPATHY. Dapsone has also been associated with a variety of neurologic adverse events. Although all of these adverse effects of dapsone are rare, the most common is a peripheral neuropathy.[96-100] Dapsone peripheral neuropathy is a primarily distal motor neuropathy, with some degree of sensory involvement. These patients present with distal motor weakness of hands and legs, often demonstrating wasting of hand muscles. Sensory symptoms are uncommon but are virtually always accompanied by motor signs and symptoms when present. Patients most frequently do not have other signs of severe dapsone toxicity (e.g., sulfone syndrome, severe anemia, and methemoglobinemia). The dosage of dapsone associated with the development of neuropathy is highly variable. Patients have been reported to develop neuropathy secondary to high-dose short-term exposure (1.2 g/day for 7 days) or chronic relatively low-dose therapy (approximately 150 mg/day for 5 years). Daily doses of dapsone ranged from 75 mg to 600 mg per day.[100] Electrophysiologic studies have revealed findings consistent with a axonal degeneration predominantly affecting motor nerves.[101] Most patients recover completely with discontinuation of the dapsone.[100] This recovery can take from several weeks to up to 2 years. Of interest, one patient with DH on high-dose, long-term dapsone with a peripheral motor neuropathy regained full function in 1 year after decreasing his dapsone dose from approximately 1 g of dapsone per day to 100 to 200 mg/day.[101a] In addition, a patient has been restarted on dapsone after complete recovery from dapsone motor neuropathy without complications.

The mechanism of dapsone neuropathy is unknown. In some cases it is clearly a dose-related phenomenon, occurring in close approximation to acute, high-dose exposure to dapsone. In other cases, however, the neuropathy has occurred after relatively short-term, low-dose therapy. There has been speculation that the acetylator phenotype of patients may play a role; however, this has not been proven.[100] Attempts to develop an animal model of dapsone neurotoxicity have not been successful. Presently no single explanation can explain the variety of cases of dapsone neuropathy reported.

OTHER NEUROLOGIC EFFECTS. Additional neurologic events have also been reported as adverse events in some patients taking dapsone. Permanent retinal damage with optic atrophy has been reported in patients with severe dapsone overdosage.[102,103] It has been proposed that this damage was secondary to severe hypoxia and the associated red blood cell fragments found in patients with dapsone overdosage. Leonard and co-workers[104] examined retinal blood flow in patients with DH taking from 50 to 100 mg daily of dapsone and found no evidence of abnormal retinal blood flow. Homeida and associates[102] reported a case of dapsone overdosage with the development of both optic atrophy and motor neuropathy. After 14 months the motor neuropathy completely resolved; however, the optic atrophy and visual impairment persisted.[105]

In addition, cases of acute psychosis after treatment with dapsone have been reported.[106-108] The vast majority of these cases have been in individuals who were treated for leprosy, but rare cases have been reported in patients being treated for skin diseases. The mental status changes generally resolved after discontinuation of the dapsone. Like dapsone motor neuropathy, the etiology of these additional neurologic complications of dapsone therapy is unknown and most likely represents idiosyncratic reactions, perhaps associated with acute exposure to high doses of dapsone.

GASTROINTESTINAL EFFECTS. A variety of gastrointestinal adverse events have been associated with dapsone, ranging from relatively benign, self-limited complaints to severe and life-threatening complications. Some patients experience mild gastrointestinal upset when taking dapsone, with symptoms such as gastric upset and anorexia. For the most part this is self-limited and can be controlled by taking dapsone with meals. Patients on dapsone have been observed to develop primary hepatocellular hepatitis and cholestatic hepatitis, which resolve with discontinuation of the drug.[109,110] Other rare adverse events associated with dapsone include severe hypoalbuminemia, gall bladder perforation, and pancreatitis.[111-113]

DAPSONE HYPERSENSITIVITY SYNDROME. A more severe adverse event associated with dapsone has also been characterized as "dapsone syndrome" and "sulfone syndrome." This rare syndrome was initially described as an infectious mononucleosis–like eruption in patients being treated for lepromatous leprosy.[114,115] Patients present with fever, a generalized cutaneous eruption, and hepatitis. The skin eruption in

these patients has ranged from maculopapular eruption to toxic epidermal necrolysis, and the hepatitis shows a mixed pattern with both hepatocellular and cholestatic features.[110,114,116] Patients often have signs of severe hypersensitivity with peripheral eosinophilia and fatalities have been reported.[114,115] Although dapsone syndrome was initially reported in patients being treated for leprosy, it has been described in patients undergoing dapsone therapy for treatment of skin diseases. Treatment with systemic corticosteroids has been undertaken; however, the rarity of the conditions makes the benefit of this treatment unclear.

CUTANEOUS HYPERSENSITIVITY ERUPTIONS. As with many drugs, dapsone has also been associated with a wide variety of skin eruptions, ranging from the typical pattern of a maculopapular drug eruption to erythema multiforme to toxic epidermal necrolysis.[114,115] In general cross-reactivity between dapsone and other sulfa-derived drugs has not been observed. Observations of patients with human immunodeficiency virus (HIV), who have developed a maculopapular rash with trimethoprim/sulfamethoxazole and were then started on dapsone, revealed an approximately 7% to 20% incidence of a similar rash on dapsone. This eruption was often mild to moderate and allowed for continuation of the dapsone.[83,84] Beumont and co-workers found no adverse events that were clearly linked to dapsone in patients with previously documented adverse events to trimethoprim/sulfamethoxazole who were subsequently treated with dapsone.[83] Although no prospective study has been done, it appears that if cross-reactivity does occur it is relatively rare and mild, suggesting that cautious use of dapsone in patients with a history of sulfa sensitivity may be attempted. Photosensitivity has been reported in some patients taking dapsone, often in the context of the dapsone hypersensitivity syndrome. In addition, these reports have for the most part been in patients who were treated for leprosy.[117-119]

CARCINOGENESIS. Dapsone has also been suggested to be a weak carcinogen. Animal studies revealed a slightly increased incidence of malignancy in some animals treated for 2 years with high doses. However, no human studies confirmed that dapsone is a carcinogen in humans.[84,120-125]

PREGNANCY AND LACTATION.   The safety of dapsone during pregnancy has also been a concern, as many patients with skin disease require treatment during pregnancy. Although dapsone has not been proved safe in pregnancy, a recent series of patients with linear IgA dermatosis and patients with leprosy, as well as anecdotal reports in the literature, suggests that dapsone can be safely used in pregnancy.[11,126,127] It should be remembered, however, that dapsone can be secreted in breast milk and rarely causes hemolytic anemia in infants breast-feeding from mothers on dapsone.[10,128]

SULFAPYRIDINE ADVERSE EFFECTS.   Sulfapyridine has a similar toxicity profile to dapsone, although the reactions are less severe. Sulfapyridine can crystallize in the urine, leading to nephrotoxicity.[129] This may be a problem in patients on relatively high doses and can be minimized by an adequate fluid intake.

DRUG INTERACTIONS

Table 11-5 lists dapsone drug interactions. Drug interactions are relatively unusual in patients taking dapsone. Probenecid can reduce the renal excretion of dapsone; however, the clinical significance of this has not been clearly established. Rifampin can also decrease the functional half-life of dapsone secondary to induction of liver enzymes that metabolize dapsone, but again the clinical significance of this interaction is not clear.[9] Potentially significant interactions may occur when patients on dapsone take other drugs that are also oxidants. The increase in oxidative stress to the erythrocyte may increase the hemolysis that is normally seen with dapsone. Such drugs include sulfonamides, sulfones, or antimalarials such as hydroxychloroquine.[87] Dapsone levels have been increased in patients with acquired immunodeficiency syndrome (AIDS) taking dapsone with trimethoprim, compared with those on dapsone alone.[130] Although some concern has been expressed regarding the absorption of dapsone when taken with magnesium-aluminum antacids present in

■ **Table 11-5**   Dapsone Drug Interactions

Interacting Drug	Mechanism
DRUGS THAT INCREASE DAPSONE LEVELS	
Trimethoprim	Documented increase in dapsone (and trimethoprim) levels in AIDS patients; both interfere with folate metabolism
Probenecid	Decreased excretion of dapsone metabolites
Folic acid antagonists	Drugs such as pyrimethamine may increase risk of hematologic reactions such as agranulocytosis
DRUGS THAT DECREASE DAPSONE LEVELS	
Activated charcoal	Decreased GI absorption and enterohepatic recirculation of dapsone
Paraamino benzoic acid	May antagonize the efficacy of dapsone, possibly through folic acid metabolic pathway
Rifampin	Rifampin is a powerful CYP 3A4 enzyme inducer
DRUGS (OXIDANTS) THAT MAY INCREASE OXIDATIVE STRESS TO RBCS	
Sulfonamides	Both are oxidants, in combination may increase the oxidation-induced hemolysis of RBCs
Hydroxychlorquine	As with sulfonamides above

Data from *CliniSphere 2.0 CD ROM*, St. Louis, June 2000, Facts & Comparisons.
GI, Gastrointestinal; *RBC,* red blood cell.

didanosine during treatment for HIV infections, prospective studies show that didanosine did not significantly affect dapsone levels.[131]

MONITORING GUIDELINES

The most important factor in minimizing the toxicity associated with dapsone therapy involves the pretreatment evaluation and close follow-up of the patient. A complete understanding of the pharmacology of dapsone and of the pathogenesis of the disease being treated allows the clinician to utilize dapsone in conditions in which the likelihood of a successful response is high and adverse effects are as low as possible. Once it is established that dapsone is an appropriate drug to treat the patient, it is important to determine that the patient does not have any underlying conditions that would increase the toxicity of the drug. A complete history and physical with particular attention to preexisting cardiac, pulmonary, hepatic, neurologic, or renal disease should be performed. Although these do not represent absolute contraindications, the presence of significant cardiopulmonary disease may change the initial dose of dapsone used. Initial laboratory evaluation should be focused in a similar manner on the potential adverse events. Complete blood count (CBC) with differential liver function tests and renal function tests should be performed.

A G6PD level should be evaluated in most if not all patients being considered for treatment with dapsone. G6PD deficiency most often occurs in African-Americans and those of Middle Eastern or Far Eastern ancestry, and all of these patients should be tested before beginning ther-

---

Dapsone Monitoring Guidelines

BASELINE
History and Examination
- Complete history and physical with emphasis on cardiopulmonary, gastrointestinal, neurologic, and renal systems

Laboratory
- Complete blood count with differential WBC count
- Liver function tests (particularly SGOT/AST and SGPT/AST)
- Renal function tests (BUN and creatinine)
- Urinalysis
- Glucose-6-phosphate dehydrogenase level (G6PD)*

FOLLOW-UP
History and Examination
- Each visit reassess peripheral motor neurologic examination
- Each visit assess for signs and symptoms of methemoglobinemia

History and Examination—cont'd
- Question for any other significant adverse effects

Laboratory
- CBC with differential WBC count every week for 4 weeks, then every 2 weeks for 8 weeks, then every 3 to 4 months†
- Reticulocyte count as needed to assess response to dapsone hemolysis
- Liver function tests initially at least monthly, then every 3 to 4 months
- Renal function tests and urinalysis every 3 to 4 months‡
- Methemoglobin levels as clinically indicated (see text)

BUN, Blood urea nitrogen; *WBC*, white blood cell.
Note: More frequent surveillance needed if laboratory values are abnormal or with high-risk patients.
*Especially important in patients of African-American, Middle Eastern, and Far Eastern ancestry.
†Closer follow-up of hematologic parameters should be done when dosage is increased significantly.
‡Renal function tests and urinalysis are most important in patients on sulfapyridine therapy.

apy with dapsone. Others with any increase risk from the adverse effects from potential pharmacologic adverse effects of dapsone should also be tested. It is also important to remember that a screening test for G6PD deficiency may be falsely normal if the patient has an elevated reticulocyte count or has a variant of the enzyme that is less capable of handling oxidative stresses in the red cell.[87,132] In those instances where the patient may be at an especially high risk for the development of the adverse effects of dapsone, a G6PD level should be obtained.

In evaluating the pretreatment laboratory evaluation, it is important to pay particular attention to the hemoglobin level. Patients that have a mild iron, folate, or B_{12} deficiency will not be able to respond with the normal increase in bone marrow activity after institution of dapsone and thus may have a more significant drop in their hemoglobin. If these deficiencies are recognized and treated before or during dapsone therapy, significant patient morbidity may be reduced.

After it has been established that the patient can reasonably take dapsone, close follow-up is required. A CBC is required at frequent intervals for the first 3 months. Initially, a weekly CBC should be obtained for 4 weeks followed by twice monthly CBCs for the next 8 weeks. This follow-up allows the clinician to quickly determine if clinically significant, adverse pharmacologic or idiosyncratic hematologic effects are going to occur. After 12 weeks of therapy on stable doses of dapsone, significant changes in hemoglobin rarely occur and agranulocytosis rarely occurs.

Long-term follow-up of patients on dapsone requires CBC every 3 to 4 months or whenever significant increases in dapsone dosage occur, with liver function and renal function being assessed every 3 to 6 months. Methemoglobin levels need not be measured unless the patient is experiencing excessive fatigue, headaches, or increasing cardiac or pulmonary symptoms. It is important to realize that patients will have increased methemoglobin levels and they should carry medication cards stating that they are taking dapsone. Patients should be instructed not to change the dose of dapsone independently since adverse effects may change dramatically with increase of dapsone dosage. Patients should be evaluated for worsening of

preexisting cardiopulmonary disease and for development of signs of a distal motor neuropathy at all follow-up visits.

Finally, at the initiation of dapsone therapy and at all follow-up visits, patients should be reminded to stop the drug if prolonged febrile illnesses occur. Patients should also be told they should not increase the dapsone without prior consultation with their physician. Patients should be instructed to consult their physician if prolonged flulike symptoms, such as nausea, vomiting, malaise, weakness, and so on, develop. Similarly, the physician should be aware of the possibility of the various dapsone toxicities that can cause these symptoms (e.g., dapsone hypersensitivity syndrome, drug-induced hepatitis, and neuropathy) and evaluate the patient accordingly. By carefully selecting the patients who are treated with dapsone, performing appropriate laboratory evaluation and follow-up, and minimizing the dose of drug used, dapsone can be an effective and safe drug for the treatment of many inflammatory skin diseases.

THERAPEUTIC GUIDELINES

Patients who are considered for treatment with dapsone should be evaluated before institution of therapy for the presence of health problems that may predispose them to significant adverse effects from dapsone. A complete history and physical with emphasis on the cardiovascular, pulmonary, neurologic, renal, and hepatic systems should be performed. Pretreatment laboratory evaluation with a CBC with differential renal and liver function tests should be performed. In addition, a G6PD level should be obtained on all individuals of Middle Eastern, African, or Asian ancestry and those at high risk for hematologic adverse events. The initial dose of dapsone should be individualized to the patient, taking into account baseline health and laboratory evaluations. Because most patients require 100 to 200 mg/day for adequate control of their skin disease, an average beginning dose is about 100 mg of dapsone per day, taken in a single daily dose. Alternatively, patients can be started on lower doses if the patient or physician desires; however, it may take a longer period of time to determine if the dapsone is effective in the treatment of the skin disease. Close follow-up of the patient with frequent laboratory monitoring is important in the early stages of therapy to minimize both pharmacologic and idiosyncratic adverse effects, and the details are shown in the monitoring guidelines. Dapsone dosage can be adjusted to obtain maximal benefit, but it must be remembered that the pharmacologic adverse effects (hemolytic anemia and methemoglobinemia) increase with the increasing dose. If patients have been under good control with few if any active skin lesions, it is recommended that the dapsone dose be gradually decreased to minimize adverse effects. Patients must be cautioned not to self-medicate and increase the dose of dapsone.

Bibliography

Coleman MD: Dapsone toxicity: some current perspectives. *Gen Pharmacol* 26:1461-1467, 1995.

Coleman MD: Dapsone: modes of action, toxicity and possible strategies for increasing patient tolerance. *Br J Dermatol* 129:507-513, 1993.

Uetrecht JP: Dapsone and sulfapyridine. *Clin Dermatol* 7:111-120, 1989.

Wozel G: The story of sulfones in tropical medicine and dermatology. *Int J Dermatol* 28:17-21, 1989.

Zuidema J, Hilbers-Modderman ESM, Merkus FWHM: Clinical pharmacokinetics of dapsone. *Clin Pharmacokinet* 11:299-315, 1986.

References

1. Costello MJ: Sulfapyridine in the treatment of dermatitis herpetiformis. *Arch Dermatol Syph* 56:614-622, 1947.

2. Kruizinga EE, Hamminga H: Treatment of dermatitis herpetiformis with diaminodiphenylsulphone (DDS). *Dermatologica* 106:386-394, 1953.

3. Battle GAH: Treatment of streptococcal infections in mice with 4,4′ diaminodiphenylsulfone. *Lancet* i:1331-1334, 1937.

4. Feldman WH, Henshaw HC, Moses HE: Treatment of experimental tuberculosis with Promin (sodium salt of P, P′-diaminodiphenyl sulfone N,N′ dextrose sulfonates): Preliminary Report. *Proc Staff Meet Mayo Clinic* 18:118-125, 1941.

5. Cornbleet T: Sulfoxone (Diasone) sodium for dermatitis herpetiformis. *Arch Dermatol Syph* 64:684-687, 1951.

6. Klotz U: Clinical pharmacokinetics of sulphasalazine, its metabolites and other prodrugs of 5-aminosalicylic acid (review). *Clin Pharmacokinet* 10:285-302, 1985.

Pharmacology

7. Mancey-Jones B: The mode of action of dapsone in leprosy and other disorders. In Ryan TJMAC, editor: *Essays on leprosy*, Oxford, 1988, Alden Press, pp 141-172.

8. Uetrecht JP: Dapsone and sulfapyridine. *Clin Dermatol* 7:111-120, 1989.

9. Zuidema J, Hilbers-Modderman ESM, Merkus FWHM: Clinical pharmacokinetics of dapsone. *Clin Pharmacokinet* 11:299-315, 1986.

10. Sanders SW, Zone JJ, Foltz RL, et al: Hemolytic anemia induced by dapsone transmitted through breast milk. *Ann Intern Med* 96:465-466, 1982.

11. Maurus JN: Hansen's disease in pregnancy. *Obstet Gynecol* 52:22-25, 1978.

12. Ellard GA, Gammon PT, Savin JA, et al: Dapsone acetylation in dermatitis herpetiformis. *Br J Dermatol* 90:441-444, 1974.

13. Swain AF, Ahmad RA, Rogers HJ, et al: Pharmacokinetic observation on dapsone in dermatitis herpetiformis. *Br J Dermatol* 108:91-98, 1983.

14. Jollow DJ, Bradshaw TP, McMillan DC: Dapsone-induced hemolytic anemia (review). *Drug Metab Rev* 27:107-124, 1995.

15. Cucinell SA, Israili ZH, Dayton PG: Microsomal N-oxidation of dapsone as a cause of methemoglobin formation in human red cells. *Am J Tropical Med Hygiene* 21:322-331, 1972.

16. Coleman MD, Scott AK, Breckenridge AM, et al: The use of cimetidine as a selective inhibitor of dapsone N-hydroxylation in man. *Br J Clin Pharmacol* 30:761-767, 1990.

17. Coleman MD, Rhodes LE, Scott AK, et al: The use of cimetidine to reduce dapsone-dependent methaemoglobinaemia in dermatitis herpetiformis patients. *Br J Clin Pharmacol* 34:244-249, 1992.

18. May DG, Arns PA, Richards WO, et al: The disposition of dapsone in cirrhosis. *Clin Pharmacol Ther* 51:689-700, 1992.

19. Wright JT, Das AK: The absorption of dapsone by patients with dermatitis herpetiformis and coeliac disease. *Clin Exp Pharmacol* 5:27-30, 1980.

Mechanisms of Action

20. Katz SI, Hertz KC, Crawford PS, et al: Effect of sulfones on complement deposition in dermatitis herpetiformis and on complement-mediated guinea-pig reactions. *J Invest Dermatol* 67:688-690, 1976.

21. Barranco VP: Inhibition of lysosomal enzymes by dapsone. *Arch Dermatol* 110:563-566, 1974.

22. Mier PD, Van Den Hurk JJM: Inhibition of lysosomal enzymes by dapsone. *Br J Dermatol* 93:471-472, 1975.

23. Stendahl O, Dahlgren C: The inhibition of polymorphonuclear leukocyte cytotoxicity by dapsone; a possible mechanism in the treatment of dermatitis herpetiformis. *J Clin Invest* 62:214-220, 1977.

24. Millar BW, Macdonald KJ, Macleod TM, et al: Dapsone and human polymorphonuclear leucocyte chemotaxis in dermatitis herpetiformis. *Acta Derm Venereol* 64:433-436, 1984.

25. Esterly NB, Furey NL, Flanagan LE: The effect of antimicrobial agents on leukocyte chemotaxis. *J Invest Dermatol* 70:51-55, 1978.

26. Harvath L, Yancey KB, Katz SI: Selective inhibition of human neutrophil chemotaxis to N-formyl-methionyl-leucyl-phenylalanine by sulfones. *J Immunol* 137:1305-1311, 1986.

27. Thuong-Nguyen V, Kadunce DP, Hendrix JD, et al: Inhibition of neutrophil adherence to antibody by dapsone: a possible therapeutic mechanism of dapsone in the treatment of IgA dermatoses. *J Invest Dermatol* 100:349-355, 1993.

28. Booth SA, Moody CE, Dahl MV, et al: Dapsone suppresses integrin-mediated neutrophil adherence function. *J Invest Dermatol* 98:135-140, 1992.

29. Debol SM, Herron MJ, Nelson RD: Antiinflammatory action of dapsone: inhibition of neutrophil adherence is associated with inhibition of chemoattractant-induced signal transduction. *J Leukoc Biol* 62:827-836, 1997.

30. Maloff BL, Fox D, Bruin E, et al: Dapsone inhibits LTB4 binding and bioresponse at the cellular and physiologic levels. *Eur J Pharmacol* 158:85-89, 1988.

31. Wozel G, Blasum C, Winter C, et al: Dapsone hydroxylamine inhibits the LTB4-induced chemotaxis of polymorphonuclear leukocytes into human skin: results of a pilot study. *Inflamm Res* 46:420-422, 1997.

32. Bonney RJ, Humes JL: Physiological and pharmacological regulation of prostaglandin and leukotriene production by macrophages. *J Leukoc Biol* 35:1-10, 1984.

33. Wozel G, Lehmann B: Dapsone inhibits the generation of 5-lipoxygenase products in human polymorphonuclear leukocytes. *Skin Pharmacol* 8:196-202, 1995.

34. Gupta AK, Ellis CN, Siegel MT, et al: Sulfasalazine improves psoriasis. A double-blind analysis. *Arch Dermatol* 126:487-493, 1990.

Dermatitis Herpetiformis and Linear IgA Bullous Dermatosis

35. Katz SI: Treatment: drugs and diet. Dermatitis herpetiformis: the skin and the gut. *Ann Intern Med* 93:857-874, 1980.

36. Fry L: The treatment of dermatitis herpetiformis (review). *Clin Exp Pharmacol* 7:633-642, 1982.

37. Leonard JN, Fry L: Treatment and management of dermatitis herpetiformis (review). *Clin Dermatol* 9:403-408, 1991.

38. Leonard JN, Haffenden GP, Ring NP, et al: Linear IgA disease in adults. *Br J Dermatol* 107:301-316, 1982.

39. Chorzelski TP, Jablonska S: IgA linear dermatosis of childhood (chronic bullous disease of childhood). *Br J Dermatol* 101:535-542, 1979.

40. Wojnarowska F, Marsden RA, Bhogal B, et al: Chronic bullous disease of childhood, childhood cicatricial pemphigoid and linear IgA disease of adults: a comparative study demonstrating clinical and immunopathologic overlap. *J Am Acad Dermatol* 19:792-805, 1988.

41. Jablonska S, Chorzelski TP, Rosinska D, et al: Linear IgA bullous dermatosis of childhood (chronic bullous dermatosis of childhood). *Clin Dermatol* 9:393-401, 1992.

Other Dermatoses—Consistent Efficacy

42. Hall RP, Lawley TJ, Smith HR, et al: Bullous eruption of systemic lupus erythematosus. Dramatic response to dapsone therapy. *Ann Intern Med* 97:165-170, 1982.

43. Anonymous. WHO Expert Committee on Leprosy (review). *World Health Organ Tech Rep Ser* 874:1-43, 1998.

44. Katz SI, Gallin JI, Hertz KC, et al: Erythema elevatum diutinum: skin and systemic manifestations, immunologic studies, and successful treatment with dapsone. *Medicine (Baltimore)* 56:443-455, 1977.

Pemphigus and Pemphigoid

45. Jeffes EWB III, Ahmed AR: Adjuvant therapy of bullous pemphigoid with dapsone. *Clin Exp Pharmacol* 14:132-136, 1989.

46. Bystryn JC: Adjuvant therapy of pemphigus (review). *Arch Dermatol* 120:941-951, 1984.

47. Beutner EH, Chorzelski TP, Wilson RM, et al: IgA pemphigus foliaceus: report of two cases and a review of the literature. *J Am Acad Dermatol* 20:89-97, 1989.

48. Basset N, Guillot B, Michel B, et al: Dapsone as initial treatment in superficial pemphigus. Report of nine cases. *Arch Dermatol* 123:783-785, 1987.

49. Honeyman JF, Honeyman AR, De la Parra MA, et al: Polymorphic pemphigoid. *Arch Dermatol* 115:423-427, 1979.

50. Bouscarat F, Chosidow O, Picard-Dahan C, et al: Treatment of bullous pemphigoid with dapsone: retrospective study of thirty-six cases. *J Am Acad Dermatol* 34:683-684, 1996.

51. Haim S, Friedman-Birnbaum R: Dapsone in the treatment of pemphigus vulgaris. *Dermatologica* 156:120-123, 1978.

52. Tauber J, Sainz de la Maza M, Foster CS: Systemic chemotherapy for ocular cicatricial pemphigoid. *Cornea* 10:185-195, 1991.

53. Terezhalmy GT, Bergfeld WF: Cicatricial pemphigoid (benign mucous membrane pemphigoid) (review). *Quintessence Int* 29:429-437, 1998.

54. Bystryn JC: Therapy of pemphigus (review). *Semin Dermatol* 7:186-194, 1988.

55. Rogers RS, Mehregan DA: Dapsone therapy of cicatricial pemphigoid (review). *Semin Dermatol* 7:201-205, 1988.

56. Venning VA, Millard PR, Wojnarowska F: Dapsone as first line therapy for bullous pemphigoid. *Br J Dermatol* 120:83-92, 1989.

Vasculitis and Neutrophilic Dermatoses

57. Fredenberg MF, Malkinson FD: Sulfone therapy in the treatment of leukocytoclastic vasculitis. Report of three cases. *J Am Acad Dermatol* 16:772-778, 1987.

58. Fortson JS, Zone JJ, Hammond ME, et al: Hypocomplementemic urticarial vasculitis syndrome responsive to dapsone. *J Am Acad Dermatol* 15:1137-1142, 1986.

59. Aram H: Acute febrile neutrophilic dermatosis (Sweet's syndrome). Response to dapsone. *Arch Dermatol* 120:245-247, 1984.

60. Prystowsky JH, Kahn SN, Lazarus GS: Present status of pyoderma gangrenosum. *Arch Dermatol* 125:57-64, 1989.

61. Sharquie KE: Suppression of Behçet's disease with dapsone. *Br J Dermatol* 110:493-494, 1984.

62. Mangelsdorf HC, White WL, Jorizzo JL: Behçet's disease. Report of twenty-five patients from the United States with prominent mucocutaneous involvement. *J Am Acad Dermatol* 34:745-750, 1996.

63. Ghate JV, Jorizzo JL: Behçet's disease and complex aphthosis (review). *J Am Acad Dermatol* 40:1-18, 1999.

Other Dermatoses—Variable Efficacy

64. McCormack LS, Elgart ML, Turner ML: Annular subacute cutaneous lupus erythematosus responsive to dapsone. *J Am Acad Dermatol* 11:397-401, 1984.

65. Callen JP: Treatment of cutaneous lesions in patients with lupus erythematosus (review). *Dermatol Clin* 12:201-206, 1994.

66. Barranco VP, Minor DB, Soloman H: Treatment of relapsing polychondritis with dapsone. *Arch Dermatol* 112:1286-1288, 1976.

67. Martin J, Roenigk HH, Lynch W, et al: Relapsing polychondritis treated with dapsone. *Arch Dermatol* 112:1272-1274, 1976.

68. Damiani JM, Levine HL: Relapsing poly-chondritis—report of ten cases. *Laryngo-scope* 89:929-946, 1979.

69. Steiner A, Pehamberger H, Wolff K: Sulfone treatment of granuloma annulare. *J Am Acad Dermatol* 13:1004-1008, 1985.

70. Rees R, Campbell D, Rieger E, et al: The diagnosis and treatment of brown recluse spider bites. *Ann Emerg Med* 16:945-949, 1987.

71. Rees RS, Altenbern DP, Lynch JB, et al: Brown recluse spider bites. A comparison of early surgical excision versus dapsone and delayed surgical excision. *Ann Surg* 202:659-663, 1985.

72. Wright SW, Wrenn KD, Murray L, et al: Clinical presentation and outcome of brown recluse spider bite. *Ann Emerg Med* 30:28-32, 1997.

73. Cole HP, Wesley RE, King LEJ: Brown recluse spider envenomation of the eyelid: an animal model. *Ophthal Plast Reconstr Surg* 11:153-164, 1994.

74. Hobbs GD, Anderson AR, Greene TJ, et al: Comparison of hyperbaric oxygen and dapsone therapy for loxosceles envenomation. *Acad Emerg Med* 3:758-761, 1996.

75. Phillips S, Kohn M, Baker D, et al: Therapy of brown spider envenomation: a controlled trial of hyperbaric oxygen, dapsone, and cyproheptadine. *Ann Emerg Med* 25:363-368, 1995.

76. van de Kerkhof P: On the efficacy of dapsone in granuloma faciale. *Acta Derm Venereol* 74:61-62, 1994.

77. Krause MH, Torricelli R, Kundig T, et al: Dapsone in granulomatous rosacea (German). *Hautarzt* 48:246-248, 1997.

78. Prendiville JS, Logan RA, Russell-Jones R: A comparison of dapsone with 13-cis retinoic acid in the treatment of nodular cystic acne. *Clin Exp Pharmacol* 13:67-71, 1988.

79. Pittelkow MR, Smith KC, Su WP: Alpha-1-antitrypsin deficiency and panniculitis. Perspectives on disease relationship and replacement therapy. *Am J Med* 84:80-86, 1988.

80. Proenca NG, Muller H: Weber-Christian panniculitis treated with sulfone. Report of 2 cases (Portuguese). *AMB Rev Assoc Med Bras* 27:309-312, 1981.

81. Uplekar MW, Antia NH: Dapsone dependent nodular panniculitis. *Indian J Lepr* 58:286-290, 1986.

82. Sanchez NP, Perry HO, Muller SA, et al: Subcorneal pustular dermatosis and pustular psoriasis. A clinicopathologic correlation. *Arch Dermatol* 119:715-721, 1983.

Contraindications—Sulfonamide Cross-Reaction

83. Beumont MG, Graziani A, Ubel PA, et al: Safety of dapsone as *Pneumocystis carinii* pneumonia prophylaxis in human immunodeficiency virus-infected patients with allergy to trimethoprim/sulfamethoxazole. *Am J Med* 100:611-616, 1996.

84. Holtzer CD, Flaherty JFJ, Coleman RL: Cross-reactivity in HIV-infected patients switched from trimethoprim-sulfamethoxazole to dapsone. *Pharmacother* 18:831-835, 1998.

Adverse Effects—Hemolytic Anemia and Methemoglobinemia

85. Jollow DJ, Bradshaw TP, McMillan DC: Dapsone-induced hemolytic anemia. *Drug Metab Rev* 27:107-124, 1995.

86. Hjelm M, DeVerdier C-H: Biochemical effects of aromatic amines-I. Methaemoglobinaemia, haemolysis and Heinz-body formation induced by 4,4'-diaminodiphenylsulphone. *Biochem Pharmacol* 14:1119-1128, 1965.

87. Motulsky AG, Yoshida A, Stametoyannopoulos G: Variants of glucose-6-phosphate dehydrogenase. *Ann NY Acad Sci* 179:636-643, 1971.

88. Eichelbaum M, Evert B: Influence of pharmacogenetics on drug disposition and response (review). *Clin Exp Pharmacol Physiol* 23:983-985, 1996.

89. Coleman MD: Dapsone toxicity: some current perspectives. *Gen Pharmacol* 26:1461-1467, 1995.

90. Prussick R, Ali MA, Rosenthal D, et al: The protective effect of vitamin E on the hemolysis associated with dapsone treatment in patients with dermatitis herpetiformis. *Arch Dermatol* 128:210-213, 1992.

91. Dawson AH, Whyte IM: Management of dapsone poisoning complicated by methaemoglobinaemia. *Med Toxicol Adverse Drug Exp* 4:387-392, 1989.

Agranulocytosis

92. Ognibene AJ: Agranulocytosis due to dapsone. *Ann Intern Med* 72:521-524, 1970.

93. Hornsten P, Keisu M, Wiholm B-E: The incidence of agranulocytosis during treatment of dermatitis herpetiformis with dapsone as reported in Sweden, 1972 through 1988. *Arch Dermatol* 126:919-922, 1990.

94. Cockburn EM, Wood SM, Waller PC, et al: Dapsone-induced agranulocytosis: spontaneous reporting data. *Br J Dermatol* 128:702-703, 1993.

95. Miyagawa S, Shiomi Y, Fukumoto T, et al: Recombinant granulocyte colony-stimulating factor for dapsone-induced agranulocytosis in leukocytoclastic vasculitis. *J Am Acad Dermatol* 28:659-661, 1993.

Peripheral Neuropathy

96. Saqueton AC, Lorincz AL, Vick NA, et al: Dapsone and peripheral motor neuropathy. *Arch Dermatol* 100:214-217, 1969.

97. Ahrens EM, Meckler RJ, Callen JP: Dapsone-induced peripheral neuropathy. *Int J Dermatol* 25:314-316, 1986.

98. Fernandez-Obregon AC, Forconi RJ: Neurologic symptoms posing as dapsone-induced polyneuropathy in two patients with dermatitis herpetiformis. *Cutis* 41:347-350, 1988.

99. Potter MN, Yates P, Slade R, et al: Agranulocytosis caused by dapsone therapy for granuloma annulare. *J Am Acad Dermatol* 20:87-88, 1989.

100. Daneshmend TK: The neurotoxicity of dapsone. *Adv Drug React Ac Pois Rev* 3:43-58, 1984.

101. Gutmann L, Martin JD, Welton W: Dapsone motor neuropathy—an axonal disease. *Neurology* 26:514-516, 1976.

101a. Hall RP, Katz SI: Personal communication.

Other Adverse Effects—Neurologic and Gastrointestinal

102. Homeida M, Babikr A, Daneshmend TK: Dapsone-induced optic atrophy and motor neuropathy. *BMJ* 281:1180, 1980.

103. Kenner DJ, Holt K, Agnello R, et al: Permanent retinal damage following massive dapsone overdose. *Br J Ophthalmol* 64:741-744, 1980.

104. Leonard JN, Tucker WF, Fry L, et al: Dapsone and the retina (letter). *Lancet* 1:453, 1982.

105. Daneshmend TK, Homeida M: Dapsone-induced optic atrophy and motor neuropathy. *Med J* 283:311, 1981.

106. Daneshmend TK: Idiosyncratic dapsone induced manic depression. *BMJ* 299:324, 1989.

107. Fine JD, Katz SI, Donahue MJ, et al: Psychiatric reaction to dapsone and sulfapyridine (letter). *J Am Acad Dermatol* 9:274-275, 1983.

108. Gawkrodger D: Manic depression induced by dapsone in patient with dermatitis herpetiformis. *BMJ* 299:860, 1989.

109. Millikan LE, Harrell ER: Drug reactions to sulfones. *Arch Dermatol* 102:220-224, 1970.

110. Johnson DA, Cattau EL Jr, Kuritsky JN: Liver involvement in the sulfone syndrome. *Arch Intern Med* 146:875-877, 1986.

111. Corp CC, Ghishan FK: The sulfone syndrome complicated by pancreatitis and pleural effusion in an adolescent receiving dapsone for treatment of acne vulgaris. *J Pediatr Gastroenterol Nutr* 26:103-105, 1998.

112. Choy AM, Lang CC: Gall-bladder perforation after long-term dapsone therapy. *J Intern Med* 228:409-410, 1990.

113. Kingham JGC, Swain P, Swarbrick ET, et al: Dapsone and severe hypoalbuminaemia. *Lancet* 2:662-664, 1979.

Dapsone Hypersensitivity

114. Prussick R, Shear NH: Dapsone hypersensitivity syndrome. *J Am Acad Dermatol* 35:346-349, 1996.

115. Frey HM, Gershon AA, Borkowsky W, et al: Fatal reaction to dapsone during treatment of leprosy. *Ann Intern Med* 94:777-779, 1981.

116. Lawrence WA, Olsen HW, Nickles DJ: Dapsone hepatitis. *Arch Intern Med* 147:175, 1987.

117. Kumar RH, Kumar MV, Thappa DM: Dapsone syndrome—a five year retrospective analysis. *Indian J Lepr* 70:271-276, 1998.

118. Rege VL, Shukla P, Mascarenhas MF: Dapsone syndrome in Goa. *Indian J Lepr* 66:59-64, 1994.

119. Dhanapaul S: DDS-induced photosensitivity with reference to six case reports. *Lepr Rev* 60:147-150, 1989.

Other Adverse Effects—Miscellaneous

120. Anonymous: Dapsone (review). *IARC Monogr Eval Carcinog Risk Chem Hum* 24:59-76, 1980.

121. Grticiute L, Tomatis L: Carcinogenicity of dapsone of mice and rats. *Int J Cancer* 25:123-129, 1980.

122. Goodman DG, Ward JM, Reichardt WD: Splenic fibrosis and sarcomas in F344 rats fed diets containing aniline hydrochloride, p-chloroaniline, azobenzene, o-toluidine hydrochloride, 4,4'-sulfonyldianiline, or D & C red No. 9. *J Natl Cancer Inst* 73:265-273, 1984.

123. Peters JH: Carcinogenic activity of Dapsone. *Int J Leprosy* 44:383-384, 1976.

124. Oleinick A: Altered immunity and cancer risk: a review of the problem and analysis of the cancer mortality experience of leprosy patients. *J Natl Cancer Inst* 43:775-781, 1969.

125. Purtilo DT, Pangi C: Incidence of cancer in patients with leprosy. *Cancer* 35:1259-1261, 1975.

126. Collier PM, Kelly SE, Wojnarowska F: Linear IgA disease and pregnancy. *J Am Acad Dermatol* 30:407-411, 1994.

127. Kahn G: Dapsone is safe during pregnancy (letter). *J Am Acad Dermatol* 13:838-839, 1985.

128. Hocking DR: Neonatal haemolytic disease due to dapsone. *Med J Austral* 1:1130-1131, 1968.

129. Erturk E, Casemento JB, Guertin KR, et al: Bilateral acetylsulfapyridine nephrolithiasis associated with chronic sulfasalazine therapy. *J Urol* 151:1605-1606, 1994.

130. Lee BL, Medina I, Benowitz NL, et al: Dapsone, trimethoprim, and sulfamethoxazole plasma levels during treatment of pneumonia in patients with the acquired immunodeficiency syndrome (AIDS). Evidence of drug interactions. *Ann Intern Med* 110:606-611, 1989.

131. Sahai J, Garber G, Gallicano K, et al: Effects of the antacids in didanosine tablets on dapsone pharmacokinetics. *Ann Intern Med* 123:584-587, 1995.

132. Todd P, Samaratunga IR, Pembroke A: Screening for glucose-6-phosphate dehydrogenase deficiency prior to dapsone therapy. *Clin Exp Pharmacol* 19:217-218, 1994.

CHAPTER 12

Jeffrey P. Callen
Charles Camisa

Antimalarial Agents

The antimalarial drugs that have been used for the treatment of dermatologic disorders include hydroxychloroquine, chloroquine, and quinacrine. Quinacrine has been difficult to obtain recently, but several individual pharmacies in the United States have been compounding the drug and made it available by mail order to individual patients. The most commonly used antimalarials (hydroxychloroquine and chloroquine) are 4-aminoquinolines (Table 12-1) and derivatives of quinine, a naturally occurring substance. Quinine is an alkaloid derived from the bark of the South American cinchona tree.[1] This bark is believed to have been used initially for its antipyretic effects, and thus the cinchona tree has also become known as the "fever" tree. In the 1800s, quinine became popular as an effective antimalarial agent.

World War I provided the impetus for the synthetic production of antimalarials. Quinacrine hydrochloride was synthesized in 1930, chloroquine phosphate in 1934, and hydroxychloroquine sulfate in 1946. The initial dermatologic use of antimalarials is attributed to Payne's use of quinine in lupus erythematosus (LE) in 1894.[2] In 1951, Page[3] used quinacrine to treat cutaneous LE.

PHARMACOLOGY

Table 12-2 lists key pharmacologic concepts for antimalarial agents.

Structure

Most antimalarials are substituted 4-aminoquinolines. Quinacrine has an extra benzene ring and is considered an acridine compound. Drug structures for hydroxychloroquine and chloroquine are shown in Figure 12-1.

Absorption and Bioavailability

Antimalarials are bitter, water-soluble, crystalline powders that are absorbed rapidly and completely from the gastrointestinal tract. Maximal plasma levels of quinacrine are achieved in 1 to 3 hours after ingestion. These drugs bind avidly to tissue protein; therefore the concentrations are highest in liver, spleen, and kidney tissues, mainly in nuclei and mitochondria.

Various single and repeated dosage regimens for hydroxychloroquine and chloroquine yield nearly identical plasma level curves with peaks at 4 and 5 hours, respectively.[4] Distributions of the two drugs in tissue are qualitatively similar; they are least found in bone, skin, fat, and brain tissues and greater in (in ascending order) muscle, eye, heart, kidney, liver, lung, spleen, and adrenal gland tissues. The absolute amounts are 2.5 times higher for chloroquine. It is possible for some tissues to accumulate concentrations of these 4-aminoquinolines several hundred times the concentrations in plasma.

Metabolism and Excretion

The major pathway of biotransformation is not known, but alterations must be extensive. About

Table 12-1 Antimalarial Agents

Generic Name	Trade Name	Generic Available	Manufacturer	Tablet/Capsule Sizes	Special Formulations	Standard Dosage Range	Price Index
Hydroxychloroquine	Plaquenil	Yes	Sanofi Winthrop	200 mg	No	200-400 mg/d Max 6.5 mg/kg/d*	$$ ($$)
Chloroquine	Aralen	Yes	Sanofi Winthrop	500 mg (scored), 250 mg (generic)	Two forms—HCl and phosphate†	250-500 mg/d Max 4.0 mg/kg/d*	$$$ ($)
Quinacrine	Must compound‡	No	None	100 mg	Yes	100-200 mg/d	—

Adapted from *CliniSphere 2.0 CD ROM*, St. Louis, June 2000, Facts & Comparisons.
$, <1.00; $$, 1.01-2.00; $$$, 2.01-5.00; $$$$, 5.01-10.00; $$$$$, >10.00; ( ), generic price; /, two different price ranges from lower dose to higher dose examples of this drug; —, no price listed for this drug.
*Maximum safe maintenance dose from an ocular standard—initial doses above this range for 1 to 2 months are acceptable.
†Injectable versions of chloroquine phosphate and chloroquine hydrochloride are available.
‡Only available in selected pharmacies in the United States via compounding.

■ **Table 12-2**   Key Pharmacologic Concepts—Antimalarial Agents

Drug	Absorption and Bioavailability			Elimination		
	Peak Levels	Bioavail-able (%)	Protein Binding	Half-life	Metabolism	Excretion
Hydroxychloro-quine	4 hrs	74%	45%	40-50 days	Desethylchloroquine and desethylhydroxy-chloroquine metabolites	50% excreted unchanged in urine; also biliary excretion
Chloroquine	5 hrs	50%	50% to 65%	40-50 days	Desethylchloroquine is main metabolite	42% to 47% excreted unchanged in urine
Quinacrine	1-3 hrs	100%	80% to 90%	5-14 days	None	Urine, bile, sweat, saliva

Adapted from Facts & Comparisons 1999 and Drug Information for the Health Care Professional.[61-63]

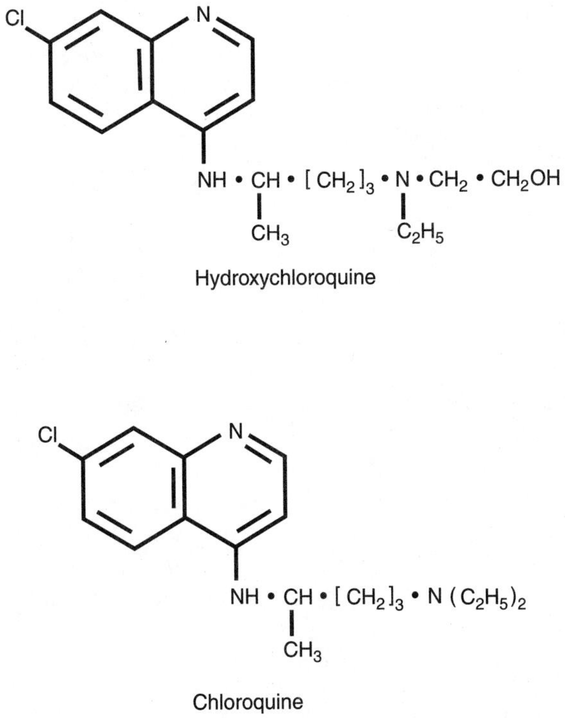

Hydroxychloroquine

Chloroquine

Figure 12-1   Antimalarial agents.

half of a daily dose is excreted in the urine, and smaller amounts are detected in feces, sweat, breast milk, saliva, and bile.[4]

The terminal half-lives of chloroquine and hydroxychloroquine are similar: 40 to 50 days.[5] The long half-lives are attributed to extensive tissue uptake and slow release into circulation. The attainment of steady-state concentrations in 3 to 4 months may account for the slow appearance of therapeutic benefit. Hydroxychloroquine can be detected in whole blood 5 months after a single dose.

Their metabolisms differ in one respect: chloroquine breaks down into one first-stage metabolite (desethylchloroquine) and hydroxychloroquine breaks down into two (desethylhydroxychloroquine and desethylchloroquine). The first-stage desethyl compounds break down in turn to the primary amine.[4]

There is also a difference in the relative amounts of drug excreted in urine and feces. After a single dose, approximately three times more chloroquine than hydroxychloroquine can be accounted for in urine, and three times more hydroxychloroquine than chloroquine can be accounted for in feces. The data suggest that hydroxychloroquine forms an ether glucuronide that is excreted in bile. The low proportion (roughly 20%) of unchanged hydroxychloroquine eliminated by the kidneys indicates that no dosage adjustment is necessary for patients with mild-to-moderate renal function impairment.[6]

Mechanism of Action

The exact mechanism by which antimalarials act to affect various diseases is not fully understood. Among the postulates for the mechanism of action are effects on light filtration, immunosuppressive actions, antiinflammatory actions, and DNA binding. Antimalarials inhibit ultraviolet-induced cutaneous reactions in LE and polymorphous light eruption and perhaps through the effects on prostaglandin metabolism, the inhibition of superoxide production, or their ability to bind to DNA.[7]

Antimalarial compounds raise intracytoplasmic pH levels, which can result in a decreased ability of macrophages to express major histocompatibility complex antigens on its cell surface. In a recent experiment, Fox and Kang[8] demonstrated a dose-dependent inhibition of the release of interleukin-2 from a CD4+ T-cell clone by both chloroquine and hydroxychloroquine. Antimalarials may inhibit the formation of antigen-antibody complexes. They have also been shown to decrease lymphocyte responsiveness to mitogens in vitro.[9]

Antiinflammatory effects of antimalarials may also be an important factor in their action. Antimalarials have been noted to decrease lysosomal size and might possibly inhibit their function.[10] These drugs also impair chemotaxis.[11]

An additional effect that may be of importance is the ability of antimalarials to inhibit platelet aggregation and adhesion and thrombus formation.[12] Wallace and colleagues[13] recently found that thromboembolic events are decreased in patients with hydroxychloroquine-treated systemic LE (SLE). Also reported were decreases in cholesterol and, after 6 weeks of therapy, decreased interleukin-2 and soluble CD8 levels. Other studies also suggested a decrease in cholesterol and possible protection from coronary artery disease in patients with SLE on prednisone.[14-15] Finally, Ornstein and Sperber[16] noted antiviral effects as demonstrated by a modest decrease in human immunodeficiency virus (HIV) load.

CLINICAL USE

Table 12-3 lists indications and contraindications for antimalarials.

FDA-Approved Indications

Except for LE, all other approved indications for antimalarials are nondermatologic. Quinacrine became obsolete for malaria and tapeworm infections as equally effective and less toxic alternatives were introduced.[17] The major indication for quinacrine is currently in the treatment of giardiasis at a dosage of 100 mg three times a day for 5 days. Microorganisms disappear from stools, and symptoms clear rapidly.

Hydroxychloroquine is used as a disease-modifying agent in rheumatoid arthritis. Improvement is seen overall in about 63% of patients, but about 12% achieve complete remission.[18]

The recommended dosages (see Table 12-1) and usage of the three antimalarials are

| Table 12-3 | Antimalarial Indications and Contraindications |

FDA-APPROVED INDICATIONS

Lupus erythematosus[3,19-25] (in selected cases)
Nondermatologic indications of interest
   include:
      Malaria (all three antimalarials)[17]
      Rheumatoid arthritis (hydroxychloroquine)[18]

OFF-LABEL USES

Photosensitivity Dermatoses
Porphyria cutanea tarda[26-34]
Polymorphous light eruption[35,36]
Solar urticaria[37]
Dermatomyositis (cutaneous features)[38-40]

Granulomatous Dermatoses
Sarcoidosis[41]
Granuloma annulare (generalized)[42]

Lymphocytic Infiltrates
Lymphocytoma cutis[43]
Lymphocytic infiltrate of Jessner[44]

Panniculitis
Panniculitis (idiopathic)[45]
Chronic erythema nodosum[46]
Lupus panniculitis[47]

Other Dermatoses
Oral lichen planus[48]
Reticular erythematous mucinosis[49-51]
Pemphigus[52]
Atopic dermatitis[53]
Urticarial vasculitis[54]
Localized scleroderma[55]
Psoriasis (Psoriatic arthritis)[56-60]

CONTRAINDICATIONS

Absolute
Hypersensitivity to the drug
(Theoretic potential for cross-reactions between
   different antimalarial agents)

Relative
Pregnancy and lactation
Severe blood dyscrasias
Significant hepatic dysfunction
Significant neurologic disorders
Retinal or visual field changes
Psoriasis (see text)

PREGNANCY PRESCRIBING STATUS CATEGORY—FDA UNRATED
(SEE CHAPTER 43)

---

closely tied to their toxicity and clinical efficacy and are discussed later in the Therapeutic Guidelines section.

LUPUS ERYTHEMATOSUS. One double-blind trial of hydroxychloroquine therapy for discoid LE demonstrated that it was more effective than placebo at 3 months and 1 year and that at cross-over it was more effective than the placebo at 3 months. Antimalarials are used in patients who fail to respond well to topical measures such as sun protection, sunscreens, and topical corticosteroids. In large, open clinical studies, 70% of patients with chronic cutaneous LE responded to antimalarials with a good-to-excellent response.[19,20] Certain subsets seem to respond less well—those patients with widespread involvement, those with hypertrophic or verrucous lesions, and those who have SLE with prominent discoid LE lesions. Similar excellent results in patients with subacute cutaneous LE have been observed in open trials.[21] Anecdotal information suggests that when hydroxychloroquine is not effective, a switch to chloroquine may result in control of the process. Before its removal from the market, quinacrine could be added to either chloroquine or hydroxychloroquine or used alone to control cutaneous LE in some patients. The onset of action for antimalarials used for cutaneous LE is between 4 and 8 weeks. Cessation of therapy during the winter months is possible with some patients.

The usefulness of antimalarials in SLE was less well documented until the Canadian Hydroxychloroquine Study Group[22] recently published their data. It had been generally accepted that arthritis, pleuritis, pericarditis, and lethargy respond to antimalarials.[23] The Canadian group found that the risk of a clinical flare of SLE was significantly greater in patients on placebo as compared with hydroxychloroquine. In the accompanying editorial, Lockshin[24] pointed out that although these data are significant, they did not address the usefulness of hydroxychloroquine in acutely ill patients with SLE, nor do they address whether all patients with SLE should have hydroxychloroquine prescribed. In a recent report, Esdaile[25] reviewed the existing data on the use of antimalarials in SLE. Although only two controlled studies exist, it appears that patients with mild-to-moderate SLE can benefit from antimalarial therapy. Esdaile also discussed a study of lupus arthritis in which objective benefits were not noted, but subjective, patient-reported benefits were statistically associated with hydroxychloroquine therapy. In addition, he discussed studies that demonstrated a corticosteroid-sparing role for antimalarials.

Antimalarials should be reserved for those patients with localized cutaneous disease who have not responded to reasonable efforts at sun avoidance, liberal use of broad-spectrum sunscreens, and potent topical or intralesional corticosteroids. Significant scalp involvement with alopecia in addition to disseminated discoid, annular, or papulosquamous skin lesions also warrants antimalarials. Systemic corticosteroids are generally not as effective as monotherapy for SLE and probably should not be used for this purpose.

Off-Label Uses

PORPHYRIA CUTANEA TARDA. Antimalarials are not the first choice of therapy for patients with porphyria cutanea tarda (PCT). After exogenous exacerbating factors are removed or discontinued, phlebotomy remains the primary therapy. In patients who are anemic or who fail to respond to phlebotomy, antimalarial therapy may be attempted. The mechanism of antimalarials is their effect on hepatocytes with release of porphyrins into the circulation and eventual excretion. The observation that antimalarials are useful was made when they were used to treat patients with LE, who may occasionally have subclinical PCT.[26] When giving hydroxychloroquine or chloroquine in usual doses, these patients developed fever, nausea, vomiting, abdominal pain, and elevated liver function tests.[27] Recovery from this acute toxic reaction could result in a prolonged remission of the PCT. To avoid the toxic reaction, low dosages of antimalarials (chloroquine, 125 mg twice weekly, or hydroxychloroquine, 100 mg three times per week) have been found to be safe and effective. Malkinson and Levitt[28] suggested that hydroxychloroquine be used as follows: 100 mg three times per week for 1 month, then 200 mg three times per week for 1 month, then 200 mg/day. Further advancement would depend on the biochemical and clinical response. This therapy should not be used in patients with renal failure on hemodialysis because the porphyrins released from the liver would not be cleared effectively. As an alternative, Petersen and Thomsen[29] used high-dose hydroxychloroquine, 250 mg three times daily for 3 days, in 72 hospitalized patients and induced a prolonged remission in a majority of them. Some remissions lasted as long as 4.5 years. Further discussion of therapy for PCT[30-34] is in the Therapeutic Guidelines section.

OTHER PHOTODERMATOSES. Photosensitivity diseases, such as polymorphous light eruption (PMLE) and solar urticaria, and photoaggravated diseases, such as dermatomyositis and reticular erythematosus mucinosis, have been successfully treated with antimalarials. PMLE can be treated intermittently with hydroxychloroquine, 200 to 400 mg daily. This treatment has been shown in a placebo-controlled trial to reduce the eruption and its attendant symptoms.[35] Another study compared chloroquine, an oral carotenoid, and placebo for the therapy of PMLE.[36] They found that both chloroquine and the oral carotenoid were significantly more effective than placebo. Only anecdotal cases of solar urticaria treated with antimalarials have been reported.[37]

In patients with dermatomyositis, cutaneous lesions may be present long after the myositic component resolves. These lesions may be extremely difficult to treat despite the use of potent topical corticosteroids, sunscreens, systemic corticosteroids, and various immunosuppressives. In an effort to reduce the cortico-steroid dosage, hydroxychloroquine was studied in an open-labeled trial in seven patients.[38] In all of the patients, improvement was noted with consequent lowering of the corticosteroid dosage in two patients, and in three a complete response occurred. Subsequently, other reports on both adults[39] and children[40] have appeared that detail similar results.

GRANULOMATOUS DERMATOSES. Anti-malarials have been used to treat various manifestations of sarcoidosis. Jones and Callen[41] recently reported on the experience with 17 patients with cutaneous sarcoidal granulomas treated with hydroxychloroquine. Patients were treated with 200 to 400 mg per day and began to note improvement after 4 to 12 weeks. Higher initial dosages were not noted to result in a more rapid response. Twelve patients were able to discontinue other therapy. Relapse was noted in six patients who had a complete response when the dosage was lowered or stopped. Maintenance therapy with hydroxychloroquine, 200 mg three times per week, was used in three patients. Hydroxychloroquine may therefore be a useful adjunctive therapy for patients with sarcoidosis. Generalized granuloma annulare has likewise responded successfully to hydroxychloroquine.[42]

LYMPHOCYTIC INFILTRATES. Stoll treated a woman 45 years of age with pseudolymphoma (lymphocytoma cutis) with hydroxychloroquine 200 mg/day initially, which was eventually increased to 400 mg/day. A complete response was noted, and a prolonged remission was reported.[43] In a study of 100 patients with Jessner's lymphocytic infiltrate of the skin, Toonstra and coauthors[44] treated 15 patients with either hydroxychloroquine or chloroquine. They observed good-to-excellent responses in only six patients. Therefore antimalarial therapy may be of benefit to some patients with lymphocytic infiltrates of the skin.

PANNICULITIS. Shelley[45] reported a woman 62 years of age with a 15-year history of a nodular panniculitis (Weber-Christian variant) who responded completely to oral chloroquine 250 mg/day. Control of the process continued even with reduction of the dosage to 250 mg every fifth day. Alloway and Franks[46] treated a woman 38 years of age with a 10-year history of recurrent erythema nodosum that worsened with menses. They began hydroxychloroquine, 200 mg/day, and within 3 months a response was noted, manifest by a decrease in the frequency and severity of the eruptions. The response was noted for at least 6 months of follow-up. Lupus panniculitis has also been effectively treated with oral antimalarial therapy as reported in a recent study of 40 patients.[47] Thirty-three of the patients were treated, and 23 (70%) of them noted a positive response. Therapy of these patients was prolonged (mean 3.6 years).

OTHER DERMATOSES. Oral lichen planus is a common disorder. Although topical or intralesional corticosteroids are effective, there are numerous patients in whom the response is incomplete or in whom secondary candidal infection may occur. Eisen[48] reported an open trial of hydroxychloroquine for 10 patients with oral lichen planus, 7 of whom had erosive disease. Of the 10 patients, 9 had an excellent response, with the onset of effect occurring as early as 1 to 2 months after therapy began. Oral erosions took 3 to 5 months to heal. None of his patients had cutaneous lichen planus. Moreover, none of the patients had an adverse reaction, but this was a short-term study.

Some patients with reticular erythematous mucinosis, a rare condition, have been successfully treated with hydroxychloroquine.[49-51]

The most recent addition to the list of conditions that may benefit from antimalarial therapy is pemphigus foliaceus. Hymes and Jordon[52] noted benefits and corticosteroid-sparing effects in two patients. The effects were noted within 2 months of therapy. Other dermatoses for which antimalarials may be beneficial include atopic dermatitis,[53] urticarial vasculitis,[54] and localized scleroderma.[55]

PSORIATIC ARTHRITIS. The use of antimalarials in patients with psoriasis has been reported to increase the severity of psoriasis, and in some cases to lead to an exfoliative erythroderma.[56,57] In addition, patients without skin disease can have the initial onset of psoriasis during therapy.[58] However, large series of patients with psoriatic arthritis have been treated successfully with hydroxychloroquine[59] or chloroquine.[60] In Kammer and associates' report[59] on hydroxychloroquine therapy, there were no patients whose psoriasis flared. Similarly, Gladman and co-workers[60] reported that the psoriasis worsened in 6 of 32 patients treated with chloroquine, as well as in 6 of 24 control patients. None of these patients had an exfoliative erythroderma.

Contraindications

The only absolute contraindication to antimalarial therapy is hypersensitivity. Also, in a patient with retinopathy further use is contraindicated.

Relative contraindications to the use of antimalarials are pregnancy and lactation because the drugs can cross the placenta and are secreted in breast milk. They are also contraindicated in patients who have myasthenia gravis. In several other situations, antimalarials may be used with caution and proper monitoring—for children, for patients with glucose-6-phosphate dehydrogenase (G6PD) deficiency, and for psychotic patients. However, routine testing for G6PD deficiency has not been deemed necessary for patients being treated with hydroxychloroquine, chloroquine, or quinacrine because hemolysis is unlikely at recommended dosages.[61-63]

Adverse Effects

Antimalarials may produce a wide array of adverse reactions (Box 12-1), some of which may be serious. With the exception of retinopathy, most of the adverse effects are reversible on discontinuation of the antimalarial agent. Several differences pertaining to the risk of certain reactions exist between the antimalarials. Yellow pigmentation is limited to quinacrine therapy. Hematologic side effects may be more common with quinacrine, but ocular toxicity is not seen with quinacrine.[61] Although both chloroquine and hydroxychloroquine have been associated with retinopathy, it appears that chloroquine is more toxic than hydroxychloroquine.[62,63]

RETINOPATHY.   Ophthalmologic toxicity is the issue of most concern to physicians who prescribe antimalarials often. Three types of ocular adverse effects may develop: corneal deposits, neuromuscular eye toxicity, and retinopathy.

Box 12-1

Selected Adverse Effects of Antimalarial Agents

OCULAR—REVERSIBLE
Corneal deposition—halos, blurred vision, photophobia (especially chloroquine)
Loss of accommodation (especially chloroquine)
Premaculopathy—usually no visual change; retinal pigment deposition, paracentral and pericentral scotoma

OCULAR—IRREVERSIBLE
True retinopathy—"bull's eye" pigment deposition, central scotoma, visual acuity changes (risk greatest with chloroquine; no risk with quinacrine)

HEMATOLOGIC
Rarely agranulocytosis or pancytopenia
Hemolysis in patients with G6PD (primarily with primaquine and other 8-aminoquinolines)

GASTROINTESTINAL
Nausea, vomiting, diarrhea (10% of chloroquine patients have intolerable GI effects)

GASTROINTESTINAL—cont'd
Liver function test changes—uncommon transaminase elevations

NEUROMUSCULAR
Irritability, nervousness, mood swings
Psychosis
Headache
Seizures (rare)
Vertigo, tinnitus, nystagmus
Skeletal muscle weakness

CUTANEOUS
Bluish-gray hyperpigmentation (especially shins, face, palate)
Bleaching of hair roots
Minor hypersensitivity reactions—morbilliform, lichenoid, eczematous
More important hypersensitivity reactions—urticaria, exfoliative erythroderma
Psoriasis—induction or exacerbation
Nails—transverse pigment bands

Only retinopathy is potentially irreversible. It has been divided into two forms—true retinopathy and premaculopathy. Premaculopathy is defined as changes on visual field or funduscopic examination that are not associated with visual loss. It is believed that premaculopathy would progress if the antimalarial agent is continued and that it is potentially reversible.[64] Rynes and Bernstein[65] recommended that the patient be evaluated for retinopathy at baseline, then reevaluated every 6 months by an ophthalmologist. They suggested that testing visual acuity and visual fields and performing a funduscopic examination are acceptable for screening practices. More expensive and cumbersome tests, such as serial photography, fluorescein angiography, and electrooculography, may remain normal even in the presence of retinopathy. Further, they point out that patient-administered Amsler grid testing has not been established as a method of screening. An interesting study in the 1980s evaluated the recommendations of rheumatologists and ophthalmologists from a Midwestern state.[66] In a review of 24 patients on hydroxychloroquine therapy, most of the physicians recommended follow-up every 6 months, although there were seven in whom no record of an ophthalmologic evaluation could be found. Fortunately, the risk of true retinopathy is very low, with chloroquine believed to be more risky than hydroxychloroquine.[64] In a retrospective study Levy and associates[67] demonstrated that hydroxychloroquine was very safe, if used in doses of <6.5 mg/kg/day for up to 10 years. Earlier recommendations for ocular monitoring in patients on long-term antimalarial therapy were proposed by Olansky[68] and Easterbrook.[69]

OTHER OCULAR EFFECTS. Antimalarials are deposited in the basal epithelium of the cornea as early as the first few weeks of therapy. Although usually asymptomatic, patients may complain of halos around lights as a result of these deposits. Visual acuity is not reduced. Corneal deposits are a frequent finding on slit-lamp examination but are not a contraindication for continued therapy. Their presence does not correlate with retinopathy. These deposits are reversible with cessation of therapy.

A reduction in the accommodative power of the eye and a change in the extraocular muscle balance may occur soon after the initiation of chloroquine therapy. If the symptoms trouble the patient, the dosage may be reduced. This finding has not been reported in patients treated with hydroxychloroquine.

USE IN CHILDREN.   Two special situations are worthy of discussion: the use of antimalarial drugs in children and in pregnant or lactating women. Until 1984 most reviews suggested that antimalarials were contraindicated in children. In a careful review of the literature, however, Rasmussen[70] pointed out that the risk of chronic toxicity was no greater than for adults. Furthermore, the main concern for children is acute toxicity usually resulting from accidental or intentional overdosage. Ziering and associates[71] examined this issue further and concluded that the antimalarials can be safely and successfully used in the treatment of children with LE, juvenile rheumatoid arthritis, dermatomyositis, panniculitis, morphea, and PCT.

For young children, the issue of administration may be important. Neither hydroxychloroquine nor chloroquine comes in a syrup. Ziering suggested that the capsules can be pulverized, weighed, and put into packets or gelatin capsules containing the desired dosage. The powder can then be mixed with jam, jelly, or applesauce to mask the bitter taste.

USE IN PREGNANCY AND LACTATION. Almost all reviews suggest that chloroquine and hydroxychloroquine are contraindicated in pregnancy. However, women of childbearing age may take chloroquine or hydroxychloroquine before pregnancy and then become pregnant. In a study of 24 women exposed to hydroxychloroquine or chloroquine during the first trimester of 27 pregnancies, there were no congenital abnormalities observed.[72] The use throughout pregnancy was not recommended by these authors because they believed that deposition in the eyes of the fetus could result in toxicity at a later date. On the other hand, Parke,[73] who followed up into their teenage years some of the infants born to mothers on antimalarials without noting any delayed toxicity, recommended that the antimalarial not be discontinued in pregnancy.

The issue of lactation and antimalarials is controversial.[73] Chloroquine is probably expressed in greater quantities in breast milk than is hydroxychloroquine, but the data are scanty.

The issue of safety relates to the effects of anti-malarials on infants. Although in small doses antimalarials are safe in children, it is not clear how large the doses would be in breast milk. Thus at the current time, either the mothers nursing infants should refrain from breast-feeding while on antimalarial therapy, or the antimalarial should be discontinued.

MISCELLANEOUS SYSTEMIC ADVERSE EFFECTS. Gastrointestinal (GI) side effects, such as nausea, vomiting, and diarrhea, are the most common reasons for early decreases in dosage or discontinuation of treatment. Approximately 10% of patients are unable to tolerate chloroquine due to these adverse GI effects. The likelihood of GI intolerance in patients receiving hydroxychloroquine is lower.[63] Infrequent central nervous system effects that may be seen in susceptible patients or with higher than recommended dosages include restlessness, excitement, confusion, headache, seizures, myasthenia, and toxic psychosis.[74] Rare but potentially fatal bone marrow toxicity has been reported, including aplastic anemia caused by quinacrine[75] and agranulocytosis caused by chloroquine.[76] Chloroquine and hydroxychloroquine have been associated with hemolysis in patients with G6PD deficiency, but not in the usual dosage range. However, hemolysis is considered more of a problem with the 8-aminoquinoline primaquine.

CUTANEOUS ADVERSE EFFECTS. A bluish-gray to black hyperpigmentation may occur in 10% to 30% of patients treated for 4 months or longer with any of the drugs. The pigmentation typically affects the shins (resembling ecchymoses), the face, the palate (with a sharp line demarcating the hard and soft palates), and the nailbeds (as transverse bands).[77,78] Biopsies show both hemosiderin around capillaries and dermal melanin. The pigmentation may take months to fade after discontinuation of therapy. Progressive bleaching of the hair roots of the scalp, the face, and the body is another unusual pigmentary disturbance that may appear in as many as 10% of patients taking chloroquine.[79] This phenomenon is also reversible.

The incidence of pruritus and dermatitis associated with antimalarial use has been reported to be 10% to 20%.[80] The rashes included ur-

ticaria, morbilliform, eczematous, lichenoid, exfoliative dermatitis, and erythema annulare centrifugum patterns.[81] Bauer[82] estimated the incidence of rashes in servicemen during World War II at 1 of 2000 and 1 of 600 for 100 and 200 mg/day of quinacrine, respectively. He also reported that three of the most severely affected servicemen with lichen planus–like histology developed the late sequela of palmar squamous cell carcinoma, two with metastases to the axilla. However, all three received prior low-dosage radiation therapy to the involved sites.

The controversial issue of whether antimalarials exacerbate preexisting psoriasis receives attention in the dermatologic and rheumatologic literature. Interestingly, these drugs are used in the treatment of psoriatic arthropathy. The incidence of flare-up actually varies from 0% to 100%.[83] Kuflik[84] studied the effect of malaria prophylaxis (200 mg/week of chloroquine and 15 mg/week of primaquine) on 48 patients with psoriasis. Psoriasis worsened in 42% of patients, but only 6% were resistant to topical treatment. For this reason, Kuflik concluded that prophylactic antimalarial treatment was not contraindicated for psoriasis patients traveling to endemic areas. Slagel and James[85] reviewed the literature and reported an overall incidence of 31% for acute generalized eruptions, including both flare-ups of psoriasis and other drug-related eruptions. Quinacrine was responsible for the greatest frequency of exfoliative erythroderma, whereas chloroquine was most commonly responsible for significant psoriasis flareups. A markedly lower incidence for both types of reactions was noted for hydroxychloroquine than for the other antimalarials. Psoriatic flareups and recalcitrance to conventional therapy are probably very low risks because hydroxychloroquine is now used almost exclusively for arthritis. In a study by Kammer and colleagues,[59] psoriatic flares were not observed in patients treated with hydroxychloroquine for psoriatic arthritis. However, Vine and associates[86] observed the onset of pustular psoriasis and again cautioned against the use of hydroxychloroquine in patients with psoriatic diathesis.

ACUTE POISONING. Fatal reactions have been reported after accidental or intentional overdosage with chloroquine. The particular sensitivity of very young children (ages 1 to 3 years) to only 1 g has been emphasized.[87,88] Irreversible cardiac arrest occurred in some patients within 1 to 2 hours of drug ingestion. Intubation, gastric lavage, and acidification of urine to increase excretion may be lifesaving measures. Rasmussen[70] pointed out that adults show the same sensitivity to chloroquine on a milligram per kilogram basis.

Although special precautions should be taken to prevent poisoning (as with any medication), antimalarials are not contraindicated for children. Malaria prophylaxis should be given according to guidelines in the Aralen and Plaquenil package inserts. Hydroxychloroquine, although not approved by the FDA for this purpose, is used in the treatment of juvenile arthritis.

MONITORING GUIDELINES

The monitoring guideline box below deals with all aspects of monitoring for adverse effects from antimalarial agents. This text section deals only with recent controversies in monitoring for retinopathy from the various antimalarial agents. Quinacrine has no significant potential for retinopathy and does not need monitoring by an ophthalmologist. The following comments pertain to hydroxychloroquine and to the less commonly used drug chloroquine.

Previously, examinations by an ophthalmologist every 6 months were considered the standard of care. Before that, eye examinations were requested as often as every 3 to 4 months. Several recent articles have called into question the current guidelines followed by most dermatologists.[89,90] In an article from the United Kingdom, Jones[89] attempted to obtain a consensus from dermatologists, rheumatologists, and ophthalmologists regarding the optimal ocular monitoring of patients on long-term antimalarial therapy. The recommendations were to obtain a baseline ophthalmologic examination for visual acuity and a funduscopic examination. Provided the dose of hydroxychloroquine was

---

Antimalarial Monitoring Guidelines[61-63,65,89-91,95]

BASELINE

Ocular
- Baseline slit-lamp and funduscopic examination, assessment of visual acuity
- Visual field testing by both static and kinetic techniques with a 3-mm red test object
- Ask patients to test themselves with the Amsler grid (see Figure 12-2) every 4 weeks; patients test each eye separately with reading glasses by occluding the opposite eye on and looking for "faded" squares

Laboratory
- Complete blood count (CBC)
- G6PD screening* (see text discussion)
- Automated chemistry profile (emphasis on liver function tests)
- Random or 24-hour urinary porphyrin screening†

FOLLOW-UP

Ocular
- Reviewing subjective visual complaints, slit-lamp and funduscopic test results, and visual acuity (every 6 months for a year; then yearly‡—see text)
- Repeating visual field testing if patients complain of difficulty in reading ("missing" words and letters) and demonstrate reproducible bilateral "fading" of Amsler grid squares (see Figure 12-2)
- Discontinuing chloroquine or hydroxychloroquine treatment if bilateral field defects are confirmed

Laboratory
CBC (monthly for 3 months, then every 4 to 6 months)
Automated chemistry profile (after 1 month, after 3 months, and then every 4 to 6 months)

Note: More frequent surveillance is needed if laboratory values are abnormal or with high-risk patients.
*G6PD testing before antimalarial therapy is somewhat controversial; probably most important with antimalarial agents rarely used in dermatology such as primaquine.
†Only performed if porphyria cutanea tarda or related porphyrias are clinically suspected (at least consider ordering).
‡Retinopathy risk is greatest for patients on antimalarials (particularly chloroquine) for at least 5 years, particularly if maximum safe maintenance doses have been exceeded.

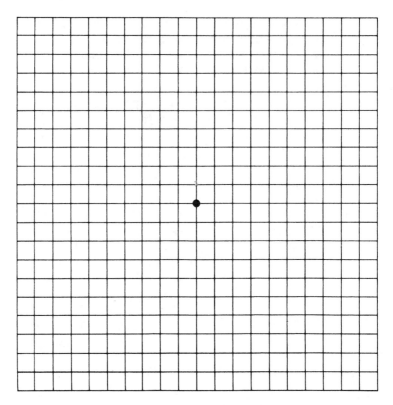

Figure 12-2   Amsler grid.

less than 6.5 mg/kg/day based on lean body weight, subsequent yearly ocular monitoring was not thought to require an ophthalmologist. Each visit should include a history for visual acuity and blurring of vision. Amsler grids were not deemed adequately reliable to be recommended for routine home use by the patients on antimalarial therapy. The consensus group recommended specific evaluation for possible retinopathy by an ophthalmologist only if the therapy exceeded 5 years.

Previously, Blyth and Lane[90] (also from the United Kingdom) had stated that after baseline assessment by an ophthalmologist, subsequent referral for ophthalmologic evaluation was needed only if antimalarial therapy exceeded 6 years. Before 6 years, the dermatologist or primary physician could evaluate yearly for new visual symptoms. Amsler grids were deemed appropriate for monthly use at home by the patient. The basic premise for both of these recommendations was the rarity of true retinopathy before 6 years of continuous antimalarial therapy as long as rec-

ommended maintenance doses are used (hydroxychloroquine <6.5 mg/kg/day; chloroquine <4.0 mg/kg/day).

The most recent North American recommendations for ophthalmologic examinations are in contrast to the United Kingdom guidelines. Easterbrook,[91] a Canadian ophthalmologist with extensive experience with antimalarial retinopathy, recommends that baseline examination, 6 month follow-up, then yearly follow-up by an ophthalmologist is indicated. The patient should utilize the Amsler grid monthly at home (Figure 12-2).

Finally, the most recent recommendations from the United States were published by Rynes and Bernstein.[65] They recommended baseline and an evaluation every 6 months by an ophthalmologist while on antimalarial therapy. Regular self-administered Amsler grid testing, albeit with absolute proof of reliability lacking, was deemed reasonable to recommend to patients.

Major differences in the health care systems in the countries from which the various afore-

■ **Table 12-4** Antimalarial Drug Interactions

Precipitant Drug	Target Drug	Mechanism
DRUGS THAT INCREASE ANTIMALARIAL DRUG LEVELS		
Cimetidine	Chloroquine	Cimetidine may decrease the oral clearance rate and metabolism of chloroquine
DRUGS THAT DECREASE ANTIMALARIAL DRUG LEVELS		
Kaolin	Chloroquine	Decreased GI absorption of chloroquine
Magnesium trisilicate	Chloroquine	Decreased GI absorption of chloroquine
DRUG LEVELS INCREASED BY ANTIMALARIALS		
Chloroquine	Digoxin	Concomitant use increases digoxin levels
Hydroxychloroquine	Digoxin	Concomitant use increases digoxin levels
POTENTIAL INCREASED TOXICITY DUE TO COMMON TARGET ORGAN		
Hydroxychloroquine (and vice versa)	Chloroquine (and vice versa)	Both share the potential for retinal toxicity; may have an additive effect when used simultaneously

Adapted from *CliniSphere 2.0 CD ROM*, St. Louis, June 2000, Facts & Comparisons and Drug Information for the Health Professional.[61-63]

mentioned authors originate make it difficult to analyze the significant differences in proposed monitoring guidelines. Until a consensus of North American experts in antimalarial therapy and ophthalmologic screening deem otherwise, the guidelines presented in this section seem to be a reasonable approach that does not create any undue financial hardship to the patient or insurer. Given that the premaculopathy (pre-retinopathy) changes are readily detectable (albeit not completely specific) and are considered reversible, the recommended protocol for monitoring with long-term yearly examinations by an ophthalmologist appears justifiable. The ophthalmologist's examination should include testing for visual acuity, careful funduscopic examination, and testing of visual fields (ideally with a red test object) at a minimum. Patient monthly utilization of an Amsler grid has virtually no cost, can be taught (and followed) by the ophthalmologist, and may be of significant value in screening for antimalarial retinopathy.

DRUG INTERACTIONS

Table 12-4 lists antimalarial drug interactions. The most significant drug interactions of con-

cern are those between antimalarials. Chloroquine and hydroxychloroquine should not be administered concurrently because of the additive retinotoxic potential. The combination of chloroquine and primaquine used for malaria prophylaxis is more likely to induce hemolysis in the G6PD-deficient patient. Although the combinations are not formally approved, rheumatologists routinely use hydroxychloroquine together with methotrexate, prednisone, and nonsteroidal antiinflammatory drugs in the treatment of SLE, rheumatoid arthritis, and psoriatic arthritis without significant drug interaction.[92] Digoxin levels may be elevated by antimalarials.

THERAPEUTIC GUIDELINES

The following dosage recommendations apply to treatment of all the dermatologic indications except PCT (see the next section). Travelers to endemic areas should contact the Centers for Disease Control for the latest recommendations for malaria prophylaxis that have been influenced by the emergence and dissemination of chloroquine-resistant strains of *Plasmodium falciparum*.

The treatment of discoid LE was reviewed in 1989.[93] The antimalarial drug of first choice is hydroxychloroquine at a maximum daily dosage of 6.5 mg/kg calculated from the patient's ideal (lean) body weight, or 400 mg, whichever is less. For sarcoidosis, it may be preferable to start with chloroquine 3.5 to 4.0 mg/kg/day or 250 mg, whichever is less.[94] It may take up to 4 to 8 weeks of therapy before a clinical response is seen and several more months for maximal benefit. Theoretically, priming a patient with an antimalarial may decrease the time necessary to reach equilibrium between plasma and tissues. An initial priming dosage of an antimalarial is used in the treatment of the acute attack of vivax or falciparum malaria. For chloroquine, this consists of 1 g followed by an additional 500 mg after 6 to 8 hours and 500 mg daily for the next 2 days, a total dosage of 2.5 g over 3 days.[95] In general, priming is not necessary for the chronic and nonlife-threatening conditions. Higher dosages may increase the risk of GI irritation and retinal toxicity. If nausea, vomiting, or diarrhea becomes problematic, stopping the drug and restarting at a lower dosage may circumvent the problem. Patients who develop a drug-related eruption must discontinue the antimalarial. However, patients who are intolerant of or allergic to hydroxychloroquine may tolerate chloroquine, and vice versa. Given a relatively low-risk cutaneous drug reaction (such as morbilliform or lichenoid reactions) such rechallenge with the alternative antimalarial agent is quite reasonable.

In patients who do not obtain maximal benefit for their skin disease after 3 months, 100 mg/day of quinacrine may be *added* to the regimen without increasing the risk of retinotoxicity. Quinacrine may be a better choice as the initial antimalarial for darkly pigmented races because the expected pigmentary alteration may be less detectable. It is also possible that a given patient may respond better to equivalent dosages of either chloroquine or hydroxychloroquine. Suggested safety monitoring tests adapted from package inserts and reviews[65,89-91,96] are shown in the Monitoring Guidelines section.

For patients who have developed retinopathy or rashes from either or both 4-aminoquinolines, or who are unreliable in keeping regular follow-up appointments, quinacrine may be used alone at a dosage of 100 to 200 mg/day.

After maximal improvement is achieved, the dosage of antimalarial should be decreased gradually by about 25% every 3 to 6 months. Relapse occurs frequently at low dosages. It therefore may be necessary to maintain some patients on one or two 200-mg tablets of hydroxychloroquine per week to suppress severe or extensive skin lesions. Some patients with seasonal, light-aggravated disease can be treated only during the problematic months; the preseasonal treatment time needed for equilibrium should then be taken into account. It has been recently documented that smokers respond less well to chloroquine than nonsmokers.[96] It is not clear if this is due to a blockade of effect of the antimalarial or to increased LE disease activity.

Treatment of PCT

For patients with PCT, ingestion of all exogenous hepatotoxins (e.g., alcohol, estrogens, and iron supplements) should first be discontinued. Assessment for possible viral infections such as HIV or hepatitis C should occur, and when identified, appropriate therapy for these infections should be part of the treatment plan. Phlebotomy is still considered the treatment of choice for PCT. Units of whole blood are removed gradually or rapidly to achieve a hemoglobin level of 10 to 11 g/dl.[43] Therefore these drugs are reserved for either patients who are already anemic or patients in whom phlebotomy is impractical or technically not feasible.

There are a variety of suggested treatments including both low-dose and high-dose therapies. Low-dose therapy might begin with a test dose of 100 or 200 mg of hydroxychloroquine or 125 mg of chloroquine. Liver function tests are performed 1 week later. This dose is then increased to two or three times per week for a month and then escalated further to 200 mg/day. Initial higher dosages may lead to hepatotoxicity as a result of rapid mobilization of hepatic porphyrin stores, but might be used in hospitalized or carefully monitored patients. Initial monitoring of liver function tests (particularly the transaminases) on a monthly basis in PCT patients is appropriate. Clinical remission and a nearly normal biochemical profile of porphyrin excretion occurs in all patients so treated. Harber and Bickers[44] recommended continued treatment until the total urinary porphyrin level is less than 300 µg/day. Relapse of the PCT generally occurs within 1 to 2 years, but some patients have remained in remission for more than 4 years.[43] The combination of phlebotomy and low dosages of chloroquine has been tried, but a convincing advantage over either treatment alone has not been shown.[45,46]

Bibliography

Ocular Monitoring

Easterbrook M: Screening for antimalarial toxicity (editorial). *Can J Ophthalmol* 28:51-52, 1993.

Jones SK: Ocular toxicity and hydroxychloroquine: guidelines for screening. *Br J Dermatol* 140:3-7, 1999.

Rynes RI, Bernstein HN: Ophthalmologic safety profile of antimalarial drugs. *Lupus* 2(Suppl 1):S17-S19, 1993.

Special Patient Groups

Parke AL, Rothfield NF: Antimalarial drugs in pregnancy—the North American experience. *Lupus* 5(Suppl 1):S67-S69, 1996.

Ziering CL, Rabinowitz LG, Esterly NB: Antimalarials for children: indications, toxicities, and guidelines. *J Am Acad Dermatol* 28:764-770, 1993.

Antimalarial Overviews

Khamashta MA, Wallace DJ: Antimalarials in rheumatology. *Lupus* 5(Suppl):S1-S74, 1996.

Luzzi GA, Peto TE: Adverse effects of antimalarials. An update. *Drug Safety* 8:295-311, 1993.

Titus ED: Recent developments in the understanding of the pharmacokinetics and mechanisms of action of chloroquine. *Ther Drug Monit* 11:369-379, 1989.

Weiss JS: Antimalarial medications in dermatology. *Dermatol Clin* 9:377-385, 1991.

Willoughby JS, Shear NH: Antimalarials. *Clin Dermatol* 7(3):60-68, 1989.

References

Introduction and Pharmacology

1. Isaacson D, Elgart M, Turner ML: Antimalarials in dermatology. *Int J Dermatol* 21:379-395, 1982.
2. Payne JF: A post-graduate lecture on lupus erythematosus. *Clin J* 4:223-229, 1894.
3. Page F: Treatment of lupus erythematosus with mepacrine. *Lancet* ii:755-758, 1951.
4. McChesney EW: Animal toxicity and pharmacokinetics of hydroxychloroquine sulfate. *Am J Med* 75(1A):11-18, 1983.
5. Tett SE, Cutler DJ, Day RO, et al: A dose-ranging study of the pharmacokinetics of hydroxychloroquine following intravenous administration to healthy volunteers. *Br J Clin Pharmacol* 26:303-313, 1988.
6. Furst DE: Pharmacokinetics of hydroxychloroquine and chloroquine during treatment of rheumatic disease. *Lupus* 5(Suppl 1):S11-S15, 1996.
7. Antimalarials. In Bickers DA, Hazen PG, Lynch WS, editors: *Clinical pharmacology of skin disease*, New York, 1984, Churchill Livingstone, pp 189-199.
8. Fox RI, Kang HI: Mechanism of action of antimalarial drugs: inhibition of antigen processing and presentation. *Lupus* 2(Suppl 1):S9-S12, 1993.
9. Dijkmans BA, deVriese E, deVreede TM, et al: Effects of anti-rheumatic drugs on in vitro mitogenic stimulation of peripheral blood mononuclear cells. *Transplant Proc* 20(Suppl 2):253-258, 1988.
10. Norris DA, Weston WL, Sams WM Jr: The effect of immunosuppressive and anti-inflammatory drugs on monocyte function in vitro. *J Lab Clin Med* 90:569-580, 1977.
11. Ward PA: The chemosuppression of chemotaxis. *J Exp Med* 7:302-307, 1964.

12. London JR: Hydroxychloroquine and postoperative thromboembolism after total hip replacement. *Am J Med* 85(Suppl 4A):57-61, 1988.

13. Wallace DJ, Linker-Israeli M, Metzger AL, et al: The release of antimalarial therapy with regard to thrombosis, hypercholesterolemia and cytokines in SLE. *Lupus* 2(Suppl 1):S13-S15, 1993.

14. Wallace DJ, Linker-Israeli M, Hynn S, et al: The effect of hydroxychloroquine therapy on serum levels of immunoregulatory molecules in patients with systemic lupus erythematosus. *J Rheumatol* 21:375-376, 1994.

15. Petri M, Lakatta C, Madger L, et al: Effect of prednisone and hydroxychloroquine on coronary artery disease risk factors in systemic lupus erythematosus? A longitudinal data analysis. *Am J Med* 96:254-259, 1994.

16. Ornstein MH, Sperber K: The anti-inflammatory and anti-viral effects of hydroxychloroquine in two patients with acquired immunodeficiency syndrome and actived inflammatory arthritis. *Arthritis Rheum* 39:157-161, 1996.

FDA-Approved Indications

17. Rollo IM: Miscellaneous drugs used in the treatment of protozoal infections. In Gilman AG, Goodman LS, Gilman A, editors: *Goodman and Gilman's the pharmacological basis of therapeutics*, ed 6, New York, 1980, Macmillan, pp 1070-1079.

18. Bell CL: Hydroxychloroquine sulfate in rheumatoid arthritis. Long-term response rate and predictive parameters. *Am J Med* 75(1A):46-51, 1983.

19. Kraak JH, VaKetel WG, Prakken JR, et al: The value of hydroxychloroquine (Plaquenil) for the treatment of chronic discoid lupus erythematosus: a double blind trial. *Dermatologica* 130:293-305, 1965.

20. Callen JP: Chronic cutaneous lupus erythematosus. *Arch Dermatol* 118:412-416, 1982.

21. Callen JP, Klein J: Subacute cutaneous lupus erythematosus: Clinical, serologic, immunogenetic, and therapeutic considerations in seventy-two patients. *Arthritis Rheum* 31:1007-1013, 1988.

22. The Canadian Hydroxychloroquine Study Group: A randomized study of the effect of withdrawing hydroxychloroquine sulfate in systemic lupus erythematosus. *N Engl J Med* 324:150-154, 1991.

23. Rynes RI (editor): Antimalarial therapy and lupus. *Lupus* 2(Suppl 1):S1-S23, 1993.

24. Lockshin MD: Therapy for systemic lupus erythematosus (editorial) *N Engl J Med* 324:189-191, 1991.

25. Esdaile JM: The efficacy of antimalarials in systemic lupus erythematosus. *Lupus* 2(Suppl):S3-S8, 1993.

26. Cram DL, Epstein JH, Tuffaneilli DL: Lupus erythematosus and porphyria. *Arch Dermatol* 108:779-784, 1973.

Off-Label Uses

27. Linden IH: Development of porphyria during chloroquine therapy for chronic discoid lupus erythematosus. *California Med* 51:235-238, 1954.

28. Malkinson FD, Levitt L: Hydroxychloroquine treatment of porphyria cutanea tarda. *Arch Dermatol* 108:779-784, 1973.

29. Petersen CS, Thomsen K: High-dose hydroxychloroquine treatment of porphyria cutanea tarda. *J Am Acad Dermatol* 26:614-619, 1992.

30. Ashton RE, Hawk JL, Magnus IA: Low-dose oral chloroquine in the treatment of porphyria cutanea tarda. *Br J Dermatol* 111:609-613, 1984.

31. Harber LC, Bickers DR: The porphyrias. In *Photosensitivity diseases. Principles of diagnosis and treatment*, ed 2, Toronto, 1989, Decker, pp 241-287.

32. Marchesi L, Di Padova C, Cainelli T, et al: A comparative trial of desferroxamine and hydroxychloroquine for treatment of porphyria cutanea tarda in alcoholic patients. *Photodermatology* 1:286-292, 1984.

33. Swanbeck G, Wennersten G: Treatment of porphyria cutanea tarda using chloroquine and phlebotomy. *Br J Dermatol* 97:77-81, 1977.

34. Horkay I, Nagy E: Combination therapy of porphyria cutanea tarda using chloroquine and bloodletting therapy. *Z Hautkr* 55:813-816, 1980.

35. Murphy GM, Hawk JLM, Magnus IA: Hydroxychloroquine in polymorphic light eruption. A controlled trial with drug and visual sensitivity monitoring. *Br J Dermatology* 116:379-386, 1987.

36. Jansen CT: Oral carotenoid treatment in polymorphous light eruption. A cross-over comparison with oxychloroquine and placebo. *Photodermatology* 2:166-8, 1985.

37. Mathews-Roth MM: Systemic photoprotection. *Dermatol Clin* 4:335-339, 1986.

38. Woo TY, Callen JP, Voorhees JJ, et al: Cutaneous lesions of dermatomyositis are improved by hydroxychloroquine. *J Am Acad Dermatol* 10:592-600, 1984.

39. James WD, Dawson N, Rodman OG: The treatment of dermatomyositis with hydroxychloroquine. *J Rheumatol* 12:1214-1216, 1985.

40. Olson NY, Lindsley CB: Adjunctive use of hydroxychloroquine in childhood dermatomyositis. *J Rheumatol* 16:1545-1547, 1989.

41. Jones EM, Callen JP: Hydroxychloroquine is effective therapy for control of cutaneous sarcoidal granuloma. *J Am Acad Dermatol* 23:487-490, 1990.

42. Carlin MC, Ratz JL: A case of generalized granuloma annulare responding to hydroxychloroquine. *Cleve Clin J Med* 54:229-232, 1987.

43. Stoll DM: Treatment of cutaneous pseudolymphoma with hydroxychloroquine. *J Am Acad Dermatol* 8:696-699, 1983.

44. Toonstra J, Wildschut A, Boer J, et al: Jessner's lymphocytic infiltration of the skin. A clinical study of 100 patients. *Arch Dermatol* 125:1525-1530, 1989.

45. Shelley WB: Chloroquine-induced remission of nodular panniculitis present for 15 years. *J Am Acad Dermatol* 5:168-180, 1981.

46. Alloway JA, Franks LK: Hydroxychloroquine in the treatment of chronic erythema nodosum. *Br J Dermatol* 132:661-673, 1995.

47. Martens PB, Moder KG, Ahmed I: Lupus panniculitis: Clinical perspectives from a case series. *J Rheumatol* 26:68-72, 1999.

48. Eisen D: Hydroxychloroquine sulfate (Plaquenil) improves oral lichen planus. An open trial. *J Am Acad Dermatol* 28:609-612, 1993.

49. Balogh E, Nagy-Vezekényi K, Fórizs E: REM syndrome. An immediate therapeutic response to hydroxychloroquine sulphate. *Acta Derm Venereol (Stockh)* 60:173-175, 1980.

50. Steigleder GK, Gartmann H, Linker U: REM syndrome: reticular erythematous mucinosis (round-cell erythematosus), a new entity? *Br J Dermatol* 91:191-199, 1974.

51. Cernea SS, Rivitti EA: Successful treatment of mucinosis with chloroquine. *J Dermatol Treat* 1:163-165, 1990.

52. Hymes SR, Jordon RE: Pemphigus foliaceus. Use of antimalarial agents as adjuvant therapy. *Arch Dermatol* 128:1462-1464, 1992.

53. Döring HF, Müllejans-Kreppel U: Chloroquine—therapy of atopic dermatitis. *Z Hautkr* 62:1205-1213, 1987.

54. Lopez LR, Davis KC, Kohler PF, et al: The hypocomplementemic urticarial-vasculitis syndrome. Therapeutic response to hydroxychloroquine. *J Allergy Clin Immunol* 73:600-603, 1984.

55. Nagy E, Ladanyi E: Treatment of circumscribed scleroderma in childhood. *Z Hautkr* 62:547-549, 1987.

56. Cornbleet T: Action of synthetic antimalarial drugs on psoriasis. *J Invest Dermatol* 26:435-436, 1956.

57. Luzar MJ: Hydroxychloroquine in psoriatic arthropathy: exacerbation of psoriatic skin lesions. *J Rheumatol* 9:462-464, 1982.

58. Gray RG: Hydroxychloroquine provocation of psoriasis. *J Rheumatol* 12:391, 1985.

59. Kammer GM, Soter NA, Gibson DJ, et al: Psoriatic arthritis. A clinical immunologic and HLA study of 100 patients. *Semin Arthritis Rheum* 9:75-95, 1979.

60. Gladman DD, Blake R, Brubacher B, et al: Chloroquine therapy in psoriatic arthritis. *J Rheumatol* 19:1724-1726, 1992.

61. United States Pharmacopeial Convention: Quinacrine. In Drug Information for the Health Care Professional, 1998, pp 2469-2470.

62. United States Pharmacopeial Convention: Chloroquine. In Drug Information for the Health Care Professional, 1998, pp 794-798.

63. United States Pharmacopeial Convention: Hydroxychloroquine. In Drug Information for the Health Care Professional, 1998, pp 1601-1604.

Adverse Effects—Ocular

64. Finbloom DS, Silver K, Newsome DA, et al: Comparison of hydroxychloroquine and chloroquine use and the development of retinal toxicity. *J Rheumatol* 12:692-694, 1985.

65. Rynes RI, Bernstein HN: Ophthalmic safety profile of antimalarial drugs. *Lupus* 2(suppl 1):S17-S19, 1993.

66. Mazzuca ST, Yung R, Brandt KD, et al: Current practices for monitoring ocular toxicity related to hydroxychloroquine (Plaquenil) therapy. *J Rheumatol* 12:692-694, 1985.

67. Levy GD, Munz SJ, Paschal J, et al: Incidence of hydroxychloroquine retinopathy in 1207 patients in a large, multicenter outpatient practice. *Arthritis Rheum* 40:1482-1486, 1997.

68. Olansky AJ: Antimalarials and ophthalmologic safety. *J Am Acad Dermatol* 6:19-23, 1982.

69. Bernstein HN: Ophthalmologic considerations and testing in patients receiving long-term antimalarial therapy. *Am J Med* 75(1A):25-34, 1983.

Other Adverse Effects

70. Rasmussen JE: Antimalarials. Are they safe to use in children? *Pediatr Dermatol* 1:89-91, 1985.
71. Ziering CL, Rabinowitz LG, Esterly NB: Antimalarials for children. Indications, toxicities and guidelines. *J Am Acad Dermatol* 28:764-770, 1993.
72. Levy M, Buskila D, Gladman DD, et al: Pregnancy outcome following first trimester exposure to chloroquine. *Am J Perinatol* 8:174-178, 1991.
73. Parks AL: Antimalarial drugs, pregnancy, and lactation. *J Rheumatol* 2(Suppl 1):S21-S23, 1993.
74. Ward WQ, Walter-Ryan WG, Shehi GM: Toxic psychosis. A complication of antimalarial therapy. *J Am Acad Dermatol* 12:863-865, 1985.
75. Schmid I, Anasetti C, Petersen FB, et al: Marrow transplantation for severe aplastic anemia associated with exposure to quinacrine. *Blut* 61:52-54, 1990.
76. Luzzi GA, Peto TE: Adverse effects of antimalarials. An update. *Drug Safety* 8:295-311, 1993.
77. Granstein RD, Sober AJ: Drug- and heavy metal-induced hyperpigmentation. *J Am Acad Dermatol* 5:1-18, 1981.
78. Daniel CR, Scher RK: Nail changes secondary to systemic drugs or ingestants. *J Am Acad Dermatol* 5:1-18, 1981.
79. Dupré A, Ortonne JP, Viraben R, et al: Chloroquine-induced hypopigmentation of hair and freckles. Association with congenital renal failure. *Arch Dermatol* 121:1164-1166, 1985.
80. Wintroub BU, Stern R: Cutaneous drug reactions. Pathogenesis and clinical classification. *J Am Acad Dermatol* 13:167-179, 1985.
81. Hudson LD: Erythema annulare centrifugum. An unusual case due to hydroxychloroquine sulfate. *Cutis* 36:129-130, 1985.
82. Bauer F: Quinacrine hydrochloride drug eruption (topical lichenoid dermatitis). *J Am Acad Dermatol* 4:239-248, 1981.
83. Abel EA, DiCicco LM, Orenberg EK, et al: Drugs in exacerbation of psoriasis. *J Am Acad Dermatol* 15:1007-1022, 1986.
84. Kuflik EG: Effect of antimalarial drugs on psoriasis. *Cutis* 26:153-155, 1980.
85. Slagel GA, James WD: Plaquenil-induced erythroderma. *J Am Acad Dermatol* 12:857-862, 1985.
86. Vine JE, Hymes SR, Warner NB, et al: Pustular psoriasis induced by hydroxychloroquine. A case report and review of the literature. *J Dermatol* 23:357-361, 1996.
87. Cann HM, Verhulst HL: Fatal acute chloroquine poisoning in children. *Pediatrics* 27:95-102, 1961.
88. Markowitz HA, McGinley JM: Chloroquine poisoning in a child. *JAMA* 189:950-951, 1964.

Monitoring and Therapeutic Guidelines

89. Jones SK: Ocular toxicity and hydroxychloroquine: guidelines for screening. *Br J Dermatol* 140:3-7, 1999.
90. Blyth C, Lane C: Hydroxychloroquine retinopathy: is screening necessary? Intensive screening is not necessary at normal doses (editorial). *BMJ* 316:716-717, 1998.
91. Easterbrook M: Screening for antimalarial toxicity (editorial). *Can J Ophthalmol* 28:51-52, 1993.
92. Rynes RI: Hydroxychloroquine treatment of rheumatoid arthritis. *Am J Med* 85(suppl 4a):18-22, 1988.
93. Lo JS, Berg RE, Tomecki KJ: Treatment of discoid lupus erythematosus. *Int J Dermatol* 28:497-509, 1989.
94. Veien NK: Cutaneous sarcoidosis. Prognosis and treatment. *Clin Dermatol* 4:75-87, 1986.
95. Rollo IM: Drugs used in the chemotherapy of malaria. In Gilman AG, Goodman LS, Gilman A, editors: *Goodman and Gilman's the pharmacological basis of therapeutics*, ed 6, New York, 1980, Macmillan, pp 1038-1060.
96. Easterbrook M: Ocular effects and safety of antimalarial agents. *Am J Med* 85(4A):23-29, 1988.
97. Rahman P, Gladman DD, Urowitz MB: Smoking interferes with efficacy of antimalarial therapy in cutaneous lupus. *J Rheumatol* 25:1716-1719, 1998.

CHAPTER 13

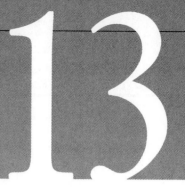

Ethan-Quan H. Nguyen
Stephen E. Wolverton

Systemic Retinoids

The term *retinoids* includes all synthetic and natural compounds that have activity like that of vitamin A, whereas the term *vitamin* A is best used to characterize a family of naturally occurring and biologic chemicals, rather than one particular compound. The initial understanding of these compounds began in the early 1900s, when Antarctic explorers experienced hypervitaminosis-A shortly after consuming polar bear liver.[1] McCollum and Davis (1913) reported that "fat soluble A" is required for maintenance of growth. The major attraction of the retinoid family in dermatology has been the effects of vitamin A on epithelial tissues. Earlier observations documented that vitamin A deficiency induced epidermal hyperkeratosis, squamous metaplasia of mucous membranes, various keratinization disorders, and certain precancerous conditions.

In mammals, vitamin A exists in interconvertible forms as retinol (vitamin A alcohol), retinal (vitamin A aldehyde), and retinoic acid (RA) (vitamin A acid). Retinol is the most potent vitamin A analog and represents the main dietary source, transport, and storage form. In 1931, vitamin A (in the form of RA) was purified from liver oil. Four years later, the role of retinal in the visual cycle was identified. Once thought of as a mere byproduct of retinol, RA is the most oxidized and water-soluble form. It is much less toxic than its parent compound, but still retains most of its biologic functions. In 1946 and 1947, retinol and RA were synthesized in vitro, respectively.

However, the first dermatologic use of vitamin A dated back to 1943 by Straumfjord for acne vulgaris.[1] Because of the narrow therapeutic index of vitamin A, the engineering of ideal synthetic retinoids having the highest therapeutic activity with the lowest possible adverse effects was initiated. In the early 1960s, Bollag[2] began testing various retinoid compounds (eventually testing about 1500 retinoids), trying to find those that had a suitable therapeutic index in the rodent papilloma model. Oral administration of all-*trans* RA (tretinoin) had initially shown promising results in the treatment of certain disorders of keratinization.[3] However, its oral use had to be abandoned because of an unsafe therapeutic index; hence only the topical tretinoin was subsequently introduced into clinical practice. In 1962, Stüttgen reported the therapeutic effectiveness of topical tretinoin in disorders of keratinization such as ichthyosis and pityriasis rubra pilaris, as well as actinic keratoses.[3] Subsequently, in 1969 Kligman and colleagues first applied topical tretinoin for acne vulgaris.[1]

Isotretinoin, first synthesized in 1955, had been studied in Europe (as RoAccutane) since 1971 for acne (Table 13-1). Unpublished data from Hoffmann-La Roche showed that oral doses of 5 to 20 mg daily yielded good results in comedonic, papulopustular, and cystic forms of

■ **Table 13-1** Systemic Retinoids

Generic Name	Trade Name	Generic Available	Manu-facturer	Tablet or Capsule Sizes	Special Formula-tions	Standard Dosage Range	Price Index
FIRST-GENERATION RETINOIDS							
Isotretinoin	Accutane	None	Roche	10, 20, 40 mg	None	0.5-2 mg/kg/day	$$$$
Tretinoin (all-trans retinoic acid)	Vesanoid	None	Roche	10 mg	Topical gel, cream, solution	45 mg/m²/d	—
SECOND-GENERATION RETINOIDS							
Etretinate	Tegison	None	Roche	10, 25 mg	None	0.25-1 mg/kg/d	—
Acitretin	Soriatane	None	Roche	10, 25 mg	None	25-50 mg/d	$$$$
THIRD-GENERATION RETINOID							
Bexarotene	Targretin	None	Ligand	75 mg	None	300 mg/m²/d	$$$$$

$, <1.00; $$, 1.01-2.00; $$$, 2.01-5.00; $$$$, 5.01-10.00; $$$$$, >10.00; ( ), generic price; /, two different price ranges from lower dose to higher dose examples of this size; —, no price listed for this drug.

acne.[3] However, further investigation was not pursued because of "the psychologic climate" engendered by the thalidomide tragedy; it was thought to be unconceivable to develop an agent with teratogenic properties for the treatment of such a common complaint as acne. Meanwhile in the United States, isotretinoin was initially tested in clinical trials for disorders of keratinization in 1972 by Peck and Yoder at the National Institutes of Health.[4] An incidental discovery during these clinical trials was a significant improvement of acne vulgaris of the nodulocystic type in patients taking oral isotretinoin.[5] In the late 1970s, isotretinoin was confirmed to be highly effective for acne vulgaris and cystic conglobate acne by the same authors and their co-workers.[6] Of the first-generation retinoids, 13-*cis* RA (isotretinoin, Accutane) was approved by the US Food and Drug Administration (FDA) in 1982 as an oral retinoid to treat severe nodulocystic acne.

The aromatic retinoids were developed because they appeared to be more effective in treating psoriasis and other keratinizing dermatoses. In 1972, Bollag[2] discovered two aromatic retinoids, etretinate and acitretin, that possessed a good therapeutic index in the chemically induced rodent papillomas. After more than a decade of research, a second-generation retinoid, etretinate (Tegison), was released in the United States in 1986 for the treatment of psoriasis. In 1998, etretinate was phased out by Roche and replaced by its metabolite, acitretin (Soriatane). This process had already taken place in Europe about a decade earlier. Because etretinate is no longer available (except in Japan), less emphasis is placed on this agent in this chapter. However, the majority of information on the mechanisms of action of the second-generation retinoids is derived from etretinate data. Current and future research is being directed toward developing third-generation retinoids with a much safer therapeutic index than the currently existing retinoids.

PHARMACOLOGY

Table 13-2 lists key pharmacologic concepts for systemic retinoids.

■ **Table 13-2**   Key Pharmacologic Concepts—Systemic Retinoids[7-14]

Drug Name	Category	Absorption and Bioavailability			Elimination		
		Peak Levels	Bioavailable (%)	Protein Binding	Half-life	Metabolism	Excretion
Tretinoin	First generation	1-2 hrs	—	Albumin 99%	48 min	Hepatic	Bile, urine
Isotretinoin	First generation	3 hrs	25%	Albumin 99%	20 hrs	Hepatic	Bile, urine
Etretinate	Second generation	4 hrs	44%	Lipoprotein 99%	120 days	Hepatic	Bile, urine
Acitretin	Second generation	4 hrs	60%	Albumin 95%	2 days	Hepatic	Bile, urine
Bexarotene	Third generation	2 hrs	No data	Plasma proteins 99%	7 hrs	Hepatic	Hepatobiliary

Vitamin A Physiology

Vitamin A is required for the development and maintenance of human life. It cannot be synthesized in vivo by the human body and thus must be acquired through the diet. To understand the mechanisms of action of retinoids, physiologic effects of different forms of vitamin A must be comprehended. The details of vitamin A physiology can be found in several complete reviews.[1-3,15,16]

The precursors of vitamin A are classified as carotenoids, function as photosensitive structures, and are synthesized by plants.[15] In the animal kingdom, ingested carotenoids are oxidized to vitamin A. Beta-carotene is primarily derived from green leafy and yellow vegetables. In the intestines, every molecule of beta-carotene is converted into two molecules of retinal before being absorbed.

Retinyl esters derived from meat and animal products, such as eggs and milk, are the primary dietary form of vitamin A. In the intestines, the retinyl esters are hydrolyzed to retinol, which is absorbed and initially stored in the ester form (particularly as retinal palmitate) in the liver. Retinol can be converted interchangeably to retinal and is irreversibly metabolized to RA.

These forms of vitamin A are important for vision, reproduction, regulation of embryogenic development and morphogenesis, promotion of general growth, and modulation of immunoresponse. Retinal, as 11-*cis* isomer and 11-*trans* isomer, is important form in the biochemical reaction of visual function, whereas retinol is essential to reproduction. Both retinal and RA play an essential role in epithelial differentiation and normal growth. Carotenoids and vitamin A may have a relatively small role as antioxidants.

Structure

All three forms of vitamin A, as well as all three generations of synthetic retinoids (see Table 13-1), come under the heading of retinoids. Beta-carotene, a precursor of retinal, is not considered a retinoid. Nonselective retinoids activate multiple pathways and are associated with a higher incidence of adverse effects. To achieve the greatest therapeutic index (highest therapeutic efficacy-to-lowest toxicity ratio), it is logical to design receptor- and function-specific retinoids that activate only desirable pathways required for the therapeutic efficacy in a specific clinical condition.[17]

Manipulation of the polar end group and the polyene side chain of vitamin A (Figure 13-1) forms the first-generation retinoids. In addition, a large number of isomers are synthesized. From this first generation of nonaromatic

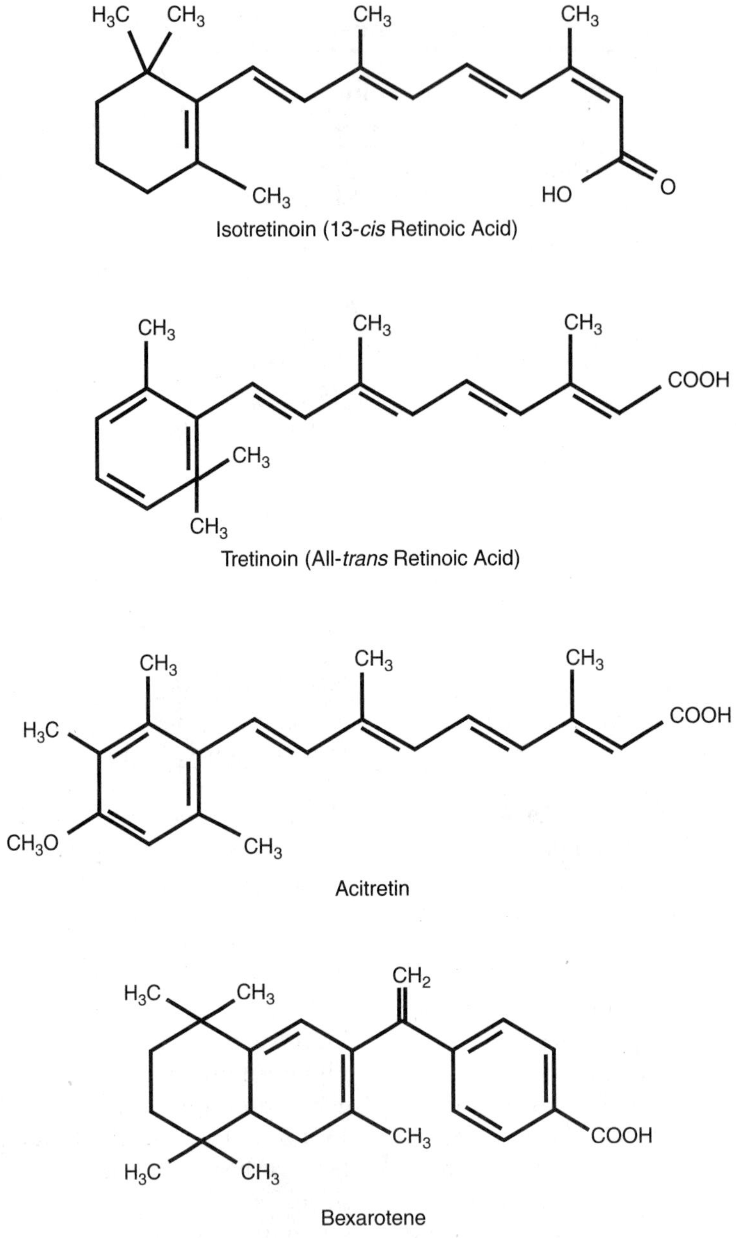

Isotretinoin (13-*cis* Retinoic Acid)

Tretinoin (All-*trans* Retinoic Acid)

Acitretin

Bexarotene

Figure 13-1   Retinoids.

retinoids, tretinoin (all-*trans* RA), isotretinoin (13-*cis* RA), and alitretinoin (9-*cis* RA), gained experimental and clinical importance in dermatology and oncology.[1]

Second-generation (monoaromatic) retinoids are synthesized by replacing the cyclic end group of vitamin A with various substituted and nonsubstituted ring systems. The therapeutically important compounds include etretinate (Tegison) and acitretin (Soriatane), which have been important drugs in treating psoriasis and other keratinizing dermatoses.

The third-generation (polyaromatic) retinoids include the arotinoids and selected other retinoids. These agents, formed through cyclization of the polyene side chain, include tazarotene (Tazorac) and adapalene (Differin), which are FDA-approved topical agents for psoriasis and acne, respectively. A third-generation oral retinoid approved by FDA for treatment of cutaneous T-cell lymphoma is bexarotene (Targretin). In contrast to the first- and second-generation retinoids, the arotinoids are constructed to interact selectively with specific receptors. This generates new methods of elucidating (1) the function of each subclass of retinoid receptors, (2) the transcriptional and subsequent biologic effects induced by activation/inhibition of different or a combination of retinoid receptors, and (3) desirable therapeutic goals. Although arotinoids are much more potent than earlier retinoids, their therapeutic index shows no significant improvement over previously developed retinoids,[17] which is why primarily topical members of third-generation retinoids have been approved to date.

Absorption and Distribution

The important physiochemical differences among the three generations of retinoids confer not only their differences in therapeutic activities and adverse effects but also in pharmacokinetic behavior. The pharmacokinetics of isotretinoin, etretinate, acitretin, and bexarotene are compared in the following text.

It is well recognized that oral bioavailability of retinoids is enhanced with food intake. The effect of fatty meals is especially great with acitretin and bexarotene.[7,8] A likely mechanism behind this observation is that there is an increase in the retinoid solubility, coupled with an increase in the lymphatic absorption and prolonged residence time of the drug in the gastrointestinal tract.[8] Mean C_{max} at steady state are not much greater than those observed after the first oral dose.

In serum, natural and synthetic retinoids are transported by plasma proteins (see Table 13-2). Bexarotene is highly bound to certain plasma proteins that have not yet been identified.[7] Similar to vitamin A storage, there is a significant accumulation of synthetic retinoids in the liver.[1] Yet the synthetic retinoids have a lesser affinity than vitamin A for storage in hepatocytes and in Ito stellate fibroblasts. When retinoid absorption exceeds liver storage capacity, symptoms of hypervitaminosis-A result.

Because isotretinoin and acitretin are water-soluble, there is very little lipid deposition. How-

ever, etretinate is approximately 50 times more lipophilic than its metabolite acitretin, resulting in increased storage in the adipose tissue from which it is slowly released.[8] This is one of the presumed advantages of using acitretin rather than etretinate in treating psoriasis, especially in fertile women. The more water-soluble retinoids (i.e., isotretinoin, acitretin, and bexarotene) are undetectable in serum within 1 month after stopping therapy. The highly lipid-soluble etretinate persists for at least several years in various fatty tissues such as subcutaneous fat.

Small amounts of the acitretin and its 13-*cis* isomer appear in breast milk; just under 20% of the corresponding serum concentration of the drug appears in breast milk. The estimated amount of drug consumed by a suckling infant corresponds to about 1.5% of the maternal dose, justifying its avoidance in breast-feeding women.[9] Based on analysis of seminal fluid from 3 male patients treated with acitretin and 6 male patients treated with etretinate, the amount of acitretin transferred in semen would be equivalent to 1/200,000 of a single 25 mg capsule.

Metabolism and Excretion

The metabolism of retinoids occurs mainly in the liver. It involves oxidation and chain shortening to biologically inactive, water-soluble products. The oxidative metabolism is induced mainly by retinoids themselves and possibly also by other agents known to induce hepatic cytochrome P-450 3A4 isoform.[18,19]

The major metabolite of isotretinoin is produced by oxidation, which forms 4-oxo-isotretinoin. Lesser amounts of tretinoin and 4-oxo-tretinoin are produced. With etretinate there is a significant first-pass hepatic metabolism by hydrolysis to the active metabolite acitretin. Acitretin metabolism differs from isotretinoin metabolism primarily in the initial metabolism, which involves isomerization instead of oxidation. The major metabolite of acitretin is its *cis* isomer. Within a few hours post dosing, isoacitretin predominates over acitretin in plasma.[9] Subsequently, both 13-*trans* and 13-*cis* acitretin are transformed by demethoxylation at the aromatic ring and are eliminated in the bile as β-glucuronide derivatives or through the kidneys as soluble metabolites with shorter side chains.

Bexarotene is oxidized to 6- and 7-hydroxy-bexarotene, then 6- and 7-oxo-bexarotene. These metabolites exhibit low activity in in vitro receptor assays, and their relative contribution to the overall drug efficacy is unknown.[7] Bexarotene-acyl-glucuronide is detected in urine but represents an insignificant fraction of the administered dose. Similar to tretinoin and alitretinoin, bexarotene induces its own metabolism/clearance without affecting the elimination half-life when given at very high dosages.

There are important differences in the terminal elimination half-lives ($T_{1/2}$) among three generations of retinoids.[7,20] Tretinoin has the shortest half-life of 40 to 60 minutes, followed by bexarotene of 7 to 9 hours, then isotretinoin of 10 to 20 hours, then acitretin of 50 hours. Etretinate has a prolonged half-life of 80 to 160 days. After etretinate therapy is discontinued, the serum levels quickly drop to very low levels. However, these levels may persist for up to 2.9 years.[8] Both isotretinoin and acitretin are completely cleared from the body within 1 month after the drug is stopped. This gives both drugs a definite advantage over etretinate for use by women of childbearing age. Based on short $T_{1/2}$ values, bexarotene probably has a clearance profile similar to isotretinoin.

All four drugs are excreted in the urine and feces.[1,7] Glucuronide conjugated metabolites appear in the bile with subsequent excretion in the feces. Isotretinoin has limited enterohepatic recirculation. On the other hand, bexarotene elimination is thought to occur primarily via the hepatobiliary route.

ACITRETIN REESTERIFICATION/"REVERSE METABOLISM."   Alcohol indirectly enhances the reesterification of acitretin to etretinate, which is detectable only after a few days of an acitretin regimen.[9] In human hepatocyte cultures, this conversion only occurs when ethanol is coadministered with acitretin.[21] Following 3-month administration of acitretin (30 mg/day) in 10 patients with psoriasis, steady-state plasma etretinate concentrations were detected at 2.5 to 56.7 ng/mL; alcohol consumption was an important contributing factor for the formation of etretinate. In another two-way crossover study,

all 10 subjects formed etretinate with concurrent ingestion of a single 100 mg dose of acitretin during a 3-hour period of ethanol ingestion. The total amount of ingested ethanol was approximately 1.4 g/kg body weight, equivalent to about 8 drinks in a 75 kg (165 lb) man. The formation of etretinate in this study was comparable to a single 5 mg oral dose of etretinate.[10] Because of this new knowledge, the recommended period for contraception after acitretin therapy has been lengthened from 2 months to 2 years in Europe.[9] In the United States, the recommended period for contraceptive use after cessation of acitretin is even longer at 3 years.[10]

In a study of 37 women of childbearing age exposed to acitretin, the levels of detectable etretinate concentration in 20 women who still used the acitretin and 17 who stopped therapy for up to 29 months revealed the prevalence of detectable etretinate concentrations to be 45% and 83% in plasma and subcutaneous tissue, respectively, among current acitretin users and 18% and 86% among those who had stopped acitretin therapy.[22] In another study, after 4 to 11 months of treatment with etretinate, its concentration in the subcutaneous fat attained equilibrium at a level of about 100 times that in plasma.[12] Even though the drug concentrations in the fat compartment are much higher than those in serum or skin tissue, it is unknown whether these persistent levels are truly enough for toxicity. Theoretically, other lipophilic drugs or agents may displace etretinate from fat. It is also possible that fat catabolism during starvation or thermogenesis accelerates the terminal elimination of the drug, although this has not been examined. Regardless, inability to detect plasma etretinate is a poor predictor of the absence of etretinate in fat. It is suggested that when monitoring acitretin and etretinate levels, both should be quantified in the subcutaneous tissue when plasma measurements are negative.[22]

Mechanisms of Retinoid Action

Tables 13-3 and 13-4 both list mechanisms of action for retinoids. Retinoids are small-molecule hormones that elicit their biologic effects by activating nuclear receptors and regulating gene transcription.[17,24,25] The majority of data presented in this section are based on ini-

Table 13-3   Mechanisms of Retinoid Action—Natural or Synthetic Retinoids[7,17,23-25]

Mechanisms	Therapeutic/Clinical Outcomes
Transactivate nuclear receptor RAR-α and RAR/RXR heterodimers that bind to RARE. Regulate gene transcription	*Direct effect:* Inducing cellular differentiation in human myeloid leukemia Differentiation therapy for human myeloid leukemia Inhibition of ovarian tumor cells
Transactivate nuclear receptor RAR/RXR heterodimers to antagonize transcription factors of genes without RARE	*Indirect effects:* Antiproliferative and antiinflammatory
Transactivate RARs (all types)	Promote wound healing: 　Increase proliferation of keratinocytes 　Increase collagen formation in the upper dermis 　Induce angiogenesis Reduction and even distribution of melanin in the epidermis Epidermal hyperplasia Clinical desquamation and peeling
Induce RAR-coactivator interactions	Increase gene transcription
Induce RAR-corepressor interactions	Decrease gene transcription
Transactivate RAR-α	Antiproliferation against breast cancer cells and T-cell/Hodgkin's lymphomas Normal development of eye and heart
Transactivate RAR-β	Antiproliferation in neuroblastoma tumor cells without differentiation Antiproliferation in lung cancer cells Control tumor growth Antiproliferation against head and neck squamous cell cancer, correlated with clinical responses
Transactivate RAR-γ	Antiproliferation and apoptosis in human melanoma cell lines Inhibition of keratinocyte differentiation and proliferation Apoptosis of acute promyelocytic cells Mucocutaneous toxicities Chondrocyte maturation Endochondral ossification Epiphyseal plate closure Induce caudal neural tube defect
Transactivate RXR-α	Induce apoptosis of human myeloid leukemia cells before committed differentiation
Transactivate RXRs (all types)	Significant hypertriglyceridemia Significant hypercholesterolemia Decreased HDL-cholesterol level
Transactivate RAR > RXR	Teratogenic effects
Induce expression of transcription factor GATA-4	Morphogenesis of the posterior heart tube and development of cardiac inflow tract

RAR, Retinoic acid receptor; *RXR,* retinoid X receptor; *RARE,* retinoic acid response elements (as part of DNA).

Table 13-4 Additional Mechanisms of Action—Specific Retinoids[1,7,9,23,26-29]

Mechanisms	Therapeutic/Clinical Outcome
ISOTRETINOIN	
Inhibition of sebaceous gland differentiation and proliferation	Reduces the amounts of sebum secreted
Reduce the size of sebaceous glands	Indirect reduction of *Propionibacterium acnes* colonization in pilosebaceous units
Suppression of sebum production	Indirect reduction of conversion of triglycerides to free fatty acids in hair follicles
Suppression of skin dihydrotestosterone production	Indirect reduction of inflammation
Down-regulation of skin androgen receptors	
Normalization of follicular epithelial desquamation	Reduction of impacted hyperkeratotic infundibula and comedones
Inhibition of neutrophil chemotaxis	Antiinflammatory
ETRETINATE	
Probably inducing cellular differentiation, antiproliferation, antiinflammation, antikeratinization	Antipsoriatic effects
Inhibition of neutrophil chemotaxis	
ACITRETIN	
Probably inducing cellular differentiation, antiproliferation, antiinflammation, antikeratinization	Antipsoriatic effects
Inhibition of neutrophil chemotaxis	
BEXAROTENE	
Transactivate RXR-α,β,γ	Differentiation and antiproliferation of cutaneous T-cell lymphomas
Regulate cellular differentiation and proliferation	

RXR, Retinoid X receptor.

tial studies of the first- and second-generation retinoids (i.e., tretinoin, isotretinoin, and etretinate). Because acitretin is the active metabolite of etretinate, it is assumed that many of its properties are similar to those of the parent compound. Selective mechanisms of action of third-generation arotinoids are discussed later.

Although vitamin A has an important role in vision, reproduction, epithelial differentiation, immune regulation, and growth, the effects of synthetic retinoids used in dermatology are mostly epithelial. It is also important to recognize the roles of other physiologic modulators (e.g., cytokines, vitamin D, steroids, and thyroid hormone) whose actions may converge with retinoids to bring about the final physiobiologic outcomes.

TRANSPORT OF RETINOIDS. A complex of retinol binding protein (RBP) and transthyretin (formerly known as prealbumin) provides transport for retinol in the serum. On hydrolysis of the ester/storage form, retinol is released from the liver. At the cellular level, retinol is bound to a surface receptor and translocated to the nucleus by cytosolic RBP (CRBP). CRBP-I is responsible for cellular uptake of retinol from plasma, solubilizes and renders retinol nontoxic in the cytoplasm, and delivers retinol to appropriate enzymes to form RA (a biologic active form) or retinyl esters (a storage form). CRBP-II and CRBP-III do

◼ Table 13-5 Ligand-Receptor Binding Selectivity Profiles of Available Retinoids[7,9,12,24,25]

Generic Name	RAR			RXR			Comments
	α	β	γ	α	β	γ	
Tretinoin (all-*trans* RA)	+	+	+	−	−	−	RAR-β ->γ >> -α RXR-β,-γ > -α
Alitretinoin (9-*cis* RA)	+	+	+	+	+	+	RXR > RAR
Isotretinoin (13-*cis* RA)	−	−	−	−	−	−	No clearly identified affinity for any retinoid nuclear receptor
Acitretin	−	−	−	−	−	−	RAR (weak interaction)
Bexarotene	−	−	−	+	+	+	RXR-α,β,γ
Adapalene	−	+	+	−	−	−	RAR-β,γ > -α Does not bind to CRABPs
Tazarotene	−	+	+	−	−	−	RAR-β,γ > -α No RXR

not have direct relevance to dermatology.[30] Interaction between CRBP and retinoids does occur, but subsequent cellular events are not clear.[31]

Physiologically, RA is predominantly in the all-*trans* form (ATRA). A small fraction is transported as 13-*cis* RA. Serum transport is by albumin. There is a separate intracellular carrier known as cytosolic retinoic acid binding protein (CRABP) that functions to transport RA to the cell nucleus.[32] CRABP-I modulates the levels of RA in various tissues. CRABP-II is the predominant form in human epidermis and is suggested to modulate the action of RA as a "morphogen."[30,33] In addition, epidermal differentiation is correlated with enhanced CRABP-II expression, and treatment with retinoids results in decreased CRABP-II expression.[33]

CRABP is present in high levels in the epidermis and is markedly elevated in lesional skin of psoriasis (by 800% compared with nonlesional skin), lamellar ichthyosis, lesional Darier's disease, pityriasis rubra pilaris, and keratosis pilaris.[31] High levels of CRABP might indicate a greater sensitivity of the lesions to retinoids. Unlike etretinate, acitretin competes with RA for CRABP.[32] During acitretin therapy, CRABP levels increase by 200% in the nonlesional skin of psoriasis patients, with little to no further increase within psoriatic plaques.[34]

In general, concentrations of these carrier proteins are central to the physiologic and pharmacologic effects of vitamin A and related synthetic retinoids. The epidermis has a much greater concentration of RBP than does dermal tissue.

RETINOID RECEPTORS/GENE TRANSCRIPTION. There are two structurally and pharmacologically distinct families of retinoid receptors, the RA receptor (RAR) family and the retinoid X receptor (RXR) family (Table 13-5). Each family has different receptor subtypes (e.g., α, β, and γ), with each encoded by different genes.[17,24,25] They belong to the large superfamily of receptors consisting also of glucocorticosteroid, thyroid hormone, and vitamin-D₃ receptors, all of which are DNA-binding proteins and functioning as *trans*-acting transcription modulating factors.

Within the cell nucleus, RARs mediate tissue-specific functions, with synthesis of at least 40 proteins influenced by retinol and related retinoids. Acitretin activates all three RAR-subtypes but binds poorly to them.[9,36] RAR-γ is predominantly expressed in human epidermis, suggesting that it is a major mediator of retinoid action in skin.[12] Cross-interaction between acitretin and vitamin-D nuclear receptor is also suggested.[37]

Retinoids can induce both direct and indirect effects on gene transcription. Their *direct* effects are mediated through retinoic acid response elements (RAREs) in the promoter regions of target genes. RAR/RXR heterodimers bind directly to RAREs. There are multiple types of RAREs that allow regulation of gene transcription by RAR/RXR heterodimers, resulting in various physiobiologic and morphogenic effects.[17] Retinoids also down-regulate certain genes that do not have RARE, thus inducing an *indirect* negative effect on gene transcription. The retinoid-receptor complex probably antagonizes various transcription factors, likely mediating many of the retinoid antiproliferative and antiinflammatory effects.[17]

Signaling by RA is mediated through a RAR-RXR heterodimer complex, in which RXR (once thought of as a transcriptionally silent partner) has distinct receptor functions from its RAR-counterpart.[38] They are unique in their ability to function as both homodimeric receptors and as obligate heterodimeric partners to receptors in multiple hormone-mediated pathways such as vitamin-D_3 receptor, thyroid hormone receptor, and peroxisome proliferator-activated receptor.[39] Alitretinoin (9-*cis* RA) has been proposed to be the physiologic ligand for RXRs,[17] whereas bexarotene selectively activates RXRs.[7]

There are three types of retinoid ligands that bind RARs to result in three different types of regulation of gene transcription.[17] Retinoids can behave as agonists, inverse agonists, and neutral antagonists in regard to gene transcription. Further discussion on gene transcription is beyond the scope of this chapter.

IMMUNOLOGIC AND ANTIINFLAMMATORY EFFECTS. Psoriasis is a useful model of retinoid pharmacodynamics. Abnormal cell proliferation is associated with (1) overexpression of IL-6 and IL-8, while IL-1 is decreased,[23,40] (2) overexpression of ICAM-1 and ELAM-1, which are important in regulating lymphocyte migration into the dermis and epidermis, and (3) increased HLA DR positivity.[40] Etretinate can correct the above overexpression of cytokine adhesion molecule and HLA DR abnormalities.[26,40,41]

Arachidonic acid metabolism is altered in psoriasis.[1] Certain retinoids, including etretinate, reduce the release of leukotrienes and hy-

droxyeicosatetraenoic acid (HETE) products, as well as the neutrophil/eosinophil chemotactic effect of these compounds.[42] In contrast, acitretin interferes with the esterification and incorporation of arachidonic acid into nonphosphorus lipids in human keratinocytes.[43]

Retinoids may exert distinct effects on various lymphocyte subsets, such as inhibiting immunoglobulin synthesis from B cells.[23,44] In addition, retinoids (except retinol) consistently reduce the lymphocyte proliferation by 20% to 30% and decrease cytotoxic T-lymphocyte induction.

EFFECTS ON PROTEIN KINASES. Two forms of cyclic adenosine monophosphate (cAMP)–dependent protein kinase A (PKA) have been reported to possess different regulatory subunits, RI and RII. RI is thought to be involved in cell proliferation, whereas RII affects differentiation and growth inhibition.[23] Compared with normal cells, the growth inhibitory activity is decreased in psoriatic fibroblasts, correlating with a deficiency in PKA.[23] Retinoids not only increase the levels and activity of PKA but also promote an increase in binding of cAMP to the RI-cAMP–binding protein.[9,23]

ANTIKERATINIZING EFFECTS. In vitro, retinoids modulate the expression of keratins. Tretinoin and isotretinoin down regulate the proliferative keratins, K6 and K16.[27] After 8 weeks of etretinate (0.75 mg/kg) therapy in 10 patients with extensive psoriasis, a 44% decrease in epidermal thickness and 62% reduction in keratinocyte proliferation were observed.[26] Keratinocyte differentiation is enhanced after etretinate therapy as indicated by increased filaggrin production, increased number and size of keratohyalin granules, greater abundance of keratin filaments, and increased Odland body secretion of intercellular lipids. Retinoids, such as etretinate and acitretin, induce differentiation and reduce hyperplasia in psoriasis.[26]

ANTIACNE AND SEBUM EFFECTS. The exact mechanism of action of retinoids on the sebaceous gland function is unclear. In vitro, tretinoin, isotretinoin, and acitretin inhibit sebocyte proliferation in a dose- and time-dependent manner.[27,28] Isotretinoin is the most potent inhibitor of lipid synthesis (48.2% reduction), followed by tretinoin (38.6% reduction), and then by acitretin (27.5% reduction). These tested retinoids markedly decrease the synthesis of triglycerides, wax/stearyl esters, and free fatty acids in cultured sebocytes; squalene synthesis remains unchanged and cholesterol synthesis slightly increases.[27]

When isotretinoin is administered at 40 mg twice daily, there is an initial reduction of sebaceous gland size accompanied by decreased differentiation to mature sebocytes. The result is a 70% to 90% decrease in sebum production. Within 1 month after cessation of therapy, sebum production returns to about 40% below baseline levels.[1]

Regulation of sebum production requires the local conversion of testosterone to the active hormone 5α-dihydrotestosterone (DHT) by the enzyme 5α-reductase. Isotretinoin can produce a 80% reduction of DHT formation and produce over a twofold reduction of androgen receptor–binding capacity.[29,45] These data show that both skin DHT and androgen receptors are sensitive to isotretinoin in acne patients.

Compared with isotretinoin, other first-generation retinoids, such as tretinoin and alitretinoin, are much less sebosuppressive.[46] Second- and third-generation retinoids produce little or no reduction in or altered composition of sebaceous gland lipids.[1]

Acne pathogenesis also includes altered follicular keratinization, which leads to microcomedo formation and subsequent inflammatory lesions. Retinoid-induced normalization of this abnormal keratinization leads to decreased follicular occlusion.[47] With the reduced sebum production, the growth of *Propionibacterium acnes* and subsequent conversion of triglycerides to free fatty acids are decreased. Inhibition of neutrophil chemotaxis is believed to be important for the beneficial effects in acne vulgaris.[1]

APOPTOSIS.   Retinoid-induced apoptosis involves regulation of the expression of apoptosis-linked gene products (BCL-2 and tissue transglutaminase), degradation of Sp1 transcription factor, and activation of tumor suppression proteins (p21, p38, p53) and caspase proteolytic activity.[48-50] Direct apoptosis of tumor and mye-

loid leukemia cells is relevant to the antineoplastic role of retinoids.

ANTITUMOR AND ANTIPROLIFERATIVE EFFECTS.   Psoriasis is associated with an overexpression of epidermal growth factor receptor (EGF-R) and transforming growth factor-α (TGF-α). In addition, ornithine decarboxylase (ODC), the rate-limiting enzyme in the biosynthesis of polyamines, is highly elevated in the hyperplastic epidermis of psoriasis.[40] Retinoids directly inhibit ODC and lessen the inflammatory hyperplasia that results from an activation of this enzyme.[23,40] Moreover, EGF-signal transduction is important in ODC gene regulation. Tazarotene normalizes EGF-R expression.[40] Certain retinoids (especially isotretinoin and arotinoic acid) inhibit EGF binding to keratinocytes and are significant modulators of this polyamine pathway.[51] This polyamine pathway has been associated with the initiation and promotion of rodent papillomas, which are a useful model of human actinic keratoses. Retinoids inhibit both ODC activation and the proliferation associated with increased polyamine synthesis.[1]

It has long been known that various epithelial structures undergo squamous metaplasia during vitamin A deficiency.[1] The subsequent replacement of vitamin A normalizes this altered keratinization.

Retinoid inhibition of expression of selected oncogenes and activation of tumor suppression genes linking to apoptosis are probably important.[50,52] The expression of RAR-β is selectively lost in premalignant oral lesions and can be restored by treatment with isotretinoin. Restoration of RAR-β expression is associated with a clinical response in these premalignant lesions.[53]

Heat shock proteins (HSP) are a group of highly conserved polypeptides that are involved in cellular response to heat, physical, or chemical stresses. In addition, HSP are important in cellular differentiation. Certain retinoids (tretinoin and alitretinoin) induce a reduction of HSP-70 in myeloid leukemia cells.[54] In addition, cyclooxygenase-2 (COX-2) expression is up regulated in transformed cells and tumors and involved in the synthesis of prostaglandins. Retinoids markedly suppress the production of COX-2 and PGE_2.[55] Inhibition of angiogenic response in tumors has been demonstrated by retinoids.[44,56]

EFFECTS ON INTERCELLULAR MATRIX COMPONENTS.

In normal skin influenced by retinoids (at physiologic concentrations), there is an increase in mucopolysaccharides, collagen, and fibronectin synthesis, and a decrease in collagenase production.[57] It is not known how retinoids stimulate fibroblasts to produce intercellular substances that also enhance wound healing. The wounded epidermis contains unusually high amounts of alitretinoin, which may be responsible for tissue regeneration.[58]

Matrix glycosaminoglycans (GAG) have been functionally implicated in cellular interactions, and have a specific role in adhesion and growth rates. Stimulation of GAG secretion in fibroblasts from psoriatic skin occurs at low concentrations of retinoids, whereas inhibition occurs at high concentrations. At nonphysiologic concentrations, retinoids inhibit the proliferation of human fibroblasts.[59,60] Moreover, synthesis of collagenous proteins, type I and type III collagen, is also decreased.[60] These findings may explain why retinoids, especially at high doses, interfere with wound healing. Retinoids are also known to inhibit collagenase activity, which suggests theoretic efficacy in recessive dystrophic epidermolysis bullosa.[1]

EFFECTS ON EMBRYONIC DEVELOPMENT AND MORPHOGENESIS.

Vitamin A and retinoids participate in the formation of diverse embryonic structures (face, heart, eye, limb, and nervous system). Studies of retinoid-deficient and retinoid-treated embryos confirm that ligand-receptor interactions are essential for embryonic development and morphogenesis.[61] In the pregnant mouse model, all RAR-agonists are strong teratogens with varying degrees of potency. A low-to-absent teratogenic response of RXR-agonists is observed. Those retinoids devoid of RAR or RXR selectivity are likely nonteratogenic.[62]

OTHER RETINOID EFFECTS.

RAR/RXR-mediated pathways can modulate infections caused by cytomegalovirus (CMV), Epstein-Barr virus (EBV), hepatitis B virus (HBV), and human papillomavirus (HPV).[63-66] RAR genes have been identified in developing follicles, with a role in hair growth and patterning.[67] Retinoids induce both synthesis and expression of connexin-43, a gap junctional protein involved in communication between cells.[68] Reduction of intracellular levels of free calcium may be one pathway for the modulation of cellular events by retinoids.[69]

ACTIVITIES OF AROTINOIDS.

The arotinoids have a 1000-fold increase in potency (dose for dose) compared with the first- and second-generation retinoids.[17] Unlike isotretinoin, arotinoids have little-to-no antiseborrheic activity. Based on both in vitro and in vivo studies of their effects on keratinocyte differentiation, arotinoids have a much higher antikeratinizing potential than second-generation retinoids. Among the third-generation retinoids, arotinoic acid is the most potent antikeratinizing agent. Although the therapeutic response of retinoids against advanced cancers is disappointing, arotinoids emerged as promising differentiation and chemopreventive agents. Particularly, the glucuronide derivatives of retinoids/arotinoids hold promising potential in this regard due to their high therapeutic indexes.

CLINICAL USE

Table 13-6 lists indications and contraindications for retinoids.

Practical Considerations

Concomitant vitamin A therapy should be limited to less than 5000 IU vitamin A per day. Oral administration with milk or fatty foods (ideally in moderation) enhances retinoid absorption. Patients should be advised not to consume alcohol and an excessively fatty diet. Potential childbearing females must not consume ethanol up to 2 months after cessation of acitretin therapy. In female patients of nonreproductive potential and in males, this conversion of acitretin to etretinate is not an issue.

FDA-Approved Indications

Three dermatoses have FDA approval for systemic retinoid use in severe subsets as outlined in Table 13-6 and in the sections that follow: (1) acitretin (Soriatane) for psoriasis, (2) isotretinoin (Accu-

Table 13-6	Retinoid Indications and Contraindications

FDA-APPROVED INDICATIONS

Psoriasis (acitretin—formerly etretinate)[9,23,70-80]
  Generalized pustular psoriasis
  Erythrodermic psoriasis
  Severe recalcitrant psoriasis
  Severe plaque-type psoriasis

Acne vulgaris (isotretinoin)[6,46,81-85,90,91]
  Nodulocystic acne
  Recalcitrant, especially if any scarring tendency
Mycosis fungoides (bexarotene)[7,92-94]
  Resistant to at least one systemic therapy

OFF-LABEL USES*

Follicular Disorders
Acne-related conditions
  Gram-negative folliculitis[86]
  HIV-associated eosinophilic folliculitis[87]
  Acne with solid facial edema[88,89]
Rosacea[97,98]
  Papulopustular
  Granulomatous rosacea
Hidradenitis suppurativa[99,100]
Dissecting cellulitis of scalp[101,102]

Disorders of Keratinization
Darier's disease[4,103,104]
Pityriasis rubra pilaris[105-108]
Ichthyosis spectrum[4,23,109,110]
Keratodermas[23,111,112]

Chemoprevention of Malignancies
Premalignant conditions[113-115]
Syndromes with increased risk of cutaneous
  malignancy
  Bazex's syndrome[116]
  Muir-Torre syndrome[117]
  Xeroderma pigmentosum[118]
Transplantation patients[119-122]
Frequent BCC or SCC[123-126]
Kaposi's sarcoma[39,127]

Other Inflammatory Dermatoses
Lupus erythematosus[9,128,130]
Lichen planus—oral erosive, palmoplantar[131]
Lichen sclerosus et atrophicus[132,133]

Miscellaneous
Graft-versus-host disease[134]
Human papillomavirus infections[135-139]
Arotinoid use (psoriasis, malignancies)[140-148]

CONTRAINDICATIONS

Absolute
Pregnancy or woman who is likely to become
  pregnant
Noncompliance with contraception
Nursing mothers
Hypersensitivity to parabens (in Accutane
  capsules)

Relative
Leukopenia
Hypothyroidism (in bexarotene patients)
Moderate-to-severe cholesterol or triglyceride
  elevation
Significant hepatic dysfunction
Significant renal dysfunction

PREGNANCY PRESCRIBING STATUS—CATEGORY X

BCC, Basal cell carcinoma; *SCC*, squamous cell carcinoma.
*Not a comprehensive list of off-label uses—see references 1,95,96 and articles in bibliography for additional dermatoses for which retinoids have had anecdotal success.

---

tane) for acne vulgaris, and (3) bexarotene (Targretin) for selected cases of mycosis fungoides.

PSORIASIS. The single indication approved by the FDA for etretinate (Tegison) was severe recalcitrant psoriasis. In 1998, etretinate was discontinued by Roche and replaced by its acid metabolite, acitretin (Soriatane). The forms most responsive to etretinate or acitretin as monotherapy include generalized pustular[1,70] and erythrodermic psoriasis.[23,71,72] Localized pustular psoriasis also improves with retinoids as monotherapy.[23,73] Acitretin use in severe plaque-type psoriasis generally leads to partial improvement and often is more effective when combined with other treatment modalities. Analysis of 385 cases of generalized pustular psoriasis (GPP) reveals that retinoid treatment is effective in 84% of patients, methotrexate in 76% of patients, cyclosporine in 71% of patients, and oral psoralen plus ultraviolet A (PUVA) in 46% of patients.[74]

Acitretin was tested in more than 1000 psoriatic patients from 1985 to 1992 as monotherapy or in combination with other conventional treatment modalities. The duration of these clinical trials ranged from 6 weeks to 12 months with administered doses of 10 to 75 mg/d in noncomparative and placebo-controlled, double-blind settings.[23] In the noncomparative studies (n = 8 to 52/study; 6 weeks to 6 months), the improvement of the psoriasis area severity index (PASI) ranged from 33% to 96%. The placebo-controlled trials (n = 20 to 53/study; 8 weeks to 6 months) showed a dose-dependent improvement of PASI of 6% to 85%.

The Canadian open multicenter study, involving 63 patients with severe psoriasis who took daily doses of 50 mg acitretin for 4 weeks that was then individually adjusted by ± 10 mg at monthly intervals thereafter during a 12-month period, showed that 70% of patients had marked improvement (based on a 7-point rating scale and PASI).[75] From these studies, acitretin at 10 to 25 mg/day conferred responses equal to those of placebo, whereas 50 to 70 mg/day significantly improved psoriasis. The result of this study was confirmed by another double-blind, controlled trial (n = 38) in the United States showing that acitretin dosages of 10 to 25 mg/day were not as effective as 50 to 75 mg/day.[23]

Acitretin induces clearance of psoriasis in a dose-dependent fashion. Overall, higher starting doses appeared to clear psoriasis faster.[23] However, severe adverse effects, such as hair loss and paronychia, occur more frequently if the initial dose was 50 mg/day. The optimal initial dose of acitretin for psoriasis was reported at 25 mg/day.[23] A maintenance dose of 20 to 50 mg/day has been recommended.[9,23] Unlike isotretinoin or etretinate, dosing of acitretin is not based on body weight. Although the recommended drug holidays are theoretically sound, most patients actually suffer relapse within 2 months after discontinuing etretinate or ac-

itretin. In our experience, a reasonable alternative is to reduce dosages to as low as 10 to 25 mg daily or 25 mg every other day for long-term maintenance therapy. Topical therapies are beneficial adjuncts during the maintenance phase.

Of historical interest, etretinate therapy was usually begun at 0.5 to 1 mg/kg/day in divided dosages. A maximal etretinate dosage of 1.5 mg/kg/day was recommended, with a maintenance dosage of 0.25 to 0.75 mg/kg/day. Etretinate improves psoriatic arthritis in 60% of patients.[1] Comparative efficacy of acitretin with etretinate for psoriatic arthritis has not been reported. In short, acitretin has been studied alone[23] and in direct comparison with etretinate for both psoriasis vulgaris and pustular psoriasis, confirming a parallel trend in their therapeutic efficacy and adverse effect profiles.[9,23,72]

Acitretin therapy is effective for psoriasis associated with human immunodeficiency virus (HIV) infection. Optimal results are reported with a dose of 75 mg/day. Acitretin does not appear to have immunosuppressive properties.[76]

ACITRETIN COMBINATION THERAPIES FOR PSORIASIS. Potential combinations include retinoids with PUVA (Re-PUVA),[1,23,77] in which retinoids are given 10 to 14 days before starting PUVA. In actual practice, patients with psoriasis with a slow response to PUVA may receive a retinoid after PUVA has been initiated. In this case, the UVA dose should be reduced by 50% 2 weeks after a retinoid is administered to prevent a photosensitivity reaction.[78] Retinoid therapy is then subsequently tapered once remission has occurred. Later PUVA doses are likewise reduced. Etretinate or acitretin, in combination with UVB, topical steroids, anthralin, or methotrexate, has been beneficial in selected patients.[1,23] The theoretic possibility of synergistic liver toxicity with methotrexate limits this particular combination.

Specific combination of acitretin with PUVA or UVB phototherapy has been assessed in several studies.[77,79,80] Most of these parallel trials ranged from 8 to 12 weeks in duration and involved 34 to 88 psoriasis patients (per study) who were taking 20 to 50 mg of acitretin per day, alone or in combination with PUVA or UVB.[23] The overall improvement rates, whether monotherapy or combination therapy was used, ranged from 50% to over 90% of patients. The response rate for acitretin (A) plus PUVA (A+PUVA) was 75% to 96% of patients with a clearance time of 40 to 57 days after 14 to 17 PUVA exposures. For acitretin plus UVB (A+UVB), response rates were 60% to 95% of patients with time to clearance of 44 to 48 days after 19 to 21 UVB exposures. When given as monotherapy, the response rates were significantly lower in patients receiving acitretin (23% to 75%), UVB (24% to 63%), or PUVA (60% to 80%) alone. The mean and cumulative UVB doses given to reach ≥75% response showed a 42% and 57% reduction, respectively, with A+UVB compared with UVB alone.[9] The mean cumulative dose given to patients receiving A+PUVA was 42% less than that required for patients in the PUVA group alone.[9] Combination therapy using A+UVB or A+PUVA offers advantages in reducing the total UVB or UVA cumulative doses and the number of irradiation exposures. Other potential combination therapies involving acitretin, including combinations with methotrexate, cyclosporine, hydroxyurea, or sulfasalazine, in treating psoriasis have not yet been reported.

ACNE AND RELATED DERMATOSES.   Of all systemic retinoids, only the first-generation agent, isotretinoin, demonstrates superior effectiveness against acne vulgaris.[1,46] After multiple clinical studies[1,6] isotretinoin was released for clinical use in the United States in September 1982. It is officially indicated for severe recalcitrant nodulocystic acne vulgaris having lesions with a tendency for scarring that has been refractory to maximal management, including several systemic antibiotics. Ideally, the isotretinoin therapy is initiated before significant scarring. Typically, 0.5 to 1 mg/kg/day is given in divided doses. An initial response is seen within 8 weeks, and improvement continues through the end of 20-week administration. Of note, the 20-week duration of therapy for acne patients was based on the original clinical trial's protocol designed to evaluate the therapeutic efficacy of isotretinoin for ichthyosis vulgaris.[4,5] More recently, some authors suggested prescribing isotretinoin until a cumulative dose of 120 mg/kg (based on 1 mg/kg/day for 120 days) is attained.[81,82]

Comparisons of 0.1, 0.5, and 1 mg/kg/day suggest similar initial efficacy at all dosages;

however, the two lower dosage options allow more frequent relapses.[47] More significant and frequent adverse effects at 1 mg/kg/day may make 0.5 mg/kg/day more suitable for less severe cases. Should another isotretinoin course be necessary, the recommendation is to wait 8 weeks after completion of the first course. There may be continuing improvement even during the 2 months after cessation of therapy. For trunk involvement and unusually recalcitrant cases, dosages from 1 to 2 mg/kg/day may be required.[1] An early flare-up of disease activity is generally due to cessation of previous systemic antibiotics in addition to the altered cutaneous barrier function that leads to increased granulation tissue and *Staphylococcus aureus* superinfection. Isotretinoin also significantly reduces total numbers of resistant *P. acnes* on the skin of acne patients.[83]

Intermittent or pulse treatment for mild-to-moderate acne has been evaluated. Suggested isotretinoin dose is 0.5 mg/kg/day for 1 week/month for 6 months. Clearance is reported in 88% of patients with a relapse of 39% (in patients with higher acne grade) 1 year after stopping treatment.[84]

Isotretinoin is reported as a drug of choice for nodulocystic acne in patients with end-stage renal disease receiving hemodialysis or renal transplant.[85] Isotretinoin has also been used for gram-negative bacterial folliculitis[86] and HIV-associated eosinophilic folliculitis.[87] Cases of solid persistent facial edema of acne successfully treated with isotretinoin[88] or the combination of isotretinoin (0.5 mg/kg/day) and ketotifen (2 mg/day) have been reported.[89]

Only a minority of patients experience complete clearing, whereas the majority of patients demonstrate marked improvement that is maintained by much less aggressive acne therapy after the discontinuation of isotretinoin. Analysis from cohort studies (n = 237) shows that closed comedonal acne and microcystic acne are the only predictive factors of resistance to isotretinoin treatment, with a relative risk of 2.7. Patients over 20 years of age and severity grade of facial acne greater than scale 3/4 are the predictive factors for relapse, with a relative risk of 0.6 and 1.5, respectively.[90] Endocrinology work-up is recommended in women with a history of acne refractory to conventional treatments and to isotretinoin, especially associated with abnormal menstruation and hirsutism. In such cases, adrenal dysfunction or 5α-reductase hyperactivity has been reported.[91]

CUTANEOUS T-CELL LYMPHOMA (MYCOSIS FUNGOIDES).

In December 1999, the U.S. FDA approved bexarotene (Targretin) for the treatment of cutaneous T-cell lymphoma (CTCL) that is refractory to at least one systemic therapy. There are multiple studies on the use of systemic retinoids in mycosis fungoides (MF), as monotherapy or combination therapy with PUVA, interferon, or systemic chemotherapy.[7,92,93] The best response has been noted in patch- and early plaque-stage disease.[7] Combination therapy of acitretin and calcitriol for MF has been reported.[94]

Bexarotene was evaluated in multicenter, open-label, historically controlled clinical trials (n = 52 to 152 per study).[7] An initial dose of 300 mg/m²/day appears to reduce associated adverse effects, compared with higher dosage options. Based on these studies, overall response (complete and partial response) in the 300 mg/m²/day initial dosing group was observed in 48% of patients (54% in early stage, 45% in advanced stage), and 58% (67% in early stage, 55% in advanced stage) in the 400 mg/m²/day initial dosing group. Time to response was noted within 4 weeks and continued until at least 28 weeks. Remission was generally durable, with a relapse rate of 28% of patients in the 300 mg/m²/day initial dosing group over a median monitoring period of 17 weeks. See the Adverse Effects section regarding a number of important bexarotene adverse effects.

In summary, the data demonstrate a dose-response antitumor efficacy of bexarotene against CTCL.[7] The recommended initial dose of bexarotene (Targretin) capsules is 300 mg/m²/day. Bexarotene should be taken as a single oral daily dose with a meal. Based on the severity of adverse effects, dosage may be down adjusted to 100 to 200 mg/m²/day or temporarily suspended if necessary. When adverse effects are controlled, doses may be carefully escalated. If there is no tumor response after 8 weeks of therapy and if the initial dose of 300 mg/m²/day is well tolerated, the dose may be increased to 400 mg/m²/day with careful monitoring. Ther-

apy with bexarotene may be continued indefinitely based on clinical response.

Off-Label Dermatologic Uses

Only a selected group of off-label uses of systemic retinoids are discussed here, and these conditions were chosen based on reasonable literature support for clinical efficacy. Reviews by Ellis and Voorhees[95] and by Dicken[96] are useful sources for uncommon, anecdotal retinoid uses.[1] Retinoid use in these conditions should be considered experimental. When pertinent, data on response of these dermatoses to etretinate are presented when comparable studies evaluating acitretin are not available.

ROSACEA.

Only a small number of studies investigated the use of isotretinoin in rosacea.[1] Therapeutic response has been greatest in treatment of the papulopustular variety and minimal in treatment of the vascular form of rosacea. At least two thirds of patients have a good response. The majority of rosacea patients sustained improvement for more than a year after isotretinoin discontinuation. Isolated cases of granulomatous rosacea respond as well. The dose range (0.5 to 1 mg/kg/day), rate of response, and duration of therapy are similar to those of isotretinoin used in acne vulgaris.[97,98] Isotretinoin should be reserved for severe cases of rosacea unresponsive to common forms of treatment.

HIDRADENITIS SUPPURATIVA AND DISSECTING CELLULITIS OF SCALP.

Only a few reports describe the use of retinoids in hidradenitis suppurativa (HS).[99,100] The response to isotretinoin is less than in acne vulgaris or rosacea. Also, higher dosages in the range of 1 to 2 mg/kg/day are required. About 50% of the patients cleared or improved significantly with 0.7 to 1.2 mg/kg/day of isotretinoin. Treatment is more successful in the milder forms of HS. Monotherapy with isotretinoin usually has a limited therapeutic effect. Dissecting cellulitis of the scalp is a related condition for which there have been a few anecdotal reports of a significant therapeutic response to isotretinoin.[101,102] An isotretinoin dosage range of at least 1 mg/kg/day is suggested; higher doses up to 2 mg/kg/day may be required for selected cases of dissecting cellulitis of the scalp.

DARIER'S DISEASE.   Since the initial report detailing retinoid use in lamellar ichthyosis, Darier's disease, and pityriasis rubra pilaris, first- and second-generation retinoids have been the innovative mainstay of treatment in most disorders of keratinization.[4] These disorders typically respond better to etretinate or acitretin than to isotretinoin.[1] A possible exception to this generalization would be isotretinoin for Darier's disease.[103] However, etretinate and acitretin are also effective in Darier's disease.[104] Episodic retinoid use, particularly in the months when the disease is expected to flare-up (warm seasons of the year), is prudent. Four- to six-month courses during these months enhance the maintenance therapy by topical measures for the remainder of the year. Although dosages of 0.5 to 1 mg/kg/day of all three drugs are generally recommended, a lower starting dose of 0.2 to 0.3 mg/kg/day may prevent the initial flare-up commonly seen in many patients treated with retinoids. Retinoids are most effective with widespread hyperkeratotic forms of Darier's disease. In such cases, acitretin may be therapeutically better than isotretinoin due to its stronger antikeratinizing property. Nevertheless, there is no existing study comparing the efficacy between first- and second-generation retinoids in Darier's disease.

PITYRIASIS RUBRA PILARIS.   Retinoid use in pityriasis rubra pilaris (PRP) has been reported.[105-108] Goldsmith and colleagues[108] evaluated 45 patients with PRP treated with isotretinoin, the largest study to date. A dosage of 1 to 1.5 mg/kg/day of isotretinoin or 1 mg/kg/day of etretinate induced significant improvement in approximately 70% of the patients in this study. A small but significant percentage of the patients achieve a sustained remission with therapy. The use of acitretin for PRP has not been reported. It is assumed that acitretin is probably effective for PRP when given within the same dose range as noted previously with etretinate.

ICHTHYOSIS.   The most frequent use of retinoids other than severe cystic acne and recalcitrant psoriasis is lamellar ichthyosis, in which management with etretinate and acitretin has distinctive advantages over isotretinoin.[109,110]

Lamellar ichthyosis associated with Sjögren-Larsson syndrome typically responds well to both etretinate and acitretin.[23] Because most cases of ichthyosis present in childhood, careful risk-benefit analysis needs to be addressed. The lower maintenance dose required of the second-generation retinoids may decrease the risk of premature epiphyseal closure and diffuse idiopathic skeletal hyperostoses (DISH)–like complications. In lamellar ichthyosis, the response to retinoid therapy and acceptance of the adverse effect profile are superior to those of other forms of ichthyosis.[4]

In ichthyosis vulgaris and recessive X-linked ichthyosis, the limited severity of the disease generally does not require retinoid use, even though these are retinoid-responsive conditions.[1,23] Acitretin at 35 mg/day provides the best efficacy with minimal adverse effects for recessive X-linked ichthyosis. Retinoid therapy for epidermolytic hyperkeratosis (bullous congenital ichthyosiform erythroderma) may lead to an initial increase in bullae. This bullous flare is less likely when the initial dosage of etretinate is 0.25 mg/kg/day and is increased gradually. Details on a number of other ichthyosis variants with case reports suggesting retinoid efficacy are beyond the scope of this chapter.

Compared with the isotretinoin dosage (≥ 2 mg/kg/day) needed to improve ichthyosis, etretinate or acitretin generally leads to good responses in the range of 0.5 to 1 mg/kg/day.[1] A significant response typically occurs during the first 2 months of therapy. After that time, the maintenance dose can be reduced to 25 mg/day. Acitretin therapy for children with inherited keratinization disorders is best started at 0.5 mg/kg/day. When basing acitretin dosages on etretinate literature reports, a 20% reduction is recommended if the etretinate dose is over 0.75 mg/kg/day or if adverse effects are dose-limiting.[109,110] As with Darier's disease, most patients with the severe forms of ichthyosis are willing to tolerate the significant adverse effects of retinoids, given the lack of efficacious alternatives.

KERATODERMAS.   The response rate and dosage range of second-generation retinoids for various forms of keratodermas are quite similar to those of ichthyosis.[1,23] Keratoderma subtypes responding well include palmoplantar hyperkeratosis of recessive hidrotic ectodermal dysplasia,[111] pachyonychia congenita tarda,[112] Unna-Thost, and punctate forms with or without epidermolytic hyperkeratosis.[1] The recessive forms with transgrediens, such as Papillon-Lefèvre syndrome and mal de Meleda, likewise respond well.[1,23] In Vohwinkel's syndrome (keratoderma hereditaria mutilans), both keratoderma and pseudoainhum improve. Caution should be exercised in patients with associated epidermolytic hyperkeratosis and the epidermolytic form of palmoplantar keratoderma because large erosions may occur with retinoid therapy. These patients should be started at low doses with a gradual increase in dosages to avoid a flare-up in the number of erosions or bullae.[1]

CHEMOPREVENTION—PREMALIGNANT CUTANEOUS DISEASES.

Despite low therapeutic responses of advanced cancers to retinoids, these drugs appear to have a promising role in chemoprevention. Patients with oral leukoplakia, actinic keratoses, arsenical keratoses, and Bowen's disease can benefit from retinoid therapy.[1,113,114] Keratoacanthomas and bowenoid papulosis are also retinoid-responsive.[1] PUVA-induced keratoses (either numerous lesions or in patients who have had prior squamous cell carcinomas [SCC]) may respond to systemic retinoids.[115] Only patients with either severe or recalcitrant versions of the above premalignant conditions should be treated with systemic retinoids. Therapy needs to be maintained indefinitely to sustain clinical improvement.[1]

CHEMOPREVENTION—SYNDROMES WITH INCREASED RISK OF CUTANEOUS MALIGNANCIES.

Successful retinoid therapy has been reported in patients with basal cell nevus syndrome, paraneoplastic acrokeratosis (Bazex's syndrome), xeroderma pigmentosum, Muir-Torre syndrome, and epidermodysplasia verruciformis.[116,117] In long-term therapy for chemoprevention of basal cell nevus syndrome and xeroderma pigmentosum, clinicians administered high-dose isotretinoin therapy, at least 2 mg/kg/day.[117,118] Isotretinoin therapeutic benefits are countered by significant adverse reactions. Second-generation retinoids will more likely be efficacious and well tolerated at ≤1 mg/kg/day.

CHEMOPREVENTION—USE IN TRANSPLANTATION PATIENTS/OTHER HIGH-RISK GROUPS.

Despite common cutaneous malignancies in all organ transplantation settings, this problem seems to be the greatest for renal transplant patients. A double-blind, placebo-controlled study evaluated the effect of acitretin 30 mg/day in 44 renal transplant recipients during a 6-month treatment period. Then acitretin group showed significantly fewer keratotic skin lesions (13% versus 28%) and new SCC lesions (11% versus 47%) as compared with the placebo group.[119]

Three other studies are important for transplantation patients receiving retinoid therapy. Acitretin was given to renal transplantation patients with frequent skin malignancies (especially SCC) at either 10 to 50 mg daily[120] or 0.3 mg/kg/day.[121] Significantly reduced rates of new cutaneous malignancies were documented in 2 of 4 patients[120] and 12 of 16 patients,[121] respectively. Etretinate dosed at 0.3 mg/kg/day in a separate study produced similar results.[122] Dosage reductions based on intolerance to acitretin are common. The bottom line is that well-controlled studies are ideally needed; in the meantime, these studies give some guidance in approaching high-risk patients.

Acitretin (60 mg/day) is effective in suppressing the occurrence of new SCC during high-dose PUVA and cyclosporine therapy.[123] In addition, premalignant lesions of the oral mucosa, larynx, trachea, bladder, and cervix have all responded to systemic retinoid therapy.[1] Retinoids also reduce the occurrence of second primaries in patients with treated head and neck cancer.[113] An important area of research would be to maximize the therapeutic benefit through proper drug and dose selection with hopes of minimizing the significant adverse effect profile that frequently limits long-term therapy of these conditions.

Systemic retinoids can be of value in a wide variety of patients at high risk for frequent cutaneous malignancies.[124] Peck and colleagues[125] demonstrated a marked reduction in formation of new basal cell carcinomas with isotretinoin at an average maintenance dose of 1.5 mg/kg/day. These patients had previously formed numerous basal cell carcinomas as a result of actinic damage without signs of basal cell nevus syndrome. In contrast, the Southwest Skin Cancer Prevention Study Group (n = 525) reported no beneficial effects after 3-year treatment with either retinol (25,000 U/day) or isotretinoin (5 to 10 mg/day) to prevent nonmelanoma skin cancers when compared with placebo.[126] However, the lack of observed beneficial effects might be due to the much lower doses of retinoids tested in this clinical trial.

KAPOSI'S SARCOMA.   Although a number of retinoids (e.g., tretinoin, isotretinoin, alitretinoin, acitretin, and Ro 13-1470) have been tested for inhibitory activity against Kaposi's sarcoma (KS),[39,127] no oral formulation is yet approved by the FDA for this condition. Only topical alitretinoin 0.1% gel (Panretin, Ligand Pharmaceuticals) is approved by the FDA for cutaneous KS.[39]

LUPUS ERYTHEMATOSUS.   Both isotretinoin and etretinate have been used successfully by patients with various cutaneous forms of lupus erythematosus.[9,128,129] A good response occurs in the hyperkeratotic variety of discoid lupus erythematosus. Patients with generalized discoid lupus (without hyperkeratosis) and subacute lupus erythematosus also responded. Both isotretinoin and etretinate have been beneficial in the range of 1 mg/kg/day with response within 4 weeks in the majority of patients. This response is typically not sustainable after discontinuation of the drug.

The efficacy of acitretin (50 mg/day; n = 28) was compared with that of hydroxychloroquine (400 mg/day; n = 30) in patients with cutaneous lupus erythematosus.[130] After 8-week therapy, overall improvement occurred in 46% of patients treated with acitretin and in 50% of patients treated with hydroxychloroquine. Incidence of adverse effects was higher in the acitretin group.

LICHEN PLANUS.   Both isotretinoin and etretinate used in the range of 1 mg/kg/day give equally mediocre results.[1] Although many patients respond within 4 weeks, the majority have insufficient improvement to warrant long-term retinoid therapy, in view of the significant adverse effects that these drugs create. Acitretin was evaluated in a multicenter, double-blind, placebo-controlled study (n = 65) for lichen planus. Af-

ter 8-week therapy with acitretin 30 mg/day, 64% of patients showed remission or marked improvement compared with placebo (13% improvement). During a subsequent 8-week open phase, 83% of previously placebo-treated patients responded favorably to acitretin therapy.[131] The important retinoid use would be for widespread, hypertrophic type or erosive oral type of lichen planus, for which retinoids alone or in combination with low-dose corticosteroids may be beneficial. In our experience, combining a systemic corticosteroid with a retinoid is much more effective to control such severe cases.

LICHEN SCLEROSUS ET ATROPHICUS. Retinoids may present as alternative to topical estrogen, testosterone, and corticosteroid for selected women with vulvar lichen sclerosus et atrophicus (LSA).[1] Moderate-to-significant improvement of LSA has been observed with etretinate therapy. In a larger, noncontrolled study (n = 20), etretinate (0.54 mg/kg/day initial dose and 0.26 mg/kg/day maintenance dose) reduced pruritus and burning symptoms as early as within 2 weeks. The disease severity was improved in 95% of patients and in 93% of severe cases, confirmed by histopathologic findings.[132] In a multicenter, randomized, placebo-controlled, double-blind trial involving 46 women with severe LSA, acitretin 20 to 30 mg/day for 16 weeks appeared effective. A significantly higher number of responders were observed in the acitretin group (64%) as compared with the placebo group (25%).[133]

GRAFT-VERSUS-HOST DISEASE.   An open study of patients with chronic graft-versus-host disease (GVHD) who have the sclerodermatous skin change, resulting from allogeneic bone marrow transplantation, showed a significant response after 3 months of therapy with etretinate.[134] Most patients failed to respond to three or more agents before etretinate treatment. Among 27 patients, 74% showed improvement including softening of skin, flattening of cutaneous lesions, increasing range of motion, and improved performance status.

HPV INFECTIONS.   Treatment of extensive warts with etretinate has been reported.[135,136] Isotretinoin is effective in the eradication of a persistent rectal ulcer associated with HPV-33 in an HIV-positive patient.[137] Combination of retinoids and IFN-α or γ can inhibit oncogene expression of HPV.[138,139] Given the role of various HPV in induction and growth of a variety of skin lesions (such as verruca, bowenoid papulosis, condyloma acuminatum, giant condyloma of Buschke-Löwenstein, verrucous carcinoma, epidermodysplasia verruciformis, oral florid papillomatosis, and Bowen's disease of the digits), systemic retinoids may have therapeutic potential in patients with these conditions.

THERAPEUTIC APPLICATIONS OF AROTINOIDS.
The sole indication for the arotinoid bexarotene by the FDA is refractory CTCL. Besides CTCL, other neoplasms also show promising results.[140-144] Successful therapeutic trials with other arotinoids have been reported for psoriasis and psoriatic arthritis.[23,145-148] In general, arotinoids are distinguished by a 1000-fold increase in potency over that of first- and second-generation retinoids, with a dosage range of 20 to 150 µg/day. In spite of this very low dosage range, their therapeutic index is similar to those of other synthetic retinoids, yet their low dosages produce serum drug levels that are difficult to measure.

FUTURE APPLICATION OF RETINOIDS.
Observations of the RAR/RXR-mediated pathway affecting CMV, EBV, HBV, and HPV infections will likely prompt future investigations of the potential role of retinoids or retinoid antagonists in antiviral therapy for infections with these viruses.[63-66]

Adverse Effects
Box 13-1 lists potentially serious adverse effects due to systemic retinoids. Acitretin may be less well tolerated than etretinate at therapeutically equivalent doses.[71] At high dosages, acitretin tends to cause more discomfort than etretinate, particularly with regard to hair loss, palmoplan-

Box 13-1

Potentially Serious Adverse Effects Due to Systemic Retinoids[149-154]

TERATOGENICITY (SEE BOX 13-2)
Retinoic acid embryopathy
Spontaneous abortions

OCULAR
Reduced night vision
Persistent dry eyes
Staphylococcus aureus infections

BONE
Diffuse interstitial skeletal hyperostosis (DISH)
Osteophyte formation
Osteoporotic changes in long bones
Premature epiphyseal closure

LIPIDS
Hypercholesterolemia*
Hypertriglyceridemia

GASTROINTESTINAL
Inflammatory bowel disease flare
Pancreatitis† (due to ↑↑ triglycerides)

HEPATIC
Transaminase elevations
Toxic hepatitis (rarely)

OTHER ENDOCRINE EFFECTS
Hypothyroidism†
Diabetes mellitus (controversial)

HEMATOLOGIC
Leukopenia†
Agranulocytosis†

NEUROLOGIC
Pseudotumor cerebri
Depression—suicidal ideation

MUSCLE
Myopathy

*Theoretically increased coronary artery disease risk with long-term therapy.
†Primarily a risk with bexarotene (Targretin).

tar peeling, and minor musculoskeletal complaints. Short-term use of isotretinoin in severe acne is generally safe and is associated with minimal, reversible adverse effects provided pregnancy is avoided.

An imposing list of potential adverse effects should be considered when the synthetic retinoids are prescribed. An individualized, careful assessment of risk-benefit ratio followed by diligent surveillance for adverse effects and careful management of the adverse effects when present are of paramount importance.

TERATOGENICITY.   Teratogenicity is the most important adverse effect of the retinoids (Box 13-2). Although doses of 10,000 IU/day or less of preformed vitamin A (retinyl esters and retinol) are considered safe, doses greater than 10,000 IU/day as supplements (without concurrent synthetic retinoid intake) were reported to cause malformations in a single epidemiologic study.[157] The recommended dietary allowance of preformed vitamin A for pregnant women is 2670 IU/day or 800 RE/day.[158]

The teratogenic threshold has not been established for synthetic retinoids in humans. Therefore there is no safe minimal dose for use during pregnancy.[7,10] The recommended duration of contraception after stopping retinoid therapy varies among different classes of retinoids (see Clinical Use section) and mainly reflects their pharmacokinetic profiles. Based on individual age, culture, religion/belief, and preference, a patient may refuse to take birth control pills or use other contraceptives. In such cases, *absolute* abstinence of sexual intercourse is required and must be enforced by parents of under-aged patients.

Common sites of retinoid-induced malformations include auditory, cardiovascular, craniofacial, axial and acral skeletal, central nervous system, and thymic abnormalities (see Box 13-2). The putative mechanism involves toxic effects on cephalic neural crest development, particularly with exposure between 3 and 6 weeks of gestation.[149] These abnormalities occur in almost 50% of full-term pregnancies in which there was first-trimester exposure to isotretinoin.[1] Spontaneous abortions occur in one

Box 13-2

Major Components of Retinoid Teratogenicity[154-156]

CARDIOVASCULAR ABNORMALITIES
Atrial/ventricular septal defects
Hypoplastic/interrupted aortic arch
Overriding aorta
Abnormal origin subclavian arteries

CRANIOFACIAL ABNORMALITIES
Cleft palate
Depressed midface
Jaw malformation
Triangular microcephalic skull

OCULAR ABNORMALITIES
Microphthalmia
Optic nerve atrophy

AUDITORY ABNORMALITIES
Microtia
Absent auditory canals
Conductive hearing loss
Sensorineural hearing loss
Vestibular dysfunction

OTHER BONE ABNORMALITIES
Absent clavicle and scapula
Aplasia/hypoplasia of long bones
Short sternum
Sternoumbilical raphe
Absent thumb

CNS ABNORMALITIES
Abnormal cortical tracts
Agenesis of cerebellar vermis
Hydrocephalus
Leptomeningeal neuroglial heterotopias
Meningomyelocele
Microcephaly

OTHER ABNORMALITIES
Thymic aplasia or hypoplasia
Anal and vaginal atresia

third of exposed pregnancies, and there is an increased number of stillbirths.[1] The incidence of acitretin- and etretinate-induced teratogenicity is lower,[149] perhaps because the patient population receiving second-generation retinoids is older and because these drugs were released much later than isotretinoin.

To date, two of six known fetal outcomes associated with acitretin use during pregnancy had malformations consistent with retinoid embryopathy.[151] In addition, numerous acral skeletal abnormalities are known to occur with exposure to retinoids during pregnancy.

Patients at greatest risk for retinoid teratogenesis are young patients, especially those who cannot comply with contraceptive measures. Of all isotretinoin-associated pregnancy reports in which contraceptive history was available, no contraception was used in 50% of patients.[1]

The conversion of acitretin to etretinate in patients consuming alcohol has been confirmed.[10,151] However, etretinate is not detected in the patient serum after administration of acitretin alone.[10] Based on these data, there is a sustained, potential risk of teratogenicity from acitretin conversion to etretinate induced by alcohol and a real justification of the 3-year delay for planning conception. If the patient absolutely does not drink alcohol, a 3-year mandated contraception is questionable because elimination of acitretin only requires a 2-month period at most. One must keep in mind that many "nonalcoholic" edibles and over-the-counter preparations actually contain some amounts of ethanol. It is not clear what quantity of ingested alcohol is required for the reesterification of acitretin to etretinate.

In men, retinoid therapy does not appear to influence spermatogenesis, sperm morphology, sperm motility, or the hypothalamic-pituitary-gonadal axis.[9] Seven pregnancies have been reported to be associated with the male partner taking acitretin at the time of conception. None of these resulted in malformations typical of retinoid embryopathy.[10] However, no conclusion can be drawn from these limited data. Because there is inadequate pharmacokinetic study of retinoids in the semen and subsequent transfer to the female, it is not known whether retinoids present in seminal fluid pose a risk to the developing fetus. Male patients taking

bexarotene (and perhaps with other synthetic retinoids) must use condoms during therapy and for 1 month after the last dose of the drug if sexually active.[91]

OCULAR EFFECTS.   The initial report of ocular adverse effects was in 1979, describing isotretinoin-induced blepharoconjunctivitis,[1] occurring in 20% to 50% of patients (Box 13-3). *S. aureus* colonization of the conjunctival sac increases significantly (7% versus 62% of patients) during isotretinoin therapy.[159] However, bacterial conjunctivitis develops in only 7% of patients. Corneal erosions leading to corneal opacities may rarely occur. These opacities slowly resolve after discontinuation of the drug. Rarely cataracts have been reported.

The mechanism responsible for dry eyes and corneal and conjunctival adverse effects is believed to be decreased tear formation, as well as decreased lipid content in the tears.[1] Abnormalities of retinal function with abnormal night vision can occur and are most likely due to interference of the retinoids with steps in the visual pigment (rhodopsin) cycle. There have been rare cases of persistent dry eyes and persistent abnormal night vision. Pseudotumor cerebri, manifested by abnormal vision with nausea, vomiting, headache, and papilledema, has been reported primarily with isotretinoin (see Central Nervous System Effects section).

In 15 of 79 patients receiving bexarotene, new cataracts or worsening of previous cataracts were found with serial slit-lamp examinations.[7] Confounding variables include the high number of elderly subjects (64% were 60 years of age or older) and the lack of a control group.

In general, management of symptoms from dry eyes is the most frequent patient intervention. Artificial tears used regularly may alleviate symptoms of blepharoconjunctivitis. Particularly with isotretinoin, topical antistaphylococcal antibiotics may be useful when clinical findings of blepharoconjunctivitis are present.

There are no specific ocular monitoring guidelines. However, any abnormality of vision that is not corrected with the use of artificial tears should be evaluated. Patients with visual abnormalities accompanied by headache, nausea, and vomiting should be promptly referred to a neurologist to rule out pseudotumor cere-

Box 13-3

Relatively Common Minor Adverse Effects Due to Systemic Retinoids[149-151,153]

CUTANEOUS
Xerosis
Palmoplantar, digital desquamation
Retinoid dermatitis
Photosensitivity
Pyogenic granulomas
Stickiness sensation—palms, soles
Staphylococcus aureus infections

HAIR
Telogen effluvium
Abnormal hair texture, dryness

NAILS
Fragility with nail softening
Paronychia
Onycholysis

OCULAR
Dry eyes with visual blurring
Blepharoconjunctivitis
Photophobia

ORAL
Cheilitis, especially lower lip
Dry mouth
Sore mouth and tongue

NASAL
Nasal mucosa dryness
Decreased mucus secretion
Epistaxis

MUSCULOSKELETAL
Arthralgias
Myalgias
Fatigue, muscle weakness
Tendinitis

NEUROLOGIC
Headache
Mild depression

GASTROINTESTINAL
Nausea
Diarrhea
Abdominal pain

---

bri. Ophthalmologic evaluation for patients with altered night vision includes dark-adaptation testing and possibly an electroretinogram or electrooculogram.[1]

BONE EFFECTS.   Adverse effects associated with synthetic retinoids closely resemble the bone findings of hypervitaminosis-A,[1] such as remodeling abnormalities of long bones, decalcification, progressive calcification of ligaments and tendon insertions, cortical hyperostosis, periosteal thickening, premature epiphyseal closure, and probably osteoporosis. Although it has been known since 1933 that vitamin A can cause bone abnormalities, the mechanism of this effect remains elusive. Recent work suggests a possible relationship between retinoids and certain cytokine actions, which result in enhanced maturation of the preosteoblast.[160]

The risk of synthetic retinoid-induced hy-perostoses and DISH syndrome–like bone changes in psoriasis, disorders of keratinization, and acne therapy has been studied by many investigators with conflicting results.[1] The initial report was by Pittsley and Yoder in 1983.[161] Findings resembling DISH syndrome are detected in up to 26% of isotretinoin-treated patients and 30% of etretinate-treated patients, respectively. Specific findings include osteophytes, with or without bridging, in the absence of disk space narrowing, along with anterior spinal ligament calcification and extraspinal calcification of other tendons and ligaments.[23] Patients are frequently asymptomatic at sites where there are calcifications.[1] High-risk patients are those taking any retinoid at high doses for long durations. Older patients and those with previous arthritis are probably at increased risk. Spinal cord compression with neurologic deficit after long-term etretinate therapy has been reported.[1]

Skeletal changes associated with acitretin deserve attention during long-term treatment. In two prospective studies (n = 63), asymptomatic osteoarticular aberrations (n = 12) with disk space narrowing at the thoracic spine levels (n = 7) and skeletal calcifications (n = 2) in the forearms and hips (not detected in the pretreatment radiographic evaluations) were found.[9] One case report of extensive extraspinal hyperostosis and bridging exostosis in the left hip occurred after 13 years of acitretin use.[9] In a noncontrolled study of 241 psoriasis patients who were treated with acitretin for as long as 2 years, skeletal hyperostosis, degenerative spondylosis, facet arthritis, and syndesmophytes occurred in only 5% of patients.[23]

Vitamin D response (VDR)/RXR heterodimers can activate VDR elements (VDRE) and may activate VDR target genes, possibly leading to accelerated bone resorption.[144] However, current data suggest but cannot confirm that osteoporosis is associated with retinoid use. After 6 months of isotretinoin treatment for cystic acne, bone density decreased by 4.4% without alteration of calcium metabolism when compared with controls.[162] Another study cited chronic therapy (2 years or longer) with etretinate was associated with decreased bone mineral density but not with isotretinoin.[163] Patients with preexisting osteoporosis or at increased risk for developing osteoporosis independent of retinoid therapy should receive preventive therapy, such as calcium and vitamin D, and possibly estrogens or bisphosphonates.

To date, five cases of premature epiphyseal closure in children have been reported, involving both isotretinoin and etretinate therapy.[1,164] The epiphyseal closure is generally partial, associated with prolonged and very high dose retinoid therapy, and accompanied by other confounding factors such as concomitant or prior vitamin A use.

There are no official guidelines for monitoring of bone-related adverse effects. Baseline x-rays are not required, although worth considering in high-risk groups described later.[9] Yearly screening x-rays (lateral thoracic spine and ankle films) of high-risk sites are optional but should be considered for patients with known pretreatment radiologic abnormalities, with prominent musculoskeletal symptoms, and with

prolonged high-dose therapy.[130,202] Radiographs of significantly symptomatic sites are considered useful. The height of children should be recorded before and during retinoid therapy.

Minor musculoskeletal complaints in the absence of radiographic changes are very common, occurring in up to 20% of retinoid-treated patients.[1] In general, musculoskeletal complaints are managed with conservative antiinflammatory drugs and rest. The retinoid dose can be reduced if the symptoms persist.[166]

LIPID EFFECTS. The most frequently detected laboratory abnormalities induced by systemic retinoids are elevated serum lipids. Bexarotene induces major lipid abnormalities in humans.[7] Approximately 70% of treated patients with initial bexarotene doses >300 mg/m²/day had fasting triglyceride levels greater than 2.5 times (800 to 1200 mg/dl) the upper normal limit. Cholesterol levels above 300 mg/dl occurred in up to 75% of patients. High-density lipoprotein (HDL) cholesterol levels <25 mg/dl were observed in up to 92% of patients (Table 13-7). Based on these findings, it is recommended that atorvastatin (a lipid-lowering agent) should be coadministered with bexarotene to lower the risk of hyperlipidemia and pancreatitis. The clinician should be aware that atorvastatin (and other "statins") are less effective in lowering triglyceride elevations than for reduction of cholesterol levels; however, the more efficacious agent for triglyceride eleva-

■ **Table 13-7**　Laboratory Test Abbreviations

ALT	Alanine aminotransferase
AST	Aspartate aminotransferase
CBC	Complete blood count
CPK	Creatine phosphokinase
HDL	High-density lipoprotein (cholesterol)
LDL	Low-density lipoprotein (cholesterol)
SGOT	Serum glutamate oxaloacetate transaminase
SGPT	Serum glutamate pyruvic transaminase
T_4	Thyroxine-4
TSH	Thyroid-stimulating hormone

tions (gemfibrozil) cannot be used concomitantly with bexarotene due to an important drug interaction.[7,167] Fenofibrate (Tricor) is a reasonable alternative to gemfibrozil.

Isotretinoin, etretinate, and acitretin elevate triglycerides in 50% and cholesterol in 30% of patients.[9,149] Although the concern regarding hyperlipidemia and atherosclerosis is greater with long-term etretinate or acitretin therapy, lipid elevations are generally higher with isotretinoin. These lipid elevations are reversible on cessation of therapy.

The exact mechanism responsible for hyperlipidemia is not known. Retinoid-induced hypertriglyceridemia is mediated, at least in part, by RARs[168] and RXRs.[7] Isotretinoin preferentially binds to serum albumin. It is not known whether retinoid-albumin interaction causing displacement of triglyceride from albumin significantly contributes to the rise of serum triglyceride during retinoid therapy.

Patients at high risk for retinoid-associated hyperlipidemia include those with diabetes mellitus, obesity, excessive alcohol intake, and patients consuming a high saturated fat, high cholesterol diet.[1,149] Although pretreatment lipid levels reportedly do not predict subsequent lipid abnormalities, the highest lipid elevations are generally seen in patients with baseline hyperlipidemia. The most important unanswered question is the long-term effect of retinoid-induced hyperlipidemia on the coronary arteries. Patients with a family history of coronary artery disease (CAD) or who have significant CAD risk factors (such as cigarette smoking and hypertension) probably should not receive long-term retinoid therapy.

High carbohydrate, low fat diets aggravate hypertriglyceridemia. Hypertriglyceridemic patients should lower their alcohol and carbohydrate intake. Significant oat bran diet can lower triglyceride levels.[169] Substituting monounsaturated fats (e.g., grains, nuts, seeds, and their oils) and fish oil (omega-3 fatty acids) for saturated animal fats lowers total cholesterol, low-density lipoprotein (LDL) fraction and increases HDL.[170]

The package insert recommendation for isotretinoin, etretinate, and acitretin is to monitor lipids every 1 to 2 weeks until they are stable, which generally occurs in 4 to 8 weeks.[1] Initial lipid determinations every month for 3 to 6 months are probably adequate for patients without risk factors for retinoid-induced hyperlipidemia *and* who have normal baseline lipids. Patients who develop triglyceride levels over 500 to 600 mg/dl or cholesterol levels over 250 to 300 mg/dl should have the retinoid therapy withdrawn until normalization of serum lipids back to pretreatment baseline occurs.

PANCREATITIS.   Acute pancreatitis has been rarely encountered in patients taking first- or second-generation retinoids. Two cases of acute pancreatitis with oral alitretinoin use and one case of fatal fulminant pancreatitis with acitretin treatment have been reported.[39,151] A high incidence of acute pancreatitis (1% to 3%) has been observed in patients treated with bexarotene >300 mg/m[2]/day and associated with marked elevations of fasting serum triglycerides.[7] The lowest triglyceride level that resulted in pancreatitis was 770 mg/dl; most patients experiencing pancreatitis had triglyceride levels well over 1000 mg/dl. One patient with advanced non-CTCL died of pancreatitis. Patients who have risk factors for pancreatitis (e.g., prior pancreatitis, uncontrolled hyperlipidemia, excessive alcohol consumption, elevated triglyceride levels associated with pancreatic toxicity) should avoid bexarotene treatment.

LIVER EFFECTS.   Routine liver function tests (LFTs) are recommended for patients receiving systemic retinoids. Transient transaminase (AST/SGOT or ALT/SGPT) abnormalities are noted in 13% to 16% of the acitretin-treated patients,[9] 20% to 30% of the etretinate-treated patients, and occur at a lower frequency (<10%) with isotretinoin and bexarotene.[7,9,149] Elevations of alkaline phosphatase, lactate dehydrogenase, and bilirubin occur much less frequently. These LFT changes usually occur between 2 and 8 weeks after treatment has begun. Severe or persistent alterations in liver enzymes are rare, occurring in about 1% of etretinate-treated patients,[1] and are even rarer in acitretin-, isotretinoin-, or bexarotene-treated patients.[7,9]

There are scattered case reports of acitretin-induced hepatotoxicity, with report liver biopsy documented fibrosis or cirrhosis.[9] The largest prospective, multicenter study (n = 83) with pretreatment and posttreatment (2 years) liver biopsies in acitretin patients demonstrated no change in 59%, improvement in 24%, and worsening in 17% of psoriasis patients. Because acitretin (25 to 75 mg/day) elicited no biopsy-proven hepatotoxicity in this 2-year study, periodic liver biopsy should not be necessary.[171] Only 2 of 504 patients taking bexarotene developed cholestasis, including 1 patient who died of liver failure.[7] For comparison purposes, liver toxicity due to etretinate has been reviewed.[172]

Although the exact mechanism of hepatotoxicity is unknown, synthetic retinoids are found stored in liver at concentrations far greater than in the serum pool. Patients at risk for liver toxicity include those with diabetes mellitus, obesity, prior or concurrent methotrexate use, excess alcohol consumption, infectious hepatitis, and abnormal baseline LFTs.

The suggested approach of monitoring LFTs is given in the Monitoring Guidelines section. Transaminase elevations greater than 3 times the upper normal range should lead to prompt retinoid discontinuation. With twofold to threefold transaminase elevations, therapy should be discontinued until the laboratory abnormalities return to normal. Subsequently, the retinoid therapy can possibly be resumed at a lower dosage, with very careful laboratory monitoring. With smaller enzyme elevations, the levels generally return to baseline while the patient is still receiving therapy without sequelae.[1,149] Liver biopsies overall do not reveal hepatotoxicity that has not been suspected on routine LFTs. At this time there is no official recommendation concerning routine liver biopsies to monitor patients treated with retinoids.

USE OF RETINOIDS IN PATIENTS WITH HEPATIC OR RENAL INSUFFICIENCY. There are no specific studies evaluating the use of retinoids in patients with hepatic insufficiency. Because retinoids are metabolized by hepatic CYP 3A4 and are partially excreted in bile, significant hepatic insufficiency may interfere with the drug elimination. Due to less than 1% of the bexarotene dose is excreted in the urine unchanged and in vitro evidence of extensive hepatic bexarotene elimination, hepatic impairment would be expected to result in de-

creased drug clearance.[7] Therefore bexarotene should be used with great caution in this population.

No formal studies have been conducted with the current retinoids in patients with renal insufficiency. One case reported probable renal impairment induced by etretinate.[173] After discontinuation of the drug, renal function normalized. Because the elimination of retinoids is partly through renal excretion, renal insufficiency may interfere with urinary elimination.

THYROID AXIS ALTERATIONS. Among the FDA-approved retinoids, only bexarotene induces biochemical evidence of clinical hypothyroidism. Approximately half of bexarotene-treated patients have reversible elevations in thyroid-stimulating hormone (TSH) (60% to 69% of patients) and reductions in total T_4 (46% to 59%) levels.[7] These laboratory changes of hypothyroidism are associated with mild symptoms of hypothyroidism in about 75% of affected patients. Over the course of CTCL study, 38% (57/152) of patients were given levothyroxine after the initiation of bexarotene. Hypothyroidism is rapidly and completely reversible with cessation of bexarotene without any clinical sequelae. The mechanism of this adverse effect is not well understood. Baseline and at least one to two follow-up laboratory evaluations of thyroid axis function should be obtained during bexarotene therapy. The ideal timing for these follow-up tests has not been delineated.[7]

HEMATOLOGIC EFFECTS. In the CTCL studies, up to 43% of patients receiving bexarotene (>300 mg/m^2/day) had reversible leukopenia (1000 to 3000 WBC/mm^3).[7] The onset of leukopenia typically ranges from 4 to 8 weeks. The leukopenia observed in most patients was dose-related and explained by neutropenia. There was no febrile neutropenia or serious infections. Leukopenia and neutropenia resolved after dose reduction or discontinuation within 30 days. The incidence of leukopenia and other hematologic abnormalities is much less frequent with first- and second-generation retinoids.[149] Frequent hematologic monitoring in patients with HIV is recommended.

CENTRAL NERVOUS SYSTEM EFFECTS.
Changes of pseudotumor cerebri, although infrequent, are the most important central nervous system adverse effects. Transient headaches are relatively common early in isotretinoin therapy. However, accompanying nausea, vomiting, and visual changes should prompt further evaluation to exclude pseudotumor cerebri.[1] In an early report on pseudotumor cerebri associated with isotretinoin use, half the patients were taking tetracycline or minocycline concomitantly.[1,174] Combined therapy with isotretinoin and tetracycline, doxycycline, or minocycline should be avoided. A single case report of pseudotumor cerebri describes a patient receiving acitretin without concomitant antibiotic use.[10]

Other uncommon neurologic adverse effects include peripheral sensory changes and vertigo.[1] There have been reports that documented severe depression, psychosis, and (rarely) suicidal attempts, mainly with isotretinoin.[175] Of the patients reporting depression, some noted the depression improved with discontinuation of therapy and recurred with reinstitution of therapy. It is probably an idiosyncratic adverse effect and not dose- or timing-dependent.

The mechanism for these neurologic changes is unknown. Patient awareness of key neurologic symptoms to report is the most important aspect of surveillance for neurologic adverse effects. These neurologic events appear to be reversible overall on discontinuation of the retinoid therapy. Patients with persistent psychiatric or neurologic symptoms should be referred for further evaluation and treatment.

MUSCLE EFFECTS.
Myalgias are noted in roughly 15% of isotretinoin-treated patients. An increased frequency and severity of these myalgias can be seen in patients undergoing physical training programs involving heavy exertion, particularly when new programs are being initiated. These symptoms have been accompanied by markedly elevated creatine phosphokinase levels but have not been accompanied by rhabdomyolysis.[1] These muscle effects are associated mostly with isotretinoin therapy. Generalized increase of muscle tone due to etretinate and acitretin-induced myopathy has been reported.[176]

The mechanism involved in adverse muscle effects is not known. High-risk patients are athletes and those whose professions or hobbies include heavy exertion. Attempts should be made to moderate these activities or avoid retinoid therapy during prolonged periods of heavy exertion. Patients with severe myalgias should have a creatine phosphokinase (and perhaps aldolase) determination. One should keep in mind that in the absence of retinoid therapy, creatine phosphokinase elevations up to 20 times baseline levels can be seen in healthy runners 24 hours after a marathon race.[1]

MUCOCUTANEOUS EFFECTS.
The most common adverse effect is cheilitis, particularly involving the lower lip; 90% of patients receiving isotretinoin for acne experience this problem. Dry skin with increased fragility occurs in 80% of patients. Etretinate and acitretin, in particular, lead to palm, sole, and fingertip desquamation and increased skin fragility.[9,75] The dermatitic changes associated with xerosis, known as "retinoid dermatitis," can at times be confused with a flare of the disease being treated.

Hypersensitivity reactions are distinctly uncommon. Both erythema multiforme and erythema nodosum have been associated with isotretinoin[1] and etretinate use.[177] Photosensitivity is noted particularly with isotretinoin and is probably due to reduction of thickness of the stratum corneum. Localized or extensive exfoliative dermatitis (in 27% of patients) is the most common cutaneous adverse effect associated with bexarotene.[7] Compared with first- and second-generation retinoids, bexarotene-related mucocutaneous and ocular toxicities are relatively infrequent and tend to be milder.

The highest incidence of dose-dependent adverse effects associated with acitretin treatment is cheilitis (87% to 100%), followed by blepharoconjunctivitis (17% to 67%), dry eyes (19% to 87%), dry nose (27% to 69%), and dryness of the oral mucosa (14% to 87%).[9,75] Persistent hematuria secondary to mucosal friability (by urologic evaluation) has been reported.[9] Many patients taking retinoids (particularly etretinate) complain of a sticky sensation of their skin, which is probably due to increased mucus deposition.[1]

S. aureus colonization tends to correlate with isotretinoin-induced reduction in sebum production and may lead to overt cutaneous infections.[178,179] These bacterial complications can possibly be prevented with pulsed intranasal mupirocin therapy.[221] One case of *S. aureus* endocarditis in a patient with chronic stable aortic insufficiency undergoing isotretinoin therapy for extensive actinic keratoses is reported.[1] Therefore patients with cardiac valve diseases may need antibiotics if they develop skin infections while receiving retinoid therapy.

In retinoid-treated patients, pyogenic granuloma–like proliferations of granulation tissue may occur early in therapy,[1] particularly within healing cystic acne lesions, nail sulci, and traumatic wounds. Similar periungual pyogenic granuloma and disseminated sarcoid-like granulomas after prolonged acitretin and etretinate treatment, respectively, have been reported.[9,75,180] The exact pathogenesis remains obscure.

Decreased sebum production, reduced stratum corneum thickness, and altered skin barrier function are all central to the mucocutaneous adverse effects. Mucosal dryness, mucositis, and cutaneous fragility are most common and most troublesome in the seasons with low humidity. Liberal use of emollients, preceded by skin hydration, and periodic use of topical corticosteroids are the mainstays of management. Oral or topical antibiotics may be necessary for staphylococcal infections. Retinoid-induced granulation tissue has been successfully treated with corticosteroids (e.g., occlusive topical, intralesional, or pulsed systemic administration), curettage, chemical cautery, and pulsed dye laser.[1,181,182]

HAIR AND NAIL EFFECTS.

The risk of telogen effluvium due to the retinoids has been reported to vary over a range of 10% to 75%.[9,75,129] The risk is greater for acitretin than etretinate therapy, and is much less common with isotretinoin and bexarotene. Hair loss is a dose-related effect and is reversible starting 2 months after either discontinuation of therapy or a significant dose reduction. Women seem to have a more noticeable hair loss, particularly if there is already a mild baseline androgenic alopecia. In general, reassurance about the reversibility of the hair loss is usually sufficient to alleviate the patient's concern. Dose reduction or even cessation of therapy may be necessary in more severe cases.

Nail fragility with onychorrhexis and onychoschizia is common. Nail dystrophy and onycholysis occur infrequently but with a higher incidence with acitretin than with etretinate use.[9,75,183]

OTHER SYSTEMIC EFFECTS.

In rare instances, patients with diabetes may have more difficult glucose control while taking a retinoid. Development of inflammatory bowel disease during retinoid therapy has been reported, although a causal relationship is uncertain.[1] Adverse effects due to bexarotene therapy not mentioned earlier include headache (34% of patients) and asthenia (46%).

A 5-year prospective study of a cohort of 956 patients with psoriasis treated with etretinate did not demonstrate an increased risk of cardiovascular disease, cancer, diabetes, or inflammatory bowel disease in association with long-term etretinate use. The study concludes that with proper patient selection and monitoring, long-term etretinate therapy up to 4 years was not associated with a significantly increased risk of the previously discussed important adverse effects.[151] Because there is not yet a similar study for acitretin, similar safety with long-term acitretin therapy has not been established. Even so, these adverse effects are unlikely to result from acitretin therapy.

Drug Interactions

Formal studies of drug interactions with retinoids have been limited. Table 13-8 lists both well-documented interactions and interactions that can be anticipated based on the CYP 3A4 metabolism of retinoids.

Monitoring Guidelines

Most urine pregnancy tests have a threshold detection limit of 20 to 50 mIU/ml. The serum pregnancy tests are more sensitive and have a better threshold detection limit of 1 to 5 mIU/ml. Concentrations of urine β-human chorionic gonadotropin (β-HCG) vary with the patient's physiology, state of hydration, and urine volume. Due to these factors, the urine pregnancy test may not be sensitive enough until 6 to 8 days postconception when the β-HCG level

Table 13-8   Retinoid Drug Interactions[7,9,10,174,185]

Interacting Drug or Group	Examples and Comments
THE FOLLOWING DRUGS MAY INCREASE THE SERUM LEVELS (AND POTENTIAL TOXICITY) OF RETINOIDS	
Vitamin A	Increased isotretinoin levels—potentiates RAR-activity, leading to hypervitaminosis A–like toxicities
Tetracycline, doxycycline, minocycline	Increased isotretinoin levels—pseudotumor cerebri risk when any of these drugs used in combination with isotretinoin, possibly other retinoids
Gemfibrozil	Increased bexarotene levels due to CYP 3A4 inhibition—result is significantly increased risk for bexarotene toxicity of various types
Macrolides, azoles, and so on	Other CYP 3A4 inhibitors may increase retinoid drug levels and resultant potential for toxicity
THE FOLLOWING DRUGS MAY DECREASE THE SERUM LEVELS OF RETINOIDS VIA CYP 3A4 INDUCTION	
Antituberculosis drugs	Rifampin, rifabutin
Anticonvulsants	Phenytoin, phenobarbital, carbamazepine
RETINOIDS MAY INCREASE THE DRUG LEVELS (AND POTENTIAL TOXICITY) OF THE FOLLOWING DRUG	
Cyclosporine	Increased cyclosporine levels via competition with retinoids for fCYP 3A4 metabolism
RETINOIDS MAY DECREASE THE DRUG LEVELS OF THE FOLLOWING DRUGS	
Progestin-only contraceptives (mini-pills—microdose progesterone)	Reduced efficacy of these contraceptives when prescribed along with acitretin or isotretinoin
OTHER POTENTIALLY IMPORTANT DRUG INTERACTIONS	
Alcohol	Acitretin "reverse metabolism" to etretinate increased when acitretin used in combination with alcohol
Methotrexate	Theoretic increased risk of liver toxicity when used concomitantly

approaches 30 mIU/ml. If the urine pregnancy test is obtained, the first void of the day should be collected.

Guidelines of contraceptive measures can be obtained from Roche's educational pamphlet, Birth Control: The Facts You Need.[187] In general, implantable, injectable, and oral birth control hormones are most effective. Diaphragm, spermicide, and condom when used together can be highly effective. No method of birth control, other than abstinence, is completely reliable. Women with a history of infertility should use contraceptives and women who have undergone tubal ligation should ideally use a second form of contraception.

Therapeutic Guidelines

Box 13-4 contains a therapeutic guidelines checklist for retinoid therapy. Two key issues influence the decision-making process regarding the selection of appropriate retinoids for therapy. First, retinoids are the single most effective category of drugs available for acne vulgaris and many disorders of keratinization and are strong contenders for therapy in severe presentations of dermatoses such as psoriasis, pityriasis rubra pilaris, and mycosis fungoides. Second, major systemic adverse effects such as teratogenicity and ocular, bone, lipid, and liver adverse effects make careful patient selection and ongoing laboratory surveillance critical. Even through addressing the items

Isotretinoin and Acitretin Monitoring Guidelines[10,154,186]

BASELINE

Examination

- Careful history and physical examination
- Identify those patients at increased risk for toxicity or adverse effects
- Document concomitant medications that may interact with retinoids (Table 13-8)

Laboratory*

- Serum or sensitive urine pregnancy test (in fertile women)†
- Complete blood count (CBC) with platelets
- Liver function tests (AST, ALT, alkaline phosphatase, bilirubin)
- Lipid profile during fasting‡ (triglycerides, total cholesterol, LDL and HDL cholesterol)
- Renal function tests (blood urea nitrogen, creatinine)
- Optional urinalysis (if patients have renal diseases, proteinuria, diabetes, or hypertension)

Special Tests

- Consider baseline x-rays of wrists, ankles, or thoracic spine if plan *long-term* retinoid therapy
- Consider ophthalmologic examination if patients have a history of cataracts or retinopathy

FOLLOW-UP

Examination

(Clinical evaluation monthly for first 3 to 6 months, then every 3 months)

- Assessment of patient response, improvement, and complaints of adverse effects

Examination—cont'd

- Routine physical examination of lesional skin
- Additional/focused physical examination of any reported adverse effects

Laboratory*

(Monthly for the first 3 to 6 months, then every 3 months)§

- Complete blood count (CBC) with platelets‖
- Liver function tests (AST, ALT)
- Fasting lipid studies‡ (triglycerides, cholesterol—order LDL and HDL cholesterol periodically)
- Renal function tests‖ (optional urinalysis)
- Serum or urine pregnancy test monthly for women of childbearing potential (and at end of therapy)

Special Tests

(Periodically as indicated by symptoms)

- Consider yearly x-rays of wrists, ankles, or thoracic spine with *long-term* retinoid therapy
- Radiographic studies of significantly symptomatic joints with long-term therapy
- Complete ophthalmologic examination if patients report visual changes (see text for components)

---

*More frequent surveillance is needed if laboratory parameters are abnormal or with high-risk patients.
†Newer guidelines request two pregnancy tests before isotretinoin therapy—isotretinoin therapy should be prescribed to begin on the second day of next normal menstrual cycle or ≥11 days after the last unprotected sexual intercourse.
‡Lipids should be drawn after a 12-hour fast and a 36-hour abstinence from ethanol.
§When isotretinoin is used for a 20-week acne course, it is reasonable to discontinue laboratory monitoring (other than pregnancy testing) after 8 to 12 weeks if laboratory results remain normal.
‖Renal function and hematologic tests are infrequently altered by these two retinoids; consider ordering these tests every other time the laboratory evaluation is done.

Bexarotene (Targretin) Monitoring Guidelines[7]

BASELINE

Examination

- Careful history and physical examination
- Identify those patients at increased risk for toxicity or adverse effects: liver disease or cirrhosis, biliary tract disease, excessive alcohol consumption, prior pancreatitis, thyroid disease, uncontrolled hyperlipidemia, uncontrolled diabetes mellitus, HIV, leukopenia, chronic infection, cataracts
- Document concomitant medications that may interact with retinoids (Table 13-8)

Laboratory*

- Serum or sensitive urine pregnancy test (in fertile women)
- Complete blood count (CBC) with platelets and differential count
- Liver function tests (AST, ALT, alkaline phosphatase, bilirubin)
- Lipid profile during fasting† (triglycerides, total cholesterol, LDL and HDL cholesterol)
- Renal function tests (blood urea nitrogen, creatinine)
- Thyroid function tests: TSH, T_4
- Optional urinalysis (if patients have renal diseases, proteinuria, diabetes, or hypertension)

Special Tests

- Baseline ophthalmologic examination if patients have a history of cataracts

FOLLOW-UP

Examination

(Clinical evaluation every 2 weeks for first 4 to 8 weeks, then monthly for the next 3 months; long-term clinical evaluation every 2 to 3 months)

- Assessment of patient clinical response and for adverse effects

Examination—cont'd

- Additional/focused physical examination of any reported adverse effects

Laboratory*

(Every 1 to 2 weeks until the lipid response to Targretin is established [usually 2 to 4 weeks], then as below)

- Lipid profile during fasting (triglycerides, total cholesterol, LDL and HDL cholesterol)

(Monthly for the first 3 to 6 months, then every 3 months)

- CBC with platelets and differential count
- Liver function tests (AST, ALT); if elevated can also order bilirubin, alkaline phosphatase
- Renal function tests‡ (optional urinalysis)
- Serum or urine pregnancy test for women of childbearing potential (continue monthly indefinitely while on therapy)
- Thyroid function tests: TSH (at least), possibly T_4 as well (reasonable to follow-up just 1 to 2 times per year)

Special Tests

- Repeat ophthalmologic examination periodically during treatment if patients have a history of abnormal ocular findings before retinoid therapy

*More frequent surveillance is needed if laboratory parameters are abnormal or with high-risk patients.

†Lipids should be drawn after a 12-hour fast and a 36-hour abstinence from ethanol.

‡Renal function tests and urinalyses are infrequently altered by bexarotene; consider performing them every other time when laboratory evaluation is done.

Box 13-4

Therapeutic Guidelines Checklist

***RISK-BENEFIT ANALYSIS* IS BEST PERFORMED WHEN CONSIDERING THE FOLLOWING ISSUES:**

✓ *Patient age and gender*—use particular caution for children and for women of childbearing potential.

✓ *Disease responsiveness*—the most specific retinoid drug choice, dose, and duration of therapy needs to be chosen; whether a sustained remission of the disease being treated is possible is of importance.

✓ *Disease severity*—systemic retinoids are best used for conditions that are severe, involve large body surface areas (over 15% to 20%), and are significantly disabling on a physical or an emotional basis.

✓ *Prior alternative therapies*—it is important to consider other topical and systemic therapies; systemic retinoids may be the treatment of choice if others are impractical, too costly, induce important adverse effects, or have worrisome drug interactions.

✓ *Adjunctive therapy*—when possible, use systemic retinoids in combination with other topical or systemic therapies to enhance efficacy and/or reduce adverse effects.

✓ *Rotational or sequential therapy*—using psoriasis as an example, long-term adverse effects *may* be minimized by alternating between retinoids and other therapeutic options such as methotrexate, cyclosporine, PUVA or UVB phototherapy.

ADDITIONAL ISSUES TO ADDRESS TO *OPTIMIZE* SYSTEMIC *RETINOID* THERAPY SAFETY:

✓ *Dose and duration*—a patient should take the lowest possible retinoid dose for the briefest possible duration that will be therapeutically beneficial; the dose can be tapered completely or more ideally reduced to the lowest effective maintenance dose to sustain adequate disease control.

✓ *Route of retinoid administration*—in many settings topical retinoid therapy can effectively treat skin conditions with limited extent, with the potential to limit both cost and adverse effects.

✓ *Laboratory surveillance*—this should be done as outlined in the Monitoring Guidelines section.

✓ *Patient education*—this education should particularly emphasize bone, ocular, central nervous system, and muscle adverse effects; these sites of potential adverse effects have no routine laboratory monitoring performed.

✓ *Management of adverse effects*—maximum patient compliance requires patient efforts directed at minimizing mucocutaneous adverse effects and awareness of expected minor hair, nail, and systemic adverse effects.

---

in Box 13-4, there are still significant potential risks with synthetic retinoid therapy. Only physicians thoroughly familiar with these risks, monitoring guidelines, and elements of patient education should prescribe the retinoids, especially bexarotene. Some of the most gratifying clinical results in dermatology can be obtained through the appropriate use of systemic retinoids.

INVESTIGATIONAL RETINOIDS

The following drugs are retinoids still under investigation and are not yet approved for use in dermatology (Box 13-5).

9-*cis* Retinoic Acid

9-*cis* RA (alitretinoin, Panretin) is a naturally occurring pan-receptor agonist. 9-*cis* RA is a metabolite of ATRA. RXRs exclusively bind to 9-*cis* RA, whereas RARs bind to both ATRA and 9-*cis* RA.

9-*cis* RA, under the name of alitretinoin (Panretin) 0.1% gel, is approved by the FDA for the topical treatment of cutaneous Kaposi's sarcoma. The capsule form (Panretin) is under clinical trial for HIV-Kaposi's sarcoma and psoriasis.[38] Compared with other retinoids, mucocutaneous reactions are mild. Because of a similar therapeutic index as tretinoin (ATRA), systemic use of 9-*cis* RA is unlikely in dermatology.

Box 13-4

Therapeutic Guidelines Checklist—cont'd

FEMALE PATIENTS SHOULD *AVOID PREGNANCY* AT ALL COSTS WHEN USING RETINOID THERAPY. ALTHOUGH THERE ARE WELL-DEFINED PATIENT GUIDELINES AND AN INFORMED CONSENT PACKET, THE FOLLOWING GUIDELINES ARE USEFUL REMINDERS:

✓ *Patient selection*—the patient's capacity to understand the risk of serious teratogenicity and the importance of complete compliance with pregnancy prevention measures is a critical determinant in retinoid therapy decisions.

✓ *Patient education*—optimal patient education involves both the physician's careful explanation and information handouts that address the important issues regarding teratogenicity. After the patient has heard and read these instructions, it is important to provide adequate opportunity to ask any questions she may have. Current retinoid packaging for isotretinoin provides an ongoing reminder of the teratogenicity potential.

✓ *Informed consent documentation*—for isotretinoin the packet, available through Roche Pharmaceuticals, is adequate from a medicolegal perspective; thorough chart documentation of the above discussion is important.

✓ *Contraception*—for all systemic retinoids there should be adequate contraception for at least 1 month before therapy; acitretin requires contraception for 3 years after cessation of therapy, whereas isotretinoin and bexarotene require contraception for just 1 month after cessation of therapy. Acceptable options include oral contraceptives, hormonal injections, intrauterine devices, and surgical sterilization.

✓ *Exclusion of pregnancy*—serum or urine pregnancy testing should be obtained within 1 week of the expected menstrual cycle, and monthly thereafter; retinoids should be started on the second or third day of a normal menstrual cycle. Frequent reminders about these issues and a limited supply of medication should be provided to encourage compliance.

✓ *Anticipating options*—before initiating retinoid therapy the female patient should consider available options if pregnancy occurs during retinoid therapy; it is helpful to document her thoughts on this subject in the medical record.

Motretinide

Motretinide (Tasmaderm) has been developed in Europe as a topical medication. Its aromatic structure is related to both acitretin and etretinate. Motretinide is less irritating than tretinoin when used topically. Motretinide is metabolized in vivo to acitretin.[188] In the United States, motretinide is not yet clinically available.

Fenretinide

Fenretinide (*N*-4-hydroxyphenyl retinamide) is an arotinoid, synthesized in the United States in the late 1960s. It is a highly selective activator of retinoid receptors. Fenretinide interacts mostly with RAR-α, RAR-β, and RXR-α.

Box 13-5

Retinoids Currently Under Investigation

Fenretinide
Motretinide
Temarotene
Arotinoids
   Arotinoic acid
   Arotinoid ethyl ester
   Arotinoid sulfones
      Sumarotene
      Etarotene
Glucuronide analogs

Topical fenretinide has been investigated to treat actinic keratoses,[189] oral lichen planus, and oral leukoplakia.[190] Systemic use of fenretinide is under clinical trial for the prevention of basal cell carcinoma[13] and chemoprevention of oral leukoplakia.[191]

Arotinoid Sulfones

Arotinoid sulfones such as the arotinoid methyl sulfone (sumarotene; Ro 14-9706) and arotinoid ethyl sulfone (etarotene; Ro 15-1570) do not bind to RARs. Sumarotene shows no teratogenic activity in pregnant hamsters.[192] On the other hand, etarotene does not cause bone alterations in rats.[193]

In a double-blind, comparative study, topical sumarotene 0.05% cream was reported as effective as tretinoin cream in treating multiple actinic keratoses. Moreover, sumarotene was better tolerated than tretinoin and caused much less local irritation, redness, and scaling.[194] Due to a better safety and adverse effect profile, including no teratogenic activity, certain arotinoid sulfones hold important potential therapeutic advantages.

Glucuronide Analogs

Glucuronide analogs of retinoids include retinoyl β-glucuronide (RBG) and N-[4-hydroxyphenyl] retinamide-O-glucuronide (4-HPROG). RBG is a naturally occurring metabolite of RA that is effective in the topical treatment of acne in humans. Unlike RA, RBG lacks the mucocutaneous signs of retinoid toxicity when applied to the skin and is nonteratogenic when administered orally to rats.[195] However, these O-glucuronide analogs are relatively unstable and deactivated by the action of β-glucuronidase. Various analogs are being evaluated to improve both stability and efficacy.[196]

Arotinoid Ethyl Ester

Arotinoid ethyl ester (Ro 13-6298) pharmacokinetics are believed to be similar to those of etretinate (an ethyl ester).[145] Its teratogenicity in mice is no better than that observed with prior generation retinoids when tested within the same relative dose-response range.[197]

In humans, arotinoid ethyl ester is highly effective in the treatment of severe etretinate-resistant dermatoses, including psoriasis and psoriatic arthritis.[146] Minimal oral doses (0.05 to 0.1 mg/day) of arotinoid ethyl ester are required. Patients with various subsets of CTCL responded as well.[141] Adverse effects similar to those caused by etretinate have been noted.[198] Although lacking improvement of the adverse effect profile and teratogenic potential, the potent antikeratinizing effect of arotinoid ethyl ester may be useful to treat second-generation retinoid-resistant disorders of keratinization.

Arotinoic Acid

Arotinoic acid (Ro 13-7410) is the carboxylic acid metabolite of arotinoid ethyl ester and is analogous to acitretin (both are carboxylic acid derivatives). Like arotinoid sulfone, it stimulates the synthesis of keratohyalin granules and has a strong antikeratinizing effect that may be useful for psoriasis therapy. Because of severe adverse effects, arotinoic acid is unlikely to be used as an oral antikeratinizing agent.

Temarotene

Temarotene (Ro 15-0778) is an arotinoid that has no effect on the human sebocyte model.[199] The temarotene metabolite (Ro 14-6113) has some immunosuppressive activities similar to cyclosporine. Ro 14-6113 inhibits proliferation of T cells and their capacity to secrete IL-2, IFN-γ, and TNF-α. It also inhibits the secretion of IgM, IgG, and IgA while stimulating IgE secretion.[200] Temarotene and its metabolite do not induce differentiation[201] and thus have no role in differentiation/antikeratinizing therapy.

Compounds With Retinoid-like Structure

Compounds with retinoid-like structure but lacking retinoid activities have been synthesized. These agents behave as analogs of vitamin D (deltanoids) and prostacyclin/prostaglandin and thromboxane (prostanoids), in addition to binding to a wide variety of other biologic receptor systems. Combination of the deltanoid and retinoid agents may be a useful synergistic approach to differentiation therapy and chemoprevention of cancers.

Bibliography

Historical Perspective

Bollag W: The development of retinoids in experimental and clinical oncology and dermatology. *J Am Acad Dermatol* 9:797-805, 1983.

Dicken CH: Retinoids: a review. *J Am Acad Dermatol* 11:541-552, 1984.

Ellis CN, Voorhees JJ: Etretinate therapy. *J Am Acad Dermatol* 16:267-291, 1987.

Drug Category Overviews

Orfanos CE, Zouboulis CC, Almond-Roesler B, et al: Current use and future potential role of retinoids in dermatology. *Drugs* 53:358-388, 1997.

Pilkington T, Brogden RN: Acitretin: a review of its pharmacology and therapeutic use. *Drugs* 43:597-627, 1992.

Adverse Effects Overviews and Monitoring Guidelines

Bigby M, Stern RS: Adverse reactions to isotretinoin. A report from the Adverse Drug Reaction Reporting System. *J Am Acad Dermatol* 18:543-552, 1988.

David M, Hodak E, Lowe NJ: Adverse effects of retinoids. *Med Toxicol* 3:273-288, 1988.

Katz IH, Waalen J, Leach EE: Acitretin in psoriasis: an overview of adverse effects. *J Am Acad Dermatol* 41:S7-12, 1999.

Meigel WN: How safe is oral isotretinoin? *Dermatology* 195(Suppl 1):22-28, 1997.

Saurat J-H: Side effects of systemic retinoids and their clinical management. *J Am Acad Dermatol* 27:S23-28, 1992.

Wolverton SE: Major adverse effects from systemic drugs: defining the risks. *Curr Prob Dermatol* 7:1-40, 1995.

References

Introduction and Pharmacology

1. Wolverton SE: Retinoids. In Wolverton SE, Wilkin JK, editors: *Systemic drugs for skin diseases*, Philadelphia, 1991, WB Saunders, pp 187-218.
2. Bollag W: The development of retinoids in experimental and clinical oncology and dermatology. *J Am Acad Dermatol* 9:797-805, 1983.
3. Bollag W, Geiger JM: The development of retinoids in dermatology. In Cunliffe WJ, Miller AJ, editors: *Retinoid therapy. A review of clinical and laboratory research*, the proceedings of an International Conference held in London, May 16-18, 1983.
4. Peck GL, Yoder FW: Treatment of lamellar ichthyosis and other keratinizing dermatoses with a synthetic retinoid. *Lancet* 2:1172-1174, 1976.
5. Yoder F: Personal communication, 1998.
6. Peck GL, Olsen TG, Yoder FW, et al: Prolonged remissions of cystic and conglobate acne with 13-cis retinoic acid. *N Engl J Med* 300:329-333, 1979.
7. Bexarotene (Targretin) package insert and product monograph. San Diego, CA. Ligand Pharmaceuticals, 2000.
8. Wiegand UW, Chou RC: Pharmacokinetics of acitretin and etretinate. *J Am Acad Dermatol* 39:S25-33, 1998.
9. Koo J, Nguyen Q, Gambla C: Advances in psoriasis therapy. *Adv Dermatol* 12:47-72, 1997.
10. Acitretin (Soriatane) package insert. Nutley, NJ. Roche Laboratories, 1997.
11. Chen C, Mistry G, Jensen B, et al: Pharmacokinetics of retinoids in women after meal consumption of vitamin A supplementation. *J Clin Pharmacol* 36:799-808, 1996.
12. Vahlquist A, Rollman O: Clinical pharmacology of 3 generations of retinoids. *Dermatologica* 175:S20-27, 1987.
13. Allen JG, Bloxham DP: The pharmacology and pharmacokinetics of the retinoids. *Pharmacol Ther* 40:1-27, 1989.
14. Sapiro SS, Latriano L: Pharmacokinetic and pharmacodynamic considerations of retinoids: tretinoin. *J Am Acad Dermatol* 39:S13-16, 1998.
15. Keddie F: Use of vitamin A in the treatment of cutaneous diseases. Relation to estrogen and the vitamin B complex. *Arch Dermatol Syphilol* 58:64-73, 1947.

16. Orfanos CE, Braun-Falco EM, Farber EM, et al, editors: *Retinoids. Advances in basic research and therapy,* New York, 1981, Springer-Verlag.

17. Chandraratna RAS: Rational design of receptor-selective retinoids. *J Am Acad Dermatol* 39:S124-128, 1998.

18. Roberts A: Microsomal oxidation of retinoic acid in hamster liver, intestine, and testis. *Ann NY Acad Sci* 359:45-53, 1981.

19. Howell SR, Shirley MA, Ulm EH: Effects of retinoid treatment of rats on hepatic microsomal metabolism and cytochromes P450. Correlation between retinoic acid receptor/retinoid x receptor selectivity and effects. *Drug Metab Dispos* 26:234-239, 1998.

20. Wiegand UW, Chou RC: The evolving role of retinoids in the management of cutaneous conditions: Pharmacokinetics of oral isotretinoin. *J Am Acad Dermatol* 39:S8-12, 1998.

21. Schmitt-Hoffmann AH, Dittrich S, Saulnier E, et al: Mechanistic studies on the ethyl-esterification of acitretin by human liver preparations in vitro. *Life Sci* 57:407-412, 1995.

22. Sturkenboom MC, de Jong-Van Den Berg LT, van Voorst-Vader PC, et al: Inability to detect plasma etretinate and acitretin is a poor predictor of the absence of these teratogens in tissue after stopping acitretin treatment. *Br J Clin Pharmacol* 38:229-235, 1994.

23. Pilkington T, Brogden RN: Acitretin: a review of its pharmacology and therapeutic use. *Drugs* 43:597-627, 1992.

Mechanisms of Action

24. Kang S, Li SY, Voorhees JJ: Pharmacology and molecular action of retinoids and vitamin D in skin. *J Invest Dermatol Symposium Proc* 1:15-21, 1996.

25. Rowe A: Retinoid X receptors. *Int J Biochem Cell Biol* 29:276-278, 1997.

26. Gottlieb S, Hayes E, Gilleaudeau P, et al: Cellular actions of etretinate in psoriasis: enhanced epidermal differentiation and reduced cell-mediated inflammation are unexpected outcomes. *J Cutan Pathol* 23:404-418, 1996.

27. Zouboulis CC, Korge B, Akamatsu H, et al: Effects of 13-cis-retinoic acid, all-trans-retinoic acid, and acitretin on the proliferation, lipid synthesis and keratin expression of cultured human sebocytes in vitro. *J Invest Dermatol* 96:792-797, 1991.

28. Doran TI, Shapiro SS: Retinoid effects on sebocyte proliferation. *Methods Enzymol* 190:334-338, 1990.

29. Boudou P, Chivot M, Vexiau P, et al: Evidence for decreased androgen 5 alpha-reduction in skin and liver of men with severe acne after 13-cis-retinoic acid treatment. *J Clin Endocrinol Metab* 78:1064-1069, 1994.

30. Okuno M, Numaguchi S, Moriwaki H, et al: Cellular retinoid-binding protein. *Nippon Rinsho* 5:879-885, 1993.

31. Siegenthaler G, Saurat JH, Salomon D, et al: Skin cellular retinoid-binding proteins and retinoid-responsive dermatoses. *Dermatologica* 173:163-173, 1986.

32. Saurat JH, Hirschel Scholz S, Salomon D, et al: Human skin retinoid-binding proteins and therapy with synthetic retinoids: a still unexplained link. *Dermatologica* 175:S13-19, 1987.

33. Sanquers S, Eller MS, Gilchrest BA: Retinoids and state of differentiation modulate CRABP II gene expression in a skin equivalent. *J Invest Dermatol* 100:148-153, 1993.

34. Siegenthaler G, Saurat JH: Therapy with a synthetic retinoid (RO 10-1670) etretin increases the cellular retinoic acid-binding protein in nonlesional psoriatic skin. *J Invest Dermatol* 87:122-124, 1986.

35. Lotan R, Clifford JL: Nuclear receptors for retinoids: Mediators of retinoid effects on normal and malignant cells. *Biomed Pharmacother* 45:145-156, 1991.

36. Tian K, Norris AW, Lin CL, et al: The isolation and characterization of purified heterocomplexes of recombinant retinoic acid receptor and retinoid X receptor ligand binding domains. *Biochemistry* 36:5669-5676, 1997.

37. Saurat JH: Retinoids and psoriasis: Novel issues in retinoid pharmacology and implications for psoriasis treatment. *J Am Acad Dermatol* 41:S2-6, 1999.

38. Chen JY, Clifford J, Zusi C, et al: Two distinct actions of retinoid-receptor ligands. *Nature* 382:819-822, 1996.

39. Redefining clinical unmet needs in the treatment of Kaposi's sarcoma. A continuing program for physicians, pharmacists, and nurses. Oxford Institute for Continuing Education, Newton, PA. August 1999.

40. Duvic M, Asano AT, Hager C, et al: The pathogenesis of psoriasis and the mechanism of action of tazarotene. *J Am Acad Dermatol* 39:S129-133, 1998.

41. Danno K, Kaji A, Mochizuki T: Alterations in ICAM-1 and ELAM-1 expression in psoriatic lesions following various treatments. *J Dermatol Sci* 13:49-55, 1996.

42. Lehman PA, Henderson WR Jr: Retinoid-induced inhibition of eosinophil LTC4 production. *Prostaglandins* 39:569-577, 1990.

43. Punnonen K, Puustinen T, Jansen CT: The antipsoriatic drug metabolite etretin (Ro 10-1670) alters the metabolism of fatty acids in human keratinocytes in culture. *Arch Dermatol Res* 280:103-107, 1988.

44. Szmurlo A, Marczak M, Jablonska S, et al: Antitumor action of retinoids: inhibition of tumor cell line-induced angiogenesis and prevention of tumors in mice. *Dermatology* 184:116-119, 1992.

45. Boudou P, Soliman H, Chivot M, et al: Effect of oral isotretinoin treatment on skin androgen receptor levels in male acneic patients. *J Clin Endocrinol Metab* 80:1158-1161, 1995.

46. Hommel L, Geiger JM, Harms M, et al: Sebum excretion rate in subjects treated with oral all-trans-retinoic acid. *Dermatology* 193:127-130, 1996.

47. Bergfeld W, et al: The evolving role of retinoids in the management of cutaneous conditions. *Clinician* 16:1-32, 1998.

48. Nagy L, Thomazy VA, Chandraratna RA, et al: Retinoid-regulated expression of BCL-2 and tissue transglutaminase during the differentiation and apoptosis of human myeloid leukemia (HL-60) cells. *Leuk Res* 20:499-505, 1996.

49. Mehta K, McQueen T, Neamati N, et al: Activation of retinoid receptors RAR alpha and RXR alpha induces differentiation and apoptosis, respectively, in HL-60 cells. *Cell Growth Differ* 7:179-186, 1996.

50. Zhang Y, Huang Y, Rishi AK: Activation of p38 and JNK/SAPK mitogen-activated protein kinase pathways during apoptosis is mediated by a novel retinoid. *Exp Cell Res* 247:233-240, 1999.

51. Zheng ZS, Xue GZ, Prystowsky JH: Regulation of the induction of ornithine decarboxylase in keratinocytes by retinoids. *Biochem J* 309:159-165, 1995.

52. Krinsky NI: Theoretical basis for anticarcinogenic effects of retinoids. *J Cut Aging Cosm Dermatol* 1:55-59, 1988.

53. Lotan R, Xu XC, Lippman SM, et al: Suppression of retinoic acid receptor-beta in premalignant oral lesions and its up-regulation by isotretinoin. *N Engl J Med* 332:1405-1410, 1995.

54. Tosi P, Visani G, Ottaviani E, et al: Reduction of heat-shock protein-70 after prolonged treatment with retinoids: biological and clinical implications. *Am J Hematol* 56:143-150, 1997.

55. Mestre JR, Subbaramaiah K, Sacks PG, et al: Retinoids suppress phorbol ester-mediated induction of cyclooxygenase-2. *Cancer Res* 57:1081-1085, 1997.

56. Rudnicka L, Marczak M, Szmurlo A, et al: Acitretin decreases tumor cell-induced angiogenesis. *Skin Pharmacol* 4:150-153, 1991.

57. Lever L, Kumar P, Marks R: Topical retinoic acid in the treatment of elastotic degeneration. *Br J Dermatol* 122:91, 1990.

58. Viviano CM, Brockes JP: Is retinoic acid an endogenous ligand during urodele limb regeneration? *Int J Dev Biol* 40:817-822, 1996.

59. Priestley GC: Proliferation and glycosaminoglycans secretion in fibroblasts from psoriatic skin: Differential responses to retinoids. *Br J Dermatol* 117:575-583, 1987.

60. Hein R, Mensing H, Muller PK, et al: Effect of vitamin A and its derivatives on collagen production and chemotactic response of fibroblasts. *Br J Dermatol* 111:37-44, 1984.

61. Smith SM, Dickman ED, Power SC, et al: Retinoids and their receptors in vertebrate embryogenesis. *J Nutr* 128:S467-470, 1998.

62. Kochhar DM, Jiang H, Penner JD, et al: Differential teratogenic response of mouse embryos to receptor selective analogs of retinoic acid. *Chem Biol Interact* 100:1-12, 1996.

63. Angulo A, Suto C, Heyman RA, et al: Characterization of the sequences of the human cytomegalovirus enhancer that mediates differential regulation by natural and synthetic retinoids. *Mol Endocrinol* 10:781-793, 1996.

64. Sista ND, Pagano JS, Liao W, et al: Retinoic acid is a negative regulator of the Epstein-Barr virus protein (BZLF1) that mediates disruption of latent infection. *Proc Natl Acad Sci USA* 90:3894-3898, 1993.

65. Raney AK, Johnson JL, Palmer CN, et al: Members of the nuclear receptor superfamily regulate transcription from the hepatitis B virus nucleocapsid promoter. *J Virol* 71:1058-1071, 1997.

66. Agarwal C, Rorke EA, Irwin JC, et al: Immortalization by human papillomavirus type 16 alters retinoid regulation of human ectocervical epithelial cell differentiation. *Cancer Res* 51:3982-3989, 1991.

67. Bergfeld WF: The evolving role of retinoids in the management of cutaneous conditions: Retinoids and hair growth. *J Am Acad Dermatol* 39:S86-89, 1998.

68. Rogers M, Berestecky JM, Hossain MZ, et al: Retinoid-enhanced gap junctional communication is achieved by increased levels of connexin 43 mRNA and protein. *Mol Carcinog* 3:335-343, 1990.

69. Fairley JA, Ewing N, Keng P: Retinoic acid decreases the free intracellular calcium level of keratinocytes (abstract). *J Invest Dermatol* 88:488, 1987.

Clinical Use—Psoriasis

70. Schroder K, Zaun H, Holzmann H, et al: Pustulosis palmo-plantaris. Clinical and histological changes during etretin (acitretin). *Acta Derm Venereol* 146:S111-116, 1989.

71. Kragballe K, Jansen CT, Geiger JM, et al: A double-blind comparison of acitretin and etretinate in the treatment of severe psoriasis. *Acta Derm Venereol* 69:35-40, 1989.

72. Gollnick H, Bauer R, Brindley C, et al: Acitretin versus etretinate in psoriasis: Clinical and pharmacokinetic results of a German multicenter study. *J Am Acad Dermatol* 19:458-469, 1988.

73. Lassus A, Geiger JM: Acitretin and etretinate in the treatment of palmoplantar pustulosis: a double-blind comparative trial. *Br J Dermatol* 119:755-759, 1988.

74. Ozawa A, Ohkido M, Haruki Y, et al: Treatment of generalized pustular psoriasis: a multicenter study in Japan. *J Dermatol* 26:141-149, 1999.

75. Murray HE, Anhalt AW, Lessard R, et al: A 12-month treatment of severe psoriasis with acitretin: Results of a Canadian open multicenter study. *J Am Acad Dermatol* 24:598-602, 1991.

76. Buccheri L, Katchen BR, Karter AJ, et al: Acitretin therapy is effective for psoriasis associated with human immunodeficiency virus infection. *Arch Dermatol* 133:711-715, 1997.

77. Saurat JH, Geiger JM, Amblard D, et al: Randomized double-blind multicenter study comparing acitretin-PUVA, etretinate-PUVA and placebo-PUVA in the treatment of severe psoriasis. *Dermatologica* 172:218-224, 1988.

78. Nguyen EQ, Koo JY, editors: *Manual of phototherapy,* Columbus, OH, 1998, Unpublished.

79. Lebwohl M: Acitretin in combination with UVB or PUVA. *J Am Acad Dermatol* 41:S22-24, 1999.

80. Roenigk HH Jr: Acitretin combination therapy. *J Am Acad Dermatol* 41:S18-21, 1999.

Clinical Use—Acne

81. Layton AM, Knaggs J, Taylor J, et al: Isotretinoin for acne vulgaris—10 years later: a safe and successful treatment. *Br J Dermatol* 129:292-296, 1993.

82. Goulden V, Layton AM, Cunliffe WJ: Long-term safety of isotretinoin as a treatment for acne vulgaris. *Br J Dermatol* 131:360-363, 1994.

83. Coates P, Adams CA, Cunliffe WJ, et al: Does oral isotretinoin prevent *Propionibacterium acnes* resistance? *Dermatology* 195:S4-9, 38-40, 1997.

84. Goulden V, Clark SM, McGeown C, et al: Treatment of acne with intermittent isotretinoin. *Br J Dermatol* 137:106-108, 1997.

85. Lin J, Shih I, Yu C: Hemodialysis-related nodulocystic acne treated with isotretinoin. *Nephron* 81:146-150, 1999.

86. Neubert U, Jansen T, Plewig G: Bacteriologic and immunologic aspects of gram-negative folliculitis: A study of 46 patients. *Int J Dermatol* 38:270-274, 1999.

87. Otley CC, Avram MR, Johnson RA: Isotretinoin treatment of human immunodeficiency virus-associated eosinophilic folliculitis. Results of an open, pilot trial. *Arch Dermatol* 131:1047-1050, 1995.

88. Humbert P, Delaporte E, Drobacheff C, et al: Solid facial edema associated with acne. Therapeutic efficacy of isotretinoin. *Ann Dermatol Venereol* 117:527-532, 1990.

89. Jungfer B, Jansen T, Przybilla B, et al: Solid persistent facial edema of acne: successful treatment with isotretinoin and ketotifen. *Dermatology* 187:34-37, 1993.

90. Lehucher-Ceyrac D, de La Salmoniere P, Chastang C, et al: Predictive factors for failure of isotretinoin treatment in acne patients: Results from a cohort of 237 patients. *Dermatology* 198:278-283, 1999.

91. Chaspoux C, Lehucher-Ceyrac D, Morel P, et al: Acne in the male resistant to isotretinoin and responsibility of androgens: 9 cases, therapeutic implications. *Ann Dermatol Venereol* 126:17-19, 1999.

Clinical Use—Cutaneous T-cell Lymphoma

92. Mielke V, Staib G, Sterry W: Systemic treatment for cutaneous lymphomas. *Recent Results Cancer Res* 139:403-408, 1995.
93. Dreno B, Celerier P, Litoux P: Roferon-A in combination with Tigason in cutaneous T-cell lymphomas. *Acta Haematol* 89:S28-32, 1993.
94. French LE, Ramelet AA, Saurat JH: Remission of cutaneous T-cell lymphoma with combined calcitriol and acitretin (letter). *Lancet* 344:686-687, 1994.

Miscellaneous Reviews—For Uncommon Indications

95. Ellis CN, Voorhees JJ: Etretinate therapy. *J Am Acad Dermatol* 16:267-291, 1987.
96. Dicken CH: Retinoids: a review. *J Am Acad Dermatol* 11:541-552, 1984.

Clinical Use—Rosacea and Hidradenitis

97. Schell H, Vogt HJ, Mack-Hennes A: Treatment of rosacea with isotretinoin. Results of a multicenter trial follow-up. *Z Hautkr* 62:1123-1124, 1129-1133, 1987.
98. Smith KW: Perioral dermatitis with histopathologic features of granulomatous rosacea: successful treatment with isotretinoin. *Cutis* 46:413-415, 1990.
99. Boer J, van Gemert MJ: Long-term results of isotretinoin in the treatment of 68 patients with hidradenitis suppurativa. *J Am Acad Dermatol* 40:73-76, 1999.
100. Dicken CH, Powell ST, Spear KL: Evaluation of isotretinoin treatment of hidradenitis suppurativa. *J Am Acad Dermatol* 11:500-502, 1984.
101. Scerri L, Williams HC, Allen BR: Dissecting cellulitis of the scalp: response to isotretinoin. *Br J Dermatol* 134:1105-1108, 1996.
102. Taylor AE: Dissecting cellulitis of the scalp: response to isotretinoin (letter). *Lancet* 2:225, 1987.

Clinical Use—Disorders of Keratinization

103. Dicken CH, Bauer EA, Hazen PG, et al: Isotretinoin treatment of Darier's disease. *J Am Acad Dermatol* 6:721-726, 1982.
104. Christophersen J, Geiger JM, Danneskiold-Samsoe P, et al: A double-blind comparison of acitretin and etretinate in the treatment of Darier's disease. *Acta Derm Venereol* 72:150-152, 1992.
105. Dicken CH: Treatment of classic pityriasis rubra pilaris. *J Am Acad Dermatol* 31:997-999, 1994.

106. Clayton BD, Jorizzo JL, Hitchcock MG, et al: Adult pityriasis rubra pilaris: a 10-year series. *J Am Acad Dermatol* 36:959-964, 1997.
107. Cohen PR, Prystowsky JH: Pityriasis rubra pilaris: a review of diagnosis and treatment. *J Am Acad Dermatol* 20:801-807, 1989.
108. Goldsmith LA, Weinrich AE, Shupack J: Pityriasis rubra pilaris response to 13-*cis* retinoic acid (isotretinoin). *J Am Acad Dermatol* 6:710-715, 1982.
109. Lacour M, Mehta-Nikhar B, Atherton DJ, et al: An appraisal of acitretin therapy in children with inherited disorders of keratinization. *Br J Dermatol* 134:1023-1029, 1996.
110. Ruiz-Maldonado R, Tamayo L: Retinoids in disorders of keratinization: their use in children. *Dermatologica* 175(Suppl 1):125-132, 1987.
111. Mashshini-Jason F, Wolff P, Pierard GE, et al: Anodontia and hidrotic ectodermal dysplasia, hyporeactive to heat. Effect of acitretin. *Ann Dermatol Venereol* 121:120-122, 1994.
112. Lucker GP, Steijlen PM: Pachyonychia congenita tarda. *Clin Exp Dermatol* 20:226-229, 1995.

Clinical Use—Chemoprevention of Malignancies

113. Sankaranarayanan R, Mathew B: Retinoids as cancer-preventive agents. *IARC Sci Publ* 139:47-59, 1996.
114. Lippman SM, Batsakis JG, Toth BB, et al: Comparison of low-dose isotretinoin with beta carotene to prevent oral carcinogenesis. *N Engl J Med* 328:15-20, 1993.
115. Hudson-Peacock MJ, Angus B, Farr PM: Response of PUVA-induced keratoses to etretinate. *J Am Acad Dermatol* 35:120-123, 1996.
116. Esteve E, Serpier H, Cambie MP, et al: Bazex paraneoplastic acrokeratosis. Treatment with acitretin. *Ann Dermatol Venereol* 122:26-29, 1995.
117. Hartig C, Stieler W, Stadler R: Muir-Torre syndrome. Diagnostic criteria and review of the literature. *Hautarzt* 46:107-113, 1995.
118. Kraemer KH, DiGiovanna JJ, Peck GL: Chemoprevention of skin cancer in xeroderma pigmentosum. *J Dermatol* 19:715-718, 1992.
119. Bavinck JN, Tieben LM, Van der Woude FJ, et al: Prevention of skin cancer and reduction of keratotic skin lesions during acitretin therapy in renal transplant recipients: A double-blind, placebo-controlled study. *J Clin Oncol* 13:1933-1938, 1995.

120. Yuan ZF, David A, Macdonald K, et al: Use of acitretin for the skin complications in renal transplant recipients. *N Z Med J* 108:255-256, 1995.

121. McKenna DB, Murphy GM: Skin cancer chemoprophylaxis in renal transplant recipients: 5 years of experience using low-dose acitretin. *Br J Dermatol* 140:656-660, 1999.

122. Gibson GE, O'Grady A, Kay EW, et al: Low-dose retinoid therapy for chemoprophylaxis of skin cancer in renal transplant recipients. *J Eur Acad Dermatol Venereol* 10:42-47, 1998.

123. van de Kerkhof PC, de Rooij MJ: Multiple squamous cell carcinomas in a psoriatic patient following high-dose photochemotherapy and cyclosporin treatment: Response to long-term acitretin maintenance. *Br J Dermatol* 136:275-278, 1997.

124. Hsu MC: Systemic treatment of neoplastic conditions with retinoids. *J Am Acad Dermatol* 39:S108-113, 1998.

125. Peck GL, DiGiovanna JJ, Sarnoff DS, et al: Treatment and prevention of basal cell carcinoma with oral isotretinoin. *J Am Acad Dermatol* 19:176-185, 1988.

126. Levine N, Moon TE, Cartmel B, et al: Trial of retinol and isotretinoin in skin cancer prevention: a randomized, double-blind, controlled trial. Southwest Skin Cancer Prevention Study Group. *Cancer Epidemiol Biomarkers Prev* 6:957-961, 1997.

127. Corbeil J, Rapaport E, Richman DD, et al: Antiproliferative effect of retinoid compounds on Kaposi's sarcoma cells. *J Clin Invest* 93:1981-1986, 1994.

Clinical Use—Other Inflammatory Cutaneous Diseases and HPV infections

128. Newton RC, Jorizzon JL, Solomon AR Jr, et al: Mechanism-oriented assessment of isotretinoin in chronic or subacute cutaneous lupus erythematosus. *Arch Dermatol* 122:170-176, 1986.

129. Shornick JK, Formica H, Parke AL: Isotretinoin for refractory lupus erythematosus. *J Am Acad Dermatol* 24:49-52, 1991.

130. Ruzicka T, Sommerburg C, Goerz G, et al: Treatment of cutaneous lupus erythematosus with acitretin and hydroxychloroquine. *Br J Dermatol* 127:513-518, 1992.

131. Laurberg G, Geiger JM, Hjorth N, et al: Treatment of lichen planus with acitretin. A double-blind, placebo-controlled study in 65 patients. *J Am Acad Dermatol* 24:434-437, 1991.

132. Romppanen U, Tuimala R, Ellmen J, et al: Oral treatment of vulvar dystrophy with an aromatic retinoid, etretinate. *Geburtshilfe Frauenheilkd* 46:242-247, 1986.

133. Bousema MT, Romppanen U, Geiger JM, et al: Acitretin in the treatment of severe lichen sclerosus et atrophicus of the vulva: A double-blind, placebo-controlled study. *J Am Acad Dermatol* 30:225-231, 1994.

134. Marcellus DC, Altomonte VL, Farmer ER, et al: Etretinate therapy for refractory sclerodermatous chronic graft-versus-host disease. *Blood* 93:66-70, 1999.

135. Boyle J, Dick DC, Mackie RM: Treatment of extensive viral warts with etretinate (Tigason) in a patient with sarcoidosis. *Clin Exp Dermatol* 8:33-36, 1983.

136. Rust O, Rufli T, Forrer J: First experience with retinoid acid derivative Ro 10-9359 in the treatment of viral epithelioma. *Schweiz Med Wochenschr* 109:1914-1920, 1979.

137. Ampel NM, Stout ML, Garewal HS, et al: Persistent rectal ulcer associated with human papillomavirus type 33 in a patient with AIDS: Successful treatment with isotretinoin. *Rev Infect Dis* 12:1004-1007, 1990.

138. Bollag W: Retinoids and interferon: A new promising combination? *Br J Haematol* 1:S87-91, 1991.

139. Bollag W: Experimental basis of cancer combination chemotherapy with retinoids, cytokines, 1,25-dihydroxyvitamin D3, and analogs. *J Cell Biochem* 56:427-435, 1994.

Clinical Use—Arotinoids

140. Sherman MI, Truitt GA: Prevention and therapy of tumors with arotinoids. *Eur J Clin Oncol* 24:359-362, 1988.

141. Hoting E, Meissner K: Arotinoid-ethylester: Effectiveness in refractory cutaneous T-cell lymphoma. *Cancer* 62:1044-1048, 1988.

142. Tousignant J, Raymond GP, Light MJ: Treatment of cutaneous T-cell lymphoma with arotinoid Ro 13-6298. *J Am Acad Dermatol* 16:167-171, 1987.

143. Costa A, Formelli F, Chiesa F, et al: Prospects of chemoprevention of human cancers with the synthetic retinoid fenretinide. *Cancer Res* 54:S2032-2037, 1994.

144. Rizvi NA, Marshall JL, Dahut W, et al: A phase I study of LGD 1069 in adults with advanced cancer. *Clin Cancer Res* 5:1658-1664, 1999.

145. Merot Y, Caminzind M, Geiger JM, et al: Arotinoid ethyl ester (Ro 13-6298): A long-term pilot study in various dermatoses. *Acta Derm Venereol* 67:237-242, 1987.

146. Ott F, Geiger JM: Therapeutic effect of arotinoid Ro 13-6298 in psoriasis. *Arch Dermatol Res* 275:257-258, 1983.

147. Tsambaos D, Orfanos CE: Antipsoriatic activity of a new synthetic retinoid. The arotinoid RO 13-6298. *Arch Dermatol* 119:746-751, 1983.

148. Saurat JH, Merot Y, Borsky M, et al: Arotinoid acid (Ro 13-7410): A pilot study in dermatology. *Dermatologica* 176:191-199, 1988.

Adverse Effects and Drug Interactions

149. David M, Hodak E, Lowe NJ: Adverse effects of retinoids. *Med Toxicol* 3:273-288, 1988.

150. Bigby M, Stern RS: Adverse reactions to isotretinoin. A report from the Adverse Drug Reaction Reporting System. *J Am Acad Dermatol* 18:543-552, 1988.

151. Katz IH, Waalen J, Leach EE: Acitretin in psoriasis: an overview of adverse effects. *J Am Acad Dermatol* 41:S7-12, 1999.

152. Meigel WN: How safe is oral isotretinoin? *Dermatology* 195(Suppl 1):22-28, 1997.

153. Saurat J-H: Side effects of systemic retinoids and their clinical management. *J Am Acad Dermatol* 27:S23-28, 1992.

154. Wolverton SE: Major adverse effects from systemic drugs: defining the risks. *Curr Prob Dermatol* 7:1-40, 1995.

155. Stern RS: When a uniquely effective drug is teratogenic: the case of isotretinoin. *N Engl J Med* 320:1007-1009, 1989.

156. Lammer EJ, Chen CT, Hoar RM, et al: Retinoic acid embryopathy. *N Engl J Med* 313:837-841, 1985.

157. Vitamin-A (Aquasol A) package insert. Westborough, MA. Astra USA; 2000.

158. Miller RK, Hendrickx AG, Mills JL, et al: Periconceptional vitamin A use: How much is teratogenic? *Reprod Toxicol* 12:75-88, 1998.

159. Egger SF, Huber-Spitzy V, Bohler K, et al: Ocular side effects associated with 13-cis-retinoic acid therapy for acne vulgaris: Clinical features, alterations of tearfilm and conjunctival flora. *Acta Ophthalmol Scand* 73:355-357, 1995.

160. McGuire J, Lawson JP: Skeletal changes associated with chronic isotretinoin and etretinate administration. *Dermatologica* 175:S169-181, 1987.

161. Pittsley RA, Yoder FW: Skeletal toxicity associated with long-term administration of 13-cis-retinoic acid for refractory ichthyosis. *N Engl J Med* 308:1012-1014, 1983.

162. Leachman SA, Insogna KL, Katz L, et al: Bone densities in patients receiving isotretinoin for cystic acne. *Arch Dermatol* 135:961-965, 1999.

163. DiGiovanna JJ, Sollitto RB, Abagan DL, et al: Osteoporosis is a toxic effect on long-term etretinate therapy. *Arch Dermatol* 131:1263-1267, 1995.

164. Nishimura G, Mugishima H, Hirao J, et al: Generalized metaphyseal modification with cone-shaped epiphyses following long-term administration of 13-cis-retinoic acid. *Eur J Pediatr* 156:432-435, 1997.

165. Paige DG, Judge MR, Shaw DG, et al: Bone changes and their significance in children with ichthyosis on long-term etretinate therapy. *Br J Dermatol* 127:387-391, 1992.

166. Ishida Y, Ozawa A, Ohkido M, et al: Joint pains with psoriasis and long-term systemic etretinate therapy: A case report and sumary of 12 cases. *J Dermatol* 20:651-653, 1993.

167. Vahlquist C, Olsson AG, Lindholm A, et al: Effects of gemfibrozil (Lopid) on hyperlipidemia in acitretin-treated patients. Results of a double-blind cross-over study. *Acta Derm Venereol* 75:377-380, 1995.

168. Standeven AM, Beard RL, Johnson AT, et al: Retinoid-induced hypertriglyceridemia in rats is mediated by retinoic acid receptors. *Fundam Appl Toxicol* 33:264-271, 1996.

169. Noakes M, Clifton PM, Nestel PJ, et al: Effect of high-amylose starch and oat bran on metabolic variables and bowel function in subjects with hypertriglyceridemia. *Am J Clin Nutr* 64:944-951, 1996.

170. Coulston AM: The role of dietary fats in plant-based diets. *Am J Clin Nutr* 70:S512-515, 1999.

171. Roenigk HH Jr, Callen JP, Guzzo CA, et al: Effects of acitretin on the liver. *J Am Acad Dermatol* 41:584-588, 1999.

172. Roenigk HH Jr: Liver toxicity of retinoid therapy. *J Am Acad Dermatol* 19:199-208, 1988.

173. Cribier B, Welsch M, Heid E: Renal impairment probably induced by etretinate. *Dermatology* 185:266-268, 1992.

174. Andersen WK, Feingold DS: Adverse drug interactions clinically important for the dermatologist. *Arch Dermatol* 131:468-473, 1995.

175. Chu A, Cunliffe WJ: The inter-relationship between isotretinoin/acne and depression. *J Eur Acad Dermatol Venereol* 12:263, 1999.

176. Lister RK, Lecky BR, Lewis-Jones MS, et al: Acitretin-induced myopathy (letter). *Br J Dermatol* 134:989-990, 1996.

177. David M, Sandbank M, Lowe NJ: Erythema multiforme-like eruptions associated with etretinate therapy. *Clin Exp Dermatol* 14:230-232, 1989.

178. Lianou P, Bassaris H, Vlachodimitropoulos D, et al: Acitretin induces an increased adherence of *S. aureus* to epithelial cells. *Acta Derm Venereol* 69:330-332, 1989.

179. Williams RE, Doherty VR, Perkins W, et al: *Staphylococcus aureus* and intra-nasal mupirocin in patients receiving isotretinoin for acne. *Br J Dermatol* 126:362-366, 1992.

180. Fernandez-Redondo V, Vazquez J, Sanchez-Aguilar D, et al: Sarcoid-like granuloma following prolonged etretinate treatment. *Dermatology* 188:226-227, 1994.

181. Friedlander SF: Effective treatment of acne fulminans-associated granulation tissue with pulsed dye laser. *Pediatr Dermatol* 15:396-398, 1998.

182. Robertson DB, Kubiak E, Gomez EC: Excess granulation tissue responses associated with isotretinoin therapy. *Br J Dermatol* 111:689-694, 1984.

183. Baran R: Therapeutic assessment and side-effects of the aromatic retinoid on the nail apparatus. *Ann Dermatol Venereol* 109:367-371, 1982.

184. *CliniSphere 2.0 CD ROM,* St. Louis, June 2000, Facts & Comparisons.

185. Cleach LL, Bocquet H, Roujeau JC: Reactions and interactions of some commonly used systemic drugs in dermatology. *Dermatol Clin* 16:421-429, 1998.

186. Wolverton SE: Monitoring for adverse effects from systemic drugs used in dermatology. *J Am Acad Dermatol* 26:661-679, 1992.

187. Cutler LE: Birth Control: The Facts You Need. Roche, Plandex 23097.

Investigational Retinoids

188. Reiners J, Lofberg B, Kraft JC, et al: Transplacental pharmacokinetics of teratogenic doses of etretinate and other aromatic retinoids in mice. *Repro Toxicol* 2:19-29, 1988.

189. Moglia D, Formelli F, Baliva G, et al: Effects of topical treatment with fenretinide (4-HPR) and plasma vitamin A levels in patients with actinic keratoses. *Cancer Lett* 110:87-91, 1996.

190. Tradati N, Chiesa F, Rossi N, et al: Successful topical treatment of oral lichen planus and leukoplakias with fenretinide (4-HPR). *Cancer Lett* 76:109-111, 1994.

191. Chiesa F, Tradati N, Marazza M, et al: Prevention of local relapses and new localizations of oral leukoplakias with the synthetic retinoid fenretinide (4-HPR). Preliminary results. *Eur J Cancer B Oral Oncol* 28B:97-102, 1992.

192. Willhite CC, Dubois A, Schindler-Horvat J, et al: Comparative disposition, receptor affinity, and teratogenic activity of sulfon arotinoids. *Teratology* 52:169-175, 1995.

193. Kistler A, Sterz H, Teelmann K: Ro 15-1570, a new sulfur-containing retinoid devoid of bone toxicity in rats. *Arch Toxicol* 56:117-122, 1984.

194. Misiewicz J, Sendagorta E, Golebiowska A, et al: Topical treatment of multiple actinic keratoses on the face with arotinoid methyl sulfone (Ro 14-9706) cream versus tretinoin cream: a double-blind, comparative study. *J Am Acad Dermatol* 24:448-451, 1991.

195. Formelli F, Barua AB, Olson JA: Bioactivities of N-[4-hydroxyphenyl]retinamide and retinoyl beta-glucuronide. *FASEB J* 10:1014-1024, 1996.

196. Curley RW, Abou-Issa H, Panigot MJ, et al: Chemopreventive activities of C-glucuronide/glycoside analogs of retinoid-O-glucuronides against breast cancer development and growth. *Anticancer Res* 16:757-763, 1996.

197. Zimmermann B, Tsambaos D, Sturje H: Teratogenicity of arotinoid ethyl ester (RO 13-6298) in mice. *Teratog Carcinog Mutagen* 5:415-431, 1985.

198. Kingston T, Gaskell S, Marks R: The effects of a novel potent oral retinoid (Ro 13-6298) in the treatment of multiple solar keratoses and squamous cell epithelioma. *Eur J Cancer Clin Oncol* 19:1201-1205, 1983.

199. Doran TI, Shapiro SS: Retinoid effects on sebocyte proliferation. *Methods Enzymol* 190:334-338, 1990.

200. Bollag W, Peck R: Modulation of human immune functions in vitro by temarotene and its metabolite. *Skin Pharmacol* 4:142-149, 1991.

201. Peck R, Bollag W: Potentiation of retinoid-induced differentiation of HL-60 and U937 cell lines by cytokines. *Eur J Cancer* 27:53-57, 1991.

CHAPTER 14

Warwick L. Morison

PUVA Photochemotherapy

Psoralen plus ultraviolet A (PUVA) photochemotherapy is the photochemical interaction between psoralen and ultraviolet A (UVA) (320 to 400 nm) radiation, which has a beneficial effect in psoriasis and over 30 other skin diseases. The term was originally used for oral methoxsalen photochemotherapy, but it is now loosely used to describe other routes of administration, such as topical and bath PUVA, as well as the use of other psoralen compounds. In this chapter, PUVA therapy refers to its original form unless otherwise stated. The drugs discussed in this chapter are listed in Table 14-1.

DRUG HISTORY

Psoralens are naturally occurring compounds, and several hundred of them occur in plants where they probably act as natural insecticides. Human contact with plants containing psoralens and subsequent exposure to sunlight results in phytophotodermatitis. This represents a phototoxic reaction in the skin manifested as erythema, blistering, and pigmentation. Significant quantities of psoralens are present in fruits and vegetables such as limes, lemons, figs, and parsnips. Thus small amounts are ingested daily as part of an ordinary diet, which might explain the extremely low incidence of allergic sensitization to this family of drugs.

Psoralens, together with sunlight as a source of UVA radiation, have been used in the Middle East and Asia for treatment of vitiligo for at least 3000 years and are still used in this original way in many countries today. El Mofty at the University of Cairo first used a purified psoralen for the treatment of vitiligo in 1947.[1] Methoxsalen (8-methoxypsoralen [8-MOP]), obtained from the seeds of a plant *Ammi majus*, was introduced to the United States in 1951. Trioxsalen (4,5',8 trimethylpsoralen), a synthetic compound, was introduced in 1964. These compounds were approved and used for treatment of vitiligo and enhancement of pigmentation; however, there was little interest in the treatment except on the part of a few dermatologists. This situation changed quite dramatically with the report[2] that oral methoxsalen in combination with a high-output source of UVA radiation was a very effective treatment for psoriasis.

PHARMACOLOGY

Therapy with most orally administered drugs aims at maintaining an adequate blood level for as long as possible. PUVA therapy is quite different because the drug psoralen has no therapeutic effect by itself and only produces an effect when exposed to UVA radiation. Therefore the aim of treatment is to consistently produce a high level of drug in the target organ, skin, only at the time of exposure to UV radiation.

■ Table 14-1 PUVA Photochemotherapy

Generic Name	Trade Name	Generic Available	Manufacturer	Formulations	Standard Dosage Range	Price Index
Methoxsalen (8-methoxypsoralen)	Oxsoralen Ultra	No	ICN Pharmaceuticals	10 mg capsule	0.4 mg/kg 1 hour before UVA	$$$ ($$$$)
	Methoxsalen	No	ICN Pharmaceuticals	10 mg capsule	0.6 mg/kg 2 hours before PUVA	$$$ ($$$$)
	Oxsoralen Lotion	No	ICN Pharmaceuticals	1 mg/ml	Topical application only	—
Trioxsalen (4,5-8 trimethylpsoralen)	Trisoralen	No	ICN Pharmaceuticals	5 mg	0.6 mg/kg 2 hours before UVA	—
Bergapten (5-methoxypsoralen)	Not available in United States	—	—	—	—	—

$, <1.00; $$, 1.01-2.00; $$$, 2.01-5.00; $$$$, 5.01-10.00; $$$$$, >10.00; ( ), generic price; /, two different price ranges from lower dose to higher dose examples of this drug; —, no price listed for this drug.

Presence of psoralen in the skin before and after exposure can be harmful through unintentional exposure to sunlight, resulting in undesirable phototoxicity.

Structure

The structure of methoxsalen is illustrated in Figure 14-1.

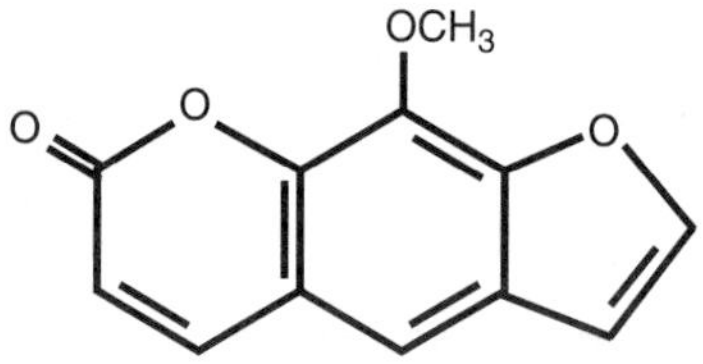

Absorption

Important features of psoralen absorption are listed in Box 14-1. Psoralens are lipophilic, non-ionized compounds and are very poorly soluble in water. This poor solubility impedes their absorption from the stomach and intestine because drugs can only cross biomembranes in a dissolved state. Solubility in water does vary in a ratio of methoxsalen:bergapten:trioxsalen (36:6:1),[3] and this is the major determinant of the relative bioavailability of these compounds. The physical formulation of the compound also alters absorption. Early formulations of methoxsalen con-

Methoxsalen

Figure 14-1 Psoralen structure.

tained large, elongated crystals that were poorly and erratically absorbed. Formulations available today contain micronized crystals of methoxsalen, which is still slowly and incompletely absorbed or dissolved psoralen (Oxsoralen Ultra) in a soft gelatin capsule that is rapidly and more completely absorbed.[4]

Intake of food before taking psoralens slows absorption and reduces the peak blood levels. This is especially significant for foods high in fat

Box 14-1

Unique Features of Psoralen Pharmacology

- Poor solubility in water
- Physical formulation influences absorption
- Food decreases absorption
- First-pass effect through liver
- Large interindividual variation in absorption

content.[5] Thus psoralens are best taken under fasting conditions, because although nausea can be a problem with a high blood level of drug, food intake can be used to alleviate this problem. Psoralens also exhibit a strong but saturable first-pass effect through the intestines and liver. This first-pass effect is accentuated if psoralen absorption is delayed. Thus a fourfold increase in methoxsalen dose (from 10 to 40 mg) resulted in a twenty-fivefold rise in peak plasma level.[6]

Presumably, because of these factors and possibly other undetermined influences, there are large interindividual and smaller intraindividual variations in absorption and bioavailability of methoxsalen and other psoralens. For example, in one study the time of peak photosensitivity after ingestion of a liquid preparation varied from 30 minutes to 3 hours in a small group of subjects and the minimum phototoxic dose (MPD) varied from 2 J/cm^2 to 15 J/cm^2 even though all subjects were fair-skinned.[7]

Bioavailability

The binding of psoralens to proteins is relatively high. In the concentration range usually obtained with oral therapy, 75% to 80% of methoxsalen is reversibly bound to serum protein and 98% to 99% of 5-methoxypsoralen is protein bound.[8] Both psoralen derivatives mainly bind to serum albumin. Epidermal tissue binding is about 90% for methoxsalen and 99% for 5-methoxypsoralen.[8] Autoradiography studies in animals demonstrate that psoralens spread rapidly to most organs, but binding seems to be short-lived and reversible, provided that there is no exposure to UVA radiation.[9,10] After 24 hours no significant radioactivity can be detected.

The best measure of the relative bioavailabilities of the three main psoralen compounds is a determination of the MPD after oral adminis-

tration of standard formulations because the MPD essentially reflects methoxsalen concentration at the target site in the skin. Methoxsalen is the most photoactive, 5-methoxypsoralen is much less photoactive, and trioxsalen is minimally photoactive.

Metabolism

Methoxsalen is metabolized in the liver rapidly and completely; only small amounts of the parent compound can be detected in urine and bile.[11] Most of the known metabolites have their origin in a metabolic attack on the furan ring. There appears to be no accumulation of metabolites. Drugs activating (inducing) cytochrome P-450 enzymes enhance and accelerate metabolism of methoxsalen.

Excretion

In man, after oral administration of 40 mg of methoxsalen, most of the radioactivity is excreted in the urine (74.2%), the fecal excretion representing 14.4% of the total radioactivity.[11] The excretion is rapid and most occurs within 12 hours.

Photochemistry

Ground state psoralen molecules are activated to the excited singlet state by absorption of photons in the UVA waveband. The peak of the absorption spectrum appears to be in the 320 to 330 nm region.[12] The singlet state undergoes decay to the triplet state, and because this is a relatively long-lived state, it is responsible for most photochemical effects. Two types of photochemical reactions occur. Type 1 (direct) photochemical reactions result in photoaddition of the compound to pyrimidines in deoxyribonucleic acid (DNA), forming monofunctional adducts and crosslinking of adjacent strands of DNA and conjugation of proteins. Type II (indirect) photochemical reactions result in production of reactive oxygen species and free radicals that cause damage to cell membranes and cytoplasmic constituents. The relative importance of these nonoxidative and oxygen-mediated pathways in the biologic and therapeutic effects of psoralens is largely undetermined.

Mechanism of Action

The mechanism by which photoactivation of psoralen results in therapeutic benefit for a very diverse group of cutaneous diseases is still speculative. Several hypotheses are suggested below.

SUPPRESSION OF DNA SYNTHESIS.   PUVA therapy suppresses DNA synthesis presumably through the formation of monoadducts and crosslinks in DNA.[13] Early on, it was suggested that this was its mechanism of action in diseases such as psoriasis that are characterized by epidermal proliferation. The main argument against this theory is that the time course of suppression of DNA synthesis is much shorter than the time course of the therapeutic effect.[14]

PHOTOIMMUNOLOGIC EFFECTS.   PUVA therapy causes selective immunosuppression,[15] and the pathogenesis of many of the diseases responding to treatment is characterized by excessive immunologic responses, many of which occur on an autoimmune basis.

SELECTIVE CYTOTOXICITY.   According to this theory, cells responsible for mediating a disease are selectively sensitive to be killed by exposure to PUVA therapy.

STIMULATION OF MELANOCYTES.   The stimulation of melanocytes theory has been invoked to explain the therapeutic effect seen in vitiligo. Although there is no doubt that PUVA therapy does stimulate melanocytes, vitiligo is an autoimmune disease, and PUVA therapy might be working by manipulating the abnormal immune response.

It is quite likely that the mechanism of action of PUVA therapy is different in various diseases. In any given case, there is likely more than one of these mechanisms, as well as other unknown mechanisms.

CLINICAL USE
Indications
Table 14-2 lists indications and contraindications for psoralens.

PSORIASIS.   PUVA therapy is successful in clearing about 90% of patients with plaque-type psoriasis in a course of up to 30 treatments.[2,16-18] The therapy is also effective as a

maintenance treatment, although long-term use has to be balanced against the potential toxicity of the therapy. Erythrodermic and pustular psoriasis can be treated with PUVA therapy alone,[19,20] but a simpler approach is to use acitretin or methotrexate first to reduce inflammation and then start PUVA therapy as a combination treatment. Psoriasis of the palms and soles responds to PUVA therapy,[21] but disease on the soles often requires several times the number of treatments required for the palms. Broadband UVB therapy is much less effective than PUVA therapy in chronic psoriasis,[2] whereas narrowband (311 nm) UVB phototherapy is almost as effective.[22] However, this form of UVB is not a suitable maintenance therapy due to the high treatment requirement of weekly or twice weekly exposures.

VITILIGO.   Vitiligo was the first indication for PUVA therapy, but it has fallen out of favor as a therapy for many dermatologists because of a low and slow response to treatment. Careful selection of patients can improve results.[23] The patient must be highly motivated because 150 to 300 treatments are usually required to produce satisfactory repigmentation. The face is the most responsive site, the torso the next most responsive, and the response diminishes down the limbs to a zero response rate on the hands and feet. Rapidly spreading, active vitiligo and segmental vitiligo rarely respond. Indoor PUVA therapy with oral methoxsalen gives the best results, whereas outdoor therapy using trioxsalen and sunlight gives fair results but is limited by climate in northern areas. Topical PUVA therapy is associated with frequent blistering phototoxic reactions, probably due to exposure to sunlight after the treatment.[24]

NEOPLASTIC DERMATOSES.   The eczematous and plaque stages of mycosis fungoides respond to PUVA therapy in almost all cases after 20 to 30 treatments.[25,26] Combination therapy with interferon alfa-2a is often effective in cases resistant to PUVA therapy alone.[27] Up to 50% of patients will remain in remission after a single course of treatment,[28,29] but due to this high relapse rate a better approach is to use long-term maintenance treatment at a frequency of once or twice a month.[23] PUVA

Table 14-2	Psoralens (PUVA) Indications and Contraindications

FDA-APPROVED INDICATIONS
Psoriasis*[2,16-22]
Vitiligo†[23,24]
Increasing tolerance to sunlight/enhancing
  pigmentation‡

OFF-LABEL USES

Neoplastic
Mycosis fungoides/Sézary syndrome[25-29]
Histiocytosis X (Langerhans' cell histiocytosis)[30]

Dermatitis/Papulosquamous
Atopic dermatitis[31,32]
Seborrheic dermatitis[33]
Chronic hand dermatitis[21]
Palmoplantar pustulosis[21]
Lichen planus[34,35]
Parapsoriasis[28]
Pityriasis lichenoides[36,37]
Lymphomatoid papulosis[38]

Photosensitivity Dermatoses
Polymorphous light eruption[39,40]
Erythropoietic protoporphyria[41]
Solar urticaria[42]
Chronic actinic dermatitis[43]

Other Pruritic Dermatoses
Dermographism[44]
Aquagenic urticaria/pruritus[45,46]
Chronic urticaria[47]
Polycythemia vera[48]
Idiopathic pruritus
Urticaria pigmentosa[49,50]
Prurigo nodularis[31]

Other Immunologic Dermatoses
Alopecia areata[51-53]
Graft-versus-host disease[54,55]
Morphea[56]
Linear scleroderma[56]

Miscellaneous Dermatoses
Transient acantholytic dermatosis (Grover's
  disease)[57]
Pigmented purpuric dermatoses[58]
Icthyosis linearis circumflexa[59]
Scleromyxedema[60]
Generalized granuloma annulare[61,62]

CONTRAINDICATIONS

Absolute
Pemphigus and pemphigoid[63,64]
Lupus erythematosus with photosensitivity
Xeroderma pigmentosum
Lactation
History of idiosyncratic reaction to psoralen
  compound

Relative
Photosensitivity/photosensitizing medications
Prior exposure to ionizing radiation or arsenic
History or family history of melanoma
History of skin cancer or chronic photodamage
Pregnancy
Severe cardiac, liver, or renal disease
Young age

PREGNANCY PRESCRIBING STATUS—CATEGORY C

*Methoxsalen capsules are approved for this indication.
†Methoxsalen solution and trioxsalen are approved for this indication.
‡Trioxsalen is approved for this indication.

therapy is usually not effective in the tumor phase of the disease unless there are only a few lesions that can be treated with adjunctive local x-irradiation. Sézary syndrome is not responsive to PUVA therapy. The skin lesions of histiocy-tosis X in two elderly patients cleared with a course of PUVA therapy, and although the lesions relapsed after cessation of treatment, repeat courses were again successful in producing a remission.[30]

DERMATITIS AND PAPULOSQUAMOUS DERMATOSES. In dermatitis and papulosquamous dermatoses PUVA therapy was first used in atopic eczema.[31] About 20 to 40 treatments are usually required to control the disease and maintenance should be given for at least 6 months. Adjunctive topical or oral corticosteroids are often required to control exacerbations of eczema during the early clearance phase of therapy, and antibiotics may be necessary to treat folliculitis or impetiginization, which can be associated features of this condition. PUVA therapy is indicated in adolescents with severe eczema so as to permit resumption of normal growth if this has been retarded by corticosteroid treatment.[32] Seborrheic dermatitis,[33] chronic hand eczema, and palmoplantar pustulosis[21] show a similar response to a regular course of PUVA therapy, and like atopic eczema require limited maintenance treatment. Lichen planus, both on the skin[34] and in the mouth,[35] responds to about 30 to 40 treatment sessions and usually maintenance treatment is not required. For oral lesions a dental UVA light source is used. Pityriasis lichenoides in both the acute and chronic forms responds to PUVA therapy, sometimes with long remissions, but more often prolonged maintenance is required.[36,37] The response in lymphomatoid papulosis is similar.[38]

PHOTOSENSITIVITY DERMATOSES. Patients with various photodermatoses·can be desensitized by prophylactic exposure to a course of PUVA therapy. Polymorphous light eruption is the most common indication for this treatment, and three exposures a week for 4 weeks in spring produce complete suppression in about 90% of patients.[39,40] About half the patients develop their eruption during treatment, but this can usually be controlled by topical corticosteroids while therapy continues. Erythropoietic protoporphyria responds in a similar manner.[41] Suppression of solar urticaria can also be achieved by PUVA therapy; however, given the risk of triggering a generalized urticarial rash with systemic collapse, this should only be attempted in a specialized center.[42] Treatment of chronic actinic dermatitis with PUVA therapy requires combined treatment with high doses of oral corticosteroids, although this therapy is not successful in controlling this challenging condition in most patients.[43]

OTHER PRURITIC DERMATOSES. PUVA therapy is effective in a variety of pruritic dermatoses, and a course of 30 to 40 treatments usually achieves a complete remission (see Table 14-2). However, in most instances symptoms return unless prolonged maintenance treatment is given, so the risks of treatment must be balanced against the need for treatment and alternative treatments available.

OTHER IMMUNOLOGIC DERMATOSES. PUVA therapy has been used in all forms of alopecia areata with moderate success,[51,52] but there have been no controlled trials, and the efficacy of the treatment has been questioned.[53] Graft-versus-host disease on the skin and in the mouth responds to PUVA therapy[54,55] and can be a very useful treatment by reducing necessity for systemic immunosuppression. Linear and generalized morphea respond to PUVA therapy, and once all activity is suppressed, maintenance therapy is unnecessary.[56]

MISCELLANEOUS DERMATOSES. Miscellaneous dermatoses, which are listed in Table 14-2, all respond to PUVA therapy, usually requiring 20 to 50 treatments to clear; maintenance treatment is usually unnecessary.

Contraindications

There are only a few absolute contraindications to PUVA therapy (see Table 14-2). Lactation is listed because psoralens are probably secreted in breast milk. If PUVA therapy is essential for the mother, lactation should stop. Treatment should be used with caution in the presence of any of the relative contraindications. When a patient is taking a potentially photosensitizing medication, this fact should be noted; however, adjustment of the dose of UVA radiation is only required when potent phototoxic agents are involved. These include doxycycline and the fluoroquinolones, in particular lomefloxacin and sparfloxacin. A 25% reduction in dose is usually adequate in these circumstances. Aphakia is often listed as a contraindication but is not, provided the patient is advised that good eye protection is essential. For the past decade all lens implants have been UV-opaque and this provides good protection for the retina.

Treatment Procedure

METHOXSALEN.   Methoxsalen is taken orally as capsules in a dose of 0.4 to 0.6 mg/kg body weight 1 or 2 hours before exposure to UVA radiation (Table 14-3). In general 0.4 mg/kg is recommended for the Oxsoralen Ultra version of methoxsalen, due to better and more predictable absorption of this specific product. The lower dose reduces the problem of nausea and the 1-hour interval is more convenient for patients. In addition, there is a cost savings with the lower methoxsalen dose allowed by using the Oxsoralen Ultra product. The medication should be taken with water only, at least 1 hour after eating. Ideally food should be avoided until after the treatment. As noted previously, selected patients can reduce the nausea associated with the methoxsalen by taking the drug with food.

UVA RADIATION.   The doses of UVA radiation (Table 14-4) are usually determined by skin type (Table 14-5). An alternative approach that is frequently used in Europe is to determine the MPD and then start at 70% of this dose. The MPD is determined by exposing eight one-inch squares on the back to increasing doses of UVA radiation 1 to 2 hours after ingestion of methoxsalen (Table 14-6). The MPD is the lowest dose resulting in erythema filling all four margins of the square, when read 48 hours later. This approach is more time-consuming but probably reduces overall exposure to radiation. Exposure to UVA radiation usually involves the

■ Table 14-3   Dose Schedule for Methoxsalen at 0.4 mg/kg Body Weight

Patient Weight		Oxsoralen Ultra Dose (mg)
Lb	Kg	
<66	>30	10
66-143	30-65	20
144-200	65-90	30
>200	>90	40

■ Table 14-4   Dose of UVA Radiation for "Induction Phase" Schedules[65]

	UVA Radiation Dose (J/cm^2)		
Skin Type	Initial Dose	Increments	Maximum Dose
I	1.5	0.5	5
II	2.5	0.5	8
III	3.5	0.5-1.0	12
IV	4.5	1.0	14
V	5.5	1.0	16
VI	6.5	1.0-1.5	20

■ Table 14-5   Sun-Reactive Skin Types[66]

Skin Type	History	Examination
I	Always burn, never tan	
II	Always burn, sometimes tan	
III	Sometimes burn, always tan	
IV	Never burn, always tan	
V		Brown skin*
VI		Black skin

*Asian, Hispanic, Middle Eastern.

■ Table 14-6   Dose Range of UVA Radiation for Determining MPD[66]

Skin Type	(J/cm^2)
I	1-8
II-IV	2-16
V-VI	10-24

whole body in a stand-up phototherapy unit. Exposure can be limited to the limbs only by wearing a gown during the treatment. If disease is present on the hands and feet, a hand and foot UVA machine can be employed. Similarly, additional treatment after a whole body exposure can be given to the hands and feet if there is marked disease at those sites.

CLEARANCE SCHEDULE.　Treatments are usually given two or three times weekly at least 48 hours apart to permit evaluation of any erythema resulting from the preceding treatment. If erythema is present and widespread, treatment should be stopped until it clears. Localized erythema, such as on the breasts or buttocks, may be shielded and treatment continued. When 95% or more of the original area of psoriasis has cleared, the patient is changed to a maintenance schedule.

MAINTENANCE SCHEDULE.　The final clearance dose of radiation is held constant and the frequency of treatment is gradually reduced as listed in Box 14-2. If a significant (>5%) amount of psoriasis begins to return, the frequency of treatment can be increased or a clearance schedule can be restarted. In most patients, an attempt to achieve and maintain a completely disease-free state results in exposure to unacceptably high cumulative UVA levels. For example, maintaining completely clear knees and elbows usually requires twice as much UVA exposure compared with that required if some disease activity is accepted at those sites.

ADJUNCTIVE TREATMENT.　Concurrent topical therapy is required for areas shielded from exposure to UVA radiation. This includes the scalp and all intertriginous areas.

COMBINATION TREATMENTS.　The advantages of using combination treatments are that they increase the success rate of therapy and potentially reduce overall exposure to UVA radiation. The most commonly employed combination treatments are listed in Box 14-3. The main indications for combination treatment are skin type 4 to 6, erythrodermic psoriasis, generalized pustular psoriasis, thick plaques, and very active, inflammatory psoriasis. In addition, UVB plus

---

Box 14-2

Maintenance Schedule for PUVA Therapy

Four treatments at weekly intervals
then
Four treatments every other week
then
Four treatments every third week
then
Four treatments every fourth week
then
Stop treatment or continue monthly
　treatments

Box 14-3

Combination Treatments Utilizing PUVA Photochemotherapy[67]

PUVA + METHOTREXATE[68]
- Methotrexate therapy initiated for 3 weeks
- Then PUVA + methotrexate until clear
- Stop methotrexate and maintain with PUVA therapy

PUVA + ACITRETIN: "REPUVA"[69]
- Acitretin therapy initiated for 2 weeks
- Then acitretin plus PUVA until clear
- Stop acitretin and maintain with PUVA therapy

PUVA + UVB[70]
- PUVA + high-dose UVB therapy (70% MED and 20% increments)
- Both treatments given at same time
- Stop UVB when clear

PUVA + TOPICAL THERAPY
- PUVA + calcipotriene[71]
- PUVA + tazarotene[72]

PUVA therapy is useful in patients showing a relatively slow response to PUVA therapy.

PROTECTION.　The main elements in protection from inadvertent exposure to UV radiation are listed in Box 14-4. When considering protection, it is important to remember that the amount of UVA radiation in sunlight does not vary much with seasons or time of day. Eye pro-

Box 14-4

Protection During PUVA Therapy[73]

WHILE IN THE PUVA UNIT PROTECT
- Eyes using small UV-opaque goggles
- Face using sunscreen or pillowcase
- Male genitalia using jock-strap or underpants

AFTER EXPOSURE TO OXSORALEN ULTRA PROTECT
- Eyes using wrap-around UV-opaque glasses when exposed to sunlight until sunset
- Eyes when exposed to sunlight through windows
- Skin using clothing, sunscreen, and avoidance of sunlight

NONTREATMENT DAYS PROTECT
- Skin avoiding sun exposure and use of sunscreens

Box 14-5

Short-Term Adverse Effects of PUVA Therapy[74]

PHOTOTOXIC REACTIONS
- Symptomatic erythema
- Pruritus
- Subacute phototoxicity
- Photoonycholysis
- Koebner phenomenon
- Friction blisters on hands and feet
- Phytophotodermatitis
- Ankle edema
- Hypertrichosis

DUE TO METHOXSALEN ALONE
- Gastrointestinal disturbance
- CNS disturbance
- Bronchoconstriction
- Hepatic toxicity
- Drug fever
- Exanthems

OTHER ADVERSE EFFECTS
- Cardiovascular stress
- Herpes simplex recurrences
- Photosensitive eruptions

tection with UVA-blocking glasses is required when the patient is using sunlight for illumination, from time of exposure to psoralen until sunset that day. In addition, regular use of UV-blocking glasses should be encouraged whenever exposed to sunlight, including exposure through windows. A sunscreen with an SPF of at least 15 and including Parsol 1789 as an ingredient is required for protection from a psoralen phototoxic reaction. Men should wear a jock strap or another means of genital protection.

Short-Term Adverse Effects

Short-term adverse effects are listed in Box 14-5. Nausea is a common adverse effect and it clearly correlates with the serum level of the drug. As a first step, nausea can usually be relieved by having the patient eat some food with ingestion of methoxsalen, given that food reduces and slows absorption. The next step is to reduce the dose by one capsule, and lastly, and very occasionally, an antiemetic is required. Symptomatic erythema is the most common phototoxic reaction and occurs in about 10% of patients.[75] There is no specific treatment; however, supportive measures, such as aspirin and cool baths, are helpful. Pruritus (the so-called PUVA itch) and subacute phototoxicity are in-

dications for stopping treatment until these problems clear, typically resuming therapy at a slightly reduced UVA dose. Central nervous system disturbances are a common adverse effect of PUVA therapy and are a "dark" effect of psoralen. They affect many patients and include headache, insomnia, hyperactivity, mild depression, and a host of other complaints.

Long-Term Adverse Effects

Long-term adverse effects are listed in Box 14-6. Photoaging of the skin occurs in all patients of skin types I through IV who have long-term exposure to the treatment. It is the most significant adverse effect for most patients. Photoaging involves freckling, loss of pigmentation, wrinkling and formation of keratoses. The so-called PUVA lentigines, which are usually large, dark, and irregularly shaped,[77] form part of this spectrum. Photoaging changes are only partially reversible on stopping treatment.

Nonmelanoma skin cancer is markedly in-

Box 14-6

Long-Term Adverse Effects of PUVA Therapy

Photoaging of the skin[76,77]
Nonmelanoma skin cancer[78-89]
Melanoma
- "Negative" studies[80-88]
- Single case reports[91-96]
- "Positive" study[90]

creased in patients who receive high cumulative UVA exposure. Again this risk is mainly confined to Caucasians. In the United States multicenter study of nearly 1400 patients treated with PUVA therapy starting in the 1970s, about one third of patients developed squamous cell carcinoma of the skin, and there have been smaller increases in basal cell carcinomas and keratoacanthomas.[78,79] This increased risk of skin cancer is dose-dependent and is particularly evident in patients receiving more than 250 treatments. These findings have been confirmed in other smaller studies.[80-88] An increased risk of squamous cell carcinoma on male genitalia has also been found in the United States multicenter study[89] but this has not been reported in other studies. Tumors have been easily treated in most instances, but metastatic spread has been reported.[79]

More recently an increased incidence of melanoma has been detected in this same study.[90] The increased incidence first appeared 15 years after the first PUVA treatment and again mainly affects patients who received more than 250 treatments. There have been isolated case reports of patients developing melanoma while on PUVA therapy,[91-96] but this has not been reported in other studies.[80-88] Continued observation of patients is required to confirm this finding.

There has been concern about other long-term adverse effects, most notably cataracts and immunosuppression. A small increase in the incidence of cataracts was reported in this multicenter study; however, there was no dose-response relationship and therefore it is likely due to the close observation of this group.[97] Similarly, there

have been no reports of any clinically important consequences from immunosuppression.

DRUG INTERACTIONS

Only two uncommon drug interactions have been observed with PUVA therapy. Phototoxic agents such as doxycycline and the fluoroquinolones may augment the action of the treatment leading to acute phototoxic erythema. Other photoactive agents such as the thiazide diuretics do not appear to cause adverse reactions of any significance.[98] Drugs that activate P-450 enzymes in the liver may decrease the effectiveness of the treatment through enhanced metabolism of methoxsalen; this is often seen with carbamazepine and phenytoin.[99]

MONITORING GUIDELINES

A complete skin examination is essential before commencing treatment and an ophthalmologic examination should be obtained close to baseline. Routine laboratory tests are not required.[73] Skin cancer is the most important adverse effect of long-term treatment. Patients should be educated about this risk; any questionable lesions must be examined by the physician, and if indicated a biopsy should be performed.

THERAPEUTIC GUIDELINES

Over 90% of unselected patients with moderate-to-severe psoriasis can be cleared with PUVA therapy.[65] Maintenance treatment prolongs remission and may be required on a long-term basis.[100] When treatment is stopped, psoriasis may return months or years later. In this case there is no rebound phenomenon as seen with some other treatments for psoriasis (see Treatment Procedure section).

Other Forms of PUVA Therapy

Topical PUVA therapy is an approved treatment for vitiligo. Methoxsalen lotion, usually diluted 1 in 10 with ethanol to give a 0.1% solution, is applied 15 minutes before exposure to UVA radiation. The initial exposure dose is 0.5 J/cm^2 with increments of 0.25 J/cm^2 until a light pink color is obtained in the vitiliginous skin. The main problem with this treatment is unexpected phototoxic reactions that are often bullous. This is typically caused by inadvertent exposure to sunlight after treatment sessions,[101] a problem that is hard to avoid.

A very dilute solution of psoralen in bath water (for whole-body exposure) or a basin (for treatment of the hands and feet) is used as an alternative to oral administration of the methox-salen in some centers. These topical routes of administration have the advantage of avoiding most systemic adverse effects of psoralens (such as nausea), although eye protection is still necessary because significant drug levels can still be detected in serum. Schedules have been published using the lotion[102] and liquid-filled capsules[103] as sources of methoxsalen. This method of treatment has not been approved by the FDA and thus has potential medicolegal consequences, which can have unfavorable outcomes for the treating physician.

Bibliography

British Photodermatology Group: British Photodermatology group guidelines for PUVA. *Br J Dermatol* 130:246-255, 1994.

Drake LA, Ceilley RI, Dorner W, et al: Guidelines of care for phototherapy and photochemotherapy. *J Am Acad Dermatol* 31:643-648, 1994.

Gupta AK, Anderson TF: Psoralen photochemotherapy. *J Am Acad Dermatol* 17:703-734, 1987.

Honig B, Morison W, Karp D: Photochemotherapy beyond psoriasis. *J Am Acad Dermatol* 31:775-790, 1994.

Morison WL: *Phototherapy and photochemotherapy of skin disease,* ed 2, New York, 1990, Raven Press.

Morison WL, Baughman RD, Day RM, et al: Consensus workshop on the toxic effects of long-term PUVA therapy. *Arch Dermatol* 134:595-598, 1998.

Studniberg HM, Weller R: PUVA, UVB, psoriasis, and nonmelanoma skin cancer. *J Am Acad Dermatol* 29:1013-1022, 1993.

References

Introduction and Pharmacology

1. El Mofty AM: A preliminary clinical report on the treatment of leukoderma with Ammi majus. *J Royal Egyptian M A* 31:651-662, 1948.
2. Parrish JA, Fitzpatrick TB, Tannenbaum L, et al: Photochemotherapy of psoriasis with oral methoxsalen and longwave ultraviolet light. *N Engl J Med* 291:1207-1211, 1974.
3. Brickl R, Schmid J, Koss FW: Clinical pharmacology of oral psoralen drugs. *Photodermatology* 1:174-186, 1984.
4. Honigsmann H, Jaschke E, Nitsche V, et al: Serum levels of 8-methoxypsoralen in two different drug preparations: correlation with photosensitivity and UV-A dose requirements for photochemotherapy. *J Invest Dermatol* 79:233-236, 1982.
5. Roelandts R, Van Boven M, Deheyn T, et al: Dietary influences on 8-MOP plasma levels in PUVA patients with psoriasis. *Br J Dermatol* 105:569-572, 1981.
6. Schmid J, Prox A, Zipp H, et al: The use of stable isotopes to prove the saturable first-pass effect of methoxsalen. *Biomed Mass Spectro* 7:560-564, 1980.
7. Levins PC, Gange RW, Momtaz-T K, et al: A new liquid formulation of 8-methoxypsoralen: bioactivity and effect of diet. *J Invest Dermatol* 82:185-187, 1984.
8. Artuc M, Stuettgen G, Schalla W, et al: Reversible binding of 5- and 8-methoxypsoralen to human serum proteins (albumin) and to epidermis in vitro. *Br J Dermatol* 101:669-673, 1979.
9. Wulf HC, Andreasen MP: Distribution of 3H-8-MOP and its metabolites in rat organs after a single oral administration. *J Invest Dermatol* 76:252-258, 1981.
10. Muni IA, Schneider H, Olsson TA, et al: Absorption, distribution, and excretion of 8-methoxypsoralen in HRA/Skh mice. *Natl Cancer Inst Monogr* 66:85-90, 1984.
11. Schmid J, Reuter A, Zipp H, et al: The metabolism of 8-methoxypsoralen in man. *Eur J Drug Metab Pharm* 5:81-92, 1980.
12. Cripps DJ, Lowe NJ, Lerner AB: Action spectra of topical psoralens: a re-evaluation. *Br J Dermatol* 107:77-82, 1982.
13. Epstein JH, Fukuyama K: Effects of 8-methoxypsoralen-induced phototoxic effects of mammalian epidermal macromolecule synthesis in vivo. *Photochem Photobiol* 24:325-330, 1975.
14. Fritsch PO, Gschnait F, Kaaserer G, et al: PUVA suppresses the proliferative stimulus produced by stripping on hairless mice. *Invest Derm* 73:188-190, 1979.
15. Morison WL: In vivo effects of psoralens plus longwave ultraviolet radiation on immunity. In Pathak MA, Dunnick JK, editors: *Photobiologic, toxicologic, and pharmacologic aspects of psoralens,* Bethesda, MD, 1986, NCI Monograph, pp 243-246.

Clinical Use—Psoriasis

16. Stern RS, Fitzpatrick TB, Honigsmann H, et al: Oral psoralen photochemotherapy. In Roenigk HH, Maibach HI, editors: *Psoriasis,* New York, 1985, Marcel Dekker, pp 475-492.
17. Anonymous: Photochemotherapy for psoriasis. A clinical cooperative study of PUVA-48 and PUVA-64. *Arch Dermatol* 115:576-579, 1979.
18. Henseler T, Wolff K, Honigsmann H, et al: Oral 8-methoxypsoralen photochemotherapy of psoriasis. *Lancet* 1:853-857, 1981.
19. Vukas A: Photochemotherapy in treatment of psoriatic variants. *Dermatologica* 55:355-361, 1977.
20. Honigsmann H, Gschnait F, Konrad K, et al: Photochemotherapy for pustular psoriasis (von Zumbusch). *Br J Dermatol* 97:119-126, 1977.
21. Morison WL, Parrish JA, Fitzpatrick TB: Oral methoxsalen photochemotherapy of recalcitrant dermatoses of the palms and soles. *Br J Dermatol* 99:297-302, 1978.
22. Tanew A, Radakovic-Fijan S, Schemper M, et al: Narrowband UV-B phototherapy vs photochemotherapy in the treatment of chronic plaque-type psoriasis. *Arch Dermatol* 135:519-524, 1999.

Vitiligo

23. Lassus A, Halme K, Eskelinen A, et al: Treatment of vitiligo with oral methoxsalen and UVA. *Photodermatology* 1:170-173, 1984.

24. Ortel B, Maytum DJ, Gange RW: Long persistence of monofunctional 8-methoxypsoralen-DNA adducts in human skin. *Photochem Photobiol* 54:645-650, 1991.

Neoplastic

25. Gilcrest BA, Parrish JA, Tanenbaum L, et al: Oral methoxsalen photochemotherapy of mycosis fungoides. *Cancer* 38:683-689, 1976.
26. Briffa DV, Warin AP, Harrington CI, et al: Photochemotherapy in mycosis fungoides. *Lancet* 2:49-53, 1980.
27. Kuzel TM, Roenigk HH, Samuelson E, et al: Effectiveness of interferon alfa-2a combined with phototherapy for mycosis fungoides and the Sezary syndrome. *J Clin Oncol* 13:257-263, 1995.
28. Honigsmann H, Brenner W, Rauschmeier, et al: Photochemotherapy for cutaneous T cell lymphoma. *J Am Acad Dermatol* 10:238-245, 1984.
29. Rosenbaum MM, Roenigk HH, Caro WA, et al: Photochemotherapy in cutaneous T cell lymphoma and parapsoriasis en plaques. *J Am Acad Dermatol* 13:613-622, 1985.
30. Iwatsuki K, Tsugiki M, Yoshizawa N, et al: The effect of phototherapies on cutaneous lesions of histiocytosis X in the elderly. *Cancer* 57:1931-1936, 1986.

Papulosquamous/Dermatitis

31. Morison WL, Parish JA, Fitzpatrick TB: Oral psoralen photochemotherapy of atopic eczema. *Br J Dermatol* 98:25-29, 1978.
32. Atherton DJ, Carabott F, Glover MT, et al: The role of psoralen photochemotherapy (PUVA) in the treatment of severe atopic eczema in adolescents. *Br J Dermatol* 118:791-795, 1988.
33. Dahl KB, Reymann F: Photochemotherapy in erythrodermic seborrheic dermatitis. *Arch Dermatol* 113:1295-1296, 1977.
34. Gonzales E, Momtaz-T K, Freedman S: Bilateral comparison of generalized lichen planus treated with psoralens and ultraviolet A. *J Am Acad Dermatol* 10:958-961, 1984.
35. Lundquist G, Forsgren H, Gajecki M, et al: Photochemotherapy of oral lichen planus. *Oral Surg Oral Med Oral Pathol Oral Radiol Endod* 79:554-558, 1995.
36. Boelen RE, Faber WR, Lambers JCCA, et al: Long-term follow-up of photochemotherapy in pityriasis lichenoides. *Acta Derm Venereol Suppl (Stockh)* 62:442-444, 1982.

37. Powell FC, Muller SA: Psoralens and ultraviolet A therapy of pityriasis lichenoides. *J Am Acad Dermatol* 10:59-64, 1984.
38. Wantzin GL, Thomas K: PUVA treatment in lymphomatoid papulosis. *Br J Dermatol* 107:687-690, 1982.

Photosensitivity Dermatoses

39. Gschnait F, Honigsmann H, Brenner W, et al: Induction of UV light tolerance by PUVA in patients with polymorphous light eruption. *Br J Dermatol* 99:293-296, 1978.
40. Parrish JA, LeVine MJ, Morison WL, et al: Comparison of PUVA and beta-carotene in the treatment of polymorphous light eruption. *Br J Dermatol* 100:187-191, 1979.
41. Ros AM: PUVA therapy for erythropoietic protoporphyria. *Photodermatology* 5:148-149, 1988.
42. Parrish JA, Jaenicke KF, Morison WL, et al: Solar urticaria: treatment with PUVA and mediator inhibitors. *Br J Dermatol* 106:575-580, 1982.
43. Yokel BK, Hood AF, Morison WL: Management of chronic photosensitive eczema. *Arch Dermatol* 126:1283-1285, 1990.

Other Off-Label Uses

44. Logan RA, O'Brien TJ, Greaves MW: The effect of psoralen photochemotherapy (PUVA) on symptomatic dermographism. *Clin Exp Dermatol* 14:25-28, 1989.
45. Martinez-Escribano JA, Quecedo E, DelaCuadra J, et al: Treatment of aquagenic urticaria with PUVA and astemizole. *J Am Acad Dermatol* 36:118-119, 1997.
46. Du H, Menage P, Norris PG, et al: The efficacy of psoralen photochemotherapy in the treatment of aquagenic pruritus. *Br J Dermatol* 129:163-165, 1993.
47. Midelfart K, Moseng D, Kavli G, et al: A case of chronic urticaria and vitiligo, associated with thyroiditis, treated with PUVA. *Dermatologica* 167:39-41, 1983.
48. Morison WL, Nesbitt JA: Oral psoralen photochemotherapy (PUVA) for pruritus associated with polycythemia vera and myelofibrosis. *Am J Hematol* 42:409-410, 1993.
49. Christophers E, Honigsmann H, Wolff K, et al: PUVA treatment of urticaria pigmentosa. *Br J Dermatol* 98:701, 1978.
50. Briffa DV, Eady RAJ, James MP, et al: Photochemotherapy (PUVA) in the treatment of urticaria pigmentosa. *Br J Dermatol* 109:67-75, 1983.

51. Claudy AL, Gagnaire D: Photochemotherapy for alopecia areata. *Acta Derm Venereol* 601:171-177, 1980.
52. Larko O, Swanbeck G: PUVA treatment of alopecia totalis. *Acta Derm Venereol* 63:546-549, 1983.
53. Healy E, Rogers S: PUVA treatment for alopecia areata—does it work? A retrospective review of 102 cases. *Br J Dermatol* 129:42-44, 1993.
54. Jampel RM, Farmer ER, Vogelsang GB, et al: PUVA therapy for chronic cutaneous graft-vs-host disease. *Arch Dermatol* 127:1673-1678, 1991.
55. Vogelsang GB, Wolff D, Altomonte V, et al: Treatment of chronic graft-versus-host disease with ultraviolet irradiation and psoralen (PUVA). *Bone Marrow Transplant* 17:1061-1067, 1996.
56. Morison WL: Psoralen UVA therapy for linear and generalized morphea. *J Am Acad Dermatol* 37:657-659, 1997.
57. Paul BS, Arndt KA: Response of transient acantholytic dermatosis to photochemotherapy. *Arch Dermatol* 120:121-122, 1984.
58. Krizsa J, Hunyadi J, Dobozy A: PUVA treatment of pigmented purpuric lichenoid dermatitis. *J Am Acad Dermatol* 27:778-780, 1992.
59. Manabe M, Yoshiike T, Negi M, et al: Successful therapy of ichthyosis linearis circumflexa with PUVA. *J Am Acad Dermatol* 8:905-906, 1983.
60. Farr PM, Ive FA: PUVA treatment of scleromyxoedema. *Br J Dermatol* 110:347-350, 1984.
61. Hindson TC, Spiro JG, Cochrane H: PUVA therapy of diffuse granuloma annulare. *Clin Exp Dermatol* 13:26-27, 1988.
62. Kerker BJ, Huang CP, Morison WL: Photochemotherapy of generalized granuloma annulare. *Arch Dermatol* 126:359-361, 1990.
63. Thomsen K, Schmidt H: PUVA-induced bullous pemphigoid. *Br J Dermatol* 95:568-569, 1976.
64. Fryer EJ, Lebwohl M: Pemphigus vulgaris after initiation of psoralen and UVA therapy for psoriasis. *J Am Acad Dermatol* 30:651-653, 1994.

Treatment Procedure

65. Melski JW, Tanenbaum L, Parrish JA, et al: Oral methoxsalen photochemotherapy for the treatment of psoriasis: a cooperative clinical trial. *J Invest Dermatol* 68:328-335, 1977.
66. Wolff K, Gschnait F, Honigsmann H, et al: Phototesting and dosimetry for photochemotherapy. *Br J Dermatol* 96:1-10, 1977.
67. Morison WL: PUVA combination therapy. *Photodermatology* 2:229-236, 1985.
68. Morison WL, Momtaz K, Parrish JA, et al: Combined methotrexate-PUVA therapy in the treatment of psoriasis. *J Am Acad Dermatol* 6:46-51, 1982.
69. Tanew A, Guggenbichler A, Honigsmann H, et al: Photochemotherapy for severe psoriasis without or in combination with acitretin: a randomized, double-blind comparison study. *J Am Acad Dermatol* 25:682-684, 1991.
70. Momtaz-T K, Parrish JA: Combination of psoralens and ultraviolet A and ultraviolet B in the treatment of psoriasis vulgaris: a bilateral comparison study. *J Am Acad Dermatol* 10:481-486, 1984.
71. Harada H, Hashimoto K, Toi Y, et al: Reduction of UV-A radiation induced by calcipotriol in the treatment of vulgar psoriasis with oral psoralen plus UV-A. *Arch Dermatol* 133:668-669, 1997.
72. Behrens S, Grundmann-Kollmann M, Peter R-U, et al: Combination treatment of psoriasis with photochemotherapy and tazarotene gel, a receptor-selective topical retinoid. *Br J Dermatol* 141:177, 1999.
73. Drake LA, Ceilley RI, Dorner W, et al: Guidelines of care for phototherapy and photochemotherapy. *J Am Acad Dermatol* 31:643-648, 1994.

Adverse Effects and Drug Interactions

74. Morison WL: *Phototherapy and photochemotherapy of skin disease*, ed 2, New York, 1990, Raven Press, pp 113-120.
75. Morison WL, Marwaha S, Beck L: PUVA-induced phototoxicity: Incidence and causes. *J Am Acad Dermatol* 36:183-185, 1997.
76. Stern RS, Parrish JA, Fitzpatrick TB, et al: Actinic degeneration in association with long-term use of PUVA. *J Invest Dermatol* 84:135-138, 1985.
77. Rhodes AR, Harrist TJ, Momtaz-T K: The PUVA-induced pigmented macule: a lentiginous proliferation of large, sometimes cytologically atypical, melanocytes. *J Am Acad Dermatol* 9:47-58, 1983.

78. Stern RS, Lange R, and Members of the Photochemotherapy Follow-up Study: Non-melanoma skin cancer occurring in patients treated with PUVA five to ten years after first treatment. *J Invest Dermatol* 91:120-124, 1988.

79. Stern RS, Laird N: The carcinogenic risk of treatments for severe psoriasis. *Cancer* 73:2759-2764, 1994.

80. Reshad H, Cahalloner F, Pollock DJ, et al: Cutaneous carcinoma in psoriatic patients treated with PUVA. *Br J Dermatol* 110:299-305, 1984.

81. Rorman AB, Roenigk HH, Caro WA, et al: Long-term follow-up of skin cancer in the PUVA-48 cooperative study. *Arch Dermatol* 125:515-519, 1989.

82. Lindelof B, Sigurgeirsson N, Tegner E, et al: PUVA and cancer: a large-scale epidemiological study. *Lancet* 338:91-93, 1991.

83. Bruynzeel I, Bergman W, Hartevelt HM, et al: 'High single-dose' European PUVA regimen also causes an excess of non-melanoma skin cancer. *Br J Dermatol* 124:49-55, 1991.

84. Chuang TY, Heinrich LA, Schultz MD, et al: PUVA and skin cancer. *J Am Acad Dermatol* 26:173-177, 1992.

85. Lever LR, Farr PM: Skin cancers or premalignant lesions occur in half of high-dose PUVA patients. *Br J Dermatol* 131:215-219, 1994.

86. McKenna KE, Patterson CC, Handley J, et al: Cutaneous neoplasia following PUVA therapy for psoriasis. *Br J Dermatol* 134:639-642, 1996.

87. Lindelof B, Sigurgeirsson B, Tegner E, et al: PUVA and cancer risk: the Swedish follow-up study. *Br J Dermatol* 141:108-112, 1999.

88. Stern RS, Lunder EJ: Risk of squamous cell carcinoma and methoxsalen (psoralen) and UV-A radiation (PUVA). *Arch Dermatol* 134:1582, 1998.

89. Stern RS, and Members of the Photochemotherapy Follow-up Study: Genital tumors among men with psoriasis exposed to psoralens and ultraviolet A radiation (PUVA) and ultraviolet B radiation. *N Engl J Med* 322:1093-1097, 1990.

90. Stern RS, Nichols KT, Vakeva LH: Malignant melanoma in patients treated for psoriasis with methoxsalen (psoralen) and ultraviolet A radiation (PUVA). *N Engl J Med* 336:1041-104, 1997.

91. Forrest JB, Forrest HJ: Case report: malignant melanoma arising during drug therapy for vitiligo. *J Surg Oncol* 13:337-340, 1980.

92. Marx JL, Auerbach R, Possick P, et al: Malignant melanoma in situ in two patients treated with psoralens and ultraviolet A. *J Am Acad Dermatol* 9:904-911, 1983.

93. Frenk E: Malignant melanoma in a patient with severe psoriasis treated by oral methoxsalen photochemotherapy. *Dermatologica* 167:152-154, 1983.

94. Johnsen J: Melanoma and psoralens and ultraviolet A. *J Am Acad Dermatol* 11:143, 1984.

95. Reseghetti A, Tribbia G, Locati F, et al: Cutaneous malignant melanoma appearing during photochemotherapy of mycosis fungoides. *Dermatology* 189:75-77, 1994.

96. Wolf P, Schollnast R, Hofer A, et al: Malignant melanoma after psoralen and ultraviolet A (PUVA) therapy. *Br J Dermatol* 138:1100, 1998.

97. Stern RS, and the Photochemotherapy Follow-up Study: Ocular lens findings in patients treated with PUVA. *J Invest Dermatol* 103:534-538, 1994.

98. Stern RS, Kleinerman RA, Parrish JA, et al: Phototoxic reactions to photoactive drugs in patients treated with PUVA. *Arch Dermatol* 116:1269-1271, 1980.

Related Topics

99. Staberg B, Hueg B: Interaction between 8-methoxypsoralen and phenytoin. *Acta Derm Venereol (Stockh)* 65:553-555, 1985.

100. Melski JW, Stern RS: Annual rate of psoralen and ultraviolet-A treatment of psoriasis after initial clearing. *Arch Dermatol* 118:404-408, 1982.

101. Gange RW, Levins P, Murray J, et al: Prolonged skin photosensitization induced by methoxsalen and subphototoxic UVA irradiation. *J Invest Dermatol* 82:219-222, 1984.

102. Lowe NJ, Weingarten D, Bourget T, et al: PUVA therapy for psoriasis: comparison of oral and bath-water delivery of 8-methoxypsoralen. *J Am Acad Dermatol* 14:754-760, 1986.

103. Vallat VP, Gilleaudeau P, Battat L, et al: PUVA bath therapy with 8-methoxypsoralen. In Weinstein GD, Gottlieb AB, editors: *Therapy of moderate-to-severe psoriasis,* Portland, OR, 1993, National Psoriasis Foundation, pp 39-56.

CHAPTER 15

Michael Girardi
Peter W. Heald

Extracorporeal Photochemotherapy

Extracorporeal photochemotherapy (ECP), also known as extracorporeal photopheresis, initially demonstrated a therapeutic impact on cutaneous T-cell lymphoma (CTCL) in the monotherapy trial for erythrodermic disease[1] and was approved in 1988 by the US Food and Drug Administration (FDA) for treatment of this condition. ECP is regarded as an immunotherapy because a small portion of the peripheral lymphocyte pool (less than 5%) is isolated, photochemically altered, and then reinfused to induce changes well beyond the effects expected by simply deleting that small portion of circulating cells. Since this therapy has become available, it has been applied in the management of several T cell–mediated cutaneous disorders, in addition to CTCL (see Indications section). ECP for noncutaneous disease, such as organ transplant rejection, is not discussed in this chapter.

TREATMENT DELIVERY AND CONSIDERATIONS

Several factors influence the decision to start ECP therapy. Currently, ECP machines (e.g., UVAR, UVAR XTS, and Therakos) are available in over 100 centers in the United States and Europe. Because most ECP therapy protocols typically require treatment schedules over months and years, the geographic constraints do limit availability of therapy. Most treatment centers perform ECP in an outpatient setting, and an individual treatment session takes 3 to 3½ hours. Such centers require a highly skilled nursing staff trained to perform such treatments.

Currently, the ECP procedure is performed after ingestion of 8-methoxypsoralen (8-MOP). (For the pharmacology of 8-MOP, see Chapter 14.) To achieve therapeutic levels of the drug (range 100 to 200 ng/ml within the isolated leukocyte compartment), patients often need to ingest 0.6 to 0.8 mg/kg, 1.5 hours before treatment. Knobler[2] developed a technique for preparing 8-MOP that can be injected directly into the treatment cassette. Such an injectable preparation of 8-MOP (UVADEX, Therakos) has recently been tested in clinical protocols in the treatment of graft-versus-host disease (GVHD), and this drug was approved by the FDA for use with ECP.

The ECP procedure (Figure 15-1) can be performed through a peripheral vein, preferably with an 18-gauge needle, which limits therapy to those patients with accessible veins. After establishing venous access, the patient undergoes discontinuous pheresis cycles to harvest the lymphocyte-rich buffy coat. These cycles may

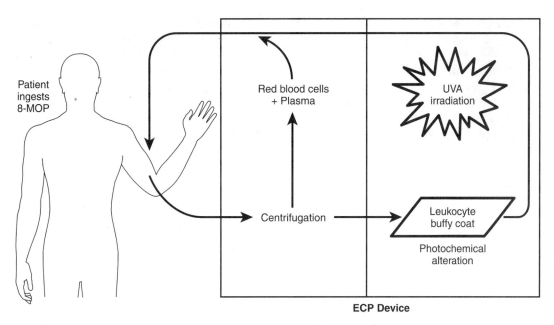

Figure 15-1 Extracorporeal photochemotherapy. The patient ingests 8-methoxypsoralen (8-MOP) 1½ hours before the initiation of treatment. Blood is accessed via an 18-gauge needle in a peripheral vein, heparinized, and collected by the ECP unit. The patient undergoes discontinuous pheresis cycles to separate out the leukocyte-rich buffy coat, which is eventually fed through a one-cell-thick transparent cassette for exposure to UVA light. These photochemically altered cells are then reinfused, as are the previously separated red blood cells and plasma. The entire procedure takes approximately 3 hours. The treatment is typically repeated a second day, and this 2-day cycle is typically repeated monthly.

deplete the patient of 200 to 400 ml of intravenous volume. Thus if the patient's cardiovascular system cannot tolerate such a rapid volume depletion, ECP is contraindicated. The separated leukocytes are held in a sterile bag, from which they are fed through a glass plate and exposed to ultraviolet A (UVA) radiation. At the completion of the treatment cycle, the reinfusion phase leaves the patient at a net gain of up to 500 ml of fluid. Again, the cardiovascular system must be able to tolerate this fluid challenge for therapy to be performed safely. In patients with mild intolerance of the fluid loading, diuretics can be simultaneously administered to avoid hypervolemia.

PHARMACOLOGY

For a complete discussion on the pharmacology of 8-MOP, see Chapter 14.

Box 15-1

ECP—Proposed Mechanisms of Action

Stimulation of anti-T cell (tumor cell) immunoresponses[1,8,23]
Induction of apoptosis of activated T cells[5-7]
Induction of immunoregulatory cytokine shifts[9,10]

Mechanisms of Action—ECP

Although the precise mechanism of ECP has yet to be fully elucidated, crucial components of ECP have been identified from clinical studies and laboratory models (Box 15-1). Mechanisms of action have been best studied for ECP in the treatment of CTCL, which likely have some relevance for therapeutic responses observed in the T cell–mediated diseases for which ECP has also been utilized.

CUTANEOUS T-CELL LYMPHOMA. CTCL is a malignancy characterized by a clonal population of $CD4^+$ T cells that show a predilection for infiltration of the skin. CTCL patients treated with ECP maintain their absolute number of normal T cells with a disproportionately greater decrease in their total body burden of malignant cells. Completely responding patients exhibit loss of all detectable signs of malignant cells, suggesting that an antitumor immunoresponse is stimulated. Tumor-infiltrating $CD8^+$ T cells (i.e., expressing a suppressor/cytotoxic T-cell phenotype) present within lesions of CTCL tend to be more plentiful in early-stage disease, and their proportion correlates positively with improved survival, strongly suggesting that they may exert an antitumor host response.[3] In CTCL patients receiving ECP, those with higher CD4/CD8 T-cell ratios in the peripheral circulation do not respond as well as those with low CD4/CD8 ratios.[4] Taken together, these findings suggest that a potential mechanism of action of ECP may be the stimulation of $CD8^+$ T-cell mediated antitumor responses.

When considering potential adjunctive therapy for ECP in the treatment of CTCL, augmentation of $CD8^+$ T-cell activity may therefore be a desirable goal. Coadministration of recombinant cytokines (e.g., interferon-γ [IFN-γ], interleukin-2 [IL-2]) may enhance $CD8^+$ T-cell responses and prove to be useful adjuncts to ECP therapy.[5] Furthermore, because antigen-presenting cells (APCs) play a critical role in the presentation of tumor-associated antigens to $CD8^+$ T cells, in the future it may prove beneficial to increase activated APCs through cytokine (e.g., GM-CSF) administration. APC stimulation of antitumor $CD8^+$ T cells may also be boosted if appropriate tumor-related peptides could be added to the therapy (i.e., to ECP treatment).

Investigators observed that CTCL patients' peripheral lymphocytes that are isolated by the ECP unit, after exposure to UVA in the presence of 8-MOP, undergo a programmed cellular death (apoptosis).[6-8] Thus an alternative, nonimmunologic theory as to the efficacy of ECP for CTCL is that repeated treatments eventually result in the exposure of nearly all peripheral tumor cells to apoptotic induction. Such an explanation may be limited by the asymptotic nature of such an exposure curve, and by the fact that many of the tumor cells are not in the peripheral circulation at any given time, although they may repeatedly migrate in and out of the skin. Nonetheless, malignant apoptotic T cells may be actively phagocytosed by macrophages, which may facilitate the presentation of relevant tumor antigens necessary to generate clone-specific, antitumor immunity.

AUTOIMMUNE DERMATOSES. Many of the so-called autoimmune disorders are likely mediated by an autoreactive population of oligoclonal T cells. Thus the apparent ability of ECP to stimulate an immunoresponse against pathogenic clones of T cells suggests a role for ECP as an immune modifier capable of inducing the down regulation of pathogenic T cells in various autoimmune disorders (see Table 15-1). This premise is supported by findings in a mouse model of ECP for lupus-like GVHD where inoculation with photochemically-attenuated effector T cells resulted in specific suppression of disease.[9,10]

In addition, ECP has demonstrated the ability to induce several nonspecific immune modifying effects. For example, Vowels and associates[11] reported the increased ability of monocytes to secrete certain cytokines (i.e., tumor necrosis factor-alpha [TNF-α] and IL-6) after ECP. Furthermore, DiRenzo and colleagues[12] demonstrated that ECP can increase the ability of peripheral blood mononuclear cells to secrete IFN-γ while decreasing IL-4 production. Such shifts in T-helper cytokine profiles have a definite role in the pathogenesis of autoimmune diseases, and may partially explain the beneficial responses observed in some patients treated for autoimmune disease with ECP.

CLINICAL USE
FDA-Approved Indications
CUTANEOUS T-CELL LYMPHOMA. As with most therapies that have undergone clinical trials to establish efficacy, the regimens for using ECP (Table 15-1) reflect the schedules used in the initial multicenter clinical trials. The first version of the lymphocyte photoinactivating device took an entire day to treat a patient, and treatments were given on 2 consecutive days.

Table 15-1	Extracorporeal Photochemotherapy Indications and Contraindications*

FDA-APPROVED INDICATIONS
Cutaneous T-cell lymphoma (Sézary syndrome)[1-24]

OFF-LABEL USES

Autoimmune Connective Tissue Diseases	GVHD
Scleroderma[27-33]	Acute GVHD[44,45,52]
Lupus erythematosus[34-36]	Chronic GVHD[45-51]
Autoimmune Bullous Dermatoses	Other Dermatoses
Pemphigus vulgaris[38-40]	Psoriatic arthritis and psoriasis[53-56]
Pemphigus foliaceus[41]	Oral erosive lichen planus[57]
Epidermolysis bullosa acquisita[42-43]	

CONTRAINDICATIONS

Absolute	Relative*
History idiosyncratic reactions to psoralen compounds	Poor venous access (may need central line)
Pregnancy and lactation	Rapidly progressing disease (such as "tumor eruptive CTCL")
Severe cardiac disease	Hematocrit <23% (should be transfused with red blood cells to hematocrit of at least 28%)
	Diastolic blood pressure <70 mm Hg (may need saline infusion and/or red blood cell transfusion)
	Congestive heart failure—compensated

PREGNANCY PRESCRIBING STATUS—FDA UNRATED

*See Chapter 14.

These 2-day treatment cycles were repeated at 4-week intervals. The results with this schedule of therapy were very effective in erythrodermic CTCL patients.[1] Based on the success of this schedule, most patients have subsequently followed the 2-day every 4-week regimen.

The results of the initial clinical trials and follow-up studies showed that as a monotherapy ECP can induce a remission in approximately one fourth of the patients treated.[13] One half of the patients with erythrodermic CTCL had a significant partial response and the remaining one fourth had no response or progressive disease. This same proportion of responses was observed in the smaller series of CTCL patients reported by Zic,[14] Armus,[15] and Bisaccia.[16]

There have been modifications in the scheduling of ECP treatments that have also met with success. Bowen[17] reported on using an every 2-week regimen at the initiation of therapy. The CTCL patient in that report had hyperleukocytic disease and after the leukemia improved the patient was put on a 4-week cycle. Several other centers have utilized this accelerated delivery schedule at the initiation of therapy.

MONITORING CTCL RESPONSE TO ECP.
Before initiating ECP, the patient should be thoroughly evaluated in terms of his tumor burden and peripheral blood status. Tumor burden can be assessed by the recording the patient's skin lesions, performing CT scans for precise measurements of palpable enlarged lymph nodes, and performing flow cytometry and/or Southern blotting of the peripheral blood for determination of clonal T-cell receptor rearrangements. Because the response to ECP is

gradual, a periodic assessment of these tumor burden measures should be conducted every 4 to 8 weeks. Goldman and co-workers[18] reported on the value of following soluble IL-2 receptor levels in the serum. These researchers demonstrated that this parameter decreased as the lymphoma responded to ECP. Patients with tumor stage skin lesions and those with hyperleukocytosis are not good candidates for monotherapy with ECP (adjuncts are discussed later). Erythrodermic patients beginning on ECP should have the disease activity be reevaluated after 3 months of therapy. By this point, a trend in their clinical status should be evident. If there are signs of improvement, the therapy should be continued to maximize the therapeutic response. Complete clearing may occur after 6 to 8 months of gradual improvement. Patients with incomplete responses at 3 to 6 months should be considered for adjunctive therapy.

ADJUVANT THERAPY IN CTCL PATIENTS. In evaluating options of adjunctive therapy for ECP, it is worthwhile to review all therapies of CTCL. The three broad categories to choose from are skin-directed therapy, biologic response modifiers, and low-dose chemotherapy (Box 15-2). In patients with significant tumor burden, a reduction of that tumor burden with

a skin-directed treatment can work synergistically with ECP. The skin-directed therapies available are radiotherapy, psoralen plus ultraviolet A (PUVA), and topical chemotherapy. Wilson and associates[19] reported that series of patients treated with ECP and total skin electron beam had improved survival when com-

---

Box 15-2

Adjunctive Therapy for ECP in Treatment of CTCL

SKIN-DIRECTED THERAPY
PUVA
Topical chemotherapy (BCNU, nitrogen mustard)
Radiation (total skin or spot electron beam radiation)[19]

BIOLOGIC RESPONSE MODIFIERS
Systemic cytokines (IL-2, IFN-γ, IFN-α)[20,21]
Monoclonal antibodies (anti-CD4)
Antibody-conjugated fusion toxins (DAB IL-2)
Retinoids (acitretin)[22]

LOW-DOSE CHEMOTHERAPY
Methotrexate[24]

ECP Monitoring—Disease Activity

CUTANEOUS T-CELL LYMPHOMA
Perform a "tumor burden assessment" before treatment and then every 4 to 8 weeks of treatment, by measuring involvement in the following:
- Skin: Clinical skin involvement (i.e., skin map recording)
- Blood: Lymphocyte count, CD4/CD8 ratio, Sézary cell count
- Lymph nodes: CT scans to measure lymph node size

In addition, molecular analysis (i.e., Southern blot and PCR) for more sensitive detection of tumor can be performed every 3 to 6 months for patients achieving clinical remission

OTHER T CELL–MEDIATED AUTOIMMUNE DERMATOSES
Perform a scoring system appropriate for the disease before treatment and then every 4 to 8 weeks of treatment
- Scleroderma: Skin map recording, joint mobility, degree of induration, vascular flow by cutaneous ultrasound
- Blistering disorders: Skin map recording, indirect immunofluorescence antibody titers
- Graft-versus-host disease: Skin map recording (see parameters for scleroderma for chronic GVHD)

pared with similarly staged patients at the same institution treated with total skin electron beam therapy alone. A relatively common occurrence is the unmasking of patch or plaque lesions of CTCL as the erythroderma fades while a patient is undergoing ECP. In that setting, these skin-directed therapies can be successful in eliminating these fixed cutaneous lesions.

In addition to ECP, therapies that are considered as biologic response modifiers include retinoids, monoclonal antibodies, interferons and other cytokines, and cytokine-based fusion toxins. Several reports presented beneficial results of combining other biologic response modifiers with ECP. Rook and colleagues[20] first reported the use of IFN-γ with ECP to establish a remission in a patient with advanced CTCL. Gottlieb and co-workers[21] reported longer term greater response rate using INF-γ as adjunctive therapy. Lim[22] utilized retinoid therapy with a resultant beneficial response in a patient receiving ECP. These preliminary results are encouraging both as being potentially beneficial for patients, and for increasing our understanding of CTCL. However, the failing immune system of CTCL patients is clearly correlated with the numbers of malignant cells, and a skin-directed therapy often provides a direct debulking effect to help reduce the tumor burden.[23]

The immunosuppressive effect of advancing CTCL is the major reason why traditional high-dose chemotherapy has been unsuccessful in treating CTCL. These high-dose regimens tend to exacerbate the immunosuppression already present in most advanced CTCL cases. However, low-dose chemotherapy has been employed with beneficial results. Methotrexate at 15 to 25 mg once weekly can safely be given to patients receiving ECP with enhanced efficacy.[24] Oral corticosteroids can be palliative in CTCL patients, but their immunosuppressive effects have been shown to negate the therapeutic effects of ECP in an experimental model.[25] Such murine systems may not adequately reflect the human system. One example of this apparent disparity between murine systems and human outcomes is a study by Rose and associates,[26] who reported that patients who had cardiac transplantations benefited from ECP while on systemic steroids and cyclosporine.

In summary, ECP can be used as monotherapy in patients with CTCL with erythrodermic disease, or as part of a multiagent regimen for patients with refractory disease or multiple tumors. The goal of therapy should be to achieve a remission and then gradually taper treatment. The taper schedule used in the majority of the initial study patients was to add a 7-day interval every three cycles of therapy. Once patients achieved 8-week intervals and their skin remained clear for a period of 6 months, they were taken off therapy. Patients with tumor stage CTCL need to continue with their maintenance schedule of skin-directed therapy (typically PUVA initially weekly, decreasing gradually to monthly therapy). Patients with an unacceptable response or progressive disease with ECP should have their next line of therapy introduced before discontinuing ECP completely. It is noteworthy that flares of CTCL occurred in patients discontinuing ECP for CTCL.

Other Dermatologic Uses— Treatment of T-Cell–Mediated Autoimmune Dermatoses

MONITORING RESPONSE OF AUTOIMMUNE DERMATOSES TO ECP.   Similar to that for CTCL previously discussed, patients with autoimmune disease being treated with ECP should have clearly defined therapeutic goals, an initial treatment evaluation, and periodic reevaluations to assess the degree of progress. For example, in patients with pemphigus vulgaris, both a recording of the skin lesions and measurements of the pemphigus antibody titer should be monitored. Scleroderma patients can have a skin sclerosis clinical score along with periodic biopsies to help monitor their disease. Adams and colleagues[27] reported on the use of imaging to document the scleroderma response to ECP. In each of these situations it is best at the start to outline the goal of ECP therapy and the guidelines for when to begin adjunctive therapy.

SCLERODERMA.   The early phase of scleroderma is characterized by an inflammatory infiltrate and edema within the dermis. It is hypothesized that activated helper T cells within the infiltrate help stimulate the production of collagen synthesis and subsequent fibrosis via the secretion of certain cytokines (e.g., transforming growth factor [TGF]-β).[28] The degree to which fibrosis is reversible in patients with scleroderma is unknown. Thus it is perhaps not surprising that ECP for scleroderma demonstrates the greatest therapeutic effect in patients with relatively recent disease onset. Current treatments for this condition include D-penicillamine (an inhibitor of collagen cross-linking and various immunosuppressive medications.

A randomized, parallel-group, single-blinded, multicenter clinical trial involving 79 patients demonstrated the safety and efficacy of ECP in the treatment of scleroderma.[29] Patients with an average 1.8 years disease duration (maximum 4 years) and a worsening of cutaneous involvement of at least 30% during the preceding 6 months were randomized to receive ECP or oral D-penicillamine (maximum dose of 750 mg/day) for 6 months. Exclusion criteria included significant renal disease (serum creatinine > 3.0 mg/dl) or pulmonary involvement (carbon monoxide diffusing capacity less than 50% of normal). Clinical examiners blinded to the treatment type delivered recorded a skin score based on skin thickness, percentage surface area involved, oral aperture diameter, and the capacity for hand closure. A significant improvement in skin score occurred in 68% (21 of 31) of patients receiving ECP and 32% (8 of 25) of patients on D-penicillamine, while significant worsening was observed in 10% (3 patients) receiving ECP and 32% (8 patients) receiving D-penicillamine. The difference between the two groups was statistically significant ($p < .02$). Furthermore, adverse reactions in the ECP study group were minimal, and all patients in the ECP group completed the study. This is in contrast to the D-penicillamine group; 24% of these patients had to permanently discontinue treatment directly due to adverse effects of this medication.

Subjects from an independent study by DiSpaltro and colleagues,[30] in which 9 patients with scleroderma in an open trial were treated with ECP for 6 to 21 months, demonstrated significant improvement in their skin, musculoskeletal system, functional index, and symptoms including Raynaud's phenomenon, dyspnea, fatigue, dysphagia, and arthralgias. Again, patients were relatively early in their disease onset,

with a history of scleroderma findings for only 6 months to 4 years. Similarly, in a third cohort, 4 of 6 patients with scleroderma who improved under ECP had a disease duration of 2 years or less, whereas only 2 of 10 patients with a disease duration greater than 2 years did better.[31] However, in separate trials reported by Zachariae[32] (8 patients) and Cribier[33] (7 patients), subjects showed little response or worsening despite treatment with ECP. Average disease duration in both trials was longer than in the randomized multicenter trial discussed above. Furthermore, patients were not excluded on the basis of severe internal organ involvement.

In summary, patients with scleroderma appear most likely to benefit from treatment with ECP if they have recent onset of the disease before there are the chronic fibrotic changes that appear irreversible. To date, patients with evidence of significant visceral disease involvement (e.g., serum creatinine > 3.0 mg/dl or carbon monoxide diffusing capacity less than 50% of normal) have been excluded from most studies, and the results with that subgroup of patients are unknown.

SYSTEMIC LUPUS ERYTHEMATOSUS. Systemic lupus erythematosus (SLE) is characterized by abnormal circulating B cells and T cells, as well as autoantibody production against various nuclear and cytoplasmic antigens. The disease is usually controlled to some degree with standard therapies, including antimalarials, corticosteroids, and other immunosuppressive agents. Experimental evidence exists that T cells are important in the skin and renal manifestations of SLE,[34] and studies in two different mouse models suggest that the down regulation of lupus-mediating T cells might be attainable through treatment with ECP.[9,35]

To test the feasibility of ECP in the treatment of SLE, a pilot study of 10 patients was conducted by Knobler and co-workers.[36] Patients satisfied the American College of Rheumatology criteria for SLE and had the disease adequately controlled with low-dose prednisone, chloroquine, azathioprine, or cyclophosphamide; however, all patients had disease flares with multiple drug tapering attempts. Strict inclusion criteria resulted in a study population with mild-to-moderate systemic involvement. Patients were treated on 2 consecutive days every month for 6 months, then every 2 months for another 6 months. In the 8 patients who completed the study, disease activity decreased, as measured by the SLE Activity Index Scoring System (SIS).[37] The SIS score, based on a combination of clinical and laboratory findings, dropped from a median 7 (range 4-9) down to 1 (range 0-5). In all patients except one, the dosages of steroids and immunosuppressive medications were reduced during this time. A marked resolution of cutaneous lesions was observed in 6 patients after 4 to 6 months of ECP. Laboratory abnormalities showed no difference from baseline values.

Thus SLE patients with mild disease who are no longer tolerating treatment or who wish to decrease treatment with systemic medications may benefit from treatment with ECP. Subsequent studies with ECP in SLE can be done based on the safety demonstrated in this pilot study. Nonetheless, the infusion of cells with photochemically modified DNA (i.e., crosslinked via 8-MOP) into patients with a disorder characterized by antinuclear and anti-DNA antibodies did not lead to any exacerbation of the autoimmune disease.

PEMPHIGUS VULGARIS AND FOLIACEUS.

In patients with pemphigus vulgaris, production of autoantibodies against the desmoglein-3 protein component of keratinocyte desmosomes leads to blister and erosion formation of cutaneous and mucosal surfaces. Although the majority of patients are adequately controlled with the use of various immunosuppressive medications (i.e., high-dose corticosteroids, azathioprine, cyclosporine, or cyclophosphamide), long-term treatment with these medications often results in adverse effects. Thus mortality remains around 5% to 15%, largely due to complications from these drugs. Because ECP has a relatively excellent short-term and long-term side-effect profile, it is a potential treatment for pemphigus patients failing drug therapy.

At least 6 patients with pemphigus vulgaris treated with ECP have been reported in the literature. Rook and associates[38] reported the efficacy of ECP in a pilot study of 4 patients (ages 61 to 78 years) with extensive and refractory pemphigus vulgaris despite large doses of immunosuppressive medications. Patients continued to receive prednisone alone or with azathioprine. All 4 patients showed clinical improvement and a drop in antidesmosomal antibody titers, despite tapering of immunosuppressive medications. After 36 to 48 months, 3 of the 4 patients demonstrated a complete remission (i.e., no clinical evidence of active disease and undetectable antidesmosome antibody titers), which lasted an average 19.3 months (range 7 to 36 months). Relapses in the 3 patients responded to reinitiation of ECP after 3 to 4 monthly cycles. Similar beneficial results of ECP for pemphigus vulgaris have been reported by Liang and colleagues[39] in the treatment of a man 31 years of age with a 4-year history of severe disease, and by Gollnick and co-workers[40] in the treatment of a woman 37 years of age with a 5-year history of severe pemphigus.

None of these patients developed serious adverse effects while receiving ECP. These case reports suggest that ECP may be a promising and relatively safe treatment for selective cases of pemphigus vulgaris. A randomized, controlled study would be helpful to define the use of ECP in less severe pemphigus vulgaris cases or possibly as a first-line therapy. ECP represents an option for patients with pemphigus vulgaris poorly controlled with, or unable to tolerate, combinations of high-dose immunosuppressive medications. More recently, Azana[41] reported a beneficial effect of ECP in the treatment of severe pemphigus foliaceus.

EPIDERMOLYSIS BULLOSA ACQUISITA.

Three patients (ages 56 to 71 years) with refractory epidermolysis bullosa acquisita (EBA) were treated with ECP, as reported by Gordon and co-workers.[42] All three demonstrated objectively measured improvement, while 2 of 3 patients had significant subjective improvement in skin fragility and clinical activity of disease. In another report, Miller[43] described a man 31 years of age with severe EBA refractory to high-dose oral and intravenous-pulsed steroids, various combinations of immunosuppressive medications, and plasmapheresis. After 3 months of ECP, the patient ceased development of new bullae. The patient's skin remained disease-free over 2 more years despite tapering of his prednisone. The patient did, however, develop an unexplained cardiomyopathy. Certainly further, more extensive studies are necessary before ECP proves to be an effective treatment option for aggressive forms of EBA.

GRAFT-VERSUS-HOST DISEASE. GVHD is a frequent complication of allogeneic bone-marrow transplantation (BMT) and peripheral blood stem cell transplantation. GVHD is mediated by donor T cells reactive against the recipient's major and minor histocompatibility antigens. That ECP is capable of eliciting an immunoregulatory response against such pathogenic T cells is suggested by results seen in mouse model systems (e.g., specific inhibition of skin graft rejection[25] and prevention of GVHD[9]), as well as a widening clinical experience (e.g., prevention of heart transplant rejection[26,44] and treatment of acute and chronic GVHD[45-53]).

The largest single-center group of patients with chronic GVHD treated with ECP was reported by Greinix and colleagues.[45] Fifteen patients with histologically proven, extensive chronic GVHD, representing a spectrum from lichenoid to sclerodermoid forms, received ECP every 2 weeks for the first 3 months and monthly thereafter. Out of the 15 patients, 12 (80%) obtained complete clearing of cutaneous findings return to normal appearing skin. Of note, 11 of 11 patients with oral mucosal involvement and 7 of 10 of patients with liver involvement demonstrated complete resolution of their extracutaneous involvement. Patients received ECP for 7 to 31 months, during which time steroid therapy could be discontinued after a median of 80 days. In an independent study by Child and colleagues,[46] 11 patients with chronic GVHD were treated with ECP twice monthly for 4 months and once monthly thereafter. Although nearly all patients initially demonstrated an improvement in skin and mucosal involvement by a blinded observer scoring at the fourth month, the effects on visceral manifestations were less impressive. For example, elevated liver enzymes improved in 1 of 6 patients but worsened in 3 patients receiving ECP. In a third study,[47] 4 of 5 patients with chronic GVHD (2 of which had extensive cutaneous involvement) demonstrated improvement on ECP, and 3 achieved complete remission and were able to eventually discontinue all treatment modalities. Although these studies and several case reports[48-51] are very encouraging, a large, randomized, multicenter controlled trial (currently underway) will more clearly delineate the role of ECP in the treatment of chronic GVHD.

Experience with ECP in the treatment of acute GVHD is more limited than for chronic GVHD, but several recently published reports are very promising. As part of the study by Greinix and associates[45] previously mentioned, 6 patients with histologic grade II to IV acute GVHD were treated with ECP twice monthly. All were unresponsive to immunosuppressive therapy with combination cyclosporin A and methylprednisolone. Four of the six patients obtained complete resolution of disease after only 2 to 3 months, at which time ECP was halted. Of note, prednisone was tapered off completely in the first 2 to 4 weeks of ECP, whereas low-dose cyclosporine was continued as a maintenance modality. Two independent published cases have also reported a rapid response of acute GVHD to ECP.[10,52]

Given the problems with the toxicity of the current standard of care therapy for GVHD (i.e., immunosuppressive medications) and the increasing incidence of GVHD as a result of an expanding use of allogeneic BMT and peripheral blood stem cell transplantation in the treatment of malignancies, the utilization of ECP in the treatment of GVHD represents the most promising potential indication other than CTCL.

PSORIATIC ARTHRITIS. Psoriatic arthritis represents a distinct inflammatory arthropathy that occurs in about 5% of patients with psoriasis. An association with certain HLA phenotypes, shifts in the CD4/CD8 ratios in the peripheral blood, and response to T-cell–targeted treatments such as cyclosporine and DAB IL-2 (partial diphtheria toxin conjugated to soluble IL-2) are some of the evidence suggesting that psoriasis is a T-cell–mediated disorder. In progressive forms of psoriatic arthritis, the disease may be poorly responsive to antiinflammatory, immunosuppressive, and cytotoxic agents.

Vahlquist[53] treated 8 patients (ages 38 to 53 years) with psoriatic arthritis with ECP for 12 weeks, followed by ECP plus PUVA for another 12 weeks. Four of these patients experienced a marked improvement in joint symptoms (74% decrease in the Ritchie articular index) that lasted over 1 year posttreatment. Wilfert and associates[54] reported on 5 patients (ages 26 to 58 years) with psoriatic arthritis who were treated with ECP after all medications except for nonsteroidal antiinflammatory agents were discontinued. The clinical results were variable. Four of the 5 patients reported a reduction in pain intensity and a decrease in morning stiffness. Objectively measured parameters of grip strength and swelling improved in three patients. However, no clear improvement in skin disease was detectable. Three patients (ages 29 to 43 years) who had psoriatic arthritis treated with ECP for 1 year were reported by de Misa and colleagues.[55] Two of the three patients demonstrated moderate improvement in spontaneous pain, morning stiffness, joint swelling, and the laboratory measured parameter of erythrocyte sedimentation rate (ESR). Skin improvement was not interpretable because patients continued to receive topical therapy. Adverse effects in these cases were minimal and included nausea and vasovagal responses.

In summary, treatment of psoriatic arthritis with ECP may help ameliorate some of the arthropathic symptoms of this disorder in patients recalcitrant to or intolerant of standard therapy. The cutaneous manifestations of psoriasis have not shown a consistent response to ECP therapy.[56]

EROSIVE ORAL LICHEN PLANUS.   A recent report by Becheral and associates[57] examined single modality ECP in the treatment of chronic erosive oral lichen planus in 7 patients resistant to multiple medications. All patients demonstrated complete remission after a mean of 12 cycles. However, follow-up in this study was short, and thus therapeutic use of ECP for this condition needs further investigation.

Adverse Effects

Box 15-3 lists adverse effects for ECP. In general, ECP is a relatively nontoxic, well-tolerated treatment. Most patients do experience some degree of

---

Box 15-3

ECP Adverse Effects*

> **RELATED TO 8-MOP***
> Nausea
> Photosensitivity
>
> **CARDIOVASCULAR EFFECTS**
> Hypotension
> Congestive heart failure
> Flushing
> Tachycardia
>
> **VENIPUNCTURE EFFECTS**
> Potential eventual loss of venous access with
>   repeated venipuncture

*See Chapter 14.

---

nausea with oral administration of 8-MOP; however, this effect is eliminated with the use of UVADEX delivery directly to the treatment cassette. In addition, use of UVADEX results in an overall postreinfusion plasma level of 8-MOP that is markedly less than that seen with oral delivery. The interval and degree of photosensitivity risk after treatment are theoretically greatly decreased.[2] Still, patients should be cautioned as to all of the potential risks associated with the systemic use of psoralens (see Chapter 14).

The major risks of ECP are related to intravascular fluid shifts associated with leukocyte isolation and reinfusion. Mild hypotensive episodes commonly respond to intravenous saline administration. However, in patients with a history of coronary artery disease or congestive heart failure, these intravascular fluid changes may exacerbate the underlying cardiac condition.

The repeated venipuncture associated with continued ECP may eventually result in loss of adequate venous access. This may be a problem in treating patients with sclerotic and edematous changes, as may be seen in patients with chronic GVHD or scleroderma, overlying antecubital fossae. A trained and highly skilled ECP unit nursing staff is crucial to handling such problems.

Bibliography

Edelson RL: Photopheresis: a new therapeutic concept. *Yale J Biol Med* 62:565-577, 1989.

Girardi M, and Heald PW: Immunomodulation through extracorporeal photochemotherapy. Burg G, Drummer R, editors: *Strategies for immunoprevention in dermatology,* Heidelberg, Germany, 1997, Springer-Verlag, pp 119-130.

Heald P, Knobler R, LaRoche L: Photoinactivated lymphocyte therapy of cutaneous T-cell lymphoma. *Dermatol Clin* 12:443-449, 1994.

Lim HW, Edelson RL: Photopheresis for the treatment of cutaneous T-cell lymphoma. *Hematol Oncol Clin North Am* 9:1117-1126, 1995.

Rook AH, Wolfe JT: Role of extracorporeal photochemotherapy in the treatment of cutaneous T-cell lymphoma, autoimmune disease, and allograft rejection. *J Clin Apheresis* 9:28-30, 1994.

References

Cutaneous T-cell Lymphoma

1. Edelson R, Berger C, Gasparro F, et al: Treatment of cutaneous T-cell lymphoma by extracorporeal photochemotherapy. Preliminary results. *N Engl J Med* 316:297-303, 1987.

2. Knobler RM, Trautinger F, Graninger W, et al: Parenteral administration of 8-methoxypsoralen in photopheresis. *J Am Acad Dermatol* 28:580-584, 1993.

3. Hoppe RT, Medeiros LJ, Warnke RA, et al: CD8-positive tumor-infiltrating lymphocytes influence the long-term survival of patients with mycosis fungoides. *J Am Acad Dermatol* 32:448-453, 1995.

4. Heald P, Rook A, Perez M, et al: Treatment of erythrodermic cutaneous T-cell lymphoma with extracorporeal photochemotherapy. *J Am Acad Dermatol* 27:427-433, 1992.

5. Rook AH, Gottlieb SL, Wolfe JT, et al: Pathogenesis of cutaneous T-cell lymphoma: implications for the use of recombinant cytokines and photopheresis. *Clin Exp Immunol* 107(Suppl 1):16-20, 1997.

6. Yoo E, Rook A, Elenitsas R, et al: Apoptosis induction by ultraviolet light A and photochemotherapy in cutaneous T-cell lymphoma: relevance to mechanism of therapeutic action. *J Invest Dermatol* 107:235-242, 1996.

7. Miracco C, Rubegni P, DeAloe G, et al: Extracorporeal photochemotherapy induces apoptosis of infiltrating lymphoid cells in patients with mycosis fungoides in early stages. A quantitative histological study. *Br J Dermatol* 137:549-557, 1997.

8. Yoo E, Rook A, Elenitsas R, et al: Apoptosis induction by ultraviolet light A and photochemotherapy in cutaneous T-cell lymphoma: relevance to mechanism of therapeutic action. *J Invest Dermatol* 107:235-242, 1996.

9. Girardi M, Herreid P, Tigelaar RE: Specific suppression of lupus-like graft-versus-host disease using extracorporeal photochemical attenuation of effector lymphocytes. *J Invest Dermatol* 104:177-182, 1995.

10. Girardi M, McNiff JM, Heald PW: Extracorporeal photochemotherapy in human and murine graft-versus-host disease. *J Dermatol Sci* 19:106-113, 1999.

11. Vowels BR, Cassin M, Boufal MH, et al: Extracorporeal photochemotherapy induces the production of tumor necrosis factor-alpha by monocytes: implications for the treatment of cutaneous T-cell lymphoma and systemic sclerosis. *J Invest Dermatol* 98:686-692, 1992.

12. Di Renzo M, Rubegni P, De Aloe G, et al: Extracorporeal photochemotherapy restores Th1/Th2 imbalance in patients with early stage cutaneous T-cell lymphoma. *Immunology* 92:99-103, 1997.

13. Heald PW, Rook A, Perez M, et al: Treatment of erythrodermic cutaneous T-cell lymphoma patients with photopheresis. *J Am Acad Dermatol* 27:427-433, 1992.

14. Zic J, Arzubiaga C, Salhany KE, et al: Extracorporeal photopheresis for the treatment of cutaneous T-cell lymphoma. *J Am Acad Dermatol* 27:729-736, 1992.

15. Armus S, Keyes B, Cahill C, et al: Photopheresis for the treatment of cutaneous T-cell lymphoma. *J Am Acad Dermatol* 23:898-902, 1995.

16. Bisaccia E, Berger C, Klainer AS: Photopheresis for the treatment of cutaneous T-cell lymphoma. *J Am Acad Dermatol* 23: 5-11, 1990.

17. Bowen GM, Steens SR, Dubin HV, et al: Diagnosis of Sezary syndrome in a patient with generalized pruritus based on early molecular study and flow cytometry. *J Am Acad Dermatol* 33:678-680, 1995.

18. Goldman BD, Oh SK, Davis B, et al: Serum soluble interleukin-2 receptor levels in erythrodermic cutaneous T-cell lymphoma correlate with response to photopheresis based treatment. *Arch Dermatol* 129:1166-1170, 1993.

19. Wilson LD, Licata AL, Braverman IM, et al: Systemic chemotherapy and extracorporeal photochemotherapy and T3 and T4 cutaneous T-cell lymphoma patients who have achieved a complete response to total skin electron beam therapy. *Int J Rad Oncol* 32:987-995, 1995.

20. Rook A, Prystowsky M, Cassin M, et al: Combined therapy for Sézary syndrome with extracorporeal photochemotherapy and low dose interferon alfa therapy. *Arch Dermatol* 127:1535-1540, 1991.

21. Gottlieb SL, Wolfe JT, Fox F, et al: Treatment of cutaneous T-cell lymphoma with extracorporeal photopheresis monotherapy and in combination with recombinant interferon alfa: a 10-year experience at a single institution. *J Am Acad Dermatol* 35:946-957, 1996.

22. Lim HW, Harris HR: Etretinate as an effective adjunctive therapy for recalcitrant palmar/plantar hyperkeratosis in patients with erythrodermic cutaneous T-cell lymphoma undergoing photopheresis. *Dermatol Surg* 21:597-599, 1995.

23. Rook A, Heald P: The immunopathogenesis of cutaneous T-cell lymphoma. *Hematol Oncol Clin North Am* 9:997-1010, 1995.

24. Zackheim HS, Epstein EH: Low dose methotrexate for Sézary syndrome. *J Am Acad Dermatol* 21:757-762, 1989.

25. Perez MI, Edelson RL, LaRoche L, et al: Inhibition of anti-skin allograft immunity by infusions with syngeneic photoinactivated effector lymphocytes. *J Invest Dermatol* 92:669-674, 1989.

26. Rose EA, Barr ML, Xu H, et al: Photochemotherapy in human heart transplant recipients at high risk for fatal rejection. *J Heart Lung Transpl* 11:746-750, 1992.

Scleroderma

27. Adams LB, Park JH, Olsen NJ, et al: Quantitative evaluation of improvement in muscle weakness in a patient receiving extracorporeal photopheresis for scleroderma: magnetic resonance imaging and magnetic resonance spectroscopy. *J Am Acad Dermatol* 33:519-522, 1995.

28. Cotton SA, Herrick AL, Jayson MI, et al: TGF-beta—a role in systemic sclerosis? *J Pathol* 184:4-6, 1998.

29. Rook AH, Freundlich B, Jegasothy BV, et al: Treatment of systemic sclerosis with extracorporeal photochemotherapy. Results of a multicenter trial. *Arch Dermatol* 128:337-346, 1992.

30. Di Spaltro FX, Cottrill C, Cahill C, et al: Extracorporeal photochemotherapy in progressive systemic sclerosis. *Int J Dermatol* 32:417-421, 1993.

31. Krasagakis K, Dippel E, Ramaker J, et al: Management of severe scleroderma with long-term extracorporeal photopheresis. *Dermatology* 196:309-315, 1998.

32. Zachariae H, Bjerring P, Heickendorff L, et al: Photopheresis and systemic sclerosis (letter). *Arch Dermatol* 128:1651-1653, 1992.

33. Cribier B, Faradji T, Le Coz C, et al: Extracorporeal photochemotherapy in systemic sclerosis and severe morphea. *Dermatology* 191:25-31, 1995.

Systemic Lupus Erythematosus

34. Peng SL, Cappadona J, McNiff JM, et al: Pathogenesis of autoimmunity in alpha beta T cell-deficient lupus-prone mice. *Clin Exp Immunol* 111:107-116, 1998.

35. Berger CL, Perez M, Laroche L, et al: Inhibition of autoimmune disease in a murine model of systemic lupus erythematosus induced by exposure to syngeneic photoinactivated lymphocytes. *J Invest Dermatol* 94:52-57, 1990.

36. Knobler RM, Graninger W, Lindmaier A, et al: Extracorporeal photochemotherapy for the treatment of systemic lupus erythematosus. A pilot study. *Arthritis Rheum* 35:319-324, 1992.

37. Brunner HI, Feldman BM, Bombardier C, et al: Sensitivity of the Systemic Lupus Erythematosus Disease Activity Index, British Isles Lupus Assessment Group Index, and Systemic Lupus Activity Measure in the evaluation of clinical change in childhood-onset systemic lupus erythematosus. *Arthritis Rheum* 42:1354-1360, 1999.

Pemphigus Vulgaris and Foliaceus

38. Rook AH, Jegasothy BV, Heald P, et al: Extracorporeal photochemotherapy for drug-resistant pemphigus vulgaris. *Ann Intern Med* 112:303-305, 1990.
39. Liang G, Nahass G, Kerdel FA: Pemphigus vulgaris treated with photopheresis. *J Am Acad Dermatol* 26:779-780, 1992.
40. Gollnick HP, Owsianowski M, Taube KM, et al: Unresponsive severe generalized pemphigus vulgaris successfully controlled by extracorporeal photopheresis. *J Am Acad Dermatol* 28:122-124, 1993.
41. Azana JM, de Misa RF, Harto A, et al: Severe pemphigus foliaceus treated with extracorporeal photochemotherapy. *Arch Dermatol* 133:287-289, 1997.

Epidermolysis Bullosa Acquisita

42. Gordon K, Chan L, Woodley D: Treatment of refractory epidermolysis bullosa acquisita with extracorporeal photochemotherapy. *Br J Dermatol* 136:415-420, 1997.
43. Miller JL, Stricklin GP, Fine JD, et al: Remission of severe epidermolysis bullosa acquisita induced by extracorporeal photochemotherapy. *Br J Dermatol* 133:467-471, 1995.

Graft-Versus-Host Disease

44. Barr ML, Meiser BM, Eisen HJ, et al: Photopheresis for the prevention of rejection in cardiac transplantation. Photopheresis Transplantation Study Group. *N Engl J Med* 339:1744-1751, 1998.
45. Greinix HT, Volc-Platzer B, Rabitsch W, et al: Successful use of extracorporeal photochemotherapy in the treatment of severe acute and chronic graft-versus-host disease. *Blood* 92:3098-3104, 1998.
46. Child FJ, Ratnavel R, Watkins P, et al: Extracorporeal photopheresis (ECP) in the treatment of chronic graft-versus-host disease (GVHD). *Bone Marrow Transplant* 23:881-887, 1999.

47. Besnier D, Chabannes D, Mahè B, et al: Treatment of graft-versus-host disease by extracorporeal photochemotherapy. *Transplantation* 64:49-54, 1997.
48. Owsianowski M, Gollnick H, Siegert W, et al: Successful treatment of chronic graft-versus-host disease with extracorporeal photopheresis. *Bone Marrow Transplant* 14:845-848, 1994.
49. Dall'Amico R, Rossetti F, Zulian F, et al: Photopheresis in paediatric patients with drug-resistant chronic graft-versus-host disease. *Br J Dermatol* 97:848-854, 1997.
50. Rossetti F, Zulian F, Dall'Amico R, et al: Extracorporeal photochemotherapy as single therapy for extensive, cutaneous, chronic graft-versus-host disease. *Transplantation* 59:49-51, 1995.
51. Konstantinow A, Balda B-R, Starz H, et al: Chronic graft-versus-host disease: successful treatment with extracorporeal photochemotherapy: a follow-up. *Br J Dermatol* 135:1003-1017, 1996.
52. Richter H, Stege H, Ruzika T, et al: Extracorporeal photopheresis in the treatment of acute graft-versus-host disease. *J Am Acad Dermatol* 36:787-789, 1997.

Psoriatic Arthritis

53. Vahlquist C, Larsson M, Ernerudh J, et al: Treatment of psoriatic arthritis with extracorporeal photochemotherapy and conventional psoralen-ultraviolet A irradiation. *Arthritis Rheum* 39:1519-1523, 1996.
54. Wilfert H, Honigsmann H, Steiner G, et al: Treatment of psoriatic arthritis by extracorporeal photochemotherapy. *Br J Dermatol* 122:225-232, 1990.
55. DeMisa RF, Azana JM, Harto A, et al: Psoriatic arthritis: one year of treatment with extracorporeal photochemotherapy. *J Am Acad Dermatol* 30:1037-1038, 1994.
56. Vonderheid EC, Kang CA, Kadin M, et al: Extracorporeal photopheresis in psoriasis vulgaris: clinical and immunologic observations. *J Am Acad Dermatol* 23:703-712, 1990.

Erosive Oral Lichen Planus

57. Bécherel PA, Bussel A, Chosidow O, et al: Extracorporeal photochemotherapy for chronic erosive lichen planus. *Lancet* 351:805, 1998.

CHAPTER 16

Brian Berman
Francisco Flores

Interferons

Interferons (IFNs) are a family of secretory glycoproteins produced by most eukaryotic cells in response to a variety of viral and nonviral inducers (Table 16-1). All IFNs display antiviral activity and also modulate other cellular functions. IFN was originally described as a product of the interaction of heat-inactivated influenza virus and isolated pieces of chick chorioallantoic membrane, which are capable of inducing interference with viral growth in fresh tissue.[1] Early in the studies on the antiviral action of IFN, it was shown that IFN did not inactivate virus directly, but rendered cells resistant to virus; in most cases these IFNs displayed "species" specificity.[2-4] Soon afterward, Ho and Enders[5] demonstrated IFN production by human primary cell cultures induced with live polio virus.

Depending on cellular source and mode of induction, human cells produce three antigenically distinct forms of human IFN that were originally described as leukocyte (α), fibroblast (β), and immune (γ). This chapter identifies IFNs such as IFN-α, IFN-β, or IFN-γ because a single cell type can produce more than one type of IFN[6] (see Table 16-1). Utilization of recombinant deoxyribonucleic acid (DNA) technology led to the production of large quantities of highly purified human IFNs in *Escherichia coli*.[7] Presently, three forms of human IFN-α have been approved by the Food and Drug Administration (FDA) for clinical use, and therefore this chapter focuses mainly on IFN-α.

PHARMACOLOGY

Table 16-2 lists key pharmacologic concepts for IFNs.

Structure
There are over 30 species of IFN-α that have a molecular weight around 20 kD with very similar sequences of 165 to 172 amino acids. IFN-α 2_a and IFN-α 2_b differ in a single amino acid and can be produced by *E. coli* utilizing recombinant DNA biotechnology. IFN-β has 29% structural homology to IFN-α; IFN-γ has no statistically significant structural homology to IFN-α or IFN-β.[9]

Absorption and Bioavailability
Systemic absorption intramuscularly (IM) and subcutaneously (SC) is greater than 80% for IFN-α and 30% to 70% for IFN-γ. Injection of 5 million IU/m^2 of IFN-α 2_b IM or SC resulted in similar peak serum levels reached in 3 to 12 hours after injection and was undetectable after 24 hours.[9] Calculated absorption and elimination half-lives were 3 to 4 hours and 6 to 7 hours, respectively. Measurable concentrations are attainable 4 to 24 hours after injection

■ Table 16-1   Interferons

Generic Name	Trade Name	Generic Available	Manu-facturer	Drug Sizes Available	Final Concentration (adding 2 ml diluent)	Price Index
IFN-α 2$_b$	Intron A	No	Schering	3, 18 million IU (SQ, IM, IV) 5, 10, 25 million IU (IM, SQ, IL)	0.015, 0.090 IU/ml* 0.025, 0.5, 0.125 IU/ml*	$$$$$
IFN-α 2$_a$	Roferon A	No	Roche	3, 6, 9, 18, 36 million IU (SQ, IM)	11.1, 22.2, 33.3, 66.7, 133.3 IU/ml	$$$$$
IFN-α N$_3$	Alferon N	No	Purdue Frederick	5 million IU (IL)	3 million IU/ 0.5 ml	$$$$$
IFN-γ†	Actimmune	No	Genentech	100 μg (3 million IU)		$$$$$

SQ, Subcutaneous; *IM*, intramuscular; *IV*, intravenous; *IL*, intralesional.
$, <1.00; $$, 1.01-2.00; $$$, 2.01-5.00; $$$$, 5.01-10.00; $$$$$, >10.00; ( ), generic price; /, two different price ranges from lower dose to higher dose examples of this drug; —, no price listed for this drug.
*After adding 2 ml diluent.
†Has FDA approval but has not been released on a widespread basis.

■ Table 16-2   Key Pharmacologic Concepts—Interferons[9]

Drug Name	Absorption and Bioavailability			Elimination		
	Peak Levels	Bioavailable (%)	Protein Binding	Half-life	Metabolism	Excretion
IFN-α 2$_b$	3-12 hrs	80%	Not pertinent	2-3 hrs (IM) 2 hrs (IV)	Proteolytic degradation during renal tubular reabsorption	Renal
IFN-α 2$_a$	3.8-7.3 hrs	80%	Not pertinent	3.7-8.5 hrs (mean 5.1)	(same as above)	Renal
IFN-α N$_3$	3-12 hrs	80%	Not pertinent	2-3 hrs (IM) 2 hrs (IV)	(same as above)	Renal
IFN-γ	4-24 hrs	30%-70%	Not pertinent	2.9 hrs (IM) 5.9 hrs (SC)	(same as above)	Renal

of IFN-α and IFN-γ. The volume of distribution is similar for both IFN-α and IFN-γ.

Metabolism and Excretion

IFN-β and IFN-γ undergo renal catabolism, but to a smaller extent than IFN-α. Human IFNs do not appear to cross the placental barrier, and although unknown for human IFNs, mouse IFNs are excreted into milk. Interferon-α 2_b was not detected in urine samples after IM, SC, or intravenous (IV) administration. Proteolytic inactivation of IFN is likely; the primary site of such inactivation is probably in the kidney.[10]

Neutralizing Antibodies

IFN-α therapy has induced the formation of neutralizing antibodies. However, resistance to IFN-α therapy does not appear to be mediated by these antibodies, given that patients who have antibodies to recombinant IFN-α still respond to natural IFN-α. Although in one study, the authors suggested that patients with cutaneous T-cell lymphoma with high titers of anti-IFN-α neutralizing antibodies had a decreased response to therapy, the clinical significance of neutralizing antibodies remains to be elucidated.[11]

Mechanisms of Action

Table 16-3 lists mechanisms of action for all IFNs. To be active, IFN requires binding to specific receptors on the surface of target cells. IFN-α and IFN-β share the same receptor encoded on chromosome 21, and IFN-γ binds to an unrelated receptor encoded on chromosome 6.[12]

The intracellular events after receptor binding that lead to gene expression are unclear. The antiviral activity of various IFNs can be explained, in part, by their ability to induce the expression of oligo-adenylate synthetase (2'-5'A synthetase). This enzyme polymerizes adenosine triphosphate (ATP) into 2'-5'-linked oligomers, some of which are capable of activating a latent cellular endonuclease that degrades both viral as well as cellular ribonucleic acid (RNA).[13] Ribonuclease L is also induced by IFNs and is activated by 2'-5'-linked poly A oligomers and degrades single stranded viral RNA.[14] Protein kinase P1, also induced by IFNs, phosphorylates serine, and threonine moieties of the subunit of elongation factor-2[15] result in the inhibition of transfer RNA (t-RNA) binding to ribosomes and the inhibition of the normal translation of viral messenger RNA (m-RNA).[16]

With respect to the antiproliferative effects of various IFNs, they affect all phases of the cell cycle. The mechanism(s) of such inhibition may involve IFN inductions of 2'-5'A synthetase with its products inhibiting mitosis, inhibiting growth factors, and the down regulating c-myc, c-fos, and certain c-ras oncogenes.

IFN-α and IFN-β are generally less potent stimulators of major histocompatibility complex (MHC) antigens required for cellular immune reactions when compared to IFN-γ; however, IFN-α and IFN-β are capable of enhancing/inducing the expression of class I or II MHC antigens on immunocompetent cells and tumor cells.[17] There are increases in natural killer (NK)

■ ## Table 16-3   Mechanisms of Action for All Interferons

Mechanisms	Clinical Result
• Induction of 2'-5'A synthetase • Induction of ribonuclease L • Induction of protein kinase P1	Antiviral
• Induction of 2'-5'A synthetase • Inhibition of various growth factors • Enhanced p53 tumor suppressor gene expression • Down regulation of c-myc, c-fos, and certain c-ras oncogenes	Antiproliferative
• Induction of class I and II MHC antigens • Increased number of natural killer cells • Inhibits production of TH-2 cytokines such as IL-4, IL-5, and IL-6	Immunoregulatory

cell numbers and activity after exposure to IFN, also leading to an enhanced immune status.

CLINICAL USE

Table 16-4 lists indications and contraindications for IFNs.

FDA-Approved Indications
CONDYLOMATA ACUMINATA (GENITAL WARTS). Condylomata acuminata are benign tumors commonly due to sexually transmitted human papillomavirus (HPV) infections, usually HPV types 6 and 11. In light of the antiviral, antiproliferative, and immunomodulatory activities of IFN, a multicenter, double-blind placebo-controlled study was undertaken. This study revealed intralesional (IL) IFN-α 2$_b$ to be safe and effective in the treatment of condylomata acuminata on the external surfaces of genital and perianal areas.[18] Compilation of three such studies yielded 487 lesions injected IL with 0.1 ml containing 1 million IU of IFN-α 2$_b$ per wart three times weekly for 3 weeks. A total of 539 lesions were similarly injected with placebo. By 17 weeks after treatment, 52% of IFN-treated warts completely cleared compared with 24% of placebo-treated lesions. Of those IFN-treated patients whose lesions cleared and were followed-up, 81% remained clear for a period of 9 to 33 months.

Table 16-4   Interferon Indications and Contraindications

FDA-APPROVED INDICATIONS
Condyloma acuminatum[18-22] (α)
AIDS-associated Kaposi's sarcoma[23-34] (α, γ)
Chronic granulomatous disease[35,36] (γ)
Malignant melanoma (adjuvant)[37-45] (α, γ)

OFF-LABEL USES
Neoplastic
Basal cell carcinoma[46-51] (α)
Squamous cell carcinoma[52-55] (α)
Keratoacanthoma[56] (α)
Cutaneous T-cell lymphoma[57-73] (α, β, γ)
Actinic keratoses[74] (α)
Keloids[75-78] (α, γ)
Hemangioma[79,80] (α)

Viral Infections
Verruca vulgaris[81-83] (α, β, γ)
Herpes zoster[84,85] (α)
Varicella[86] (α)
Herpes simplex[87-89] (α)

Papulosquamous and Dermatitis
Atopic dermatitis[90-99] (α, γ)
Psoriasis[100,101] (γ)

Other Dermatoses
Lupus erythematosus[102] (α)
Follicular mucinosis[103] (α, γ)
Behçet's disease[104-106] (α)
Progressive systemic sclerosis[107-111] (γ)

CONTRAINDICATIONS
Absolute
Hypersensitivity to IFN-α and IFN-γ formulations
Hypersensitivity to mouse immunoglobulin

Relative
Pregnancy
Organ transplant recipient
Cardiac dysrhythmias
Depression or other psychiatric disorders
Leukopenia
Patients under 18 years of age

PREGNANCY PRESCRIBING STATUS—CATEGORY C (same rating for all types of IFN currently available)

Furthermore, in one study, at 1 week after the completion of therapy, IFN-α 2$_\beta$ produced a 62.4% decrease in mean wart area, which was a significantly ($p<0.001$) greater reduction than the 1.2% increase in area in the placebo group.[19] Thirteen weeks after the completion of therapy, the mean wart area was still decreased 39.9% from baseline in the IFN group, whereas the wart surface area increased by 46% in the placebo group ($p<0.001$). Reduction in wart area may allow for other therapeutic modalities to be used subsequently, such as surgical excision. The results of combining IFN treatment of condylomata with cryosurgery or podophyllin resin have been promising.

Recombinant IFN-γ SC once daily (100 μg) for two separate 1-week courses spaced by a therapy-free 3-week interval failed to show response, supporting that short-term systemic IFN-γ therapy is ineffective for condylomata. No major difference in cure rate was observed when surgical excision alone was compared with surgical excision and adjuvant recombinant IFN-γ SC for 1 week.[20]

It has been suggested that the data on systemic, intralesional, and topical IFN therapy for condylomata acuminata do not prove this modality to be superior to other therapies available for this condition.[21,22] Many of the data on IFN, however, are on patients who have failed other treatment modalities in the past. Given the cost of treatment and the multiple visits required, IFN therapy should be reserved for highly motivated patients who have failed other simpler and less costly modes of therapy.

ACQUIRED IMMUNODEFICIENCY SYNDROME ASSOCIATED WITH KAPOSI'S SARCOMA.   Recently the FDA has approved the use of IFN-α 2$_a$ and IFN-α 2$_b$ in the treatment of Kaposi's sarcoma (KS) in patients with acquired immunodeficiency syndrome (AIDS) due to human immunodeficiency virus (HIV). Those who responded to IFN therapy tended to develop fewer opportunistic infections and appeared to have a distinct survival advantage over the nonresponders.[23] Interferon has been shown to increase β_2-macroglobulin expression, a component of MHC I molecules involved in antigen expression; however, such an increase is noted not only on responders but also in non-

responders to IFN therapy, indicating a more complex mechanism of action.[24,25]

The overall objective response rates with IFN-α 2$_a$ and IFN-α 2$_b$ equaled or surpassed those achieved with conventional cytotoxic chemotherapy. However, IFN provides only a palliative approach to KS/AIDS because even in patients in whom complete KS tumor regression was achieved, the underlying immunodeficiency was not reversed. The beneficial cosmetic effects of IFN in the treatment of KS/AIDS were evident and had a dramatic impact on the patient's quality of life. The recommended dosages of IFN-α 2$_a$ and IFN-α 2$_b$ are 36 and 30 million IU SC, respectively, administered daily. As a single agent, IFN-α induces approximately a 75% response rate in those patients with greater than 400 CD4 T cells/mm^3, whereas only 13% of patients with fewer than 200 CD4 cells/mm^3 respond.

Given the antiviral activity of IFN-α and zidovudine (AZT), both drugs have been used in combination for HIV-related KS.[26] The combination of AZT (100 mg every 4 hours) and IFN-α 2$_b$ (4 to 6 million IU daily) appears to increase tumor regression to 50% in those patients with less than 200 CD4 cells /mm^3. Therapy is continued until no remaining tumor is evident unless severe adverse effects develop (reduce dose by 50% or discontinue therapy for a week) or until evidence of opportunistic organisms is detected (discontinue therapy). The average response rate of KS to high dose IFN-α therapy has been approximately 30%.[27] Currently, the optimal duration of IFN treatment of KS is not known. In many cases, tumor recurrence occurs within 6 months in complete responders and the response for second treatment is not reliable. These facts lead to a current recommendation of maintenance treatment as long as adverse effects are tolerated.[26-29] Several authors recommend a dose of 100 mg of AZT every 4 hours combined with 5 to 10 million IU of IFN-α to limit toxicity and adverse effects.[29]

Dupuy and co-workers[30] claim a high response rate when AZT was combined with 1 million IU of IFN-α 2$_b$ three times weekly; nevertheless, there was no demonstrable superiority over placebo-treated lesions. It is possible that the close proximity of some IFN- and placebo-treated lesions and the low number of placebo-treated lesions could have led to such results.[30] IFN's antiretroviral action is speculated to be at the level of viral particle assembly and release of intact virions.[29,31] Interestingly, it has been suggested that lesions of KS have genomic evidence of human herpes virus 8 infection.[32,33]

Although KS is not an FDA-approved indication for IFN-γ, this form of IFN has been used in doses ranging from 0.3 to 3 mg/m² IV twice weekly with response rates lower than those for IFN-α. Heagy and coauthors[34] reported a response of 18%. The responders in this study all had CD4 counts over 200 and many patients in the study had prior histories of opportunistic infection, which could have resulted in a lower response.[34]

CHRONIC GRANULOMATOUS DISEASE.
IFN-γ has been shown to enhance bactericidal activity and superoxide production in macrophages of patients with chronic granulomatous disease of childhood who lack proper phagocyte function.[35] Clinical studies have proven IFN-γ to decrease the frequency of serious infections and thus lead to fewer hospitalizations in patients with chronic granulomatous disease. The recommended dosage for children with affected surface area of greater than 0.5 m² is 50 μg/m² SC three times weekly for life.[36]

MALIGNANT MELANOMA.
IFN-α as a single agent in doses as high as 100 million IU daily IV results in a response rate (complete and partial response) of 4% to 29%, depending on the individual study. A study found that DTIC 800 mg/m² IV in a single dose resulted in a 17% response rate, but when combined with IFN-α 2ᵦ (2 million IU/m² IV for 5 days) and repeated in 3-week intervals until progression or for 6 months in complete responders, resulted in a 27% response rate and had significantly better survival.[37] A phase II trial of 191 patients with disseminated malignant melanoma compared the effects of 50 million IU/m² IM three times weekly of IFN-α 2ₐ; 12 million IU/m² IFN-α 2ₐ IM three times weekly; IFN-α 2ₐ with cimetidine; IFN-γ; IFN-α 2ₐ with IFN-γ; IFN-α 2ₐ with BCNU; and IFN-α 2ₐ with DFMO. The objective regression rates were 23%, 20%, 23%, 10%, 5%, 7%, and 0%, respectively.[38] Although IFN-α at the higher dose resulted in higher re-

sponse rates, there was no statistically significant survival advantage when compared with any of the other regimens.

A statistically significant difference between IFN-α 2ᵦ-treated patients with stage I and II melanoma versus controls was found in a recent study.[39] Median overall survival was increased by 1.04 years using adjuvant IFN-α 2ᵦ. The greatest patient response was in patients with nodal disease. Similar increased survival time of 1.6 years in patients treated with IFN-α 2ᵦ has been reported by Creagan.[40] The overall 5 year survival in stage IIIb melanoma patients treated with IFN-α 2ᵦ was 62% versus 36% in non-treated patients.[41] In patients with disease limited to the skin and lymph nodes, the combination of isotretinoin and IFN-α has been useful (5 of 20 patients with a partial to complete response).[42,43] These data support the use of high-dose IFN-α 2ᵦ for patients at high risk of recurrence.[44] Overall, the use of IFN as a single agent in metastatic malignant melanoma is beneficial in a minority of cases. In general, the combined use of IFN and chemotherapeutic agents such as dacarbazine and vindesine are the most effective regimens.[45]

Off-Label Uses
See Table 16-4.

BASAL CELL CARCINOMA.
Basal cell carcinoma (BCC) is the most common form of skin cancer and constitutes about one eighth of all cancers diagnosed in the United States. Buechner[46] reported complete cure of nodular BCC when given at low doses (1.5 million IU IFN-α 2ᵦ) three times weekly for 4 weeks in four patients. The most recent results of a multicenter, placebo-controlled, randomized study of 172 patients with biopsy-proven BCC confirmed the findings of earlier pilot studies that the optimal intralesional dose of IFN-α 2ᵦ was 1.5 million IU administered three times weekly for 3 weeks. This IFN regimen resulted in an 86% complete response rate including no histologic evidence of residual BCC, compared with a 29% rate in the placebo group ($p < 0.0001$). Nodular and superficial BCCs were treated at the same dose but for 3 weeks.[47] Similar doses, however, when used for aggressive (recurrent or morpheaform) BCC resulted in a complete cure in only 27% of patients.[48]

Studies completed to date have not led to FDA approval of the use of IFN in nodular and superficial BCC. These studies do indicate that the dose and duration of treatment are important in achieving cures. For example, a dose of 13.5 million IU if given in divided doses for only 1 week produced a 38% cure rate, compared with a 74% cure rate when divided over a 2-week period.[49] A study compared the efficacy of sustained release preparation of IFN-α 2$_b$ (10 million IU) when given only once, to once a week for 3 weeks (recurrent and morpheaform BCC were excluded). The different dosing regimens resulted in no significant difference between the cure rates of nodular and superficial lesions; however, there was a significant difference between single dose (52% cure rate) and multiple dose therapy (80% cure rate).[50] Eighty-two percent of patients experienced at least one adverse severe reaction and most developed mild inflammation at the site of injection, probably due to excessive nonlinear release of IFN. The enhancement of tumor-associated antigen expression may account for IFN's success in treating BCCs.[50] Ikic[51] reported 106 patients with BCC treated with natural IFN-α or recombinant IFN-α 2$_c$ IL for 3 to 6 weeks. Overall, 13 of 86 patients with BCC treated with natural IFN were cured and 14 of 20 patients with BCC treated with recombinant IFN-α 2$_c$ were cured. In addition, there was significant reduction in the size of the tumor in many of the lesions that did not completely resolve. The predominant locations of the tumors were in the face, lips, and ears, and therefore IL IFN provides an alternative for cosmetically difficult surgical locations.[51] Based on these results, the IFN treatment of patients with BCC can be regarded as an alternative to surgery in a number of selected cases with nodular or superficial BCCs.

SQUAMOUS CELL CARCINOMA.
Squamous cell carcinoma (SCC) of skin constitutes 10% to 25% of nonmelanoma skin cancers. In a study by Edwards and associates,[52] patients with biopsy proven SCC in sun-exposed areas were treated IL three times weekly with 1.5 million IU IFN-α 2$_b$ for 3 weeks. At the end of the study, the treated area was excised and examined histologically for residual SCC. Thirty-three of 34 lesions revealed histologic absence of SCC.[52]

In addition, papillomavirus infections with malignant transformation to SCC appear to respond to IFN therapy.[53] An open-label study designed to evaluate the effectiveness and cosmetic result of IL recombinant IFN-α 2$_b$ on actinically induced primary cutaneous SCCs was carried out.[54] In this study, 27 patients with invasive SCC and 7 patients with in situ SCC, ranging in size from 0.5 to 2.0 cm in the longest dimension, were treated with 1.5 million IU IL three times a week for 3 weeks. The treatment sites were excised 18 weeks after therapy and examined for histologic evidence of remaining tumor. Over 97% of the patients with SCC were cured both clinically and histologically. This excellent cure rate was not due simply to successful treatment of in situ lesions, in that the majority of these lesions were indeed invasive and resulted in 96.2% cure rate of the 27 invasive lesions. The investigators and patients independently judged 93.9% of the cases to have a "very good" or "excellent" cosmetic result.

In a larger study, 32 patients received 0.4 million IU of natural IFN-α 2$_b$ IL into SCC, including lesions on the lip and at least one on the tonsil. Patients received 20 to 30 injections over a 3 to 6 week period of time, and the lesion was excised within 72 hours of the final treatment. Altogether, 59% of these patients had both a clinical and a histologic cure.[55] As with BCC therapy, IFN-α 2$_b$ therapy can be considered for patients with SCC who are not candidates for surgical excision or who are not amenable to surgery.

KERATOACANTHOMA.
Grob and co-workers[56] reported regression in 5 out of 6 large keratoacanthomas (greater than 2 cm in diameter) treated with intralesional IFN-α 2$_a$, 9 to 20 injections per patient with total resolution in 4 to 7 weeks. Whether keratoacanthomas are low-grade SCCs is unclear; however, avoiding the scarring after surgery may prompt the selective use of IFN in this condition.[56] Appropriate prospective sites for IFN injection of keratoacanthomas on the face can include forehead, perinasal, and auricular areas.

CUTANEOUS T-CELL LYMPHOMA.
Cutaneous T-cell lymphoma (mycosis fungoides [MF]) is a malignant proliferation of T cells,

typically helper/inducer (CD4) lymphocytes with initial presentation in the skin. Olsen and colleagues[57] treated 22 patients with stage Ia to IVa (without visceral involvement) histologically confirmed cutaneous T-cell lymphoma patients with a daily 3 to 36 million IU IFN-α 2_a escalating–IM induction dose for 10 weeks. This was followed by a maintenance dose dependent on the response at the end of induction. A total of 13 of 22 patients had a complete (3) or partial (10) response with remissions lasting 4 to 27½ months. The overall complete response rate with further treatment was 6/22 (27%), four patients with extensive plaque stage MF and two patients with erythrodermic disease, suggesting IFN-α 2_a to be an effective single agent therapy for both early and advanced cutaneous T-cell lymphoma.

Intralesional injection of plaques of MF with IFN-α 2_b (1 million IU three times weekly for 4 weeks) produced substantial localized clinical and histologic improvement with 10 of 12 plaques demonstrating complete regression localized to the IFN injected sites.[58] A review of the literature on MF by Bunn and coauthors[59] revealed an overall response rate of 55% and complete response of 17% in 207 patients. There was no apparent therapeutic difference between IFN-α 2_a and IFN-α 2_b. The response rate of IFN-β and IFN-γ was 41% with a 15% complete response rate, which suggests that they may offer no therapeutic advantage over IFN-α.[59-61] Kuzel and co-workers[62] reported response rates of 93%, with 80% complete response. Analysis of responders by stage of their disease was not reported. A similarly high response was reported by other authors.[63,64] In a study of 23 patients treated with SC IFN-α 2_a, 3 to 18 million IU for 12 weeks, 74% of the patients had objective tumor response, with 35% having a complete response and 39% having a partial response.[65] Using the same protocol, Simoni[66] reported a complete response in 42% and a partial response in 50% of patients treated with IFN-α 2_a.

The addition of PUVA to IFN-α 2_a appeared to increase the number of complete responses (62%) in stage IB to IVB patients.[67] Similar high response rates have been reported by Stadler and associates.[68] Interferon-α and PUVA appear to be a highly effective combination for the treatment of cutaneous T-cell lymphoma.[67-69] The effectiveness of combining retinoids with IFN-α has been studied.[70-73] Better results are obtained in patients with plaque stage disease versus Sézary syndrome, with an overall response rate of 56% to 63%.[70-73] Overall, the mode of IFN delivery does not appear to affect the therapeutic outcome. More studies, however, need to be performed to determine the optimal duration and dose of treatment.

ACTINIC KERATOSES. Up to 93% of actinic keratoses completely cleared after IL injection of 0.5 million IU of IFN-α 2_b three times weekly for 2 to 3 weeks with no clearing in the placebo-injected group.[74] Because of practical considerations and the availability of other effective treatments, the clinical usefulness of this modality for treatment of actinic keratoses is quite limited.

KELOIDS. Berman and Duncan[58] injected a keloid IL with 1.5 million IU IFN-α 2_b (0.15 ml) twice over 4 days. The area of the keloid reduced by approximately 50% by day 9. In vitro testing of the fibroblasts before and after the two injections of IFN revealed that the original increased collagen and glycosaminoglycan production and the reduced collagenase activity were normalized. After short-term treatment of a keloid with two IL injections (7 days apart) of IFN-α 2_b (1.5 million IU/injection) the lesional area of a formerly progressively enlarging keloid was initially reduced by 41% and was undetectable 2 years later.[75]

Granstein and co-workers[76] performed a placebo-controlled, double-blind trial of IL recombinant IFN-γ in the treatment of the keloids of 10 patients. Eight of the 10 patients completed the course of treatment with injections of either 0.1 or 0.01 mg IFN-γ and injection of diluent alone three times per week for 3 weeks. The average percent reduction in keloidal height 22 days after the initial injection was 30.4% for IFN-γ treated keloids and only 1.1% for diluent treated keloids ($p<0.002$). No statistically significant difference was found between the percentage reduction in lesional height of keloids treated with the low versus high dose of IFN-γ. IFN-γ at doses of 0.5 μg once per week for 10 weeks decreased the linear dimension by at least 50% in 5 out of 10 scars studied with minimal adverse effects reported.[77]

A postoperative adjunctive advantage of IL IFN-α 2$_b$ over keloid excision alone and over postoperative triamcinolone acetonide (TAC) injections was reported. Only 3 of 16 (19%) IFN-α 2$_b$ treated sites recurred after excision, compared with 22 of 43 (51%) recurrences in lesions excised alone and 38 of 65 (58%) recurrences in lesions excised and treated with TAC. One million IU per 0.1 ml was injected into the incision site after surgical excision of the keloid at intervals of 1 cm of sutured defect (up to 0.5 ml total). Patients had a repeat injection at the same site at the same dose 1 week after suture removal. Follow-up ranged from 7 to 47 months. These studies demonstrated the efficacy of IL IFN-α and IFN-γ in situ. Furthermore, significant efficacy over IL corticosteroid injections in reduction of keloid recurrences makes IFN-α 2$_b$ an excellent postoperative therapy, particularly in patients who received multiple corticosteroid injections that failed.[78]

HEMANGIOMA.   Blei[79] reported significant involution of debilitating perioral hemangiomas in a young patient treated with daily subcutaneous injections of 1.5 million IU IFN-α 2$_a$ for 22 months. IFN-α 2$_a$ IM has been used for diffuse neonatal hemangiomatosis at doses of 3 million IU per day. This daily dose for 18 months resulted in 20% to 40% reduction in skin lesions and decrease in liver size in a young girl who had prior steroid therapy that failed.[80]

VERRUCA VULGARIS.   Nimura and colleagues[81] reported a "good response" in 81% of common warts treated with nonrecombinant IFN-β compared with 17% in controls. Berman and co-workers[82] reported a mean reduction of 86% in the lesional area of common warts treated with 0.1 million IU IFN-α 2$_b$ compared with a 38% improvement in the placebo-injected group. Reports of success in the treatment of common warts with a needleless injector need to be further evaluated in a controlled fashion because this may provide a less painful alternative mode of treatment.[83]

HERPES ZOSTER.   The multiplication of varicella-zoster virus within infected cells in tissue culture is inhibited by human IFN. Although little or no circulating IFN could be demonstrated in varicella-zoster infections, high titers are detected in resolving vesicle fluid.[84] The development of detectable IFN in vesicular fluid is delayed in those patients with dissemination beyond the primary dermatome. These findings suggest that IFN might be involved in the recovery process of varicella-zoster infection. The most comprehensive study was performed by Merigan and co-workers[85] in which 90 patients with malignancies and herpes zoster in a single dermatome were treated with either placebo (45 patients) or nonrecombinant human IFN-α 0.48 − 5.1 × 10^5 IU/kg per day in two divided doses for 4 to 8 days. They found a significant decrease ($p<0.01$) in cutaneous dissemination in patients receiving IFN, and no dissemination occurred in those receiving the highest dosage. The number of days of new vesicle formation within the primary dermatome was decreased to a mean of 2.3 days in this group ($p<0.05$). Early treatment was required to show the therapeutic effect of IFN on new lesion formation due to the short overall duration of days in the placebo recipients. Treated patients had a trend toward less severe pain, and at higher doses the severity of postherpetic neuralgia was significantly ($p<0.05$) diminished. Interestingly, no difference was observed in the time to complete healing between the IFN-treated group (50 ± 7 days) and the placebo recipients (49 ± 8 days). Six visceral complications, meningoencephalitis, postherpetic segmental paresis, keratitis, and hemorrhagic vesicles with consumption coagulopathy, occurred in placebo recipients with only one complication of postherpetic segmental paresis occurring in the IFN recipient group ($p<0.05$). The increased number of complications in placebo-treated patients underscores the effect of IFN in preventing viral dissemination in cancer patients.

A comparison of patients treated with 5 mg/kg three times daily of IV acyclovir or 10 million IU of recombinant leukocyte derived IFN SC for 5 days was completed. This study showed equal therapeutic efficacy for both drugs, when comparing the rate of healing and inhibition of viral dissemination. Although statistical significance was not detected, the IFN-treated group developed a higher distant cutaneous spread compared with the acyclovir-treated group. Also, a higher number of patients in the IFN group developed adverse effects, but neither drug had any effect on postherpetic neuralgia.[50]

VARICELLA. Arvin and coauthors[86] treated children having malignancies and early varicella with nonrecombinant IFN-α (4.2×10^4 to 2.55×10^5 U/kg/day for an average of 6.4 days) or with placebo. Six of nine placebo treated patients, compared with two of nine IFN treated patients, developed serious complications with the development of fever as a prominent side effect of the IFN treatment. Two placebo treated patients and one patient receiving IFN died.

HERPES SIMPLEX. After surgical treatment of trigeminal neuralgia there is frequent reactivation of herpes labialis in patients with a history of such lesions. Pazin and co-workers[87] recognized this and initiated a double-blind, placebo-controlled prospective study of 37 patients with a history of herpes labialis who were to undergo surgical treatment of trigeminal neuralgia. Starting 1 day before surgery, 19 patients received either nonrecombinant IFN-α (7×10^4 IU/kg/day IM in divided doses of 12 hours for 5 days) or placebo. Five of 19 IFN-treated patients versus 10 of 18 placebo treated patients had reactivation of herpes labialis. In addition, a statistically significant reduction in both frequency and duration of oropharyngeal herpes simplex virus shedding was detected in the IFN treated group. A similar study of 387 patients utilizing IFN-α n_3 at a concentration of 6 million IU/g four times daily for 4 days revealed a decrease in viral shedding and pain, itching, and time to crusting for males. Interestingly, although the time of viral shedding also decreased for females, symptomatic improvement did not occur.[88] A controlled comparison of 20 patients treated with 10^5 IU/g of human leukocyte IFN-α with dimethylsulfoxide (DMSO) revealed fewer recurrences of genital herpes compared with DMSO alone; however, this reduction in recurrences was not statistically significant.[89]

ATOPIC DERMATITIS (AD). Evidence of reduced production of IFN-γ in vitro by mononuclear cells of patients with atopic dermatitis (AD) and the suppression of IL 4-mediated IgE stimulation by IFN-γ prompted evaluation the use of IFN in atopic disease.[90] A randomized, placebo-controlled, double-blind, multicenter trial studied the effects of SC ($50 \mu g/m^2$) recombinant IFN-γ versus placebo for 12 weeks in 78 patients. Altogether, 45% of the recombinant IFN-γ treated group and 21% of placebo treated patients achieved a significant response (>50% improvement) by a physicians' evaluations. Similarly, there was significant improvement in the IFN group by patients' accounts and also a decrease in other symptoms such as conjunctivitis, pruritus, and erythema.[91] Interestingly, there was a nonsignificant increase in serum IgE, in spite of a significant reduction of mean eosinophil count.

An open trial of 14 patients treated with SC IFN-γ in doses of $100 \mu g$ given 5 days weekly for the first week then 3 days weekly for 3 weeks followed by twice weekly for the last 2 weeks reported a 57% clinical improvement. No statistically significant reduction in serum IgE levels was observed; however, there was a reduction in spontaneous IgE production in vitro after 6 weeks of therapy.[92] Another study showed that although no significant effect on IgE production was observed, overall clinical improvement was noted after treatment with 0.01 mg/m^2 to 0.1 mg/m^2.[93] Similar findings were reported by Muscial and associates.[94] A separate study failed to demonstrate any difference in overall response to IFN-γ versus controls in AD-treated patients.[95] The results of these and other studies indicate that the pathogenesis of AD is much more complex than merely a reduction of IFN-γ in atopic patients.[96,97]

Therapy with IFN-α has also been attempted in patients with AD, with varied and contradictory results; thus larger controlled trials to establish its efficacy are required. Torrelo[98] reported a satisfactory response (investigator and patient global assessment) in 5 of 13 patients treated with 3 million IU IFN-α 2_a SC three times per week for 4 weeks. Mackie[99] reported no benefit from the same regimen for a total duration of 12 to 14 weeks of treatment. Further clinical trials are warranted to demonstrate the clinical effectiveness of this expensive treatment.

PSORIASIS. Initial reports,[100] documenting improvement of psoriatic plaques and psoriatic arthritis, have not been confirmed by later trials. A double-blind randomized study of 24 patients treated with $100 \mu g$ IFN-γ SC daily in 28 days and one open trial of 56 patients treated with the same dose daily for 2 weeks and three times weekly for almost 9 months[101] failed to show improvement in psoriatic arthritis. The arthritis actually worsened in those patients initially classified as responders in the first 3 months. Interestingly, a report of induction of psoriatic lesions at sites of IFN injection, which were not seen in placebo injection sites, supports the theory that IFN-γ plays a causative role in induction of local psoriasis.

LUPUS ERYTHEMATOSUS. A study of 10 patients with either discoid lupus erythematosus (DLE) or subacute cutaneous lupus erythematosus (SCLE), treated systemically with IFN-α 2_a, revealed rapid clearing of lesions within 6 weeks, with DLE patients responding more than SCLE. Unfortunately, all patients relapsed on stopping the treatments.[102]

FOLLICULAR MUCINOSIS. Meissner and coauthors[103] also found combinations of IFN-α and IFN-γ to be effective in the treatment of primary progressive follicular mucinosis unrelated to cutaneous T-cell lymphoma.

BEHÇET'S DISEASE. Fourteen patients with either oral ulcers, genital ulcers, pustular vasculitis, erythema nodosum, or thrombophlebitis were treated with IFN-α 2_a million IU three times per week escalating to 12 million IU for a 2 month period. It was observed that all patients were symptom free at 2 months and had decreased number of recurrences in the posttreatment period.[104] High response rates have also been reported by Mahrle and coauthors[105] (3 of 4 with complete remission) and Fierlbeck and coauthors[106] (90% response rate) at doses of 100 μg/day for 2 to 3 weeks. Maintenance doses once or twice weekly, however, were required to prevent early relapses.

PROGRESSIVE SYSTEMIC SCLEROSIS. The ability of IFNs to inhibit in vitro the activated functions of dermal fibroblasts derived from the involved skin of patients with scleroderma, morphea, or keloids has been demonstrated in several laboratories.[107-110] The elevated collagen production by scleroderma, morphea, and keloid fibroblasts has been inhibited by IFN-α, IFN-β, and IFN-γ.[107-110] IFN-α, IFN-β, and IFN-γ also inhibit the proliferation of sclero-

derma fibroblasts, although the inhibition does not persist.[107] All three classes of IFN also inhibit the proliferation and glycosaminoglycan production of keloid fibroblasts while enhancing their production of collagenase activity.[110]

Progressive systemic sclerosis is a disease of unknown etiology characterized by excessive deposition of connective tissue matrix components, primarily collagen, in multiple organs including skin, kidneys, heart, lung, and gastrointestinal tract. This disease is also associated with microvascular and immunologic abnormalities. Kahan and co-workers[111] assessed the clinical therapeutic efficacy of recombinant IFN-γ IM daily for 6 months in nine patients with stable or worsening systemic sclerosis. Escalating doses of IFN-γ, initially at 10 μg per day, were administered and patients achieved a constant dose of 100 μg per day for the final 5 months of the study. Significant ($p<0.05$) improvement from baseline values was observed in total skin thickening score, maximal oral opening, range of motion of wrists and elbows, grip strength, functional index, dysphagia, and creatinine clearance. Although the results of this pilot study are promising, there were a number of study limitations including a lack of placebo controls, the use of concurrent medications (including up to 10 mg of prednisone daily), and a limited number of patients. There was also the acute development of pericarditis and renal crisis in a patient who was removed from the study after 6 weeks. These confounding variables all point to the need for additional clinical trials.

Adverse Effects

Table 16-5 lists the frequency of adverse effects associated with IFN therapy. The adverse effects of IFNs are dose-dependent and generally remit either during continued therapy or after dose reduction. In addition, the adverse effects are generally rapidly reversible on cessation of therapy.

INFLUENZA-LIKE SYMPTOMS. The most commonly associated adverse effects after IFN therapy are the influenza-like symptoms of fever, chills, myalgias, headache, and arthralgia. It is our experience that in generally healthy individuals, SC administration of IFN in doses of 3 million units or less every other day induced nominal and tolerable flu-like symptoms or no adverse effects

▪ Table 16-5 Frequency of Adverse Effects Associated With Interferon Therapy*[112]

Fatigue	137 (96%)
Neutropenia/Leukopenia†	132 (92%)
Fever	116 (81%)
Myalgia	107 (75%)
Anorexia	99 (69%)
Vomiting/Nausea	95 (66%)
Increased LFTs‡	90 (63%)
Headache	89 (62%)

LFT, Liver function tests.
*N = 143; dose not specified.
†Agranulocytosis or pancytopenia very uncommon—primarily in setting of hepatitis C or when combined with cytotoxic drugs.
‡Magnitude of LFT changes not specified.

at all. Prophylactic (1 to 2 hours before injection) administration of acetaminophen (650 mg), aspirin (650 mg), or nonsteroidal agents (400 mg ibuprofen) helps to prevent these effects.

RHABDOMYOLYSIS. Fatal rhabdomyolysis and multiple organ failure occurred in a patient treated with high-dose IFN-α 2$_b$ (20 million IU IV twice daily).[113] The patient developed generalized myalgias and subsequent hemodynamic shock on the fifth day of therapy. Two other cases of rhabdomyolysis have been reported.[114,115] The authors propose monitoring of creatine kinase and urinary myoglobin concentrations and discontinuation of treatment in patients with evidence of muscle damage.

CARDIOVASCULAR EFFECTS. Significant hypotension, dysrhythmia, or tachycardia (150 beats/min or greater) associated with IFN use has been reported.[116] Hypotension may occur during administration or for up to 2 days posttherapy and may require supportive therapy, including fluid replacement to maintain intravascular volume. These adverse experiences were controlled by modifying dosages or by discontinuing treatment but may require specific additional therapy. Closely monitor patients

with a recent history of myocardial infarction or a history of a dysrhythmic disorder.

NEUROLOGIC AND PSYCHIATRIC EFFECTS. Spastic diplegia was reported in 5 of 26 patients with hemangiomas treated with 1.02 to 3.60 million IU/day of IFN-α 2$_b$.[117] Presumably, preservatives such as benzyl and phenol alcohol in the commercially injectable solution are the culprits, and preservative-free saline solution is recommended. Depression and suicidal behavior including suicidal ideation, attempts, and completed suicides have been reported in association with IFN-α therapy.[8]

OTHER ADVERSE EFFECTS. Gastrointestinal disturbances such as nausea and diarrhea can occur.[8,118] Neutralizing antibodies can develop in patients receiving IFN-α 2$_a$ and IFN-α 2$_b$ that appear to be specific to the recombinant IFN and not natural IFN. In the case of long-term use of IFN-α 2$_a$, the development of neutralizing antibodies in hairy cell leukemic patients was correlated with the development of resistance to IFN-α 2$_a$ and subsequent disease progression.[119] These patients responded to subsequent treatment with natural IFN-α.

DRUG INTERACTIONS

In one study, a single IM injection of IFN-α 2$_a$ and a single injection of aminophylline in 9 subjects had a variable effect on clearance of aminophylline (Table 16-6) and showed a 50% reduction in median clearance probably due to inhibition of the cytochrome P-450 enzyme system.

MONITORING GUIDELINES

Refer to the IFN monitoring guidelines box.

THERAPEUTIC GUIDELINES

Moderate-to-severe adverse experiences may require modification of the patient's dosage regimen, or in some cases, termination of therapy with IFN.

■ Table 16-6 Interactions Between Interferons and Other Medications[8,9,120]

Interacting Drug	Comments
Aminophylline	Reduced cytochrome P-450 activity, resulting in decreased clearance of aminophylline (possibly a CYP 1A2 interaction)
Zidovudine	Use with zidovudine or other myelosuppressive agents may increase the risk of hematologic complications
Interleukin-2	Roferon A in conjunction with IL-2 may increase risk of renal failure

Interferon Monitoring Guidelines[8]

In addition to tests normally required for monitoring AIDS patients, the following are recommended for all patients on IFN therapy (see *Note* below):

MONITORING FREQUENCY
- Before beginning treatment
- 2 weeks after initiation of therapy
- Then perform examination and do laboratory monitoring monthly thereafter while on therapy

LABORATORY TESTING
- CBC and differential including platelet counts*

LABORATORY TESTING—cont'd
- Blood chemistries (including electrolytes and CPK)
- Liver function tests—particular emphasis on transaminases (AST/SGOT and ALT/SGPT)
- TSH at baseline *only*†

SPECIAL TESTING
- Patients with preexisting cardiac abnormalities, or in advanced stages of cancer, should have ECGs taken before and during treatment

CBC, Complete blood count; *CPK*, creatine phosphokinase; *TSH*, thyroid-stimulating hormone; *ECG*, electrocardiogram.
Note: These monitoring guidelines *may not* be medically necessary for otherwise healthy patients receiving 1 or 2 intralesional injections of <5 million IU IFN.
*In malignant melanoma patients, CBCs should be done weekly during the induction phase and monthly during the maintenance phase of therapy.
†If the patient is hyperthyroid, there is an increased risk of dysrhythmia and IFN would be contraindicated.

Because of the fever and other flu-like symptoms associated with IFN administration, various IFNs should be used cautiously in patients with debilitating medical conditions. For example, patients with a history of cardiovascular disease (e.g., unstable angina, uncontrolled congestive heart failure), pulmonary disease (e.g., chronic obstructive pulmonary disease), or diabetes mellitus prone to ketoacidosis should be carefully followed. Caution should also be observed in patients with coagulation disorders (e.g., thrombophlebitis, pulmonary embolism) or severe myelosuppression (leukopenic or anemic patients). Administer IFN SC and not IM to patients with platelet counts <50,000/mm³ (see Monitoring Guidelines section). IFN-α has been shown to affect the menstrual cycle and decrease serum estradiol and progesterone levels in females. At doses higher than those used in humans, IFN-α has abortifacient activity in animals. Careful consideration should be given as to whether the pregnant or adolescent patient should be treated.

Bibliography

Berman B, Sequeira M: Dermatologic uses of interferons. *Dermatol Clin* 13:699-711, 1995.

Kassas H, Kirkwood JM: Adjuvant application of interferons. *Semin Oncol* 23:737-743, 1996.

Knop J: Immunologic effects of interferon. *J Invest Dermatol* 95:72S-74S, 1990.

Memar OM, Tyring SK: Antiviral agents in dermatology: current status and future prospects. *Int J Dermatol* 34:597-606, 1995.

Olsen EA, Bunn PA: Interferon in the treatment of cutaneous T-cell lymphoma. *Hematol Oncol Clin North Am* 9:1089-1107, 1995.

Stadler R: Interferons in dermatology: present-day standard. *Dermatol Clin* 16:377-398, 1998.

Stadler R, Ruszczak Z: Interferons: new additions and indications for use. *Dermatol Clin* 11:187-199, 1993.

References

Pharmacology

1. Isaacs A, Lindenmann J: Virus interference. I. The interferon. *Proc Royal Soc London (Biol)* 147:258-272, 1957.

2. Isaacs A, Lindenmann J, Valentine RC: Virus interference II. Some properties of interferon. *Proc Royal Soc London (Biol)* 147: 268-273, 1957.

3. Lindenmann J, Burke D, Isaacs A: Studies on the production, mode of action and properties of interferon. *Br J Exp Path* 38:551-552, 1957.

4. Vilcek J: The action of interferon. *Interferon,* New York, 1969, Springer-Verlag, pp 72-73.

5. Ho M, Enders JF: An inhibitor of viral activity appearing in infected cell cultures. *Proc Natl Acad Sci USA* 45:385, 1959.

6. Havell EA, Berman B, Ogburn CA, et al: Two antigenically distinct species of human interferon. *Proc Natl Acad Sci USA* 72:2185-2187, 1975.

7. Streuli M, Nagata S, Weissman C: At least three human type interferons: Structure of 2. *Science* 209:1343-1346, 1980.

8. Interferon-β1a, -β1b, α 2a, α 2b, α n3. In *Physicians' desk reference,* ed 52, Montvale, 1998, Medical Economics Company, pp 305-307,1290-1292, 2489-2494, 2637-2644.

9. Wills RJ: Clinical pharmacokinetics of interferons. *Clin Pharmacokinet* 19:390-399, 1990.

10. Bino JR, Madar Z, Gertler A, et al: The kidney is the main site of interferon degradation. *J Interferon Res* 2:301-308, 1982.

11. Rajan GP, Seifert B, Prummer O, et al: Incidence of in-vivo relevance of anti-interferon antibodies during treatment of low-grade cutaneous T-cell lymphomas with interferon alpha-2a combined with acitretin or PUVA. *Arch Dermatol Res* 288:543-548, 1996.

12. Stadler R, Ruszczak Z: Interferons. New additions and indications for use. *Dermatol Clin* 11:187-199, 1993.

13. Chebath J, Benech P, Hovanessian A, et al: Four different forms of interferon-induced 1',5'-Oligo(A) synthetase identified by immunoblotting in human cells. *J Bio Chem* 262:3852-3857, 1987.

14. Ratner L, Sen GC, Brown GE, et al: Interferon, double stranded RNA and RNA degradation: Characteristics of an endonuclease activity. *Eur J Biochem* 79:565-577, 1977.

15. Lebleu B, Sen GC, Shaila S, et al: Interferon, double stranded RNA, and protein phosphorylation. *Proc Natl Acad Sci USA* 73:3107-3111, 1976.

16. Sen GC: Biochemical pathways in interferon action. *Pharmacol Therap* 24:235-257, 1984.

17. Rhodes J, Ivanyi J, Cozens P: Antigen presentation by human monocytes: Effects of modifying major histocompatibility complex class II antigen expression and interleukin-1 production by using recombinant interferons and corticosteroids. *Eur J Immunol* 16:370-375, 1986.

Condyloma Acuminatum

18. Vance JC, Brit BJ, Hassen RC, et al: Intralesional recombinant alfa-2a interferon for the treatment of patients with condyloma acuminatum or verruca plantaris. *Arch Dermatol* 122:272-277, 1986.

19. Eron LJ, Judson F, Tucker S, et al: Interferon therapy for condylomata acuminata. *N Engl J Med* 315:1059-1064, 1986.

20. Zouboulis CC, Buttner P, Orfanos CE: Systemic interferon gamma as adjuvant therapy for refractory anogenital warts. A randomized clinical trial and meta-analysis of the available data. *Arch Dermatol* 128:1413-1414, 1992.

21. Kraus S, Stone K: Management of genital infection caused by human papillomavirus. *Rev Infect Dis* 12:620S-632S, 1990.

22. Ling M: Therapy of genital papillomavirus infections, Part II: Methods of treatment. *Int J Dermatol* 32:769-776, 1992.

AIDS-Associated Kaposi's Sarcoma

23. Abrams DI, Volberding PA: Interferon therapy in AIDS-associated Kaposi's sarcoma. *Semin Oncol* 14:43-47, 1987.

24. De Wit R, Bakker PJM, Reiss P, et al: Temporary increase in serum beta$_2$-microglobulin during treatment with interferon-alfa for AIDS-associated Kaposi's sarcoma. *AIDS* 4:459-462, 1990.

25. De Wit R: AIDS-associated Kaposi's sarcoma and the mechanism of interferon's activity; a riddle within a puzzle. *J Intern Med* 231:321-325, 1992.

26. Hartshorn KL, Vogt MW, Chout C, et al: Synergistic inhibition in human immunodeficiency virus in vitro by azidothymidine and recombinant A interferon. *Antimicrob Agents Chemother* 31:168-172, 1987.

27. Krown SE: Interferon and other biological agents for the treatment of Kaposi's Sarcoma. *Hem Oncol Clin North Am* 5:311-322, 1991.

28. Krown SE, Gold JWM, Niedzwiecki D, et al: Interferon-α with zidovudine: Safety, tolerance, and clinical and virologic effects in patients with Kaposi's sarcoma associated with the acquired immunodeficiency syndrome. *Ann Intern Med* 112:812-821, 1990.

29. Lane HC, Clifford H: The role of α-interferon in patients with human immunodeficiency virus infection. *Semin Oncol* 18:46-52, 1991.

30. Dupuy J, Price M, Lynch G, et al: Intralesional interferon-α and zidovudine in epidemic Kaposi's sarcoma. *J Am Acad Dermatol* 18:966-972, 1993.

31. De Maeyer E, De Maeyer-Guignard J: The antiviral activity of interferons. In *Interferons and other regulatory cytokines*, New York, 1988, Wiley and Sons, pp 114-133.

32. Noel JC, Their F, Dobbeleer G, Heenen M: Demonstration of herpes virus 8 in a lymphangioma-like Kaposi's sarcoma occurring in a non-immunosuppressed patient (letter). *Dermatology* 194:90-91, 1997.

33. Maiorana A, Luppi M, Barozzi P, et al: Detection of human herpes virus type 8 DNA sequences as a valuable aid in the differential diagnosis of Kaposi's sarcoma. *Mod Pathol* 10:182-187, 1997.

34. Heagy W, Groopman J, Schindler J, et al: Use of IFN-γ in patients with AIDS. *J Acq Immune Def Synd* 3:584-590, 1990.

Chronic Granulomatous Disease

35. Sechler JMG, Malceh HL, White CJ, et al: Recombinant human interferon-γ reconstitutes defective phagocyte function in patients with chronic granulomatous disease of childhood. *Proc Natl Acad Sci USA* 85:4874-4878, 1988.

36. Bolinger AM, Taeubel MA: Recombinant interferon gamma for treatment of chronic granulomatous disease and other disorders. *Clin Pharm* 11:834-850, 1992.

Melanoma

37. Rudolf Z, Strojan P: DTIC vs. IFN-alpha plus DTIC in the treatment of patients with metastatic malignant melanoma. *Neoplasma* 43:93-97, 1996.

38. Creagan ET, Scheid DJ, Ahmann DL, et al: Disseminated malignant melanoma and recombinant interferon: Analysis of seven consecutive phase II investigations. *J Invest Dermatol* 95:185S-187S, 1990.

39. Rusciani L, Petraglia S, Alotto M, et al: Postsurgical adjuvant therapy for melanoma. Evaluation of a 3-year randomized trial with recombinant interferon-alpha after 3 and 5 years of follow-up. *Cancer* 79:2354-2360, 1997.

40. Creagan ET, Dalton RJ, Ahmann DL, et al: Randomized, surgical adjuvant clinical trial of recombinant interferon alfa-2a in selected patients with malignant melanoma. *J Clin Oncol* 13:2776-2783, 1995.

41. Doveil GC, Fierro MT, Novelli M, et al: Adjuvant therapy of stage IIIb melanoma with interferon alfa-2b: clinical and immunological relevance. *Dermatology* 191:234-239, 1995.
42. Triozzi PL, Walker MJ, Pellegrini AE, et al: Isotretinoin and recombinant interferon alfa-2a therapy or metastatic malignant melanoma. *Cancer Invest* 14:293-298, 1996.
43. Eisenhauer EA, Lippman SM, Kavanagh JJ, et al: Combination 13-cis-retinoic acid and interferon alpha-2a in the therapy of solid tumors. *Leukemia* 8:1622-1625, 1994.
44. Kirkwood JM, Resnick GD, Cole BF: Efficacy, safety, and risk-benefit analysis of adjuvant interferon alfa-2b in melanoma. *Semin Oncol* 24:16S-23S, 1997.
45. Barth A, Morton DL: The role of adjuvant therapy in melanoma management. *Cancer* 75:726S-734S, 1995.

Basal Cell Carcinoma

46. Buechner S: Intralesional interferon-alfa 2b in the treatment of basal cell carcinoma. *J Am Acad Dermatol* 24:731-734, 1991.
47. Greenway HT, Cornell RC, Tanner DJ, et al: Treatment of basal cell carcinoma with intralesional interferon. *J Am Acad Dermatol* 15:437-443, 1986.
48. Stenquist B, Wennberg AM, Gisslen H, et al: Treatment of aggressive basal cell carcinoma with intralesional interferon: evaluation of efficacy by Mohs surgery. *J Am Acad Dermatol* 27:65-69, 1992.
49. Cornell RC, Greenway HT, Tucker SB, et al: Intralesional interferon therapy for basal cell carcinoma. *J Am Acad Dermatol* 23:694-700, 1990.
50. Edwards L, Tucker SB, Perednia D, et al: The effect of an intralesional sustained-release formulation of interferon-alfa 2b on basal cell carcinoma. *Arch Dermatol* 126:1029-1032, 1990.
51. Ikic D, Padovan I, Pipic N, et al: Interferon therapy for basal cell carcinoma and squamous cell carcinoma. *Int J Clin Pharmacol Ther* 29:342-346, 1991.

Squamous Cell Carcinoma

52. Edwards L, Berman B, Rapini RP, et al: Treatment of cutaneous squamous cell carcinoma by intralesional interferon-alfa 2b therapy. *Arch Dermatol* 128:1486-1489, 1992.
53. Andophy EJ, Dvoretzky I, Malaish AE, et al: Response of warts in epidermodysplasia verruciformis to treatment with systemic and intralesional interferon. *J Am Acad Dermatol* 11:197-202, 1984.
54. Edwards L, Berman B, Rapini RP, et al: Treatment of cutaneous squamous cell carcinomas by intralesional interferon-2b therapy. *Arch Dermatol* 128:1486-1489, 1992.
55. Ikic D, Padovan I, Pipic N, et al: Treatment of squamous cell carcinoma with interferon. *Int J Dermatol* 30:58-61, 1991.

Keratoacanthoma

56. Grob JJ, Suzini F, Richard A, et al: Large keratoacanthomas treated with intralesional interferon-alfa 2a. *J Am Acad Dermatol* 29:237-241, 1993.

Cutaneous T-cell Lymphoma

57. Olsen EA, Rosen ST, Vollmer RT, et al: Interferon-alfa 2a in the treatment of cutaneous T cell lymphoma. *J Am Acad Dermatol* 20:395-407, 1989.
58. Vonderheid EC, Thompson R, Smiles KA, et al: Recombinant interferon-2b in plaque-phase mycosis fungoides—intralesional and low-dose intramuscular therapy. *Arch Dermatol* 123:757-763, 1987.
59. Bunn PA Jr, Hoffman SJ, Norris D, et al: Systemic therapy of cutaneous T-cell lymphomas (mycosis fungoides and the Sézary syndrome). *Ann Intern Med* 121:592-602, 1994.
60. Kaplan EH, Rosen ST, Norris D, et al: Phase II study of recombinant interferon gamma for treatment of cutaneous T-cell lymphoma. *J Natl Cancer Inst* 82:208-212, 1990.
61. Zinzani PL, Mazza P, Tura S: Beta interferon in the treatment of mycosis fungoides International Symposium on Cutaneous Lymphoma. *Haematologica* 73:547-548, 1988.
62. Kuzel TM, Gilyon K, Springer E, et al: Interferon-alfa 2a combined with phototherapy in the treatment of cutaneous T-cell lymphoma. *J Natl Cancer Inst* 82:203-207, 1990.
63. Otte HG, Herges A, Stadler R: Kombinations Therapri mit interferon-alfa 2a and PUVA bei Kutanen T-cell lymphomen. *Hautarzt* 43:695-699, 1992.
64. Papa G, Tura S, Mandelli F, et al: Is interferon alpha in cutaneous T-cell lymphoma a treatment of choice? *Br J Haematol* 79:48S-51S, 1991.

65. Vegna ML, Papa G, Defazio D, et al: Interferon alpha-2a in cutaneous T-cell lymphoma. *Eur J Hematol* 52:32S-35S, 1990.

66. Simoni R, Cavalieri R, Coppola G, et al: Recombinant leukocyte interferon alfa-2a in the treatment of mycosis fungoides. *J Biol Reg Homeostast Ag* 1:93-99, 1987.

67. Kuzel TM, Roenigk HH, Samuelson E, et al: Effectiveness of interferon alfa-2a combined with phototherapy for mycosis fungoides and the Sézary syndrome. *J Clin Onc* 13:257-263, 1995.

68. Stadler R, Otte HG: Combination therapy of cutaneous T cell lymphoma with interferon alpha-2a and photochemotherapy. *Recent Results Cancer Res* 139:391-401, 1995.

69. Roenigk HH, Kuzel TM, Skoutelis AP, et al: Photochemotherapy alone or combined with interferon alpha-2a in the treatment of cutaneous T-cell lymphoma. *J Inv Dermatol* 95:198S-205S, 1990.

70. Dreno B: Roferon-A (interferon alpha 2a) combined with Tegison (etretinate) for treatment of cutaneous T cell lymphomas. *Stem Cells* 11:269-275, 1993.

71. Knobler RM, Trautinger F, Radaszkiewicz T, et al: Treatment of cutaneous T cell lymphoma with a combination of low dose interferon alfa-2b and retinoids. *J Am Acad Dermatol* 24:247-252, 1991.

72. Dreno B, Claudy A, Meynadier J, et al: The treatment of 45 patients with cutaneous T-cell lymphoma with low doses of interferon-alpha 2a and etretinate. *Br J Dermatol* 125:456-459, 1991.

73. Zachariae H, Thestrup-Pedersen K: Interferon-alpha and etretinate combination treatment of cutaneous T-cell lymphoma. *J Inv Dermatol* 95:206S-208S, 1990.

Other Neoplastic Disorders

74. Edwards L, Levine N, Weidner M, et al: Effect of intralesional interferon in actinic keratoses. *Arch Dermatol* 122:779-782, 1986.

75. Berman B, Duncan MR: Short-term keloid treatment in vivo with human interferon-α 2_β results in a selective and persistent normalization of keloidal fibroblast collagen, glycosaminoglycan and collagenase production in vitro. *J Am Acad Dermatol* 21:694-702, 1989.

76. Granstein RD, Rook A, Flotte TJ, et al: A controlled trial of intralesional recombinant interferon-γ in the treatment of keloidal scarring. *Arch Dermatol* 126:1295-1302, 1990.

77. Larrabee WF Jr, East CA, Jaffe HS, et al: Intralesional interferon gamma treatment for keloids and hypertrophic scars. *Arch Otolaryngol Head Neck Surg* 116:1159-1162, 1990.

78. Berman BB, Flores F: Recurrence rates of excised keloids treated with postoperative triamcinolone acetonide injections or interferon-α 2b injections. *J Am Acad Dermatol* 37:755-757, 1997.

79. Blei F, Orlow SJ, Geronemus R: Interferon-alfa 2a therapy for extensive perianal and lower extremity hemangioma. *J Am Acad Dermatol* 29:98-99, 1993.

80. Spiller JC, Sharma V, Woods GM, et al: Diffuse neonatal hemangiomatosis treated successfully with interferon-alfa-2a. *J Am Acad Dermatol* 27:102-104, 1992.

Verruca Vulgaris

81. Nimura M: Intralesional human fibroblast interferon in common warts. *J Dermatol* 10:217-220, 1983.

82. Berman B, Davis-Reed L, Silverstein L, et al: Treatment of verruca vulgaris with α-2 interferon. *J Infect Dis* 154:328-330, 1986.

83. Naples SP, Brodell RT: Verruca vulgaris. Treatment with natural interferon-alfa using a needleless injector. *Arch Dermatol* 129:698-700, 1993.

Herpesvirus Infection

84. Stevens DA, Merigan TC: Interferon, antibody, and other host factors in herpes zoster. *J Clin Invest* 51:1170-1176, 1972.

85. Merigan TC, Rand KH, Pollard RB: Human leukocyte interferon for the treatment of herpes zoster in patients with cancer. *N Engl J Med* 298:981-987, 1978.

86. Arvin AM, Kushner JH, Feldman S, et al: Human leukocyte interferon for the treatment of varicella in children with cancer. *N Engl J Med* 306:761-765, 1982.

87. Pazin GJ, Armstrong SA, Lam MT, et al: Prevention of reactivated herpes simplex infection by human leukocyte interferon after operation on the trigeminal root. *N Engl J Med* 301:225-230, 1979.

88. Lebwohl M, Sacks S, Conant M, et al: Recombinant α-2 interferon gel treatment of recurrent herpes genitalis. *Antiviral Res* 17:235-243, 1992.

89. Shupack J, Stiller M, Davis M, et al: Topical α-interferon ointment with dimethyl sulfoxide in the treatment of recurrent genital herpes simplex. *Dermatology* 184:40-44, 1992.

Atopic Dermatitis

90. Reinhold U, Wehrmann W, Kukel S, et al: Evidence that defective interferon-gamma production in atopic dermatitis patients is due to intrinsic abnormalities. *Clin Exp Immunol* 79:374-379, 1990.
91. Hanifin SM, Schneider LC, Leung DY, et al: Recombinant interferon gamma therapy for atopic dermatitis. *J Am Acad Dermatol* 28:189-197, 1993.
92. Reinhold U, Kukel S, Brzoska J, et al: Systemic interferon gamma treatment in severe atopic dermatitis. *J Am Acad Dermatol* 29:58-63, 1993.
93. Boguniewicz M, Jaffe HS, Izu A, et al: Recombinant gamma interferon in treatment of patients with atopic dermatitis and elevated IgE levels. *Am J Med* 88:365-370, 1990.
94. Musial J, Milewski M, Undas A, et al: Interferon-gamma in the treatment of atopic dermatitis: influence on T-cell activation. *Allergy* 50:520-523, 1995.
95. Nishioka K, Matsunaga T, Katayama I: Gamma-interferon therapy for severe cases of atopic dermatitis of the adult type. *J Dermatol* 22:181-185, 1995.
96. Horneff G, Dirksen U, Wahn V: Interferon-gamma for treatment of severe atopic eczema in two children. *Clin Inv* 72:400-403, 1994.
97. Pung YH, Vetro SW, Bellanti JA: Use of interferons in atopic (IgE-mediated) diseases. *Ann Allergy* 71:234-238, 1993.
98. Torrelo A, Horto A, Sendagorta E, et al: Interferon-α therapy in atopic dermatitis. *Acta Derm Venereol* 75:370-372, 1992.
99. Mackie RM: Interferon-α for atopic dermatitis. *Lancet* 335:1282-1283, 1990.

Eczematous/Papulosquamous Disorders

100. Morhenn VB, Pregerson-Rodan K, Mullen RH, et al: Use of recombinant interferon gamma administered intramuscularly for the treatment of psoriasis. *Arch Dermatol* 123:1633-1637, 1987.
101. Fierlbeck G, Rassner G: Treatment of psoriasis and psoriatic arthritis with interferon gamma. *J Invest Dermatol* 95:138S-141S, 1990.

Other Dermatoses

102. Thiovelt J, Nicolas JF, Kanitakis J, et al: Recombinant interferon-α 2a is effective in the treatment of discoid and subacute cutaneous lupus erythematosus. *Br J Dermatol* 122:405-409, 1990.

103. Meissner K, Weyer U, Kowalzick L, Altenhoff J: Successful treatment of primary progressive follicular mucinosis with interferons. *J Am Acad Dermatol* 24:848-850, 1991.
104. Alpsoy E, Yilmaz E, Basaran E: Interferon therapy for Behçet's disease. *J Am Acad Dermatol* 31:617-619, 1994.
105. Mahrle G, Schulze HJ: Recombinant interferon-gamma (rIFN-gamma) in dermatology. *J Inv Dermatol* 95:132S-137S, 1990.
106. Fierlbeck G, Rassner G: Rekombinantes Interferon-gamma bei psoriasis arthropathica, progressiv systemischer Skerlodermie und Morbus behcet. *Med Klin* 83:695-699, 1988.

Scleroderma

107. Rosenbloom J, Feldman G, Freundlich B, Jimenez SA: Inhibition of excessive scleroderma fibroblast collagen synthesis by recombinant gamma interferon. *Arthritis Rheum* 29:851-856, 1966.
108. Duncan MR, Berman B: Persistence of a reduced collagen producing phenotype in cultured scleroderma fibroblasts after short-term exposure to interferons. *J Clin Invest* 79:1318-1324, 1987.
109. Kahari V-M, Heino J, Vuoriot T, et al: Interferon-alfa and interferon-gamma reduce excessive collagen synthesis and procollagen mRNA levels of scleroderma fibroblasts in culture. *Biochem Biophys Acta* 968:45-50, 1988.
110. Berman B, Duncan MR: Short-term keloid treatment in vivo with human interferon-α 2_b results in a selective and persistent normalization of keloidal fibroblast collagen, glycosaminoglycan and collagenase production in vitro. *J Am Acad Dermatol* 21:694-702, 1989.
111. Kahan A, Amor B, Menkes CJ, et al: Recombinant interferon-γ in the treatment of systemic sclerosis. *Am J Med* 87:273-277, 1989.

Adverse Effects

112. Greenway H, Kosty M, Papadopoulos D, et al: Recent advances in the use of interferon in dermatology. A presentation summary of the roundtable discussion for dermatologists. Annenberg Center for Health Sciences at Eisenhower, p 14.

113. Reinhold U, Hartl C, Hering R, et al: Fatal rhabdomyolysis and multiple organ failure associated with adjuvant high dose interferon alfa in malignant melanoma (letter). *Lancet* 349:540-541, 1997.

114. Anderlini P, Buzaid AC, Legha SS: Acute rhabdomyolysis after concurrent administration of interleukin-2, interferon-alfa, and chemotherapy for metastatic melanoma. *Cancer* 76:678-679, 1995.

115. Greenfield SM, Harvey RS, Thompson RPH: Rhabdomyolysis after treatment with interferon alfa. *BMJ* 309:512, 1994.

116. Deyton LR, Walker RE, Kovac JA, et al: Reversible cardiac dysfunction associated with interferon-alfa therapy in AIDS patients with Kaposi's sarcoma. *N Engl J Med* 321:1246-1249, 1989.

117. Barlow CF: Spastic diplegia as a complication of interferon alfa-2a treatment of hemangiomas of infancy. *J Pediatr* 132:527-530, 1998.

118. Ruszczak Z, Schwartz RA: Interferons in dermatology: biology, pharmacology, and clinical applications. In *Advances in dermatology,* New York, 1998, Mosby-Year Book, pp 235-288.

119. Steis RG, Smith JW, Urba WJ, et al: Resistance to recombinant interferon-alfa 2a in hairy-cell leukemia associated with neutralizing anti-interferon antibodies. *N Engl J Med* 318:1409-1413, 1988.

120. Williams SJ, Baird-Lambert JA, Farrell GC: Inhibition of theophylline metabolism by interferon. *Lancet* 2:939-941, 1987.

PART IV

Miscellaneous Systemic Drugs

CHAPTER 17

Malcolm W. Greaves

Antihistamines

IMPORTANCE OF HISTAMINE IN SKIN DISEASES

Histamine acts on a wide range of target cells within the skin, including endothelial cells, neurons, and immunocompetent cells. Diseases in which histamine plays a pivotal role include most forms of urticaria, cutaneous mastocytosis, and acute insect bite reactions. Histamine is also important in the pathogenesis of the pruritus in patients with atopic eczema.

Histamine is synthesized and stored by human cutaneous mast cells. These cells, which are mainly of the chymase-tryptase expressing type, synthesize histamine from histidine via the enzyme histidine decarboxylase. The histamine product is bound noncovalently in metachromatically staining granules composed of glycosaminoglycans. Released histamine undergoes rapid local degradation catalyzed by enzymatic N-methylation or oxidative deamination.[1] Histamine secretion or release occurs as a consequence of immunologic or nonimmunologic stimuli. Cutaneous mast cells characteristically express the high affinity immunoglobulin E (IgE) receptor (FcεRI) on the cell surface. Cross linking of adjacent IgE receptors by antigen triggers an intracellular stimulus-secretion coupling process. This process culminates in the release of histamine and other mediators including proteases, eicosanoids (e.g., prostaglandins and leukotrienes), and a variety of cytokines. Other immunoreactants, which trigger mast cell activation and histamine release via dimerized FcεRI, include immunoglobulin G (IgG) anti-FcεRIα–autoantibodies (in about a third of patients with chronic urticaria[2,3]) and IgG anti-IgE.[4] However, cutaneous mast cells can also be activated by nonimmunologic stimuli, including substance P and other neuropeptides, complement components (including C5a), and stem cell factor. These nonimmunologic stimuli act via receptors distinct from FcεRI.

Both histamine H_1 and H_2 subclasses of receptors are expressed in human skin.[5] Histamine-induced itching and the axon reflex flare are mediated by H_1 receptors. Both H_1 and H_2 receptors participate in histamine-evoked vasodilation and increased vascular permeability. Histamine also regulates T-lymphocyte activity via H_2 receptors. Histamine suppresses T-lymphocyte proliferation and cytotoxicity of allogenic target cells. A cytokine termed *histamine suppressor factor (HSF)* has also been reported to be produced by a subpopulation of T cells via H_2 receptors.[6,7] Other recently described subclasses of histamine receptors have not been positively identified in skin. These subclasses include both H_3 autoreceptors (which mediate negative feedback actions on histamine biosynthesis and release) and the Hic receptors (which are associated with the tissue growth-promoting actions of histamine).

Elevated tissue histamine levels have been demonstrated in involved skin of chronic urticaria.[8] The histamine-mediated erythema, local edema, and a surrounding axon reflex flare were described in the pioneering work of Lewis.[9] This three-part sequence of cutaneous changes has subsequently been called the "triple response of Lewis." The wheals of chronic "idiopathic" urticaria are unlikely to be due solely to histamine because the duration of the wheal is measured in hours rather than minutes. However, the itching of chronic idiopathic urticaria is largely histamine-mediated. The involvement of other mediators besides histamine in the vascular pathology of chronic urticaria is also suggested by the incomplete suppression of redness and wheals by orally administered H_1 antihistamines. Nevertheless, the itching is usually substantially relieved by H_1 antihistamines. Histamine also plays a role in urticarial vasculitis. Local histamine release from leukocytes and platelets increases the permeability of postcapillary venules, which in turn permits the extravasation of circulating immunoreactants leading to local complement activation. The cellular consequences include leukocyte diapedesis, chemotaxis and activation of neutrophils, and subsequent degranulation leading to vessel wall damage.

Attempts to lower tissue histamine levels by interference with histamine biosynthesis using histidine decarboxylase inhibitors have to date been unsuccessful. Likewise, pharmacologic attempts to prevent mast cell degranulation and suppress secretion of histamine and other mediators by mast cells have largely been unsuccessful.[10,11] Ketotifen allegedly is able to suppress histamine secretion through prevention of mast cell degranulation; however, the drug is probably ineffective in this regard.[12] Thus for amelioration of the clinical effects of histamine, reliance has to be placed on the H_1 antihistamines.

HISTORICAL OVERVIEW

The first generation of antihistamines were ethers based on the imidazole ring structure of histamine. The first clinically useful synthetic derivative was mepyramine (Neoantergan).[13,14] Its successor, diphenhydramine hydrochloride, was the first antihistamine formally investigated in North America.[15] In Britain, mepyramine and other antihistamine congeners were evaluated in a series of articles by Bain, Warin, and others.[16,17] Subsequently, drugs were developed and marketed with a variety of relatively minor refinements of these archetypal antihistamines, primarily based on modification of the side chain of the imidazole ring. No further major innovations emerged until attempts were made to alter the configuration of the imidazole ring structure itself.

It had long been recognized that the original first-generation antihistamines were ineffective in blocking histamine-evoked gastric acid secretion. Ash and Schild[18] were the first to provide experimental evidence for the existence of a second class of histamine receptors, named H_2 receptors. A new type of antihistamine, selective for H_2 receptors, was based on modification of the imidazole ring by Black and colleagues.[19] The first drug in this new class was cimetidine. Although H_2 receptors are known to be expressed by skin blood vessels,[20] H_2-receptor antagonists have proven disappointing in the treatment of chronic urticaria, either alone or in combination with H_1 antihistamines.[21] This clinical reality was particularly disappointing in view of the H_2 antihistamines being relative free from adverse effects typically associated with the H_1 antihistamines. Itching due to histamine is mediated by H_1 receptors (and not H_2-histamine receptors)[20] and is therefore unresponsive to H_2 antihistamines. However, the ability of H_2 antihistamines to block H_2-receptor–mediated down regulation of T-lymphocyte activation has encouraged use of these compounds as adjunctive therapy for chronic infections associated with impaired T-lymphocyte function, including chronic mucocutaneous candidiasis.[22]

The clinical value of the first-generation H_1 antihistamines is significantly limited by their adverse effects (sedation, weight gain, and atropine-like complications including dry mouth, blurred vision, constipation, and dysuria). The introduction of H_2 antihistamines markedly improved this adverse effect profile but were less effacious for cutaneous disorders than their predecessors.

The late 1980s through the 1990s brought on a new generation (second-generation) of H_1 antihistamines, with negligible propensity to induce drowsiness and other troublesome adverse effects of the first-generation H_1 antihistamines. These "low-sedation" antihistamines have greatly

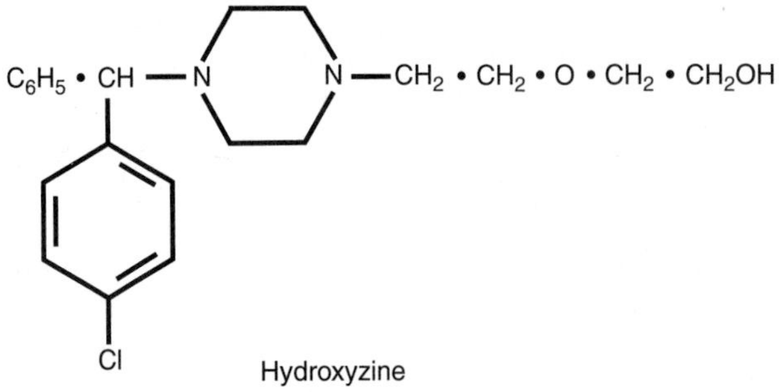

Hydroxyzine

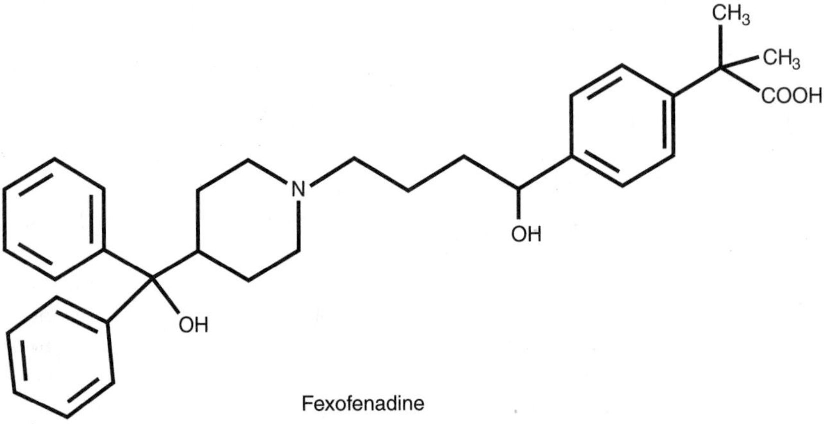

Fexofenadine

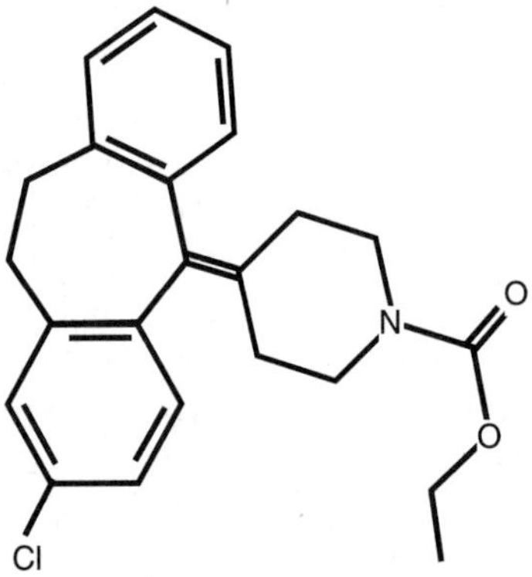

Loratadine

Figure 17-1 H_1 Antihistamines.

improved prospects for effective treatment of chronic urticaria, allergic conjunctivitis, and rhinitis.

The sedative action of first-generation H_1 antihistamines is related to the function of histamine as a neurotransmitter. At least three classes of histamine receptors (H_1, H_2, and H_3) have been identified in the central nervous system and are highly expressed in the cerebral cortex. They are thought to serve the level of arousal; hence traditional (first-generation) H_1 antihistamines reduce alertness and cause cognitive impairment. Some of these effects may also be attributable to atropine-like adverse effects.[23]

The selectivity of action for second-generation H_1 antihistamines determines their relative freedom from toxicity. In addition, these second-generation drugs show a low capacity to cross the blood-brain barrier, thus greatly reducing sedation and cognitive impairment. It is important to note that for certain dermatoses (such as atopic eczema), the sedative attributes of first-generation H_1 antihistamines may actually be beneficial. However, low-sedation antihistamines represent the preferred option for most cutaneous disorders due to improved safety margins and superior patient compliance.

Alternative pharmacologic approaches to drug therapy of histamine-mediated skin disorders have been explored. Sodium cromoglycate is effective in suppressing release of histamine from mast cells of lung, mucous membranes, and intestine. Unforunately this drug is largely inactive against skin mast cells.[10] Use of β-adrenergic agonists, with or without xanthine phosphodiesterase inhibitors,[11] has so far been clinically disappointing due to lack of specificity of action. Ketotifen, an H_1 antihistamine with the alleged additional capacity to suppress mast cell degranulation in the skin,[24] provides modest benefit to patients with urticaria pigmentosa.[25] In urticaria and urticaria pigmentosa, ketotifen does not significantly reduce urinary excretion of histamine and its metabolites. Attempts to lower tissue histamine levels by interference with histamine biosynthesis using histidine decarboxylase inhibitors have to date been unsuccessful.[12] Thus two generations of H_1 antihistamines remain the mainstay of therapy in most histamine-mediated disorders.

MAJOR GROUPS OF ANTIHISTAMINES
First-Generation Antihistamines
PHARMACOLOGY.　The structure of a representative H_1 antihistamine (hydroxyzine) is shown in Figure 17-1. H_1 antihistamines are competitive antagonists of histamine by binding to H_1 receptors, preventing histamine from combining with and activating these receptors. These drugs do not bind significantly to H_2 or H_3 receptors. This group comprises all H_1 antihistamines introduced before 1981. The first-generation H_1 antihistamines can be divided into five classes (Table 17-1). Further de-

■ **Table 17-1**　First-Generation H_1 Antihistamines— Major Categories and Representative Examples

Category	Representative Antihistamine
Ethanolamine	Diphenhydramine
Piperidine	Cyproheptadine
Phenothiazine	Promethazine
Alkylamine	Chlorpheniramine
Piperazine	Hydroxyzine

tails for available drugs in this group are listed in Table 17-2.

As a class, the first-generation H_1 antihistamines are lipophilic. In vitro these drugs may decrease mediator release from mast cells and basophils, although the concentrations required for this effect greatly exceed those achieved during therapeutic administration, and are independent of their H_1-antagonistic properties.[26]

Because of their lipophilicity, they generally readily cross the blood-brain barrier and cause significant sedation. They usually reach plasma peak concentrations in about 2 hours, and are substantially protein-bound. Metabolism occurs via the hepatic cytochrome P-450 (CYP) system. Thus in patients with liver disease, or in patients who are currently receiving CYP 3A4 inhibitors such as erythromycin or ketoconazole, the plasma half-life may be greatly prolonged.

The important pharmacologic features of five H_1 antihistamines, representative of the first-generation H_1 antihistamines as a class, are given in Table 17-3. All H_1 antagonists suppress the wheal and flare caused by intradermal histamine injection in a dose-related fashion. Evidence of suppression is manifest 1 to 2 hours after oral administration, and maximum wheal and flare suppression occurs later than the time to maximum plasma level. Thus oral antihistamine administered during or after the onset of an allergic response in the skin may be less effective than expected. These antihistamines should be

▌ Table 17-2　Antihistamines

FIRST-GENERATION SEDATING H$_1$ ANTIHISTAMINES

Generic Name	Trade Name	Generic Available	Manufacturer	Tablet/Capsule Sizes	Special Formulations	Adult Dosage Range	Price Index
Diphenhydramine	Benadryl*	Yes	WarnerWellcome, others	25, 50 mg (Chew Tabs 12.5 mg)	Elixir 12.5 mg/5 ml syrup 6.25 mg/5 ml	25-50 mg q6-8 hrs†	$ ($)
Cyproheptadine	Periactin	Yes	Merck, others	4 mg	2 mg/5 ml	4-8 mg q8-12 hrs	$ ($)
Promethazine	Phenergan	Yes	Wyeth-Ayerst, others	12.5, 25, 50 mg	6.25 and 25 mg/5 ml (also suppositories)	12.5-25 mg q6-8 hrs†	$ ($)
Chlorpheniramine	Chlor-Trimeton	Yes	Schering, others	4, 12 mg‡	None	4-8 mg bid†	($)
Hydroxyzine	Atarax, Vistaril*	Yes	Pfizer, others	10, 25, 50, 100 mg	Syrup 10 mg/5 ml susp. 25 mg/5 ml	12.5-25 mg q6-8 hrs†	$/$$ ($)

SECOND-GENERATION H$_1$ ANTIHISTAMINES (BOTH LOW-SEDATING AND NONSEDATING)

Loratadine	Claritin, Claritin D	Schering	No	10 mg	Syrup 5 mg/ 5 ml	10 mg qd (Claritin D 5 mg bid)	$$$
Cetirizine	Zyrtec	Pfizer	No	5, 10 mg	Syrup 5 mg/ 5 ml	10 mg qd	$$/$$$
Fexofenadine	Allegra, Allegra D	Aventis	No	60, 180 mg	None	60 mg bid, 180 mg qd (Allegra D 60 mg bid)	$$

TRICYCLIC ANTIHISTAMINE

Doxepin	Sinequan	Roerig, others	Yes	10, 25, 50, 75 mg	Liquid 10 mg/ml	10-75 mg qhs†	$ ($)

MAST CELL DEGRANULATION INHIBITOR

Cromolyn sodium	Gastrochrome	Medeva	No	200 mg	Inhaler	200 mg q6 hrs	$$

Note: The "D" with Claritin D and Allegra D represents the antihistamine/decongestant combination formulation of these drugs.
$, <1.00; $$, 1.01-2.00; $$$, 2.01-5.00; $$$$, 5.01-10.00; $$$$$, >10.00; ( ), generic price; /, two different price ranges from lower dose to higher dose examples of this drug; —, no price listed for this drug.
*Injectable formulations of this drug are available (Vistaril is the injectable form of hydroxyzine).
†In general with sedating first-generation antihistamines and doxepin—start with lower end of dosage range and slowly titrate to higher doses if necessary; always warn patient regarding potential sedation and its impact on driving, cognitive function.
‡Sustained-release formulation available in the 12 mg dosage of this product.

■ Table 17-3   Key Pharmacologic Concepts—Antihistamines

| Drug | Absorption and Bioavailability | | | Elimination | | |
	Peak Levels (hours)	Bioavail-able (%)	Protein Binding	Half-life (hours)	Metabolism	Excretion
FIRST-GENERATION SEDATING H_1 ANTIHISTAMINES						
Diphenhydramine	0.6-2.8	40%-60%	75%-81%	4	Significant hepatic metabolism	
Cyproheptadine	2-3	??	??	??	Extensive hepatic metabolism	
Promethazine	2-3	25%	??	10-14		
Chlorpheniramine	2.0-3.6	25%-57%	67%-73%	15-25		
Hydroxyzine	1.7-2.5	??	??	20	Acid metabolite is cetirizine	
SECOND-GENERATION H_1 ANTIHISTAMINES						
Fexofenadine	1-3	??	60%-70%	14.4	Excreted largely unchanged	80% in feces, 12% in urine
Loratadine	1-2.5	??*	97 (73%-77%)†	8-11	Active metabolite descarboethoxy-loratadine	Negligible urinary excretion
Cetirizine	0.5-1.5	??	93%	8.3	Minimal metabolism	Excreted largely unchanged in urine
TRICYCLIC ANTIHISTAMINES						
Doxepin	1-2	17%-37%	80%-84%	11-23	CYP 2D6, active metabolite is desmethyldoxepin	Not found in urine

Note: Multiple major sources of pharmacokinetic data present incomplete information regarding this group. Second-generation H_1 antihistamines data adapted from Simons FER, Simons KJ: *N Engl J Med* 330:1663-1670, 1994, and Paton DM, Webster DR: *Clin Pharmacokinet* 10(6):477-497, 1985.
*Extensive first pass hepatic metabolism.
†For the active metabolite of this drug.

given as a preventative, rather than on a "as required" basis.

Due to the persistence of the antihistamines at tissue sites despite apparent complete clearance from plasma, the therapeutic half-life in the skin is frequently considerably in excess of the plasma half-life. This may explain why many patients find that a single dose of an antihistamine with a short plasma half-life controls symptoms in a relatively sustained fashion.

CLINICAL USE.   The formulations and doses of the five representative first-generation anti-histamines are given in Table 17-2. The recognized adverse effects of the first-generation H_1 antihistamines are listed in Table 17-4. The reader is encouraged to consult antihistamine reviews listed in the Bibliography section for further information on clinical use of these first-generation H_1 antihistamines.

SPECIAL POINTS.   Cyproheptadine is claimed to have antiserotonin (5-hydroxytryptamine) as well as H_1 antihistaminic properties. It has been alleged to be the preferred antihistamine for cold urticaria and other physical urticarias, al-

■ **Table 17-4**   First-Generation H$_1$ Antihistamines Systemic Adverse Effects

Category	Adverse Effects
Central nervous system	Sedation
	Hyperexcitability*
	Impaired cognitive function
	Increased appetite
Gastrointestinal	Dry mouth
	Constipation
Genitourinary	Dysuria
	Erectile dysfunction
Cardiac	Tachycardia
	Dysrhythmias
Other	Blurred vision

*May occur with high doses in children.

though this specific benefit has never been substantiated. Cyproheptadine interferes with hypothalamic function, may cause increased appetite and weight gain, and may retard growth in children. These adverse effects may also occasionally occur with other H$_1$ antihistamines.

Second-Generation H$_1$ Antihistamines

The second-generation antihistamines, like their predecessors, are antagonists of histamine at H$_1$ receptors. They are normally competitive antagonists but may be noncompetitive at higher doses. The most important feature of this group is their high therapeutic index (ratio of the minimum toxic dose and the minimum therapeutic dose). They are, as a group, poorly lipophilic and do not readily traverse the blood-brain barrier, such that somnolence and cognitive impairment are less troublesome. Their actions are also highly selective, with little or no atropine-like activity.

Three second-generation antihistamines are currently available for clinical use—fexofenadine, loratadine, and cetirizine. These three drugs will be considered in significant detail. There will only be a brief discussion regarding terfenadine and astemizole, which have been withdrawn from the market in the United States due to serious drug interactions involving Q-T interval prolongation with resultant torsades de pointes.

Overall, the general pharmacologic characteristics of the second-generation H$_1$ antihistamines resemble those of the first generation.[26] However, important differences will be highlighted for each antihistamine individually. The formulations and dosages of three currently available second-generation antihistamines in the United States are listed in Table 17-2.

FEXOFENADINE
Pharmacology

Terfenadine is a prodrug that can cause serious cardiotoxicity. Terfenadine is transformed via the cytochrome P-450 system to its pharmacologically active acid metabolite, fexofenadine, which is a substituted benzene acetic acid (see Figure 17-1). Fexofenadine is not metabolized by the liver and is excreted essentially unchanged. Fexofenadine is readily absorbed by the oral route with peak plasma levels being achieved at 1 to 3 hours after administration. Eighty percent of a single dose is recovered unchanged in the feces and 12% is excreted in the urine. The elimination half-life is 11 to 15 hours.[27] Fexofenadine is a selective histamine H$_1$-receptor competitive antagonist with few or no sedative or anticholinergic adverse effects. Extensive studies in man and laboratory animals have failed to reveal evidence of cardiotoxicity for fexofenadine.

In a single dose of 40 mg or more, fexofenadine produces greater than 79% inhibition of a histamine wheal and flare response, lasting up to 12 hours.[28] There is no evidence of tolerance after repeated administration. Coadministration of fexofenadine with macrolide antibiotics and imidazole antifungals failed to reveal evidence of interactions, with no prolongation of the electrocardiographic Q-T interval (Table 17-5). Furthermore, there is no evidence of back metabolism of fexofenadine to the parent compound terfenadine (manufacturer's personal communication to author).

Clinical Use

INDICATIONS.   Currently fexofenadine is not licensed in the United States for any dermatologic indications. Present evidence indicates, however, that fexofenadine in an oral single dosage of 180 mg daily in adults is as effective as

■ **Table 17-5**   Antihistamine Drug Interactions

Interacting Drug	Examples and Comments
THESE DRUGS MAY INCREASE THE SERUM LEVELS OF ANTIHISTAMINES— POSSIBLE MAJOR CARDIOVASCULAR RISK	
Macrolide antibiotics	Erythromycin > clarithromycin (CYP 3A4 inhibitors) ↑ risk for torsades de pointes (especially with terfenadine or astemizole; possible risk loratadine*)
Azole antifungal agents	Ketoconazole >> itraconazole, ? fluconazole (CYP 3A4 inhibitors) ↑ risk for torsades de pointes (especially terfenadine or astemizole; possible risk loratadine)
HIV-1 protease inhibitors	Ritonavir, indinavir > saquinavir, nelfinavir (CYP 3A4 inhibitors) ↑ risk for torsades de pointes (especially with terfenadine or astemizole; possible risk loratadine)
SSRI antidepressants	All five members of this drug group have the potential to ↑ risk for torsades de pointes (especially with terfenadine or astemizole; possible risk loratadine)
Foods	Grapefruit juice contains a substance (CYP 3A4 inhibitor) that ↑ risk for torsades de pointes (especially with terfenadine or astemizole; possible risk loratadine)
H_2 antihistamines	Cimetidine is a relatively weak CYP 3A4 inhibitor, ↑ loratidine levels
Quinine	Increased levels of astemizole and its metabolites; uncertain mechanism
Zileuton	Increased levels of astemizole and its metabolites; uncertain mechanism
THESE DRUGS MAY INCREASE THE TOXICITY OF ANTIHISTAMINES (INDEPENDENT OF SERUM LEVELS)	
CNS depressants	Alcohol and other CNS depressants may produce an additive sedating effect when used in combination with first-generation H_1 antihistamines
MAO inhibitors	Various members of this group may prolong/intensify the sedating and anticholinergic effects (especially with first-generation antihistamines)

Adapted from *CliniSphere 2.0 CD ROM*, St. Louis, June 2000, Facts & Comparisons.
*Loratidine may prolong Q-T interval, although no risk of torsades de pointes has been documented.

terfenadine 60 mg twice daily in the treatment of chronic urticaria (manufacturer's data). However, the currently recommended dosage of fexofenadine is 60 mg twice daily. Present evidence also suggests that there is no need for dosage adjustment in the elderly or in patients with mild renal or hepatic impairment.

SUMMARY.   Fexofenadine is the pharmacologically active metabolite of the prodrug terfenadine. There is no evidence for cardiotoxicity of fexofenadine. However, the product has only recently been licensed in the United States (for nondermatologic indications) and in the United Kingdom. More clinical experience evaluating the safety and efficacy of long-term administration is required.

LORATADINE
Pharmacology
Loratadine is a piperidine tricyclic selective long-acting H_1 antihistamine with minimal sedative and anticholinergic adverse reactions with the recommended dosage. Loratadine undergoes rapid transformation in humans. The major metabolite, descarboethoxy-loratadine, is likewise biologically active. Maximum plasma levels are reached 1 to 1.5 hours (2.5 hours for the active metabolite) after administration with a mean elimination half-life of 8 to 11 hours for loratadine (17 hours for the active metabolite). Renal and hepatic impairment as well as old age appear to have no major influence on the drug pharmacokinetics.[29] However, a lower dosage is officially recommended for patients with

chronic renal or hepatic disease. After a single 10 mg dose, suppression of whealing due to intradermal histamine is detected for 12 hours. This suppression may last considerably longer after a larger dosage.[30] Tolerance to repeated doses does not appear to be a clinical problem.

Clinical Use

INDICATIONS.   Loratadine is administered as 10 mg capsules and syrup (1 mg/ml). "Reditabs" are available in a 10 mg tablet that rapidly disintegrates in the mouth. Loratadine is indicated for the treatment of chronic urticaria in adults. Several clinical trials[31,32] attest to the effectiveness of loratadine 10 mg daily in the treatment of chronic urticaria.

DRUG INTERACTIONS AND CONTRAINDICATIONS.   Loratadine has some effect on the function of myocardial potassium channels, but does not cause cardiac dysrhythmias.[33] Coadministration of drugs that interfere with CYP 3A4 inhibitors (e.g., macrolide antibiotics and azole antifungal agents such as ketoconazole and itraconazole) does not interact adversely with loratadine.

SUMMARY.   Loratadine is a long-acting, minimally sedating selective H_1 antihistamine. Although loratadine is not contraindicated in patients with chronic liver or renal disease, cautious administration of reduced dosage is advisable. There are no significant adverse drug interactions, and loratadine appears to be free of cardiotoxicity. The drug's main dermatologic indication is chronic urticaria.

CETIRIZINE
Pharmacology

Cetirizine is the carboxylic acid metabolite of the first-generation H_1 antihistamine hydroxyzine. This drug undergoes only minimal metabolic transformation in humans to an inactive metabolite and is primarily excreted unchanged in the urine. It is rapidly absorbed after oral administration. Maximum plasma levels are achieved in about 1 hour, and the plasma half-life is about 7 hours.[34] A single 10 mg oral dose causes significant histamine wheal suppression in 20 to 60 minutes and lasts for

24 hours.[35] Steady-state plasma levels are achieved after 3 consecutive days of treatment. There is little or no tolerance after repeated dosage. Minimal anticholinergic activity occurs after administration of the recommended dosage; however, 13.7% of patients noticed drowsiness after a 10 mg dose, compared with only 6.3% who received placebo. Plasma levels are higher in patients with chronic renal or liver disease. Although these higher plasma levels are of doubtful clinical significance, a reduced dosage (5 mg daily) is recommended in these patients.

In addition to the drug's H_1-histamine antagonistic activity, cetirizine appears to have an inhibitory action on eosinophil accumulation in tissues, including the skin. Administration of 10 mg cetirizine orally caused a significant reduction in migration of eosinophils in response to challenge by a specific antigen using a skin window technique.[36] Additionally, cetirizine causes inhibition of eosinophil chemotaxis in vitro.[37] The clinical inportance of these observations is unclear.

Clinical Use
INDICATIONS.   Cetirizine is licensed for the indication of chronic urticaria in the United States. Several studies support the effectiveness of cetirizine for this indication,[38,39] and it has also been found to be effective in cold urticaria. It is formulated as 10 mg tablets and a 1 mg/ml syrup. The recommended adult dose is 10 mg daily, although 5 mg daily is advised in patients with chronic renal or hepatic impairment.

DRUG INTERACTIONS AND CONTRAINDICATIONS.   No clinically significant drug interactions have been reported (see Table 17-5). As previously indicated, reduced dosage is recommended in patients with impaired liver and kidney function. No significant cardiac adverse effects have been reported to date.

SUMMARY.   Cetirizine is a long-acting, low-sedation H_1 antihistamine. Reduced dosage is recommended in patients with chronic hepatic or renal disease. There are no significant adverse drug interactions and there is no significant cardiotoxicity. The main dermatologic indication is chronic urticaria.

SECOND-GENERATION H₁ ANTIHISTAMINES— CURRENTLY NOT AVAILABLE FOR CLINICAL USE

To provide the reader with a broader historical perspective of the second-generation antihistamines, there will be a brief discussion on two H₁ antihistamines withdrawn from the market in the late 1990s due to cardiotoxicity. The importance of clinicians maximizing their understanding of drug interactions is illustrated by terfenadine and astemizole.

Terfenadine

A substituted piperidine derivative, terfenadine is a prodrug.[40] First pass metabolism results in extensive transformation via cytochrome P-450 isoforms to one of its two major metabolites, a carboxylic acid transformation product (fexofenadine). This active metabolite, fexofenadine, is responsible for terfenadine's clinical activity. Terfenadine has little or no action on cholinergic or histamine H₂ receptors and does not penetrate the blood-brain barrier.

Terfenadine (Seldane) was the first nonsedating H₁ antihistamine that received Food and Drug Administration (FDA) approval in the United States. The drug was widely used for chronic urticaria, with reasonable levels of success and excellent patient acceptance, due to the lack of sedation.

The downfall of terfenadine was the potentially serious drug interactions that related to the drug being a CYP 3A4 substrate (see Table 17-5). This enzyme is responsible for converting the prodrug (terfenadine) to the active form (fexofenadine). CYP 3A4 enzyme inhibitors, such as ketoconazole and erythromycin, led to inhibition of conversion to fexofenadine, with resultant sustained terfenadine levels leading to electrocardiographic Q-T interval prolongation and tachydysrhythmias due to the parent prodrug, terfenadine. Terfenadine was withdrawn from the market in the late 1990s after multiple reports of potentially fatal torsades de pointes.[41,42]

Astemizole

Although based structurally on the piperazine ring, astemizole does not fit into the traditional H₁-antihistamine subclasses. There have been several reviews of the drug's pharmacology.[43,44] Metabolism occurs by oxidative hydroxylation and glucuronidation, with the main metabolic product being desmethylastemizole. There is little evidence of sedation in response to doses ranging from 10 to 60 mg and the sedative actions of alcohol, and benzodiazepines are not potentiated. Anticholinergic adverse effects did not differ significantly from placebo.

Astemizole (Hismanal) was the second nonsedating H₁ antihistamine licensed for clinical use. The drug was approved in the United States and the United Kingdom for the indication of chronic urticaria.[45]

Astemizole is likewise a CYP 3A4 substrate, subject to drug interactions involving 3A4 inhibitors such as ketoconazole and erythromycin (see Table 17-5). As with terfenadine, astemizole was withdrawn from the market in the late 1990s due to relatively frequent reports of Q-T interval prolongation and resultant tachydysrhythmias associated with torsades de pointes.[42,46] The metabolite, desmethylastemizole, is believed to be central to the pathogenesis of these tachydysrhythmias.

H₁-ANTIHISTAMINE THERAPY— SPECIAL POINTS

H₁ Antihistamines in Pregnancy

No antihistamine is entirely safe for administration in pregnancy. However, antihistamines occasionally have to be prescribed and the risk-benefit balance must be considered for both mother and unborn child. It should be borne in mind that withdrawal of an effective antihistamine may have a negative overall impact on pregnancy in a woman with severe urticaria. In such a case, chlorpheniramine, which has been prescribed in the United Kingdom for 33 years, is considered to be unassociated with increased risk of fetal malformation.[47] Diphenhydramine (Benadryl) likewise has a relatively long track record of safety with use in pregnancy. With regard to the newer low-sedation antihistamines, data are inadequate to draw conclusions on safety in pregnancy. A prospective case-control study of 114 women, who took astemizole during the first trimester of pregnancy, and their offspring were compared with a similar group of untreated mothers. Two instances of fetal malformation occurred in both groups,[48] a frequency of 1.9%, which is well within the expected range of 1% to 3% in the general population.

Tolerance (Tachyphylaxis and Subsensitivity)

Development of tolerance after continued regular administration of H_1 antihistamines is frequently perceived as a problem by patients and physicians alike. However, clear evidence substantiating such tolerance is hard to come by, and recent reviews omitted mention of the problem. In a comparison of several antihistamines administered daily for 3 weeks, hydroxyzine (75 mg/day) proved to be the most effective in suppressing intracutaneously injected histamine wheals. In addition, hydroxyzine also showed the greatest degree of tolerance, not only to itself, but also to the other H_1 antihistamines.[49] In contrast, chlorpheniramine showed little or no tendency to produce subsensitivity. Whether any tolerance manifest after repeated antihistamine dosage occurs (1) at the receptor level, (2) to increased tissue clearance, (3) through induction of metabolic pathways, or (4) through alteration in protein binding is unclear. Some patients who develop a perceived "tolerance" to first-generation H_1 antihistamines have done so because of poor compliance due to adverse effects. The consequent intermittent dosage is less effective.

Topical Antihistamine Therapy

Doxepin is a tricyclic antidepressant drug with potent H_1- and H_2-antihistamine activity. It has proved useful when given systemically in the treatment of severe urticaria.[50-52] Recently doxepin has been formulated as a 5% cream with the indication of allaying pruritus in eczematous dermatitis.[53] Although effective, 5% doxepin cream may cause significant drowsiness due to percutaneous absorption. There is also concern about the risk of allergic contact dermatitis (dermatitis medicamentosa).[54] Topical doxepin should be used for 8 days at the most, according to the package insert. Doxepin should not be administered topically or systemically concurrently with terfenadine. Although other topical antihistamine preparations (such as those containing diphenhydramine) still survive as over-the-counter products on the pharmacist's shelves, they are of doubtful efficacy and constitute a significant risk for allergic contact dermatitis.

Therapy of Chronic Urticaria and Angioedema

Notwithstanding recent advances in understanding of the etiology, immunopathology, and molecular basis of some patients with chronic "idiopathic" urticaria, H_1 antihistamines remain the cornerstone of drug treatment. Whether or not patients with chronic urticaria can be shown to have anti-$Fc\varepsilon RI\alpha$ or anti-IgE functional autoantibodies, antihistamines are the preferred treatment. For patients with physical urticarias (e.g., symptomatic dermographism, delayed pressure urticaria, cholinergic urticaria, cold urticaria), there are few reasonable alternatives to antihistamine treatment. Angioedema is frequently associated with chronic idiopathic urticaria and with some physical urticarias. Angioedema usually responds adequately to H_1-antihistamine treatment. When mucocutaneous surfaces are involved, additional treatment by adrenaline or other adrenergic drugs (given locally or systemically) may be required.

Chronic urticaria is pruritic, and simple physical measures including cooling the skin by tepid showering and the use of cooling salves such as menthol 1% cream may be helpful. Avoiding factors that enhance pruritus (e.g., aspirin ingestion, alcohol consumption, wearing of tight elasticized apparel, or coarse woolen fabrics) is also important. In prescribing antihistamines, it is also important to take into account the times of the day when urticaria is most troublesome. Many patients in employment find pruritus to be most intense in the evenings after returning from work, such that administration of antihistamines should be timed accordingly. For patients with daytime and nighttime symptoms a sedative H_1 antihistamine at night, coupled with a low-sedation antihistamine in the morning, is a reasonable choice. A reasonable strategy would, for an average adult, be to prescribe loratadine 10 mg or fexofenadine 60 to 120 mg each morning together with hydroxyzine 25 mg at night. Some patients suffer considerable anxiety and depression associated with chronic urticaria and angioedema. In these circumstances, oral doxepin 25 to 75 mg each night may be a preferred substitute for hydroxyzine.

The initial dose should be 10 to 25 mg, gradually titrating up to the previously mentioned dosage range. With regard to the choice of low-sedation antihistamines for daytime use, the options are loratadine, cetirizine, and fexofenadine.

An urticaria self-assessment diary[55] may assist both patient and physician in optimization of an antihistamine combination regimen. Combination therapy with H_1 and H_2 antihistamines (e.g., cimetidine) is probably of only marginal value, although occasional patients are convinced of the added benefits of cimetidine.[21]

Bibliography

Genovese A, Spadaro G: Highlights in cardiovascular effects of histamine and H_1-receptor antagonists. *Allergy* 52(Suppl 34):67-78, 1997.

Goldsmith P, Dowd PM: The new H_1 antihistamines. Treatment of urticaria and other clinical problems. *Dermatol Clin* 11:87-95, 1993.

Gonzalez MA, Estes KS: Pharmacokinetic overview of second-generation H_1 antihistamines. *Int J Clin Pharmacol Ther* 36:292-300, 1998.

Greaves MW, Sabroe RA: Histamine: the quintessential mediator. *J Dermatol* 23:735-740, 1996.

Herman LE, Bernhard JD: Antihistamine update. *Dermatol Clin* 9:603-610, 1991.

Juhlin L: Nonclassical clinical indications for H_1-receptor antagonists in dermatology. *Allergy* 50:36-40, 1995.

Monroe EW: Nonsedating H_1 antihistamines in chronic urticaria. *Ann Allergy* 71:585-591, 1993.

Simons FER, Simons KJ: The pharmacology and use of H_1-receptor-antagonist drugs. *N Engl J Med* 330:1663-1670, 1994.

References

Importance of Histamine in Skin Disease

1. Francis DM, Thompson MF, Greaves MW: The kinetic properties and reaction mechanism of histamine methyltransferases from human skin. *J Biochem* 18:819-828, 1980.

2. Hill M, Francis DM, Grattan CE, et al: Auto antibodies against the high affinity IgE receptor as a cause for histamine release in chronic urticaria. *N Engl J Med* 328:1599-1604, 1993.

3. Fieiger E, Maurer D, Holub H: Serum IgG autoantibodies directed against the α-chain of Fcε RI a selective marker and pathogenetic factor for a distinct subset of chronic urticaria patients. *J Clin Invest* 96:2606-2612, 1995.

4. Niimi N, Francis DM, Kermani F, et al: Dermal mast cell activation by autoantibodies against the high affinity IgE receptor in chronic urticaria. *J Invest Dermatol* 106:1001-1006, 1996.

5. Greaves MW, Marks R, Robertson I: Receptors for histamine in human skin blood vessels in review. *Br J Dermatol* 97:225-228, 1997.

6. Bach J-F, Chatenoud L, Dy M: Lymphocytes and histamine—a new entry to immunoregulation. In Ganellin CR, Schwartz J-C, editors: *Frontiers in histamine research,* Oxford, 1985, Pergamon, pp 353-356.

7. Rocklin RE: Histamine induced cell response in normal and atopic subjects. In Ganellin CR, Schwartz J-C, editors: *Frontiers in histamine research,* Oxford, 1985, Pergamon, pp 357-364.

8. Kaplan AP, Horakova Z, Katz I: Assessment of tissue fluid histamine levels in patients with urticaria. *J Allergy Clin Immunol* 61:350-354, 1978.

9. Lewis T, editor: *The blood vessels of the human skin and their responses,* London, 1927, Shaw & Sons, p 288.

10. Pearce CA, Greaves MW, Plummer VM, et al: Effect of disodium cromoglycate on antigen—evoked histamine release from human skin. *Clin Exp Immunol* 17:437-440, 1974.

11. Keahey TM, Greaves MW: Cold urticaria: disassociation of cold evoked histamine release and urticaria following cold challenge. *Arch Dermatol* 116:174-177, 1980.

12. Mallet AI, Norris PR, Tendell NB, et al: The effect of disodium cromoglycate and ketotifen on the excretion of histamine and *N*-methyl imidazole acetic acid in urine of patient with mastocytosis. *Br J Clin Pharmacol* 27:88-91, 1989.

Historical Overview

13. Bovet D: Introduction to antihistamine agents and antergan derivatives. *Ann N Y Acad Sci* 50:1089-1126, 1950.

14. Lowe ER, Kaiser ME, Moore V: Synthetic benzhydryl alkamine ethers effective in preventing fatal experimental asthma in guinea pigs exposed to atomized histamine. *J Pharmacol Exp Ther* 83:120-129, 1945.

15. Curtis AC, Owens BB: β-Dimethylamino–ethyl benzhydryl ether hydrochloride (Benadryl) in the treatment of acute and chronic urticaria. *Univ Hosp Bull Ann Arbor* 11:25-26, 1945.

16. Bain WA, Hellier FF, Warin RP: Some aspects of the action of histamine antagonists. *Lancet* 11:964-969, 1948.

17. Bain WA, Broadbent JL, Warin RP: Comparison of anthisan (mepyramine maleate) and phenergan as histamine antagonists. *Lancet* 11:47-52, 1949.

18. Ash ASF, Schild HO: Receptors mediating some actions of histamine. *Br J Pharmacol* 27:427-439, 1966.

19. Black JW, Duncan WAD, Durant CJ, et al: Definition and antagonism of histamine H$_2$ receptors. *Nature* 236:385-390, 1972.

20. Greaves MW, Marks R, Robertson J: Receptors for histamine in human skin blood vessels: a review. *Br J Dermatol* 97:225-228, 1977.

21. Bleehen SS, Thomas SE, Greaves MW: Cimetidine and chlorpheniramine in the treatment of chronic idiopathic urticaria: a multicentre randomized double blind study. *Br J Dermatol* 117:81-88, 1987.

22. Rocklin RE: Modulation of cellular immune responses in vivo and in vitro by histamine receptor–bearing lymphocytes. *J Clin Invest* 57:1051-1058, 1976.

23. Gengo FM: Reduction of central nervous system adverse effects associated with antihistamines in the management of allergic disorders. *J Allergy Clin Immunol* 98:319-325, 1996.

24. Huston DP: Prevention of mast cell degranulation by ketotifen in patients with physical urticaria. *Ann Intern Med* 104:507-510, 1986.

25. Czarnetzki BM: A double-blind cross-over study of the effect of ketotifen in urticaria pigmentosa. *Dermatologica* 166:44-47, 1983.

Traditional H$_1$ Antihistamines

26. Simons FER, Simons KJ: Pharmacological use of H$_1$ receptor–antagonist drugs. *N Engl J Med* 330:1663-1670, 1994.

Nonsedating H$_1$ Antihistamines—Fexofenadine, Loratadine, and Cetirizine

27. Lippert C, Ling C, Brown P, et al: Mass balance and pharmacokinetics of fexofenadine HCl in healthy male volunteers. *Pharmaceut Res* 12(Suppl 9):F390, 1995.

28. Russell T, Stolz M, Eller M, et al: Acute and subchronic dose tolerance of fexofenadine HCl in healthy male subjects (Abs p 41). British Society of Allergy and Clinical Immunology meeting. Sept 1996.

29. Clissold SP, Sorkin EM, Goa KL: Loratadine, a preliminary review of its pharmacodynamic properties and therapeutic efficacy. *Drug Eval* 37:42-57, 1989.

30. Kassem N, Roman I, Gural R, et al: Effects of loratadine (SCH 29851) in suppression of histamine–induced skin wheals. *Ann Allergy* 60:505-507, 1988.

31. Bernstein IL, Bernstein DI: The efficiency and safety of loratadine in the management of chronic idiopathic urticaria. *J Allergy Clin Immunol* 81:211, 1988.

32. Palmeiri G, Savasta C, DeBartolo G, et al: Loratadine in the management of chronic idiopathic urticaria. *Acta Therapeut* 18:193-202, 1992.

33. Delpon E, Valenzuela C, Tamargo J: Blockade of cardiac potassium and other channels by antihistamines. *Drug Saf* 21(Suppl 1):11-18, 81-87, 1999.

34. Wood SG, John BA, Chasseaud LF, et al: The metabolism and pharmacokinetics of 14 C—cetirizine in humans. *Ann Allergy* 59:31-34, 1987.

35. Juhlin L, Devos C, Rihous J-P: Inhibiting effect of cetirizine on histamine induced and 48/80–induced wheals and flares, experimental dermagraphism and cold-induced urticaria. *J Allergy Clin Immunol* 80:599-602, 1987.

36. Michel L, DeVos C, Rihoux JP, et al: In-
    hibitory effect of oral cetirizine on in vivo
    antigen–induced histamine and PAF–acether
    release and eosinophil recruitment in human
    skin. *J Allergy Clin Immunol* 82:101-109,
    1988.
37. DeVos C, Joseph M, Leprevost C, et al: Inhi-
    bition of eosinophil chemotaxis by a new
    anti-allergic compound (cetirizine). *Int Arch
    Allergy Appl Immunol* 87:9-13, 1988.
38. Breneman D, Bronsky EA, Bruce S, et al: Cet-
    irizine and astemizole therapy for chronic
    idiopathic urticaria. A double blind placebo
    controlled comparative trial. *J Am Acad
    Dermatol* 33:192-198, 1995.
39. Alomar A, De la Cuadra J, Fernandez J: Ceti-
    rizine versus astemizole in the treatment of
    chronic idiopathic urticaria. *J Intern Med Res*
    18:358-365, 1990.

**Nonsedating H$_1$ Antihistamines—
Terfenadine and Astemizole**

40. Sorkin GM, Heel RC: Terfenadine: a review of
    its pharmacodynamic properties and thera-
    peutic efficiency. *Drugs* 29:34-56, 1985.
41. Woosley RL, Chen Y, Freeman JP, et al: Me-
    chanics of cardiotoxic effects of terfenadine.
    JAMA 269:1532-1536, 1993.
42. Genovese A, Spadaro G: Highlights in car-
    diovascular effects of histamine and H$_1$-re-
    ceptor antagonists. *Allergy* 52(Suppl 34):67-
    78, 1997.
43. Richards DM, Grogden RN, Heal RC, et al:
    Astemizole. A review of its pharmacody-
    namic properties and therapeutic efficacy.
    Drugs 28:38-61, 1984.
44. Anonymous. Astemizole—another non-se-
    dating antihistamine. *Med Lett Drugs Ther*
    31:43-44, 1989.
45. Kailasam V, Mathews KP: Controlled clinical
    assessment of astemizole in the treatment of
    chronic idiopathic urticaria and angioedema.
    J Am Acad Dermatol 16:797-804, 1987.

46. Sakemi H, VanNatta B: Torsade de pointes
    induced by astemizole in a patient with pro-
    longation of the QT interval. *Am Heart J*
    125:1436-1438, 1993.

Special Topics—Including Doxepin

47. Pratt W: Allergic diseases in pregnancy and
    breast feeding. *Ann Allergy* 47:355-361,
    1981.
48. Pastausak A, Schick B, D'Alimonte D, et al:
    The safety of astemizole in pregnancy. *J Al-
    lergy Clin Immunol* 98:748-750, 1996.
49. Long WF, Taylor RJ, Wagner CJ, et al: Skin
    test suppression by antihistamines and the
    development of subsensitivity. *J Allergy Clin
    Immunol* 76:113-117, 1985.
50. Goldsobel AB, Rohr AS, Siegel SC: Efficacy
    of doxepin in the treatment of chronic idio-
    pathic urticaria. *J Allergy Clin Immunol*
    78:867-873, 1986.
51. Greene SL, Reed CE, Schroeter AL: Double-
    blind crossover study comparing doxepin
    with diphenhydramine for the treatment of
    chronic urticaria. *J Am Acad Dermatol*
    12:669-675, 1985.
52. Sullivan TJ: Pharmacologic modulation of
    the whealing response to histamine in hu-
    man skin: identification of doxepin as a po-
    tent in vivo inhibitor. *J Allergy Clin Immunol*
    69:260-267, 1982.
53. Drake LA, Millikan LE: Antipruritic effect of
    doxepin 5% cream in patients with eczema-
    tous dermatitis. *Arch Dermatol* 131:1403-
    1408, 1995.
54. Shelley WB, Shelley E, Talanin NY: Self po-
    tentiating allergic contact dermatitis caused
    by doxepin hydrochloride cream. *J Am Acad
    Dermatol* 34:143-144, 1996.
55. Greaves MW: Antihistamine treatment: a pa-
    tient self-assessment method in chronic ur-
    ticaria. *BMJ* 283:1435-1437, 1981.

CHAPTER 18

Verity Blackwell
Pauline M. Dowd

Vasoactive and Antiplatelet Agents

PATHOPHYSIOLOGY

The cutaneous vasculature must both provide nutrients for the metabolism of the skin and control body temperature. To respond to changing requirements, vessels of the skin have a great capacity to moderate the flow of blood, ranging from 0.3 to 150 ml/100 mg/min. Blood flow through a vessel depends on the diameter of the tube and the viscosity of the blood (Poiseuille's law). Physiologic control depends largely on changes in vessel diameter. These variations are controlled by muscular elements in the arterial tree and by the contractile activity of pericytes and endothelial cells. Vascular tone is controlled by both nervous stimuli and local release of chemical mediators.

The cutaneous vasculature is innervated by both the somatic and autonomic nervous systems. The somatic nerves are unmyelinated C fibers or finely myelinated A-δ fibers. In peripheral vasculature, nonadrenergic, noncholinergic sensorimotor neurons are important in the skin's local vascular response to environmental temperature differences and chemical stimuli. Skin vasculature is capsaicin sensitive and has peptide neurotransmitters, largely calcitonin gene–related peptide (CGRP) and substance P (Table 18-1). The net result of these mediators is vasodilation,

which is endothelium dependent and mediated by nitric oxide (NO).[1] It has been shown that patients with Raynaud's phenomenon have a deficiency of perivascular CGRP-containing neurons.[2,3] Autonomic fibers have α_1 and α_2 receptor vasoconstrictor effects and there is evidence for β receptor–mediated vasodilation. However, in addition to responding to vasoactive stimuli, the vasculature also produces vasoactive mediators. This led to the concept of vascular tone being a function of control from without and within. A number of vasoactive mediators are released by the vessels themselves, including prostaglandin E_2 (PGE_2) and PGI_2, along with endothelium-derived relaxing factor (EDRF), which was recently identified as NO.[4] Diffusion of NO from endothelial cells results in vascular smooth muscle relaxation and hence vasodilation. Endothelium-dependent vasodilation also occurs in response to adenosine triphosphate (ATP), adenosine diphosphate (ADP), arachidonic acid, substance P, CGRP, 5-hydroxytryptamine (5-HT), bradykinin, histamine, neurotensin, vasopressin, angiotensin II, and thrombin, although the site of synthesis of many of these mediators is yet to be elucidated.[1] It has also been shown that endothelin-1 (ET-1), a potent vasoconstrictor, is synthesized by human cutaneous microvascular endothelial cells and has autocrine

■ **Table 18-1** Some Controls of Cutaneous Vasodilation and Vasoconstriction

Vasodilation	Vasoconstriction
EXOGENOUS FACTORS—SOURCES OTHER THAN ENDOTHELIAL CELLS	
Capsaicin*	α_1 adrenergic
CGRP*	α_2 adrenergic
Substance P*	
Histamine	
Bradykinin	
5-Hydroxytryptamine	
β_1 adrenergic	
ENDOGENOUS FACTORS—DERIVED FROM ENDOTHELIAL CELLS	
Prostaglandins—PGE_2 and PGI_2	Endothelin-1 (ET-1)
Endothelial-derived relaxation factor (same as NO)	

CGRP, Calcitonin gene–related peptide; NO, nitric oxide.
*Vasodilation induced by these mediators is mediated by NO.

Box 18-1

Vasoactive and Antiplatelet Agents

MAJOR DRUGS
Calcium channel blockers
   Nifedipine
   Diltiazem
   Amlodipine
Ketanserin
Aspirin
Dipyridamole
Pentoxifylline

ADDITIONAL DRUGS
NO donors
Iloprost (PGI_2 analog)
Minoxidil
Hexylnicotinate
CGRP
Tamoxifen

NO, Nitric oxide; CGRP, calcitonin gene–related peptide.

and paracrine activity.[5] It has been shown that ET-1 causes both direct vasoconstriction and a neurogenically mediated flare.[6]

Resting vascular tone is therefore thought to be a product of spontaneously released NO in opposition to ET-1 and α-adrenergic sympathetic activity. Thus under normal circumstances adjustments to blood flow in response to environmental changes are largely brought about by perivascular nerves, and endothelial cells respond to changes from within, as with hypoxia. Studies in blood flow in patients with primary Raynaud's phenomenon suggest impairment in neurogenic regulation of blood flow[2] and myogenic function.[7]

Changes in plasma viscosity are less often implicated in cutaneous vascular problems. Many factors are responsible for the viscosity of blood, including platelet function, clotting factors, and red cell concentration and flexibility. The viscosity of blood may vary widely under different physiologic and pathologic conditions, especially changes in plasma proteins or envi-

ronmental temperature. Cold may increase the viscosity of blood.

An intact vascular epithelium and continuous blood flow inhibit activation of clotting and platelets. The endothelium produces PGI_2, which inhibits platelet activation and is vasodilatory. Platelets do not bind to normal endothelial cells. Damage to vessel walls from either atheroslerosis or vasculitis associated with connective tissue disorders may pathologically initiate clotting. In addition, some acquired disorders of platelet function may present with cutaneous disease such as paraproteinemias and myeloproliferative diseases. Fibrinolytic therapy has been used for cutaneous vascular disorders and has largely concentrated on modifying the complex role played by platelets.

Box 18-1 lists vasoactive and antiplatelet agents.

CALCIUM CHANNEL BLOCKERS
Pharmacology
All calcium channel blockers are well absorbed orally. Bioavailability varies between drugs: 50% to 70% for nifedipine, 20% to 40% for diltiazem, and 50% to 88% for amlodipine. Peak

plasma levels after oral administration are reached at 30 minutes with diltiazem, 1 to 2 hours with nifedipine, and 7 to 8 hours with amlodipine. These drugs are largely protein bound. Nifedipine is principally excreted via the kidney (70% to 80%), whereas 60% to 65% of diltiazem is excreted via the feces after extensive deacetylation. The plasma half-life for nifedipine and diltiazem is 4 hours, whereas the plasma half-life of amlodipine is much greater at 35 hours after a single oral dose.

MECHANISM OF ACTION.   Calcium channel blockers prevent the transport of Ca^{++} across the plasma cell membrane of smooth muscle cells, which contain little stored intracellular Ca^{++} and thus inhibit excitation contraction coupling and muscle constriction. The drugs within this class have varying effects on atrioventricular (AV) conduction and heart rate. Verapamil is a strong depressor of AV conduction, is predominantly used for dysrhythmias, and hence is not indicated for cutaneous vascular diseases. Nifedipine has also been demonstrated to increase red cell deformability and to have synergistic platelet antiaggregation activity with prostacyclin in vitro.[8] In vivo, nifedipine has antiplatelet effects in patients with systemic sclerosis.[9]

Clinical Use

OFF-LABEL USES.   Box 18-2 lists drugs with established efficacy in treating Raynaud's phenomenon.

   Raynaud's Phenomenon and Chilblains. The agent of choice for peripheral vascular disorders is nifedipine; however, diltiazem and nicardipine have also been used successfully.[10] Verapamil has been shown to be ineffective.[11] Nifedipine has been shown in controlled double-blind studies to be effective in the treatment of primary and secondary Raynaud's phenomenon.[10-15] Nifedipine can be effective in the treatment of recalcitrant chilblains.[16]

   Diltiazem has also been shown to be effective in the treatment of primary and secondary Raynaud's phenomenon in randomized controlled trials.[17,18] Additionally, diltiazem has been effective in the treatment of occupational Raynaud's phenomenon (i.e., vibration white finger) in an open study.[19] A case report of a single patient with CREST syndrome suggested that diltiazem may reduce the progression of calcinosis.[20] Amlodipine may also be helpful in the treatment of Raynaud's phenomenon.[21]

Box 18-2

Drugs With Established Efficacy in Treating Raynaud's Phenomenon

> Calcium channel blockers
>   Nifedipine
>   Diltiazem
>   Amlodipine
> Ketanserin
> Pentoxifylline
> NO donors*
> Iloprost
> Hexylnicotinate*
> CGRP*

NO, Nitric oxide; *CGRP*, calcitonin gene–related peptide.
*Proprietary forms are not currently available.

ADVERSE EFFECTS.   Nifedipine's main action is vasodilation. Adverse effects are frequent; however, they rarely require cessation of therapy. Most of the adverse effects are due to vasodilation and include dizziness, headache, peripheral edema, nausea, and flushing. Few patients are troubled by symptomatic hypotension. Diltiazem and amlodipine have similar but less severe adverse effects.

THERAPEUTIC GUIDELINES.   Treatment with nifedipine can be initiated at 10 mg three times daily or 20 mg twice daily of sustained-release preparations. A reasonable maximum dose is 90 mg daily of a sustained-release form of nifedipine. The dose can be increased, titrating symptom control with side effects. High doses may be required for patients with severe peripheral vasospasm and are usually then well tolerated. Patients may vary their drug doses and many are able to stop therapy during the summer months. One study has suggested that 5 mg of nifedipine sublingually may be effective when used 15 to 30 minutes before predictable cold exposure.[22] Diltiazem treatment should be commenced at 60 mg three times daily, increasing to 120 mg three times daily if tolerated.

KETANSERIN
Pharmacology

Ketanserin is rapidly absorbed from the gastrointestinal tract but undergoes extensive first-pass metabolism with a bioavailability of 50%. This drug is largely bound to platelets in the circulation and has a half-life after a single oral dose of 10 to 18 hours. This half-life increases to between 19 and 29 hours after multiple doses.[23]

MECHANISM OF ACTION.
Ketanserin blocks serotonin (5-HT) inhibitors with a high affinity for peripheral serotonin-2 (5-HT2) receptors and thus inhibits 5-HT–induced vasoconstriction, bronchoconstriction, and platelet aggregation. In addition, it binds to histamine-1 receptors and dopamine receptors. It also binds to α-adrenergic receptors, which may result in vasodilation, although studies showed that this is unlikely to be the mechanism involved in digital vasodilation.[24] Ketanserin has been shown in some studies to inhibit platelet aggregation in patients with Raynaud's phenomenon. This appears to be short-lived because inhibition of platelet aggregation could not be demonstrated 12 hours after administration.[25]

Clinical Use

OFF-LABEL USES.
Ketanserin is used in the treatment of hypertension but has also been used in peripheral vascular disorders.

Raynaud's Phenomenon. Many studies have shown ketanserin to be of benefit in Raynaud's phenomenon. Open trials showed a decrease in the number and duration of attacks in patients with primary Raynaud's phenomenon,[26] and these findings have largely been confirmed by double-blind controlled studies.[27-30] Patients with secondary Raynaud's phenomenon have also been extensively investigated with similar results of decreased frequency and severity of attacks with oral ketanserin, with one study involving 222 patients from 10 countries.[29,31-33] One study of 9 patients with scleroderma, however, failed to show any benefit with ketanserin versus placebo.[34] Intravenous ketanserin has also been used in patients with primary and secondary Raynaud's phenomenon and has resulted in improved skin color and temperature and in healing of trophic changes.[35]

ADVERSE EFFECTS.
Ketanserin may cause sedation, dizziness, headache, dry mouth, and nausea. Profound hypotension has been reported in patients taking concomitant propranolol.

THERAPEUTIC GUIDELINES.
Ketanserin therapy may be started at 40 mg twice daily, although a number of studies used 40 mg three times daily. Experimental data suggest that this higher dose may be more effective.[32,36]

ASPIRIN
Pharmacology

Aspirin (acetylsalicylic acid) is rapidly absorbed from the stomach and small intestine and is widely distributed throughout the body. Peak plasma levels are reached after 2 hours and then slowly decline. The majority of salicylates (50% to 80%) are protein bound, largely to plasma albumin, and only the free drug is active. This occurs to a lesser extent for aspirin, although it may acetylate plasma albumin, which may change its antigenicity and may be responsible for aspirin hypersensitivity. Salicylates are metabolized by the liver, and the amount metabolized depends on the rate of urinary excretion, which depends on urinary pH (being greater in alkaline urine).

MECHANISM OF ACTION.
Low-dose aspirin acetylates platelet enzymes responsible for the synthesis of prostaglandins and thromboxane A_2 and as such inhibits the aggregation and activation of platelets, inflammation, and fever. Higher doses of aspirin inhibit synthesis of prostacyclin, an endogenous inhibitor of platelet aggregation produced by the vessel wall, and hence may lose the antiplatelet effect at these doses.

Clinical Use

OFF-LABEL USES.
Aspirin is used in greatest quantities for the prevention of stroke and transient ischemic attacks[37] but also has indications for some dermatoses.

Atrophie Blanche (Livedoid Vasculitis). Low-dose aspirin in combination with dipyridamole has been reported to improve atrophie blanche in two studies.[38,39] The aspirin dose should be no higher than 325 mg daily. Titrating with baby aspirin between one and four daily may be tried if one adult aspirin (325 mg) is not successful. A reduction of pain frequently precedes the ulcer healing; full reepithelialization of the ulcer may take up to several months.

Malignant Atrophic Papulosis (Degos' Disease).   Aspirin has been shown to be helpful in controlling cutaneous symptoms in patients with Degos' disease both alone and in combination with dipyridamole.[40,41] Many patients have various abnormalities in platelet aggregation. Tests reflecting this abnormal thrombosis may normalize with the aspirin therapy. Again, low-dose aspirin (325 mg or less), with or without dipyridamole, is the key to successful therapy of this condition.

Necrobiosis Lipoidica.   Seven diabetic patients with ulcerative necrobiosis lipoidica responded to treatment with aspirin and dipyridamole.[42] Elevated thromboxane levels may occur in these patients. Therapy with aspirin and dipyridamole may normalize these thromboxane abnormalities as the patient's ulcer heals.

Niacin-induced Cutaneous Changes.   Patients who receive nicotinic acid experience side effects of flushing and pruritus. A randomized, controlled trial showed that this may be suppressed by concomitant treatment with aspirin 325 mg daily.[43]

ADVERSE EFFECTS.   These include hypersensitivity reactions in susceptible patients (e.g., angioedema, urticaria, asthma, and rhinitis), exacerbation of asthma, and dyspepsia.

THERAPEUTIC GUIDELINES.   Aspirin should be used in low dose (75 mg daily) because as previously described, higher doses result in suppression of prostacyclin and reduce the antiplatelet benefits. Aspirin tablets crushed, dissolved in chloroform, and applied topically resulted in significantly reduced pain in patients with pain due to herpes zoster and postherpetic neuralgia.[44]

DIPYRIDAMOLE
Pharmacology
Dipyridamole is absorbed orally and reaches peak plasma levels after 75 minutes. The half-life is approximately 10 hours. Dipyridamole is largely bound to plasma proteins and metabolized in the liver to be excreted in the bile.

MECHANISM OF ACTION.   Dipyridamole inhibits platelet aggregation and in combination with aspirin prolongs the survival of platelets in thrombotic diseases. It is thought that this occurs via interaction with thromboxane A_2 and prostacyclin. The drug is also a vasodilator.

Clinical Use
OFF-LABEL USES.   Dipyridamole is used orally as an adjunct to oral anticoagulation for prophylaxis of thromboembolism associated with prosthetic heart valves. It has been used in combination with aspirin in a number of dermatologic conditions: Degos' disease,[40] necrobiosis lipoidica,[42] and atrophie blanche[39] (see previous section).

ADVERSE EFFECTS.   Dipyridamole can cause gastric upset, dizziness, headache, hypotension, tachycardia, and worsening of coronary heart disease. It is contraindicated after recent myocardial infarction and in rapidly worsening angina.

THERAPEUTIC GUIDELINES.   Dipyridamole should be given at a dose of 300 to 400 mg daily in three to four divided doses. Slow-release preparations also exist for twice daily dosage. There is a newly released formulation (Aggrenox) that combines low-dose aspirin with a sustained-release version of dipyridamole. Even though this new product has no official indications in dermatology, its use in those disorders for which aspirin and dipyridamole are used is reasonable.

PENTOXIFYLLINE
Pharmacology
Pentoxifylline is a methyl xanthine derivative. It is well absorbed orally but undergoes extensive first-pass metabolism in the liver before being excreted in the urine. Peak plasma levels occur within 2 hours, and the half-life is 4 to 6 hours.

MECHANISM OF ACTION.   Pentoxifylline increases erythrocyte and leukocyte deformability and inhibits neutrophil adhesion and activation. It also reduces platelet aggregation and activation.

Clinical Use

OFF-LABEL USES. Pentoxifylline has been used for many years for the treatment of intermittent claudication in patients with occlusive arterial disease.

Raynaud's Phenomenon. Pentoxifylline has been used successfully both as single-agent and combination therapy for the treatment of Raynaud's phenomenon.[29,45,46] These anecdotal reports typically use pentoxifylline at a dosage of 400 mg three to four times daily. A full therapeutic response may take up to several months.

Atrophie Blanche. Clinical improvement in atrophie blanche was observed in two small studies of 5 and 8 patients.[47,48] In one of these studies, patients who had this condition between 4 and 20 years received pentoxifylline therapy. Overall, 3 of 8 patients completely healed and 4 of 8 had marked improvement with therapy.

Necrobiosis Lipoidica. One patient with long-standing necrobiosis lipoidica diabeticorum responded well to pentoxifylline therapy.[49] In another case report, pentoxifylline 400 mg twice daily led to ulcer healing by 8 weeks in a patient whose ulcer had been refractory to a variety of therapies for 13 months before therapy.

ADVERSE EFFECTS. Pentoxifylline should be avoided in patients intolerant of methyl xanthine derivatives and should be used with caution in patients with severe cardiac disease. It may cause nausea, gastrointestinal disturbances, dizziness, and headache.

THERAPEUTIC GUIDELINES. The usual dose is 400 mg three to four times daily. The dose should be reduced in renal impairment. Most clinicians believe that it may take up to 2 to 4 months to obtain the maximal therapeutic benefit from pentoxifylline.

NITRIC OXIDE DONORS

NO has many properties. It is produced by the endothelium and induces vasodilation (see Pathophysiology section). It is produced by two isoforms of NO synthetase (NOS) enzyme; both use L-arginine as a substrate. NO can be induced by a number of factors including tumor necrosis factor (TNF)-α, interferon-λ, and IL-1, IL-2, and IL-6. Various treatments have been developed to increase the concentration of NO.

A topical acidified nitrite cream has been used in the treatment of tinea pedis.[51] A topical NO-generating system (5% sodium nitrite in K-Y jelly) was used in a randomized placebo crossover trial in patients with Raynaud's phenomenon and was shown to increase microcirculatory volume and flux.[52] Intraarterial infusions of L-arginine and sodium nitroprusside improved Raynaud's symptoms that were induced in a laboratory in patients with scleroderma.[53] This was not shown when oral L-arginine was used in patients with Raynaud's phenomenon.[54]

ILOPROST

Iloprost is a prostacyclin (PGI$_2$) analog and is a vasodilator (see Pathophysiology section). Iloprost has been used successfully as an intravenous infusion in the treatment of Raynaud's phenomenon. Twenty-five patients with Raynaud's phenomenon in association with systemic sclerosis were treated with iloprost; 88% showed objective improvement.[55]

Adverse effects are dose dependent and include flushing, headache, nausea, hypotension, and bradycardia. Epoprostenol is the formulation available in the United Kingdom and is actually licensed as an inhibitor of platelet aggregation in hemodialysis. An effective dose consists of 5- to 10-day infusions of 1 to 10 ng/kg/min for up to 8 hours daily (a total dose of 500,000 ng daily). The infusion rate is gradually increased every 30 minutes until the maximum dose is achieved.

MINOXIDIL

Minoxidil is a potent peripheral vasodilator of arterioles. Topical formulations of minoxidil are available (2% and 5%). There appears to be little systemic absorption from topical application.[56] Topical minoxidil can be prescribed for use in androgenic alopecia where the mechanism of action is not fully elucidated. Topical minoxidil 5% was used as a single application to the fingers of patients with primary Raynaud's phenomenon and did not appear to increase baseline digital blood flow and cold tolerance.[57]

HEXYLNICOTINATE

Hexylnicotinate has been shown to increase blood flow when applied topically in patients with Raynaud's phenomenon.[58] This preparation has been very useful in our patients who are unable to take or intolerant of oral vasodilators. It has also been used in patients with acrocyanosis and perniosis with good effect (PM Dowd—personal observation). A 2% cream should be applied three times daily in patients with Raynaud's phenomenon.

CALCITONIN GENE–RELATED PEPTIDE

CGRP is a potent endogenous vasodilator (see Pathophysiology section) and has been shown to cause peripheral vasodilation when given intravenously. Intravenous CGRP was given to patients with severe Raynaud's phenomenon in association with connective tissue diseases and increased acral blood flow and healing of digital ulcers.[59] (Human CGRP is unlicensed in the United Kingdom. It is manufactured by a company called Clinalfa in Switzerland and distributed in the United Kingdom by Calbiochem-Novabiochem.)

Patients report flushing, headache, and gastrointestinal disturbances. The regimen used is based on the study by Bunker and associates.[59] A total of 100 μg daily are given for 5 consecutive days. This dose is administered as an infusion at 0.6 μg/min for 3 hours daily.

TAMOXIFEN

Tamoxifen is an estrogen antagonist. It binds to peripheral estrogen receptors, and the tamoxifen receptor complex is translocated to the nucleus. This reduces the number of free estrogen receptors and also prevents the normal feedback inhibition control of estrogen synthesis by the hypothalamus and pituitary. After the oral administration peaks, concentrations of tamoxifen are found in the blood after 4 to 7 hours. Plasma clearance is biphasic and the terminal half-life may be as long as 7 days. It is extensively metabolized, undergoes enterohepatic circulation, and is excreted in the feces. Patients with anorexia accompanied by acrocyanosis and perniosis intolerant of other treatments responded to low-dose (5 mg daily) tamoxifen (PM Dowd—unpublished data).

The most frequent adverse effects include hot flashes, nausea, and vomiting. Excessive enlargement of the ovaries has been seen in premenopausal patients treated with high doses (100 to 200 mg daily). There is an increased incidence of endometrial changes, including hyperplasia, polyps, and carcinoma.

Bibliography

Burnstock G: Integration of factors controlling vascular tone. Overview. *Anesthesiology* 79:1368-1380, 1993.

Dowd PM: The treatment of Raynaud's phenomenon. *Br J Dermatol* 114:527-533, 1986.

Ely H: Pentoxifylline therapy in dermatology. *Dermatol Clin* 6:585-608, 1988.

Ho M, Belch JJ: Raynaud's phenomenon: state of the art. *Scand J Rheumatol* 27:319-322, 1998.

Pope J, Fenlon D, Thompson A, et al: Ketanserin for Raynaud's phenomenon in progressive systemic sclerosis. *Cochrane Database Systems Review* 2:CD000954, 2000.

Sacco RL, Elkind MS: Update on antiplatelet therapy for stroke prevention. *Arch Intern Med* 160:1579-1582, 2000.

References

Pathophysiology

1. Burnstock G: Integration of factors controlling vascular tone. Overview. *Anesthesiology* 79:1368-1380, 1993.
2. Bunker CB, Terenghi G, Springall DR, et al: Deficiency of calcitonin gene-related peptide in Raynaud's phenomenon. *Lancet* 336:1530-1533, 1990.
3. Goldsmith PC, Molina FA, Bunker CB, et al: Cutaneous nerve fibre depletion in vibration white finger. *J R Soc Med* 87:377-381, 1994.
4. Palmer RMJ, Ferrige AG, Moncada S: Nitric oxide release accounts for the biological activity of endothelium-derived relaxing factor. *Nature* 327:524-526, 1987.
5. Bull HA, Bunker CB, Terenghi G, et al: Endothelin-1 in human skin: immunolocalization, receptor binding MRNA expression and effects on microvascular endothelial cells. *J Invest Dermatol* 97:618-623, 1991.
6. Bunker CB, Coulson ML, Hayes NA, et al: Further studies on the actions of endothelin-1 on blood flow in human skin. *Br J Dermatol* 127:85-90, 1992.
7. Stefanovska A, Leger P, Bracic T, et al: Linear and non-linear analysis of blood flow in healthy subjects and in subjects with Raynaud's phenomenon. *Technol Health Care* 7:225-241, 1999.

Calcium Channel Blockers

8. Onada JM, Sloan BF, Honn KV: Antithrombogenic effects of calcium channel blockers: synergism with prostacyclin and thromboxane synthetase inhibitors. *Throm Res* 34:367-378, 1984.
9. Rademaker M, Meyrick Thomas RH, Kirby JD, et al: The anti-platelet effect of nifedipine in patients with systemic sclerosis. *Clin Exp Rheumatol* 10:57-62, 1992
10. Dowd PM: The treatment of Raynaud's phenomenon. *Br J Dermatol* 114:527-533, 1986.
11. Smith CR, Rodeheffer RJ: Treatment of Raynaud's phenomenon with calcium channel blockers. *Am J Med* 78(2B):39-42, 1985.
12. Belch JJ, Ho M: Pharmacotherapy of Raynaud's phenomenon. *Drugs* 52:682-695, 1996.
13. Ho M, Belch JJ: Raynaud's phenomenon: state of the art. *Scand J Rheumatol* 27:319-322, 1998.

14. Sturgill MG, Seibold JR: Rational use of calcium-channel antagonists in Raynaud's phenomenon. *Curr Opin Rheumatol* 10:584-588, 1998.
15. Anonymous: Comparison of sustained-release nifedipine and temperature biofeedback for treatment of primary Raynaud's phenomenon. Results from a randomized clinical trial with 1-year follow up. *Arch Intern Med* 160:1101-1108, 2000.
16. Rustin MHA, Newton JA, Smith NP, et al: The treatment of chilblains with nifedipine: The results of a pilot study, a double-blind placebo-controlled randomized study and a long term open trial. *Br J Dermatol* 120:267-275, 1989.
17. Kahan A, Amor B, Menkes CJ: A randomized double-blind trial of diltiazem in the treatment of Raynaud's phenomenon. *Ann Rheum Dis* 44:30-33, 1985.
18. Rhedda A, McCans J, Willan AR, et al: A double blind placebo controlled crossover randomized trial of diltiazem in Raynaud's phenomenon. *J Rheumatol* 12:724-727, 1985.
19. Matoba T, Ciba M: Effects of diltiazem on occupational Raynaud's syndrome (vibration disease). *Angiology* 36:850-856, 1985.
20. Farah MJ, Palmieri GM, Sebes JI, et al: The effect of diltiazem on calcinosis in a patient with the CREST syndrome. *Arthritis Rheum* 33:1287-1293, 1990.
21. La Civita L, Pitaro N, Rossi M, et al: Amlodipine in the treatment of Raynaud's phenomenon. *Br J Rheumatol* 32:524-525, 1993.
22. Weber A, Bounameaux H: Effects of low-dose nifedipine on a cold provocation test in patients with Raynaud's disease. *J Cardiovasc Pharmacol* 15:853-855, 1990.

Ketanserin

23. Robertson JI: Serotonergic type-2 (5-HT2) antagonists: a novel class of cardiovascular drugs. *J Cardiovasc Pharmacol* 17(Suppl 5): S48-53, 1991.
24. Brouwer RM, Wenting GJ, Schalekamp MA: Acute effects and mechanism of action of ketanserin in patients with Raynaud's phenomenon. *J Cardiovasc Pharmacol* 15:868-876, 1990.

25. Marasini B, Biondi ML, Mollica R: Effect of chronic ketanserin treatment on serotonin-induced platelet aggregation in patients with Raynaud's phenomenon. *Eur J Pharmacol* 39:289-290, 1990.

26. Arioso E, Montesi G, Zannoni M, et al: Efficacy of ketanserin in the therapy of Raynaud's phenomenon: thermometric data. *Angiology* 42:408-413, 1991.

27. Van de Wal HJ, Wijn PF, van Lier HJ, et al: The effectiveness of ketanserin in patients with primary Raynaud's phenomenon. A randomized, double-blind, placebo controlled study. *Int Angiol* 6:313-333, 1987.

28. Marasini B, Biondi ML, Bianchi E, et al: Ketanserin treatment and serotonin in patients with primary and secondary Raynaud's phenomenon. *Eur J Clin Pharmacol* 35:419-421, 1988.

29. Arioso E, Montesi G, Zannoni M, et al: Comparative efficacy of ketanserin and pentoxifylline in treatment of Raynaud's phenomenon. *Angiology* 40:633-638, 1989.

30. Tooke JE, Williams SA, Rawlinson DW, et al: Ketanserin and capillary flow in Raynaud's phenomenon. *Int J Microcirc Clin Exp* 9:249-255, 1990.

31. Arneklo-Nobin B, Elmer O, Akesson A: Effect of long term ketanserin treatment on 5-HT levels, platelet aggregation and peripheral circulation in patients with Raynaud's phenomenon. A double-blind, placebo-controlled cross-over study. *Int Angiol* 7:19-25, 1988.

32. Coffman JD, Clement DL, Greager MA, et al: International study of ketanserin in Raynaud's phenomenon. *Am J Med* 87:264-268, 1989.

33. Pope J, Fenlon D, Thompson A, et al: Ketanserin for Raynaud's phenomenon in progressive systemic sclerosis. *Cochrane Database Systems Review* 2:CD000954, 2000.

34. Engelhart M: Ketanserin in the treatment of Raynaud's phenomenon associated with generalized scleroderma. *Br J Dermatol* 119:751-754, 1988.

35. Caputi CA, De Carolis G, Tomasetti C: Regional intravenous ketanserin and guanethidine therapy in Raynaud's phenomenon. *Angiology* 42:473-480, 1991.

36. Marasini B, Bassani C: Digital blood flow and 5-hydroxytryptamine receptor blockade after ketanserin in patients with Raynaud's phenomenon. *Br J Pharmacol* 30:847-851, 1990.

Aspirin and Dipyridamole

37. Sacco RL, Elkind MS: Update on antiplatelet therapy for stroke prevention. *Arch Intern Med* 160:1579-1582, 2000.

38. Drucker CR, Duncan WC: Anti-platelet therapy in atrophie blanche and livedo vasculitis. *J Am Acad Dermatol* 7:359-363, 1982.

39. Kern AB: Atrophie blanche. Report of two patients treated with aspirin and dipyridamole. *J Am Acad Dermatol* 6:1048-1053, 1982.

40. Stahl D, Thomsen K, Hou-Jensen K: Malignant atrophic papulosis: treatment with aspirin and dipyridamole. *Arch Dermatol* 114:1687-1689, 1978.

41. Farrell AM, Moss J, Costello C, et al: Benign cutaneous Degos' disease. *Br J Dermatol* 139:708-712, 1998.

42. Heng MC, Song MK, Heng MK: Healing of necrobiotic ulcers with antiplatelet therapy. Correlation with plasma thromboxane levels. *Int J Dermatol* 28:195-197, 1989.

43. Jungnickel PW, Maloley PA, Vander Tiun EL, et al: Effect of two aspirin pre-treatment regimens on niacin-induced cutaneous reactions. *J Gen Intern Med* 12:591-596, 1997.

44. King RB: Topical aspirin in chloroform and the relief of pain due to herpes zoster and post herpetic neuralgia. *Arch Neurol* 50:1046-1053, 1993.

Pentoxifylline

45. Goldberg J: Successful treatment of Raynaud's phenomenon with pentoxifylline. *Arthritis Rheum* 29:1055-1056, 1980.

46. Ely H: Pentoxifylline therapy in dermatology. *Dermatol Clin* 6:585-608, 1988.

47. Sauer GC: Pentoxifylline (Trental) therapy for vasculitis of atrophie blanche (letter). *Arch Dermatol* 122:380-381, 1986.

48. Sams WM Jr: Livedo vasculitis. *Arch Dermatol* 124:684-687, 1988.

49. Littler CM, Tschen EH: Pentoxifylline for necrobiosis lipoidica diabeticorum. *J Am Acad Dermatol* 17:314-316, 1987.

50. Noz KC, Korstanje MJ, Vermeer BJ: Ulcerating necrobiosis lipoidica effectively treated with pentoxifylline. *Clin Exp Dermatol* 18:78-79, 1993.

Other Drugs

51. Weller R, Ormerod AD, Hobson RP, et al: A randomized trial of acidified nitrite cream in the treatment of tinea pedis. *J Am Acad Dermatol* 38:559-563, 1998.

52. Tucker AT, Pearson RM, Cooke ED, et al: Effect of nitric oxide generating system on microcirculatory blood flow in skin of patients with severe Raynaud's phenomenon: a randomized trial. *Lancet* 13;354(9191):1670-1675, 1999.

53. Freedman RR, Grigis R, Mayes MD: Acute effect of nitric oxide on Raynaud's phenomenon in scleroderma. *Lancet* 354:739, 1999.

54. Khan F, Litchfield SJ, McLaren M, et al: Oral L-arginine supplementation and cutaneous vascular responses in patients with primary Raynaud's phenomenon. *Arthritis Rheum* 40:352-357, 1997.

55. Dowd PM, Martin MFR, Cooke ED, et al: Treatment of Raynaud's phenomenon by intravenous infusion of prostacyclin (PGI$_2$). *Br J Dermatol* 106:81-89, 1982.

56. Franz TJ: Percutaneous absorption of minoxidil in man. *Arch Dermatol* 121:203, 1985.

57. Whitmore SE, Wigley FM, Wise RA: Acute effect of topical minoxidil on digital blood flow in patients with Raynaud's phenomenon. *J Rheumatol* 22:50-54, 1995.

58. Bunker CB, Reavley C, O'Shaughnessey D, et al: Intravenous calcitonin gene-related peptide in severe Raynaud's phenomenon. *Lancet* 342:80-83, 1993.

59. Bunker CB, Lanigan S, Rustin MH, et al: The effects of topically applied hexyl nicotinate lotion on the cutaneous blood flow in patients with Raynaud's phenomenon. *Br J Dermatol* 119:771-776, 1988.

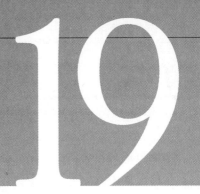

CHAPTER 19

Marty E. Sawaya

Antiandrogens and Androgen Inhibitors

Historically, the term *antiandrogen* has been used for "compounds that block the synthesis or action of androgens."[1] Most, if not all such agents have been androgen receptor (AR) blocking agents, hence the term *antiandrogens*.

More recently, drugs that inhibit the biologic effect of androgens by mechanisms other than AR blockade have emerged. These drugs include finasteride and GI 198745 (which are 5α-reductase inhibitors), as well as leuprolide, which is a gonadotropin-releasing hormone (GnRH) agonist. Leuprolide works at the level of the ovary and pituitary. Many experts prefer to designate these newer drugs as "androgen inhibitors," because they have no direct effect in blocking or binding to the AR. In this chapter, *antiandrogens* is the term utilized for AR inhibitors, with *androgen inhibitors* the standard term for all other modes of action.[2] The 5α-reductase inhibitors, such as finasteride (Box 19-1), are most important to dermatology.

Androgens have a profound influence in cutaneous structures such as hair follicles and sebaceous glands. Androgens, such as testosterone and dihydrotestosterone (DHT), are the biologically active androgens at various target tissues such as the pilosebaceous unit. Testosterone and DHT have a central role in the pathogenesis of androgenetic alopecia (AGA), acne vulgaris, and hirsutism. Antiandrogens, such as

spironolactone, flutamide, and cyproterone acetate, are not Food and Drug Administration (FDA)–approved for these indications, although various clinical studies provide data that support the use of these drugs for selected patients with the aforementioned disorders of androgen excess.

In contrast, the androgen inhibitor finasteride (Propecia, 1 mg) has FDA approval for men with AGA. Another 5α-reductase inhibitor designated as GI 198745 is now in clinical trial testing for use in AGA.

This chapter provides an overview of how various antiandrogens and androgen inhibitors work, their approved and off-label indications, dosing, and adverse effects. Particular emphasis is given to spironolactone and finasteride, with a lesser emphasis on the other drugs listed in Box 19-1.

PHYSIOLOGIC ROLE OF ANDROGENS
Males
Androgens have different biologic effects at different stages of life. In embryonic life, virilization of the urogenital tract occurs between 8 and 12 weeks in the male embryo, at which time androgens are essential for the development of the male phenotype.[3] Developmental influence of androgens may also involve the central nervous

Box 19-1

A List of Antiandrogens and Androgen Inhibitors

ANTIANDROGENS
Spironolactone*
Flutamide
Progesterone
Cyproterone acetate
Cimetidine

ANDROGEN INHIBITORS
Finasteride*
Ketoconazole
Oral contraceptives
Leuprolide
Nafarelin
GI 198745†
Saw Palmetto Plus‡

*Drugs of greatest current practical importance in the chapter.
†Investigational drug—currently not available for prescription use.
‡Herbal remedy discussed in chapter due to product's recent "publicity."

system. Before puberty, minimal androgen secretion from the testis and adrenal cortex suppresses secretion of gonadotropins. At puberty, the gonadotropins becomes less sensitive to feedback inhibition and the testes start to enlarge.[4,5] Thereafter the penis and scrotum enlarge and pubic hair appears. Growth-promoting properties of androgens cause an increase in height and the development of a more masculine skeletal musculature, which increases overall body weight.

When androgen secretion increases at puberty, the skin becomes thicker and more oily due to the proliferation of sebaceous glands. As this proliferation occurs, the pilosebaceous units can become prone to follicular plugging and bacterial colonization, increasing the likelihood of acne vulgaris. Subcutaneous fat is reduced, and veins become more prominent. Axillary hair grows, and hair on the trunk and limbs develops into a pattern typical of a man. Voice changes occur due to growth of the larynx. Increased growth of beard and body hair, due to the conversion of vellus to terminal hairs, occurs later as a secondary sex characteristic. Those males who inherit the genes for AGA may start to show signs of recession of the frontal hairline and ver-

tex areas of scalp later in puberty.[2] The last spurt of growth comes to an end in later puberty as the epiphyses of the larger long bones begin to close.[1]

In adult men, production of testosterone by the adrenal cortex alone is not sufficient to maintain spermatogenesis or secondary sex characteristics. In certain adrenal conditions, such as adrenal tumors or congenital adrenal hyperplasia, the adrenal cortex can secrete large quantities of androstenedione. Testosterone can be formed from this androgen precursor in extraglandular locations, including cutaneous sites.[1]

Females

The ovary and the adrenal cortex are the primary sources of testosterone and other androgens in women. Androstenedione and dehydroepiandrosterone (DHEA) are likewise produced by the ovary and adrenal gland and can be converted either to more potent androgens (e.g., testosterone) or to estrogens in peripheral organs and skin[2] (Figure 19-1). The average daily rate of testosterone production in women is approximately 0.25 mg. About one half of this daily output of testosterone is derived from the metabolic conversion of androstenedione to testosterone at extraglandular sites, including skin.[1,2]

Fluctuations in plasma concentrations of testosterone and androstenedione occur during the menstrual cycle.[1] The concentration of testosterone in the plasma of women ranges from 15 to 65 ng/dl (0.5 to 2.3 nM). Two peaks of androgen concentration parallel the peaks of plasma estrogens at the preovulatory and luteal phases of the menstrual cycle.[6] In certain ovarian disorders, such as polycystic ovary syndrome, increased quantities of androgens are secreted by the ovary, resulting in signs of cutaneous virilization such as scalp hair loss, acne, and hirsutism.[7]

Mechanism of Action

To understand the role of antiandrogens and androgen inhibitors in cutaneous disease, it is important to understand the mechanism of androgen actions and how antiandrogens and androgen inhibitors work to inhibit various androgen actions.[2]

At the pilosebaceous unit and the prostate, testosterone has minimal biologic activity un-

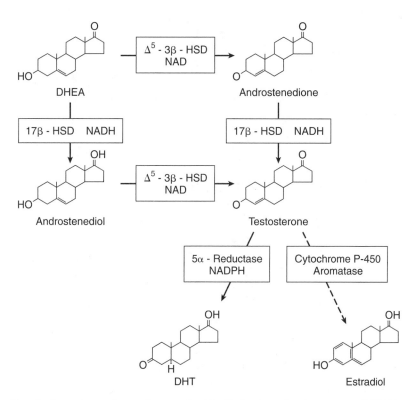

Figure 19-1 Metabolic pathway for androgens in skin. Dehydroepiandrosterone (DHEA) converts to potent androgens, such as testosterone and dihydrotestosterone (DHT), via the 3β- and 17β-hydroxysteroid dehydrogenase enzymes and 5α-reductase, as well as the conversion of androgens to estrogens, via cytochrome P-450. Aromatase enzyme converts testosterone to estradiol and also may have androstenedione as a substrate.

til it is converted to DHT by the enzyme 5α-reductase. There are two isoenzyme forms of 5α-reductase: type I and type II. The biochemical characteristics, amino acid sequence, enzyme distribution, and amounts of these two isoenzyme forms vary.[1,8-10] Type I 5α-reductase is located largely in nongenital skin primarily sebaceous glands lobules, hair follicles, and other organs such as the liver, spleen, and kidney. Type II 5α-reductase is located in hair follicles on top of the scalp from frontal scalp to vertex. In addition, this isoenzyme is largely found in sebaceous gland ducts, genital skin of both men and women, and the urogenital tract of men (especially prostate, seminal vesicles, and epididymis).

Both testosterone and DHT bind to a specific intracellular receptor, the AR. This hormone-receptor complex subsequently binds to specific nuclear hormone regulatory elements in DNA and acts to increase or decrease the synthesis of specific mRNAs and resultant proteins. The human AR is a member of the steroid and

Box 19-2

Disorders With Androgen Excess in Varying Percentages of Patients

> Acne vulgaris
> Androgenetic alopecia (AGA)
>   Female pattern
>   Male pattern
> Hirsutism
> Hidradenitis suppurativa

thyroid hormone receptor superfamily. The AR is encoded by a gene on the X chromosome and contains androgen binding, DNA binding, and functional domains.[1]

The net biologic effect of testosterone and DHT is to promote virilization of the male. Clinical conditions such as AGA, hirsutism, and acne can be induced by systemic or local abnormalities of androgens (Box 19-2). The patho-

Table 19-1 Antiandrogens and Androgen Inhibitors*

Generic Name	Trade Name	Generic Available	Manufacturer	Tablet/ Capsule Sizes	Special Formulations	Standard Dosage Range	Price Index
ANTIANDROGENS							
Spironolactone	Aldactone	Yes	Searle	25, 50† mg	Topical‡	100-200 mg/d (bid)	$ ($)
Flutamide	Eulexin	No	Schering	250 mg	Topical‡	125-250 mg bid	$$$
Medroxyprogesterone acetate	Provera	Yes	Various	2.5, 5, 10 mg	Topical‡	Not established	—
Cimetidine	Tagamet	Yes	SK Beecham	100, 200, 300, 400, 800 mg	Oral solution	400 mg bid-qid	$/$$ ($/$$)
ANDROGEN INHIBITORS							
Finasteride	Propecia Proscar	No	Merck	1 mg 5 mg	None	1 mg qd (for AGA)	$$

$, <1.00; $$, 1.01-2.00; $$$, 2.01-5.00; $$$$, 5.01-10.00; $$$$$, >10.00; ( ), generic price; /, two different price ranges from lower dose to higher dose examples of this drug; —, no price listed for this drug.

*The drugs listed in this table are those products that have specific oral proprietary formulations available in the United States.

†The 50-mg formulation is only available as the trade name product Aldactone.

‡Topical formulations have been studied in clinical research settings; aside from progesterone gel, no topical proprietary formulations are available.

genesis of various disorders of androgen excess can be either increased circulating androgen levels or abnormal/increased androgen activity at cutaneous sites, due to either 5α-reductase or AR abnormalities. Antiandrogens and androgen inhibitors can be utilized to reverse the biologic effects androgens at the cutaneous level (Table 19-1).

ANTIANDROGENS
Spironolactone
PHARMACOLOGY.　Table 19-2 lists key pharmacologic concepts for antiandrogens and an-

drogen inhibitors. Spironolactone is an aldosterone antagonist that acts as a relatively weak antiandrogen, working both by blocking the AR and by inhibiting androgen biosynthesis. Spironolactone may be converted to other active metabolites via progesterone 17-hydroxylase, which reversibly inhibits adrenal and ovarian cytochrome P-450 enzymes, with the net result of decreased testosterone and DHT production. The progestational activity of spironolactone is variable. The drug influences the ratio of luteinizing hormone (LH) to follicle-stimulating hormone (FSH) by decreasing the response of LH to GnRH.[11,12]

■ **Table 19-2**　Key Pharmacologic Concepts—Antiandrogens and Androgen Inhibitors

Drug	Absorption and Bioavailability			Elimination		
	Peak Levels	Bioavailable (%)	Protein Binding	Half-life	Metabolism	Excretion
ANTIANDROGENS						
Spironolactone	2-4 hrs*	>90%	98%*	10-35 hrs* (19.4 hrs avg.)	Canrenone is the active metabolite	Predominantly hepatobiliary route
Flutamide	2 hrs	??	94%-96%	6-8 hrs	α-hydroxylate metabolite also has activity	Predominantly renal
Medroxyproges-terone acetate	1-2 hrs	??	??	8-9 hrs	Prompt hepatic degradation	Especially renal, also hepatobiliary
Cimetidine	0.75-1.5 hrs	60%-70%	13%-25%	2 hrs	30%-40% of drug metabolized by liver	Predominantly renal
ANDROGEN INHIBITORS						
Finasteride	1-2 hrs	64%	90%	4.8 hrs	Extensive liver metabolism to inactive metabolites	39% in urine, 57% in feces
Ketoconazole	1-2 hrs	Uncertain†	95%-99%	8 hrs	Extensive liver metabolism to inactive metabolites	85%-90% in feces, 10%-15% in urine

Adapted from *CliniSphere 2.0 CD ROM,* St. Louis, June 2000, Facts & Comparisons.
*These values are for canrenone, the active metabolite of spironolactone.
†Bioavailability is highly variable and highly dependent on an acid pH in the GI tract.

Spironolactone is a steroid molecule, containing the basic steroid nucleus of four rings (Figure 19-2). This drug has the greatest resemblance to the mineralocorticoids, possessing an esterified lactone ring. The bioavailability from oral administration is at least 90% but varies depending on the manufacturer. Spironolactone is 98% protein bound, and the primary metabolite, canrenone, is at least 90% protein bound.[13] Canrenone is the active aldosterone antagonist and is the primary metabolite contributing to the diuretic activities of spironolactone.

Food increases the absorption of spironolactone. Spironolactone is rapidly metabolized by the liver. The primary metabolite, canrenone, can be interconverted enzymatically to its hydrolytic product, canrenoate. The unmetabolized drug does not appear in the urine.[13] Metabolites of spironolactone are excreted in urine and bile.[1]

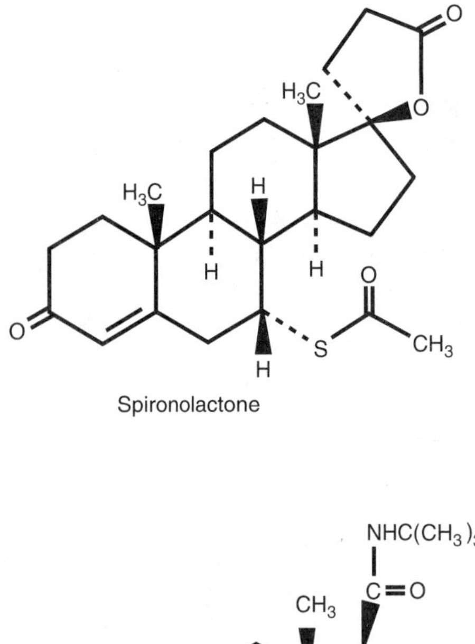

In a dose range of 25 to 200 mg, a linear relationship between a single dose of spironolactone and plasma levels of canrenone occurs within 96 hours. The half-life is approximately 19.2 hours for canrenone; for spironolactone it is 12.5 hours.[13]

CLINICAL USE.   Table 19-3 lists indications and contraindications for spironolactone.

Off-Label Uses.   There are currently no FDA-approved dermatologic indications for spironolactone. The drug has approval as a diuretic for a wide variety of medical conditions.

Spironolactone has been used to treat hirsutism,[14-24] acne,[25-29] and androgenetic alopecia.[30,31] Spironolactone is a logical choice for selected cases of hidradenitis suppurativa, although there are no published reports for this use of the drug. In many women with hirsutism, the spironolactone gradually decreases the

Spironolactone

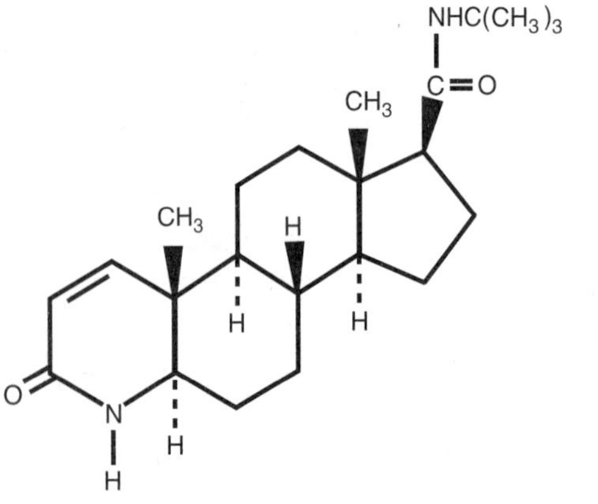

Finasteride

Figure 19-2   Antiandrogens and androgen inhibitors.

Table 19-3	Spironolactone Indications and Contraindications

FDA-APPROVED DERMATOLOGIC INDICATIONS
None specific to dermatology

OFF-LABEL USES
Acne vulgaris[25-29,34,35]
Androgenetic alopecia[30,31]
Hirsutism[14-24,32,33]
Hidradenitis suppurativa

CONTRAINDICATIONS
Renal insufficiency—acute or chronic
Anuria
Hyperkalemia
Pregnancy
Abnormal uterine bleeding
Family or personal history of estrogen-
    dependent malignancy*

PREGNANCY PRESCRIBING STATUS—CATEGORY X

*This would include breast, ovarian, or uterine malignancies.

growth rate and mean diameter of facial hair.[32] In clinical studies, spironolactone is less effective in improving hirsutism scores than flutamide[33]; however, spironolactone was shown to be more effective than finasteride.[14]

Common doses range between 50 and 200 mg/day, with 100 mg/day typically being better tolerated than higher dosages.[18] Even at this dose, menorrhagia or other menstrual dysfunction is common. These menstrual problems may resolve after 2 to 3 months of therapy. If menstrual abnormalities do not improve with time, the options include[20] (1) decreasing the spironolactone dose to the 50 to 75 mg/day range, (2) adding an oral contraceptive (OC) to reduce the menstrual dysfunction, or (3) "cycling" the spironolactone (as done with OCs), giving spironolactone 21 consecutive days, followed by 7 days when the drug is not administered. Patients less than 35 years of age are usually given OCs, whereas women at least 35 years of age may be treated with conjugated estrogens alone.[20]

In Europe, topical 5% spironolactone lotion and cream have been used to treat grade II acne, which has similar efficacy to topical antibiotic therapy in acne.[34] Topical 5% spironolactone gel produced a significant reduction in sebum secretion in young adults, supporting a potential role in acne patients.[35]

Adverse Effects. The most potentially serious common adverse effect of spironolactone is hyperkalemia.[36] This complication is most likely to occur when spironolactone is given concomitantly with a thiazide diuretic or to patients with severe renal insufficiency. Other important adverse effects include gynecomastia and minor gastrointestinal symptoms.

The potential for spironolactone to induce estrogen-dependent malignancies has been long debated.[37,38] Many authors suggest caution in prescribing spironolactone for women with a personal or family history of breast cancer and other estrogen-dependent malignancies; however, definitive proof of a causal role in such malignancies is lacking. The FDA gives a warning in the package insert that states tumors found in chronic toxicity studies of rats, in which 25 to 250 times the usual human dose (on a body weight basis) was given to rats. These doses resulted in benign adenomas of the thyroid and testes, malignant mammary tumors, and proliferative changes in the liver. Because of these and other changes reported in the rat, it has been recommended that spironolactone not be given to women with a genetic predisposition to breast cancer.[37,38]

Spironolactone and metabolites may cross the placental barrier. Studies in rats have demonstrated feminization of the male rat fetus. When women have taken spironolactone while nursing, canrenone has been detected in breast milk.[13]

Drug Interactions. Spironolactone has a relatively small list of potential drug interactions.[39] Spironolactone may have a reduced diuretic effect when taken with salicylates. Angiotensin-converting enzyme inhibitors, such as captopril and enalapril, further decrease aldosterone production, increasing the likelihood of hyperkalemia. Concomitant use of spironolactone and potassium supplements may also lead to hyperkalemia. Concurrent use of spironolactone and digoxin may increase the absorption of digoxin, producing increased digoxin blood levels and resultant increased potential for toxicity. Spironolactone may also interfere with radioimmunoassay measurement of digoxin, which can give falsely elevated serum digoxin values.

Monitoring Guidelines. Laboratory monitoring of the abnormal circulating androgen (testosterone or DHEA-S) every 3 to 4 months is recommended to ensure successful androgen suppression. Complete suppression usually takes 4 to 12 months of therapy. This androgen follow-up testing is not necessary if the values are normal at baseline. This therapeutic benefit may also plateau after 1 year and it may be necessary to add either an adjunctive antiandrogen or an androgen inhibitor. It is important to note here that the various androgen-induced disorders discussed in this chapter commonly have normal circulating androgen levels.

It is reasonable to periodically monitor serum potassium levels, especially early in therapy. The reality is that hyperkalemia from spironolactone is quite uncommon in the absence of the aforementioned risk factors for this complication. Blood pressure and weight should also be monitored periodically.

Flutamide

PHARMACOLOGY. See Tables 19-1 and 19-2 for general information and key pharmacologic concepts of flutamide. Flutamide is a nonsteroidal antiandrogen that is devoid of other hormonal activity. The drug becomes pharmacologically active after conversion to 2-hydroxyflutamide, which is a potent competitive inhibitor of DHT binding to the AR.[1,7,40] Flutamide causes regression of androgen target tissues such as prostate and seminal vesicles in mature rats. The drug also blocks the inhibitory feedback of testosterone on LH production, which results in a profound increase in plasma concentrations of LH and testosterone.[1] Similar effects on the prostate and seminal vesicles were noted in adult men when treated with flutamide 750 mg/day.[1,41] The predominant pituitary effect appears to be enhancement of the frequency of pulses of LH secretion. Therefore the drug may be effective in vitro as an antiandrogen; however, in vivo elevations of plasma testosterone levels limit clinical use of flutamide in disorders of androgen excess.

Flutamide can inhibit the action of adrenal androgens in castrated men or in men receiving GnRH blockade via leuprolide therapy. The latter effect of leuprolide is possible because LH production is not subject to negative feedback control by androgens such as the feedback regulation in women.

CLINICAL USE.   Flutamide is indicated for prostatic cancer. Flutamide has been used in conjunction with OCs for treating hirsutism.[14-16,23,42-44] Further studies are needed to evaluate its efficacy as a topical agent in treating hirsutism. Topical flutamide has shown potential for significant reduction of androgen levels in animal models.[45]

Flutamide crosses the placenta; therefore it would be expected to produce pseudohermaphroditism if a male fetus is exposed to the drug. The most important adverse effect is hepatotoxicity, which may progress to fulminant liver failure.[46,47] This potential complication serves to limit the drug's usefulness in dermatology.

Progesterone

See Tables 19-1 and 19-2 for general information and key pharmacologic concepts of progesterone. Progesterone is a hormone that is structurally similar to testosterone. As a result of this structural similarity, progesterone can inhibit 5α-reductase and can bind to the AR, thus acting both as an antiandrogen and an androgen inhibitor. Various progestins may have inherent estrogenic or androgenic effects.[1] Although progesterone binds to its own intracellular transcription receptor, it also has affinity for the AR. After 5α-reduction of progesterone, the metabolite becomes 5α-pregnane-3,20-dione, which is similar overall to DHT.

Progesterone is secreted by the ovary (mainly from the corpus luteum) primarily during the second half of the menstrual cycle, leading to the development of a secretory endometrium. Progesterone is essential for sustaining pregnancy through the normal gestational duration. This hormone is vital to the developing mammary gland. Progesterone also has a known thermogenic effect during the luteal phase of the menstrual cycle.

Progesterone can be given intramuscularly or orally, with both routes readily absorbed but at a rate that may be too rapid for optimal therapeutic efficiency. Biotransformation takes place largely in the liver. Many progestins are conjugated by glucuronidation or sulfonation to more hydrophilic metabolites for excretion in the urine. A small amount can be stored in body fat. There are multiple analogs of progesterone that are less susceptible to hepatic metabolism and therefore may have a more sustained therapeutic effect compared with progesterone. Approximately 50% to 60% of administered radioactive progesterone appears in the urine and about 10% in feces.

The most common oral formulation used in clinical practice is medroxyprogesterone acetate (Provera). Most therapeutic indications for progesterone are for ovarian disorders and contraception. Off-label uses include variable effectiveness as a topical agent for treating AGA at 2% to 5% progesterone concentrations.[48]

Cyproterone Acetate

Cyproterone acetate is a progestin with well-known antiandrogen properties. The drug has a long track record in several European countries but is currently not available in the United States. In the search for progestins that had antiandrogenic activity, a 1,2-α-methylene substitution led to the discovery of cyproterone. In addition to potent antiandrogen effects, the drug also possesses strong progestational activity with resultant suppression of gonadotropin secretion.[40] The primary action of cyproterone is competition with DHT for the AR binding site.[49] When given to pregnant animals, cyproterone acetate blocks the actions of androgens in the male fetus and induces a form of pseudohermaphroditism.[49]

Cyproterone acetate administered at 100 mg/day to normal young men causes a 50% decrease in plasma concentrations of LH and FSH and a 75% decrease in plasma testosterone. These hormonal effects are due to the inhibition of testosterone production, as well as interference with androgen action at the AR.[50] Cyproterone is available in most European countries for the indication of prostatic cancer and benign prostatic hypertrophy, as well as inhibition of libido in patients with deviations of sexual behavior. Off-label uses include AGA, hirsutism, and virilizing syndromes.[7,40,41] Cyproterone is available in Europe as the progestin in an OC named Diane.

Cimetidine

See Tables 19-1 and 19-2 for general information and key pharmacologic concepts of cimetidine. Cimetidine was the first H_2 antihistamine to be introduced for treatment of duodenal ulcers and other gastric hypersecretory conditions. Cimetidine also has antiandrogen effects through binding to AR. It follows that adverse effects may include loss of libido, impotence, or gynecomastia (stimulated prolactin). Cimetidine is also a relatively weak cytochrome P-450 3A4 inhibitor with the potential for relatively minor elevations of drug substrates metabolized by this isoform (see Chapter 44).

There have been anecdotal reports of cimetidine use for acne,[29] hirsutism,[51] and AGA.[52] A small amount of benefit was noted particularly for acne and AGA. The preferred dose range is 800 to 1600 mg/day, given as 400 mg by mouth up to four times daily.[7] In general, most other antiandrogens and androgen inhibitors have significantly greater efficacy for disorders of androgen excess.

ANDROGEN INHIBITORS
Finasteride

Finasteride (Propecia, 1 mg) is the only oral FDA-approved product available for use in men with AGA (see Table 19-1). Minoxidil (in a topical formulation) is the only other drug that has received FDA approval for AGA. Proscar (the 5 mg version of finasteride) is indicated for the treatment of benign prostatic hypertrophy.

PHARMACOLOGY.   See Table 19-2 for key pharmacologic concepts of finasteride. Finasteride is a specific inhibitor of type II 5α-reductase, which catalyzes conversion of testosterone to DHT (see Figure 19-2). As discussed earlier, type II 5α-reductase predominates in hair follicles on the top of the scalp and in the sebaceous gland ducts. The drug does not bind to the AR and therefore is not a traditional antiandrogen. The fact that male pseudohermaphrodites with genetic deficiency of 5α-reductase type II do not lose their scalp hair correlates well with the distribution of type II 5α-reductase.[1,10,53,54]

After finasteride administration in 1 mg doses, serum concentration of DHT decreases by 65% within 24 hours.[55] Serum concentrations of testosterone and estradiol increase about 15% but remain within normal limits. Prostate concentrations of testosterone increase about sixfold.[55] Finasteride is well absorbed in the gastrointestinal tract, metabolized in the liver, and excreted in urine and feces. The serum half-life is 5 to 6 hours. Minute quantities (nanogram levels) of the drug are detectable in human semen, and therefore the drug is not thought to have any adverse consequences in female partners of men receiving finasteride who are exposed to the drug by sexual contact.

CLINICAL USE
FDA-Approved Indication. Table 19-4 lists indications and contraindications for finasteride. Three double-blind multicenter trials conducted in men 18 to 41 years of age have been reported in abstract form.[56-58] In one trial, 1553 men with mild-to-moderate AGA predominantly in the vertex area took either finasteride 1 mg/day or placebo for 1 year.[58] Hairs were systemically counted in a 1-inch diameter circle on the scalp. There was a mean baseline hair count of 876 hairs. After 3 months of treatment, the men who took finasteride were significantly more satisfied with the appearance of their hair. At the end of 1 year, patients receiving finasteride had an average of 107 more hairs than those individuals who took placebo. Hair counts were maintained for up to 24 months in men who continued to take the drug.[58]

Table 19-4	Finasteride Indications and Contraindications

FDA-APPROVED DERMATOLOGIC INDICATION
Male pattern androgenetic alopecia[56-60]

OFF-LABEL USES
Acne vulgaris[44]
Female pattern androgenetic alopecia
Hirsutism[61-65]
Hidradenitis suppurativa[44]

CONTRAINDICATIONS

Absolute	Relative
Hypersensitivity to finasteride or any component of product	Use in women of childbearing potential
Use in children	

PREGNANCY PRESCRIBING STATUS—CATEGORY X

Another study evaluating 326 men with mild-to-moderate frontal hair loss found that after 1 year, finasteride-treated men had statistically significantly higher hair counts in the frontal scalp.[59] About 50% of treated men and 30% of those who took placebo thought that the appearance of their hair had improved.[58,59] Hair regrowth was not reported in older men taking 5 mg finasteride tablets (Proscar) for prostatic hypertrophy.[60] This lack of observed scalp hair improvement was either from lack of focus on cutaneous findings by these investigators or due to an innate reduced response of scalp pilosebaceous units to finasteride in older men.

Off-Label Uses.   There are several off-label uses of finasteride for which there are supporting data. To date, studies evaluating finasteride for hirsutism utilized the 5 mg dosage form.[61-65] Acne and hidradenitis in women are other theoretic indications for this drug.[44] Further studies evaluating finasteride for these disorders of androgen excess are in order.

Adverse Effects.   Infrequent adverse effects with 5 mg finasteride (Proscar) in older men were found to be loss of libido, erectile and ejaculatory dysfunction, hypersensitivity reactions, gynecomastia, and severe myopathy.[58] The drug also causes a 50% decrease in prostate-specific antigen (PSA) in clinical trials with the 1 mg tablets in men 18 to 41 years old. Decreased libido, erectile dysfunction, or a decreased volume of ejaculate have been reported in less than 4% of younger patients receiving 1 mg daily of finasteride (Propecia). Because DHT primarily has a central role in the pilosebaceous unit and in the prostate, only decreased volume of ejaculate is likely to be causally related to finasteride use.

Finasteride has teratogenic effects in animals, causing genitourinary abnormalities in the male offspring. The concentration of the drug in the semen of men who took 1 mg/day was lower than the concentration associated with teratogenic effects in monkeys.[66] The Merck manufacturers warn that women who are or may be pregnant should not take finasteride or handle crushed or broken tablets. Unless there is a cutaneous barrier abnormality in the women handling the crushed or broken tablets, significant percutaneous absorption is unlikely. Reasonable caution is in order.

Drug Interactions.   No significant drug interactions have been demonstrated with finasteride.

Monitoring Guidelines.   There are no laboratory monitoring guidelines required for following therapy with finasteride for male pattern androgenetic alopecia. A baseline PSA value is appropriate for older men *before* receiving finasteride. A reasonable timeframe to consider ordering a PSA value before prescribing finasteride would be for men over 50 years of age.

Ketoconazole

PHARMACOLOGY.   See Table 19-2 for key pharmacologic concepts of ketoconazole. Ketoconazole is an azole antifungal agent in the imidazole subgroup, which is available in oral and topical formulations. Ketoconazole has broad therapeutic potential for treatment of superficial cutaneous and systemic fungal infections. The drug has a secondary pharmacologic effect of inhibiting cytochrome P-450 enzymes involved in steroid hormone biosynthesis.[67] The net result can be reduced production of both glucocorticoids and androgenic steroids. Ketoconazole studies in animals showed inhibition of testicular synthesis of androgens and displacement of sex steroids from sex hormone–binding globulin. This secondary effect has been turned into a therapeutic advantage to pharmacologically induce androgen deprivation in selected patients with prostate cancer.[68]

CLINICAL USE.   Ketoconazole is available as 200 mg tablets and is generally administered once daily for mycologic indications. Typically, higher doses in the range of 400 to 800 mg daily are necessary to inhibit androgen production. An off-label use of ketoconazole is in the treatment of hirsutism.[69] There are no published reports regarding the use of this drug for acne or AGA.

Adverse effects include gastrointestinal irritation leading to nausea and vomiting, headache, epigastric pain, and thrombocytopenia.[1] Gynecomastia has been reported. It is likely that the previously mentioned inhibition of the biosynthesis of adrenal glucocorticoids limits the clinical utility of ketoconazole as an oral agent for treating AGA or hirsutism. Furthermore, hepatic dysfunction manifest by mild elevation of transaminases in 5% to 10% of patients and toxic hepatitis in at least 1/10,000 patients is an important issue.[70]

Ketoconazole is available in shampoo formulations as Nizoral Shampoo in a 2% formulation (only by prescription) and is available as an over the counter 1% formulation. Given ketoconazole's androgen inhibitory properties, it has been hypothesized that this drug may potentially have topical effects in retarding hair loss.

Oral Contraceptives

PHARMACOLOGY.   There are two kinds of OCs[71]—the "minipill," which may contain a progestin alone, and the "combination pill," which contains an estrogen and progestin. There are two types of combination pills—"monophasic," in which there is no variation in the daily dose of estrogen or progestin, and "multiphasic," in which the daily dose of estrogen and progestin varies.

The estrogen in the OCs is generally ethinyl estradiol, although mestranol is occasionally used.[71] Mestranol is one-half to two-thirds as potent as ethinyl estradiol, when compared on a microgram to microgram basis. It is important to know that women taking exogenous estrogens may still produce endogenous estrogens from the ovaries and from adipose tissues. Endogenous estrogen production may vary in the presence of exogenous estrogens in OCs but correlates inversely to a degree with the dose of exogenous estrogen given.

Synthetic progestins for OCs are derived from 19-nortestosterone. As previously stated in the Progesterone section, these progestins can have androgenic properties, estrogenic properties, or function as antiandrogens. Given that more androgenic progestins (norgestrel, levonorgestrel) may induce acne, AGA, and hirsutism, it is interesting to note that OCs with less androgenic progestins (norgestimate, desogestrel) may be useful clinically for treatment of these same disorders.

CLINICAL USE

Indications.   The androgenic potency of progestins in OCs varies as shown in Box 19-3. Desogestrel, norgestimate, and gestodene are the newest progestins in OCs and have the lowest androgenic index.[71] Gestodene has not been released in OCs in the United States to date. In one study of over 11,000 women taking OCs with either gestodene or desogestrel, nearly 80% had a decrease in acne, with desogestrel having a lower androgenic index than norgestimate.[72] Ortho-Tricyclen, which contains norgestimate, has an official FDA indication for use in acne vulgaris in women after several clinical

Box 19-3

Oral Contraceptives and Relative Androgenicity of the Progestins in Specific Products[71]

LOW ANDROGENICITY
*Desogestrel**
Desogen
Ortho-Cept

Gestodene
(None available yet)

Norgestimate
Ortho-Cyclen
Ortho Tri-Cyclen

MODERATE ANDROGENICITY
Norethindrone
Micronor†
Ovcon-35
Brevicon
Modicon
Ortho-Novum 7/7/7‡
Ortho-Novum 10/11‡
Tri-Norinyl‡
Norinyl 1/35
Ortho-Novum 1/35

Ethynodiol diacetate
Ovulen
Demulen 1/35

HIGH ANDROGENICITY
Levonorgestrel
Triphasil‡
Tri-Levlen‡
Nordette‡

Norgestrel
Lo/Ovral
Ovrette†
Ovral

Norethindrone

Acetate
Loestrin 1/20
Loestrin 1.5/30

*The generic drug name for desogestrel and other progestins is capitalized; within each column, the specific progestins and trade name contraceptives are listed in order of gradually increasing androgenicity.
†These contraceptives are progestin only products.
‡These contraceptives are multiphasic as defined in text.

trials demonstrated significant benefit for women receiving this drug.[73,74] Other disorders of androgen excess may benefit from contraceptives containing these newer progestins.[75]

Women with acne, AGA, or hirsutism, who are either currently taking or plan on taking an OC, should be advised to avoid those OCs that contain progestins with a higher androgenic index. Individual responses to OCs can vary; therefore it may depend on an individual's genetic predisposition in regard to how they respond to the specific OC being prescribed.

Adverse Effects. Well-known adverse effects of estrogens include nausea, increased breast size and tenderness, cyclic weight gain, headaches, and thromboemboli.[71] Current OCs contain 50 μg or less of mestranol or ethinyl estradiol. Other adverse effects include vaginal bleeding and mood swings, which may necessitate changes of OCs for individual tolerance.

Also, there should be an awareness that taking other drugs may cause failure of the OCs to prevent pregnancy.[76,77] Several of these drugs are hepatic cytochrome P-450 enzyme inducers, including rifampin and griseofulvin. In addition, there is the controversial reported association of contraceptive failure with antibiotics such as penicillins, sulfonamides, and tetracyclines. OC failure may also be due to inconsistent usage or significant physical illnesses (Box 19-4).

Gonadotropin-Releasing Hormone Analogs

Potent analogs of GnRH can inhibit secretion of gonadotropins, such as LH and FSH, with resultant effect on androgen production by the ovaries. GnRH agonists, such as leuprolide or nafarelin, initially increase LH and FSH production for 2 to 4 weeks, before a sustained inhibition of the secretion of these two go-

Box 19-4

Drugs That May Cause Failure of Oral Contraceptives[76,77]

HEPATIC-ENZYME INDUCERS—WELL ESTABLISHED

Anticonvulsants
  Carbamazepine
  Phenobarbital
  Primidone
Antimicrobial agents
  Griseofulvin
  Rifampin
Other drugs
  Phenylbutazone
  Alcohol

DRUGS AFFECTING ENTEROHEPATIC RECIRCULATION OF ESTROGENS*

Antimicrobial agents
  Penicillins (especially ampicillin)
  Sulfonamides
  Tetracyclines

*It is highly controversial whether there is a true causal relationship with these drugs and OC failure. The physician must always consider the OC background failure rate even with ideal use of contraceptives.

nadotropins. Leuprolide and nafarelin are now being studied for potential indications of hirsutism and AGA.[78,79] These drugs have been utilized for contraception in postpartum women who are not candidates for OCs. Some authors have reported that 1 to 2 mg of leuprolide can be given for disorders of androgen excess. Daily leuprolide injections of 1 mg reduces ovarian function by about 50%, and the 2-mg dose reduces ovarian function to prepubertal levels.

Two studies evaluated these GnRH agonists for therapy of hirsutism.[78,79] Leuprolide (Lupron-Depot) given intramuscularly 3.75 mg/month in addition to daily 0.625 mg conjugated estrogens and cyclic medroxyprogesterone acetate (10 mg on days 1 to 12 of each month) was compared with the estrogen/progesterone therapy alone.[78] Nafarelin (400 μg given intranasally twice daily) plus Norinyl 1/35 tablets daily for 21 of 28 days of the menstrual cycle was compared with Norinyl 1/35 monotherapy.[79] In both studies, the addition of the GnRH agonist (leuprolide or nafarelin) to the hormonal regimens showed significantly greater improvement in the hirsute women, compared with the estrogen/progesterone hormone therapy alone. Further studies with these agents are needed to assess safety, efficacy, and practicality for use in dermatologic disorders of androgen excess because these drugs are expensive and need careful monitoring on a regular basis by gynecologists experienced with their use.

GI 198745

Glaxo-Wellcome is currently investigating this 5α-reductase inhibitor in a multicenter clinical trial for males with AGA. To date, there are no published reports regarding this potential indication. Structurally, GI 198745 is similar to the parent structure of finasteride, maintaining the core four ring steroid nucleus; however, on the C-21 branch is a trifluorophenyl group that renders the molecule highly electronegative and perhaps gives greater binding affinity for both the type I and type II isoenzyme forms of 5α-reductase.[2] In contrast to finasteride, GI 198745 is an inhibitor of both type I and type II 5α-reductase. This investigational drug inhibits serum DHT levels by over 90% within 24 hours after oral administration.

It is postulated that given this relatively complete DHT reduction, this investigational androgen inhibitor may be more effective than finasteride in promoting hair growth on the scalp in men. GI 198745 may also be effective in treating acne, where type I 5α-reductase predominates in the distal sebaceous gland lobules, with type II 5α-reductase residing in the sebaceous proximal duct.[2] The results of future studies will be eagerly awaited regarding the potential clinical benefits for disorders of androgen excess from this new compound.

Herbal Remedies

Saw Palmetto Plus (*Serenoa repens* extract) is an over-the-counter herbal remedy that has recently been promoted by various health food stores. This herbal product reportedly provides nutritional support for the health of the prostate gland with resultant improvement in urinary function.[80-83] There are implications that the product promotes hair growth on the scalp.[84] This herbal product is postulated to act by irreversibly inhibiting the conversion of testosterone to dihydrotestosterone, suggesting that 5α-reductase inhibition (type I, type II, or possibly both) is responsible for the theoretic benefits. Another active ingredient, *Pygeum africanum* compound, is added to this extract and is speculated to influence testosterone metabolism. Again the mechanism of action is not clear.

    An overall criticism of herbal remedies, such as Saw Palmetto Plus, is that there are not strict guidelines regarding purity or consistency of drug concentration from batch to batch. In addition, the producer's therapeutic claims regarding safety and efficacy are not validated by clinical trials. Therefore there should be tremendous caution regarding recommending such herbal agents until more careful clinical evaluation is undertaken.

Bibliography

Burkman RT Jr: The role of oral contraceptives in the treatment of hyperandrogenic disorders. *Am J Med* 98(1A):130S-136S, 1995.

Chen W, Zouboulis CC, Orfanos CE: The 5α-reductase system and its inhibitors. *Dermatology* 193:177-184, 1996.

Price VH: Treatment of hair loss. *N Engl J Med* 341:964-973, 1999.

Redmond GP: Androgenic disorders of women: diagnostic and therapeutic decision making. *Am J Med* 98(Suppl 1A):120S-128S, 1995.

Rittmaster RS: Finasteride. *N Engl J Med* 330:120-125, 1994.

Sawaya ME, Hordinsky MK: The antiandrogens: when and how they should be used. *Dermatol Clin* 11:65-72, 1993.

Shaw JC: Antiandrogen and hormonal treatment of acne. *Dermatol Clin* 14:803-811, 1996.

Shaw JC: Spironolactone in dermatologic therapy. *J Am Acad Dermatol* 24:236-243, 1991.

References

Introduction and Androgen Physiology

1. Wilson J: Androgens. In Hardman JG, Limbird LE, Molinoff PB, et al, editors: *Goodman & Gilman's the pharmacological basis of therapeutics*, ed 9, New York, 1996, McGraw-Hill, pp 1441-1457.

2. Sawaya ME: Alopecia—the search for novel agents continues. *Expert Opinion in Therapeutic Patents* 7:859-872, 1997.

3. Jost A: Embryonic sexual differentiation. In Jones HW, Scott WW, editors: *Hermaphroditism, genital anomalies and related endocrine disorders*, ed 2, Baltimore, 1971, Williams & Wilkins, pp 16-64.

4. Franchimont P: Pituitary gonadotropins. *J Clin Endocrinol Metab* 6:101-116, 1977.

5. Boyar RM: Control of the onset of puberty. *Ann Rev Med* 29:509-520, 1978.

6. Judd HL, Yen SSC: Serum androstenedione and testosterone levels during the menstrual cycle. *J Clin Endocrinol Metab* 36:475-481, 1973.

7. Sawaya ME: Clinical updates in hair. *Dermatol Clin* 15:37-43, 1997.

8. Sawaya ME, Price VH: Different levels of 5α-reductase type I and II, aromatase, androgen receptor in hair follicles of women and men with androgenetic alopecia. *J Invest Dermatol* 109:295-300, 1997.

9. Andersson S, Russell DW: Structural and biochemical properties of cloned and expressed human and rat steroid 5α-reductases. *Proc Natl Acad Sci USA* 87:3640-3644, 1990.

10. Andersson S, Berman DM, Jenkins EP, et al: Deletion of steroid 5α-reductase gene in male pseudohermaphroditism. *Nature* 354:159-161, 1991.

Antiandrogens—Spironolactone

11. Vellacott ID, O'Brien PM: Effect of spironolactone on premenstrual syndrome symptoms. *J Reprod Med* 32:429-434, 1987.

12. Young RL, Goldzieher JW, Elkind-Hirsch K: The endocrine effects of spironolactone used as an antiandrogen. *Fertil Steril* 48:223-228, 1987.

13. Beermann B, Groschinsky-Grind M: Clinical pharmacokinetics of diuretics. *Clin Pharmacokinet* 5:221-245, 1980.

Spironolactone—Hirsutism

14. Erenus M, Yucelten D, Durmusoglu F, et al: Comparison of finasteride versus spironolactone in treatment of idiopathic hirsutism. *Fertil Steril* 68:1000-1003, 1997.
15. Moghetti P, Tosi F, Tosti A, et al: Comparison of spironolactone, flutamide, and finasteride efficacy in the treatment of hirsutism: a randomized, double blind, placebo-controlled trial. *J Clin Endocrinol Metab* 85:89-94, 2000.
16. Venturoli S, Mareschalchi O, Colombo FM, et al: A prospective randomized trial comparing low dose flutamide, finasteride, ketoconazole and cyproterone acetate-estrogen regimens in the treatment of hirsutism. *J Clin Endocrinol Metab* 84:1304-1310, 1999.
17. Zemstov A, Wilson L: Successful treatment of hirsutism in HAIR-AN syndrome using flutamide, spironolactone, and birth control therapy. *Arch Dermatol* 133:431-433, 1997.
18. Barch JH, Cherry CA, Wojnaroivska I, et al: Spironolactone is an effective and well-tolerated systemic antiandrogen therapy for hirsute women. *J Clin Endocrinol Metab* 66:966-970, 1989.
19. Kelestimur F, Sahin Y: Comparison of Diane 35 and Diane 35 plus spironolactone in the treatment of hirsutism. *Fertil Steril* 69:66-69, 1998.
20. Helfer EL, Miller JL, Rose LI: Adverse effects of spironolactone therapy in the hirsute woman. *J Clin Endocrinol Metab* 66:208-211, 1988.
21. Vetr M, Sobek A: Low dose spironolactone in the treatment of female hyperandrogenemia and hirsutism. *Acta Univ Palack Olomucensis Facultatis Medicae* 135:55-57, 1993.
22. Crosby PD, Rittmaster RS: Predictors of clinical response in hirsute women treated with spironolactone. *Fertil Steril* 55:1076-1081, 1991.
23. Yulceten D, Erenus M, Gurbuz O, et al: Recurrence rate of hirsutism after 3 different antiandrogen therapies. *J Am Acad Dermatol* 41:64-68, 1999.
24. Wong IL, Morris RS, Chang L, et al: A prospective randomized trial comparing finasteride to spironolactone in the treatment of hirsute women. *J Clin Endocrinol Metab* 80:233-238, 1995.

Spironolactone—Acne and Alopecia

25. Shaw JC: Antiandrogen and hormonal treatment of acne. *Dermatol Clin* 14:803-811, 1996.
26. Hughes BR, Cunliffe WJ: Tolerance of spironolactone. *Br J Dermatol* 118:687-691, 1988.
27. Muhlemann MF, Carter GD, Cream JJ, et al: Oral spironolactone: an effective treatment of acne vulgaris in women. *Br J Dermatol* 115:227-232, 1986.
28. Goodfellow A, Alaghband-Zadeh J, Carter G, et al: Oral spironolactone improves acne vulgaris and reduces sebum excretion. *Br J Dermatol* 111:209-214, 1984.
29. Hatwai A, Bhatt RP, Agrawal JK, et al: Spironolactone and cimetidine in treatment of acne. *Acta Dermatol Venereol* 68:84-87, 1988.
30. Adamopoulos DA, Karamertzanis M, Nicopoulou S, et al: Beneficial effect of spironolactone on androgenic alopecia. *Clin Endocrinol* 47:759-760, 1997.
31. Callan AW, Montalto J: Female androgenetic alopecia: an update. *Australas J Dermatol* 36:51-55, 1995.
32. Dorrington-Ward P, McCartney ACE, Holland S, et al: The effect of spironolactone on hirsutism and female androgen metabolism. *Clin Endocrinol* 23:161-167, 1985.
33. Cusan L, Dupont A, Gomez JL, et al: Comparison of flutamide and spironolactone in the treatment of hirsutism: a randomized controlled trial. *Fertil Steril* 61:281-287, 1994.
34. Califano L, Cannavo S, Siragusa M, et al: Experience in the therapy of acne with topical administration of spironolactone as an antiandrogen. *Clinica Terapeutica* 135:193-199, 1990.
35. Yamamoto A, Ito M: Topical spironolactone reduces sebum secretion rates in young adults. *J Dermatol* 23:243-246, 1996.

Spironolactone—Adverse Effects and Interactions

36. Greenberg A: Diuretic complications. *Am J Med Sci* 319:10-24, 2000.
37. Cumming DC: Use of spironolactone in treatment of hirsutism. *Cleveland Clin J Med* 57:285-287, 1990.
38. Danielson DA, Jick H, Hunter JR, et al: Nonestrogenic drugs and breast cancer. *Am J Epidemiol* 116:329-332, 1982.
39. *CliniSphere 2.0 CD ROM*, St. Louis, June 2000, Facts & Comparisons.

Flutamide

40. Neri RO: Antiandrogens. *Adv Sex Horm Res* 2:233-262, 1976.
41. Knuth UA, Hano R, Nieschlag E: Effect of flutamide or cyproterone acetate on primary and testicular hormones in normal men. *J Clin Endocrinol Metab* 59:963-969, 1984.
42. Muderris II, Bayram F, Sahin Y, et al: A comparison between two doses of flutamide in the treatment of hirsutism. *Fertil Steril* 68:644-667, 1997.
43. Falsetti L, Gambera A, Legrenzi L, et al: Comparison of finasteride versus flutamide in the treatment of hirsutism. *Eur J Endocrinol* 141:361-367, 1999.
44. Diamanti-Kandarakis E: Current aspects of antiandrogen therapy in women. *Curr Pharmaceut Design* 5:707-723, 1999.
45. Sintov A, Serafimovich S, Gilhar A: New topical antiandrogenic formulations can stimulate hair growth in human bald scalp grafted onto mice. *Int J Pharmaceut* 194:125-134, 2000.
46. Dankoff JS: Near fatal liver dysfunction secondary to administration of flutamide for prostate cancer. *J Urol* 148:1914, 1991.
47. Wysowski DK, Freiman JP, Tourtelot JB, et al: Fatal and nonfatal hepatotoxicity associated with flutamide. *Ann Intern Med* 118:860-864, 1993.

Other Antiandrogens

48. Tromovitch TA, Glogau RG, Stegman SJ: Medical treatment of male pattern alopecia (androgenic alopecia). *Head Neck Surg* 7:336-339, 1985.
49. Neumann F, Topert M: Pharmacology of antiandrogens. *J Steroid Biochem* 25:885-895, 1986.
50. Brown TR, Rothwell SW, Sultan C, et al: Inhibition of androgen binding in human foreskin fibroblasts by antiandrogens. *Steroids* 37:635-648, 1981.
51. Golditch IM, Price VH: Treatment of hirsutism with cimetidine. *Obstet Gynecol* 75:911-913, 1990.
52. Aram H: Treatment of female androgenetic alopecia with cimetidine. *Int J Dermatol* 26:128-130, 1987.

Androgen Inhibitors—Finasteride

53. Imperato-McGinley J, Guerrero L, Gautier T, et al: Steroid 5α-reductase deficiency in man: an inherited form of male pseudohermaphroditism. *Science* 186:1213-1215, 1974.
54. Dallob AL, Sadick NS, Unger W, et al: The effect of finasteride, a 5α-reductase inhibitor, on scalp skin testosterone and dihydrotestosterone concentrations in patients with male pattern baldness. *J Clin Endocrinol Metab* 79:703-706, 1994.
55. McConnell JD, Wilson JD, George FW, et al: Finasteride, an inhibitor of 5α-reductase, suppresses prostatic dihydrotestosterone in men with benign prostatic hyperplasia. *J Clin Endocrinol Metab* 74:505-508, 1992.
56. Kaufman KD, DeVillez R, Roberts J, et al: A 12-month pilot clinical study of the effects of finasteride on men with male pattern baldness. *J Invest Dermatol* 102:615, 1994.
57. Drake L, Hordinsky M, Fiedler V, et al: The effects of finasteride on scalp skin and serum androgen levels in men with androgenetic alopecia. *J Am Acad Dermatol* 41:550-554, 1999.
58. Anonymous: Propecia and Rogaine Extra Strength for alopecia. *Med Lett Drugs Ther* 40:25-27, 1998.
59. Leyden J, Dunlap F, Miller B, et al: Finasteride in the treatment of men with frontal male pattern hair loss. *J Am Acad Dermatol* 40:930-937, 1999.
60. Brenner S, Matz H: Improvement of androgenetic alopecia in 53-76 year old men using oral finasteride. *Int J Dermatol* 38:928-930, 1999.
61. Bayram F, Muderris II, Sahin Y, et al: Finasteride treatment for one year in 35 hirsute patients. *Exp Clin Endocrinol Diabetes* 107:195-197, 1999.
62. Petrone A, Civitillo RM, Galante L, et al: Usefulness of a 12 month treatment with finasteride in idiopathic and polycystic ovary syndrome associated hirsutism. *Clin Exp Obstet Gynecol* 26:213-216, 1999.
63. Faloia E, Filippone S, Mancini V, et al: Effect of finasteride in idiopathic hirsutism. *J Endocrinol Invest* 21:694-698, 1998.
64. Castello R, Tosi F, Perrone F, et al: Outcome of long term treatment with the 5α-reductase inhibitor, finasteride in idiopathic hirsutism: clinical and hormonal effects during a 1 year course of therapy and 1 year follow up. *Fertil Steril* 66:734-740, 1996.
65. Moghetti P, Castello R, Magnani CM, et al: Clinical and hormonal effects of the 5α-reductase inhibitor finasteride in idiopathic hirsutism. *J Clin Endocrinol Metab* 79:1115-1121, 1994.

66. Overstreet JW, Fuh VL, Gould J, et al: Chronic treatment with finasteride daily does not affect spermatogenesis or semen production in young men. *J Urol* 162:1295-1300, 1999.

Ketoconazole

67. Feldman D: Ketoconazole and other imidazole derivatives as inhibitors of steroidogenesis. *Endocrinol Rev* 7:409-420, 1986.
68. Mahler C, Verhelst J, Denis L: Ketoconazole and liarozole in the treatment of advanced prostatic cancer. *Cancer* 71(Suppl 3):1068-1073, 1993.
69. Isik AZ, Gokmen O, Zeyneloglu HB, et al: Low dose ketoconazole is an effective and a relatively safe alternative in the treatment of hirsutism. *Aust N Z J Obstet Gynaecol* 36:487-489, 1996.
70. Lewis JH, Zimmerman HJ, Benson GD, et al: Hepatic injury associated with ketoconazole therapy: analysis of 33 cases. *Gastroenterology* 86:503-513, 1984.

Oral Contraceptives and Gonadotropin-Releasing Hormone Agonists

71. Reed BR: The pill. *Fitzpatrick's J Clin Dermatol* 2(5):41-44, 1994.
72. Mango D, Ricci S, Manna P, et al: Clinical and hormonal effects of ethinyl estradiol combined with gestodene and desogestrel in young women with acne vulgaris. *Contraception* 53:163-170, 1996.
73. Lucky AW, Henderson TA, Olson WH, et al: Effectiveness of norgestimate and ethinyl estradiol in treating moderate acne vulgaris. *J Am Acad Dermatol* 37:746-754, 1997.
74. Redmond GP, Olson WH, Lippman JS, et al: Norgestimate and ethinyl estradiol in the treatment of acne vulgaris: a randomized, placebo-controlled trial. *Obstet Gynecol* 89:615-622, 1997.

75. Burkman RT Jr: The role of oral contraceptives in the treatment of hyperandrogenic disorders. *Am J Med* 98(1A):130S-136S, 1995.
76. Helms SE, Bredle DL, Zajic J, et al: Oral contraceptive failure rates and oral antibiotics. *J Am Acad Dermatol* 36:705-710, 1997.
77. Fleischer AB, Resnick SD: The effect of antibiotics on the efficacy of oral contraceptives. A controversy revisited. *Arch Dermatol* 125:1562-1564, 1989.
78. Azziz R, Ochoa TM, Bradley EL, et al: Leuprolide and estrogen versus oral contraceptives for the treatment of hirsutism. A prospective randomized study. *J Clin Endocrinol Metab* 80:3406-3411, 1995.
79. Heiner JS, Greendale GA, Kawakai AK, et al: Comparison of a gonadotropin-releasing hormone agonist and a low dose oral contraceptive given alone or together in the treatment of hirsutism. *J Clin Endocrinol Metab* 80:3412-3418, 1995.

Herbal Remedies

80. McKinney DE: Saw palmetto for benign prostatic hyperplasia. *JAMA* 281:1699, 1999.
81. Marks LS, Tyler VE: Saw palmetto extract: newest (and oldest) treatment alternative for men with symptomatic benign prostatic hyperplasia. *Urology* 53:457-461, 1999.
82. Goepel M, Hecker U, Krege S, et al: Saw palmetto extracts potently and noncompetitively inhibit human alpha-1-adrenoceptors in vitro. *Prostate* 38:208-215, 1999.
83. Wilt TJ, Ishani A, Stark G, et al: Saw palmetto extracts for treatment of benign prostatic hyperplasia: a systemic review. *JAMA* 280:1604-1609, 1998.
84. Sawaya ME, Shapiro J: Androgenetic alopecia: new approved and unapproved treatments. *Dermatol Clin* 18:47-61, 2000.

John Y. M. Koo
Chai Sue Lee

Psychotropic Agents

A significant proportion of patients seen in an average dermatologic practice have psychosocial issues associated with their skin diseases. Sometimes, the psychopathology plays an etiologic role in the skin manifestations of patients who have no real skin disease, such as in delusions of parasitosis or trichotillomania. In other patients, psychologic factors, such as emotional stress, can exacerbate bona fide skin disorders, such as psoriasis or atopic dermatitis. Furthermore, many patients develop emotional problems as a result of having a disfiguring skin disease.

To address the psychologic issues, the most obvious course of action would be to refer psychodermatologic patients to a psychiatrist or another mental health professional. However, these patients frequently refuse such a referral. Some of these patients refuse a referral to a psychiatrist because of the perceived stigma associated with psychiatric illness, whereas others may refuse the referral because they lack the insight to recognize the psychologic component of their skin complaint. Faced with these patients, a dermatologist has two choices. The first choice is to try to "look the other way" and pacify the patient by providing relatively benign but minimally effective treatments. The other option is to try to address the psychologic/psychiatric problems. The idea of using psychotropic medications may seem foreign to many dermatologists, given that dermatology residencies and postgraduate courses have limited emphasis on principles of psychopharmacotherapy. Patients with psychodermatologic problems who refuse referral to a psychiatrist can still be greatly helped by a dermatologist who has an adequate knowledge base and the experience to prescribe psychotropic medications. This knowledge and experience are especially important when the alternative is for these problems to be left unattended. Although a nonpharmacologic approach to psychiatric illness may be beneficial, most dermatologists have neither the time nor the training to conduct such treatment modalities. In this chapter, a clinically useful way of classifying psychodermatologic cases is presented, followed by a discussion of the treatments for the major categories of psychopathologic conditions encountered in a dermatology practice. These categories include anxiety, depression, psychosis, and obsessive-compulsive disorder (OCD). The drugs discussed in this chapter pertinent to each of these diagnostic categories are listed in Table 20-1.

CLASSIFICATION OF PSYCHODERMATOLOGIC DISORDERS

There are at least two ways to classify psychodermatologic cases: first, by the category of psychodermatologic disorder, and second, by the nature of the underlying psychopathologic conditions.

■ Table 20-1 Psychotropic Agents

Generic Name	Trade Name	Generic Name	Trade Name
ANXIOLYTIC MEDICATIONS		ANTIPSYCHOTIC MEDICATIONS	
Alprazolam	Xanax	Pimozide	Orap
Buspirone	BuSpar	Risperidone	Risperdal
		Olanzapine	Zyprexa
ANTIDEPRESSANT MEDICATIONS		Quetiapine	Seroquel
Doxepin	Sinequan		
Fluoxetine	Prozac	ANTIOBSESSIVE-COMPULSIVE	
Paroxetine	Paxil	MEDICATIONS	
Sertraline	Zoloft	Fluoxetine	Prozac
Citalopram	Celexa	Paroxetine	Paxil
Venlafaxine	Effexor	Sertraline	Zoloft
Nefazodone	Serzone	Fluvoxamine	Luvox
Bupropion	Wellbutrin	Citalopram	Celexa
		Clomipramine	Anafranil

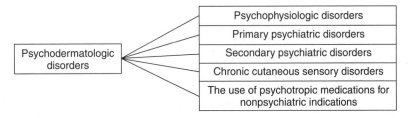

Figure 20-1 Classification of psychodermatologic disorders. (*Adapted from Koo J:* Curr Probl Dermatol *VII(6):203-232, 1995.*)

Five Categories of Psychodermatologic Disorders

Most psychodermatologic conditions can be classified into five categories. These are psychophysiologic disorders, primary psychiatric disorders, secondary psychiatric disorders, cutaneous sensory disorders, and the use of psychopharmacologic agents for purely dermatologic (i.e., nonpsychiatric) cases (see later section) (Figure 20-1).

PSYCHOPHYSIOLOGIC DISORDERS. Psychophysiologic disorders refer to psychodermatologic cases where a bona fide skin disorder is exacerbated by emotional factors such as stress. Some examples of psychophysiologic conditions in dermatology include atopic dermatitis, psoriasis, acne vulgaris, lichen simplex chronicus, and hyperhidrosis. With each of these conditions,

there are patients who experience a close chronologic association between psychologic stress and exacerbation of their skin condition, and other patients for whom their emotional state has negligible influence on the natural course of their disease (Table 20-2).

PRIMARY PSYCHIATRIC DISORDERS. Primary psychiatric disorders are conditions in which the patient has no real skin disease but presents instead with serious psychopathology; all the skin manifestations are self-induced. Some examples of primary psychiatric disorders include neurotic excoriations, delusions of parasitosis, factitial dermatitis, onychotillomania, and trichotillomania.

SECONDARY PSYCHIATRIC DISORDERS. Secondary psychiatric disorders describe pa-

■ **Table 20-2**   Incidence of Emotional Triggering of Common Dermatoses

Diagnosis	Proportion With Emotional Trigger (%)	Biologic Incubation Between Stress and Clinical Change
Hyperhidrosis	100	Seconds
Lichen simplex chronicus	98	Days
Rosacea	94	2 days
Dyshidrosis	76	2 days for vesicles
Atopic dermatitis	70	Seconds for itching
Urticaria	68	Minutes
Psoriasis	62	Days
Papular acne vulgaris	55	2 days
Seborrheic dermatitis	41	Days
Fungus infection	9	Days
Nevi	0	
Basal cell carcinoma	0	
Keratoses	0	

Adapted from Griesemer RD: *Psychiatr Ann* 8:49-56, 1978.

tients in whom emotional problems are the result of having a disfiguring skin disease such as vitiligo, alopecia areata, or cystic acne.

CUTANEOUS SENSORY DISORDERS.   Cutaneous sensory disorders refer to conditions in which the patients have only cutaneous sensory disturbances, such as itching, burning, stinging, crawling, biting, or any other disagreeable sensations on the skin, in the absence of a primary skin disorder or an identifiable underlying medical or neurologic condition. A psychiatric diagnosis may or may not coexist. Moreover, in some clinical situations, psychotropic medications may be preferentially used to treat purely dermatologic conditions, such as in postherpetic neuralgia where one of the best treatment options is the antidepressant amitriptyline (Elavil) because of its well-known analgesic effect.

These distinctions are important because they help guide physicians to select the optimal therapeutic approach for a given patient. For example, patients with psychophysiologic disorders or secondary psychiatric disorders usually welcome the opportunity to discuss their psychologic status. In contrast, some patients with primary psychiatric disorders are extremely resistant to talking about their situation in psychologic terms. In addition, because the clini-

cian is dealing with the skin and the mind simultaneously in psychophysiologic cases, the simultaneous use of both somatic (i.e., dermatologic) and psychotropic therapeutic modalities may be more effective than either one alone. In dealing with primary psychiatric cases, somatic modalities are at best supportive and are more likely therapeutically useless. For secondary psychiatric cases, the approach may be somatic such as resorting to a more powerful therapeutic option because of the great emotional distress suffered by the patient. An example would be the use of isotretinoin (Accutane) for borderline acne. The approach used may also be psychologically helpful, such as referral to a support group like the National Psoriasis Foundation or the National Alopecia Areata Foundation. Last, with cutaneous sensory disorders, successful treatment often involves a highly empiric approach to therapy with therapeutic trials with various psychotropic medications having analgesic or antipruritic effect or both.

Four Major Underlying Psychopathologic Conditions

In the first four categories of psychodermatologic disorders, the choice of a psychotropic medication is based on the nature of the underlying psychopathology involved. Most psychodermato-

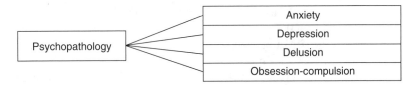

Figure 20-2   Common psychopathologies underlying psychodermatologic disorders. (*Adapted from Koo J: Curr Probl Dermatol VII(6):203-232, 1995.*)

logic patients fall into four underlying psychiatric diagnoses: anxiety, depression, psychosis, and OCD (Figure 20-2). For example, if the underlying psychopathology involves depression, an antidepressant would be a logical choice. It does not matter whether the patient presents with a primary psychiatric disorder (e.g., neurotic excoriations resulting from depression), a psychophysiologic disorder (e.g., psoriasis exacerbated by depression), or secondary depression resulting from disfigurement. As long as the underlying psychopathology is depression, an antidepressant would be the most appropriate choice. The same holds for anxiety, psychosis, and OCD where the use of antianxiety agents, antipsychotic agents, and antiobsessive-compulsive agents, respectively, may be indicated.

Any one of the psychopathologic conditions, such as anxiety, depression, psychosis, or OCD, can be found in any one of the five previously discussed categories of psychodermatologic disorders. The determination of the category of psychodermatologic disorders and the decision about the underlying psychiatric diagnosis are made independently. Also, it is important to recognize that dermatologic labels used to diagnose psychodermatologic patients may not give any information as to the true nature of the underlying psychopathology involved. For example, when a patient presents with self-induced skin lesions, the diagnosis of "neurotic excoriations" may be given. Even though this term contains the word "neurotic," the nature of the underlying psychopathologic condition may not involve neurosis. Patients may excoriate their skin in response to a variety of other psychopathologies such as anxiety, depression, or OCD. Therefore for each individual case, it is important to move beyond the dermatologic label to assess the exact nature of the underlying

Box 20-1

Symptoms and Signs of Generalized Anxiety Disorder

- Excessive anxiety and worry
- Restlessness or feeling "keyed up" or "on edge"
- Difficulty concentrating or mind going blank
- Irritability
- Muscle tension
- Stress
- Sleep disturbance (difficulty falling or staying asleep; or restless, unsatisfying sleep)
- Dizziness
- Sweating
- Palpitations
- Abdominal complaints
- Frequent urination

psychopathology involved to guide the psychopharmacologic therapy.

DIAGNOSIS AND TREATMENT OF ANXIETY DISORDER IN DERMATOLOGY

An anxiety disorder can manifest itself either as subjective feelings or as physiologic symptoms and signs. Subjective manifestations of anxiety include feelings of tension, agitation, stress, and an inability to relax. The physiologic manifestations of anxiety include muscle tension, sweating, shortness of breath, palpitations, and frequent urination (Box 20-1).

In general, psychodermatologic cases involving anxiety can be divided into two groups—

acute anxiety disorder and chronic anxiety disorder. The acute and time-limited episodes of anxiety usually involve specific situational stress such as increasing demands at work, interpersonal difficulties, or a financial crisis. Unlike patients with chronic anxiety, many of these patients with acute situational anxiety have a good premorbid functional level in society and have adequate coping skills; consequently, these patients usually recover from the crisis after a few weeks. However, this period of stress can be long enough to exacerbate their skin disorder. The use of an antianxiety medication (Table 20-3) may be indicated short-term to improve their psychodermatologic condition, especially if the nonpharmacologic measures are either not feasible or not adequate to control the patient's anxiety.

Specific Medications

Table 20-4 lists key pharmacologic concepts for anxiolytic medications.

ALPRAZOLAM.   For the treatment of acute and self-limited stress, an antianxiety agent with a quick onset of action is indicated. Alprazolam (Xanax) is a prototypical quick-acting benzodiazepine that is used to treat anxiety. Usually a half or a whole 0.5 mg tablet four times daily on an "as needed" basis appears to be adequate for most patients with acute anxiety. Because of the possible risk of addiction with long-term use, the physician should try to limit the duration of the treatment to no more than 3 to 4 weeks. In many cases, the situational stress resolves within this time period. For short-term usage, sedation is usually the only adverse effect encountered, and this can eas-

■ Table 20-3   Anxiolytic Medications

Generic Name	Trade Name	Generic Available	Manufacturer	Drug Category	Tablet/ Capsule Sizes	Standard Dosage Range	Price Index
Alprazolam	Xanax	Yes	Pharmacia Upjohn	Benzodiazepine	0.25, 0.5, 1, 2 mg	0.25-0.5 mg tid	$/$$ ($)
Buspirone	BuSpar	No	Bristol-Myers Squibb	Nonbenzodiazapine	5, 10, 15, 30 mg	15-60 mg/d (divided bid to tid)	$$/$$$

$,<1.00; $$, 1.01-2.00; $$$, 2.01-5.00; $$$$, 5.01-10.00; $$$$$,>10.00; ( ), generic price; /, two different price ranges from lower dose to higher dose examples of this drug; —, no price listed for this drug.

■ Table 20-4   Key Pharmacologic Concepts—Anxiolytic Medications

	Absorption and Bioavailability			Elimination		
Drug	Peak Levels	Bioavailable (%)	Protein Binding	Half-life	Metabolism	Excretion
Alprazolam	1-2 hrs	—	80%	12-15 hrs	Hepatic, active metabolite is alpha-hydroxy-alprazolam	Primarily renal
Buspirone	40-90 min	90%	86%	2-3 hrs	Hepatic CYP3A4, active metabolite is 1-pyrimidinylpiperazine	Renal 29%-63%, fecal 18%-38%

ily be controlled by dosage adjustment. Alprazolam differs from the older benzodiazepines, such as diazepam (Valium) or chlordiazepoxide (Librium), because the half-life is short and predictable, whereby most of the previous dose is metabolically inactivated or eliminated before the patient takes the next dose. Even though this feature of the newer benzodiazepines makes them much safer in terms of the reduced likelihood of accumulation of the medication in the patient's body, it also requires tapering the medication when the therapeutic course is complete. Even though the risk of physical dependency is extremely small with short-term usage, patients who stop alprazolam "cold turkey" may experience the recurrence of anxiety or even rebound anxiety. Alprazolam also has another advantage over the older benzodiazepines in that it may have an antidepressant effect, whereas most other benzodiazepines generally have a depressant effect.[1-5]

BUSPIRONE.   If the patient has chronic anxiety, buspirone (BuSpar) may be a safer choice for long-term use because it is an antianxiety medication that is nonsedating and does not cause dependency. Buspirone is not a benzodiazepine. The major drawback of this drug is that its onset of action may be delayed for 2 to 4 weeks so that buspirone cannot be used on an as needed basis. Buspirone has to be taken on a regular basis in dosages ranging from 5 to 10 mg 3 or 4 times daily to exert its most optimal effect. Because of the slow onset of action over 2 to 4 weeks, this agent is not appropriate for the treatment of acute anxiety such as in cases of acute situational stress. Therefore buspirone is not useful for the treatment of acute anxiety because the therapeutic effect may not become evident until after the stressful event has been resolved. Buspirone is generally well tolerated. Most patients experience no adverse effects.

DIAGNOSIS AND TREATMENT OF DEPRESSION IN DERMATOLOGY

Depression is frequently encountered in a dermatology practice. It can have subjective and physiologic manifestations. Subjective manifestations of depression include depressed mood, crying spells, anhedonia, and excessive guilt along with feelings of helplessness, hopelessness, and worthlessness. The physiologic manifestations of depression include insomnia, hypersomnia, loss of appetite, hyperphagia, difficulty with concentration, memory loss, fatigue, psychomotor agitation or retardation, and especially in older individuals constipation (Box 20-2). The easiest way to make the diagnosis of depression is to ask the patient questions such as "Are you depressed?" or "Have you been feeling very discouraged?" It is not unusual, however, for many patients to deny the fact that they are experiencing depression because they use denial as the primary method for coping with their depression. Frequently, this denial takes the form of somatization where they consciously or unconsciously focus on a physical complaint to diminish their awareness that they are feeling depressed.

When one encounters patients who deny their depression, it is frequently helpful to change the line of questioning to general medical inquiries. Patients are usually not defensive in responding to such questions. Consequently, one can obtain supporting evidence in making the diagnosis of depression by confirming the

---

Box 20-2

Symptoms and Signs of a Major Depressive Episode

- Very depressed mood
- Anhedonia (i.e., markedly diminished interest or pleasure in activities)
- Significant weight loss when not dieting, weight gain, or decrease or increase in appetite
- Insomnia or hypersomnia
- Psychomotor agitation or retardation
- Fatigue, lack of energy
- Helplessness, hopelessness, worthlessness
- Excessive guilt
- Difficulty with concentration, memory loss
- Suicidal ideation/plan
- Crying spells (i.e., finding oneself tearful for no reason or with minimal provocation)
- Somatization (i.e., preoccupation with vague, nonspecific, or exaggerated physical concerns but not of delusional intensity)

■ **Table 20-5**   Antidepressant Medications

Generic Name	Trade Name	Generic Available	Manufacturer	Drug Category	Tablet/Capsule Sizes	Standard Dosage Range	Price Index
Doxepin	Sinequan	Yes	Pfizer, Lotus, various	Tricyclic	10, 25, 50, 75, 100, 150 mg*	100 mg qhs (depression) 10-50 mg qhs (pruritus)	$ ($)
Amitriptyline	Elavil	Yes	Zeneca, various	Tricyclic	10, 25, 50, 75, 100, 150 mg	100 mg qhs (depression) 25-75 mg qhs (PHN)	$ ($)
Bupropion	Wellbutrin Wellbutrin SR	No	Glaxo-Wellcome	Atypical antidepressant	Wellbutrin: 75, 100 mg Wellbutrin SR: 100, 150 mg	200-450 mg/d bid	$$/$
Venlafaxine	Effexor	No	Wyeth-Ayerst	Atypical antidepressant	25, 37.5, 50, 75, 100 mg	150-225 mg/d bid	$$/$$$
Nefazodone	Serzone	No	Bristol-Myers Squibb	Atypical antidepressant	50, 100, 150, 200, 250 mg	300-500 mg/d bid	$$

PHN, Postherpetic neuralgia; $, <1.00; $$, 1.01-2.00; $$$, 2.01-5.00; $$$$, 5.01-10.00; $$$$$, >10.00; ( ), generic price; /, two different price ranges from lower dose to higher dose examples of this drug; —, no price listed for this drug.
*Doxepin also has a liquid formulation of 10 mg/ml.

![] **Table 20-6**   Key Pharmacologic Concepts—Antidepressant Medications

Drug	Absorption and Bioavailability			Elimination		
	Peak Levels	Bioavail-able (%)	Protein Binding	Half-life	Metabolism	Excretion
Doxepin	1-4 hrs	13%-45%	80%-85%	28-52 hrs*	Hepatic, active metabolite is desmethyldoxepin	Renal
Amitriptyline	1-4 hrs	30%-60%	90%-97%	9-25 hrs	Hepatic, active metabolite is nortriptyline	Primarily renal
Bupropion	2 hrs	N/A in humans; in animals (rats and dogs) 5%-20%	85%	Initial 1.5 hrs Second 14 hrs	Hepatic, active metabolites are hydroxybupropion, threo-hydrobu-propion, erythro-hydrobupropion	Renal 87%
Venlafaxine	Parent 2 hrs Metab-olite 4 hrs	N/A	Parent 25%-30% Metabolite 18%-42%	Parent 3-5 hrs Metabolite 9-11 hrs	Hepatic CYP 2D6, active metabolite is O-desmethyl-venlafaxine	Renal 87%
Nefazodone	1 hr	20%	>99%	2-4 hrs	Hepatic, active metabolites are hy-droxynefazodone, metachlorophenyl-piperazine, and triazoledione	Renal 55%, fecal 20%-30%

*Half-life of doxepin major metabolite.

presence of physiologic manifestations of depression such as insomnia and loss of appetite. Once the clinician is quite certain that the patient is suffering from depression, one should ask the patient open-ended questions regarding his or her personal, occupational, or financial situation in a sympathetic, nonjudgmental way. It is not unusual for depressed patients to come to realize the presence of depression as they talk about the difficulties in their lives. Once such an understanding is reached, it is much easier to obtain the patient's cooperation in treating underlying depression.

There are several antidepressant agents to choose from. Currently available antidepressants are generally equally effective, with 60% to 80% of patients responding adequately. Full clinical response is typically gradual. The initial

response to antidepressants usually begins in about 2 to 3 weeks after the optimal therapeutic dosage is reached. A minimum of 6 weeks of full-dose treatment is required before full therapeutic effectiveness is reached. Side effect profiles and toxicity vary substantially, so the choice of an antidepressant medication depends primarily on tolerability and safety. The antidepressants can be broadly separated into tricyclic and nontricyclic antidepressants (Table 20-5).

Specific Medications

Table 20-6 lists key pharmacologic concepts for antidepressant medications (Figure 20-3).

DOXEPIN.   The tricyclic antidepressant doxepin (Sinequan) is probably the ideal agent for the treatment of depressed patients with neu-

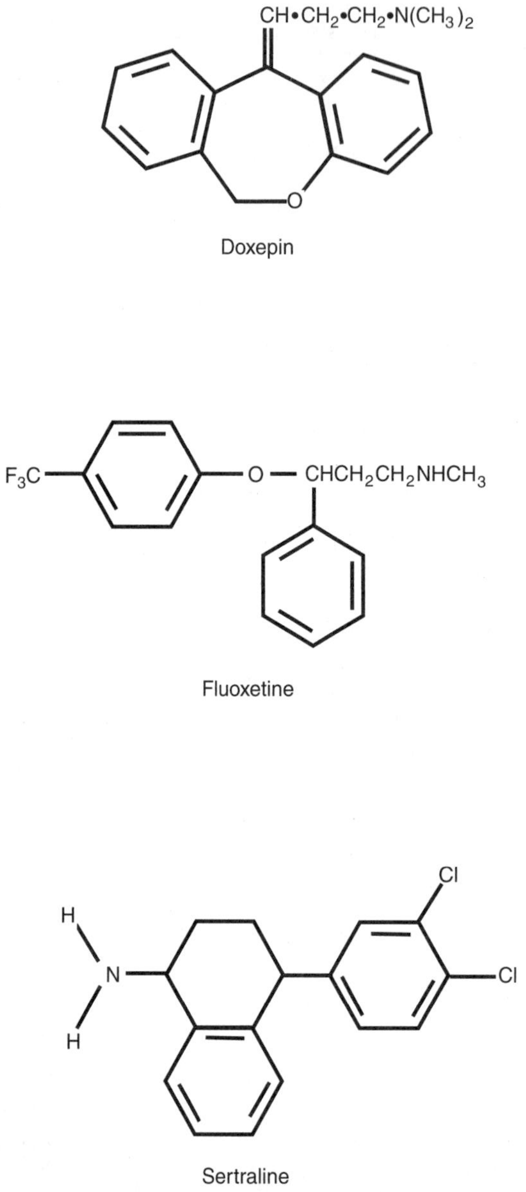

CH•CH$_2$•CH$_2$•N(CH$_3$)$_2$

Doxepin

F$_3$C— O — CHCH$_2$CH$_2$NHCH$_3$

Fluoxetine

Sertraline

Figure 20-3 Psychotropic agents.

rotic excoriations. In addition to its antidepressant effects, doxepin has strong antipruritic effects because it is a very powerful H$_1$ antihistamine. To stop the excoriating behavior, it is important to treat the patient's depression and to put an end to the itch/scratch cycle. Moreover, the majority of depressed patients who present with excoriations appear to be suffering from an agitated depression in which the patient paradoxically becomes more rest-

less, angry, and argumentative when depressed. For these patients, the most common adverse effect of doxepin, sedation, can actually be therapeutic.

The usual starting dosage of doxepin for depression is 25 mg at bedtime. The dosage can be titrated with 25 mg increments every 5 to 7 days, as tolerated, up to the usual therapeutic range for depression, which is anywhere from 100 to 300 mg. For depression, as stated previously, it generally takes at least 2 weeks after the therapeutic dosage is reached before the antidepressant effect can be observed. However, the other therapeutic effects of doxepin, such as the antipruritic effect, analgesic effect, and effects in calming the patient down and improving insomnia, generally occur right away. There can be up to twentyfold difference in serum blood levels among individuals who are taking the same dose of doxepin. Given this wide interindividual variation, patients who fail to show a therapeutic response despite taking a relatively large dose of doxepin for several weeks should have a serum doxepin level tested to see if it is within the therapeutic range for depression.[6] Table 20-7 lists drug interactions for tricyclic antidepressants.

The most common side effect of doxepin is sedation. The sedative effect of doxepin can usually be avoided by taking it at bedtime. More persistent sedation may require lowering the dose or changing the time of administration of doxepin. For example, if the patient complains of difficulty waking in the morning, this can usually be overcome by taking doxepin earlier than bedtime or by dividing the dose so that the patient takes some of the dose when he or she gets home and takes the rest at least 1 to 2 hours before bedtime. This way the patient is less likely to experience excessively high peak serum level and the resultant sedation the next morning. The other adverse effects of doxepin are similar to those of other older tricyclic antidepressants (TCA), including cardiac conduction disturbances, weight gain, orthostatic hypotension, and anticholinergic adverse effects such as dry mouth, blurry vision, constipation, and urinary retention. In terms of the cardiac conduction disturbance, the most prominent effect of a TCA such as doxepin is to prolong the QT interval. Thus older patients or any patient with a history of cardiac conduction disturbance should have a

Table 20-7   Drug Interactions—Tricyclic Antidepressants

Interacting Drug Group	Examples and Comments
THESE DRUGS MAY INCREASE THE SERUM LEVELS (AND POTENTIAL TOXICITY) OF TRICYCLIC ANTIDEPRESSANTS	
Anticonvulsants	Valproic acid
Antidepressants—other	Bupropion (various tricyclics), venlafaxine (desipramine)
Antipsychotic agents	Haloperidol may increase levels of tricyclic antidepressants
H_2 antihistamines	Cimetidine may significantly increase levels; no interaction with other H_2 blockers
MAO inhibitors	Concurrent therapy may induce a hyperpyretic crisis with CNS and cardiovascular complications as well
SSRI antidepressants	Various SSRIs, especially fluvoxamine (Luvox)
THESE DRUGS MAY DECREASE THE SERUM LEVELS OF TRICYCLIC ANTIDEPRESSANTS—CYP INDUCERS	
Anticonvulsants	Carbamazepine, phenobarbital both may decrease tricyclic levels and efficacy
Charcoal*	Administration may reduce tricyclic toxicity in an overdose
Rifamycins	Rifampin and rifabutin with similar effect due to enzyme induction
TRICYCLIC ANTIDEPRESSANTS MAY INCREASE THE DRUG LEVELS (AND POTENTIAL TOXICITY) OF THESE DRUGS	
Antiadrenergic agents	Clonidine
Anticholinergic agents	Various
Anticoagulants	Dicumarol
Anticonvulsants	Carbamazepine
Fluoroquinolones	Grepafloxacin, sparfloxacin (torsades de pointes—life threatening)
TRICYCLIC ANTIDEPRESSANTS DECREASE THE DRUG LEVELS OF THESE DRUGS	
Antiparkinson therapy	Levodopa absorption delayed and bioavailability decreased; may result in hypertensive crisis
Sympathomimetic agents	Various

Adapted from *CliniSphere 2.0 CD ROM*, St. Louis, June 2000, Facts & Comparisons.
*Charcoal reduces tricyclic levels but is not a CYP inducer.

pretreatment electrocardiogram (ECG) to rule out the presence of prolonged QT interval. In addition, an ECG should be repeated to rule out dysrhythmia if doxepin is used in dosages of 100 mg daily or higher. Doxepin should also be used with caution in patients with a history of seizure disorder or manic-depressive disorder because it can lower the seizure threshold and precipitate a manic episode. Because of the possibility of suicide with an overdose of TCA, it is good practice for dermatologists to see these types of patients frequently, at times as often as on a weekly basis. This follow-up interval allows the clinician to closely monitor the patient and titrate the dosage and reduces the number of pills the patient receives at one time.

SSRI ANTIDEPRESSANTS. The newer, non-tricyclic antidepressant agents known as the selective serotonin reuptake inhibitors (SSRIs) are the most widely prescribed class of antidepressants. The SSRIs include fluoxetine (Prozac), sertraline (Zoloft), paroxetine (Paxil), and fluvoxamine (Luvox). Recently, citalopram (Celexa) has been approved as well. All of the above SSRIs are Food and Drug Administration (FDA) approved for the treatment of depression except for fluvoxamine (Luvox). Fluvoxamine is FDA approved for OCD in children and adults but is just as effective as the other SSRIs for depression. However, many drug interactions with cytochrome P450–metabolized medications have been reported with fluvoxamine. Therefore it is not commonly used to treat depression because the other SSRIs are just as effective. Table 20-8 lists drug interactions for SSRI antidepressants.

 Table 20-8 Drug Interactions—SSRI Antidepressants

Interacting Drug Group	Examples and Comments
THESE DRUGS MAY INCREASE THE SERUM LEVELS (AND POTENTIAL TOXICITY) OF VARIOUS SSRI ANTIDEPRESSANTS	
Antidepressants—MAO inhibitors	Serious reactions occurred when various SSRIs used concurrently
Azole antifungal agents	Particularly ketoconazole (also itraconazole) may increase citalopram levels
H$_2$ antihistamines	Cimetidine may increase paroxetine and sertraline levels
Macrolide antibacterial agents	Erythromycin coadministration may increase citalopram levels
Other drugs	L-tryptophan (fluoxetine, fluvoxamine, paroxetine), dextromethorphan (fluoxetine) increase drug levels
THESE DRUGS MAY DECREASE THE SERUM LEVELS OF VARIOUS SSRI ANTIDEPRESSANTS	
Anticonvulsants	Phenytoin and phenobarbital both may decrease paroxetine levels
SSRI ANTIDEPRESSANTS MAY INCREASE THE DRUG LEVELS (AND POTENTIAL TOXICITY) OF THESE DRUGS	
Anticoagulants	Warfarin activity may be potentiated by all SSRIs
Anticonvulsants	Carbamazepine levels increased by fluoxetine, fluvoxamine, and citalopram
Antidepressants—tricyclic, other	Tricyclic antidepressants (by all SSRIs), buspirone by fluoxetine
Antipsychotic agents	Clozapine and haloperidol levels increased by fluvoxamine and fluoxetine; pimozide levels increased by fluoxetine
Benzodiazepines	Risk probably greatest with alprazolam in combination with SSRIs
Beta-blockers	Most noteworthy is fluvoxamine or citalopram effect on propranolol and metoprolol levels
Bronchodilators	Theophylline clearance may be decreased by up to threefold with fluvoxamine and paroxetine coadministration
Calcium channel blockers	Diltiazem and fluvoxamine concurrent use may induce a bradycardia
Lithium	Both increased and decreased levels reported with various SSRIs
Other drugs	Digoxin, methadone, sumatriptan, tolbutamide
OTHER POTENTIALLY IMPORTANT DRUG INTERACTIONS	
Alcohol	No clear cut interaction proven; however, concurrent use is discouraged
Alternative medical therapies	Concurrent use with St. John's wort may increase sedative-hypnotic effects
Smoking	Smoking significantly increases fluvoxamine metabolism

Adapted from *CliniSphere 2.0 CD ROM*, St. Louis, June 2000, Facts & Comparisons.

The SSRIs are as effective as the TCA in the treatment of depression but as a class have a much more favorable side effect profile. They are potent and selective inhibitors of serotonin (5-HT) reuptake at the presynaptic terminal. This pharmacologic characteristic results in an increase in 5-HT availability at serotonergic synapses. Unlike the TCA, SSRIs have no activity against the muscarinic/cholinergic receptors and are virtually free of anticholinergic adverse effects such as urinary retention, blurry vision, dry mouth, or constipation. They also have no activity against α-adrenergic receptors and are generally not associated with orthostatic hypotension, dizziness, and cardiotoxicity. They do not block histamine receptors in the CNS and are generally not associated with sedation, drowsiness, and weight gain. Instead of weight gain, patients on SSRIs tend to experience weight loss.[7] Because the SSRI antidepressants are typically better tolerated, compliance may be better, which may result in improved overall therapeutic outcome. Another significant advantage of the SSRIs is that a therapeutic effect may be achieved earlier because they require less dosage titration. For example, the starting dose for fluoxetine (Prozac) is 20 mg daily, which is within the usual effective dose, compared with TCA in which, due to the concerns regarding side effects, one has to titrate the dose over several weeks before the therapeutic dose is reached. The SSRIs are also safer in overdose situations than the TCA.[8]

The side effect profiles of the SSRIs are more alike than different, given their similar mechanism of action. Gastrointestinal effects, such as nausea and diarrhea, are the most common adverse reactions. Giving the medication with food often alleviates the nausea. Nausea usually improves after several days. Insomnia may occur with any of the SSRIs, but fluoxetine (Prozac) is more likely to produce anxiety and insomnia than the other SSRIs. The SSRI should be given in the morning if insomnia occurs. Sedation is more likely to occur with paroxetine (Paxil) and fluvoxamine (Luvox). If sedation occurs, the medication should be given at bedtime. Sertraline (Zoloft) is less activating compared with fluoxetine (Prozac) and less sedating compared with paroxetine (Paxil) or fluvoxamine (Luvox). The SSRIs can be associated with sexual dysfunctions. Most SSRI studies reveal an incidence of about 40% for sexual difficulties, most commonly involving difficulties with orgasm.[9] A variety of treatments have been used to alleviate antidepressant drug–associated sexual problems such as yohimbine, cyproheptadine, amantadine, and stimulants. However, none of these treatments have been demonstrated to work predictably or reliably,[10] and patients are generally reluctant to take a drug to treat the side effect of another drug, especially when dealing with sexual function side effects. When sexual side effects occur, switching to another class of antidepressants that causes less sexual dysfunctions than the SSRIs, such as nefazodone or bupropion, is recommended.

Like other antidepressant treatments, full clinical response to SSRIs is gradual. The onset of response to SSRIs usually begins in about 2 to 3 weeks, and 4 to 6 weeks is required before the full therapeutic effect is achieved. There is no linear relationship between SSRI dose and response. For partial responders, however, the dosage may be increased to maximize therapeutic effect. The lack of response to one SSRI or inability to tolerate one SSRI is not predictive of the same reaction to another SSRI. Patients showing no improvement after 6 weeks of SSRI treatment at the usual effective dose should switch to another SSRI or to another class of antidepressants (i.e., nefazodone, venlafaxine, bupropion).

On discontinuation, some patients may experience dizziness, lethargy, nausea, irritability, and headaches. These symptoms can be prevented by slowly tapering the medication over several weeks when discontinuing the drug.

VENLAFAXINE. It has been recognized for many years that most antidepressants are either potent reuptake blocking agents for noradrenergic receptors (i.e., many TCA) or serotonergic receptors (i.e., SSRIs). Previously in clinical practice, when a particular case of depression proved unresponsive to a norepinephrine reuptake inhibitor, the patient was tried on medications that preferentially block the reuptake of neurotransmitters in the serotonergic system and vice versa. Venlafaxine (Effexor) is a novel antidepressant that is believed to act by selectively inhibiting *both* norepinephrine and serotonin reuptake with little effect on other neurotransmitter systems.[11] It is an effective antidepressant, and a number of clinical studies provide evidence that venlafaxine may offer advantages over conventional therapy in terms of an increased number of responders and improved long-term efficacy.[12-14] In addition, clinical trials demonstrate that venlafaxine has anxiolytic effect and may be particularly useful in patients with mixed symptoms of depression and anxiety.[15-18]

Venlafaxine comes in two formulations—immediate release and extended release. Immediate release treatment begins with 75 mg in two divided doses with food. The dose can be increased by 75 mg/day after several weeks of treatment for partial responders. The usual effective dose is 75 to 225 mg/day on a twice-daily schedule. Extended release treatment begins with 37.5 to 75 mg daily with food. The usual effective dose is 150 to 175 mg/day. Venlafaxine has a relatively benign side effect profile. The most common side effects are insomnia and nervousness. Nausea, sedation, fatigue, sweating, dizziness, headache, loss of appetite, constipation, and dry mouth are also common. Like the SSRIs, venlafaxine may cause sexual dysfunctions after several weeks of treatment. Venlafaxine has been reported to cause hypertension in about 3% of patients and appears to be dose related. Blood pressure should be monitored during venlafaxine therapy, and venlafaxine-induced hypertension may be managed with standard antihypertensives. Venlafaxine can produce dizziness, insomnia, dry mouth, nausea, nervousness, and sweating with abrupt discontinuation. Consequently, it should be slowly tapered over several weeks.

NEFAZODONE.   Nefazodone (Serzone) has been shown to have the same efficacy as the SSRIs in the treatment of depression. However, it has little to no adverse effect on sexual functioning.[19] In addition to its antidepressant effect, clinical trials with nefazodone demonstrate that this drug significantly improves comorbid anxiety symptoms associated with depression.[20,21]

Nefazadone is different from the other antidepressants because of its dual actions on the serotonin system. It is a selective serotonin (5-HT2A) receptor antagonist, as well as a serotonin reuptake inhibitor of moderate potency. Treatment begins with 100 mg twice daily and increase dose after several days to weeks by 50 to 100 mg/day in partial responders. The usual effective dose is 300 to 500 mg/day on a twice-daily schedule. In general, nefazodone is a well-tolerated medication. The most common side effects are nausea, dry mouth, dizziness, sedation, agitation, constipation, weight loss, and headaches. Neither the incidence nor the severity of these effects is high. Historically, coadministration of nefazodone with terfenadine (Seldane), astemizole (Hismanal), or cisapride (Propulsid) is contraindicated due to the potential risk of toxicity that may result in life-threatening dysrhythmia (e.g., torsades de pointes). All three of these drugs have been removed from the market in the United States.

BUPROPION.   Bupropion (Wellbutrin) has been shown to be as effective as the SSRIs in the treatment of depression but causes very few sexual side effects.[22,23] Bupropion differs from all other types of antidepressants in its chemical structure and in its proposed mechanism of action. Bupropion is a relatively weak inhibitor of dopamine reuptake, with modest effects on norepinephrine reuptake and no effect on serotonin reuptake.[24] Bupropion comes in two formulations—regular release and sustained release. For regular release, treatment begins with 100 mg twice daily. After 4 to 7 days, the dose is increased to 100 mg three times daily. The usual effective dose is 300 to 750 mg/day divided into three equal daily doses. For sustained release, treatment begins with 150 mg daily. After 4 to 7 days, the dose is increased to 150 mg twice daily. In general, bupropion is a well-tolerated medication. The most common side effects are insomnia, agitation, headache, constipation, dry mouth, nausea, and tremor. A rare but serious adverse effect of bupropion is seizure induction. The incidence of seizures in patients receiving bupropion at therapeutic dosages of 450 mg/day or less ranges from 0.33% to 0.44%.[25] Bupropion should not be used in patients with a history of seizure or with conditions, such as bulimia, that may potentially lower the seizure threshold. This medication should be avoided in drug/alcohol abusers.

THE MANAGEMENT OF PSYCHOTIC DISORDERS IN DERMATOLOGY

Psychosis is defined by the presence of delusions or hallucinations. Patients with monosymptomatic hypochondriac psychosis (MHP) (Box 20-3) are psychologically "normal" in every way except for the presence of an "encapsulated"

Box 20-3

Symptoms and Signs of Monosymptomatic Hypochondriac Psychosis (MHP)

Presence of a *delusion* defined by
- A false belief
- The patient is absolutely convinced that the "idea" is true

The *delusion* is characterized by:
- Being "encapsulated"—i.e., has a very narrow and specific focus such as concerns about a particular parasite
- Somatic (physical) and hypochondriac in nature
- Differs from schizophrenia in that psychologic capacity outside of the chief complaint remains largely intact (e.g., proper affect, sociability, proper manners when discussing other aspects of life)
- Treatment of choice is pimozide (Orap)

delusional ideation that revolves around one particular hypochondriac concern and, possibly, hallucinatory experiences that are compatible with the delusion.[26-28] For example, many patients with delusions of parasitosis also experience formication, which is manifested as cutaneous sensations of crawling, biting, and stinging. MHP is very different from schizophrenia in which in addition to the delusional ideation, patients with schizophrenia often exhibit symptoms of other major psychologic disturbances.

Specific Medications

Tables 20-9 and 20-10 list antipsychotic medications and their key pharmacologic concepts.

PIMOZIDE. The most common type of MHP seen by dermatologists is delusions of parasitosis. The treatment of choice for delusions of parasitosis is the antipsychotic medication pimozide (Orap).[29-31] As with anxiolytics and antidepressants, careful titration of pimozide dosage is the key to safe use of this medication. Because of the possibility of extrapyramidal side effects, such as stiffness and restlessness, the clinician can start with a dose of 1 mg daily. The dosage of pimozide can be increased gradually by 1 mg increments every 4 to 7 days until the optimal clinical response is attained. Most patients experience significant improvement in delusional preoccupation, agitation, and formi-

◼ Table 20-9   Antipsychotic Medications

Generic Name	Trade Name	Generic Available	Manufacturer	Drug Category	Tablet/ Capsule Sizes	Standard Dosage Range	Price Index
Pimozide	Orap	No	Gate	Traditional antipsychotic	2 mg (scored)	1-6 mg qd	$
Risperidone	Risperdal	No	Janssen	"Atypical" antipsychotic	1, 2, 3, 4 mg (Liquid) 1 mg/ml	2-3 mg/d bid	$$$
Olanzapine	Zyprexa	No	Lilly	"Atypical" antipsychotic	2.5, 5, 7.5, 10 mg	5-20 mg qhs	$$$$
Quetiapine	Seroquel	No	Zeneca	"Atypical" antipsychotic	25, 100, 200 mg	300-400 mg/d bid	$$$

$,<1.00; $$, 1.01-2.00; $$$, 2.01-5.00; $$$$, 5.01-10.00; $$$$$, >10.00; ( ), generic price; /, two different price ranges from lower dose to higher dose examples of this drug; —, no price listed for this drug.

■ **Table 20-10**   Key Pharmacologic Concepts—Antipsychotic Medications

Drug	Absorption and Bioavailability			Elimination		
	Peak Levels	Bioavailable (%)	Protein Binding	Half-life	Metabolism	Excretion
Pimozide	6-8 hrs	N/A	N/A	55 hrs	Hepatic CYP3A	Primarily renal
Risperidone	1 hr	70%	90%	20 hrs	Hepatic CYP2D6 active metabolite is 9-hydroxy resperidone	N/A
Olanzapine	6 hrs	N/A	93%	21-54 hrs	Hepatic	Renal 57%, fecal 30%
Quetiapine	1.5 hrs	100%	83%	6 hrs	Hepatic	Renal 73%, fecal 20%

cation by the time the dosage of 4 to 6 mg per day is reached.

In Europe, there have been case reports of sudden death in patients with chronic schizophrenia who were treated with high-dose pimozide, possibly resulting from pimozide's potential for cardiac toxicity.[32] So far, we have never seen any ECG changes from low-dose pimozide used to treat MHP. However, a pretreatment ECG is recommended for all patients before starting pimozide to make sure that the patient does not have a dysrhythmia or prolonged QT interval. An ECG should be repeated after the patient reaches the dosage range of 4 to 6 mg daily.

Once the patient shows improvement in his or her clinical state and becomes nondelusional or "quietly delusional" (where the delusion or formication no longer significantly interferes with the capacity to work or enjoy life), this clinically effective dosage is maintained for at least 1 month. Should the patient persist in his or her improvement, the dosage of pimozide can be gradually decreased by 1 mg decrements every 1 to 2 weeks until either the minimum effective dosage is determined or the patient is successfully tapered off pimozide altogether. If the patient subsequently has an exacerbation of a delusional belief system and formication, the patient can be restarted on pimozide and once again treated in a time-limited fashion to control that particular episode. A minority of patients require long-term treatment with pimozide. Most patients with delusions of parasitosis can be treated on an "as needed" basis and can be successfully tapered off pimozide after 2 to 3 months of treatment. Long-term use of pimozide is best avoided to minimize the risk of tardive dyskinesias developing in these patients. Apart from tardive dyskinesia, there is an extremely rare condition called "withdrawal dyskinesia" in which the patient develops involuntary movements, especially around the mouth, when an antipsychotic medication such as pimozide is discontinued. Withdrawal dyskinesia is a benign, self-limited condition. Knowledge of this clinical entity avoids unnecessary concern on the part of the clinician about the possibility of tardive dyskinesia.

Because pimozide differs from the chemical structure of haloperidol (Haldol) by only one methyl group, the adverse effects of pimozide are almost identical to those of haloperidol.[29,30] The most common adverse effects encountered are the acute forms of extrapyramidal side effects manifested by stiffness and a subjective feeling of restlessness called akathisia. Akathisia is characterized by fidgeting, pacing, foot tapping, and an overall inability to sit quietly. Repetitive stereotyped movements, such as stroking the face, may also occur. Patients may also experience feelings of anxiety and an inability to relax.

Even though only a minority of patients treated with pimozide experience any extrapyramidal side effects, it is advisable for the clinician to explain the possibility of developing such adverse effects and to write a prescription for benztropine mesylate (Cogentin) 1 to 2 mg daily or diphenhydramine hydrochloride (Benadryl) 25 mg four times daily before starting pimozide. These medications can be initiated promptly so that should stiffness or restlessness occur, patients can promptly control these adverse effects. The advantage of benztropine mesylate over diphenhydramine hydrochloride is that the former agent is not sedating. As long as the extrapyramidal side effects can be controlled with one of the two medications as described, it is fine to continue with treatment with pimozide and even increase the dose until the optimal dosage is reached.

The most challenging aspect of managing patients with delusions of parasitosis or any other cases of MHP is to get them to agree to take pimozide. Truly delusional patients have little or no insight regarding the psychogenic nature of their condition and therefore are vehemently opposed to even the slightest suggestion that their condition may be psychologic. In addition, paranoid patients are typically suspicious and mistrustful of physicians. Moreover, if the MHP patient previously had negative experiences in their encounters with other physicians, they may be defensive and hostile. The question "How do you get someone with delusions of parasitosis to take pimozide?" is one of the most frequently asked questions in psychodermatology. One particular approach is presented here, providing a reference point to be utilized by other clinicians.

The first step in trying to manage patients with delusions of parasitosis successfully is to establish rapport with the patient. In trying to establish rapport with the patient, it is important to recognize that the patient with delusions of parasitosis is expecting the clinician to treat him or her as having a bona fide skin disease, not just as a psychiatric case. Therefore the most effective approach may be to spend relatively little time talking with the patient about psychologic issues. Instead, such patients need the clinician to take his or her chief complaint seriously. A careful and complete skin examination is critical not only in ruling out the presence of a true dermatologic diagnosis but also to demonstrate to the patient that his or her concerns are being taken seriously. If the patient brings in various specimens as proof of "infestation," it is important to at least look at them, once again to demonstrate to the patient that his or her con-

cerns are being taken seriously. At the same time, it is important to avoid any statement that may inadvertently reinforce the patient's delusional ideation such as commenting (falsely) that an organism responsible for his or her condition was actually found. Delusional patients are much more difficult to deal with if they believe that a clinician agrees with them about the delusion.

The process of establishing therapeutic rapport may take several visits. Once the clinician senses that a reasonable working relationship has developed between them, a therapeutic trial of pimozide can be gently introduced. There are many different ways to introduce pimozide. Even when these patients develop a trust in the dermatologist, they will most likely refuse the medication if the dermatologist presents pimozide bluntly and tactlessly as an antipsychotic medication. The dermatologist might irrevocably damage the therapeutic rapport in that setting. A more pragmatic approach would be to present pimozide as a medication that can help the patient by decreasing his or her formication (i.e., crawling, biting, and stinging sensations), agitation, and mental preoccupation. Patients usually experience significant symptomatic relief once they start taking pimozide, and this improvement can work as a further incentive for them to continue with the medication.

ATYPICAL ANTIPSYCHOTIC AGENTS. The use of pimozide and other traditional antipsychotic medications by nonpsychiatrists has been limited by serious adverse effects, most notably extrapyramidal side effects (EPS) and tardive dyskinesia (TD). A new generation of antipsychotic agents referred to as "atypical" antipsychotics entered clinical practice, which are as effective as conventional agents, such as pimozide and haloperidol (Haldol), yet better tolerated with a significantly lower incidence of EPS and TD, as well as less sedation and less weight gain. Three atypical antipsychotic medications are now the most prescribed agents for the treatment of psychosis. They are risperidone (Risperdal), olanzapine (Zyprexa), and quetiapine (Seroquel). These atypical antipsychotics are both dopamine (D_2) and serotonin ($5HT_2$) receptor antagonists. Atypical antipsychotics have greatly reduced risk for side effects such as EPS and TD because they are much more selective in binding to these receptors, which are thought to be related to its antipsychotic effects but not to other receptors that are related to side effects.[33-36]

Differing side effect profiles may guide the use of a particular agent for an individual patient. None of these newer agents have been compared to one another in "head-to-head" clinical trials. In addition, studies comparing pimozide with the new atypical antipsychotics in the treatment of delusions of parasitosis and other MHP have not yet been done. More research is needed to place these new drugs into clinical perspective.

RISPERIDONE. Risperidone (Risperdal) has been administered to over 1 million patients during its postmarketing period, and it appears to be generally well tolerated at therapeutic doses. Treatment begins with 1 mg twice daily, and the dose should slowly be increased every 5 to 7 days to the usual effective dose of 4 to 6 mg/day on a twice-daily schedule. After titration, the patient may take the entire dose at bedtime. The most common side effects are anxiety, dizziness, and rhinitis. Dose-related side effects include sedation, fatigue, and accommodation disturbance. Risperidone is known to prolong the QT interval and should be used with caution in patients with abnormal baseline QT intervals or those taking other medications that can prolong the QT interval (e.g., antidysrhythmics such as quinidine or procainamide). Risperidone-induced EPS are often negligible at a dose of 6 mg/day or less, but their incidence rises with higher doses.[34,35,37,38]

OLANZAPINE. Olanzapine (Zyprexa) is generally well tolerated, with a very low incidence of EPS. Start treatment with 5 to 10 mg daily. The usual effective dose is 10 to 15 mg/day. The most common side effects are sedation, anticholinergic effects (e.g., dry mouth, blurry vision, urinary hesitation, and constipation), and weight gain.

QUETIAPINE. Quetiapine (Seroquel) is a novel antipsychotic drug belonging to a unique chemical class, the dibenzothiazepines. Like the other atypical antipsychotic drugs, it binds to both D_2 and 5 HT_2 receptors in the brain, with a higher affinity for the 5 HT_2 site. Quetiapine also blocks histamine H_1 and α-1 adrenergic receptors. Some patients who fail to respond to other atypical antipsychotics respond to quetiapine. Treatment starts with 25 mg twice daily. The usual effective dose is 150 to 750 mg/day. Quetiapine is well tolerated in doses up to 750 mg/day. The most common side effects are mild somnolence and mild anticholinergic effects such as dry mouth, blurry vision, urinary hesitation, and constipation. Quetiapine is associated more often with orthostatic hypotension than the other newer atypical antipsychotics but is usually manageable with careful dose adjustment, and patients frequently become partially or fully tolerant of it.[39] Quetiapine does not seem to cause EPS.[40-42]

THE MANAGEMENT OF OBSESSIVE-COMPULSIVE DISORDER IN DERMATOLOGY

An obsession is a repugnant thought that repetitively intrudes into the thought process of the patient, whereas a compulsion refers to repetitious, stereotyped behavior that is very difficult for the patient to suppress (Box 20-4). The di-

---

Box 20-4

Symptoms and Signs of Obsessive-Compulsive Disorder (OCD)

- Presence of *obsession*—Obsession is a recurrent, intrusive, ego-dystonic (i.e., feeling foreign to oneself) idea.
- Presence of *compulsion*—Compulsion is a behavioral response to obsession. If suppressed, compulsive urge may build up.
- Obsession and compulsion need *not* both be present. The presence of one or the other is sufficient to make the diagnosis.
- Presence of varying degrees of insight (in contrast to psychosis, where, by definition, there is no insight).
- Six *approved medications* with antiobsessive-compulsive effect
    Fluoxetine (Prozac)
    Sertraline (Zoloft)
    Paroxetine (Paxil)
    Fluvoxamine (Luvox)
    Citalopram (Celexa)
    Clomipramine (Anafranil)

agnosis of OCD may be justified when either the obsession or the compulsion is of sufficient intensity to interfere with the patient's lifestyle or cause significant subjective distress. It should be emphasized that the diagnosis of OCD can be made without the presence of both obsession and compulsion because some patients present only with obsessions, whereas others present only with compulsive behaviors. For example, one patient may obsess about the "unsightly greasiness" of his or her face without engaging in any special activity to try to correct this "greasy complexion," whereas another patient may present with an irresistible compulsion to excoriate his or her acne without having any special thought process associated with the compulsion.

An obsession can be mistaken for a delusion because in both cases the patient presents with a mental preoccupation involving an overvalued idea. However, the key distinction between obsession and delusion is the presence or absence of insight on the part of the patient. Obsessive patients can usually acknowledge the bizarre, meaningless, or destructive nature of their obsessions and compulsions and yet be unable to stop the obsessive thought or the compulsive behavior. In contrast, delusional patients truly believe in the validity of their delusional thoughts. Frequently, patients with obsessive-compulsive behavior are even apologetic for their obsession or compulsion. For example, a patient with acne excoriée may say "I know I am not supposed to be doing this, and I know that if I keep picking on my acne I might really scar myself, but I can't stop picking on it because when I try to stop, I feel this tremendous urge to pick on my acne." The presence of such a compulsive urge intensifies until the patient finally gives in and engages in the compulsive activity, despite the presence of good insight, which helps differentiate OCD from a delusional disorder. There are many different manifestations of OCD or tendencies in dermatologic practice. These include trichotillomania, onychotillomania, onychophagia, acne excoriée, and some cases of factitial dermatitis and neurodermatitis.

Specific Medications

Tables 20-11 and 20-12 list SSRIs and their key pharmacologic concepts. In a dermatologic setting, a pharmacologic approach may be most feasible for patients who refuse to be referred to a psychiatrist. Currently, five SSRIs—fluoxetine (Prozac), paroxetine (Paxil), sertraline (Zoloft), and fluvoxamine (Luvox)—are the first-line therapy for the management of patients with OCD. Recently, citalopram (Celexa) has been approved as well. Clomipramine (Anafranil), a

▮ Table 20-11 Selective Serotonin Reuptake Inhibitors

Generic Name	Trade Name	Generic Available	Manu-facturer	Drug Category	Tablet/ Capsule Sizes	Standard Dosage Range	Price Index
Fluoxetine	Prozac	No	Lilly	SSRI	10, 20 mg*	20-60 mg/d (bid if >20 mg/d)	$$$
Paroxetine	Paxil	No	SmithKline Beecham	SSRI	20, 30 mg	20-50 mg qd	$$$
Sertraline	Zoloft	No	Pfizer	SSRI	25, 50, 100 mg	50-200 mg qd	$$$
Fluvoxamine	Luvox	No	Solvay	SSRI	25, 50, 100 mg	100-300 mg/d bid	$$$
Citalopram	Celexa	No	Forest	SSRI	20, 40 mg	20-60 mg/d	$$/$$$

SSRI, Selective serotonin reuptake inhibitors; $, <1.00; $$, 1.01-2.00; $$$, 2.01-5.00; $$$$, 5.01-10.00; $$$$$, >10.00; ( ), generic price; /, two different price ranges from lower dose to higher dose examples of this drug; —, no price listed for this drug.
*Fluoxetine also has a liquid formulation available in 20 mg/5 ml.

■ **Table 20-12**   Key Pharmacologic Concepts—Selective Serotonin Reuptake Inhibitors

Drug	Absorption and Bioavailability			Elimination		
	Peak Levels	Bioavail-able (%)	Protein Binding	Half-life	Metab-olism	Excretion
Fluoxetine	6-8 hrs	N/A	94.5%	1-3 days after acute administration and 4-6 days after chronic administration; norfluoxetine 4-16 days	Hepatic	Renal
Paroxetine	5.2 hrs	N/A	93%-95%	21 hrs	Hepatic	Renal 64%, fecal 36%
Sertraline	4.5-8.4 hrs	N/A	98%	26 hrs	Hepatic	Renal 40%-45%, fecal 40%-45%
Fluvoxamine	3-8 hrs	53%	80%	15.6 hrs	Hepatic	Renal 94%
Citalopram	4 hrs	80%	80%	35 hrs	Hepatic	Renal 20%

TCA with specificity for serotonin, also has well-demonstrated efficacy for OCD.[43-47] However, because head-to-head comparisons of SSRIs to clomipramine generally show the former to be equally effective but much better tolerated and safer when taken in overdose,[48,49] it is generally recommended that dermatologists use an SSRI to treat OCD rather than clomipramine. Like other TCA, the side effect profile of clomipramine, especially sedation and anticholinergic effects, such as blurry vision, dry mouth, constipation, and urinary retention, often prevents patients from achieving an adequate dosage. SSRIs may also cause cardiac conduction disturbance, orthostatic hypotension, and weight gain and be toxic in overdose.

SSRI ANTIDEPRESSANT CHOICE. The choice of a particular SSRI depends primarily on the individual side effect profiles, although they are more alike than different (see previous section on SSRIs). Many clinicians find that patients with OCD often require higher doses of SSRIs when treating obsessive-compulsive symptoms and take longer to respond than when treating depression. In OCD, initial response to SSRIs can take 4 to 8 weeks, and maximal response may take as long as 20 weeks. Af-

ter 6 weeks of therapy, the response should be assessed and the dose increased for patients with partial response. Complete remission is unusual. A 10- to 12-week trial with an SSRI at therapeutic dosage is the minimum necessary to confirm failure to respond. A failure to respond to one SSRI does not predict failure to respond to another.[50] For nonresponders, a 10-week trial of an SSRI followed by a switch to another SSRI is the most recommended current practice if a psychiatric referral is not feasible. Therapy should be continued for at least 6 months to 1 year once a therapeutic response is achieved.[51] Medications should be tapered slowly during discontinuation and should be restarted if symptoms worsen.

No matter which medication one chooses to use, it is important to tell the patient that these medications are not "magic bullets." They can be very helpful in overcoming one's obsessive thoughts or compulsive behaviors, but these medications are no substitute for the patient's own motivation to stop the destructive behavior. Therefore patients should be encouraged to keep up their own efforts and vigilance in controlling their compulsive behavior while they undergo treatment with antiobsessive-compulsive medications.

PSYCHOPHARMACOLOGIC MEDICATIONS FOR TREATING PURELY DERMATOLOGIC CONDITIONS

Certain psychopharmacologic agents are known to be useful in treating purely dermatologic conditions. The class of medications with the most well-documented analgesic effect is the older tertiary TCA such as doxepin (Sinequan) and amitriptyline (Elavil).[52-57] If pruritus is the primary problem, doxepin is the preferred agent. On the other hand, if various manifestations of pain, such as burning, stinging, biting, or chafing, are the primary sensations, amitriptyline is the preferred agent.

Doxepin is frequently used to treat pruritus when more conventional antipruritic agents, such as diphenhydramine (Benadryl) or hydroxyzine (Atarax), prove inadequate. There are several advantages of using doxepin for the control of pruritus compared with the conventional antipruritic agents. First, doxepin has a much higher affinity for histamine receptors than do the traditional antihistamines and may therefore exert a much more powerful antipruritic effect. The affinity of doxepin for histamine (H_1) receptor in vitro is approximately 56 times that of hydroxyzine and 775 times that of diphenhydramine.[58] Second, the therapeutic effect of doxepin is much longer-lasting than either of these H_1-antihistamine medications. Because of its long half-life, doxepin taken once per day, usually at bedtime, is adequate to provide therapeutic benefit for up to 24 hours. With diphenhydramine and hydroxyzine, patients with severely pruritic conditions, such as atopic dermatitis, frequently wake up in the middle of the night from pruritus when blood levels of these medications are no longer in the therapeutic range. Third, doxepin normalizes sleep curves. When the patient spends more time in a deeper state of sleep, the amount of nighttime excoriation often dramatically diminishes.[59] Doxepin can also be helpful in treating patients with chronic urticaria or other disorders mediated by histamines who have failed treatment with traditional antihistamines.[60,61] There are no good data regarding the optimal therapeutic blood level of doxepin for treatment of conditions such as pruritus or urticaria. A wide dosage range may be adequate depending on the individual patient. For example, the dosage of doxepin adequate for control of pruritus may range from as little as 10 mg nightly to as much as 300 mg nightly, which is the maximum recommended dose according to the package insert. If a patient is not showing an initial desirable therapeutic response, the clinician should gradually titrate the doxepin dose upward as tolerated until the desired therapeutic response is seen.

Amitriptyline is the treatment of choice for postherpetic neuralgia. When TCA are used as analgesics, the dosage required tends to be much less than the dosage required for its antidepressant effect. Therefore when amitriptyline is used to treat postherpetic neuralgia, the effective dosage range is from 25 to 75 mg at bedtime, which is much less than the usual antidepressant dosage of 100 mg at bedtime or higher.[52-54]

The efficacy of TCA as analgesics is most well established with the older TCA such as doxepin or amitriptyline. These medications are also the most difficult TCA to tolerate because of the relative frequency of sedative, cardiac, anticholinergic, and α-adrenergic adverse effects, including orthostatic hypotension, which can be particularly problematic in elderly patients. These adverse effects can be minimized by the use of a lowest possible effective dose. If the patient cannot tolerate these agents, other TCA, such as imipramine (Tofranil) or desipramine (Norpramin, Pertofrane), may be used.[62] The dosage range for these medications is very similar to that of amitriptyline in that the patient can be started at 25 mg at bedtime and titrated to the maximally effective dose. For use as an analgesic, a dosage of 100 mg per day or less should suffice. If the patient still cannot tolerated the newer TCA, then an SSRI antidepressant, such as fluoxetine (Prozac), can be tried. There are some reports of SSRI antidepressants usefulness as analgesic agents.[63]

SUMMARY

This chapter presents relatively detailed explanations regarding the use of selected psychopharmacologic agents along with their psychodermatologic indications. For a more complete description regarding the use of these medications, the reader is advised to consult standard textbooks on psychopharmacology and the *Physicians' Desk Reference*. It should be emphasized that psychiatric consultation should be obtained whenever feasible. For a significant proportion of patients who refuse psychiatric referral, the judicious use of these medications may still provide the much-needed assistance in the recovery of these patients from various psychodermatologic disorders.

Bibliography

Casey DE: Side effect profiles of new antipsychotic agents. *J Clin Psychiatry* 57(Suppl 11):40-45, 1996.

Gupta MA, Gupta AK: Psychodermatology: an update. *J Am Acad Dermatol* 34:1030-1046, 1996.

Koo J: Psychodermatology: a practical manual for clinicians. *Curr Prob Dermatol* 7:203-225, 1995.

Koo J, Gambla C: Delusions of parasitosis and other forms of monosymptomatic hypochondriacal psychosis. General discussion and case illustrations. *Dermatol Clin* 14:429-438, 1996.

Koo J, Gambla C: Psychopharmacology for dermatologic patients. *Dermatol Clin* 14(3):509-524, 1996.

Mourilhe P, Stokes PE: Risks and benefits of selective serotonin reuptake inhibitors in the treatment of depression. *Drug Saf* 18:57-82, 1998.

Rasmussen SA, Eisen JL: Treatment strategies for chronic and refractory obsessive-compulsive disorder. *J Clin Psychiatry* 58(Suppl 13):9-13, 1997.

Ritchelson E: Pharmacokinetic drug interactions of new antidepressants: a review of the effects on the metabolism of other drugs. *Mayo Clin Proc* 72:835-847, 1997.

References

Drugs for Anxiety Disorder

1. Remick RA, Keller FD, Buchanan RA, et al: A comparison of the efficacy and safety of alprazolam and desipramine in depressed outpatients. *Can J Psychiatry* 33:590-594, 1988.
2. Rickels K, Chung HR, Csanalosi IB, et al: Alprazolam, diazepam, imipramine, and placebo in outpatients with major depression. *Arch Gen Psychiatry* 44:862-866, 1987.
3. Schatzberg AF, Cole JO: Benzodiazepines in depressive disorders. *Arch Gen Psychiatry* 35:1359-1365, 1978.
4. Singh AN, Nair NP, Suranyi-Dadotte B, et al: A double blind comparison of alprazolam and amitriptyline hydrochloride in the treatment of nonpsychotic depression. *Can J Psychiatry* 33:218-222, 1988.
5. Warner MD, Peabody CA, Whiteford HA, et al: Alprazolam as an antidepressant. *J Clin Psychiatry* 49:148-150, 1988.

Drugs for Depression

6. Friedel RO, Raskind MA: Relationship of blood levels of Sinequan to clinical effects in the treatment of depression in aged patients. In Mendels J, editor: *A monograph of recent clinical studies*, Lawrenceville, NJ, 1975, Excerpta Medica.
7. Richelson E: Antidepressants and brain neurochemistry. *Mayo Clin Proc* 65:1227-1236, 1990.
8. Grimsley SR, Jann MW: Paroxetine, sertraline, and fluvoxamine: new selective serotonin reuptake inhibitors. *Clin Pharm* 11:930-957, 1992.
9. Settle EC Jr: Antidepressant drugs: disturbing and potentially dangerous adverse effects. *J Clin Psychiatry* 59(Suppl 16):25-30, 1998.
10. Gitlin MJ: Psychotropic medications and their effects on sexual function: diagnosis, biology, and treatment approaches. *J Clin Psychiatry* 55:406-413, 1994.

11. Montgomery SA: Venlafaxine: a new dimension in antidepressant pharmacotherapy. *J Clin Psychiatry* 54:119-126, 1993.

12. Clerc GE, Ruimy P, Verdeau-Pailles J: A double-blind comparison of venlafaxine and fluoxetine in patients hospitalized for major depression and melancholia. *Int Clin Psychopharmacol* 9:139-143, 1994.

13. Lecrubier Y, Bourin M, Moon CAL, et al: Efficacy of venlafaxine in depressive illness in general practice. *Acta Psychiatr Scand* 95:485-493, 1997.

14. Shrivastava RK, Cohn C, Crowder J, et al: Long-term safety and clinical acceptability of venlafaxine and imipramine in outpatients with major depression. *J Clin Psychopharmacol* 14:322-329, 1994.

15. Silverstone PH, Ravindran A, for the Venlafaxine XR 360 Canadian Study Group: Once-daily venlafaxine extended release (XR) compared with fluoxetine in outpatients with depression and anxiety. *J Clin Psychiatry* 60:22-28, 1999.

16. Haskins JT, Aguiar L, Pallay A, et al, for the Venlafaxine XR 210 Study Group: Double-blind, placebo-controlled study of once daily venlafaxine XR in outpatients with generalized anxiety disorder (abstract). Presented at the 11th Congress of the European College of Neuropsychopharmacology; Oct 31-Nov 4, 1998; Paris, France.

17. Haskins JT, Rudolph R, Aguiar L, et al, for the Venlafaxine XR 214 Study Group: Double-blind, placebo-/comparator-controlled study of once daily venlafaxine XR and buspirone in outpatients with generalized anxiety disorder (abstract). Presented at the 11th Congress of the European College of Neuropsychopharmacology; Oct 31-Nov 4, 1998; Paris, France.

18. Haskins JT, Rudolph R, Aguiar L, et al, for the Venlafaxine XR 218 Study Group: Venlafaxine XR is an efficacious short- and long-term treatment for generalized anxiety disorder (abstract). Presented at the 11th Congress of the European College of Neuropsychopharmacology; Oct 31-Nov 4, 1998; Paris, France.

19. Feiger A, Kiev A, Shrivastava RK, et al: Nefazodone versus sertraline in outpatients with major depression: focus on efficacy, tolerability, and effects on sexual function and satisfaction. *J Clin Psychiatry* 57(Suppl 2):53-62, 1996.

20. Zajecka JM: The effect of nefazodone on co-morbid anxiety symptoms associated with depression: experience in family practice and psychiatric outpatient settings. *J Clin Psychiatry* 57:10-14, 1996.

21. Fawcett J, Marcus RN, Anton SF, et al: Response of anxiety and agitation symptoms during nefazodone treatment of major depression. *J Clin Psychiatry* 56:37-42, 1995.

22. Modell JG, Katholi CR, Modell JD, et al: Comparative sexual side effects of bupropion, fluoxetine, paroxetine, and sertraline. *Clin Pharmacol Ther* 61:476-487, 1997.

23. Kavoussi RJ, Segraves RT, Hughes AR, et al: Double-blind comparison of bupropion sustained release and sertraline in depressed outpatients. *J Clin Psychiatry* 58:532-537, 1997.

24. Richelson E: Biological basis of depression and therapeutic relevance. *J Clin Psychiatry* 52(Suppl):4-10, 1991.

25. Davidson J: Seizures and bupropion: a review. *J Clin Psychiatry* 50:256-261, 1989.

Drugs for Psychotic Disorders

26. Munro A: Monosymptomatic hypochondriacal psychosis. *Br J Psychiatry* 153(Suppl):37-40, 1988.

27. Munro A, Chmars J: Monosymptomatic hypochondriacal psychosis: a diagnostic checklist based on 50 cases of the disorder. *Can J Psychol* 27:374-376, 1982.

28. Bishop ER Jr: Monosymptomatic hypochondriacal syndromes in dermatology. *J Am Acad Dermatol* 9:152-158, 1983.

29. Damiani JT, Flowers FP, Pierce DK: Pimozide in delusions of parasitosis. *J Am Acad Dermatol* 22:312-313, 1990.

30. Hamann K, Avnstorp L: Delusions of infestation treated by pimozide: a double-blind crossover clinical study. *Acta Derm Venereol (Stockh)* 62:55-58, 1982.

31. Holmes VF: Treatment of monosymptomatic hypochondriacal psychosis with pimozide in an AIDS patient (letter). *Am J Psychiatry* 146:554-555, 1989.

32. *Physicians' desk reference*, ed 43, Oradell, NJ, 1989, Medical Economics Company.

33. Meltzer HY: New drugs for the treatment of schizophrenia. *Psychiatr Clin North Am* 16:365-385, 1993.

34. Deutch AY, Moghaddam B, Innis RB, et al: Mechanisms of action of atypical antipsychotic drugs: implications for novel therapeutic strategies for schizophrenia. *Schizophr Res* 4:121-156, 1991.

35. Gerlach J: New antipsychotics: classifications, efficacy and adverse effects. *Schizophr Bull* 17:289-309, 1991.

36. Davis KL, Kahn RS, Ko G, et al: Dopamine in schizophrenia: a review and reconceptualization. *Am J Psychiatry* 148:1474-1486, 1991.

37. Lieberman JA: Prediction of outcome in first-episode schizophrenia. *J Clin Psychiatry* 54(Suppl):13-17, 1993.

38. Meltzer HY: New drugs for the treatment of schizophrenia. *Psychiatr Clin North Am* 16:365-385, 1993.

39. Hansen TE, Casey DE, Hoffman WF: Neuroleptic intolerance. *Schizophr Bull* 23:567-582, 1997.

40. Arvanitis LA, Miller BG: ICI 204, 636, an atypical antipsychotic: results from a multiple fixed-dose, placebo-controlled trial (abstract). *Psychopharmacol Bull* 32:391, 1996.

41. Hong WW, Arvanitis LA, Miller BG, et al: The atypical profile of ICI 204, 636 is supported by its lack of induction of extrapyramidal symptoms (abstract). *Psychopharmacol Bull* 32:458, 1996.

42. Arvanitis LA, Miller BG, and the Seroquel Trial 13 Study Group: Multiple fixed doses of "Seroquel" (quetiapine) in patients with acute exacerbation of schizophrenia: a comparison with haloperidol and placebo. *Biol Psychiatry* 42:233-246, 1997.

Drugs for Obsessive-Compulsive Disorder

43. DeVeaugh-Geiss J, Katz R, Landau P, et al: Clinical predictors of treatment response in obsessive-compulsive disorder; exploratory analyses from multicenter trials of clomipramine. *Psychopharmacol Bull* 26:54-59, 1990.

44. Insel TR: New pharmacologic approaches to obsessive-compulsive disorder. *J Clin Psychiatry* 51(Suppl):47-51, 56-58, 1990.

45. Katz RJ, DeVeaugh-Geiss J, Landau P: Clomipramine in obsessive-compulsive disorder. *Biol Psychiatry* 28:401-414, 1990.

46. Swedo SE, Leonard HL, Rapoport JL: A double-blind comparison of clomipramine and desipramine in the treatment of trichotillomania (hair pulling). *N Engl J Med* 321:497-501, 1989.

47. Trimble MR: Worldwide use of clomipramine. *J Clin Psychiatry* 51(Suppl):27-31, 55-58, 1990.

48. Pigott TA, Pato MT, Bernstein SE, et al: Controlled comparisons of clomipramine and fluoxetine in the treatment of obsessive-compulsive disorder: behavioral and biological results. *Arch Gen Psychiatr* 47:926-932, 1990.

49. Zohar J, Judge R: Paroxetine versus clomipramine in the treatment of obsessive-compulsive disorder. OCD Paroxetine Study Investigators. *Br J Psychiatry* 169:468-474, 1996.

50. Leonard HL: New developments in the treatment of obsessive-compulsive disorder. *J Clin Psychiatry* 58(Suppl 14):39-45, 1997.

51. Rasmussen SA, Eisen JL: Treatment strategies for chronic and refractory obsessive-compulsive disorder. *J Clin Psychiatry* 58(Suppl 13):9-13, 1997.

52. Watson CP, Evans RJ, Reed K, et al: Amitriptyline versus placebo in postherpetic neuralgia. *Neurology* 32:671-673, 1982.

53. Max MB, Schafer SC, Culnane M, et al: Amitriptyline, but not lorazepam, relieves postherpetic neuralgia. *Neurology* 38:1427-1432, 1988.

54. Watson CPN, Chipman M, Reed K, et al: Amitriptyline versus maprotiline in postherpetic neuralgia: a randomized, double-blind crossover trial. *Pain* 48:29-36, 1992.

55. Feinmann C, Harris M, Cawley R: Psychogenic facial pain: presentation and treatment. *BMJ* 288:436-438, 1984.

56. Urban BJ, France FD, Maltbie AA, et al: Long-term use of narcotic/antidepressant medication in the management of phantom limb pain. *Pain* 24:191-196, 1986.

57. Eberhard G, von Knorring L, Nilsson HL, et al: A double-blind randomized study of clomipramine versus maprotiline in patients with idiopathic pain syndromes. *Neuropsychobiology* 19:25-34, 1988.

58. Bernstein JE, Whitney DH, Soltani K: Inhibition of histamine-induced pruritus by topical tricyclic antidepressants. *J Am Acad Dermatol* 5:582-585, 1981.

59. Savin JA, Paterson WD, Adam K, et al: Effects of trimeprazine and trimipramine on nocturnal scratching in patients with atopic eczema. *Arch Dermatol* 115:313-315, 1979.

60. Figueiredo A, Ribeiro CA, Goncalo M, et al: Mechanism of action of doxepin in the treatment of chronic urticaria. *Fund Clin Pharmacol* 4:147-158, 1990.

61. Lawlor F, Greaves MW: The development of recent strategies in the treatment of urticaria as a result of clinically oriented research. *Zeitschrift fur Hautkrankheiten* 65:17-27, 1990.

62. Kishore-Kumar R, Max MB, Schafer SC, et al: Desipramine relieves postherpetic neuralgia. *Clin Pharmacol Ther* 47:305-312, 1990.

63. Boyer WI: Potential indications for the selective serotonin reuptake inhibitors. *Int J Clin Psychopharmacol* 6(Suppl 5):5-12, 1992.

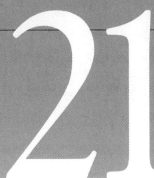
Loretta S. Davis

Newer Uses of Older Drugs—An Update

A number of systemic drugs used in dermatology have no dermatologic indications formally approved by the Food and Drug Administration (FDA). Still, many of these older drugs are being increasingly used for a wide variety of dermatologic conditions. This chapter reviews a number of these unrelated drugs and their potential dermatologic indications. Primary emphasis is given to colchicine, gold, potassium iodide, the attenuated androgens, and nicotinamide. The chapter concludes with brief discussions on nonsteroidal antiinflammatory drugs (NSAIDs) and potassium para-aminobenzoate (Table 21-1).

COLCHICINE

Colchicine is an alkaloid extracted from seeds and tubers of *Colchicum autumnale* (autumn crocus, meadow saffron). Since as far back as the 6th century A.D., the *Colchicum* species has been used for the treatment of acute gout. Not only is colchicine the most efficacious antiinflammatory agent for gout, but it is the drug of choice for treatment of familial Mediterranean fever.[1,2] In addition, colchicine is developing a therapeutic niche in the treatment of dermatologic diseases characterized by polymorphonuclear leukocyte (PMN) infiltration.[1]

Pharmacology

Colchicine has the formula $C_{22}H_{25}O_6N$ (Figure 21-1). Although it was synthesized in 1965, commercial preparations are still derived from extracts of *C. autumnale*, a widely available flowering plant. Colchicine must be shielded from ultraviolet light exposure, which degrades it into therapeutically inactive products. Peak plasma levels are reached between 30 and 120 minutes after oral administration of the drug. The drug is metabolized in the liver; the majority is eliminated through bile in the feces. Overall, 10% to 20% of the dose is eliminated unchanged in the urine.[1]

MECHANISM OF ACTION. Colchicine concentrates extremely well in leukocytes. It effectively binds to the dimers of tubulin, preventing the assembly of tubulin subunits into microtubules. Microtubular toxicity results in mitotic arrest at metaphase and interference with cell motility. Thus the drug is both antimitotic and antiinflammatory. Specifically, colchicine has been shown to decrease PMN motility, adhesiveness, and chemotaxis and to interfere with lysosomal degranulation. In addition to tubulin, colchicine binds to a number of other proteins. This protein binding may contribute to its ability in vitro to inhibit histamine release from mast cell granules, inhibit parathormone and in-

■ Table 21-1 New Uses of Older Drugs (An Update)

Generic Name	Trade Name	Generic Available	Manu-facturer	Tablet/Capsule Sizes	Special Formulations	Standard Dosage Range	Price Index
Colchicine	Various	Yes	Various	0.5 mg, 0.6 mg tablets	—	0.6 mg bid	($)
Nicotinamide	Various	Yes	Various	50, 100, 125, 250, 500 mg tablets	—	300-500 mg tid	—
Auranofin	Ridaura	No	Smith Kline Beecham	3 mg capsule	—	3 mg bid	$$
Potassium iodide	SSKI	Yes	Upshear-Smith	300 mg	Solution: 1g/ml	5 drops tid increasing up to ≥15 drops tid	—
Danazol	Danocrine	Yes	Sanofi Winthrop	50, 100, 200 mg capsules	—	200 mg bid-tid and taper	$$$ ($$$)
Stanozolol	Winstrol	No	Sanofi Winthrop	2 mg tablets	—	2 mg tid and taper	$
Para-amino-benzoic acid	Potaba, others	No	Glenwood Palasades	500 mg tablets; 500 mg capsules	Envules (powder) 2 g	3 g qid	—

$, <1.00; $$, 1.01-2.00; $$$, 2.01-5.00; $$$$, 5.01-10.00; $$$$$, >10.00; ( ), generic price; /, two different price ranges from lower dose to higher dose examples of this drug; —, no price listed for this drug.

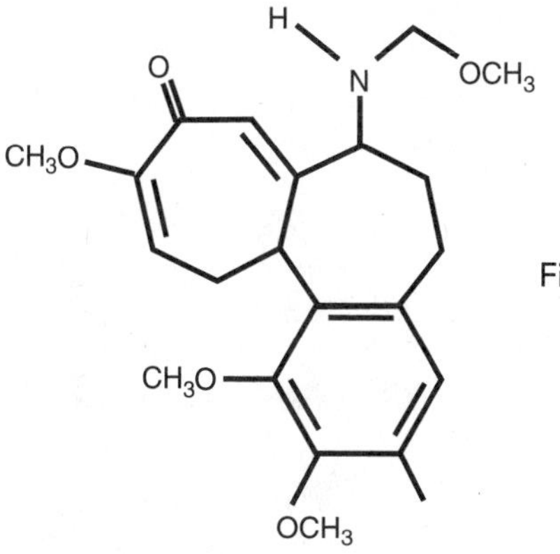

Figure 21-1 Colchicine.

sulin release, and inhibit melanosome movements in melanophores (i.e., dermal melanocytes of amphibians).[1,2]

Clinical Use

Table 21-2 lists indications and contraindications for colchicine.

OFF-LABEL USES

Neutrophilic Dermatoses. Colchicine's value in the treatment of acute gouty arthritis and familial Mediterranean fever is well established. Because Behçet's disease shares features with familial Mediterranean fever, it follows that colchicine might be efficacious in the treatment of this disease as well. Several uncontrolled studies and case reports document improvement in oral, genital, and ocular lesions of Behçet's disease with some benefit in associated erythema nodosum and articular complaints.[2-4] However, not all reports are as encouraging; one double-blind study revealed no difference in most parameters measured.[5] The intensely neutrophilic inflammatory infiltrate and enhanced leukocyte chemotaxis of Behçet's disease are also seen in recurrent aphthous stomatitis, for which colchicine has also been noted to have therapeutic efficacy.[6,7] Case reports suggest that colchicine may be useful in treating dermatitis herpetiformis[8] and Sweet's syndrome.[9] It has also been reported to be an effective treatment for linear immunoglobulin A (IgA) bullous dermatosis in both children and adults.[10-12]

Vasculitis. The use of colchicine in the treatment of cutaneous leukocytoclastic vasculitis is controversial. One prospective, randomized, controlled trial showed no significant therapeutic effect with colchicine compared with placebo but identified several patients who cleared with colchicine and relapsed with its discontinuation.[13] Many uncontrolled reports advocate the use of colchicine for treating chronic cutaneous leukocytoclastic vasculitis, citing a majority of patients achieving complete disease

Table 21-2	Colchicine Indications and Contraindications

FDA-APPROVED INDICATIONS
None specific to dermatology

OFF-LABEL USES	
Neutrophilic Dermatoses/Bullous Dermatoses	Papulosquamous Dermatoses
Behçet's disease[2-5]	Psoriasis[19,20]
Aphthous stomatitis[6,7]	Palmoplantar pustulosis[21]
Dermatitis herpetiformis[8]	
Sweet's syndrome[9]	Autoimmune Connective Tissue Diseases
Linear IgA bullous dermatosis[10-12]	Dermatomyositis[22,23]
	Scleroderma[23]
	Relapsing polychondritis[24]
Vasculitis	
Leukocytoclastic vasculitis[13-16]	Other Dermatoses
Urticarial vasculitis[17,18]	Pachydermoperiostosis[25]
	Type II lepra reaction[26]

CONTRAINDICATIONS	
Absolute	Relative
Hypersensitivity to colchicine	Serious GI, renal, hepatic, or cardiac disorders
Blood dyscrasias	

PREGNANCY PRESCRIBING STATUS—CATEGORY C (PARENTERAL FORMS CATEGORY D)

Contraindications from *CliniSphere 2.0 CD ROM*, St. Louis, June 2000, Facts & Comparisons.

control or being able to taper their concurrent steroid dose.[14-18] A beneficial effect on associated arthritis has also been observed.[15]

Papulosquamous Dermatoses. Logic dictates that colchicine, with its PMN suppression and antimitotic activity, would be beneficial in treating psoriasis and palmoplantar pustulosis. In many patients, favorable results have been observed.[19-21] Colchicine may work best for thin psoriatic lesions and as maintenance therapy after remission is obtained through another modality.[17]

Autoimmune Connective Tissue Disorders. Colchicine's suppression of local inflammation due to calcinosis in dermatomyositis and due to progressive systemic sclerosis has been reported.[22,23] Although colchicine was considered to be a possible therapy for the other cutaneous manifestations of progressive systemic sclerosis, prolonged colchicine therapy has not been shown to halt disease progression.[1]

Other Dermatoses. Anecdotal reports suggest that colchicine may be efficacious for a host of other diseases, including relapsing polychondritis,[24] pachydermoperiostosis with acro-osteolysis,[25] and mild-to-moderate type II lepra reactions.[26]

ADVERSE EFFECTS

Gastrointestinal Effects. The colchicine dosage for dermatologic conditions is typically 0.6 mg twice or three times daily; the dosage is subsequently tapered as disease activity allows. Therapeutic doses of colchicine alter both jejunal and ileal function in such a way that abdominal cramping, hyperperistalsis, and watery diarrhea can occur.[1] Most patients can tolerate 0.6 mg twice daily, whereas three times daily dosing often leads to these adverse effects. Diarrhea can be controlled with aluminum-containing antacids or specific oral antidiarrheal medications such as loperamide.

Colchicine Overdose. Overdosage can lead to a cholera-like syndrome with dehydration, hypokalemia, hyponatremia, metabolic acidosis, renal failure, and ultimately shock.[1,27] Respiratory distress syndrome, disseminated intravascular coagulation, and bone marrow failure may ensue. Other toxic manifestations include hepatic failure and late central nervous system disorders. Myopathy, hypocalcemia,

alopecia, stomatitis, and porphyria cutanea tarda have been reported in acutely intoxicated patients who ultimately survived.[1,27]

Symptoms of chronic intoxication may occur after prolonged therapy with at least 1 mg/day. Chronic complications include leukopenia, aplastic anemia, myopathy, and alopecia. Azoospermia and megaloblastic anemia secondary to vitamin B_{12} malabsorption have also been described.[1]

MONITORING GUIDELINES. It is suggested that complete blood counts, platelet count, serum multiphasic analysis, and urinalysis be performed at least every 3 months.[10] Monthly laboratory monitoring for the first few months of therapy is a reasonable protocol. Colchicine should not be used during pregnancy[16] (pregnancy category C).

GOLD

Chrysotherapy refers to the therapeutic use of gold. Chrysotherapy is a well-established modality for the treatment of rheumatoid arthritis. Gold therapy has especially been used in dermatologic practice to treat discoid lupus erythematosus and pemphigus.

Pharmacology

Gold remained a parenterally administered medication until 1985, when oral auranofin became available. The two parenteral agents, aurothioglucose and aurothiomalate, are completely absorbed; each has a half-life of about 6 days, and 70% of each is excreted in the urine. In contrast, auranofin is only 25% absorbed, has a longer half-life of approximately 21 days, and is excreted primarily via the hepatobiliary tract. Gold accumulates in highest concentrations in the reticuloendothelial system (i.e., bone marrow, liver, and spleen), as well as in the kidneys and the adrenal glands. Such tissue accumulation of the parenterally administered forms is much greater.[28]

MECHANISM OF ACTION. Gold compounds exert multiple biologic effects. In vitro, gold inhibits phagocytic and chemotactic responses of macrophages and PMNs.[28,29] Gold compounds inhibit the first component of complement and interfere with prostaglandin synthesis. They also inhibit lysosomal enzymes that may propagate inflammation.[28] It has been hypothesized that the beneficial effect of gold in treating pemphigus may relate to interference of blister formation by inhibition of degradative epidermal lysosomal enzymes.[30] Although anti-epithelial antibody titers decrease with chrysotherapy, gold compounds neither directly suppress antibody synthesis nor impair binding of pemphigus antibody to epidermal antigens.[30] A normalization of defective Langerhans' cell antigen presentation has been noted after chrysotherapy for pemphigus.[31]

Clinical Use

Table 21-3 lists indications and contraindications for gold.

INDICATIONS

Autoimmune Disorders. Chrysotherapy is FDA-approved for use in treating rheumatoid arthritis. However, it has also been used to treat psoriatic arthritis, as well as discoid lupus erythematosus and pemphigus.[28] Parenteral gold salts were commonly used for therapy of discoid lupus erythematosus until the advent of synthetic antimalarials, which were felt to be less toxic. Gold does remain a therapeutic option for patients with severe chronic discoid lupus erythematosus when other forms of therapy are ineffective or not tolerated.[32,33] Gold therapy for systemic lupus erythematosus has not been adequately examined.[34]

Bullous Dermatoses. Gold has been advocated as an adjunctive agent in treating pemphigus vulgaris and pemphigus foliaceus. Several case reports and small series argue for its efficacy in permitting reduction in steroid dose, concurrently decreasing antiskin-antibody titers, and inducing remissions of disease activity.[35-43] However, although most reports support the adjunctive use of gold in pemphigus, controlled studies have never been performed.[44] Gold compounds have also been advocated for use in treating cicatricial pemphigoid and acquired epidermolysis bullosa.[45]

ADVERSE EFFECTS

Mucocutaneous Effects. Unfortunately, chrysotherapy is associated with a high prevalence of adverse reactions. The incidence of mucocutaneous reactions is 40% with parenteral

---

Table 21-3	Gold Indications and Contraindications

FDA-APPROVED INDICATIONS
None specific to dermatology

OFF-LABEL USES

Autoimmune Connective Tissue Diseases	Bullous Dermatoses
Discoid lupus erythematosus[28]	Pemphigus vulgaris[34-43]
Systemic lupus erythematosus[33]	Cicatricial pemphigoid[44]
	Epidermolysis bullosa acquisita (EBA)[44]

CONTRAINDICATIONS

Absolute (for Ridaura)	Relative
Prior anaphylactic reaction to gold	None
Exfoliative dermatitis	
Aplastic anemia or other severe hematologic disorder	
Necrotizing enterocolitis	
Pulmonary fibrosis	

PREGNANCY PRESCRIBING STATUS—CATEGORY C

Contraindication specific to oral gold—auranofin.

gold therapy and 10% to 30% with auranofin.[45] A variety of cutaneous eruptions can occur; variants such as lichen planus–like or pityriasis rosea–like eruptions are well recognized.[28,46] These cutaneous eruptions may persist for several months after gold therapy is discontinued. Gold cheilitis and stomatitis may occur with or without accompanying dermatitis. When significant dermatitis does occur, therapy should be withheld but may often be resumed at lower dosages without triggering recurrent cutaneous toxicity.[28,46]

Gastrointestinal and Renal Effects. Of patients taking auranofin, 35% to 40% have diarrhea, which is typically managed by a decrease in the dosage. Gold-induced enterocolitis and intrahepatic cholestasis have been rarely reported.[28]

Proteinuria occurs with a frequency of 2% to 10%, more commonly with injectable gold than with auranofin.[45] The prognosis of gold-induced nephropathy is usually good if it is recognized early. Therapy is withheld until urinary changes resolve and may then be cautiously reinstituted at lower dosages. More severe nephrotoxicity is rare.[28,29]

Hematologic Effects. Hematologic side effects, occurring in approximately 1% to 2% of patients, include leukopenia, thrombocytopenia, eosinophilia, and in rare instances, aplastic anemia. Either direct bone marrow toxicity or allergic hypersensitivity phenomena are responsible for these reactions.[28,45] Significant leukopenia ($<4000/mm^3$) or thrombocytopenia ($<100,000/mm^3$) requires cessation of gold therapy until the role of gold in causing the abnormality is clarified. Eosinophilia has been noted to be a harbinger of gold dermatitis.[29]

Other Adverse Effects. Sudden dyspnea with diffuse bilateral pulmonary infiltrates is another rare reaction that can progress to chronic pulmonary fibrosis. Infrequent neurologic complications include acute progressive polyneuropathy and diffuse fasciculations.[28] Intrahepatic cholestasis and rare hepatonecrosis have been reported.[47]

Gold compounds can cause keratitis with corneal ulceration and can be deposited in both cornea and lens, producing chrysiasis.[28,29]

The nitritoid reaction is a vasomotor response characterized by flushing, dizziness, metallic taste, hypotension, and syncope occurring within 10 minutes of gold injection. The nitritoid reaction occurs almost exclusively with the aqueous gold sodium thiomalate formulation.[48]

There are several notable differences in the incidence of adverse effects of injectable and oral gold. Proteinuria occurs almost six times more frequently with injectable gold. Diarrhea is over three times more common with auranofin. Stomatitis and various cutaneous eruptions are slightly more frequent with injectable gold. Hematologic and liver adverse effects occur at a similar rate with both methods of administration (see the Ridaura package insert).

MONITORING GUIDELINES. When gold therapy is used, clinical and laboratory surveillance is mandatory. Initial screening should include a complete blood count with differential, platelet count, liver function tests, and urinalysis. Thereafter complete blood count with differential, platelets, and urinalysis should be checked before each parenteral injection and monthly with auranofin. Liver enzymes and bilirubin should be monitored every 1 to 2 months.[45]

THERAPEUTIC GUIDELINES. Dosage regimens for gold are those used for patients with rheumatoid arthritis. Parenteral therapy in adults begins with a 10 mg intramuscular injection. This is followed 1 week later by a 25 mg injection and subsequent biweekly 50 mg injections. Once a clinical response is obtained, the interval between dosages may be lengthened or the weekly dosage decreased. Children initially receive 1 mg/kg weekly, and the interval between dosages is subsequently lengthened to 2 to 4 weeks.[28]

In adults, auranofin therapy is initiated at 3 mg twice daily.[28] A total daily dosage of 9 mg may be required for selected patients. When disease control is attained, a daily dosage of 3 mg may maintain adequate control. Observations have been made regarding a longer "lag" time between institution of therapy and response with auronafin when compared with parenteral gold.[43] A cumulative dose of greater than 1000 mg of parenteral gold and a therapeutic course of at least 6 months for auranofin may be necessary to determine the efficacy of gold therapy in various cutaneous diseases.[45]

Relative contraindications to gold therapy include preexisting renal or liver disease, inflammatory bowel disease, prior gold-induced dermatitis, and bone marrow suppression. The safety of gold during pregnancy has not been determined. Gold does cross the placenta in significant quantities. It can be teratogenic in animals, and although teratogenicity has yet to be reported in humans, it must be assumed that gold is potentially teratogenic[45] (pregnancy category C).

POTASSIUM IODIDE

Potassium iodide has been in the physician's armamentarium for about 150 years. In *Diseases of the Skin*, Radcliffe-Crocker in 1908 listed syphilis, lupus vulgaris, eczema, and psoriasis as diseases in which iodine and iodide treatment were indicated.[49] Although more modern medications have been developed for the treatment of these diseases, potassium iodide remains useful in treating several dermatologic conditions. It is effective for cutaneous sporotrichosis and has found renewed enthusiasm as a treatment for a variety of dermatoses regarded as probable hypersensitivity reactions.[49]

Pharmacology

MECHANISM OF ACTION.   Potassium iodide has no effect on *Sporothrix schenckii* in vitro. Rather, its efficacy is probably mediated through alteration in the host's immunologic or nonimmunologic response to the organism.[50] Iodides concentrate in infected granulomas and necrotic tissue and have been shown to inhibit granuloma formation.[51]

Schulz and Whiting[51] speculated that the mechanism of action of potassium iodide in hypersensitivity disorders is due to an immunosuppressive effect mediated through heparin. Heparin, which is released in large quantities from mast cells by iodide administration, has been shown to suppress delayed hypersensitivity reactions.[51] Potassium iodide can also suppress the generation of inflammatory oxygen intermediates from activated PMNs and thus may confer protection from auto-oxidative tissue injury.[49]

Clinical Use

Table 21-4 lists indications and contraindications for potassium iodide.

| Table 21-4 | Potassium Iodide Indications and Contraindications |

FDA-APPROVED INDICATIONS
None specific to dermatology

OFF-LABEL USES

Fungal Infections	Hypersensitivity Reactions
Sporotrichosis[51,52]	Erythema multiforme[48]
	Sweet's syndrome[57-59]
	Pyoderma gangrenosum[60]
Panniculitis	
Subacute nodular migratory panniculitis[53]	
Erythema nodosum[48,50,54-56]	**Granulomatous Dermatoses**
Nodular vasculitis/erythema induratum[50,54]	Wegener's granulomatosis[61]
	Granuloma annulare[62-64]

CONTRAINDICATIONS

Absolute	Relative
Hypersensitivity to iodides	Hypothyroidism
	Cardiac disease
	Renal insufficiency
	Addison's disease

PREGNANCY PRESCRIBING STATUS—CATEGORY D

Concomitant use of potassium iodide and potassium-sparing diuretics can result in hyperkalemia.

OFF-LABEL USES

Sporotrichosis.   Although newer oral anti-fungals, specifically itraconazole, will most likely supplant its use, potassium iodide remains an effective agent for lymphocutaneous sporotrichosis.[52] The initial dose for sporotrichosis is 5 drops of the saturated solution (a drop contains 67 mg) three times daily in milk or juice. This is increased by 3 to 5 drops daily until a dosage of at least 15 drops three times daily is reached. Dosages up to 50 drops three times daily may be required. Lesions usually heal within 2 to 4 weeks, and therapy is continued for an additional 2 to 4 weeks.[53,54]

Panniculitis.   Reports of excellent results with potassium iodide in subacute nodular migratory panniculitis[55] prompted Schulz and Whiting[51] to use this drug for erythema nodosum and nodular vasculitis. Of their 45 patients, 40 responded; symptoms were relieved within 2 days, and lesion resolution occurred in an average of 2 weeks. Subsequent uncontrolled studies supported the beneficial role of potassium iodide therapy in these diseases.[49,56-58] Clinical response tended to be better in those who received treatment shortly after the onset of their disease. Improvement was most dramatic in patients with systemic symptoms such as fever and joint pains.[56] Dosages ranged from 360 to 900 mg/day; most patients received 900 mg/day.

Other Dermatoses.   Potassium iodide has also been advocated for use in treating erythema multiforme, Sweet's syndrome, and pyoderma gangrenosum. Although their studies were uncontrolled, these advocates reported prompt and dramatic improvement correlating with initiation of therapy.[49,59-61] Potassium iodide was also used with prednisolone to successfully treat a single patient with a limited form of Wegener's granulomatosis.[63] Treatment of granuloma annulare with potassium iodide is controversial, with a few reports of improvement after months of therapy and one double-blind report showing no significant advantage of potassium iodide over placebo.[64-66]

ADVERSE EFFECTS.

Overall, potassium iodide therapy is considered quite safe. Adverse reactions are usually associated with chronic therapy and are dosage-related.

Systemic Adverse Effects.   Chronic intoxication begins with an unpleasant brassy taste, a burning sensation in the mouth, and increased salivation. Coryza, sneezing, and eye irritation are common. Mild iodism simulates a head cold. Parotid and submaxillary glands may become enlarged and tender. Gastric irritation is common. Diarrhea, fever, anorexia, and depression may occur.[67] Vasculitic syndromes have been reported.[68]

Cutaneous Adverse Effects.   Skin lesions are remarkably common and varied and include acneiform, dermatitic, and vascular eruption patterns.[49,67,68] A distinctive vegetating eruption known as iododerma may occur with chronic low-dose ingestion or after one large dose of iodide radiocontrast dye, typically in the setting of impaired kidney function.[69] Paradoxically, both erythema multiforme and erythema nodosum have been attributed to iodide ingestion. Iodides are known to cause flare-ups of certain coexistent skin disorders, namely dermatitis herpetiformis, pyoderma gangrenosum, and pustular psoriasis.[70]

MONITORING GUIDELINES.

Iodide goiter, with or without hypothyroidism, may occasionally be induced by high-dosage, long-term potassium iodide therapy. Patients typically have an underlying thyroid disease. In these patients, there is impairment of the autoregulatory mechanism required to escape from the Wolff-Chaikoff effect (i.e., cessation of thyroid hormone synthesis caused by excess iodide inhibiting organic binding of iodide in the thyroid gland).[71] Thus before initiating potassium iodide therapy, patients should be closely questioned regarding previous history of thyroid disease. Thyroid gland size should be assessed. Note should be taken of concurrent medications, such as lithium and amiodarone, that can also affect thyroid function. Baseline thyroid-stimulating hormone (TSH), T_4, antithyroglobulin, and antimicrosomal antibodies should be checked in patients suspected of having an underlying thyroid disease.[71] Within several weeks of potassium iodide therapy, the autoregulatory mechanism of a normal thyroid gland should allow escape from the Wolff-Chaikoff effect. A TSH should then be drawn on all patients after 1 month of therapy.[71] Iodide-induced hypothyroidism is typically reversible with discontinuation of the iodide.[65,71] Finally, large doses should not be given to pregnant women because iodide goiter and hypothyroidism are commonly induced in the fetus.[65]

ATTENUATED ANDROGENS— DANAZOL AND STANOZOLOL

Synthetic derivatives of testosterone, danazol and stanozolol, have impressive anabolic properties with markedly attenuated androgenic properties.[72-75] These drugs are used to treat hereditary angioedema. Danazol has been used in gynecology for the treatment of endometriosis and fibrocystic breast disease. Both danazol and stanozolol have potent fibrinolytic activity and have been used for treatment of lipodermatosclerosis, cryofibrinogenemia, and livedoid vasculitis.

Pharmacology

Danazol and stanozolol are attenuated androgens alkylated in position 17-α. This alkylation causes a marked decrease in hepatic degradation of these hormones, permitting oral administration. A pyrazole ring attached to the steroid nucleus is felt to enhance the anabolic properties of these drugs, resulting in very large anabolic/androgenic ratios. Consequently, these drugs have very markedly attenuated masculinizing activity in comparison with their anabolic properties.[75]

MECHANISM OF ACTION.

The biologic properties of the 17-α alkylated androgens are exceedingly complex. They are known to increase concentrations of several plasma glycoproteins synthesized in the liver, including several clotting factors and the inhibitor of the first component of complement. Thus the beneficial effect of danazol and stanozolol in hereditary angioneurotic edema is a result of their direct effect on production of select hepatic-derived proteins.[76]

These drugs also alter the synthesis of hepatic proteins involved in the fibrinolytic process and thus have potent fibrinolytic properties. This stimulation of fibrinolysis is a property of oral (and not parenteral) anabolic steroids.[75]

Clinical Use
INDICATIONS

Hereditary Angioedema. Hereditary angioedema, an autosomal-dominant disease, is characterized by low antigenic or functional levels of the serum inhibitor of the activated first component of complement (C1 INH). This deficiency results in unopposed activation of the complement system with release of C2 kinin-like mediators and resultant episodic bouts of edema. Subcutaneous tissues, the intestinal wall, and the upper airway can be affected. Intestinal involvement typically presents as abdominal colic and may cause intussusception. Laryngeal edema can be fatal. Both danazol and stanozolol are FDA approved for the prevention of attacks of angioedema in patients with this disease.

Stanozolol therapy is initiated at a dose of 2 mg three times daily; danazol at a dose of 200 mg two or three times daily (see respective package inserts). After edematous episodes are successfully prevented, the dosages are slowly titrated downward. Long-term prophylaxis is typically obtained with doses not exceeding 2 mg daily of stanozolol or 200 mg daily of danazol. Alternate-day dosing regimens can also be effective. Dosages must be individualized; optimally, the lowest dose that will suppress life-threatening bouts of the disease should be used. Plasma C1 INH and C4 levels rise with therapy but need not totally normalize for clinical disease control to be achieved.[77-82]

Other Dermatoses. Additional therapeutic applications for the attenuated androgens take advantage of their substantial fibrinolytic properties. They have been shown to rapidly relieve the pain and heal the cutaneous ulcerations of cryofibrinogenemia.[83] They have been shown to improve the spectrum of lipodermatosclerosis,[84] as well as to effectively treat livedoid vasculitis.[85,86]

Some researchers suggest that attenuated androgens may have an ameliorative effect on mildly active systemic lupus erythematosus, decreasing immunoglobulins and improving thrombocytopenia.[87] In contrast, other researchers warn that in patients with hereditary angioedema, attenuated androgens may actually exacerbate or induce lupus erythematosus.[88,89] These authors and others speculate that attenuated androgens may either increase immune complex production or increase complement levels, providing additional substrate for ongoing immune complex disease.[90]

The use of attenuated anabolic steroids has been reported in a variety of other skin diseases including Melkersson-Rosenthal syndrome,[79] familial cold urticaria,[91] chronic urticaria,[92] Raynaud's phenomenon,[93,94] refractory pruritus associated with myeloproliferative disorders and several other diseases,[95] and pityriasis rubra pilaris.[96-98] The efficacy of such therapy in pityriasis rubra pilaris remains controversial.

One double-blind crossover study showed objective, but not subjective, improvement of peripheral microcirculation in systemic sclerosis with stanozolol therapy. In this same study, patients with primary Raynaud's phenomenon did not show the same improvement with stanozolol, probably reflecting a different pathogenesis of primary and secondary Raynaud's phenomenon.[94]

ADVERSE EFFECTS.   Adverse effects of danazol and stanozolol are clearly related to dosage and duration of therapy. When the lowest possible dosages are used, virilizing adverse effects are usually minimal. Nevertheless, mild hirsutism, deepening of the voice, alopecia, and acne have been reported to occur in female patients.[75,78,99] Weight gain and menstrual irregularities, including amenorrhea and menometrorrhagia, are well known to occur. Neuromuscular dysfunctions manifested as muscle cramps, myalgias, and elevations in serum creatine phosphokinase have also been described.[96-99] Reports of microscopic hematuria and actual hemorrhagic cystitis with attenuated androgen therapy are worrisome.[78,100,101] Exacerbation of symptomatic prostatic hypertrophy can be problematic.[75] Insulin resistance and mild deterioration of glucose tolerance may occur.[102] Episodes of anxiety and tremulousness, as well as exacerbations of underlying migraine headaches, have been described.[78] Because of the sodium-retaining effects of these drugs, worsening of hypertension and congestive heart failure may occur. Lipid profiles can be altered with an increase in low-density lipoproteins and a decrease in high-density lipoproteins. These drugs can also cause increased sensitivity to anticoagulants necessitating close monitoring of the international normalized ratio (INR).[75]

Because androgen derivatives can cause cholestatic jaundice, peliosis hepatis, and liver tumors, monitoring of liver function is advised.[103-107] Transient, mild elevations in hepatocellular enzymes typically return to normal with dosage reduction.[78] Hosea and colleagues[78] followed 69 patients on long-term danazol therapy and documented mild hepatocellular enzyme elevations in 14%. These elevations were usually less than twice normal and often normalized without altering the therapy.[78] Finally, danazol should not be used during pregnancy or childhood because of its possible interference with the child's normal sexual development.[72,74]

NICOTINAMIDE
Pharmacology
Nicotinic acid (niacin, vitamin B_3) is an essential dietary constituent, the lack of which leads to pellagra. In the body, nicotinic acid is converted to nicotinamide (niacinamide), which functions as a crucial coenzyme that accepts hydrogen ions in oxidation-reduction reactions that are essential for tissue respiration.[108] Both nicotinic acid and nicotinamide are readily absorbed from the gastrointestinal tract and distributed to all tissues.

MECHANISM OF ACTION.   The rationale for nicotinamide's diverse clinical trials has centered on its potent suppression of antigen- and mitogen-induced lymphoblast transformation. This suppression may be explained by its potent inhibitory effect on serum phosphodiesterase, with resultant increase in cyclic adenosine monophosphate (cAMP). Increasing cAMP concentration decreases the release of proteases from leukocytes.[109] For example, nicotinamide's use in treating granuloma annulare focuses on the increased activity of a cytokine found in this disease, macrophage migration inhibition factor. Accumulation of macrophages and granuloma formation in granuloma annulare may be inhibited by this drug.[109]

Other reports show nicotinamide to be effective in inhibiting antigen-immunoglobulin-E–induced histamine release; this inhibition blocks mast cell-mediator release in actively sensitized tissue in vitro. Thus in bullous pemphigoid, nicotinamide may work partly through mast cell stabilization, prohibiting the release of eosinophil chemotactic factor and other mediators of inflammation.[110]

Clinical Use

OFF-LABEL USES.   Both can be used for prophylaxis and treatment of pellagra that is due to poor nutrition, to Hartnup disease, or to carcinoid tumors.[108] In addition, nicotinamide has been used to treat a variety of seemingly unrelated cutaneous disorders. There have been anecdotal reports about the use of niacinamide in treating erythema multiforme,[111] dermatitis herpetiformis,[112,113] linear IgA dermatosis,[114,115] erythema elevatum diutinum,[116] polymorphous light eruption,[117] granuloma annulare,[109] necrobiosis lipoidica,[118] pemphigus,[115] and bullous pemphigoid.[110,119]

One randomized, open-label trial suggested comparable efficacy and fewer adverse effects using the combination of nicotinamide and tetracycline compared with prednisone as first-line therapy for bullous pemphigoid.[119] Another small review suggested that the combination of nicotinamide and tetracycline may be an effective alternative to steroids (e.g., in pemphigus foliaceus and pemphigus erythematosus) and a steroid-sparing adjuvant rather than steroid alternative (e.g., in pemphigus vulgaris).[115] Assessment of clinical response to niacinamide in treating autoimmune blistering disorders and erythema elevatum diutinum has clearly been complicated by concomitant tetracycline or erythromycin use in these studies. It has been proposed that the antiinflammatory properties of these antibiotics may function synergistically with nicotinamide in the treatment of diseases with excessive neutrophil chemotaxis.[110,116] Because tetracycline alone has been reported to clear bullous pemphigoid, it is difficult to assess nicotinamide's exact contribution in treatment of bullous diseases.[120,121]

Some researchers believe that nicotinamide has a beneficial effect in the prevention of polymorphous light eruption.[117] However, using phototesting, others failed to document this favorable response.[122]

In treatment of bullous pemphigoid[110,119] and the granulomatous diseases,[109,118] the dosage of nicotinamide has averaged 500 mg three times daily. Most clinicians initiate therapy at 200 to 300 mg three times daily. The concurrent tetracycline dose has typically been 500 mg four times daily although lower doses proved to be efficacious. Minocycline 100 mg twice daily has been substituted in patients with gastrointestinal distress attributed to tetracycline.[110,119]

ADVERSE EFFECTS.   Nicotinamide is considered a very safe medication with few adverse effects. Extensive information regarding adverse effects is available through the older literature on schizophrenia, for which the drug was used in dosages of 3 to 12 g/day. Headache and gastrointestinal complaints occasionally occur. Hepatotoxicity is considered extremely rare but may justify the monitoring of liver function tests in patients receiving long-term, high-dosage therapy.[123,124] Whereas nicotinic acid is a potent vasodilator, nicotinamide is not and thus is not typically associated with flushing and other prostaglandin-triggered side effects.[124] Also, whereas nicotinic acid adversely affects glucose tolerance curves, nicotinamide does not typically have the same effect. Diabetic patients should perhaps still be monitored.[124,125]

NONSTEROIDAL ANTIINFLAMMATORY DRUGS

NSAIDs refer to compounds whose molecular formula is based on a substituted phenolic or benzene ring that inhibits cyclooxygenase- or lipoxygenase-transformations of arachidonic acid.[126] At the present time, NSAIDs have limited clinical utility in dermatology; the cyclooxygenase inhibitors, aspirin and indomethacin, are the ones most commonly used historically.

Aspirin has been used in the treatment of erythema nodosum, although reports suggest that indomethacin may be a better drug for this problem.[127,128] Naproxen has also been shown to be efficacious.[129] Indomethacin is typically given as 100 to 150 mg daily in divided doses.

Aspirin has also been shown to be effective therapy for erythromelalgia.[130] This disease is characterized by severe burning pain, erythema, and warmth of the extremities (particularly the feet), typically provoked by environmental heat, exercise, and dependency. A single daily dose of aspirin is said to result in a dramatic relief of symptoms. Relief obtained with aspirin is reported to last for days, in comparison with improvement with indomethacin, which lasts for less than 24 hours. This difference is attributed to aspirin's irreversible inactivation of platelet cyclooxygenase, in comparison with indomethacin's reversible inhibition of this enzyme.[130] Unfortunately, therapeutic failures have been reported.[131,132]

Although indomethacin has been reported to help relieve the pruritus of late-stage HIV-1 infection,[133] NSAIDs are typically ineffective in alleviating the pruritus associated with common dermatoses.[134] In contrast, the pruritus of polycythemia vera is often responsive to aspirin therapy. There are increased numbers of skin mast cells in this disease. By directly suppressing mast cell prostaglandin metabolism, aspirin inhibits pruritus due to mast cell degranulation.[135]

Systemic mastocytosis may also be managed best with the cautious addition of aspirin after adequate H_1- and H_2-antihistamine blockade therapy. Aspirin effectively inhibits formation of prostaglandin D_2, an important mediator of systemic mastocytosis. The institution of aspirin therapy should be carried out with extreme caution because severe hypotensive episodes culminating in death have been described.[136]

The NSAIDs have been used with some benefit in treating several types of urticaria. Aspirin has been beneficial in nonimmunologic contact urticaria.[137] Aspirin, indomethacin, and ibuprofen all may improve delayed pressure urticaria.[138] Aspirin has also been used to desensitize patients with aspirin-induced urticaria and angioedema.[139] Indomethacin was found to be helpful in conjunction with heat desensitization for localized heat-induced urticaria.[140] Finally, indomethacin has been shown to be a therapeutic option in urticarial vasculitis.[141]

Significant but incomplete suppression of ultraviolet B (UVB) erythema has been documented with aspirin, as well as with oral and topical indomethacin.[142-145] Such observations suggest a possible role for these drugs in minimizing sunburn potential. In contrast to earlier studies, one report documented similar suppression of UVA-induced and psoralens plus UVA (PUVA)–induced inflammation with topical indomethacin.[145]

Clearly, the NSAIDs are better known within the realm of dermatology for their cutaneous adverse reactions rather than for their clinical utility in treatment of the aforementioned dermatoses. There are several complete reviews on this subject.[146-148] The cutaneous drug reactions commonly induced by NSAIDs include potentially serious entities such as Stevens-Johnson syndrome, toxic epidermal necrolysis, and anaphylactoid reactions.

POTASSIUM PARA-AMINOBENZOATE

Potassium para-aminobenzoate (Potaba) has been used to treat diseases of fibrosis, including progressive systemic sclerosis, morphea, linear scleroderma, Peyronie's disease, Dupuytren's contracture, and dermatomyositis.[149-152] The FDA has classified this drug as "possibly" effective for these conditions (see Potaba package insert). It has also been reported as effective therapy for lichen sclerosus et atrophicus.[153]

Potassium para-aminobenzoate is a member of the vitamin B complex; small amounts are found in cereal, eggs, milk, and meats. The mode of action of this drug is unknown. In early research on the drug, its antifibrotic effect was felt to be mediated through increased monoamine oxidase activity, which permitted increased oxygen uptake at the tissue level.[154] Later investigation documented the drug's ability to reduce acid mucopolysaccharide synthesis and glycosaminoglycan secretion.[155,156] Further studies evaluating the drug's mechanisms of action are clearly warranted.

The average daily adult dose of potassium para-aminobenzoate is 12 g given in four to six divided doses. Children receive 225 mg/kg (1 g/10 lb) in divided doses. Side effects are infrequent and include anorexia, nausea, fever, and skin rash. Hypoglycemia may ensue if the drug is administered through a period of inadequate food intake.[149] Hepatotoxicity has been described but is thought to be extremely rare.[157,158] Sulfonamides should not be concurrently administered because they are metabolic antagonists of para-aminobenzoic acid and its salts.[149]

Bibliography

Overview of Multiple Drugs in Chapter

Fivenson DP: Nonsteroidal treatment of autoimmune skin diseases. *Dermatol Clin* 15:695-705, 1997.

Colchicine

Ben-Chetrit E, Levy M: Colchicine: 1998 update. *Semin Arthritis Rheum* 28:48-59, 1998.

Sullivan TP, King LE Jr, Boyd AS: Colchicine in dermatology. *J Am Acad Dermatol* 39:993-999, 1998.

Gold

Papp KA, Shear NH: Systemic gold therapy. *Clin Dermatol* 9:535-551, 1992.

Thomas I: Gold therapy and its indications in dermatology. *J Am Acad Dermatol* 16:845-854, 1987.

Potassium Iodide

Heymann WR: Potassium iodide and the Wolff-Chaikoff effect: relevance for the dermatologist. *J Am Acad Dermatol* 42:490-492, 2000.

Kauffman CA: Old and new therapies for sporotrichosis. *Clin Infect Dis* 21:981-985, 1995.

Sterlin JB, Heymann WR: Potassium iodide in dermatology: a 19th century drug for the 21st century—Uses, pharmacology, adverse effect, and contraindications. *J Am Acad Dermatol* 43:691-697, 2000.

Danazol and Stanozolol

Donaldson VH: Danazol. *Am J Med* 87:49N-55N, 1989.

Helfman T, Falanga V: Stanozolol as a novel therapeutic agent in dermatology. *J Am Acad Dermatol* 32:254-258, 1995.

Nicotinamide

(See Fivenson review.)

Nonsteroidal Antiinflammatory Drugs

Lichtenstein J, Flowers F, Sherertz EF: Nonsteroidal anti-inflammatory drugs: their use in dermatology. *Int J Dermatol* 26:80-87, 1987.

References

Colchicine

1. Famaey JP: Colchicine in therapy: state of the art and new perspectives for an old drug. *Clin Exp Rheumatol* 6:305-317, 1988.
2. Harper RM, Allen BS: Use of colchicine in the treatment of Behçet's disease. *Int J Dermatol* 21:551-554, 1982.
3. Sander HM, Randle HW: Use of colchicine in Behçet's syndrome. *Cutis* 37:344-348, 1986.
4. Jorizzo JL, Hudson RD, Schmalstieg FC, et al: Behçet's syndrome: immune regulation, circulating immune complexes, neutrophil migration, and colchicine therapy. *J Am Acad Dermatol* 10:205-214, 1984.
5. Aktulga E, Altac M, Müftüoglu A, et al: A double blind study of colchicine in Behçet's disease. *Haematologica (Pavia)* 65:399-402, 1980.
6. Gatot A, Tovi F: Colchicine therapy in recurrent oral ulcers (letter). *Arch Dermatol* 120:994, 1984.
7. Ruah CB, Stram JR, Chasin WD: Treatment of severe recurrent aphthous stomatitis with colchicine. *Arch Otolaryngol Head Neck Surg* 114:671-675, 1988.

8. Silvers DN, Juhlin EA, Berczeller PH, et al: Treatment of dermatitis herpetiformis with colchicine. *Arch Dermatol* 116:1373-1384, 1980.
9. Suehisa S, Tagami H: Treatment of acute febrile neutrophilic dermatosis (Sweet's syndrome) with colchicine (letter). *Br J Dermatol* 105:483, 1981.
10. Aram H: Linear IgA bullous dermatosis: successful treatment with colchicine. *Arch Dermatol* 120:960, 1984.
11. Zeharia A, Hodak E, Mukamel M, et al: Successful treatment of chronic bullous dermatosis of childhood with colchicine. *J Am Acad Dermatol* 30:660-661, 1994.
12. Banodkar DD, Al-Suwaid AR: Colchicine as a novel therapeutic agent in chronic bullous dermatosis of childhood. *Int J Dermatol* 26:213-216, 1997.
13. Sais G, Vidaller A, Jucglà A, et al: Colchicine in the treatment of cutaneous leukocytoclastic vasculitis: results of a prospective, randomized controlled trial. *Arch Dermatol* 131:1399-1402, 1995.

14. Hazen PG, Michel B: Management of necrotizing vasculitis with colchicine: improvement in patients with cutaneous lesions and Behcet's syndrome. *Arch Dermatol* 115:1303-1306, 1979.

15. Callen JP: Colchicine is effective in controlling chronic cutaneous leukocytoclastic vasculitis. *J Am Acad Dermatol* 13:193-200, 1985.

16. Callen JP, af Ekenstam E: Cutaneous leukocytoclastic vasculitis: clinical experience in 44 patients. *South Med J* 80:848-851, 1987.

17. Muramatsu C, Tanabe E: Urticarial vasculitis: response to dapsone and colchicine (letter). *J Am Acad Dermatol* 13:1055, 1985.

18. Wiles JC, Hansen RC, Lynch PJ: Urticarial vasculitis treated with colchicine. *Arch Dermatol* 121:802-805, 1985.

19. Wahba A, Cohen H: Therapeutic trials with oral colchicine in psoriasis. *Acta Derm Venereol (Stockh)* 60:515-520, 1980.

20. Baker H: Pustular psoriasis. *Dermatol Clin* 2:455-470, 1984.

21. Takigawa M, Miyachi Y, Uehara M, et al: Treatment of pustulosis palmaris et plantaris with oral doses of colchicine. *Arch Dermatol* 118:458-460, 1982.

22. Fuchs D, Ruchter L, Fishel B, et al: Colchicine suppression of local inflammation due to calcinosis in dermatomyositis and progressive systemic sclerosis. *Clin Rheumatol* 5:527-530, 1986.

23. Taborn J, Bole GG, Thompson GR: Colchicine suppression of local and systemic inflammation due to calcinosis universalis in chronic dermatomyositis. *Ann Intern Med* 89:648-649, 1978.

24. Askari AD: Colchicine for treatment of relapsing polychondritis. *J Am Acad Dermatol* 10:507-510, 1984.

25. Matucci-Cerinic M, Fattorini L, Gerini G, et al: Colchicine treatment in a case of pachydermoperiostosis with acroosteolysis. *Rheumatol Int* 8:185-188, 1988.

26. Kar HK, Roy RG: Comparison of colchicine and aspirin in the treatment of type 2 lepra reaction. *Lepr Rev* 59:201-203, 1988.

27. Simons RJ, Kingma DW: Fatal colchicine toxicity. *Am J Med* 86:356-357, 1989.

Gold

28. Thomas I: Gold therapy and its indications in dermatology. *J Am Acad Dermatol* 16:845-854, 1987.

29. Penneys NS: Gold therapy: dermatologic uses and toxicities. *J Am Acad Dermatol* 1:315-320, 1979.

30. Penneys NS, Ziboh V, Gottlieb NL, et al: Inhibition of prostaglandin synthesis and human epidermal enzymes by aurothiomalate in vitro: possible actions of gold in pemphigus. *J Invest Dermatol* 63:356-361, 1974.

31. Blitstein-Willinger E: Behavior of cutaneous Langerhans' cells and skin reactivity after gold sodium thiomalate treatment of pemphigus vulgaris. *Dermatologica* 174:68-75, 1987.

32. Dalziel K, Going G, Cartwright PH, et al: Treatment of chronic discoid lupus erythematosus with an oral gold compound (auranofin). *Br J Dermatol* 115:211-216, 1986.

33. Haxthausen H: Treatment of lupus erythematosus by intravenous injections of gold chloride. *Arch Derm* 22:77-90, 1930.

34. Weisman MH, Albert D, Muelle MR, et al: Gold therapy in patients with systemic lupus erythematosus. *Am J Med* 75:157-164, 1983.

35. Penneys NS, Eaglstein WH, Indgin S, et al: Gold sodium thiomalate treatment of pemphigus. *Arch Dermatol* 108:56-60, 1973.

36. Penneys NS, Eaglstein WH, Frost P: Management of pemphigus with gold compounds: a long-term follow-up report. *Arch Dermatol* 112:185-187, 1976.

37. Paltzik RL, Laude TA: Childhood pemphigus treatment with gold. *Arch Dermatol* 114:768-769, 1978.

38. Poulin Y, Perry HO, Muller SA: Pemphigus vulgaris: results of treatment with gold as a steroid-sparing agent in a series of thirteen patients. *J Am Acad Dermatol* 11:851-857, 1984.

39. Frumkin A: Low-dose aurothioglucose in pemphigus vulgaris. *Isr J Med Sci* 22:903-905, 1986.

40. Walton S, Keczkes K: Pemphigus foliaceus—successful treatment with adjuvant gold therapy. *Clin Exp Dermatol* 12:364-365, 1987.

41. Kielwasser S, Heid E, Grosshans E, et al: Gold and pemphigus vulgaris (letter). *Dermatologica* 174:258, 1987.

42. Piamphongsant T, Ophaswongse S: Treatment of pemphigus. *Int J Dermatol* 30:139-146, 1991.

43. Murdock DK, Lookingbill DP: Immunosuppressive therapy of pemphigus vulgaris complicated by nocardia pneumonia: gold as an alternate therapy. *Arch Dermatol* 126:27-28, 1990.

44. Bystryn JC: Adjuvant therapy of pemphigus. *Arch Dermatol* 120:941-951, 1984.

45. Papp KA, Shear NH: Systemic gold therapy. *Clin Dermatol* 9:535-551, 1992.

46. Wilkinson SM, Smith AG, David MJ, et al: Pityriasis rosea and discoid eczema: dose related reactions to treatment with gold. *Ann Rheum Dis* 51:881-884, 1992.

47. Rye B, Krusinski PA: Hepatonecrosis resulting from parenteral gold therapy in pemphigus vulgaris. *J Am Acad Dermatol* 28:99-101, 1993.

48. Rapini RP: Gold treatment of pemphigus (letter). *J Am Acad Dermatol* 13:310, 1985.

Potassium Iodide

49. Horio T, Danno K, Okamoto H, et al: Potassium iodide in erythema nodosum and other erythematous dermatoses. *J Am Acad Dermatol* 9:77-81, 1983.

50. Shelley WB, Sica PA: Disseminated sporotrichosis of skin and bone cured with 5-fluorocytosine: Photosensitivity as a complication. *J Am Acad Dermatol* 8:229-235, 1983.

51. Schulz EJ, Whiting DA: Treatment of erythema nodosum and nodular vasculitis with potassium iodide. *Br J Dermatol* 94:75-78, 1976.

52. Kauffman CA: Old and new therapies for sporotrichosis. *Clin Infect Dis* 21:981-985, 1995.

53. Anderson PC: Cutaneous sporotrichosis. *Am Fam Physician* 27:201-204, 1983.

54. Urabe H, Honbo S: Sporotrichosis. *Int J Dermatol* 25:255-257, 1986.

55. Vilanova X, Aguade JP: Subacute nodular migratory panniculitis. *Br J Dermatol* 71:45-50, 1959.

56. Horio T, Imamura S, Danno K, et al: Potassium iodide in the treatment of erythema nodosum and nodular vasculitis. *Arch Dermatol* 117:29-31, 1981.

57. Ozols II, Wheat LJ: Erythema nodosum in an epidemic of histoplasmosis in Indianapolis. *Arch Dermatol* 117:709-712, 1981.

58. Marshall JK, Irvine EJ: Successful therapy of refractory erythema nodosum associated with Crohn's disease using potassium iodide. *Can J Gastroenterol* 11:501-502, 1997.

59. Myatt AE, Baker DJ, Byfield DM: Sweet's syndrome: a report on the use of potassium iodide. *Clin Exp Dermatol* 12:345-349, 1987.

60. Horio T, Imamura S, Danno K, et al: Treatment of acute febrile neutrophilic dermatosis (Sweet's syndrome) with potassium iodide. *Dermatologica* 160:341-347, 1980.

61. Leibovici V, Yaacov M, Lijovetzky G: Sweet's syndrome. *Int J Dermatol* 26:178-180, 1987.

62. Richardson JB, Callen JP: Pyoderma gangrenosum treated successfully with potassium iodide. *J Am Acad Dermatol* 28:1005-1007, 1993.

63. Torinuki W: Wegener's granulomatosis successfully treated with prednisolone and potassium iodide. *J Dermatol* 21:693-695, 1994.

64. Giessel M, Graves E, Kalivas J: Treatment of disseminated granuloma annulare with potassium iodide (letter). *Arch Dermatol* 115:639-640, 1979.

65. Caserio RJ, Eaglstein WH, Allen CM: Treatment of granuloma annulare with potassium iodide (letter). *J Am Acad Dermatol* 10:294-295, 1984.

66. Smith JB, Hansen CD, Zone JJ: Potassium iodide in the treatment of disseminated granuloma annulare. *J Am Acad Dermatol* 30:791-792, 1994.

67. Farwell AP, Braverman LE: Iodide. In Hardman JG, Limbird LE, Molinoff PB, et al, editors: *Goodman and Gilman's the pharmacological basis of therapeutics*, ed 9, New York, 1996, McGraw-Hill, pp 1402-1404.

68. Eeckhout E, Willemsen M, Deconinck A, et al: Granulomatous vasculitis as a complication of potassium iodide treatment for Sweet's syndrome. *Acta Derm Venereol (Stockh)* 67:362-364, 1987.

69. Soria C, Allegue F, España A, et al: Vegetating iododerma with underlying systemic diseases: report of three cases. *J Am Acad Dermatol* 22:418-422, 1990.

70. Shelley WB: Generalized pustular psoriasis induced by potassium iodide: a postulated role for dihydrofolic reductase. *JAMA* 201:133-138, 1967.

71. Heymann WR: Potassium iodide and the Wolff-Chaikoff effect: relevance for the dermatologist. *J Am Acad Dermatol* 42:490-492, 2000.

Attenuated Androgens

72. Gelfand JA, Sherins RJ, Alling DW, et al: Treatment of hereditary angioedema with danazol: Reversal of clinical and biochemical abnormalities. *N Engl J Med* 295:1444-1448, 1976.

73. Dmowski WP: Danazol—a steroid derivative with multiple and diverse biological effects. *Br J Clin Pract* 42:343-347, 1988.

74. Darbieri RL: Danazol treatment of angio-edema (letter). *J Allergy Clin Immunol* 71:257-258, 1982.

75. Helfman T, Falanga V: Stanozolol as a novel therapeutic agent in dermatology. *J Am Acad Dermatol* 33:254-258, 1995.

76. Wilson JD: Androgens. In Hardman JG, Limbird LE, Molinoff PB, et al, editors: *Goodman and Gilman's the pharmacological basis of therapeutics,* ed 9, New York, 1996, McGraw-Hill, p 1452.

77. Cicardi M, Bergamaschini L, Cugno M, et al: Long-term treatment of hereditary angioedema with attenuated androgens: a survey of a 13-year experience. *J Allergy Clin Immunol* 87:768-773, 1991.

78. Hosea SW, Santaella ML, Brown EJ, et al: Long-term therapy of hereditary angioedema with danazol. *Ann Intern Med* 93:809-812, 1980.

79. Madanes AE, Farber M: Danazol. *Ann Intern Med* 96:625-630, 1982.

80. Warin AP, Greaves MW, Gatecliff M, et al: Treatment of hereditary angio-oedema by low dose attenuated androgens: disassociation of clinical response from levels of C1 esterase inhibitor and C4. *Br J Dermatol* 103:405-409, 1980.

81. Sheffer AL, Fearon DT, Austen KF: Clinical and biochemical effects of impeded androgen (oxymetholone) therapy of hereditary angioedema. *J Allergy Clin Immunol* 64:275-280, 1979.

82. Spath PJ, Wuthrich B, Butler R: C1 inhibitor functional activities in hereditary angioedema plasma of patients under therapy with attenuated androgens. *Dermatologica* 169:310-304, 1984.

83. Kirsner RS, Eaglstein WH, Katz MH, et al: Stanozolol causes rapid pain relief and healing of cutaneous ulcers caused by cryofibrinogenemia. *J Am Acad Dermatol* 28:71-74, 1993.

84. Kirsner RS, Pardes JB, Eaglstein WH, et al: The clinical spectrum of lipodermatosclerosis. *J Am Acad Dermatol* 28:623-627, 1993.

85. Hsiao G-H, Chiu H-C: Livedoid vasculitis: response to low-dose danazol. *Arch Dermatol* 132:749-751, 1996.

86. Hsiao G-H, Chiu H-C: Low-dose danazol in the treatment of livedoid vasculitis. *Dermatology* 194:251-255, 1997.

87. Agnello V, Pariser K, Gell J, et al: Preliminary observations on danazol therapy of systemic lupus erythematosus: effects on DNA antibodies, thrombocytopenia and complement. *J Rheumatol* 10:682-687, 1983.

88. Fretwell MD, Altman LC: Exacerbation of a lupus-erythematosus-like syndrome during treatment of non-C1-esterase-inhibitor-dependent angioedema with danazol. *J Allergy Clin Immunol* 69:306-310, 1982.

89. Guillet G, Sassolas B, Plantin P, et al: Anti-Ro-positive lupus and hereditary angioneurotic edema: a 7-year follow-up with worsening of lupus under danazol treatment. *Dermatologica* 177:370-375, 1988.

90. Hory B, Blanc D, Boillot A, et al: Guillain-Barré syndrome following danazol and corticosteroid therapy for hereditary angioedema. *Am J Med* 79:111-114, 1985.

91. Ormerod AD, Smart L, Reid TMS, et al: Familial cold urticaria. *Arch Dermatol* 129:343-346, 1993.

92. Brestel EP, Thrush LB: The treatment of glucocorticosteroid-dependent chronic urticaria with stanozolol. *J Allergy Clin Immunol* 82:265-269, 1988.

93. Jarrett PEM, Morland M, Browse NL: Treatment of Raynaud's phenomenon by fibrinolytic enhancement. *BMJ* 2:523-525, 1978.

94. Jayson MIV, Holland CD, Keegan A, et al: A controlled study of stanozolol in primary Raynaud's phenomenon and systemic sclerosis. *Ann Rheum Dis* 50:41-47, 1991.

95. Kolodny L, Horstman LL, Sevin B-U, et al: Danazol relieves refractory pruritus associated with myeloproliferative disorders and other diseases. *Am J Hematol* 51:112-116, 1996.

96. Bergamaschini L, Tucci A, Colombo A, et al: Effect of stanozolol in patients with pityriasis rubra pilaris and retinol-binding protein deficiency (letter). *N Engl J Med* 306:346-347, 1982.

97. Pavlidakey GP, Hashimoto K, Savoy LB, et al: Stanozolol in the treatment of pityriasis rubra pilaris. *Arch Dermatol* 121:546-548, 1985.

98. van Voorst Vader PC, van Oostveen F, Houthoff HJ, et al: Pityriasis rubra pilaris, vitamin A and retinol-binding protein: a case study. *Acta Derm Venereol (Stockh)* 64:430-432, 1984.

99. Sheffer AL, Fearon DT, Austen KF: Clinical and biochemical effects of stanozolol therapy for hereditary angioedema. *J Allergy Clin Immunol* 68:181-187, 1981.

100. Andriole GL, Brickman C, Lack EE, et al: Danazol-induced cystitis: an undescribed source of hematuria in patients with hereditary angioneurotic edema. *J Urol* 135:44-46, 1986.

101. Sweet LC, Jackson CE, Yanari SS, et al: Danazol therapy in hereditary angioedema. *Henry Ford Hosp Med J* 28:31-35, 1980.

102. Wynn V: Metabolic effects of danazol. *J Int Med Res* 5(Suppl):25-35, 1977.

103. Bagheri SA, Boyer JL: Peliosis hepatis associated with androgenic-anabolic steroid therapy: a severe form of hepatic injury. *Ann Intern Med* 81:610-618, 1974.

104. Pearson K, Zimmerman JH: Danazol and liver damage (letter). *Lancet* 1:645-646, 1980.

105. Søe KL, Søe M, Gluud C: Liver pathology associated with the use of anabolic-androgenic steroids. *Liver* 12:73-79, 1992.

106. Haupt HA, Rovere GD: Anabolic steroids: a review of the literature. *Am J Sports Med* 12:469-484, 1984.

107. Cicardi M, Bergamaschini L, Tucci A: Morphologic evaluation of the liver in hereditary angioedema patients on long-term treatment with androgen derivatives. *J Allergy Clin Immunol* 72:294-298, 1983.

Nicotinamide

108. Marcus R, Coulston AM: Nicotinic acid. In Hardman JG, Limbird LE, Molinoff PB, et al, editors: *Goodman and Gilman's the pharmacological basis of therapeutics*, ed 9, New York, 1996, McGraw-Hill, pp 1559-1561.

109. Ma A, Medenica M: Response of generalized granuloma annulare to high-dose niacinamide. *Arch Dermatol* 119:836-839, 1983.

110. Berk MA, Lorincz AL: The treatment of bullous pemphigoid with tetracycline and niacinamide: a preliminary report. *Arch Dermatol* 122:670-674, 1986.

111. Weisberg A, Rosen E: Erythema exudativum multiforme. *Arch Dermatol Syphilol* 53:99-106, 1946.

112. Johnson HH, Binkley GW: Nicotinic acid therapy of dermatitis herpetiformis. *J Invest Dermatol* 14:233-238, 1950.

113. Zemtsov A, Neldner KH: Successful treatment of dermatitis herpetiformis with tetracycline and nicotinamide in a patient unable to tolerate dapsone. *J Am Acad Dermatol* 28:505-506, 1993.

114. Peoples D, Fivenson DP: Linear IgA bullous dermatosis: successful treatment with tetracycline and nicotinamide. *J Am Acad Dermatol* 26:498-499, 1992.

115. Chaffins ML, Collison D, Fivenson DP: Treatment of pemphigus and linear IgA dermatosis with nicotinamide and tetracycline: a review of 13 cases. *J Am Acad Dermatol* 28:998-1000, 1993.

116. Kohler IK, Lorincz AL: Erythema elevatum diutinum treated with niacinamide and tetracycline. *Arch Dermatol* 116:693-695, 1980.

117. Neumann R, Rappold E, Pohl-Markl H: Treatment of polymorphous light eruption with nicotinamide: a pilot study. *Br J Dermatol* 115:77-80, 1986.

118. Handfield-Jones S, Jones SK, Peachey R: High dose nicotinamide in the treatment of necrobiosis lipoidica. *Br J Dermatol* 118:693-696, 1988.

119. Fivenson DP, Breneman DL, Rosen GB, et al: Nicotinamide and tetracycline therapy of bullous pemphigoid. *Arch Dermatol* 130:753-758, 1994.

120. Pereyo NG, Davis LS: Generalized bullous pemphigoid controlled by tetracycline therapy alone. *J Am Acad Dermatol* 32:138-139, 1995.

121. Thornfeldt CR, Menkes AW: Bullous pemphigoid controlled by tetracycline. *J Am Acad Dermatol* 16:305-310, 1987.

122. Ortel B, Wechdorn D, Tanew A, et al: Effect of nicotinamide on the phototest reaction in polymorphous light eruption. *Br J Dermatol* 118:669-673, 1988.

123. Zackheim HS, Vasily DB, Westphal ML, et al: Reactions to niacinamide (letter). *J Am Acad Dermatol* 4:736-737, 1981.

124. Ranchoff RE, Tomecki KJ: Niacin or niacinamide? Nicotinic acid or nicotinamide? What is the difference? (letter). *J Am Acad Dermatol* 15:116-117, 1986.

125. Handfield-Jones S, Jones SK, Peachey RD: Nicotinamide treatment in diabetes (letter). *Br J Dermatol* 116:277, 1987.

Nonsteroidal Antiinflammatory Drugs

126. Greaves MW: Pharmacology and significance of nonsteroidal anti-inflammatory drugs in the treatment of skin diseases. *J Am Acad Dermatol* 16:751-764, 1987.

127. Ubogy Z, Persellin RH: Suppression of erythema nodosum by indomethacin. *Acta Derm Venereol (Stockh)* 62:265-266, 1982.

128. Elizaga FV: Erythema nodosum and indomethacin (letter). *Ann Intern Med* 96:383, 1982.

129. Lehman CW: Control of chronic erythema nodosum with naproxen. *Cutis* 26:66-67, 1980.

130. Kurzrock R, Cohen PR: Erythromelalgia and myeloproliferative disorders. *Arch Intern Med* 149:105-109, 1989.

131. Thompson GH, Hahn G, Rang M: Erythromelalgia. *Clin Orthop* 144:249-254, 1979.

132. Cohen IJK, Samorodin CS: Familial erythromelalgia. *Arch Dermatol* 118:953-954, 1982.

133. Smith KJ, Skelton HG, Yeager J, et al: Pruritus in HIV-1 disease: therapy with drugs which may modulate the pattern of immune dysregulation. *Dermatology* 195:353-358, 1997.

134. Daly BM, Shuster S: Effects of aspirin on pruritus. *BMJ* 293:907, 1986.

135. Jackson N, Burt D, Crocker J, et al: Skin mast cells in polycythaemia vera: relationship to the pathogenesis and treatment of pruritus. *Br J Dermatol* 116:21-29, 1987.

136. Crawhall JC, Wilkinson RD: Systemic mastocytosis: management of an unusual case with histamine (H1 and H2) antagonists and cyclooxygenase inhibition. *Clin Invest Med* 10:1-4, 1987.

137. Lahti A, Väänänen A, Kokkonen EL, Hannuksela M: Acetylsalicylic acid inhibits nonimmunologic contact urticaria. *Contact Dermatitis* 16:133-135, 1987.

138. Sussman GL, Harvey RP, Schocket AL: Delayed pressure urticaria. *J Allergy Clin Immunol* 70:337-342, 1982.

139. Grzelewska-Rzymowska I, Roznlecki J, Szmidt M: Aspirin "desensitization" in patients with aspirin-induced urticaria and angioedema. *Allergol Immunopathol (Madr)* 16:305-308, 1988.

140. Koro O, Dover JS, Francis DM, et al: Release of prostaglandin D2 and histamine in a case of localized heat urticaria, and effect of treatments. *Br J Dermatol* 115:721-728, 1986.

141. Millns JL, Randle HW, Solley GO, et al: The therapeutic response of urticarial vasculitis to indomethacin. *J Am Acad Dermatol* 3:349-355, 1980.

142. Miller WS, Ruderman FR, Smith JG Jr: Aspirin and ultraviolet light-induced erythema in man. *Arch Dermatol* 95:357-358, 1967.

143. Kobra-Black A, Greaves MV, Hensby CN, et al: Effects of indomethacin on prostaglandins E_2, F_2 alpha and arachidonic acid in human skin 24 hours after UV-B and UV-C irradiation. *Br J Clin Pharmacol* 6:261-266, 1978.

144. Søndergaard J, Bisgaard H, Thorsen S: Eicosanoids in skin UV inflammation. *Photodermatology* 2:359-366, 1985.

145. Imodaka G, Tejima T: A possible role of prostaglandins in PUVA-induced inflammation: implication by organ cultured skin. *J Invest Dermatol* 92:296-300, 1989.

146. Bigby M, Stern R: Cutaneous reactions to nonsteroidal anti-inflammatory drugs. *J Am Acad Dermatol* 12:866-876, 1985.

147. Roujeau JC: Clinical aspects of skin reactions to NSAIDs. *Scand J Rheumatol* 65(Suppl):131-134, 1987.

148. O'Brien N, Bagby GF: Rare adverse reactions to nonsteroidal antiinflammatory drugs. *J Rheumatol* 12:13-20, 1985.

Potassium Para-aminobenzoate

149. Zarafonetis CJD: Antifibrotic therapy with Potaba. *Am J Med Sci* 248:550-561, 1964.

150. Zarafonetis CJD, Curtis AC, Gulick AE: Use of para-aminobenzoic acid in dermatomyositis and scleroderma: report of 6 cases. *Arch Int Med* 85:27-43, 1950.

151. Zarafonetis CJD, Dabich L, Negri D, et al: Retrospective studies in scleroderma: effect of potassium para-aminobenzoate on survival. *J Clin Epidemiol* 41:193-205, 1988.

152. Zarafonetis CJD, Dabich L, Skovronski JJ, et al: Retrospective studies in scleroderma: skin response to potassium para-aminobenzoate therapy. *Clin Exp Rheumatol* 6:261-268, 1988.

153. Penneys NS: Treatment of lichen sclerosus with potassium para-aminobenzoate. *J Am Acad Dermatol* 10:1039-1042, 1984.

154. Zarafonetis CJD: The treatment of scleroderma: results of potassium para-aminobenzoate therapy in 104 cases. In Mills LC, Moyer JH, editors: *Inflammation and diseases of connective tissue*, Philadelphia, 1961, WB Saunders, pp 688-696.

155. Priestley GC, Brown JC: Effects of potassium para-aminobenzoate on growth and macromolecule synthesis in fibroblasts cultured from normal and sclerodermatous human skin, and rheumatoid synovial cells. *J Invest Dermatol* 72:161-164, 1979.

156. Gillon M, Priestley GC, Heyworth R: Effects of para-aminobenzoate on skin fibroblasts from lichen sclerosus et atrophicus and from morphoea (abstract). *Br J Dermatol* 116:454, 1987.

157. Kantor GR, Ratz JL: Liver toxicity from potassium para-aminobenzoate (letter). *J Am Acad Dermatol* 13:671-672, 1985.

158. Zarafonetis CJD, Dabich L, DeVol EB, et al: Potassium para-aminobenzoate and liver function test findings. *J Am Acad Dermatol* 15:144-149, 1986.

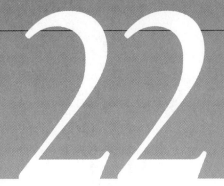

CHAPTER 22

Alfred L. Knable, Jr.

Miscellaneous Systemic Drugs

The drugs discussed in this chapter (Table 22-1) have unique structures and mechanisms of action and are used in relatively unique circumstances in dermatologic care after more familiar remedies failed. Some of these medications can be found over-the-counter at the corner grocery store. Others carry such significant risks for severe adverse effects that they are available only under strictly controlled circumstances. Some cost only pennies per month's supply, whereas cost is a limiting factor for others in their prescription. Although many of these drugs have limited US Food and Drug Administration (FDA) indications for dermatologic use, they are increasingly being utilized as data accumulate to support their efficacy. Detailed discussions are devoted to thalidomide, clofazimine, and intravenous immunoglobulin (IVIg). Brief sections focus on the use of penicillamine, representative anticholinergic agents, biotin, oral vitamin E, and zinc sulfate.

The views expressed in this chapter are those of the author and do not reflect the official position of the United States Air Force, the Department of Defense, or the U.S. Government.
I would like to thank Lt. Dea Brueggemeyer, Pharmacist, WPMC, and SrA Tina Whytal for their help in compiling literature for this chapter.

THALIDOMIDE

Arguably, no pharmacologic agent in history acquired the notoriety to equal thalidomide (Figure 22-1).

Thalidomide was introduced to Western Europe in the late 1950s as a "safe" sleeping aid with negligible adverse effects. The drug never obtained approval from the FDA and did not enter the American market. Dramatic reports soon began to appear of an association between use of thalidomide during pregnancy and infant limb defects (phocomelia), often accompanied by internal deformities. In 1961, the drug was rapidly withdrawn from world markets as its teratogenicity was confirmed, and its ability to cause irreversible peripheral nerve damage became apparent. Unfortunately, before its disappearance, thalidomide-related cases of phocomelia were estimated in the thousands.[1,2] The world's shock on viewing those afflicted with phocomelia sparked a renewed vigilance with regard to drug safety issues. The word *thalidomide* became symbolic of our former naiveté.

Thalidomide's exile was short lived. In 1965, it was reported to dramatically alleviate the symptoms associated with erythema nodosum leprosum (ENL).[3] Since then, clinical researchers gradually reported its beneficial effects for a variety of conditions; its use was limited to a "named patient" basis. In 1997, the FDA

Table 22-1 Miscellaneous Systemic Drugs

Generic Name	Trade Name	Generic Available	Manu-facturer	Tablet/Capsule Sizes	Special Formulations	Standard Dosage Range	Price Index
Thalidomide	Thalomid	No	Celgene	50 mg	None	50-300 mg/d	$$$$
Clofazimine	Lamprene	No	Geigy	50 mg	None	50-100 mg/d, plus monthly bolus 300 mg	$
Immunoglobulin (IV)	Various	Yes	Various	None	IV 1, 3, 6, 12 g vials	2 g/kg/month	$$$$$
Penicillamine	Cuprimine	Yes	Merck	250 mg	None	250 mg/d, slowly ↑ to 750-1500 mg/d	$$
Glycopyrrolate	Robinul (Forte)	Yes	Wyeth	1 mg (2 mg)	IV form available as preop med	1-2 mg bid-tid	$
Propantheline	Pro-Banthine	Yes	Roberts	15 mg	None	15 mg bid-tid	—
Biotin	Various	Yes	Various	300 µg	None	2500 µg/d	—
Vitamin E	Various	Yes	Various	100-1000 IU	Drops 50 mg/ml	200-1600 IU/d	—
Zinc sulfate	Various	Yes	Various	220 mg	IV form for TPN*	1-2 mg/kg/d	—

$, <1.00; $$, 1.01-2.00; $$$, 2.01-5.00; $$$$, 5.01-10.00; $$$$$, >10.00; ( ), generic price; /, two different price ranges from lower dose to higher dose examples of this drug; —, no price listed for this drug.
*TPN, Total parenteral nutrition.

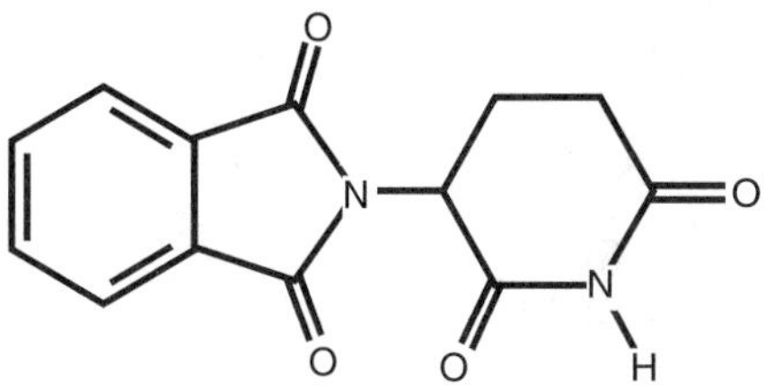

Figure 22-1   Thalidomide.

granted thalidomide "approvable" status for the treatment of ENL, opening the door for its use in off-label indications. Although its exile has ended, the thalidomide image requires extensive rehabilitation and its probation in the public's mind may never end. Those electing to prescribe thalidomide must be mindful of its potential hazards and ever respectful of those whose lives have been irrevocably altered by this medication.

Pharmacology

Table 22-2 lists key pharmacologic concepts for thalidomide and other systemic drugs.

STRUCTURE.   Thalidomide is a nonpolar glutamic acid derivative, specifically, alpha-*N*-phthalimidoglutarimide. Being a piperidine-dione hypnotic, it is structurally similar to glutethimide, methyprylon, and bemegride. It consists of a left-sided phthalimide ring and a right-sided glutaramide ring with a single asymmetric carbon atom centrally; this feature allows for its rapid conversion between two isomeric forms in vivo.[1,4]

ABSORPTION AND BIOAVAILABILITY. Thalidomide is available for oral administration only. There is little difference in absorption whether taken with or without meals. Because thalidomide displays poor solubility in water and there is no intravenous formulation, the absolute bioavailability of thalidomide in humans has not been calculated. Animal studies yielded values ranging from 67% to 93%.[5] The drug is absorbed relatively slowly, reaching peak plasma levels usually within 2 to 6 hours.[5] Its onset of action varies according to the condition being treated (see Clinical Use section).

A volume of distribution of 120 liters has been estimated.[5,6] Protein-binding studies have not been performed in humans. Given thalido-

mide's nonpolar nature, however, protein binding in the plasma is speculated to be significant. Even so, thalidomide readily crosses the placental membrane due to the drug's lipid solubility.[3]

METABOLISM AND EXCRETION.   Extensive study of thalidomide metabolism has not been carried out in humans. In animal studies the major degradative pathway appears to be nonenzymatic hydrolysis.[7] At physiologic pH, thalidomide undergoes rapid hydrolytic degradation into most of its twelve theoretically possible cleavage products.[8] There is also evidence that hepatic metabolism of the parent compound involves the cytochrome P-450 family. Even though P-450 inhibitors have been shown to prevent hepatic degradation of thalidomide, to date, no specific drug interaction warnings have been posted on this basis.[1,9]

The half-life of thalidomide has been determined to be approximately 9 hours. Its excretion appears to be predominantly nonrenal, with less than 1% of a dose found unchanged in the urine after 24 hours. The total body clearance of the drug was calculated to be approximately 10 L/hour.[5,6]

MECHANISMS OF ACTION.   Table 22-3 lists drug mechanisms for thalidomide and other systemic drugs. Very few of the multiple biologic activities attributed to thalidomide have been explained at the molecular level. For such a simple molecule, it exerts myriad effects. The task of sorting out how the drug works is in no small way complicated by its twelve cleavage products. Most of the known mechanisms of action can be included under one of the following headings: hypnosedative effects, immunomodulatory and antiinflammatory effects, and neural or vascular tissue effects.

Hypnosedative Effects.   Thalidomide readily penetrates the central nervous system (CNS) where it exerts hypnosedative effects comparable with barbiturates. Despite similar potencies even at large doses, acute toxicity is almost negligible.[1,3] Thalidomide acts via an independent, still undetermined mechanism from the barbiturates. It is thought that this sedating property may in part explain thalidomide's effectiveness in the treatment of pruritic conditions such as prurigo nodularis and actinic prurigo.[10]

■ **Table 22-2**   Key Pharmacologic Concepts—Miscellaneous Systemic Drugs

Drug Name	Absorption and Bioavailability			Elimination		
	Peak Levels	Bioavail-able (%)	Protein Binding	Half-life	Metabolism	Excretion
Thalidomide[5-9]	2-6 hrs	67%-93%	No data	9 hrs	Nonenzymatic hydrolytic cleavage	Predominantly nonrenal, precise mechanism unknown
Clofazimine[84,85]	1-6 hrs*	20%-70%	Negligible	70 days†	Hepatic	Small amounts excreted in urine, smaller amounts via sebum, sweat and tears
IV Immunoglobulin[127,131]	Days	40%-50%	Not pertinent	3-5 wks	General protein catabolism	Small percentage excreted unchanged in urine
Penicillamine[159]	1-3 hrs	40%-70%	~80 %	1-3 hrs	Hepatic	Renal >> fecal
Glycopyrrolate[81]	5 hrs	10%-25%	No data	~1.7 hrs	Minimal	Renal and bile, most excreted as unchanged drug
Propantheline[81]	1 hr	Poor/variable	No data	~1.6 hrs	Minimal	Renal, most excreted as unchanged drug

*After steady state is obtained—approximately 70 days.
†With long course of therapy—when a short course is given the half-life is about 7 days.

■ **Table 22-3**   Drug Mechanisms—Miscellaneous Systemic Drugs

Drug Name	Mechanism	Resultant Clinical Effects
Thalidomide	1. Hypnosedative[1]	Erythema nodosum leprosum therapy (Mech 1, 2)
	2. Immunomodulatory/antiinflammatory effect*[1,10,15]	Cutaneous lupus erythematosus therapy (Mech 2)
	3. Effects on neural tissue[10]	Stomatitis/Behçet's disease therapy (Mech 2)
	4. Effects on vascular tissue[19]	Prurigo nodularis/actinic prurigo therapy (Mech 1, 2, 3)
	(Mechanism for teratogenicity is unknown)	Kaposi's sarcoma therapy (Mech 4)
	(Mechanism for peripheral neuropathy is unknown)	
Clofazimine	1. Antimicrobial effects[81,82]	Leprosy/atypical mycobacterial infection therapy (Mech 1, 2, 3)
	2. Antiinflammatory effects[81,82]	Chronic cutaneous lupus erythematosus therapy (Mech 2, 3)
	3. Selective immunomodulation[82-84]	Pyoderma gangrenosum therapy (Mech 2, 3)
	4. Lipophilicity of drug and deposition of metabolites in crystalline form	Hyperpigmentation: due to deposition of clofazimine, as well as stimulated hypermelanosis (Mech 4)
		Xerosis and possible progression to ichthyosis (Mech unknown)
		Abdominal pain, transient GI disturbances, rarely splenic infarction (Mech 4)
		Possible cardiotoxicity (Mech unknown)
IV Immunoglobulin[124]	1. Blockade of Fc receptors	GVHD, diabetes mellitus, autoimmune bullous dermatoses therapy (Mech 1, 2, 3)
	2. Prevention of complement-mediated damage	Atopic dermatitis therapy (Mech 4, possibly 3)
	3. Reduction of circulating pathogens and antibodies	
	4. Alteration of cytokine/cytokine antagonist ratios	

Mech, Mechanism; *GVHD,* graft-versus-host disease.
*Through inhibition of TNF-α release and activity.

Immunomodulatory and Antiinflammatory Effects.   Multiple studies, some yielding contradictory results, have focused on thalidomide's influence on the immune system. The drug exhibits specific inhibition of tumor necrosis factor-alpha (TNF-α).[11] When given to healthy volunteers, the drug induced a drop in their helper T-cell counts and a corresponding, though relatively small, rise in their suppresser T-cell number.[12]

The drug has been observed to potently suppress the production of interleukin-12 (IL-12), which plays a crucial role in the development of cellular immunoresponses.[13] Disease-specific influences of these molecular effects remain to be worked out. However, these studies provide insight into thalidomide's possible modes of action in disorders characterized by undesirable cellular immune reactions such as ENL, sarcoidosis, and chronic graft-versus-host disease (GVHD). Humoral immunity is also affected as evidenced by the selective enhanced production of IL-4 and IL-5 (B-cell activators) with simultaneous interferon-gamma (IFN-γ) inhibition.[14] Paradoxically, both enhanced and diminished humoral responses have been experimentally observed with thalidomide administration.

Thalidomide's success in treating other diseases, such as chronic cutaneous lupus erythematosus (CCLE) and pyoderma gangrenosum (PG), can perhaps best be understood by examining its antiinflammatory properties. Thalidomide has been shown to decrease neutrophil chemotaxis and phagocytosis.[15,16] Monocyte phagocytosis is also decreased.[17] In addition, antagonism of inflammatory mediators such as histamine, acetylcholine, prostaglandins, and 5-hydroxytryptamine (serotonin) has been

demonstrated.[15] Given these qualities, the drug might theoretically be expected to work for a great number of inflammatory disorders.

Effects on Neural and Vascular Tissues. It has been hypothesized that thalidomide has direct effects on nervous tissue.[10] Whether or not the drug's effectiveness in treating prurigo nodularis in one patient is mediated by the same mechanism that causes peripheral neuropathy in another is still to be determined. Some evidence indicates that two distinct mechanisms may be at work, one leading to desirable the other to undesirable effects. For example, in cases of prurigo nodularis, abnormal or proliferating neural tissue seems to be preferentially affected.[18] Definitive studies remain to be done.

Preliminary work has demonstrated thalidomide's ability to inhibit angiogenesis by an as

Table 22-4	Thalidomide Indications and Contraindications

FDA-APPROVED INDICATIONS
Erythema nodosum leprosum*[15,20]

OFF-LABEL USES

HIV-related Dermatoses	Lymphocytic Infiltrates
AIDS-associated oral stomatitis*[29-32]	Cutaneous features lupus erythematosus[49-57]
AIDS-related Kaposi's sarcoma[33]	Jessner's lymphocytic infiltrate of the skin[58,59]
	Cutaneous lymphoid hyperplasia[60]
Neutrophilic Dermatoses	
Giant aphthous stomatitis[35-38]	Other Dermatoses
Behçet's disease[39-42]	Chronic GVHD*[61-63]
Pyoderma gangrenosum[43-45]	Prurigo nodularis/actinic prurigo[51,64-66]
	Sarcoidosis[67-69]
Vesiculobullous Dermatoses	Langerhans cell histiocytosis[70]
Erosive lichen planus[46]	Weber-Christian disease[71]
Bullous pemphigoid[47]	Palmoplantar pustulosis[42]
Cicatricial pemphigoid[47]	Uremic pruritus[72]
Recurrent erythema multiforme[48]	Postherpetic neuralgia[10]

CONTRAINDICATIONS

Absolute	Relative
Sensitivity to thalidomide	Patients with significant hepatic or renal
Pregnancy	impairment
Women of childbearing potential	Patients with history of neuritis or other
Patients with existing peripheral neuropathy	neurologic disorders
Men engaging in sexual intercourse with	Congestive heart failure or hypertension
women of childbearing potential (must use	Constipation, other GI disorders
barrier method of contraception)	Hypothyroidism

PREGNANCY PRESCRIBING STATUS—CATEGORY X

*Thalidomide is generally considered the drug of choice for this disorder.

yet unknown mechanism.[19] This discovery may partially explain its teratogenic potential. It may also lead to future research using the drug as an antineoplastic agent.

Clinical Use

Table 22-4 lists indications and contraindications for thalidomide.

FDA-APPROVED INDICATION

Erythema Nodosum Leprosum. Although no direct effect against *Mycobacterium leprae* has been demonstrated, thalidomide is the drug of choice for ENL (type 2 leprosy reaction).[15,20] This reaction occurs in approximately 50% of patients with lepromatous leprosy but only occasionally in those with borderline forms. Over a decade after his initial work began the drug's resurrection, Sheskin[21] surveyed over 4500 cases of ENL treated with thalidomide from around the world and reported an amazing response rate of 99%. The drug is ineffective in reversal (type 1) leprosy reactions.[22]

For milder cases of ENL, thalidomide has been administered alone. In controlled studies, 100 mg was given four times daily for 7 days. The course was repeated for an additional 7 days for nonresponders and for relapses, which can be frequent.[23-25] Others have successfully used an initial dose of 100 mg three to four times daily with reduction to a 50 to 100 mg maintenance dose over 2 weeks.[26,27] Attempts to discontinue the drug should be made periodically.

Resolution of cutaneous ENL lesions almost uniformly begins within 24 to 48 hours.[21] Systemic signs and symptoms of ENL tend to resolve within a few days as well.

More severe cases of ENL, involving progressive neural degeneration, significant ocular involvement, or severe skin ulceration, require the combined use of thalidomide and corticosteroids. Pfaltzgraff[28] reported on the concomitant use of these two medications. In general, antileprosy chemotherapy should continue throughout treatment of the leprosy reaction.[22]

OFF-LABEL USES—WELL-DOCUMENTED BENEFITS

Human Immunodeficiency Virus–Related Conditions. Thalidomide's effective use in treating human immunodeficiency virus (HIV)–associated mucosal ulceration is well docu-

mented and will likely gain specific FDA approval in the future. Doses of 100 to 300 mg/day generally result in control of symptoms within 2 weeks and dramatic healing of ulceration within 2 to 4 weeks.[29-32] Unfortunately, the drug's effect appears to be suppressive rather than curative; relapse commonly occurs within 1 month of discontinuing therapy. There is also a case report discussing thalidomide's successful use in treating Kaposi's sarcoma.[33] Helper T-cell counts are evidently unaffected by therapy within the HIV-positive population.[34]

Neutrophilic Dermatoses. Thalidomide has also proven valuable in treating a number of neutrophilic dermatoses. Several controlled studies and case reports attest to its efficacy in the therapy of chronic and giant aphthous stomatitis.[35-38] Dosages of 100 to 300 mg/day generally resulted in more rapid pain reduction than observed among the HIV-positive population, followed by remission of ulcers within only 1 to 2 weeks. Again, relapse is commonly observed shortly after cessation of therapy. Smaller series and individual case reports of the drug's potential use in the treatment of Behçet's syndrome have been published.[39-42] In most of these reports, the dosing regimen was similar to that previously mentioned. Some suggest more aggressive initial dosing at 400 mg/day for the first 5 days, tapering as rapidly as possible while maintaining desired clinical effect. Unfortunately, ocular lesions have not been shown to respond as well to thalidomide as have mucocutaneous lesions. Less substantial evidence exists to support the use of thalidomide for the treatment of pyoderma gangrenosum.[43-45]

Vesiculobullous Dermatoses. There is a paucity of reports discussing the use of thalidomide for various vesiculobullous disorders. Citations can be found for its successful employment in patients with erosive lichen planus,[46] bullous and cicatricial pemphigoid,[47] and recurrent erythema multiforme.[48] Given the limited data available, it is hard to predict if thalidomide will have significant impact on the treatment of this challenging category of disorders.

Lupus Erythematosus. Thalidomide has been successfully used to treat the cutaneous manifestations of the various forms of lupus erythematosus (LE).[49-57] The response rate in CCLE is estimated between 75% and 90%.[49,51] Compared with other conditions, CCLE usually responds to smaller initial doses, in the range of 50 to 200 mg/day. Response is usually seen within 2 to 4 weeks. Thereafter the dose may be tapered, with a maintenance dose requirement of 25 to 50 mg/day required for most patients.[49,51,52] Within this dose range (50 to 200 mg/day), similar response rates have been documented in subacute cutaneous LE (SCLE).[49,54] In systemic LE (SLE), larger initial doses are required with longer periods of time until response may be expected. Atra[55] reported a response rate of 90% for cutaneous lesions of SLE and also described the steroid-sparing attributes of the medication. Unfortunately, systemic features of SLE do not respond as well. Thalidomide has also been successfully used in the treatment of lupus profundus (lupus panniculitis).[56] Perhaps by similar mechanisms, reports detail the success of using thalidomide to treat Jessner's lymphocytic infiltrate of the skin[58,59] and cutaneous lymphoid hyperplasia.[60]

Graft-Versus-Host Disease. Numerous citations can be found describing thalidomide's utility in treating chronic GVHD.[61-63] The dosages and length of time required to obtain a clinical response in chronic GVHD tend to be greater than for many other dermatoses discussed in this section. Dosages as high as 800 mg/day used over several weeks were required to obtain complete or partial response rates in 20% to 59% of patients. A significant number of patients discontinued therapy secondary to various adverse effects common at such dosages. Even though less dramatic in its effects in chronic GVHD than in other conditions, thalidomide offers hope for many patients with recalcitrant or more severe forms of the disease. The exact mechanism is unknown, but its immunosuppressive and antiinflammatory actions are presumed to be central in its benefit to patients with chronic GVHD.

Prurigo Nodularis. Actinic prurigo and prurigo nodularis have been shown to respond to thalidomide in case reports and small series.[51,64-66] Initial doses of 300 to 400 mg/day yielded good response rates within 3 months in most instances. Tapering to a dose as low as 50 mg/day is possible; however, complete cessation of the drug leads to recurrence of symptoms in most cases.[66]

Other Dermatologic Uses. Anecdotal evidence exists to support a trial of thalidomide in the following conditions: cutaneous sarcoidosis,[67-69] Langerhans' cell histiocytosis,[70] Weber-Christian disease,[71] palmoplantar pustulosis,[42] uremic pruritus,[72] and postherpetic neuralgia.[10] In addition to the dosages discussed for these specific conditions, pediatric dosing has been reported by Cole[62] and Atra.[55] The former used an initial dosage of 12 mg/kg/day to the nearest 50 mg divided two to four times daily. Blood levels were recommended in an effort to maintain drug concentrations of 6 to 12 µmol/L.

CONTRAINDICATIONS.   Thalidomide is absolutely contraindicated in individuals with a known sensitivity to the drug. It is also absolutely contraindicated during pregnancy, in women of childbearing potential (without strict contraception), and in men actively engaging in sexual relations with women who may become pregnant. It should also not be given to individuals with existing peripheral neuropathy.

The use of thalidomide is relatively contraindicated for patients with any of the following preexisting conditions: significant hepatic or renal impairment, neuritis or other neurologic disorders, congestive heart failure, hypertension, significant constipation, other gastrointestinal disorders, or hypothyroidism.

ADVERSE EFFECTS
Teratogenicity.   Despite intense scrutiny over almost 4 decades, the exact mechanism of thalidomide's teratogenic potential remains unknown. Speculation has focused on the drug's affinity for nerve tissue, as well as its ability to suppress angiogenesis, but no definitive results have been obtained. It is known that peak vulnerability to the drug occurs between days 21 to 36 of gestation; during this critical window a single 100 mg dose of thalidomide results in nearly a 100% incidence of birth defects.[1,3] The most common defect is phocomelia (deformity with underdevelopment of the arms, legs, or both), which may be accompanied by ear malformation. Abnormalities of the gastrointestinal, renal, and urogenital systems have also been reported.[1,3]

Peripheral Neuropathy.   The reported incidence of thalidomide-induced peripheral neuropathy varies from 1% among patients treated for ENL to over 70% for those treated for prurigo nodularis.[1,73] The most common presentation of the syndrome consists of mild proximal muscle weakness with symmetric painful paresthesias of the hands and feet frequently associated with a lower limb sensory loss.[74] Although motor weakness usually recovers rapidly after drug cessation, sensory dysfunction improves slowly if at all.[1] Electrophysiologic studies demonstrate a pattern consistent with axonal neuropathy with reduction in sensory nerve action potential (SNAP) amplitude. There is relative sparing of conduction velocities.[74,75]

Although a dose- or duration-dependent relationship between the drug and the development of neuropathy has been suggested by some, Ochonisky[73] and colleagues found no such relationship in their retrospective study of 42 patients treated for various dermatologic disorders. In fact, they found neuropathy developing in patients with cumulative doses as low as 3 to 6 g. They reported an incidence of 21% to 50%, with women and the elderly experiencing the greatest risk. They concluded that individual susceptibility, possibly due to a genetic predisposition, was more important than cumulative dose of the drug with regard to the development of neuropathy. One possible predisposing factor may be slow acetylation.[76]

Other Adverse Effects. Endocrine effects, specifically hypothyroidism, hypoglycemia, and adrenocorticotropic hormone (ACTH) stimulation, have been rarely reported.[1] Other, less common adverse effects with potentially severe complications include leukopenia[77] and exfoliative or erythrodermic reactions.[78,79] A hypersensitivity reaction taking various clinical forms has been described in the HIV-positive population.[80]

More commonly encountered adverse effects of less consequence include the following: drowsiness (very common), mood changes, xerostomia, brittle fingernails, nausea, constipation (common), increased appetite, peripheral edema, xerosis, pruritus, irregular menses, hyperglycemia, bradycardia, red palms, decreased libido, and dizziness.[1,75]

Drug Interactions

Table 22-5 lists drug interactions for thalidomide. Thalidomide has additive effects with other sedative agents, such as (but not limited to) alcohol, barbiturates, chlorpromazine, or reserpine, with resultant increased CNS depres-

sion. It has been shown to antagonize the effects of histamine, serotonin, acetylcholine, and the prostaglandins in vitro.[6] To date, there are no reports documenting thalidomide's concomitant use with various cytochrome P-450 inducers or inhibitors. Extreme caution must be used when patients receiving thalidomide are also taking medications with the potential to interfere with hormonal contraceptives.

Monitoring Guidelines

As of mid 1999, thalidomide has been approved for marketing under a special restricted distribution progam developed by the manufaturer (Celgene) and the FDA (see Thalidomide Monitoring Guidelines box). Only physicians and pharmacists registered with the system for thalidomide education and prescribing safety (S.T.E.P.S) are permitted to prescribe and dispense the product. Registration may be initiated by contacting the Celgene Corporation at 1-888-4-CELGENE.

After mutual agreement has been reached between the physician and the patient regarding the medical necessity for thalidomide, informed consent must be formally registered. Standard-

 Table 22-5   Thalidomide Drug Interactions*

Interacting Drugs	Comments
Alcohol Barbiturates Chlorpromazine Reserpine	Drugs with additive sedative effects when used in combination with thalidomide
Acetylcholine Histamine Prostaglandins Serotonin	Drugs that thalidomide may antagonize
HIV-1 protease inhibitors Griseofulvin Rifampin Rifabutin Phenytoin Carbamazepine	Various cytochrome P-450 enzyme inducers that may interfere with hormonal contraception (increasing the risk of teratogenicity)

*1974-1998 Micromedix Inc., Vol. 95.

Thalidomide Monitoring Guidelines[2,73,82,83]

BASELINE

- Determine the patient's ability to comprehend the drug risks and willingness to sign the consent form, as well as willingness to participate in ongoing monitoring programs

Laboratory Testing

- Pregnancy test: serum (or urine test of adequate sensitivity) in women of childbearing potential
- Complete blood count (CBC) with platelets

Neurologic Evaluation

- Clinical neurologic examination*
- At least one, preferably two, measurements of sensory nerve action potential (SNAP) amplitudes† if indicated by history of peripheral nervous disease or positive history or physical findings

FOLLOW-UP

Laboratory Testing

- Pregnancy tests: weekly for first 4 weeks, then monthly for women of childbearing potential with regular menses, or every 2 weeks for irregular menses and as clinically indicated
- Monthly CBC with platelet determination and liver transaminase testing until dose is stable, then every 2-3 months

Neurologic Evaluation

- Clinical evaluation to include neurologic examination, at least monthly for the first 3 months, thereafter every 1 to 6 months as indicated
- Consider SNAP measurements after every 6 months or when clinically indicated

Note: More frequent surveillance is needed if laboratory values are abnormal or with high-risk patients.
*Clinical neurologic examination should include a subjective review of sensory and motor function as well as an objective search for distal hypesthesia or paresthesia, muscle weakness, or ankle jerk reflex depression.
†SNAP amplitudes should be measured from at least three nerves. Two measurements allow a confidence interval to be calculated for an individual patient. A fall of 40% or more from baseline should be considered significant. A fall of 30% to 40% from baseline indicates the need for more frequent neurologic examination and SNAP measurement, as well as requiring reevaluation of the necessity for continued thalidomide therapy.

ized informed consent forms and important product information are provided after registering with the S.T.E.P.S. program.[82] A sample consent form and package insert can also be obtained by contacting the FDA or the Celgene Corporation.[83] Before the first dose, a complete history and physical examination should be performed with emphasis on detecting preexisting neurologic defects. Obtaining at least one and preferably two SNAP amplitudes as a baseline should be considered if indicated by significant historical or physical findings suggesting possible peripheral neuropathy.[2,73] In women, effective birth control must be in place for at least 1 month before and a negative pregnancy test (minimum sensitivity of 50 mIU/ml) should be obtained within 24 hours of beginning therapy. Fertile men should be advised to wear a condom during sexual intercourse because thalidomide has been detected in semen. In addition, a baseline complete blood count (CBC) with platelets should be obtained.[2,73,83]

After therapy is initiated, clinical evaluation with emphasis on neurologic findings, such as numbness, tingling, or pain in the hands and feet, should be carried out at least monthly for the first 3 months and every 1 to 6 months thereafter as indicated. SNAP measurements should at least be considered when clinically warranted and after every 6 months of therapy, whichever is sooner, in an effort to detect asymptomatic neuropathy. A negative pregnancy test with a sensitivity of at least 50 mIU/ml must be performed within 24 hours before initiating thalidomide. Pregnancy tests are then required weekly for the first 4 weeks then monthly for women with regular menses and every 2 weeks for those with irregular menses and as otherwise indicated. A CBC with platelet count should be obtained monthly, monitoring for neutropenia.[2,73,82,83]

CLOFAZIMINE

Clofazimine (Lamprene or B663) is the most active antimycobacterial riminophenazine dye known. This class of agents was developed in 1944, as the result of an effort to chemically imitate diploicin (a compound naturally occurring in lichens, that had demonstrated the ability to inhibit *Mycobacterium tuberculosis* in vitro.[84] In clinical trials, clofazimine proved more effective in treating leprosy than tuberculosis and this is still the drug's major clinical use. Given this agent's antimicrobial and antiinflammatory properties, however, it has been used in a number of conditions. Clofazimine has been successfully employed to treat infectious, inflammatory, and granulomatous diseases of the skin.

Pharmacology

See Table 22-2 for key pharmacologic concepts of clofazimine. Under normal conditions, clofazimine, $C_{27}H_{22}Cl_2N_4$, is deep red-to-orange in color. Chemically it belongs to the group of phenazine molecules known as riminophenazines, distinguished by substitution on the N2, N3, and C7 positions. It is most commonly synthesized today by the reduction of anilino-aposafranines.[84]

The absorption of clofazimine after oral intake is variable. When taken with food, absorption is increased and the t_{max} is significantly decreased.[84,85] The drug is highly lipophilic and concentrates in lipid-rich tissues, particularly within the reticuloendothelial system, but also in the breasts, intestines, and liver. Because of this the drug is slowly eliminated with a half-life of approximately 70 days.[85] There have been three proposed routes of hepatic metabolism, the clinical relevance of which is unknown. Only small amounts of the drug are found in urine. Minimal, but clinically significant, elimination occurs via the sebum, sputum, tears, and sweat. Formal studies of fecal/biliary elimination have not been carried out.[84,85]

MECHANISMS OF ACTION. See Table 22-3 for drug mechanisms of clofazimine. To date there is no single theory to fully explain clofazimine's antimicrobial effects. In vitro, clofazimine selectively binds to DNA guanine residues, which are in higher concentration in mycobacteria than in humans. Whether or not this explains its in vivo activity is uncertain. Other proposed mechanisms of action involve the drug's inhibition of the mitochondrial respiratory chains and inhibition of the increased production of free radicals within various cell lines.[84,85] Recent in vitro work has shown that the antimycobacterial effects of clofazimine can be augmented by IFN-γ or TNF-α under certain circumstances.[86] Perhaps cytokine-enhanced clofazimine therapy will someday be a reality for the treatment of human mycobacterial infection.

Within the immune system, clofazimine exerts its effects mainly by altering the functions of monocytes and neutrophils.[84,85] Among other effects on monocytes, the drug has been shown to increase the size and number of lysosomes and phagolysosomes. Neutrophil motility and lymphocyte transformation are inhibited in a dose-dependent manner, and superoxide production is enhanced.[84] Although phospholipase A_2 production is also enhanced, the overall effect of the drug is usually antiinflammatory.[87]

Clinical Use

Table 22-6 lists indications and contraindications for clofazimine.

FDA-APPROVED INDICATIONS

Leprosy and Other Mycobacterial Infections. Clofazimine is approved for the treatment of lepromatous leprosy. It has also been used in the treatment of ENL.[85] In multibacillary leprosy, combination drug therapy has been advocated as initial therapy to decrease the development of resistance. The drug has been used extensively in combination with dapsone and rifampin. In the most commonly used regimen, 50 mg of clofazimine is taken daily along with an additional bolus of 300 mg monthly for at least 2 years. Different amounts of dapsone and rifampin have been recommended for concurrent use during this course.[85,88] It has been suggested that the addition of ofloxacin to this regimen may decrease the length of therapy.[89] In addition to leprosy, clofazimine has been used to treat tuberculosis and other atypical mycobacterial infections.[85,90-93]

OFF-LABEL USES

Inflammatory Skin Diseases. Within the realm of inflammatory diseases, multiple reports discuss the use of clofazimine in the treatment of pyoderma gangrenosum in both its classic and malignant forms.[94-97] Small series and case reports exist to support a trial of clofazimine in a number of other inflammatory, granulomatous, and infectious processes (see Table 22-6). The

Table 22-6	Clofazimine Indications and Contraindications

FDA-APPROVED INDICATIONS
Lepromatous leprosy—including drug resistant cases and cases complicated by erythema nodosum leprosum[79,84,85]

OFF-LABEL USES

Inflammatory and Autoimmune Dermatoses
Pyoderma gangrenosum[94-97]
Chronic cutaneous lupus erythematosus[52,98]
Chronic GVHD[99]
Pustular psoriasis[100]
Erythema dyschromicum perstans (ashy dermatosis)[101,102]
Vitiligo[103]
Erythema elevatum diutinum[104]
Acute febrile neutrophilic dermatosis (Sweet's syndrome)[105]
Acne fulminans[106-108]

Granulomatous Dermatoses (including infectious)
Atypical mycobacterial infections[90-92]
Tuberculosis[85,93]
Leishmaniasis[84,109]
Malakoplakia[110,111]
Rhinoscleroma[112]
Melkersson-Rosenthal syndrome[113,114]
Necrobiosis lipoidica[115]
Granuloma annulare, disseminated[115]
Annular elastolytic giant cell granuloma[84]
Granuloma faciale[116]

CONTRAINDICATIONS

Absolute
Sensitivity to clofazimine

Relative
Pregnancy or lactation
Existing gastrointestinal disease
Preexisting electrolyte disturbance[116]

PREGNANCY PRESCRIBING STATUS—CATEGORY C

likelihood of successful therapeutic outcome, as gauged by response and remission rates, is highly variable. Although clofazimine is used for a host of dermatoses, it does not appear to be the drug of choice for any one condition.

Clofazimine is seldom used as a solitary agent. It is most often used in combination with other antimicrobial or antiinflammatory drugs. It does not affect the bioavailability of dapsone.[84] It slightly alters the pharmacodynamics of rifampin, and its levels in urine and plasma are slightly elevated with simultaneous isoniazid use; the clinical significance of these alterations is presumed negligible.[85] Usually 50 to 300 mg is given daily; doses as high as 400 mg daily have been reported by some authors. Larger doses are usually divided three to four times daily. Attempts to taper the drug to a maintenance dose should be made after clinical response occurs.

ADVERSE EFFECTS. Clofazimine is usually safe and well tolerated. The most common adverse effect seen with its use is a reversible or-ange-brown discoloration of the skin beginning within 2 to 4 weeks of initiating use. The cause is not only direct drug deposition but is also due to an induced hypermelanosis. Tears, sweat, hair, sputum, milk, urine, and feces can also have this discoloration. This usually resolves spontaneously within a few months of stopping therapy. Approximately 30% of patients experience a generalized xerosis, although progression to frank ichthyosis is not uncommon.[84,85]

Rare and more serious adverse effects can result from crystal deposition within the viscera. This usually occurs in a dose- and duration-dependent manner. Deposition within the small bowel may rarely cause a fatal enteropathy.[117] Splenic infarction and eosinophilic enteritis have also been reported.[118-120] One case reporting cardiac dysrhythmia related to clofazimine use and a preexisting electrolyte disturbance exists.[121] Common effects of less significance include abdominal cramping, nausea, and diarrhea. Nail changes, pedal edema, and exacerbation of vitiligo have also been reported.[122-124]

Table 22-7   Clofazimine Drug Interactions

Interacting Drug	Comments
Dapsone[84]	*No effect on the bioavailability of dapsone*
Rifampin[85]	Clofazimine slightly alters the pharmacodynamics of rifampin but does not alter risks or benefits
Isoniazid[84]	Clofazimine levels are increased in urine and plasma by this drug, unknown mechanism, or significance

Clofazimine Monitoring Guidelines

BASELINE

Clinical Evaluation
- Review of systems and examination with emphasis on baseline pigmentation, preexisting gastrointestinal conditions, and preexisting depression*

Laboratory Testing
- Electrolyte panel[116]†
- Liver function tests to include serum bilirubin and AST if doses over 100 mg/day are anticipated[85]

FOLLOW-UP
- Frequency—at least monthly for first 3 to 4 months, thereafter at least every 3 to 6 months

Clinical Evaluation
- Review of systems and examination with emphasis on cutaneous pigmentation and possible signs and symptoms of clinical depression
- Also focus on gastrointestinal symptomatology

Laboratory Testing
- Electrolyte panel with each visit‡
- Liver function tests with each visit for those patients on clofazimine doses over 100 mg/day

Note: More frequent surveillance needed if laboratory values are abnormal or with high-risk patients.
*Depression may occur secondary to cutaneous discoloration; two suicides have been reported.
†Cardiotoxicity, in the form of torsades de pointes, has been reported in one person with preexisting low serum levels of magnesium.[121]
‡An electrocardiogram should be considered for patients on clofazimine who develop electrolyte disturbances or other symptoms of clofazimine toxicity to rule out the presence of coexisting cardiotoxicity.[121]

Drug Interactions

The relatively few drug interactions involving clofazimine are listed in Table 22-7. Note that the concomitant use of dapsone with clofazimine is acceptable.

Monitoring Guidelines

The drug is absolutely contraindicated for those with sensitivity to clofazimine. It is relatively contraindicated during pregnancy (category C) and lactation and for patients with preexisting gastrointestinal (GI) disease or individuals prone to electrolyte disturbances. Monitoring should focus on GI symptomatology. Patients receiving doses in excess of 100 mg daily should have

liver function tests evaluated periodically.[85] Baseline electrolyte panels may be prudent. Continuing evaluation of skin discoloration and its possible psychologic effects on the patient may also be necessary.

INTRAVENOUS IMMUNOGLOBULIN

Immunoglobulins are produced by mature plasma cells, which are derived from activated B cells. IVIg is extracted from pooled plasma, requiring between 10,000 and 20,000 donors per production cycle. Numerous measures are in place to ensure the safety of IVIg. Even though comprehensive screening for infectious diseases occurs, the possibility of transmitting unforeseen pathogens via IVIg must be considered during the risk/benefit analysis of therapeutic options. Nevertheless, the improved quality of IVIg is leading to its more frequent use as availability and economics allow. IVIg offers new hope for the treatment of certain dermatoses, such as the bullous autoimmune diseases, where only a decade ago few treatment alternatives existed.[125] Its use in the field of dermatology continues to expand beyond the treatment of dermatomyositis and was recently the subject of an excellent review by Jolles and colleagues.[126]

Pharmacology

See Table 22-2 for key pharmacologic concepts of IVIg. Of the existing classes of immunoglobulins (IgM, IgD, IgE, IgA, and IgG), IVIg products are composed primarily of the IgG class, of which a normal subclass distribution is desired. IgA is eliminated as much as possible to decrease the possibility of anaphylaxis in patients with isolated IgA deficiency. IFN-γ, soluble CD4, and class II human leukocyte antigens (HLA) are also present in small quantities.[126] IgG anti-

bodies are readily available after infusions with peak levels occurring almost instantaneously.[127] Due primarily to its distribution between intravascular and extravascular compartments, serum levels of IVIg drop to between 40% and 50% of their peak within 1 week of administration.[128-130] The half-life of IVIg appears to be between 3 and 5 weeks and may be decreased among those with fever or active infection.[127,131]

MECHANISMS OF ACTION. See Table 22-3 for drug mechanisms of IVIg. Mouthon[132] suggested several mechanisms by which IVIg may exert its immunoregulatory effects via the IgG molecule. These include the blockade of reticuloendothelial fragment crystallizable (Fc) receptors, impedance of complement-mediated damage, alteration of cytokine and cytokine antagonist levels, reduction of circulating autoantibodies, and elimination of pathogens, which may trigger autoantibody production. In addition to IgG, IVIg contains other immunologically active components, which have been hypothesized to mediate its beneficial effects.[133]

Clinical Use

Table 22-8 lists indications and contraindications for IVIg.

Table 22-8	IV Immunoglobulin Indications and Contraindications

FDA-APPROVED INDICATIONS
GVHD[125,126]

OFF-LABEL USES

Connective Tissue Diseases	Hypersensitivity Dermatoses
Dermatomyositis[126,134-138]	Erythema multiforme[149]
	Chronic urticaria[126]
Autoimmune Bullous Dermatoses	
Pemphigus vulgaris and foliaceus[139-142]	**Other Dermatoses**
Bullous pemphigoid[144,148]	Atopic dermatitis[147,148]
Epidermolysis bullosa acquisita[144-146]	Pyoderma gangrenosum[150,151]
Pemphigoid gestationis (herpes gestationis)[152]	

CONTRAINDICATIONS

Absolute	Relative
History of severe systemic reaction to immune globulin or anti-IgA	Progressive renal dysfunction
Sensitivity to thimerosal	Pregnancy
IgA deficiency	

PREGNANCY PRESCRIBING STATUS—NOT LISTED

FDA-APPROVED INDICATIONS

Graft-Versus-Host Disease.   At present the only illness a dermatologist is likely to encounter for which FDA approval of IVIg use exists is GVHD. In this setting, IVIg is sometimes used to prophylactically decrease the occurrence of acute GVHD and systemic infection in the first 100 days after bone marrow transplantation.[125]

OFF-LABEL USES

Dermatomyositis.   The best documented off-label dermatologic use for the agent is in the treatment of dermatomyositis (DM). An adequate number of studies have now been published to establish IVIg as an appropriate adjunctive therapy in cases of DM in which conventional therapy is ineffective or poorly tolerated.[123,131-134] Its effective use in juvenile DM is also documented.[135] The off-label use of IVIg has been reported for several other challenging dermatologic conditions having an immunologic component to their pathogenesis (see Table 22-8).

ADVERSE EFFECTS.   Adverse effects associated with the use of IVIg are rare and usually self-limiting. The most frequently encountered symptoms occur within an hour of infusion and may include headache, flushing, chills, myalgia, wheezing, tachycardia, lower back pain, nausea, or hypotension. If encountered, infusion should be slowed or stopped. If symptoms are anticipated, the patient may be premedicated with either IV hydrocortisone or an antihistamine.[153] Anaphylaxis occurs rarely.[126] Hematologic events, such as disseminated intravascular coagulation with associated serum sickness and transient neutropenia, have been reported.[154,155] An aseptic meningitis syndrome is listed in the warning sections in the various manufacturers' package inserts. Cutaneous adverse effects reported include eczematous eruptions and alopecia.[156,157]

The use of IVIg is contraindicated in those with a history of severe reaction to either immunoglobulin or anti-IgA, or a known sensitivity to thimerosal. Patients with isolated IgA deficiency are at higher risk for anaphylaxis. The use of IVIg can also diminish the effectiveness of measles/mumps/rubella, varicella, and yellow fever vaccines. The individual vaccine package insert should be consulted before the use of IVIg.

Monitoring Guidelines

Before therapy, baseline liver and renal functions must be assessed. Patients with progressive renal disease may not be appropriate candidates for IVIg therapy. Screening for hepatitis and IgA deficiency is necessary, and high titers of rheuma-

---

Intravenous Immunoglobulin Monitoring Guidelines[126]

BASELINE	FOLLOW-UP
Clinical Evaluation	• Frequency—as indicated and before each subsequent infusion
• Complete history and physical examination with emphasis on preexisting liver or renal disease or history of reaction to previous infusion of blood products	
	Clinical Evaluation
	• Directed history and physical focusing on adverse effects with past infusions
Laboratory Testing	
• Liver and renal function tests and complete blood cell count (CBC) with platelets[121]	**Laboratory Testing**
• Screen for HIV antibodies	• Liver and renal function tests and CBC with platelets
• Screen for hepatitis antibodies A, B, and C	• For those on long-term therapy with known risk factors, HIV and hepatitis screening should probably be repeated annually
• Immunoglobulin levels to exclude IgA deficiency*	
• Rheumatoid factor and cryoglobulin levels	
• Store small sample of serum used before each infusion†	

Note: More frequent surveillance is needed if laboratory values are abnormal or with high-risk patients.
*If no IgA antibodies are found, anti-IgA antibody titers should be obtained.
†For future analysis in the event of infectious disease transmission.

toid factor and cryoglobulins must be excluded. A small amount of the serum used should be stored for future examination should the question of an acquired infectious disease arise.[126]

Therapeutic Guidelines

In general, the dose of IVIg used in the treatment of inflammatory or autoimmune diseases is much greater than the dose used for immunodeficiencies. In this context, the term "high-dose" IVIg is used. The most common dose used is 2 g/kg/month, divided into either two doses of 1 g/kg daily or five doses of 0.4 g/kg daily.[126] The rate of response varies from within a matter of days to several months. In most cases, however, it is possible to reduce the amount of other medications, such as corticosteroids or azathioprine, necessary to benefit the patient. The typical duration of clinical benefit from IVIg and a maintenance schedule for its use have not been adequately established to date.

IVIg is expensive. Jolles[126] estimated the cost of the drug alone for the treatment of a theoretical patient with DM to be $42,000 per year (in 1997). Given the drug's cost and complexity of administration, which usually requires hospital admission, IVIg is unlikely to become the drug of choice for any dermatologic condition. However, when improvement in quality of life for highly selected dermatoses is factored into the equation, it becomes clear that this drug will be used more frequently in the future. Except for DM, controlled studies have not been published to date. Anyone proposing to use IVIg for any other indication should seek out an ongoing study in which to enroll their patient so that the clinical utility and safety of this promising therapy can be better established.

PENICILLAMINE

Penicillamine is a breakdown product of penicillin. It is a potent chelator of heavy metals (i.e., copper, gold, lead, mercury, and zinc), promoting their excretion in urine. Nondermatologic indications for its use include the treatment of heavy metal poisoning, cystinuria, Wilson's disease, primary biliary cirrhosis, and rheumatoid arthritis.[158] The use of penicillamine in cutaneous disease seems to be declining; historically, penicillamine

has primarily been used in the treatment of various forms of scleroderma. This is undoubtedly due to its long list of commonly induced adverse effects, its dubious track record of efficacy, and the availability of better therapeutic options. In fact, given its propensity to cause cutaneous adverse effects, the practicing dermatologist is more likely to encounter eruptions induced by penicillamine than to prescribe this medication.

Pharmacology

See Table 22-2 for key pharmacologic concepts of penicillamine. The oral absorption of penicillamine ranges between 40% and 70% and is diminished by food and antacids containing magnesium-aluminum salts and diminished in patients with gastrointestinal manifestations of scleroderma. The peak plasma concentration of the parent compound occurs within 1 to 3 hours after a dose; its half-life also approximates 1 to 3 hours.[159] Hepatic metabolism occurs, transforming most penicillamine to disulfides and inorganic sulfate. The disulfides play major roles in both therapeutic and toxic effects. The disulfide products readily bind to plasma proteins and are not excreted renally. These metabolic products accumulate during the first few weeks of therapy and are slowly eliminated once therapy is stopped.[158] Unmetabolized drug is primarily eliminated via the kidneys with unabsorbed drug found in the feces.[159]

MECHANISMS OF ACTION. The binding of penicillamine to copper has been utilized in patients with Menkes' syndrome being simultaneously treated with intramuscular copper.[160] However, a different mechanism of action, inhibition of collagen maturation, is important in the treatment of scleroderma.

Clinical Use

INDICATIONS. Adult dosing is initiated at 250 mg/day with increases of 125 to 250 mg/day occurring incrementally every 1 to 3 months until satisfactory remission or toxicity occurs (usually at levels between 750 and 1500 mg/day). Therapy is commonly required for several months, with time to response and remission varying widely. The dose should be slowly decreased as possible while maintaining remission. Using such a regimen, Jimenez[161] reported a cutaneous response rate of over 90% in a 15-year prospective study of the drug's use in progressive systemic sclerosis. The dose must be adjusted during renal failure, pregnancy, and for children.

CONTRAINDICATONS.   The drug should be used with extra caution during pregnancy and in those allergic to penicillin or with renal dysfunction. There is a relative contraindication to pencillamine therapy in patients simultaneously undergoing therapy with gold, phenylbutazone, oxyphenbutazone, or antimalarial agents and cytotoxic agents.

ADVERSE EFFECTS.   Common adverse effects of therapy include nausea, vomiting, abdominal pain, and diarrhea. The list of noncutaneous adverse effects reported with the use of penicillamine is exhaustive. Bialy-Golan and Brenner[158] included a thorough discussion of this topic in their recent review. Among other unpleasant possibilities, the clinician must be aware of the possibility of proteinuria, blood and platelet dyscrasias, and hepatotoxicity.[161] Established adverse cutaneous effects related to the use of penicillamine are well known to anyone ever having the pleasure of taking a dermatology board examination and include the bullous dermatoses (including several forms of pemphigus, cicatricial and bullous pemphigoid, and possibly epidermolysis bullosa acquisita),[158,162] a lupus-like syndrome,[163,164] lichen planus,[165] elastosis perforans serpiginosa,[166-169] and pseudoxanthoma elasticum.[170] Some have even described characteristic nail changes and a unique dermatopathy related to penicillamine use.[171,172]

ANTICHOLINERGIC AGENTS (GLYCOPYRROLATE AND PROPANTHELINE)

The use of systemic anticholinergic drugs for the symptomatic treatment of hyperhidrosis has been established since at least the 1950s.[173] There are multiple atropine-like agents available; however, atropine itself is seldom used due to its relatively frequent ophthalmic adverse effects. Glycopyrrolate and propantheline bromide appear to be the most frequently used anticholinergic agents in the sparse literature available on this topic.

Absorption after oral administration is poor and variable. This may explain in part why clinical effects from these medications vary so much from one patient to the next. Individual sensitivity to a given drug's anticholinergic effects is also likely to be partially responsible. It is often necessary for multiple drugs from this class to be used before finding one that adequately controls a given patient's symptoms. Anticholinergic agents ultimately work by blocking the effect of acetylcholine on sweat glands, thus decreasing perspiration.[174,175]

Glycopyrrolate is usually prescribed in doses of 1 to 2 mg, two to three times daily. Propantheline's initial dose is usually 15 mg, two to three times daily. These medications can be gradually titrated to higher doses if symptoms are tolerated. Reduction in hyperhidrosis often occurs within a matter of days; unfortunately adverse effects are common at effective drug levels. Less serious symptoms include dryness of the mouth and blurred vision. More serious adverse effects are rare but include glaucoma, hyperthermia, and seizures.[173-177] The coadministration of these drugs with several medications, such as the tricyclic antidepressants, may lead to increased anticholinergic adverse effects. In addition, the pharmacologic effects of atenolol and digoxin may be increased by the simultaneous use of anticholinergic agents. The antipsychotic effects of the phenothiazines may be decreased. The package inserts for these medications should be consulted before their prescription for a more thorough discussion of possible drug interactions.

Although these agents are often poorly tolerated, a significant number of patients' symptoms are adequately controlled at doses low enough as to induce no appreciable adverse effects. Given the reasonable possibility of success, a trial with anticholinergic medication is often warranted before pursuing more invasive therapies for hyperhidrosis.

BIOTIN

Biotin (vitamin H) is a water soluble, B-complex vitamin essential for the function of a number of carboxylase enzymes. Food sources of biotin include organ meats, egg yolk, milk, fish, and nuts; biotin may also be synthesized by intestinal flora. Biotin is readily available as a supplement without a prescription. Dietary deficiency of biotin is rare. More frequently, deficiencies have been reported in association with total parenteral nutrition. Cutaneous signs of biotin deficiency are similar to those seen in multiple carboxylase deficiency. These signs include thinning of the hair and loss of hair pigmentation. Seborrheic dermatitis or other eczematous eruption frequently occurs around the eyes, nose, and mouth, which may mimic the rash seen in zinc deficiency.[178,179]

The practicing physician is unlikely to encounter a patient with true biotin deficiency. When discovered, response to supplementation is rapid. The cutaneous findings in the deficient state, however, along with reports regarding hoof and mane development from the veterinary literature, led to the use of biotin in patients without a documented biotin deficiency. Biotin has been used with reported success in the treatment of brittle nails,[180,181] atopic dermatitis,[182] uncombable hair syndrome,[183] and Unna-Thost syndrome.[184] Other physicians prescribed supplementation for patients' subjective concerns of thinning or brittleness of the hair, with anecdotal success.

The daily requirement of biotin for an adult is between 100 and 200 μg. The most frequently used dosage for hair and nail problems is 2500 to 3000 μg daily. Higher doses have been used for treating dermatitic eruptions (5 mg/day) and keratodermas (50 mg/day). Duration of therapy ranges from several weeks to months.[180-184] Time to response is variable and supplementation must be continued indefinitely to maintain improvement. Toxicity due to biotin intake has not been reported to date. The only reported side effect is the rare occurrence of GI upset. Controlled studies are necessary to determine the true clinical utility of biotin.

VITAMIN E

Vitamin E (tocopherol) is a fat-soluble vitamin whose exact biochemical mechanisms are unclear. Many of this vitamin's actions have been attributed to its antioxidant properties. Sources of vitamin E include vegetable oils, leafy vegetables, milk, eggs, meat, and some nuts. Clinical deficiency of vitamin E is exceedingly rare; however, supplements are readily available and widely used. In the industrialized world, no cutaneous signs or symptoms have been reported from vitamin E deficiency.[181]

Keller and Fenske[186] recently reviewed potential dermatologic uses for oral vitamin E. Conditions for which there is evidence of vitamin E efficacy include epidermolysis bullosa, CCLE, yellow nail syndrome, granuloma annulare, and claudication contributing to skin ulceration. There have also been reports discussing the possible role of vitamin E in skin cancer prevention.[185,187,188] Although some studies have been promising, it would be premature to conclude there is a beneficial effect in this regard at present. Recently, its utility in reducing side effects associated with oral retinoid therapy has been anecdotally reported.[189] There is a wide range of reported dosages for the therapeutic use of vitamin E. Ingestion of vitamin E may augment the effects of oral anticoagulants.

Cutaneous conditions for which vitamin E is ineffective include psoriasis, atopic dermatitis, dermatitis herpetiformis, porphyria, and subcorneal pustular dermatosis.[185]

ZINC SULFATE

Zinc is a trace element involved in many cellular processes. Deficiency has been reported secondary to dietary inadequacy, especially among those dependent on total parenteral nutrition and in breast-fed infants.[190] The classic cutaneous findings associated with zinc deficiency are circumorificial and acral dermatitis and accompanying diarrhea. Zinc deficiency is mimicked by acrodermatitis enteropathica (AE), an autosomal-recessive disorder of zinc metabolism that presents in infancy.[191,192] AE and dietary zinc deficiency can each be readily confirmed with serum zinc levels, and both rapidly respond to zinc supplementation. Usual doses of zinc replacement are in the range of 1 to 2 mg/kg/day of elemental zinc in three divided doses.

In the past, zinc was used with inconsistent success to treat acne vulgaris and alopecia. The mineral's utility in these conditions now seems circumspect at best. Recent work has shown zinc sulfate in combination with cimetidine to be effective in the therapy of common variable immunodeficiency.[193] Other publications recently discounted associations between low zinc levels and seborrheic dermatitis among people who are HIV-positive and among women with recurrent vulvovaginal candidiasis.[194,195]

Bibliography

Thalidomide

Barnhill RL, McDougall AC: Thalidomide: Use and possible mode of action in reactional lepromatous leprosy and in various other conditions. *J Am Acad Dermatol* 7:317-323, 1982.

System for thalidomide education and prescribing safety: Thalomid (thalidomide)—balancing the benefits and the risks. Copyright 1998, Celgene Corporation, Warren, NJ 07059 USA (1-888-4-CELGENE).

Tseng S, Pak G, Washenik K, et al: Rediscovering thalidomide: A review of its mechanism of action, side effects, and potential uses. *J Am Acad Dermatol* 35:969-979, 1996.

Clofazimine

Arbiser JL, Moschella SL: Clofazimine: A review of its medical uses and mechanisms of action. *J Am Acad Dermatol* 32:241-247, 1995.

O'Connor R, O'Sullivan JF, O'Kennedy R: The pharmacology, metabolism, and chemistry of clofazimine. *Drug Metab Rev* 27:591-614, 1995.

Intravenous Immunoglobulin

Dwyer JM: Manipulating the immune system with immune globulin. *Drug Ther* 326:107-116, 1992.

Jolles S, Hughes J, Whittaker S: Dermatological uses of high-dose intravenous immunoglobulin. *Arch Dermatol* 134:80-86, 1999.

Mouthon L, Kaveri SV, Spalter SH, et al: Mechanisms of action of intravenous immune globulin in immune mediated diseases. *Clin Exp Immunol* 104(Suppl 1):3-9, 1996.

Penicillamine

Bialy-Golan A, Brenner S: Penicillamine-induced bullous dermatoses. *J Am Acad Dermatol* 35:732-742, 1996.

Jimenez SA, Sigal SH: A 15-year prospective study of treatment of rapidly progressive systemic sclerosis with D-penicillamine. *J Rheumatol* 18:1496-1503, 1991.

Netter P, Bannwarth B, Pere P, et al: Clinical pharmacokinetics of D-penicillamine. *Clin Pharmacol* 13:317-333, 1987.

Anticholinergic Agents

Herxheimer A: Excessive sweating. *Trans St. John's Hosp Dermatol Soc* 40:20-25, 1958.

Biotin

Mock DM: Skin manifestations of biotin deficiency. *Semin Dermatol* 10:296-302, 1991.

Vitamin E

Pehr K, Forsey RR: Why don't we use vitamin E in dermatology? *Can Med Assoc J* 149:1247-1253, 1993.

Zinc Sulfate

Sandstrom B, Cederblad A, Lindblad BS, et al: Acrodermatitis enteropathica, zinc metabolism, copper status, and immune function. *Arch Pediatr Adolesc Med* 148:980-985, 1994.

References

Thalidomide—Pharmacology

1. Tseng S, Pak G, Washenik K, et al: Rediscovering thalidomide: a review of its mechanism of action, side effects, and potential uses. *J Am Acad Dermatol* 35:969-979, 1996.

2. Powell RJ, Gardner-Medwin JMM: Guideline for the clinical use and dispensing of thalidomide. *Postgrad Med J* 70:901-904, 1994.

3. Stirling D, Sherman M, Strauss S: Thalidomide—A surprising recovery. *J Am Pharm Assoc* NS37:306-313, 1997.

4. Eriksson T, Bjorkman S, Roth B, et al: Stereospecific determination, chiral inversion in vitro and pharmacokinetics in humans of the enantiomers of thalidomide. *Chirality* 7:44-52, 1995.

5. Chen TL, Vogelsang GB, Petty BG, et al: Plasma pharmacokinetics and urinary excretion of thalidomide after oral dosing in healthy male volunteers. *Drug Metab Dispos* 17:402-405, 1989.

6. Gunzler V: Thalidomide in human immunodeficiency virus (HIV) patients: a review of safety considerations. *Drugs* 7:116-134, 1992.

7. Schumacher H, Smith RL, Williams RT: The metabolism of thalidomide: the fate of thalidomide and some of its various hydrolysis products in various species. *Br J Pharmacol* 25:338-351, 1965.

8. Robertson J: Thalidomide revisited. *Okla St Med Assoc J* 65:45, 1972.

9. Braun AG, Harding FA, Weinreb SL: Teratogen metabolism: thalidomide activation is mediated by cytochrome P-450. *Toxicol Appl Pharmacol* 82:175-179, 1986.

10. Barnhill RL, McDougall AC: Thalidomide: Use and possible mode of action in reactional lepromatous leprosy and in various other conditions. *J Am Acad Dermatol* 7:317-323, 1982.

11. Sampaio EP, Sarno EN, Galilly R, et al: Thalidomide selectively inhibits tumor necrosis factor-alpha production by stimulated human monocytes. *J Exp Med* 173:699-703, 1991.

12. Gad SM, Shannon EJ, Krotoski WA, et al: Thalidomide induces imbalances in T-lymphocyte sub-populations in the circulating blood of healthy males. *Lepr Rev* 56:35-39, 1985.

13. Moller DR, Wysocka M, Greenlee BM, et al: Inhibition of IL-12 production by thalidomide. *J Immunol* 159:5157-5161, 1997.

14. McHugh SM, Rifkin IR, Deighton J, et al: The immunosuppressive drug thalidomide induces T helper cell type 2 (Th2) and concomitantly inhibits Th1 cytokine production in mitogen- and antigen-stimulated human peripheral blood mononuclear cell cultures. *Clin Exp Immunol* 99:160-167, 1995.

15. Hastings RC: Kellersberger Memorial Lecture 1979: Immunosuppressive/anti-inflammatory thalidomide analogues. *Ethiop Med J* 18:65-71, 1980.

16. Faure M, Thivolet J, Gaucherand M: Inhibition of PMN leukocyte chemotaxis by thalidomide. *Arch Dermatol Res* 269:275-280, 1980.

17. Barnhill RL, Doll NJ, Millikan LE, et al: Studies on the anti-inflammatory properties of thalidomide: effects on polymorphonuclear leukocytes and monocytes. *J Am Acad Dermatol* 11:814-819, 1984.

18. Van den Broek H: Treatment of prurigo nodularis with thalidomide. *Arch Dermatol* 116:571-572, 1980.

19. D'Amato RJ, Loughnan MS, Flynn E, et al: Thalidomide is an inhibitor of angiogenesis. *Proc Natl Acad Sci USA* 91:4082-4085, 1994.

Thalidomide—Clinical Use

20. Marwick C: Thalidomide back under strict control. *JAMA* 278:1135-1137, 1997.

21. Sheskin J: The treatment of lepra reaction in lepromatous leprosy: fifteen years' experience with thalidomide. *Int J Dermatol* 19:318-322, 1980.

22. AMA Department of Drugs: *Drug evaluation subscription*, Chicago, 1991, Am Med Association.

23. Sheshkin J, Convit J: Results of a double-blind study of the influence of thalidomide on the lepra reaction. *Int J Lepr* 37:135-146, 1969.

24. Iyers CGS, Languillon J, Ramanujam K, et al: WHO coordinated short-term double-blind trial with thalidomide in the treatment of acute lepra reactions in male lepromatous patients. *Bull World Health Org* 45:719-732, 1971.

25. Jew LJ: Thalidomide in erythema nodosum leprosum. DICP. *Ann Pharmacother* 24:482-483, 1990.

26. Reynolds JEF, editor: *Martindale: The Extra Pharmacopoeia* (electronic version), Denver, CO, 1993, Micromedix, Inc.

27. Levis WR: Treatment of leprosy in the United States. *Bull NY Acad Med* 60:696-711, 1984.

28. Pfaltzgraff RE: The management of reaction in leprosy. *Int J Leprosy* 57:103-109, 1989.

29. Alexander LN, Wilcox CM: A prospective trial of thalidomide for the treatment of HIV-associated idiopathic esophageal ulcers. *AIDS Res Hum Retrovir* 13:301-304, 1997.

30. Youle M, Clarbour J, Farthing C, et al: Treatment of resistant aphthous ulceration with thalidomide in patients positive for HIV antibody. *BMJ* 298:432, 1989.

31. Radeff B, Kuffer R, Samson J: Recurrent aphthous ulcer in patient infected with human immunodeficiency virus: successful treatment with thalidomide. *J Am Acad Dermatol* 23:523-525, 1990.

32. Ghigliotti G, Repetto T, Farris A, et al: Thalidomide: treatment of choice of aphthous ulcers in patients seropositive for human immunodeficiency virus. *J Am Acad Dermatol* 28:271-272, 1993.

33. Soler RA, Howard M, Brink NS, et al: Regression of AIDS-related Kaposi's sarcoma during therapy with thalidomide. *CID* 23:501-503, 1996.

34. Paterson DL, Georghiou PR, Allworth AM, et al: Thalidomide as treatment of refractory aphthous ulceration related to human immunodeficiency virus infection. *Clin Infect Dis* 20:250-254, 1995.

35. Mascaro JM, Lecha M, Torras H: Thalidomide in the treatment of recurrent, necrotic, and giant mucocutaneous aphthae and aphthosis (letter). *Arch Dermatol* 115:636-637, 1979.

36. Grinspan D: Significant response of oral aphthosis to thalidomide treatment. *J Am Acad Dermatol* 12:85-90, 1985.

37. Revuz J, Guillaume JC, Janier M, et al: Crossover study of thalidomide vs placebo in severe recurrent aphthous stomatitis. *Arch Dermatol* 126:923-927, 1990.

38. Menni S, Imondi D, Brancaleone W: Recurrent giant aphthous ulcers in a child: protracted treatment with thalidomide. *Ped Dermatol* 10:283-285, 1993.

39. Mangelsdorf HC, White WL, Jorizzo JL: Behçet's disease: Report of twenty-five patients from the United States with prominent mucocutaneous involvement. *J Am Acad Dermatol* 34:745-750, 1996.

40. Lewis DA, Amerasinghe CN, Murphy SM: Successful treatment of Behçet's syndrome in an African female patient with thalidomide. *Int J STD AIDS* 7:518-520, 1996.

41. Saylan T, Saltik I: Thalidomide in the treatment of Behçet's syndrome (letter). *Arch Dermatol* 118:536, 1982.

42. Hamza M: Behçet's disease, palmoplantar pustulosis and HLA-B27: treatment with thalidomide (CG-217). *J Int Med* 228:405-407, 1990.

43. Hecker MS, Lebwohl MG: Recalcitrant pyoderma gangrenosum: treatment with thalidomide. *J Am Acad Dermatol* 38:490-491, 1998.

44. Rustin MHA, Gilkes JJH, Robinson TWE: Pyoderma gangrenosum associated with Behçet's disease: Treatment with thalidomide. *J Am Acad Dermatol* 23:941-944, 1990.

45. Munro CS, Cox NH: Pyoderma gangrenosum associated with Behçet's syndrome: response to thalidomide. *Clin Exp Dermatol* 13:408-410, 1988.

46. Dereure O, Basset-Seguin N, Guilhou JJ: Erosive lichen planus: dramatic response to thalidomide. *Arch Dermatol* 132:1392-1393, 1996.

47. Naafs B, Faber WR: Thalidomide therapy: an open trial. *Int J Dermatol* 24:131-134, 1985.

48. Bahmer FA, Zaun H, Luszpinski P: Thalidomide treatment of recurrent erythema multiforme. *Acta Derm Venereol (Stockh)* 62:449-450, 1982.

49. Stevens RJ, Andujar C, Edwards CJ, et al: Thalidomide in the treatment of the cutaneous manifestations of lupus erythematosus: experience in sixteen consecutive patients. *Br J Rheum* 36:353-359, 1997.

50. Holm AL, Bowers KE, McMeekin TO, et al: Chronic cutaneous lupus erythematosus treated with thalidomide. *Arch Dermatol* 129:1548-1550, 1993.

51. Grosshans E, Illy G: Thalidomide therapy for inflammatory dermatoses. *Int J Dermatol* 23:598-602, 1984.

52. Lo JS, Berg RE, Tomecki KJ: Treatment of discoid lupus erythematosus. *Int J Dermatol* 28:497-507, 1989.

53. Knop J, Bonsmann G, Happle R, et al: Thalidomide in the treatment of sixty cases of chronic discoid lupus erythematosus. *Br J Dermatol* 108:461-466, 1983.

54. Naafs B, Bakkers EJM, Flinterman J, et al: Thalidomide treatment of subacute cutaneous lupus erythematosus. *Br J Dermatol* 107:83-86, 1982.

55. Atra E, Sato EI: Treatment of the cutaneous lesions of systemic lupus erythematosus with thalidomide. *Clin Exp Rheum* 11:487-493, 1993.

56. Burrows NP, Walport MJ, Hammond AH, et al: Lupus erythematosus profundus with partial C4 deficiency responding to thalidomide. *Br J Dermatol* 125:62-67, 1991.

57. Warren KJ, Nopper AJ, Crosby DL: Thalidomide for recalcitrant discoid lesions in a patient with systemic lupus erythematosus. *J Am Acad Dermatol* 39:293-295, 1998.

58. Moulin G, Bonnet F, Barrut D, et al: Traitement de la maladie de Jessner-Kanoff par la thalidomide. *Ann Dermatol Venereol* 119:611-614, 1983.

59. Guillaume JC, Moulin G, Dieng MT, et al: Crossover study of thalidomide vs placebo in Jessner's lymphocytic infiltration of the skin. *Arch Dermatol* 131:1032-1035, 1995.

60. Benchikhi H, Bodemer C, Fraitag S, et al: Treatment of cutaneous lymphoid hyperplasia with thalidomide: Report of two cases. *J Am Acad Dermatol* 40:1005-1007, 1999.

61. Parker PM, Chao N, Nademanee A, et al: Thalidomide as salvage therapy for chronic graft-versus-host disease. *Blood* 86:3604-3609, 1995.

62. Cole CH, Rogers PCJ, Pritchard S, et al: Thalidomide in the management of chronic graft-versus-host disease in children following bone marrow transplantation. *Bone Marrow Transplant* 14:937-942, 1994.

63. Vogelsang GB, Farmer ER, Hess AD, et al: Thalidomide for the treatment of chronic graft-versus-host disease. *N Engl J Med* 326:1055-1058, 1992.

64. Grabczyska SA, Hawk JL: Managing PLE and actinic prurigo. *Practitioner* 241:74-79, 1997.

65. Berger TG, Hoffman C, Thieberg MD: Prurigo nodularis and photosensitivity in AIDS: treatment with thalidomide. *J Am Acad Dermatol* 33:837-838, 1995.

66. Londono F: Thalidomide in the treatment of actinic prurigo. *Int J Dermatol* 12:326-328, 1973.

67. Carlesimo M, Giustini S, Rossi A, et al: Treatment of cutaneous and pulmonary sarcoidosis with thalidomide. *J Am Acad Dermatol* 32:866-869, 1995.

68. Rousseau L, Beylot-Barry M, Doutre MS, et al: Cutaneous sarcoidosis successfully treated with thalidomide. *Arch Dermatol* 134:1045-1046, 1998.

69. Lee JB, Koblenzer PS: Disfiguring cutaneous manifestation of sarcoidosis treated with thalidomide: a case report. *J Am Acad Dermatol* 39:835- 838, 1998.

70. Misery L, Larbre B, Lyonnet S, et al: Remission of Langerhans cell histiocytosis with thalidomide treatment. *Clin Exp Dermatol* 15:487, 1993.

71. Eravelly J, Waters MF: Thalidomide in Weber-Christian disease (letter). *Lancet* 1:251, 1977.

72. Silva S, Viana PC, Lugon NV, et al: Thalidomide for the treatment of uremic pruritus: a crossover randomized double-blind trial. *Nephron* 67:270-273, 1994.

Thalidomide—Adverse Effects

73. Ochonisky S, Verroust J, Bastuji-Garin S, et al: Thalidomide neuropathy incidence and clinico electrophysiologic findings in 42 patients. *Arch Dermatol* 130:66-69, 1994.

74. De Iongh RU: A quantitative ultrastructural study of motor and sensory lumbosacral nerve roots in the thalidomide-treated rabbit fetus. *J Neuropathol Exp Neurol* 49:564-581, 1990.

75. Clemmensen OJ, Olsen PZ, Andersen KE: Thalidomide neurotoxicity. *Arch Dermatol* 120:338-341, 1984.

76. Hess CW, Hunzicker T, Kupfer A, et al: Thalidomide-induced peripheral neuropathy: a prospective clinical neurophysiological and pharmacogenetic evaluation. *J Neurol* 233:83-89, 1986.

77. Anonymous: Thalidomide: important patient information. Health and Human Services, Public Health Service, http://www.fda.gov/cder/news/thalidomide.htn.

78. Salafia A, Kharkar RD: Thalidomide and exfoliative dermatitis. *Ann Dermatol Venereol* 117:313-321, 1990.

79. Bielsa I, Teixido J, Ribera M, et al: Erythroderma due to thalidomide: report of two cases. *Dermatology* 189:179-181, 1994.

80. Williams I , Weller IVD, Malin A, et al: Thalidomide hypersensitivity in AIDS. *Lancet* 337:436-437, 1991.

81. 1974-1998 Micromedix, Inc., all rights reserved, Vol. 95.

82. System for Thalidomide Education and Prescribing Safety: Thalomid (thalidomide)—balancing the benefits and the risks. Copyright 1998, Celgene Corporation, Warren, NJ, 07059 USA.

83. U.S. Food and Drug Administration Center for Drug Evaluation and Research, public communication. http://www.fda.gov/cder/foi/label/1998/20785lbl.htm.

Clofazimine

84. O'Connor R, O'Sullivan JF, O'Kennedy R: The pharmacology, metabolism, and chemistry of clofazimine. *Drug Metab Rev* 27:591-614, 1995.

85. Arbiser JL, Moschella SL: Clofazimine: A review of its medical uses and mechanisms of action. *J Am Acad Dermatol* 32:241-247, 1995.

86. Gomez-Flores R, Tucker SD, Kansal R, et al: Enhancement of antibacterial activity of clofazimine against *Mycobacterium avium-Mycobacterium intracellulare* complex infection induced by IFN-gamma is mediated by TNF-alpha. *J Antimicrob Chemother* 39:189-197, 1997.

87. Krajewska MM, Andersin R: An in vitro comparison of the effects of the prooxidative riminophenazines clofazimine and B669 on neutrophil phospholipase A2 activity and superoxide generation. *J Infect Dis* 167:899-904, 1993.

88. Gallo ME, Alvim MF, Nery JA, et al: Two multidrug fixed-dosage treatment regimens with multibacillary leprosy patients. *Indian J Lepr* 68:235-245, 1996.

89. Rao PS, Ramachandran A, Sekar B, et al: Ofloxacin-containing combined drug regimens in the treatment of lepromatous leprosy. *Lepr Rev* 65:181-189, 1994.

90. Bodemer C, Durand C, Blanche S, et al: Disseminated *Mycobacterium marinum* infection. *Ann Dermatol Venereol* 116:842-843, 1989.

91. Yarrish RL, Shay W, Labombardi VJ, et al: Osteomyelitis caused by *Mycobacterium haemophilum:* successful therapy in two patients with AIDS. *AIDS* 6:557-561, 1992.

92. Vurma-Rapp U, Colla F, Flepp M: *Mycobacterium kansasii* and *Pneumocystis carinii* pneumonia in a patient with acquired immunodeficiency syndrome. *Infection* 17:88-89, 1989.

93. Reddy VM, Nadadhur G, Daneluzzi D, et al: Antituberculosis activities of clofazimine and its new analogs B4154 and B4157. *Antimicrob Agents Chemother* 40:633-636, 1996.

94. Goihman-Yahr M: Malignant pyoderma gangrenosum responding to clofazimine. *Int J Dermatol* 35:757-758, 1996.

95. Erdi H, Anadolu R, Piskin G, et al: Malignant pyoderma: A clinical variant of pyoderma gangrenosum. *Int J Dermatol* 35:811-813, 1996.

96. Kaplan B, Trau H, Sofer E, et al: Treatment of Pyoderma gangrenosum with clofazimine. *Int J Dermatol* 31:591-593, 1992.

97. Michaelsson G, Molin L, Ohman S, et al: Clofazimine: a new agent for the treatment of pyoderma gangrenosum. *Arch Dermatol* 112:344-349, 1976.

98. Mackey JP, Barnes J: Clofazimine in the treatment of discoid lupus erythematosus. *Br J Dermatol* 91:93-96, 1974.

99. Lee SJ, Wegner SA, McGarigle CJ, et al: Treatment of chronic graft-versus-host disease with clofazimine. *Blood* 89:2298-2302, 1997.

100. Chuprapaisilp T, Piamphongsant T: Treatment of pustular psoriasis with clofazimine. *Br J Dermatol* 99:303-305, 1978.

101. Baranda L, Torres-Alvarez B, Cortes-Franco R, et al: Involvement of cell adhesion and activation molecules in the pathogenesis of erythema dyschromicum perstans (ashy dermatitis): The effect of clofazimine therapy. *Arch Dermatol* 133:325-329, 1997.

102. Piquero-Martin J, Perez-Alfonzo R, Abrusci V, et al: Clinical trial with clofazimine for treating erythema dyschromicum perstans: Evaluation of cell-mediated immunity. *Int J Dermatol* 28:198-199, 1989.

103. Kumar B, Kaur S, Kaur I, et al: More about clofazimine—3 years experience and review of literature. *Indian J Lepr* 59:63-74, 1987.

104. Farella V, Lotti T, Difonzo EM, et al: Erythema elevatum diutinum. *Int J Dermatol* 33:638-640, 1994.

105. Saxe N, Gordon W: Acute febrile neutrophilic dermatosis (Sweet's syndrome): four case reports. *S Afr Med J* 32:253-256, 1978.

106. Helander I, Aho HJ: Solid facial edema as a complication of acne vulgaris: treatment with isotretinoin and clofazimine. *Acta Derm Venereol* 67:535-537, 1987.

107. Cros D, Gamby T, Serratrice G: Acne rheumatism: report of a case. *J Rheumatol* 8:336-339, 1981.

108. Prendiville J, Cream JJ: Clofazimine responsive acne vulgaris. *Br J Dermatol* 109:90-91, 1983.

109. Evans AT, Croft SL, Peters W, et al: Antileishmanial effects of clofazimine and other antimycobacterial agents. *Ann Trop Med Parasitol* 83:447-454, 1989.

110. Herrero C, Torras H, Palou J, et al: Successful treatment of a patient with cutaneous malacoplakia with clofazimine and trimethoprim-sulfamethoxazole. *J Am Acad Dermatol* 23:947-948, 1990.

111. Palou J, Torras H, Baradad M, et al: Cutaneous malakoplakia: report of a case. *Dermatologica* 176:288-292, 1988.

112. Shehata MA, Salama AM: Clofazimine in the treatment of scleroma. *J Laryngol Otol* 103:856-860, 1989.

113. Mahler VB, Hornstein OP, Boateng BI, et al: Granulomatous glossitis as an unusual manifestation of Melkersson-Rosenthal syndrome. *Cutis* 55:244-249, 1995.

114. Sussman GL, Yang WH, Steinberg S: Melkersson-Rosenthal syndrome: clinical, pathologic, and therapeutic considerations. *Ann Allerg* 69:187-194, 1992.

115. Mensing H: Clofazimine-therapeutische alternative bei necrobiosis lipoidica und granuloma annulare. *Hautarzt* 40:99-103, 1989.

116. Wollina U, Karte K, Geyer A, et al: Clofazimine in inflammatory facial dermatosis: Granuloma faciale and lipogranulomatosis subcutanea (Rothmann-Makai). *Acta Dermatol Venereol* 76:77-79, 1996.

117. Belaube P, Devaux J, Pizzi M, et al: Small bowel deposition of crystals associated with the use of clofazimine in the treatment of prurigo nodularis. *Int J Lepr Other Mycobact Dis* 51:328-330, 1983.

118. McDougall AC, Horsfall WR, Hede JE, et al: Splenic infarction and tissue accumulation of crystals with the use of clofazimine (Lamprene; B663) in the treatment of pyoderma gangrenosum. *Br J Dermatol* 102:227-230, 1980.

119. Ravi S, Holubka J, Veneri R, et al: Clofazimine-induced eosinophilic gastroenteritis in AIDS. *Am J Gastroenterol* 88:612-613, 1993.

120. Mason GH, Ellis-Pegler RB, Arthur JF: Clofazimine and eosinophilic enteritis. *Lepr Rev* 48:175-180, 1977.

121. Choudri SH, Harris L, Butany JW, et al: Clofazimine induced cardiotoxicity—a case report. *Lepr Rev* 66:63-68, 1995.

122. Dixit VB, Chaudhary SD, Jain VK: Clofazimine induced nail changes. *Indian J Lepr* 61:476-478, 1989.

123. Tyagi PY, Oommen T: Pedal edema following clofazimine therapy; a case report. *Int J Lepr* 61:636, 1993.

124. Brown-Harrel V, Nitta AT, Goble M: Apparent exacerbation of vitiligo syndrome in a patient with pulmonary *Mycobacterium avium* complex disease who received clofazimine therapy. *Clin Infect Dis* 22:581-582, 1996.

Intravenous Immunoglobulin

125. Dwyer JM: Manipulating the immune system with immune globulin. *Drug Ther* 326:107-116, 1992.

126. Jolle S, Hughes J, Whittaker S: Dermatological uses of high-dose intravenous immunoglobulin. *Arch Dermatol* 134:80-86, 1998.

127. Product information: Gammagard S/D®, immune globulin intravenous. Baxter Healthcare, Glendale, CA, 1996.

128. Product information: Iveegam®, immune globulin intravenous. Immuno US, Inc, Rochester, MI, 1996.

129. Product Information: Venoglobulin®-I, immune globulin. Alpha Therapeutic Corporation, Los Angeles, CA, 1996.

130. Morell A, Schurch B, Ryser D, et al: In vivo behavior of gamma globulin preparations. *Vox Sang* 38:272, 1980.

131. Morell A, Riesen W, Nydegger UE, editor: *Structure, function and catabolism of immunoglobulins in immunotherapy,* London, 1981, Academic Press, pp 17-26.

132. Mouthon L, Kaveri SV, Spalter SH, et al: Mechanisms of action of intravenous immune globulin in immune mediated diseases. *Clin Exp Immunol* 104(Suppl 1):3-9, 1996.

133. Lam L, Whitsett CF, McNicholl JM, et al: Immunologically active proteins in intravenous immunoglobulin. *Lancet* 342:678, 1993.

134. Dalakas MC, Illa I, Dambrosia JM, et al: A controlled trial of high-dose intravenous immune globulin infusions as treatment for dermatomyositis. *N Engl J Med* 329:1993-2000, 1993.

135. Cherin P, Herson S, Wechsler B, et al: Efficacy of intravenous gammaglobulin therapy in chronic refractory polymyositis and dermatomyositis: An open study with 20 adult patients. *Am J Med* 91:162-168, 1991.

136. Lang BA, Laxer RM, Murphy G, et al: Treatment of dermatomyositis with intravenous gammaglobulin. *Am J Med* 91:169-172, 1991.

137. Bodemer C, Teillac D, Le Bourgeois M, et al: Efficacy of intravenous immunoglobulins in sclerodermatomyositis (letter). *Br J Dermatol* 123:545-551, 1990.

138. Collet E, Dalac S, Maerens B, et al: Juvenile dermatomyositis: treatment with intravenous gammaglobulin. *Br J Dermatol* 130:231-234, 1994.

139. Beckers RCY, Brand A, Vermeer BJ, et al: Adjuvant high-dose intravenous gammaglobulin in the treatment of pemphigus and bullous pemphigoid: experience in six patients. *Br J Dermatol* 133:289-293, 1995.

140. Bewley AP, Keefe M: Successful treatment of pemphigus vulgaris by pulsed intravenous immunoglobulin therapy. *Br J Dermatol* 135:128-129, 1996.

141. Messer G, Sizmann N, Feucht H, et al: High-dose intravenous immunoglobulins for immediate control of severe pemphigus vulgaris (letter). *Br J Dermatol* 133:1014-1015, 1995.

142. Humbert P, Derancourt C, Aubin F, et al: Effects of intravenous gamma-globulin in pemphigus (letter). *J Am Acad Dermatol* 22:326, 1990.

143. Godard W, Roujeau JC, Guillot B, et al: Bullous pemphigoid and intravenous gammaglobulin. *Ann Intern Med* 103:964-965, 1985.

144. Mohr C, Sunderkotter C, Hildebrand A, et al: Successful treatment of epidermolysis bullosa acquisita using intravenous immunoglobulins. *Br J Dermatol* 132:824-826, 1995.

145. Meier F, Sonnichsen K, Schaumburg-Lever G, et al: Epidermolysis bullosa acquisita: Efficacy of high-dose intravenous immunoglobulins. *J Am Acad Dermatol* 29:334-337, 1993.

146. Caldwell JB, Yancey KB, Engler JM, et al: Epidermolysis bullosa acquisita: Efficacy of high-dose intravenous immunoglobulins (letter). *J Am Acad Dermatol* 31:827-828, 1994.

147. Kimata H: High-dose gammaglobulin treatment for atopic dermatitis. *Arch Dis Child* 70:335-336, 1994.

148. Pons-Guiraud A: Value of alleroglobulin in the treatment of atopic dermatitis in children and young adults: a double-blind randomized study. *Rev Med Interne* 7:537-542, 1986.

149. Schofield JK, Tatnall FM, Leigh IM: Recurrent erythema multiforme: clinical features and treatment in a large series of patients. *Br J Dermatol* 128:542-545, 1993.

150. Dirschka T, Kastner U, Beherns S, et al: Successful treatment of pyoderma gangrenosum with intravenous human immunoglobulin. *J Am Acad Dermatol* 39:789-90, 1998.

151. Gupta AK, Shear NH, Sauder DN: Efficacy of human intravenous immune globulin in pyoderma gangrenosum. *J Am Acad Dermatol* 32:140-142, 1995.

152. Matthiesem L, Andersson T, Vahlquist C, et al: Intravenous immunoglobulin in gestational pemphigoid: the itching disappeared and skin changes healed. *Lakartidningen* 92:409-410, 1995.

153. Misbah SA, Chapel HM: Adverse effects of intravenous immunoglobulin. *Drug Saf* 9:254-262, 1993.

154. Comenzo RL, Malachowski ME, Meissner HC, et al: Immune hemolysis, disseminated intravascular coagulation, and serum sickness after large doses of immune globulin given intravenously for Kawasaki disease. *J Peds* 120:926-928, 1992.

155. Grebenau MD: Transient neutropenia induced by intravenous immune globulin (letter). *N Engl J Med* 325:270-271, 1992.

156. Barucha C, McMillan JC: Eczema after intravenous infusion of immunoglobulin (letter). *BMJ* 295:1141, 1987.

157. Chan-Lam D, Fitzsimons EJ, Douglas WS: Alopecia after immunoglobulin infusion (letter). *Lancet* 1:1436, 1987.

Penicillamine

158. Bialy-Golan A, Brenner S: Penicillamine-induced dermatoses. *J Am Acad Dermatol* 35:732-742, 1996.

159. Netter P, Bannwarth B, Pere P, et al: Clinical pharmacokinetics of D-penicillamine. *Clin Pharmacol* 13:317-333, 1987.

160. Nadal D, Baerlocher K: Menkes' disease: long-term treatment with copper and D-penicillamine. *Eur J Pediatr* 147:621-625, 1988.

161. Jimenez SA, Sigal SH: A 15-year prospective study of treatment of rapidly progressive systemic sclerosis with D-penicillamine. *J Rheumatol* 18:1496-1503, 1991.

162. Weller R, White MI: Bullous pemphigoid and penicillamine. *Clin Exp Dermatol* 21:121-122, 1996.

163. Yung RL, Richardson BC: Drug-induced lupus. *Rheum Dis Clin N Am* 20:61-86, 1994.

164. Fritzler MJ: Drugs recently associated with lupus syndromes. *Lupus* 3:455-459, 1994.

165. Thompson DF, Skaehill PA: Drug-induced lichen planus. *Pharmacotherapy* 14:561-571, 1994.

166. Amichai B, Rotem A, Metzker A: D-penicillamine-induced elastosis perforans serpiginosa and localized cutis laxa in a patient with Wilson's disease. *Isr J Med Sci* 30:667-669, 1994.

167. Iozumi K, Nakagawa H, Tamaki K: Penicillamine-induced degenerative dermatoses: Report of a case and brief review of such dermatoses. *J Dermatol* 24:458-465, 1997.

168. Sahn EE, Maize JC, Garen PD, et al: D-penicillamine-induced elastosis perforans serpiginosa in a child with juvenile rheumatoid arthritis. *J Am Acad Dermatol* 20:979-988, 1989.

169. Ratnavel RC, Norris PG: Penicillamine-induced elastosis perforans serpiginosa treated successfully with isotretinoin. *Dermatology* 189:81-83, 1994.

170. Bolognia JL, Bravernab I: Pseudoxanthoma-elasticum-like skin changes induced by penicillamine. *Dermatology* 184:12-18, 1992.

171. Bjellerup M: Nail changes induced by penicillamine. *Acta Derm Venereol* 69:339-341, 1989.

172. Goldstein JB, McNutt NS, Hambrick GW, et al: Penicillamine dermatopathy with lymphangiectases. *Arch Dermatol* 125:92-97, 1989.

Anticholinergic Agents

173. Herxheimer A: Excessive sweating. *Trans St. John's Hosp Dermatol Soc* 40:20-25, 1958.
174. Rook A, Wilkinson DS, Ebling FJG, editors: *Textbook of dermatology*, vol 3, ed 5, Oxford, 1992, Blackwell Scientific Publications, p 1754.
175. Sato K, Ohtsuyama M, Samman G: Eccrine sweat gland disorders. *J Am Acad Dermatol* 24:1010-1014, 1991.
176. Sato K, Kang WH, Saga K, et al: Biology of sweat glands and their disorders. II. Disorders of sweat gland function. *J Am Acad Dermatol* 20:713-726, 1989.
177. Dobson RL: Treatment of hyperhidrosis (editorial). *J Am Acad Dermatol* 123:883-884, 1987.

Biotin

178. Prendiville JS, Manfredi LN: Skin signs of nutritional disorders. *Semin Dermatol* 11:88-97, 1992.
179. Mock DM: Skin manifestations of biotin deficiency. *Semin Dermatol* 10:296-302, 1991.
180. Hochman LG, Scher RK, Meyerson MS: Brittle nails: response to daily biotin supplementation. *Cutis* 51:303-305, 1993.
181. Colombo VE, Gerber F, Bronhofer M, et al: Treatment of brittle fingernails and onychoschizia with biotin: Scanning electron microscopy. *J Am Acad Dermatol* 23:1127-1132, 1990.
182. Ikura Y, Odajima Y, Nagakura T, et al: Oral biotin treatment is effective for atopic dermatitis in children with low biotinidase activity. *Acta Paediatr Scand* 77:762-763, 1988.
183. Shelley WB, Shelley ED: Uncombable hair syndrome: Observations on response to biotin and occurrence in siblings with ectodermal dysplasia. *J Am Acad Dermatol* 13:97-102, 1985.
184. Menni S, Saleh F, Piccinno R, et al: Palmoplantar keratoderma of Unna-Thost: Response to biotin in one family. *Clin Exp Dermatol* 17:337-338, 1992.

Vitamin E

185. Pehr K, Forsey RR: Why don't we use vitamin E in dermatology? *Can Med Assoc J* 149:1247-1253, 1993.
186. Keller KL, Fenske NA: Uses of vitamins A, C, and E and related compounds in dermatology: a review. *J Am Acad Dermatol* 39:611-625, 1998.
187. Sahl WJ, Glore S, Garrison P, et al: Basal cell carcinoma and lifestyle characteristics. *Int J Dermatol* 34:398-402, 1995.
188. Stryker WS, Stampfer MJ, Stein EA, et al: Diet, plasma levels of beta-carotene and alphatocopherol, and risk of malignant melanoma. *Am J Epid* 131:597-611, 1990.
189. Lebwohl M: Clinical pearl: Vitamin E (alphatocopherol), 800 IU daily, may reduce retinoid toxicity. *J Am Acad Dermatol* 41:260, 1999.

Zinc Sulfate

190. Bilinski DL, Ehrenkranz RA, Cooley-Jacobs J, et al: Symptomatic zinc deficiency in a breast-fed, premature infant. *Arch Dermatol* 123:1221-1224, 1987.
191. Sandstrom B, Cederblad A, Linblad BS, et al: Acrodermatitis enteropathica, zinc metabolism, copper status, and immune function. *Arch Pediatr Adolesc Med* 148:980-985, 1994.
192. Kumar S, Sehgal VN, Sharma RC: Acrodermatitis enteropathica (letter). *J Dermatol* 24:135-136, 1997.
193. Della Bella S, Vanoli M, Bazzi S: Successful treatment of common variable immunodeficiency and related disorders with cimetidine and zinc sulfate (letter). *Int J Clin Lab Res* 27:79-80, 1997.
194. Basset-Seguin N, Sotto A, Guillot B, et al: Zinc status in HIV-infected patients: Relation to the presence or absence of seborrhic dermatitis. *J Am Acad Dermatol* 38:276-278, 1998.
195. Bohler K, Meisinger V, Klade H, et al: Zinc levels of serum and cervicovaginal secretion in recurrent vulvovaginal candidiasis. *Genitourin Med* 70:308-310, 1994.

PART V

Topical Drugs for Infectious Diseases

Sylvia Hsu
Long Thang Quan

Topical Antibacterial Agents

The major advantage in the topical use of an antibiotic (Figure 23-1) is the ability to achieve high local drug concentrations with minimal systemic absorption, thus minimizing the risk of systemic adverse effects. This chapter summarizes the current data on popular topical antibiotics and their role in skin diseases. In addition, the potential of allergic contact sensitivity is discussed from several of the topical antibacterial agents. The chapter is divided into two broad categories of topical antibacterial agents: drugs used primarily for wound care and drugs used primarily for acne and rosacea. Popular topical antiseptic agents are briefly discussed at the end of the chapter.

DRUGS USED FOR WOUND CARE
Bacitracin
PHARMACOLOGY. Bacitracin is a polypeptide antibiotic produced by the Tracey I strain of *Bacillus subtilis*. This strain was originally isolated from the damaged tissue and street debris in a compound fracture of a girl 7 years of age. The patient's name was Tracey, hence the name bacitracin.[1] Originally intended for parenteral use, this route of administration was abandoned due to severe nephrotoxicity.

The molecule consists of a thiazolidine ring and a polypeptide chain. It inhibits bacterial cell wall synthesis by complexing with the carrier protein C55-prenol pyrophosphatase, which is involved in the transfer of polysaccharides, liposaccharides, and peptidoglycans to a growing cell wall.[2] Of the three recognized subgroups of bacitracin (i.e., A, B, or C), commercial preparations contain mainly subgroup A.[3]

Bacitracin is available as a water-soluble form that has a shelf life of 2 years. The drug is also complexed with zinc (about 7%) to form a more stable, less water-soluble form with a shelf life as long as 5 years.[4] Both forms of bacitracin can be incorporated into creams or ointments, either alone or in combination with polymyxin B and possibly also neomycin to provide a wider spectrum of bacterial coverage (Table 23-1).

MICROBIOLOGIC ACTIVITY. Bacitracin is active against *Staphylococcus aureus*, *Streptococcus pneumoniae*, *Neisseria* organisms, *Haemophilus influenzae*, and *Treponema pallidum* at concentrations of 0.1 unit (or less)/ml. At concentrations ranging from 0.5 to 5 units/ml, bacitracin is effective against *Actinomyces* organisms and *Fusobacterium* organisms. It has minimal gram-negative coverage and is not active against *Pseudomonas* organisms, *Nocardia* organisms, Enterobacteriaceae, *Candida* organisms, or *Cryptococcus* organisms.[5]

INDICATIONS. Because of its low cost and minimal toxicity, bacitracin became popular for treating minor wounds and topical infections.

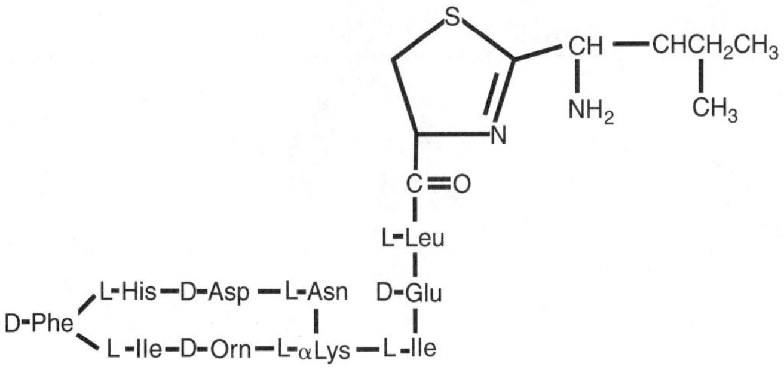

Bacitracin

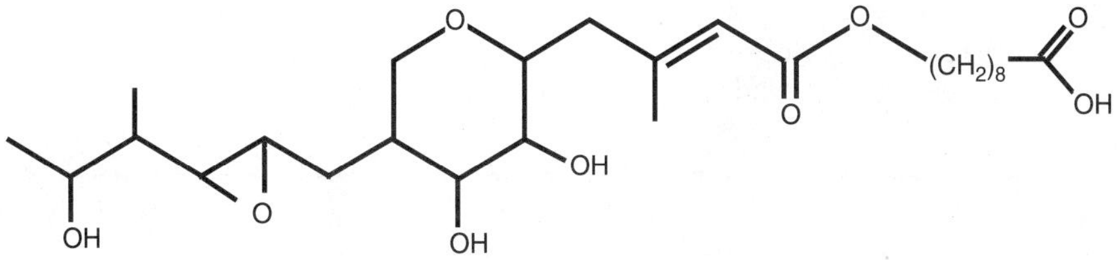

Mupirocin

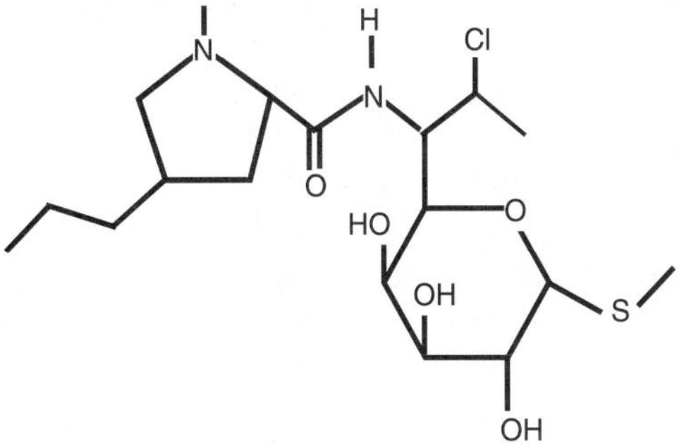

Clindamycin

Figure 23-1   Topical antibacterial agents.

There are very few controlled studies on the effectiveness of bacitracin on skin infections. One study demonstrated that a gel containing cetrimide, bacitracin, and polymyxin B significantly decreased the amount of *S. aureus* on artificially inoculated skin in healthy volunteers.[6] In another study, a bacitracin-polymyxin B-neomycin combination effectively eliminated *S. aureus* contamination from experimentally induced wounds compared with a wound protectant and several antiseptics.[7] In the previous two studies, bacitracin was evaluated only in combination therapy; however, as monotherapy, bacitracin is ineffective for eliminating nasal carriage of *S. aureus*.[8]

In a double-blind study comparing bacitracin with white petrolatum in 922 ambulatory dermatologic surgery patients, there were no statistical differences between the postoperative infection rates or healing times of the two groups. Ninety percent of the wound infections

Table 23-1　Topical Antibacterial Agents Used for Wound Care

Generic Name	Trade Name	Manu-facturer	Generic Available	Cream Tube Sizes	Ointment Tube Sizes	Special Formulations
Bacitracin Polymyxin (B)	Bacitracin Polysporin,* others	Various Warner Wellcome, others	Yes Yes		15, 30 g 15, 30 g	Powder—10 g
Neomycin	Neosporin,† others	Warner Wellcome, others	Yes	15 g	15, 30 g	
Mupirocin	Bactroban	SmithKline Beecham	No	15, 30 g	15, 30 g	
Gentamicin	Garamycin	Schering	Yes	15 g	15 g	
Silver sulfadiazine	Silvadene, others	Hoechst Marion Roussel	Yes	20, 80 g		

*Polysporin and generic "double antibiotics" contain bacitracin and polymyxin B; polymyxin B is not available as an individual product.
†Neosporin and generic "triple antibiotics" contain bacitracin, polymyxin B, and neomycin; neomycin is not available as an individual product.

in the petrolatum group were due to *S. aureus*, which was sensitive to dicloxacillin. The patients treated with bacitracin grew ciprofloxacin-sensitive gram-negative bacteria. Due to the higher cost of treating gram-negative infections, the 0.9% rate of contact allergy, and the higher cost of bacitracin, it was deemed less expensive to treat clean dermatologic surgical wounds with white petrolatum. In fact, these authors calculated that the bacitracin group cost four times more to treat than the petrolatum group. It should be noted that this study compared only clean surgery wounds.[9]

ADVERSE EFFECTS. There have been no published reports on the topical absorption of bacitracin into skin. However, one study reported no significant systemic absorption when used in bladder irrigation.[10] Common side effects of topical application include localized itching and burning. Allergic contact sensitivity is relatively uncommon in the North American population overall.[11] However, bacitracin is a frequent allergen in patients with chronic stasis dermatitis, conjunctivitis, or keratoconjunctivitis.[12] One recent study described 12.3% of 73 patients with stasis dermatitis who had positive patch

tests to bacitracin.[13] A previous study quoted that 13.1% of 192 patients with stasis dermatitis were allergic to bacitracin.[14] Barrier disruption in several of these clinical settings may allow the development of contact dermatitis.[15-17] Thus long-term use on nonintact skin, such as a stasis ulcer or chronic inflammatory conditions, may lead to an increased risk of contact allergy. Occlusion with dressings or stockings may contribute to the increased rate of sensitization in patients with stasis dermatitis as well. Bacitracin, as with other topical antibiotics, is recommended for short-term use on minor wounds.

Although rare, contact sensitivity can occur with sporadic use of the drug.[4] An example is a patient who presents with a vesicular pruritic dermatitis around a wound being treated with a topical antibiotic. A diagnosis of eczema may have been applied but the patient failed a course of topical steroids.[18] At this time it is appropriate to perform a patch test. This is done with 20% bacitracin in petrolatum. It should be noted that zinc bacitracin is less soluble than bacitracin and may provide false-negative test results. In addition, a 48-hour patch test reading may miss a positive reaction, which may not be manifest until 96 hours.[4]

■ **Table 23-2**   Key Concepts—Topical Antibacterial Agents Used for Wound
Care

Name	Comments
Bacitracin	• Relatively common sensitizer, especially with stasis dermatitis • Common coreactions with neomycin (not a true cross-reaction) • Anaphylaxis possible with application in an ulcer bed
Polymyxin B	• Available in combination with bacitracin as polysporin; combination is often called a "double antibiotic" • Good gram (−) bacterial coverage, including *Pseudomonas* organisms
Neomycin	• Also a relatively common sensitizer, especially with stasis dermatitis • In combination with bacitracin and polymyxin B is known as Neosporin or a "triple antibiotic" • Good gram (+) bacterial coverage—notably *S. aureus*
Mupirocin	• Very uncommon sensitizer • Very effective in eradicating nasal staphylococci carriage state • Resistant strains of *S. aureus* are possible
Gentamicin	• Uncommon sensitizer • Good gram (−) bacterial coverage, notably *Pseudomonas* organisms
Silver sulfadiazine	• Very effective in setting of burn patients, including when MRSA or *P. aeruginosa* present on culture • Can cross-react with patients having sulfonamide allergy

To date, there have been six reported cases of anaphylactic shock due to topical bacitracin.[12,19-24] Several of the cases involved patients who had been using the antibiotic on nonintact skin such as ulcers. However, one case involved small areas of dermatitic skin on the dorsal surface of the feet.[12] Bacitracin often coreacts but does not cross-react with neomycin, so patch testing to both may uncover a neomycin allergy. It is felt that the co-reaction is due to coincidental sensitization because bacitracin is chemically unrelated to neomycin and both antibiotics are commonly found in combination topical antibiotic ointments[25] (Table 23-2).

Polymyxin B
PHARMACOLOGY.   Polymyxin B is a cationic branched cyclic decapeptide isolated from the aerobic gram-positive rod *Bacillus polymyxa* (Table 23-3). The antibiotic destroys bacterial membranes with a surface detergent-like mechanism.[26]

Polymyxin B may be administered intravenously or intramuscularly. However, in dermatology, it is commonly added to topical formulations with bacitracin and possibly neomycin as well to broaden coverage against gram-negative bacteria, especially *P. aeruginosa.*

MICROBIOLOGIC ACTIVITY.   Polymyxin B is bactericidal in vitro against gram-negative bacteria including *Proteus mirabilis, P. aeruginosa,* and *Serratia marcescens.* This antibiotic is not effective against gram-positive bacteria nor against fungi.[26]

INDICATIONS.   Polymyxin B is usually combined with other topical antibiotics to broaden its bacterial coverage. For example, the "triple antibiotic" combination of neomycin, bacitracin, and polymyxin B is a popular, inexpensive, over-the-counter formulation for the treatment of minor skin wounds.

ADVERSE EFFECTS.   Despite its widespread use, contact allergy is rare. Polymyxin B was deemed a very weak sensitizer on testing in a guinea pig model.[27] Indeed, there are very few case reports of polymyxin allergy in the literature. In spite of the widespread use of the triple antibiotic combination, there has been only one report of two patients who developed a simultaneous contact allergy to all three antibiotics: neomycin, bacitracin, and polymyxin B.[28] Because polymyxin B binds avidly to cell membranes, there is little systemic absorption and

■ **Table 23-3**   Spectrum of Coverage and Mechanisms of Action—Topical Antibacterial Agents Used for Wound Care

Name	Bacterial Coverage	Mechanism of Action	Origin
Bacitracin	Bactericidal against gram (+) and *Neisseria* species	Interferes with bacterial wall synthesis; occurs by inhibition of phospholipid receptors involved in peptidoglycan synthesis	*Licheniformis* group of *B. subtilis* var. Tracey I
Polymyxin B	Bactericidal against gram (−) bacteria only; effective against *P. aeruginosa*	Increases permeability of bacterial cell membrane; occurs by interacting with phospholipid components of membrane	*B. polymyxa, B. subtilis*
Neomycin	Bactericidal against gram (+) and gram (−) bacteria; good *S. aureus* coverage	Inhibits protein synthesis; occurs by binding to 30s subunit of ribosomal RNA; end result is misreading of bacterial genetic code	Aminoglycoside antibiotic derived from *S. fradiae*
Mupirocin	Bactericidal against methicillin-resistant *S. aureus;* streptococci	Inhibits bacterial RNA and protein synthesis; occurs by reversibly binding to bacterial isoleucyl transfer RNA synthetase	*P. fluorescens*
Gentamicin	Bactericidal against gram (+) and gram (−) organisms; coverage includes *P. aeruginosa*	Inhibits bacterial protein synthesis; occurs by irreversibly binding to 30s ribosomal subunits	Aminoglycoside antibiotic derived from *M. purpurea*
Silver sulfadiazine	Bactericidal against gram (+) and gram (−) organisms	Binds to bacterial DNA and inhibits its replication	Synthesized from reaction of silver nitrate and sodium sulfadiazine

few systemic reactions even when applied to open wounds.[2] Still, there has been one reported case of acute renal failure in a man 67 years of age treated with an ointment containing polymyxin B for leg ulcers. His renal function returned to normal 13 days after the drug was discontinued.[29] When contact allergy is suspected, patch testing may be done with 3% polymyxin B in petrolatum.

Neomycin

PHARMACOLOGY.   Neomycin is a bactericidal aminoglycoside antibiotic first isolated from *Streptomyces fradiae* in 1949 by Waksman and Lechevalier.[30] It binds to the 30s subunit of the bacterial ribosome to inhibit protein synthesis. It may also inhibit bacterial DNA polymerase.[31] Neomycin sulfate, the usual commercial preparation, contains a mixture of two active stereoisomers: neomycin B and C. A degradation product, neomycin A, is present in minute quantities.[32]

MICROBIOLOGIC ACTIVITY.   Neomycin has good coverage against most clinically important gram-negative and some gram-positive organisms including *Escherichia coli, H. influenzae, Klebsiella* organisms, *Proteus* organisms, *S. aureus,* and *Serratia* organisms. It does not cover *P. aeruginosa* nor anaerobic bacteria such as *Bacteroides* organisms. Moreover, neomycin has only weak activity against streptococci.[26,32] Resistance to neomycin has been reported in both gram-positive and gram-negative bacteria. To reduce the emergence of resistant strains, neomycin is virtually always used in combination with other topical antibiotics. For example, bacitracin is typically added for its gram-positive coverage and to bolster the weak streptococcal coverage of neomycin. Another popular combination is the triple antibiotic combination with bacitracin, neomycin, and polymyxin B. The third antibiotic (polymyxin B) adds better gram-negative coverage including *Pseudomonas* organisms.

INDICATIONS. Neomycin is useful for treating minor wounds and topical infections. It is used in combination with bacitracin to achieve optimal staphylococcal and streptococcal coverage.

ADVERSE EFFECTS. As with other aminoglycosides, systemic toxicity to neomycin includes ototoxicity and nephrotoxicity. Systemic absorption and toxicity do not occur when the antibiotic is used topically on minor skin lesions. Neomycin-related deafness has been reported, usually involving a neomycin solution to irrigate a large wound.[33] One example described a 3-week application of gauze soaked with1% neomycin to a decubitus ulcer on a patient with renal failure.[34] There have been rare reported cases of deafness from using ear drops containing neomycin. Ear drops containing an ototoxic agent should not be used in patients with tympanic membrane perforation.[35,36] For application on skin, it is recommended that no more than 1 g per day of a topical preparation containing neomycin be used for a maximum of 7 days.[32] Following this guideline should reduce the potential for developing allergic contact sensitivity, bacterial resistance, or systemic toxicity.

The overall prevalence of allergic contact sensitivity to neomycin the United States has been reported to range from 0.09% to 1.1%.[37,38] However, this figure rises in patients with chronic use. For example, in a study of 192 patients suffering from stasis dermatitis and leg ulcers, 24% of patients patch tested positive to neomycin.[39] Patch testing is done by applying 20% neomycin sulfate in petrolatum under occlusion for 48 hours. Although the majority of tests are positive in 96 hours, it may take 7 days to become positive.[32] Neomycin potentially cross-reacts with streptomycin, kanamycin, gentamicin, paromomycin, spectinomycin, and tobramycin.[40] As previously mentioned, neomycin often co-reacts but does not cross-react with bacitracin. Therefore patch testing to both may uncover a bacitracin allergy. Beore the increasing

awareness about bacitracin allergy potential, many patients allergic to a triple antibiotic preparation were assumed allergic to only neomycin. The coreaction is due to coincidental sensitization because neomycin is chemically unrelated to bacitracin and both antibiotics are commonly found in combination topical antibiotic ointments.[25]

Mupirocin

PHARMACOLOGY. Mupirocin, formerly pseudomonic acid, is a major metabolite of *P. fluorescens*. It inhibits bacterial isoleucyl-tRNA synthetase, thereby hindering bacterial RNA synthesis, protein synthesis, and cell wall synthesis.[41] Due to its unique structure and mechanism of action, mupirocin does not cross-react with other topical antibiotics.

Parenteral administration results in rapid metabolism into inactive monic acid, which is excreted in the urine. Consequently, mupirocin is limited to topical use.[42] The drug is bacteriostatic at low concentrations but is bactericidal at concentrations achieved by topical administration.

Topical absorption is minimal. Topical application on rats resulted in 1.3% of the mupirocin reaching the systemic circulation in 72 hours.[43] Any mupirocin that is absorbed into the skin is converted into monic acid and excreted in the urine. The skin is also able to metabolize mupirocin; however, the amount is below 3%. This leaves most of the drug available on the skin surface for antibacterial activity.[26] Mupirocin is less effective in the presence of serum and may be less effective on weeping wounds because 95% of the drug is protein bound.[44]

Mupirocin is available with a prescription as a 2% ointment in a polyethylene glycol base (Bactroban ointment, Beecham Laboratories)[42] or in a white soft paraffin/Softisan 649 base (Bactroban Nasal) and as a 2% cream in a mineral oil cream base (Bactroban cream). The nasal formulation does not contain polyethylene glycol, thus it is less irritating on mucosal surfaces. All forms are relatively expensive compared with other topical antibiotics.

MICROBIOLOGIC ACTIVITY. Mupirocin has excellent activity against *S. aureus*, *S. epidermidis*, *S. pyogenes*, and β-hemolytic streptococci. In addition, it covers methicillin-resistant *S. aureus*

(MRSA).[42] However, mupirocin-resistant MRSA has increased substantially due to increased use of the medication. As many as 65% of MRSA were resistant to mupirocin in one study.[45] Mupirocin is not active against anaerobic bacteria, *P. aeruginosa*, *S. faecalis*, *S. faecium*, *S. bovis*, or fungi.[26,42] In addition, it has minimal activity against normal skin flora such as corynebacteria, micrococci, and *Propionibacterium* organisms.[42]

INDICATIONS. Mupirocin is used for the treatment of skin infections frequently initiated by staphylococci and streptococci, including impetigo, folliculitis, impetiginized eczema, burns, lacerations, and leg ulcers. Mupirocin ointment has been shown to be equivalent to oral erythromycin for the treatment of impetigo. Moreover, it has been approved as a monotherapy for impetigo.[44] The higher cost of treatment with mupirocin is offset by the increased incidence of adverse effects and days lost from school and work with erythromycin.[46] It is important to treat the underlying condition leading to the impetigo simultaneously, particularly in the setting of an impetiginized eczema.

Nasal Staphylococcal Carriage. Intranasal mupirocin is effective for the elimination of staphylococci, even MRSA, from chronic carriers.[47-49] Most recent studies advocate twice daily application for 5 days. Prolonged suppression of nasal staphylococcal carriage may be achieved by either weekly dosing or a 5-day course once a month. Prolonged use of intranasal mupirocin over a year has been shown to decrease the rate of skin infections in immunocompetent patients experiencing recurrent skin infections.[50] Intranasal mupirocin has been shown to decrease the incidence of *S. aureus* bacteremia in hemodialysis patients.[51] One study of intranasal mupirocin-treated hemodialysis patients showed that recolonization was 0% at 1 month after treatment but increased to 66% at 10 months. Therefore retreatment is often necessary.[52] An unblinded intervention trial with historical controls on cardiac surgery patients demonstrated a lower rate of surgical-site infections in patients pretreated with intranasal mupirocin compared with the historical controls.[53]

It is unclear whether additional use of an antibacterial soap in conjunction with mupirocin is necessary. One study compared mupirocin ointment with and without chlorhexidine baths in the eradication of *S. aureus* nasal carriage in nursing home residents. There was no significant difference between eradication of nasal carriage and prevention of recolonization with *S. aureus* in the two groups.[54]

Methicillin-resistant S. aureus. To date, there have been no published reports of systemic toxicity due to topical application of mupirocin. In cell culture, the drug is not cytotoxic to keratinocytes or fibroblasts.[55] For these reasons, mupirocin may be advantageous for topical treatment of staphylococcus-infected burns, especially those colonized with MRSA. One study showed that a twice daily application of mupirocin under occlusion was effective in eliminating MRSA in all 59 burn wounds. These authors recommend that mupirocin be used on burns encompassing less than 20% of body surface and for less than 5 days.[56] The safety of mupirocin on burns exceeding 20% of body surface area has not been addressed.

ADVERSE EFFECTS. Most reactions are local and include pain, burning, and itching. This is attributed to the vehicle base (polyethylene glycol) because the incidence is no greater than the vehicle alone.[42] True allergic contact sensitivity to mupirocin is extremely rare. To date, there have been only two reported cases.[57,58]

Gentamicin

Gentamicin is an aminoglycoside antibiotic derived from cultures of *Micromonospora purpurea*. It inhibits protein synthesis by irreversibly binding to 30s ribosomal subunits. Gentamicin is bactericidal against some gram-positive bacteria, such as *S. aureus*, and gram-negative bacteria, such as *Escherichia coli*, *Proteus* organisms, and *P. aeruginosa*. It is not effective against streptococci.[59] Topical gentamicin is most commonly used for treatment of eye infections such as bacterial conjunctivitis.

Allergic contact dermatitis to gentamicin is rare. Because cross-reactivity between gentamicin and neomycin is common, 40% of patients who were allergic to neomycin in one study also had positive patch tests to gentamicin even though they had not been exposed to gentamicin previously.[60] It is patch tested as 20% gentamicin in petrolatum.

Silver Sulfadiazine

Silver sulfadiazine has been the most commonly used topical antimicrobial agent for the treatment of burns for the past two decades. It is bactericidal against gram-positive and gram-negative bacteria including MRSA and *P. aeruginosa*, respectively.[61] It is a compound synthesized from a reaction of silver nitrate and sodium sulfadiazine. The agent binds to bacterial deoxyribonucleic acid (DNA) and inhibits its replication.

The most frequent clinical use of silver sulfadiazine preparations is in a burn unit, in which the drug's coverage against *Pseudomonas* organisms is important.[62] Silver sulfadiazine has a low toxicity profile. Silver sulfadiazine has a theoretically contact sensitizing potential in patients who are allergic to sulfonamides.[63] However,

there have been reports of significant absorption of silver from extensive burn sites.[64] Rarely, silver sulfadiazine can cause a brown-gray hyperpigmentation of the skin.[65]

DRUGS USED FOR ACNE AND ROSACEA
Benzoyl Peroxide
PHARMACOLOGY.   Benzoyl peroxide is available in washes, lotions, creams, and gels ranging from 2.5% to 20%[66] (Tables 23-4 and 23-5). The stability of benzoyl peroxide is very dependent on its vehicle. It is least stable in propylene glycol.[67,68] Gels are generally more active, with the water-based gels being less irritating than alcohol- or acetone-based formulations.[69,70] Approximately 5% of topically applied benzoyl peroxide is absorbed through the skin. The drug is completely metabolized to benzoic acid in the skin. Systemically absorbed benzoic

■ Table 23-4   Topical Antibacterial Agents Used for Acne and Rosacea

Generic Name	Trade Name	Manu-facturer	Generic Available	Cream* Tube Sizes	Special Formulations
Benzoyl peroxide†	Various	Various	Yes	Various	Lotion—various sizes Gel—various sizes Solution—various sizes
Clindamycin phosphate (1%)	Cleocin T Lotion	Pharmacia Upjohn	No		Lotion—60 ml Gel—30, 60 g Solution—30, 60 ml
	Cleocin T Gel		No		
	Cleocin T Solution		Yes		
Erythromycin‡	Various	Various	Yes		Gel—30, 60, 65 g pads, 60/box Solution—60, 120 ml
Metronidazole	Metrogel (0.75%)	Galderma Galderma	No		Gel—45 g
	MetroCream	Dermik		Cream—45 g	
	Noritate (1%)		No	Cream—30 g	
Azelaic acid	Azelex	Allergan	No	Cream—30 g	
Sodium sulfacetamide	Sulfacet R	Dermik	Yes		Lotion—25 g
	Novacet	GenDerm			Lotion—30 g
	Klaron	Dermik			Lotion—60 g

*None of these topical antibiotics are available in ointment formulations.
†For full spectrum of benzoyl peroxide options see Table 23-5.
‡For full spectrum of topical erythromycin options see Table 23-9.

■ Table 23-5   Common Benzoyl Peroxide Formulations

Name	Manufacturer	Formulations	Sizes
Benzac	Galderma	5%, 10% gel	60 g
Benzac AC	Galderma	2.5%, 5%, 10% gel	60 g
Benzac W*	Galderma	2.5%, 5%, 10% gel	60, 90 g
Benzagel	Dermik	5%, 10% gel	45, 90 g
Benzashave	Medicis	5%, 10% shaving cream	120 g
Brevoxyl	Stiefel	4% gel	42.5 g
Desquam-E	Westwood-Squibb	2.5%, 5%, 10% gel	45 g
Desquam-X*	Westwood-Squibb	2.5% gel	45 g
		5%, 10% gel	45, 90 g
PanOxyl	Stiefel	5%,10% gel	60, 120 g

*These formulations are also available as "washes."

■ Table 23-6   Key Concepts—Topical Antibiotics Used in Treatment of Acne and Rosacea

Name	Comments
Benzoyl peroxide	• Antibacterial effects >> keratolytic effects for acne • Beneficial effects can be "neutralized" with simultaneous tretinoin use • Has not been associated with induction of bacterial resistance • Rare potential for contact allergy
Clindamycin	• Good gram (+) and anaerobic bacterial coverage • Antibiotic-associated colitis very unlikely with topical use of clindamycin phosphate
Erythromycin	• Resistance of some *P. acnes* strains • A significant component of long-term acne benefit through erythromycin antiinflammatory effects
Metronidazole	• Has coverage for both aerobic and anaerobic bacteria • Also has some parasitic coverage—uncertain role of *D. folliculorum* in rosacea patients
Azelaic acid	• Broad antimicrobial coverage, including *P. acnes* • Also useful for certain disorders of pigmentation
Sodium sulfacetamide	• Available in several rosacea products in combination with sulfur

acid is so rapidly cleared by the kidneys that no systemic toxicity due to drug accumulation can be expected.[71,72]

MICROBIOLOGIC ACTIVITY.   Benzoyl peroxide is a broad-spectrum bactericidal agent that functions through its powerful oxidizing activity.[73] In vitro studies on skin microflora show that benzoyl peroxide is lethal to *P. acnes, S. capitis, S. epidermidis, S. hominis, P. avidum, P. granulosum,* and *Pityrosporum ovale.*[73] In vivo studies show that topical benzoyl peroxide produces a 1 to 3 $\log_{10}$ reduction in the cutaneous microflora during treatment.[74,75]

INDICATIONS

Acne Vulgaris—Monotherapy.   Topical benzoyl peroxide is indicated for the treatment of mild-to-moderate acne vulgaris. It is bactericidal for *P. acnes*, inhibits triglyceride hydrolysis, and decreases inflammation of acne lesions.[70,76-81] The drug has keratolytic and comedolytic activities[82] (Table 23-6). Benzoyl peroxide is available in a range of concentrations from 2.5% to 20% in many different vehicles (see Table 23-5). In the United States, the highest concentration available is 10%. In a small study, twice daily application of 2.5% benzoyl peroxide was as effective as the 5% or 10% formulations but with much fewer adverse effects.[77] Although the vehicle of the 2.5% formulation was different from the 5% and 10% formulations, one must consider that a higher concentration is not always better. Choosing a correct formulation should be a balance between the desired concentration, the vehicle base, and the risk of adverse effects.

Benzoyl peroxide has been compared with other topical drugs used to treat acne. It is as effective on inflammatory lesions (pustules and papules) but is more effective on noninflamed lesions when compared with erythromycin[83] or clindamycin.[80,81] Benzoyl peroxide is comparable to topical tretinoin in treating noninflammatory lesions; however, it is superior to tretinoin for inflammatory lesions.[84,85]

Acne Vulgaris—Combination Therapy. Although benzoyl peroxide is a capable single drug therapy, its activity is enhanced when used in combination with other medication. A benzoyl peroxide 5% and erythromycin 3% combination was found to be more effective than either drug alone.[86] This combination was also more effective than a 4% erythromycin/1.2% zinc formulation.[87] In a 1983 study, researchers compared application of benzoyl peroxide 5% in the morning and 1% clindamycin solution in the evening with twice daily application of either clindamycin or benzoyl peroxide. They concluded that combination therapy consistently showed a lower, although not statistically significant, acne severity index throughout the study.[81] A repeat study with a greater number of subjects comparing once daily application of these drugs showed that combination therapy with benzoyl peroxide and clindamycin was statistically superior to either monotherapy in scores for noninflammatory lesions, inflammatory lesions, and mean global improvement.[80] In both studies, combination therapy produced less irritation than benzoyl peroxide monotherapy.[80,81] Theoretically, combination treatments are superior because benzoyl peroxide can suppress antibiotic-resistant bacteria during treatment.[88] Benzoyl peroxide has not been associated with induction

of resistance in *Propionibacterium acnes*.[89] Another alternative is to use short intervening courses of benzoyl peroxide (7 days) during long-term antibiotic acne treatment.[75]

Combination treatment with benzoyl peroxide and topical tretinoin has been shown to be superior to monotherapy with either drug.[90,91] Because benzoyl peroxide may oxidize tretinoin if applied simultaneously, it is recommended that one be used in the morning and one at night. A topical or oral antibiotic may be added to these regimens for an additive effect.[70]

ADVERSE EFFECTS. The main adverse effect of topical benzoyl peroxide is an irritant dermatitis with symptoms of burning, erythema, peeling, and dryness.[66,67] If this occurs, one may decrease the dose by using a lower concentration, changing to a less irritating vehicle, or using every other day dosing. There is a 0.2% to 1% incidence of true contact allergy.[92,93] Patch testing may be done with 5% gel (15% false-positive reactions) or with 2% benzoyl peroxide in petrolatum (3% false-positive reactions).[93] Patients should be advised that the drug can bleach fabric, hair, and other colored materials.[66]

When the drug was first released there was concern that it may be carcinogenic in humans due to studies in mice that demonstrated it as a tumor promoter.[94-96] However, subsequent human studies have not found any link between benzoyl peroxide and skin cancer.[95,97,98] It is unclear whether these mice tumor promotion studies apply to humans.[95] Presently, clinical evidence supports benzoyl peroxide safety in humans.[99]

Clindamycin

PHARMACOLOGY. Clindamycin is a synthetic derivative of the antibiotic lincomycin, which is isolated from the *Streptomyces* species. For topical application, it is available as a 1% alcohol-based solution, 1% lotion, and 1% gel. Although all formulations are as efficacious for the treatment of acne vulgaris, the lotion is less irritating with fewer reports of dryness.[100] Topical application of a 1% solution for acne resulted in undetectable levels of the drug in the serum, although low levels were detected in the urine. These authors estimate that about 4% to 5% of the drug is systemically absorbed.[101]

MICROBIOLOGIC ACTIVITY. The drug is a broad-spectrum antibiotic that functions by irreversibly binding to the 50s subunit of the bacterial ribosome[102] (Table 23-7). This inhibits bacterial protein synthesis and may produce bactericidal or bacteriostatic effects in susceptible bacteria. The drug is effective against most aerobic gram-positive cocci and anaerobic gram-positive and gram-negative organisms.[103] Clindamycin (topically or systemically) is effective against *P. acnes*.[104]

INDICATIONS. The main indication for topical clindamycin is the treatment of acne vulgaris. It is more efficacious than topical tetracycline.[105] Two 8-week double-blind studies showed that it is superior to 500 mg/day and 1 g/day oral tetracycline for treating inflammatory lesions,[106,107] whereas one 12-week double-blind study found no significant differences between topical clindamycin and 1g/day of oral tetracycline.[108] Twice daily application of 1% clindamycin is as effective as oral minocycline 50 mg twice daily for the treatment of moderate-to-severe acne vulgaris.[109] When compared with topical 1.5% erythromycin, 1% clindamycin showed a greater improvement in pustules but less improvement in noninflammatory lesions and comedones.[110] However, in a later study both 1% clindamycin and 1.5% erythromycin were equally more effective against inflammatory lesions (~60% reduction) than noninflammatory lesions (~40% reduction).[111] A third study showed that a 4% erythromycin-zinc formulation was superior to 1% clindamycin solution for inflammatory and noninflammatory lesions.[112] Of note, the third study used a higher concentration of erythromycin than the previous two studies. It is also unclear what effect the zinc has in the formulation since a small study comparing 4% erythromycin with 1.2% zinc (n = 20) to 4% erythromycin without zinc (n = 25) found no statistical difference in the reduction of mean inflamed and noninflamed lesion count after 12 weeks of treatment.[113] Another study showed that 2% zinc sulfate was no different than placebo for the

■ **Table 23-7**   Spectrum of Coverage and Mechanisms of Action—Topical Antibacterial Agents Used for Acne and Rosacea

Name	Bacterial Coverage	Mechanism of Action	Origin
Benzoyl peroxide	Bactericidal, broad spectrum	Nonspecific oxidizing activity	Organic peroxide
Clindamycin	Broad spectrum (*S. aureus*, streptococci, pneumococci, *B. fragilis*, *P. acnes*)	Reversibly binds to 50s subunit of ribosomal RNA subunit; net result is inhibition of protein synthesis	7-deoxy-7-chloro semisynthetic derivative of lincomycin from *Streptomyces* species
Erythromycin	Bactericidal against most gram (+) bacteria and *P. acnes*	Reversibly binds to 50s subunit of ribosomal RNA subunit; net effect is inhibition of protein synthesis	*S. erythraeus*
Metronidazole	Gram (+) and gram (−) bacterial coverage as well as anaerobic coverage	Disruption of DNA and inhibition of nucleic acid synthesis	Synthetic nitro imidazole
Azelaic acid	Bacteriostatic and bactericidal against *P. acnes*	Disruption of mitochondrial respiration and DNA synthesis	Naturally occurring dicarboxylic acid
Sodium sulfacetamide	*P. acnes*	Inhibits proinflammatory enzymes	Synthetic molecule derived from aniline

treatment of acne.[114] Clindamycin is compared with benzoyl peroxide previously in this chapter. Topical clindamycin has also been reported successful for treatment of erythrasma, folliculitis, periorificial facial dermatitis, rosacea, and Fox-Fordyce disease.[115,116]

ADVERSE EFFECTS.   Mild local reactions include itching, burning, stinging, excessive dryness, peeling, oily skin, and erythema.[66] These reactions are usually due to the vehicle.[107] Contact allergy to clindamycin is very rare even though use of the drug is widespread (Table 23-8). To date, only a few cases have been reported.[117-123] Patch testing can be done with a 1% clindamycin suspension in water. Gram-negative folliculitis has been associated with topical clindamycin use.[124] Although extremely rare, a few cases of pseudomembranous colitis have been reported in association with topical clindamycin.[125,126] Only one report[125] described this complication with topical clindamycin phosphate used in current proprietary formulations.

Erythromycin
PHARMACOLOGY.   Erythromycin is a macrolide antibiotic isolated from a strain of *S. erythraeus*.[103] The drug, which has poor aqueous solubility, is available in various vehicles and concentrations from 1% to 4%. In the United States, it is available in concentrations from 2% to 3%. A recent study that compares the various vehicles showed the following effective permeation of erythromycin: liposomal formulations > conventional emulsions > hydroalcoholic solutions.[127] When applied to skin, erythromycin is distributed in the stratum corneum with a decreasing gradient from the upper layers.[128] To date, there are no published data on systemic absorption from topical erythromycin.

MICROBIOLOGIC ACTIVITY.   The drug is bactericidal and inhibits bacterial protein synthesis by irreversibly binding to the 50s subunit of the bacterial ribosome. The binding site is either identical to or very close to that of clindamycin.[102] Erythromycin is effective against gram-positive cocci, *Corynebacterium diphtheriae*, *H. influenzae*, *Legionella pneumophila*, *Chlamydia* organisms, *Treponema pallidum*, *Mycoplasma pneumoniae*, and *Ureaplasma urealyticum*.[102] Topical use in the treatment of acne vulgaris is dependent on its activity against *P. acnes*.[129,130]

INDICATIONS.   The main indication for topical erythromycin is the treatment of acne vulgaris. Topical erythromycin is available in concentrations of 2% and 3%, in a variety of vehicles (Table 23-9). Although the literature is full of review articles, there are relatively few original reports for this indication, and many of the studies use different concentrations of the drug in different vehicles. Thus care should be taken when comparing the different studies.

■ **Table 23-8**   Patch Testing for Contact Dermatitis from Topical Antibacterial Agents[60]

Name	Patch Testing Ingredients	Contact Sensitization
Bacitracin	20% in petrolatum	0.9%
Polymyxin	3% in petrolatum	Rare
Neomycin	20% in petrolatum	0.09%-1.1%
Mupirocin	2% in petrolatum	Rare
Gentamicin	20% in petrolatum	Rare
Silver sulfadiazine	5% in petrolatum	Rare
Benzoyl peroxide	5% gel, 2% in petrolatum	0.2%-1%
Clindamycin	1% aqueous solution	Rare
Erythromycin	1%-5% in petrolatum	Rare
Metronidazole	1% in petrolatum	Rare
Azelaic acid	20% in cream	Rare

■ **Table 23-9**   Common Topical Erythromycin Formulations

Name	Manufacturer	Formulations	Sizes
A/T/S	Hoechst Marion Roussel	2% solution	60 ml
		2% gel	30 g
Benzamycin	Dermik	3% erythromycin *plus* 5% benzoyl peroxide gel	23.3, 46.6 g
Erycette	Ortho Dermatological	2% swabs	60/box
Erygel	Allergan	2% gel	30, 60, 65 g
Theramycin Z	Medicis	2% solution	60 ml
T-stat	Westwood-Squibb	2% solution	60 ml
		2% pads	60/box

Erythromycin (1.5% to 2%) is more effective than placebo for treatment of inflammatory lesions and overall acne grade.[131,132] A 4% erythromycin/1.2% zinc acetate solution is more effective than placebo[133,134] and oral tetracycline (250 mg twice daily) in reducing severity grade and papules.[134] The role of zinc is unclear because a small study comparing 4% erythromycin with 1.2% zinc acetate (n = 20) with 4% erythromycin without zinc (n = 25) found no statistical difference in the reduction of mean inflamed and noninflamed lesion count after 12 weeks of treatment.[113] Another study showed that topical 2% zinc sulfate was no different than placebo for the treatment of acne.[114] For a comparison to clindamycin or benzoyl peroxide, please refer to the section on acne vulgaris combination therapy under benzoyl peroxide.

ADVERSE EFFECTS. Over the years, the use of topical erythromycin has led to a greater prevalence of erythromycin-resistant *P. acnes*. In 1993, 25% of antibiotic-treated acne patients harbored the resistant bacteria, regardless of treatment history.[135] Bacterial resistance has been associated with therapeutic failure with erythromycin.[136] One strategy to circumvent this problem is to use a higher concentration of erythromycin. A small study found that 4% erythromycin with 1.2% zinc (Zineryt) or without zinc was equally effective in decreasing erythromycin-resistant propionibacteria in vivo.[113] This higher concentration of erythromycin is not commercially available in the United States. These authors concluded that higher concentrations of topical erythromycin

should be effective in treating patients who carry erythromycin-resistant propionibacteria. Another tactic is to use an erythromycin/benzoyl peroxide combination, which has been found effective in reducing erythromycin-resistant propionibacteria and in decreasing the acne grade in these patients.[118]

Mild symptoms, such as erythema, scaling, tenderness, burning, itching, irritation, oiliness, and dryness, have been reported.[131,137] Erythromycin is a weak sensitizer[138] and only sporadic cases of contact dermatitis to topical erythromycin have been reported.[139-141] Patch testing can be done with erythromycin base 1% to 5% in petrolatum.

Metronidazole
PHARMACOLOGY. Metronidazole is a synthetic nitroimidazole antibiotic of which the exact mechanism of action has yet to be elucidated. The drug is readily taken up by anaerobic organisms and various cells. Inside these cells and susceptible organisms, metronidazole is reduced to unidentified polar products that lack the nitro group. It is thought that these reduction products are responsible for the cytotoxic and antimicrobial effects of this drug. Activity includes DNA disruption and inhibition of nucleic acid synthesis in anaerobic cells and organisms.[142]

Oral administration results in 80% absorption. Distribution is to most body tissues and fluids. Metronidazole readily crosses the placenta and is distributed in breast milk after oral or parenteral administration. Both oral and topical metronidazole are classified as pregnancy risk category B.[103]

For topical application, this drug is available in the United States as a 0.75% gel or cream and a 1% cream. When applied to skin, systemic absorption is negligible.[143-145] Due to poor systemic absorption, studies on the distribution and elimination of metronidazole after topical application have not been published.[141]

MICROBIOLOGIC ACTIVITY. Metronidazole is active against most anaerobic bacteria and protozoa including *B. fragilis*, *B. melaninogenicus*, *Fusobacterium* organisms, *Veillonella* organisms, *Clostridium* organisms, *Peptococcus* organisms, *Peptostreptococcus* organisms, *Entamoeba histolytica*, *Trichomonas vaginalis*, *Giardia lamblia*, and *Balantidium coli*.[142] This drug is not active against *P. acnes*, staphylococci, streptococci, fungi, or *Demodex folliculorum*.[141,145] In addition to the antimicrobial effects, metronidazole has antiinflammatory effects that include suppression of cell-mediated immunity and impeding leukocyte chemotaxis.[144]

The mechanism of action of metronidazole for the treatment of rosacea is uncertain. After one month of treatment, skin microflora of topical metronidazole-treated patients were no different than those in untreated patients.[146] In vitro studies show that *D. folliculorum* can survive in as much as 1 mg/ml of metronidazole. Thus it seems unlikely that the effect of metronidazole stems from direct killing of the mite.[147] Antibiotics used for the treatment of rosacea (tetracyclines, erythromycin) have antiinflammatory properties. Presumably, metronidazole exerts a similar effect in the treatment of rosacea.

INDICATIONS

Rosacea. The main indication for topical metronidazole is the treatment of rosacea. The link between metronidazole and rosacea was discovered serendipitously when patients with rosacea improved during treatment with oral metronidazole for other indications. Based on this, a double-blind trial with 29 patients showed that oral metronidazole (200 mg twice daily) was superior to placebo for the treatment of rosacea. Metronidazole is effective against pustules, papules, and to a lesser degree, erythema. However, it is ineffective against telangiectasias and rhinophyma.[148]

Clinical trials of 4 weeks to 15 weeks duration with metronidazole 0.75 topical gel or 1% topical cream showed an improvement of inflammatory lesions in 68% to 96% of patients.[142,149] In two double-blind split-face trials on patients with moderate rosacea, twice daily application of 0.75% metronidazole gel resulted in a 51% to 65% reduction of papules and pustules after 9 weeks compared with 0% to 15% for vehicle alone. Erythema was also reduced in both studies.[143,150] Telangiectasias were unaffected in one study,[143] while they were slightly increased in both the placebo- and metronidazole-treated sides in the second study.[150] It was unclear whether this was due to the vehicle or whether the decrease in active disease unmasked the underlying telangiectasias.[150]

Topical metronidazole is not effective for rhinophyma.[142] Previous experience has shown that this drug does not improve the ocular effects of rosacea. However, a small study with 10 patients showed that topical metronidazole applied to lid margin with lid hygiene improved rosacea blepharitis over lid hygiene alone.[151] Topical metronidazole can be effective for severe and recalcitrant rosacea.[152] The 1% metronidazole cream has been shown to be as effective as oral tetracycline.[153] There have been no published studies comparing topical against oral metronidazole for the treatment of rosacea.

Acne Vulgaris. It is unclear whether topical metronidazole has a role in treating acne vulgaris. One study using 2% metronidazole with 5% benzoyl peroxide showed a significant improvement over benzoyl peroxide alone and placebo.[154] A more recent study showed that 0.75% metronidazole gel had no beneficial effect on acne vulgaris.[155] Studies comparing higher concentrations of metronidazole have yet to be done.

Cutaneous Ulcers. Several reports demonstrated that topical metronidazole can be used to eliminate the odor of putrid smelling ulcers.[156-158] There have also been several reports of using topical metronidazole for controlling odor in ulcerated or fungating tumors.[159,160] Witowski and Parish[161] treated 10 sacral decubitus ulcers with metronidazole gel and eliminated odor after 36 hours of treatment. This was correlated with negative anaerobic cultures and Wood's light examination after treatment.[161]

ADVERSE EFFECTS. Adverse effects of topical metronidazole are very rare and include dryness, itching, burning, and stinging. To date, there has only been one reported case of contact allergy to topical metronidazole[162] (see Table 23-8). Patch testing can be done with 1% metronidazole in petrolatum. Another author reported a case of contact allergy to tioconazole with cross-reactivity to metronidazole.[163]

Azelaic Acid

PHARMACOLOGY.   Azelaic acid is a naturally occurring saturated nine-carbon dicarboxylic acid. Interest in this drug arose from studies of hypochromia produced by pityriasis versicolor infection. Researchers demonstrated that dicarboxylic acids of various lengths were competitive inhibitors of tyrosinase.[164] Longer molecules had more activity than shorter ones. Azelaic acid was chosen for further study due to its moderate activity against tyrosinase, low cost, and solubility.

In cell culture, normal cells are not damaged by azelaic acid at concentrations toxic to tumor cells. Azelaic acid can inhibit mitochondrial respiration, anaerobic glycolysis, and DNA synthesis in tumor cell lines. Tumor cell lines not containing tyrosinase are equally affected.[165-167] Azelaic acid penetrates tumor cells at two to three times the level of normal cells of the corresponding cell lines.[168] It is postulated that the toxicity is due to increased uptake of azelaic acid in tumor cells or hyperactive cells, which could lead to an excess of the azelaic acid beyond the cell's ability to fully metabolize the drug.[169]

Application of 1g of 20% azelaic acid cream results in a serum level of 0.038 μg/ml. The percentage of topical dose absorbed is calculated to be about 3%. Percutaneous absorption is governed by the formulation employed. A 15% gel has been shown to result in higher absorption (8%) than the 20% cream (3%).[170] In the United States, azelaic acid is available only as a 20% cream.

MICROBIOLOGIC ACTIVITY.   The antimicrobial activity of azelaic acid is attributable to inhibition of protein synthesis in susceptible organisms. The exact mechanism of action is unclear. Azelaic cream (20%) is roughly equivalent to 1.0 M. In vitro, azelaic acid is bacteriostatic against *S. epidermidis, S. aureus, S. capitis, S. hom-*

inis, P. acnes, P. granulosum, P. avidum, Proteus mirabilis, E. coli, P. aeruginosa, and *C. albicans* with the minimum inhibitory concentrations (MIC) varying from 0.03 M to 0.25 M.[166] In vitro activity against bacteria is enhanced under nutrient depletion and low pH; the latter factor favors uptake of azelaic acid into the cell.[167] Consequently, the MIC may vary in different studies depending on the experimental conditions.

INDICATIONS

Acne Vulgaris.   Azelaic acid is indicated for the treatment of acne. This was discovered by serendipity when patients who were being treated for melasma noticed an improvement in their acne.[171] When applied twice daily for 8 weeks, azelaic acid reduces the concentration of *P. acnes* on the skin surface and follicles.[172,173] Azelaic acid inhibits the division and differentiation of human keratinocytes but does not reduce the rate of sebum production.[173] Nevertheless, patients often subjectively report gradual and progressive reduction in skin greasiness after 1 to 2 months of treatment.[171,175]

Azelaic acid is more effective than placebo[172,176] but is comparable with topical 0.05% tretinoin cream,[176] topical 5% benzoyl peroxide,[177] and topical 2% erythromycin cream[166] in reducing comedonal, papular, and pustular lesions in mild-to-moderate acne. In addition, azelaic acid is equivalent to, or only slightly less effective than, oral tetracycline.[173,178]

Patients should apply the drug to affected areas and the surrounding areas to prevent further lesions. The cream should be rubbed well into the skin until absorbed. If dryness occurs, an emollient cream may be added.[179] Higher penetration into lesions may be achieved by applying the cream three to four times daily.[165] Improvement in acne is detectable after 1 to 2 months[172,178] and is maximal at about 4 months of use.[176,178]

Pigmentation Disorders.   Azelaic acid was originally researched as a treatment for pigmentary disorders. However, this drug has no depigmenting activity on normal skin, solar freckles, senile freckles, lentigines, pigmented seborrheic keratoses, and nevi.[166] Azelaic acid has some activity against hypermelanosis caused by physical and chemical agents, postinflammatory hyperpigmentation, melasma, lentigo maligna, and lentigo malignant melanoma.[165-167,169] These conditions are characterized by either hyperactivity or abnormal proliferation of melanocytes. Thus increased uptake by these hyperactive cells leads to their toxicity.

Azelaic acid is superior to 2% hydroquinone[180] and equivalent to 4% hydroquinone for the treatment of melasma.[181,182] In addition, there is no risk of exogenous ochronosis, which can be associated with higher concentrations of hydroquinone. Azelaic acid, together with tretinoin, produced more skin lightening than azelaic acid alone.[183] Patients should be advised to use a sunscreen concurrently.

ADVERSE EFFECTS.   Tests on rats and rabbits verify that azelaic acid is nontoxic, nonmutagenic, and nonteratogenic.[184-186] In humans, azelaic acid had been considered a possible substrate for total parenteral nutrition. Continuous parenteral infusion for up to a week resulted in no adverse effects.[184]

To date, there have been no reported cases of allergic hypersensitivity to azelaic acid. Thus topically applied azelaic acid does not seem to be sensitizing and is well tolerated. Up to 10% of patients may report itching, burning, or scaling, which may last 1 to 4 weeks. These local adverse reactions may be decreased by initiating treatment with once daily azelaic application during the first 1 to 2 weeks of treatment.[179]

Sodium Sulfacetamide
Sodium sulfacetamide is commonly incorporated in a formulation with sulfur for use in the treatment of acne and rosacea. Both sulfacetamide and sulfur minimize the formation of new lesions by inhibiting proinflammatory enzymes.[187] One 12-week study of 60 women with acne, who had failed other topical agents, such as tretinoin or topical antibiotics, showed a 78% decrease in total acne lesion count and an 83% decrease in inflammatory lesion count. The most common side effects were mild-to-moderate dryness and transient pruritus in over half of the patients.[187]

ANTISEPTICS

Antiseptics are most commonly used for surgical skin sterilization and for personal hygiene. They are found in products such as skin care preparations, mouthwashes, and toothpastes. They have a broad antimicrobial spectrum with low incidence of irritant or allergic contact dermatitis (Table 23-10).

Triclosan
Triclosan (2,4,4'-trichloro-2'-hydroxydiphenyl ether) is a broad-spectrum antimicrobial agent found in many personal care products such as deodorants, deodorant soaps, toothpaste, mouth rinses, and handwashes. It has antibacterial activity against staphylococci and coliform bacteria. In addition, triclosan has antiinflammatory properties. Several in vitro studies show that triclosan inhibits the cyclooxygenase and lipoxygenase pathways of prostaglandin and leukotriene production.[188] Thus triclosan inhibits the formation of several important mediators of inflammation and has been beneficial in minimizing the for-

◼ Table 23-10   Key Concepts—Common Topical Antiseptics

Name	Comments
Triclosan	• Primary antibacterial soap ingredient available today
	• Active ingredient in Lever 2000, Dial, pHisoderm, Safeguard, Softsoap, others
Chlorhexidine	• Primarily used as a surgical scrub
	• Active ingredient in Hibiclens
	• Also in liquid hand cleansers, toothpastes, and contact lens care products
Povidone/iodine	• Primarily used as a surgical scrub
	• Active ingredient in Betadine solution

mation of aphthous ulcers,[189] treating gingivitis, and reducing the effects of topical irritants such as sodium lauryl sulfate.[190,191] The addition of triclosan reduces the side effects of mouthwashes containing sodium lauryl sulfate alone.[192]

Triclosan has a very low incidence of irritant and allergic contact dermatitis even when used on eczematized skin.[189] It is tested as 2% triclosan in petrolatum.

Of historical interest, soaps with halogenated salicylanilide antibacterial agents have been discontinued because of association with sustained photocontact dermatitis.[193]

Chlorhexidine

Chlorhexidine (1,1-hexamethylenebis[5-(P-chlorophenyl) biguanide]) is an antimicrobial agent that has broad-spectrum coverage, including *S. aureus*, *P. aeruginosa*, *S. marcescens*, and facultative anaerobes.[194] It is commonly used preoperatively in handwashing and on surgical sites. Chlorhexidine is also commonly used by dentists for caries and gingivitis.[195]

Allergic reactions to chlorhexidine are rare. Patch testing is usually performed with a 1% aqueous solution of chlorhexidine gluconate.[196] When using chlorhexidine for skin sterilization near the ear, it is prudent to ensure that none of the disinfectant trickles into the ear as chlorhexidine has been associated with ototoxicity resulting in deafness.[197]

Povidone-iodine

Povidone-iodine is an antimicrobial agent that is active against gram-positive and gram-negative bacteria. It is commonly used as an antiseptic perioperatively and for skin wounds.

The incidence of irritant and allergic contact dermatitis is rare. However, there have been reports of irritant contact dermatitis and tissue necrosis after prolonged contact with large quantities of povidone-iodine.[198]

Bibliography

Hirschmann JV: Topical antibiotics in dermatology. *Arch Dermatol* 124:1691-1700, 1988.

Leyden, JJ: Therapy for acne vulgaris. *N Engl J Med* 336:1156-1162, 1997.

Leyden JJ, Sulzberger MB: Topical antibiotics and minor skin trauma. *Am Fam Phys* 23:121-125, 1981.

Toyoda M, Morohashi M: An overview of topical antibiotics for acne treatment. *Dermatology* 196:130-134, 1998.

Winkelman W, Gratton D: Topical antibacterials. *Clin Dermatol* 7:156-162, 1989.

References

Bacitracin

1. Meleney FL, Johnson BA: Bacitracin. *Am J Med* 7:794-806, 1949.
2. Sleytr UB, Oliver TC, Thorne KJ: Bacitracin-induced changes in bacterial plasma membrane structure. *Biochimica et Biophysica Acta* 419:570-573, 1976.
3. Chambers HF, Sande MA: Antimicrobial agents: general considerations. In Hardman JG, Limbird LE, Molinoff PB, et al, editors: *Goodman & Gilman's the pharmacological basis of therapeutics*, ed 9, New York, 1996, McGraw-Hill, p 1147.
4. Katz BE, Fisher AA: Bacitracin: a unique topical antibiotic sensitizer. *J Am Acad Dermatol* 17:1016-1024, 1987.
5. Goodman LS, Gilman AG: *The pharmacological basis of therapeutics*, New York, 1985, Macmillan.
6. Langford JH, Benrimoj S: Clinical investigation of topical antimicrobials in healthy volunteers. *Ann Pharmacother* 31:34-38, 1997.
7. Leyden JJ, Bartelt NM: Comparison of topical antibiotic ointments, a wound protectant, and antiseptics for the treatment of human blister wounds contaminated with *Staphylococcus aureus*. *J Fam Pract* 24:601-604, 1987.

8. McAnally TP, Lewis MR, Brown DR: Effect of rifampin and bacitracin on nasal carriers of *Staphylococcus aureus*. *Antimicrob Agents Chemother* 25:422-426, 1984.

9. Smack DP, Harrington AC, Dunn C, et al: Infection and allergy incidence in ambulatory surgery patients using white petrolatum vs bacitracin ointment. A randomized controlled trial. *JAMA* 276:972-977, 1996.

10. Chamberlain G, Needham P: The absorption of antibiotics from the bladder. *J Urology* 116:172-173, 1976.

11. Fisher AA: Adverse reactions to bacitracin, polymyxin, and gentamicin sulfate. *Cutis* 32:510-512, 520, 1983.

12. Elsner P, Pevney I, Burg G: Anaphylaxis induced by topically applied bacitracin. *Am J Contact Derm* 1:162-164, 1990.

13. Lindemayr H, Drobil M: Eczema of the lower leg and contact allergy (German). *Hautarzt* 36(4):227-231, 1985.

14. Fraki JE, Peltonen L, Hopsu-Havu VK: Allergy to various components of topical preparations in stasis dermatitis and leg ulcer. *Contact Dermatitis* 5:97-100, 1985.

15. Wilhelm KP, Maibach HI: Factors predisposing to cutaneous irritation. *Dermatol Clin* 8:17-22, 1990.

16. Allenby CF, Basketter DA: An arm immersion model of compromised skin (II). Influence on minimal eliciting patch test concentrations of nickel. *Contact Dermatitis* 28:129-133, 1993.

17. McLelland J, Shuster S, Matthews JN: "Irritants" increase the response to an allergen in allergic contact dermatitis. *Arch Dermatol* 127:1016-1019, 1991.

18. Sherertz EF: Chronic finger dermatitis after trauma. Diagnosis: posttraumatic eczema with allergic contact dermatitis to neomycin, bacitracin, and topical corticosteroids. *Arch Dermatol* 132:461-464, 1996.

19. Comaish JS, Cunliffe WJ: Absorption of drugs from varicose ulcers: a cause of anaphylaxis. *Br J Clin Prac* 21:97-98, 1967.

20. Roupe G, Strannegard O: Anaphylactic shock elicited by topical administration of bacitracin. *Arch Dermatol* 100:450-452, 1969.

21. Schechter JF, Wilkinson RD, Del Carpio J: Anaphylaxis following the use of bacitracin ointment. Report of a case and review of the literature. *Arch Dermatol* 120:909-911, 1984.

22. Vale MA, Connolly A, Epstein AM, et al: Bacitracin-induced anaphylaxis. *Arch Dermatol* 114:800, 1978.

23. Elsner P, Pevney I, Burg G: Anaphylaxis induced by topically applied bacitracin. *Am J Contact Dermatits* 1:162-164, 1990.

24. Dyck ED, Vadas P: Anaphylaxis to topical bacitracin. *Allergy* 52:870-871, 1997.

25. Binnick AN, Clendenning WE: Bacitracin contact dermatitis. *Contact Dermatitis* 4:180-181, 1978.

Polymyxin B

26. Winkelman W, Gratton D: Topical antibacterials. *Clin Dermatol* 7:156-162, 1989.

27. Goh CL: Contact sensitivity to topical antimicrobials. (II) Sensitizing potentials of some topical antimicrobials. *Contact Dermatitis* 21:166-171, 1989.

28. Grandinetti PJ, Fowler JF Jr: Simultaneous contact allergy to neomycin, bacitracin, and polymyxin. *J Am Acad Dermatol* 23:646-647, 1990.

29. Pedersen RS, Lonka L, Hansen HE: Acute renal failure caused by polymyxin B containing ointment. *Scand J Urol Nephrol* 21:153-154, 1987.

Neomycin

30. Waksman SA, Lechevalier HA: Neomycin, a new antibiotic active against streptomycin-resistant bacteria, including tuberculosis organisms. *Science* 109:305-307, 1949.

31. Lechevalier HA: The 25 years of neomycin. *CRC Critical Reviews in Microbiology* 3:359-397, 1975.

32. Macdonald RH, Beck M: Neomycin: a review with particular reference to dermatological usage. *Clin Exp Dermatol* 8:249-258, 1983.

33. Manuel MA, Kurtz I, Saiphoo CS, et al: Nephrotoxicity and ototoxicity following irrigation of wounds with neomycin. *Can J Surg* 22:274-277, 1979.

34. Johnson CA: Hearing loss following the application of topical neomycin. *J Burn Care Rehab* 9:162-164, 1988.

35. Podoshin L, Fradis M, Ben D Jr: Ototoxicity of ear drops in patients suffering from chronic otitis media. *J Laryngol Otol* 103:46-50, 1989.

36. Lind O, Kristiansen B: Deafness after treatment with ear drops containing neomycin, gramicidin and dexamethasone. A case report. *ORL J Otorhinolaryngol Relat Spec* 48:552-554, 1986.

37. Leyden JJ, Kligman AM: Contact dermatitis to neomycin sulfate. *JAMA* 242:1276-1278, 1979.

38. Prystowsky SD, Nonomura JH, Smith RW, et al: Allergic hypersensitivity to neomycin. Relationship between patch test reactions and 'use' tests. *Arch Dermatol* 115:713-715, 1979.
39. Fraki JE, Peltonen L, Hopsu-Havu VK: Allergy to various components of topical preparations in stasis dermatitis and leg ulcer. *Contact Dermatitis* 5:97-100, 1979.
40. Fisher AA: Topical medicaments which are common sensitizers. *Annals Allergy* 49:97-100, 1982.

Mupirocin

41. Ward A, Campoli-Richards DM: Mupirocin. A review of its antibacterial activity, pharmacokinetic properties and therapeutic use. *Drugs* 32:425-444, 1986.
42. Parenti MA, Hatfield SM, Leyden JJ: Mupirocin: a topical antibiotic with a unique structure and mechanism of action. *Clin Pharm* 6:761-770, 1987.
43. Wuite J, Davies BI, Go MJ, et al: Pseudomonic acid, a new antibiotic for topical therapy. *J Am Acad Dermatol* 12:1026-1031, 1985.
44. Leyden JJ: Review of mupirocin ointment in the treatment of impetigo. *Clin Pediatr* 31:49-53, 1992.
45. Miller MA, Dascal A, Portnoy J, et al: Development of mupirocin resistance among methicillin-resistant *Staphylococcus aureus* after widespread use of nasal mupirocin ointment. *Infect Control Hosp Epidemiol* 17:811-813, 1996.
46. Rice TD, Duggan AK, DeAngelis C: Cost-effectiveness of erythromycin versus mupirocin for the treatment of impetigo in children. *Pediatrics* 89:210-214, 1992.
47. Redhead RJ, Lamb YJ, Rowsell RB: The efficacy of calcium mupirocin in the eradication of nasal *Staphylococcus aureus* carriage. *Br J Clin Pract* 45:252-254, 1991.
48. Kauffman CA, Terpenning MS, He X, et al: Attempts to eradicate methicillin-resistant *Staphylococcus aureus* from a long-term-care facility with the use of mupirocin ointment. *Am J Med* 94:371-378, 1993.
49. Fernandez C, Gaspar C, Torrellas A, et al: A double-blind, randomized, placebo-controlled clinical trial to evaluate the safety and efficacy of mupirocin calcium ointment for eliminating nasal carriage of *Staphylococcus aureus* among hospital personnel. *J Antimicrob Chemother* 5:399-408, 1995.

50. Raz R, Miron D, Colodner R, et al: A 1-year trial of nasal mupirocin in the prevention of recurrent staphylococcal nasal colonization and skin infection. *Arch Intern Med* 156:1109-1112, 1996.
51. Kluytmans JA, Manders MJ, Van Bommel E, et al: Elimination of nasal carriage of *Staphylococcus aureus* in hemodialysis patients. *Infect Contr Hosp Epidemiol* 17:793-797, 1996.
52. Perez-Fontan M: Treatment of *Staphylococcus aureus* nasal carriers in CAPD with mupirocin. *Adv Perit Dial* 8:242-245, 1992.
53. Kluytmans JA, Mouton JW, VandenBergh MF, et al: Reduction of surgical-site infections in cardiothoracic surgery by elimination of nasal carriage of *Staphylococcus aureus*. *Infect Contr Hosp Epidemiol* 17:780-785, 1996.
54. Watanakunakorn C, Axelson C, Bota B, et al: Mupirocin ointment with and without chlorhexidine baths in the eradication of *Staphylococcus aureus* nasal carriage in nursing home residents. *Am J Infect Contr* 23:306-309, 1995.
55. Boyce ST, Warden GD, Holder IA: Cytotoxicity testing of topical antimicrobial agents on human keratinocytes and fibroblasts for cultured skin grafts. *J Burn Care Rehab* 16:97-103, 1995.
56. Rode H, Hanslo D, de Wet PM, et al: Efficacy of mupirocin in methicillin-resistant *Staphylococcus aureus* burn wound infection. *Antimicrob Agents Chemother* 33:1358-1361, 1989.
57. Eedy DJ: Mupirocin allergy in the setting of venous ulceration. *Contact Dermatitis* 32:240-241, 1995.
58. Zappi EG, Brancaccio RR: Allergic contact dermatitis from mupirocin ointment. *J Am Acad Dermatol* 36:266, 1997.

Gentamicin

59. Winkelman W, Gratton D: Topical antibacterials. *Clin Dermatol* 7:156-162, 1989.
60. Marks JG Jr, DeLeo VA: *Contact and occupational dermatology*, St Louis, 1997, Mosby-Year Book, Inc.

Silver Sulfadiazine

61. Marone P, Monzillo V, Perversi L, et al: Comparative in vitro activity of silver sulfadiazine, alone and in combination with cerium nitrate, against staphylococci and gram-negative bacteria. *J Chemother* 10:17-21, 1998.

62. Nagaesha CN, Shenoy KJ, Chandrashekar MR: Study of burn sepsis with special reference to *Pseudomonas aeruginosa*. *J Indian Med Assoc* 94:230-233, 1996.

63. Degreef H, Dooms-Goossens A: Patch testing with silver sulfadiazine cream. *Contact Dermatitis* 12:33-37, 1985.

64. Tsipouras N, Rix CJ, Brady PH: Solubility of silver sulfadiazine in physiological media and relevance to treatment of thermal burns with silver sulfadiazine cream. *Clin Chem* 41:87-91, 1995.

65. Dupus LL, Shear NH, Zucker RM: Hyperpigmentation due to topical application of silver sulfadiazine cream. *J Am Acad Dermatol* 12:1112-1114, 1985.

Benzoyl Peroxide

66. *Physicians' desk reference*. Montvale, 1992, Medical Economics Data.

67. Das Gupta V: Effect of some formulation adjuncts on the stability of benzoyl peroxide. *J Pharmaceut Sciences* 71:585-587, 1982.

68. Chellquist EM, Gorman WG: Benzoyl peroxide solubility and stability in hydric solvents. *Pharmaceutical Res* 9:1341-1346, 1982.

69. Fyrand O, Jakobsen HB: Water-based versus alcohol-based benzoyl peroxide preparations in the treatment of acne vulgaris. *Dermatologica* 172:263-267, 1986.

70. Hurwitz S: *Clinical pediatric dermatology: a textbook of skin disorders of childhood and adolescence*, Philadelphia, 1993, WB Saunders.

71. Nacht S, Yeung D, Beasley JN Jr, et al: Benzoyl peroxide: percutaneous penetration and metabolic disposition. *J Am Acad Dermatol* 4:31-37, 1981.

72. Yeung D, Nacht S, Bucks D, et al: Benzoyl peroxide: percutaneous penetration and metabolic disposition. II. Effect of concentration. *J Am Acad Dermatol* 9:920-924, 1983.

73. Cove JH, Holland KT: The effect of benzoyl peroxide on cutaneous micro-organisms in vitro. *J Applied Bacteriol* 54:379-382, 1983.

74. Nacht S, Gans EH, McGinley KJ, et al: Comparative activity of benzoyl peroxide and hexachlorophene. In vivo studies against *Propionibacterium acnes* in humans. *Arch Dermatol* 119:577-579, 1983.

75. Bojar RA, Cunliffe WJ, Holland KT: The short-term treatment of acne vulgaris with benzoyl peroxide: effects on the surface and follicular cutaneous microflora. *Br J Dermatol* 132:204-208, 1995.

76. Kligman AM, Leyden JJ, Stewart R: New uses for benzoyl peroxide: a broad-spectrum antimicrobial agent. *Int J Dermatol* 16:413-417, 1977.

77. Mills OH Jr, Kligman AM, Pochi P, et al: Comparing 2.5%, 5%, and 10% benzoyl peroxide on inflammatory acne vulgaris. *Int J Dermatol* 25:664-667, 1986.

78. Belknap BS: Treatment of acne with 5% benzoyl peroxide gel or 0.05% retinoic acid cream. *Cutis* 23:856-859, 1979.

79. Smith EB, Padilla RS, McCabe JM, et al: Benzoyl peroxide lotion (20 percent) in acne. *Cutis* 25:90-92, 1980.

80. Lookingbill DP, Chalker DK, Lindholm JS, et al: Treatment of acne with a combination clindamycin/benzoyl peroxide gel compared with clindamycin gel, benzoyl peroxide gel and vehicle gel: combined results of two double-blind investigations. *J Am Acad Dermatol* 37:590-595, 1997.

81. Tucker SB, Tausend R, Cochran R, et al: Comparison of topical clindamycin phosphate, benzoyl peroxide, and a combination of the two for the treatment of acne vulgaris. *Br J Dermatol* 110:487-492, 1984.

82. Oh CW, Myung KB: Retention hyperkeratosis of experimentally induced comedones in rabbits: the effects of three comedolytics. *J Dermatol* 23:169-180, 1996.

83. Burke B, Eady EA, Cunliffe WJ: Benzoyl peroxide versus topical erythromycin in the treatment of acne vulgaris. *Br J Dermatol* 108:199-204, 1983.

84. Belknap BS: Treatment of acne with 5% benzoyl peroxide gel or 0.05% retinoic acid cream. *Cutis* 23:856-859, 1979.

85. Lyons RE: Comparative effectiveness of benzoyl peroxide and tretinoin in acne vulgaris. *Int J Dermatol* 17:246-251, 1978.

86. Chalker DK, Shalita A, Smith JG Jr, et al: A double-blind study of the effectiveness of a 3% erythromycin and 5% benzoyl peroxide combination in the treatment of acne vulgaris. *J Am Acad Dermatol* 9:933-936, 1983.

87. Chu A, Huber FJ, Plott RT: The comparative efficacy of benzoyl peroxide 5%/erythromycin 3% gel and erythromycin 4%/zinc 1.2% solution in the treatment of acne vulgaris. *Br J Dermatol* 136:235-238, 1997.

88. Eady EA, Bojar RA, Jones CE, et al: The effects of acne treatment with a combination of benzoyl peroxide and erythromycin on skin carriage of erythromycin-resistant propionibacteria. *Br J Dermatol* 134:107-113, 1996.

89. Gollnick H, Schramm M: Topical drug treatment in acne. *Dermatology* 196:119-125, 1998.

90. Hurwitz S: The combined effect of vitamin A acid and benzoyl peroxide in the treatment of acne. *Cutis* 17:585-590, 1976.

91. Handojo I: The combined use of topical benzoyl peroxide and tretinoin in the treatment of acne vulgaris. *Int J Dermatol* 18:489-496, 1979.

92. Cunliffe WJ, Burke B: Benzoyl peroxide: lack of sensitization. *Acta Derm Venereol* 62:458-459, 1982.

93. Balato N, Lembo G, Cuccurullo FM, et al: Acne and allergic contact dermatitis. *Contact Dermatitis* 34:68-69, 1996.

94. Reiners JJ Jr, Nesnow S, Slaga TJ: Murine susceptibility to two-stage skin carcinogenesis is influenced by the agent used for promotion. *Carcinogenesis* 5:301-307, 1984.

95. Kraus AL, Munro IC, Orr JC, et al: Benzoyl peroxide: an integrated human safety assessment for carcinogenicity. *Reg Toxicol Pharmacol* 21:87-107, 1995.

96. Slaga TJ, Klein-Szanto AJ, Triplett LL, et al: Skin tumor-promoting activity of benzoyl peroxide, a widely used free radical-generating compound. *Science* 213:1023-1025, 1981.

97. Elwood JM, Gallagher RP, Stapleton P: No association between malignant melanoma and acne or psoriasis: results from the Western Canada Melanoma Study. *Br J Dermatol* 115:573-576, 1986.

98. Cartwright RA, Hughes BR, Cunliffe WJ: Malignant melanoma, benzoyl peroxide and acne: a pilot epidemiological case-control investigation. *Br J Dermatol* 18:239-242, 1988.

99. Liden S, Lindelof B, Sparen P: Is benzoyl peroxide carcinogenic? *Br J Dermatol* 123:129-130, 1990.

Clindamycin

100. Goltz RW, Coryell GM, Schnieders JR, et al: A comparison of Cleocin T 1 percent solution and Cleocin T 1 percent lotion in the treatment of acne vulgaris. *Cutis* 36:265-268, 1985.

101. Barza M, Goldstein JA, Kane A, et al: Systemic absorption of clindamycin hydrochloride after topical application. *J Am Acad Dermatol* 7:208-214, 1982.

102. Mycek MJ, Gertner SB, Perper MM: *Lippincott's illustrated review: pharmacology,* New York, 1992, JB Lippincott.

103. Moreau D: *Physician's drug handbook,* Springhouse, 1995, Springhouse Corporation.

104. Nishijima S, Kurokawa I, Kawabata S: Sensitivity of *Propionibacterium acnes* isolated from acne patients: comparative study of antimicrobial agents. *Acta Derm Venereol* 24:473-477, 1996.

105. Padilla RS, McCabe JM, Becker LE: Topical tetracycline hydrochloride vs. topical clindamycin phosphate in the treatment of acne: a comparative study. *Int J Dermatol* 20:445-448, 1981.

106. Braathen LR: Topical clindamycin versus oral tetracycline and placebo in acne vulgaris. *Scand J Infect Dis (Suppl)* 43:71-75, 1984.

107. Stoughton RB, Cornell RC, Gange RW, et al: Double-blind comparison of topical 1 percent clindamycin phosphate (Cleocin T) and oral tetracycline 500 mg/day in the treatment of acne vulgaris. *Cutis* 26:424-425, 429, 1980.

108. Katsambas A, Towarky AA, Stratigos J: Topical clindamycin phosphate compared with oral tetracycline in the treatment of acne vulgaris. *Br J Dermatol* 116:387-391, 1987.

109. Sheehan-Dare RA, Papworth-Smith J, Cunliffe WJ: A double-blind comparison of topical clindamycin and oral minocycline in the treatment of acne vulgaris. *Acta Derm Venereol* 70:534-537, 1990.

110. Thomas DR, Raimer S, Smith EB: Comparison of topical erythromycin 1.5 percent solution versus topical clindamycin phosphate 1.0 percent solution in the treatment of acne vulgaris. *Cutis* 29:624-625, 628-632, 1982.

111. Shahlita AR, Smith EB, Bauer E: Topical erythromycin vs clindamycin therapy for acne. A multicenter, double-blind comparison. *Arch Dermatol* 120:351-355, 1984.

112. Schachner L, Pestana A, Kittles C: A clinical trial comparing the safety and efficacy of a topical erythromycin-zinc formulation with a topical clindamycin formulation. *J Am Acad Dermatol* 22:489-495, 1990.

113. Bojar RA, Eady EA, Jones CE, et al: Inhibition of erythromycin-resistant propionibacteria on the skin of acne patients by topical erythromycin with and without zinc. *Br J Dermatol* 130:329-336, 1990.

114. Cochran RJ, Tucker SB, Flannigan SA: Topical zinc therapy for acne vulgaris. *Int J Dermatol* 24:188-190, 1985.

115. Rosen T, Waisman M: Topically administered clindamycin in the treatment of acne vulgaris and other dermatologic disorders. *Pharmacotherapy* 1:201-205, 1981.

116. Feldmann R, Masouye I, Chavaz P, et al: Fox-Fordyce disease: successful treatment with topical clindamycin in alcoholic propylene glycol solution. *Dermatology* 184:310-313, 1992.

117. de Groot AC: Contact allergy to clindamycin. *Contact Dermatitis* 8:428, 1982.

118. Vejlstrup E, Menne T: Contact dermatitis from clindamycin. *Contact Dermatitis* 32:110, 1995.

119. Conde-Salazar L, Guimaraens D, Romero LV: Contact dermatitis from clindamycin. *Contact Dermatitis* 9:225, 1983.

120. Coskey RJ: Contact dermatitis due to clindamycin. *Arch Dermatol* 114:446, 1978.

121. Yokoyama R, Mizuno E, Takeuchi M, et al: Contact dermatitis due to clindamycin. *Contact Dermatitis* 25:125, 1991.

122. Garcia R, Galindo PA, Feo F, et al: Delayed allergic reactions to amoxicillin and clindamycin. *Contact Dermatitis* 35:116-117, 1996.

123. Herstoff JK, Bogaars HA: Sensitization to topical antibiotics. *Arch Dermatol* 114:1402, 1978.

124. Piamphongsant T: Pustular acne. *Int J Dermatol* 24:441-443, 1985.

125. Parry MF, Rha CK: Pseudomembranous colitis caused by topical clindamycin phosphate. *Arch Dermatol* 122:583-584, 1986.

126. Milstone EB, McDonald AJ, Scholhamer CF Jr: Pseudomembranous colitis after topical application of clindamycin. *Arch Dermatol* 117:154-155, 1981.

Erythromycin

127. Jayaraman SC, Ramachandran C, Weiner N: Topical delivery of erythromycin from various formulations: an in vivo hairless mouse study. *J Pharmaceut Sciences* 85:1082-1084, 1996.

128. van Hoogdalem EJ: Assay of erythromycin in tape strips of human stratum corneum and some preliminary results in man. *Skin Pharmacol* 5:124-128, 1992.

129. Puhvel SM: Effects of treatment with erythromycin 1.5 percent topical solution or clindamycin phosphate 1.0 percent topical solution on *P. acnes* counts and free fatty acid levels. *Cutis* 31:339-342, 1983.

130. Rapaport M, Puhvel SM, Reisner RM: Evaluation of topical erythromycin and oral tetracycline in acne vulgaris. *Cutis* 30:122-126, 130, 132-135, 1982.

131. Dobson RL, Belknap BS: Topical erythromycin solution in acne. Results of a multiclinic trial. *J Am Acad Dermatol* 3:478-482, 1980.

132. Lesher JL Jr, Chalker DK, Smith JG Jr, et al: An evaluation of a 2% erythromycin ointment in the topical therapy of acne vulgaris. *J Am Acad Dermatol* 12:526-531, 1985.

133. Strauss JS, Stranieri AM: Acne treatment with topical erythromycin and zinc: effect of *Propionibacterium acnes* and free fatty acid composition. *J Am Acad Dermatol* 11:86-89, 1984.

134. Feucht CL, Allen BS, Chalker DK, et al: Topical erythromycin with zinc in acne. A double-blind controlled study. *J Am Acad Dermatol* 3:483-491, 1980.

135. Eady EA, Jones CE, Tipper JL, et al: Antibiotic resistant propionibacteria in acne: need for policies to modify antibiotic usage. *BMJ* 306:555-556, 1993.

136. Eady EA, Cove JH, Holland KT, et al: Erythromycin resistant propionibacteria in antibiotic treated acne patients: association with therapeutic failure. *Br J Dermatol* 121:51-57, 1989.

137. Jones EL, Crumley AF: Topical erythromycin vs blank vehicle in a multiclinic acne study. *Arch Dermatol* 117:551-553, 1981.

138. Fisher AA: The safety of topical erythromycin. *Contact Dermatitis* 2:43-44, 1976.

139. van Ketel WG: Immediate- and delayed-type allergy to erythromycin. *Contact Dermatitis* 2:363-364, 1976.

140. Fernandez Redondo V, Casas L, Taboada M, et al: Systemic contact dermatitis from erythromycin. *Contact Dermatitis* 30:43-44, 1994.

141. Martins C, Freitas JD, Goncalo M, et al: Allergic contact dermatitis from erythromycin. *Contact Dermatitis* 33:360, 1995.

Metronidazole

142. Schmadel LK, McEvoy GK: Topical metronidazole: a new therapy for rosacea. *Clin Pharm* 9:94-101, 1990.
143. Aronson IK, Rumsfield JA, West DP, et al: Evaluation of topical metronidazole gel in acne rosacea. *Drug Intell Clin Pharm* 21:346-351, 1987.
144. Gamborg Nielsen P: Metronidazole treatment in rosacea. *Int J Dermatol* 27:1-5, 1988.
145. Gamborg Nielsen P: Treatment of rosacea with 1% metronidazole cream. A double-blind study. *Br J Dermatol* 108:327-332, 1983.
146. Eriksson G, Nord CE: Impact of topical metronidazole on the skin and colon microflora in patients with rosacea. *Infection* 15:8-10, 1987.
147. Persi A, Rebora A: Metronidazole and *Demodex folliculorum*. *Acta Derm Venereol* 61:182-183, 1981.
148. Pye RJ, Burton JL: Treatment of rosacea by metronidazole. *Lancet* 1:1211-1212, 1976.
149. Maddin S: A comparison of topical azelaic acid 20% cream and topical metronidazole 0.75% cream in the treatment of patients with papulopustular rosacea. *J Am Acad Dermatol* 40:961-965, 1999.
150. Bleicher PA, Charles JH, Sober AJ: Topical metronidazole therapy for rosacea. *Arch Dermatol* 123:609-614, 1987.
151. Barnhorst DA Jr, Foster JA, Chern KC, et al: The efficacy of topical metronidazole in the treatment of ocular rosacea. *Ophthalmology* 103:1880-1883, 1996.
152. Lowe NJ, Henderson T, Millikan LE, et al: Topical metronidazole for severe and recalcitrant rosacea: a prospective open trial. *Cutis* 43:283-286, 1989.
153. Gamborg Nielsen P: A double-blind study of 1% metronidazole cream versus systemic oxytetracycline therapy for rosacea. *Br J Dermatol* 109:63-65, 1983.
154. Gamborg Nielsen P: Topical metronidazole gel. Use in acne vulgaris. *Int J Dermatol* 30:662-666, 1991.
155. Tong D, Peters W, Barnetson RS: Evaluation of 0.75% metronidazole gel in acne—a double-blind study. *Clin Exp Dermatol* 19:221-223, 1994.
156. Jones PH, Willis AT, Ferguson IR: Treatment of anaerobically infected pressure sores with topical metronidazole. *Lancet* 1:213-214, 1978.
157. Pierleoni EE: Topical metronidazole therapy for infected decubitus ulcers. *J Am Geriatr Soc* 32:775, 1984.
158. Herman J: Metronidazole for a malodorous pressure sore. *Practitioner* 227:1595-1596, 1983.
159. Finlay IG, Bowszyc J, Ramlau C, et al: The effect of topical 0.75% metronidazole gel on malodorous cutaneous ulcers. *J Pain Symptom Manage* 11:158-162, 1996.
160. Kuge S, Tokuda Y, Ohta M, et al: Use of metronidazole gel to control malodor in advanced and recurrent breast cancer. *Japan J Clin Oncol* 26:207-210, 1996.
161. Witkowski JA, Parish LC: Topical metronidazole gel. The bacteriology of decubitus ulcers. *Int J Dermatol* 30(9):660-661, 1991.
162. Vincenzi C, Lucente P, Ricci C, et al: Facial contact dermatitis due to metronidazole. *Contact Dermatitis* 36:116-117, 1997.
163. Izu R, Aguirre A, Gonzalez M, et al: Contact dermatitis from tioconazole with cross-sensitivity to other imidazoles. *Contact Dermatitis* 26:130-131, 1992.

Azelaic Acid

164. Caprilli F, Mercantini R, Nazzaro-Porro M, et al: Studies of the genus *Pityrosporum* in submerged culture. *Mycopathologia et Mycologia Applicata* 51:171-189, 1973.
165. Nazzaro-Porro M: Azelaic acid. *J Am Acad Dermatol* 17:1033-1041, 1987.
166. Nguyen QH, Bui TP: Azelaic acid: pharmacokinetic and pharmacodynamic properties and its therapeutic role in hyperpigmentary disorders and acne. *Int J Dermatol* 34:75-84, 1995.
167. Fitton A, Goa KL: Azelaic acid. A review of its pharmacological properties and therapeutic efficacy in acne and hyperpigmentary skin disorders. *Drugs* 41:780-798, 1991.
168. Picardo M, Passi S, Sirianni MC, et al: Activity of azelaic acid on cultures of lymphoma- and leukemia-derived cell lines, normal resting and stimulated lymphocytes and 3T3 fibroblasts. *Biochem Pharmacol* 34:1653-1658, 1985.
169. Breathnach AC, Nazzaro-Porro M, Passi S, et al: Azelaic acid therapy in disorders of pigmentation. *Clin Dermatol* 7:106-119, 1989.
170. Maru U, Michaud P, Garrigue J, et al: In vitro diffusion and skin penetration of azelaic preparations: study of correlations. *J de Pharmacie de Belgique* 37:207-213, 1982.

171. Nazzaro-Porro M, Passi S, Picardo M, et al: Beneficial effect of 15% azelaic acid cream on acne vulgaris. *Br J Dermatol* 109:45-48, 1983.

172. Cunliffe WJ, Holland KT: Clinical and laboratory studies on treatment with 20% azelaic acid cream for acne. *Acta Derm Venereol Suppl (Stockh)* 143:31-34, 1989.

173. Bladon PT, Burke BM, Cunliffe WJ, et al: Topical azelaic acid and the treatment of acne: a clinical and laboratory comparison with oral tetracycline. *Br J Dermatol* 114:493-499, 1986.

174. Mayer-da-Silva A, Gollnick H, Detmar M, et al: Effects of azelaic acid on sebaceous gland, sebum excretion rate and keratinization pattern in human skin. An in vivo and in vitro study. *Acta Derm Venereol Suppl (Stockh)* 143:20-30, 1989.

175. Marsden JR, Shuster S: The effect of azelaic acid on acne. *Br J Dermatol* 109:723-724, 1983.

176. Katsambas A, Graupe K, Stratigos J: Clinical studies of 20% azelaic acid cream in the treatment of acne vulgaris. Comparison with vehicle and topical tretinoin. *Acta Derm Venereol Suppl (Stockh)* 143:35-39, 1989.

177. Cavicchini S, Caputo R: Long-term treatment of acne with 20% azelaic acid cream. *Acta Derm Venereol Suppl (Stockh)* 143:40-44, 1989.

178. Hjorth N, Graupe K: Azelaic acid for the treatment of acne. A clinical comparison with oral tetracycline. *Acta Derm Venereol Suppl (Stockh)* 143:45-48, 1989.

179. Anonymous: Azelaic acid—a new topical treatment for acne. *Drug Therapeutics Bull* 31:50-52, 1993.

180. Verallo-Rowell VM, Verallo V, Graupe K, et al: Double-blind comparison of azelaic acid and hydroquinone in the treatment of melasma. *Acta Derm Venereol Suppl (Stockh)* 143:58-61, 1989.

181. Balina LM, Graupe K: The treatment of melasma. 20% azelaic acid versus 4% hydroquinone cream. *Int J Dermatol* 30:893-895, 1991.

182. Piquero Martin J, Rothe de Arocha J, Beniamini Loker D: Double-blind clinical study of the treatment of melasma with azelaic acid versus hydroquinone. *Medicina Cutanea Ibero-Latino-Americana* 16:511-514, 1988.

183. Breathnach AS: Melanin hyperpigmentation of skin: melasma, topical treatment with azelaic acid, and other therapies. *Cutis* 57(1 Suppl):36-45, 1996.

184. Bertuzzi A, Gandolfi A, Salinari S, et al: Pharmacokinetic analysis of azelaic acid disodium salt. A proposed substrate for total parenteral nutrition. *Clin Pharmacokin* 20:411-419, 1991.

185. Topert M, Rach P, Siegmund F: Pharmacology and toxicology of azelaic acid. *Acta Derm Venereol Suppl (Stockh)* 143:14-19, 1989.

186. Mingrone G, Greco AV, Nazzaro-Porro M, et al: Toxicity of azeleic acid. *Drugs Exp Clin Res* 9:447-455, 1983.

Sodium Sulfacetamide

187. Breneman DL, Ariano MC: Successful treatment of acne vulgaris in women with a new topical sodium sulfacetamide/sulfur lotion. *Int J Dermatol* 32:365-367, 1993.

Antiseptics

188. Gaffar A, Scherl D, Afflitto J, et al: The effect of triclosan on mediators of gingival inflammation. *J Clin Periodontol* 22:480-484, 1995.

189. Skaare AB, Herlofson BB, Barkvoll P: Mouthrinses containing triclosan reduce the incidence of recurrent aphthous ulcers (RAU). *J Clin Periodontol* 23:778-781, 1996.

190. Jackson EM: Triclosan in leave-on products. *Cosmetic Dermatol* 11:23-24, 26, 1998.

191. Sporik R, Kemp AS: Topical triclosan treatment of atopic dermatitis. *J Allergy Clin Immunol* 99:861, 1997.

192. Waaler SM, Rolla G, Skjorland KK, et al: Effects of oral rinsing with triclosan and sodium lauryl sulfate on dental plaque formation: a pilot study. *Scand J Dent Res* 101:192-195, 1993.

193. Freeman RG, Knox JM: The action spectrum of photocontact dermatitis caused by halogenated salicylanilide and related compounds. *Arch Dermatol* 97:130-136, 1968.

194. Gusberti FA, Sampathkumar P, Siegrist BE, et al: Microbiological and clinical effects of chlorhexidine digluconate and hydrogen peroxide mouth rinses on developing plaque and gingivitis. *J Clin Periodontol* 15:60-67, 1988.

195. Fisher AA: *Contact Dermatitis*, Baltimore, 1995, Williams & Wilkins.

196. Knudsen BB, Avnstorp C: Chlorhexidine gluconate and acetate in patch testing. *Contact Dermatitis* 24:45-49, 1991.

197. Aursnes J: Cochlear damage from chlorhexidine in guinea pigs. *Acta Otolaryngol (Stockh)* 92:259-271, 1981.

198. Corazza M, Bulciolu G, Spisani L, et al: Chemical burns following irritant contact with povidone-iodine. *Contact Dermatitis* 36:115-116, 1997.

CHAPTER 24

Rhea M. Phillips
Theodore Rosen

Topical Antifungal Agents

Fungal infections are among the most common diseases of the skin and are second to acne as the most common condition treated by dermatologists. Topical antifungals (Figure 24-1) are generally considered as first-line therapy for uncomplicated, superficial, relatively localized dermatomycoses due to their high efficacy and low potential for systemic adverse effects.

In the 1830s Robert Remak and Johann Schonlein first identified fungi as the etiologic agent of human dermatomycoses and revealed the infectious nature of these microorganisms.[1] David Gruby and Raimond Sabouraud were two influential mycologists who later published extensive research on the clinical, microscopic, and cultural nature of fungi and their relationship to human disease. These developments marked the beginning of the science of medical mycology. Effective therapies for human dermatomycoses were slow to evolve, and it was not until 100 years after Remak's initial findings that the first therapies with specific antimycotic actions were developed.[1,2]

World War II marked a pivotal transition in the development of antifungal medications. Soldiers experienced a major problem with athlete's foot that was exacerbated by poor living conditions, inadequate hygiene, communal showers, and lack of appropriate bedding and facilities. Before the 1940s, antifungal therapy was limited to Castellani's paint, Whitfield's ointment, and gentian violet. For the most part, these agents were irritating, staining, nonspecific, and minimally effective.[2,3] The explosive increase in fungal infections and widespread treatment failures during World War II led to a more aggressive search for improved therapeutic measures and prompted the development of new training facilities, research institutions, and federal agencies specializing in medical mycology.[1,2,4]

Today, there are multiple modern topical antimycotics capable of achieving clinical and mycologic eradication of human dermatomycoses. The most commonly employed topical antifungals are among three main classes: the polyenes, the azoles, and the allylamines/benzylamines (Table 24-1). Other topical antimycotics (not among these major drug classes) include a hydroxypyridone (ciclopirox olamine), selenium sulfide, and a thiocarbonate (tolnaftate).

POLYENES

Developed in the late 1950s, polyene antimycotics were the first agents to have specific antifungal properties. Polyene antifungals are characterized by a macrolide ring of carbon atoms containing a number of conjugated double bonds ($-C=C-C=C-$), hence the name "polyene."[5-8] The polyene macrolide ring is closed by an internal ester or lactose.[5] The two clinically significant and readily available polyenes are nystatin and amphotericin B. Topical amphotericin

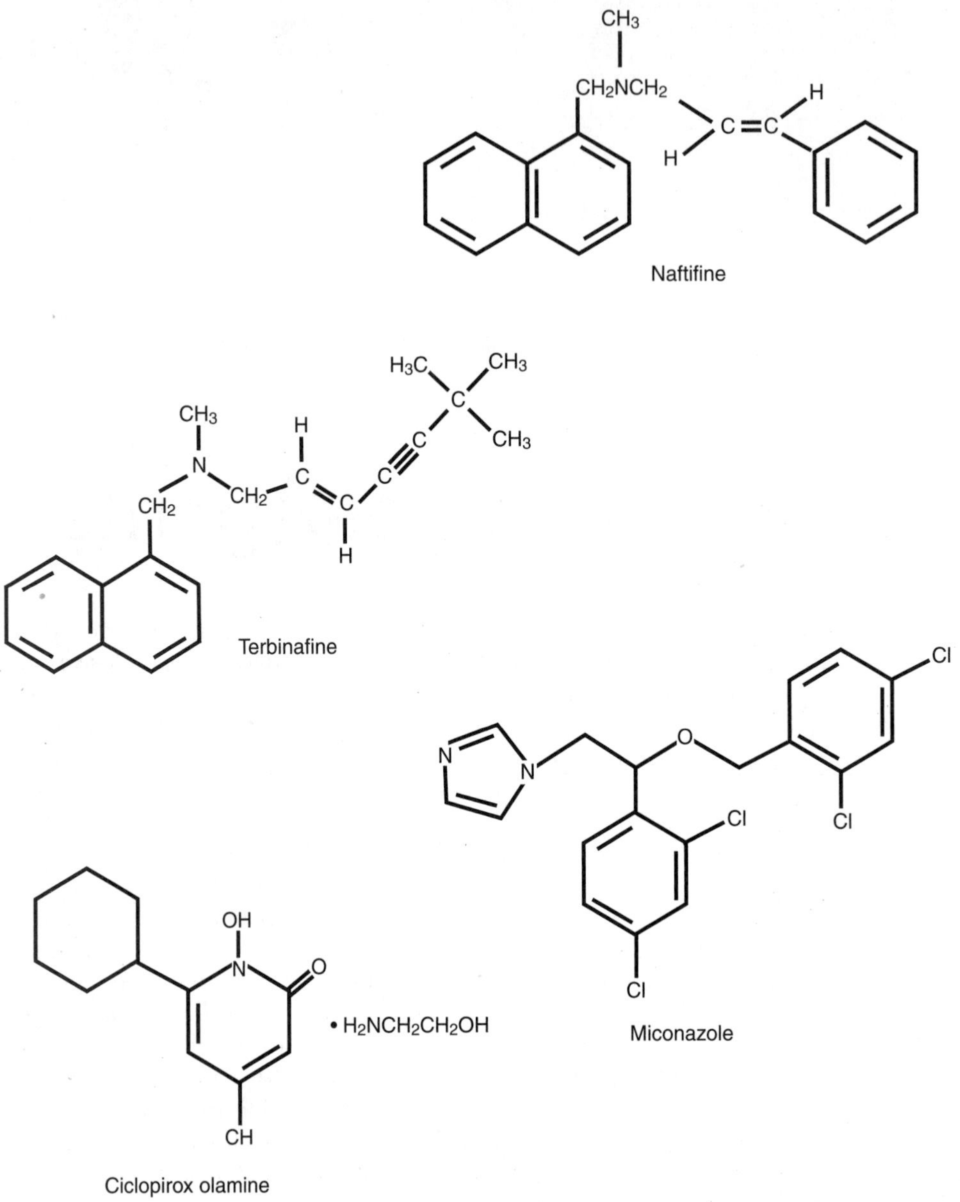

Naftifine

Terbinafine

Miconazole

Ciclopirox olamine

• H$_2$NCH$_2$CH$_2$OH

Figure 24-1 Topical antifungal agents.

B is rarely used in the United States anymore but is still available on request from the manufacturer.

Nystatin

Nystatin was the first specific antimycotic to become available for human use and was discovered in 1949 by Hazen and Brown in the New York State Health Laboratory, hence the name, nystatin.[9,10]

PHARMACOLOGY.   Nystatin is a polyene antibiotic produced by *Streptomyces noursei* and *S. albidus*.[8-10] It is a tetraene antibiotic with both a conjugated diene and a conjugated tetraene moiety in the molecule. It also contains a sugar moiety, mycosamine, as part of its composition.[5,7] It has a structure and mode of action similar to that of amphotericin B, but associated systemic toxicity limits its use to topical applications.

Table 24-1 Topical Antifungal Agents

Generic Name	Trade Name	Manufacturer	Generic	Cream	Ointment	Special Formulations	PPS
POLYENES							
Nystatin	Mycostatin, Mytrex, Nystop, others	Westwood-Squibb, Others	Yes	Cream*	Yes	Powder, suspension, pastille	B
Amphotericin B	Fungizone	Bristol-Myers Squibb	Yes	None	No	Oral suspension 100 mg/ml (also IV)	B
AZOLES							
Miconazole	Monistat-Derm, Micatin	Ortho	Yes	2% cream	No	Spray, powder (Also IV)	B
Clotrimazole	Lotrimin, Mycelex	Schering-Plough, Bayer	Yes	1% cream	No	1% solution/lotion Oral troches (Mycelex) Also powder, spray	B
Ketoconazole	Nizoral	Janssen	No	1% cream,† 2% cream	No	1%,† 2% shampoos	B
Oxiconazole	Oxistat	Glaxo-Wellcome	No	1% cream	No	1% lotion	B
Econazole	Spectazole	Ortho	No	1% cream	No	None	B
Sulconazole	Exelderm	Westwood-Squibb	No	1% cream	No	1% solution	B
ALLYLAMINES AND BENZYLAMINES							
Naftifine	Naftin	Allergan	No	1% cream	No	1% gel	B
Terbinafine	Lamisil	Novartis	No	1% cream	No	250 mg tablets	B
Butenafine	Mentax	Penederm	No	1% cream	No	None	B
OTHER ANTIFUNGAL AGENTS							
Ciclopirox	Loprox (Penlac)	Hoechst-Marion Roussel (Penlac Dermik)	No	1% cream	No	1% lotion (8% nail lacquer)	B
Selenium sulfide	Selsun, Exsel, others	Allergan, Ross	Yes	None	No	1%, 2.5% shampoos	C
Tolnaftate	Tinactin	Alpharma	Yes	1% cream	No	Spray, solution	C

PPS, Pregnancy prescribing status—U.S. FDA.
*Not expressed as a percentage; 100,000 USP units/g.
†OTC strength for ketoconazole products.

Absorption. Nystatin is essentially insoluble in water and not absorbed from intact skin, the gastrointestinal tract, or the vagina.[11]

Mechanism of Action. Nystatin is an antifungal antibiotic, with both fungistatic and fungicidal activity in vitro. It acts by binding irreversibly to membrane sterols of susceptible species of *Candida*, resulting in a change in membrane permeability and the subsequent leakage of essential intracellular components[5,8,12,13] (Table 24-2).

CLINICAL USE

Indications. Nystatin is a topical antimycotic agent that is clinically and mycologically effective in the treatment of cutaneous or mucocutaneous mycotic infections caused by *C. albicans* and other susceptible candidal species such as *C. parapsilosis*, *C. krusei*, and *C. tropicalis*. However, nystatin is clinically ineffective in the treatment of common mycoses due to dermatophyte species. Nystatin shows no appreciable activity against bacteria, protozoa, or viruses.[5,14] Nystatin is available in cream, ointment, and powder formulations for twice daily cutaneous application. Nystatin is also available in suspension and slowly dissolving pastille (a medicated disk used for a local action on the mucosa of the throat and mouth) formulations for the treatment of oral candidiasis (thrush). Four to five times daily use is recommended in the latter situation.

Adverse Effects. Nystatin is well tolerated by patients, with less than 0.1% of patients reporting adverse effects; the more common adverse effects include burning, rash, eczema, and pain on application.[13] Very rare occurrences of hypersensitivity reactions have been reported.[15-21]

AZOLES

The introduction of the azole antimycotics presented a new class of compounds with a broader spectrum of activity, including activity against the common dermatophytes that were not susceptible to the polyenes. Azoles act by blocking the biosynthesis of ergosterol, the primary sterol derivative of the fungal cell membrane[22,23] (see Table 24-2). Depletion of ergosterol results in membrane permeability changes incompatible with fungal growth and survival. The azoles block sterol synthesis by interfering with the cytochrome P-450–dependent enzyme, lanosterol 14α-demethylase, which catalyzes the conversion of lanosterol to ergosterol. The binding of the azoles proceeds primarily by a direct link of an azole nitrogen to the heme iron located in a binding domain of the cytochrome P-450 molecule. These antifungals bind to the heme iron of the cytochrome at the same site that oxygen is bound. In this manner, the azole compounds compete with oxygen and inhibit its binding and

---

■ **Table 24-2**   In Vitro and In Vivo Activity of Common Antifungal Agents

Class	Drug(s)	Mechanism of Action	Organisms Treated
Polyene antibiotics	Nystatin	Binds to cell membrane sterols causing cell leakage and permeability changes	Yeast (*Candida*)
Azoles	Miconazole Clotrimazole Ketoconazole Econazole	Inhibits ergosterol synthesis blocking, 14α-demethylation of lanosterol	Dermatophytes, *M. furfur*, *Candida*
Azoles (subset)	Oxiconazole Sulconazole	Same as azoles above	Dermatophytes, *M. furfur*, *Candida**
Allylamines	Naftifine Terbinafine	Inhibits sterol synthesis by blocking action of squalene epoxidase	Dermatophytes (both drugs) *Candida** (only terbinafine)
Benzylamines	Butenafine	Same as allylamines above	Dermatophytes, *Candida**

*Activity against *Candida* species is relatively weak compared with the other azole antifungal agents.

activation. This results in inhibition of the cytochrome P-450 catalysis of lanosterol to ergosterol. Decreased availability of ergosterol and accumulation of intracellular 14α-methylsterols result in increased membrane rigidity, membrane permeability changes, alterations in critical membrane-bound enzymes, inhibition of growth, and cell death.[22,24-26]

The human skin is an efficient barrier to most azole compounds. On intact skin, percutaneous absorption is generally less than 1%. The absorption may be increased up to 4% on inflamed or damaged skin, which can be mimicked by abrasion or stripping of the stratum corneum.[27]

Miconazole
PHARMACOLOGY.   Miconazole is a synthetic β-substituted 1-phenethyl imidazole derivative with the chemical name 1-[2,4-dichloro-β-{(2,4-dichlorobenzyl)oxyl}phenethyl] imidazole mononitrate. It is very slightly soluble in water and slightly soluble in most common organic solvents and diluted inorganic acids.[28]

Absorption.   Miconazole penetrates the stratum corneum well and can be detected there up to 4 days after a single application. Systemic absorption is minimal, with less than 1% of the drug absorbed after topical application.[11,29]

Mechanism of Action.   The principal mode of action of miconazole is the inhibition of cytochrome P-450–dependent 14α-demethylation in the formation of ergosterol, which is an essential constituent of the fungal cell membrane.[22,23]

CLINICAL USE
Indications.   Miconazole is active in vitro against the common dermatophytes *Trichophyton rubrum*, *T. mentagrophytes*, and *Epidermophyton floccosum*. It also has inhibitory activity against *C. albicans* and *Malassezia furfur.*[28,30,31] Miconazole cream is effective in the treatment of tinea pedis, tinea corporis, tinea cruris, and tinea versicolor, and in the treatment of cutaneous candidiasis.[32-38] Miconazole also demonstrated activity against some gram-positive bacteria; it has proven modestly effective in the treatment of erythrasma, impetigo, or ecthyma caused by Group A β-hemolytic streptococci or pathogenic staphylococci.[28,39,40] However, antibacterial activity is not sufficient to make this agent a drug of choice for such infections. A

benzoyl peroxide and miconazole combination has also been used successfully in the treatment of acne vulgaris and was superior to benzoyl peroxide alone in the treatment of inflammatory acne after 30 days of treatment[41]; unfortunately, this product is not commercially available. Twice daily application is recommended in all clinical situations except tinea versicolor in which once daily application is effective.

Adverse Effects.   Topical application of miconazole is well tolerated, with rare adverse effects, including irritation, burning, maceration, and allergic dermatitis at application sites.[13]

Clotrimazole
PHARMACOLOGY.   First synthesized in 1967, clotrimazole is a broad-spectrum chlorinated trityl imidazolyl antimycotic with the chemical name bis-phenyl(2-chlorophenyl)-1-imidazole methane.[42]

Absorption.   After topical application of clotrimazole 1% cream and clotrimazole 1% solution to intact and acutely inflamed skin, the concentration of clotrimazole was measured as 100 μg/cm^3 in the stratum corneum, 0.5 to 1 μg/cm^3 in the dermis, and 0.1 μg/cm^3 in the subcutis. During routine topical application, systemic absorption of clotrimazole is extremely low; after topical application of clotrimazole cream and solution under occlusive dressing for 48 hours, no measurable amount of clotrimazole was found in the serum and only 0.5% or less of the applied product was recovered in the urine.[43]

Mechanism of Action.   Like the other azoles, clotrimazole acts by inhibiting 14α-demethylase in the ergosterol biosynthetic pathway. Depletion of ergosterol by clotrimazole results in changes in the cell membrane permeability, efflux of critical cell constituents, breakdown of cellular nucleic acids, and cessation of cell growth.[22,23]

CLINICAL USE
Indications.   In in vitro studies, clotrimazole exhibits a broad spectrum of activity against most strains of *Trichophyton*, *Epidermophyton*, and *Microsporum* species.[44] It is also active against gram-positive bacteria and exhibits efficacy slightly less than that of nystatin in *Candida* inhibition.[29,45] Clotrimazole is effective in the treatment of tinea pedis, tinea corporis, tinea

cruris, tinea versicolor, and cutaneous candidiasis.[44-56] The agent is available in cream, lotion, and solution formulations for twice daily application. It is also used in the treatment of oropharyngeal (troches) and vaginal (intravaginal tablet, cream) candidiasis.[50] Oral troches are designed to slowly dissolve in the mouth and should be administered four to five times daily for 2 weeks. Intravaginal clotrimazole may be effective after once daily tablet insertion for 1 to 2 days.

Adverse Effects. Clotrimazole is generally well tolerated, with isolated reports of erythema, burning, irritation, stinging, peeling, blistering edema, pruritus, and urticaria at the site of application.[43]

Ketoconazole

PHARMACOLOGY. Ketoconazole is a water-soluble imidazole derivative with the chemical name *cis*-1-acetyl-4-[4-[2-(2,4,-dichlorophenyl)-2-(1H-imidazol-1-ylmethyl)-1,3-dioxolan-4-methoxylphenyl] piperazine. First synthesized in 1977, ketoconazole is a synthetic antimycotic with a broad spectrum of activity against dermatophytes and yeasts.[57-60]

Absorption. After a single topical application to the trunk and upper extremities of healthy volunteers, there were no detectable plasma levels of ketoconazole at a sensitivity level of 5 μg/L over a 72-hour period after application.[57] In infants treated with topical ketoconazole to the scalp, no plasma levels were detected over a 10-day treatment period.[61]

Mechanism of Action. Like the other azole antimycotics, ketoconazole inhibits the cytochrome P-450–dependent 14α-demethylation of lanosterol in the ergosterol biosynthesis pathway, resulting in depletion of ergosterol, a lipid component critical to membrane integrity.[62] Ergosterol depletion and intracellular accumulation of 14α-methylsterols result in alterations in membrane permeability and cessation of cell growth.[22,23,59,60,62]

CLINICAL USE

Indications. Ketoconazole is a broad-spectrum antimycotic that exhibits a wide spectrum of activity against dermatophytes, *C. albicans*, and *M. furfur* in vitro.[58-60] In clinical trials, ketoconazole 2% cream has been shown to be

effective in the treatment of tinea pedis, tinea cruris, and tinea corporis. Lester and colleagues[63] reported that 82% of patients with tinea pedis, tinea cruris, or tinea corporis had an excellent response to 4 weeks of therapy with once daily applications of topical ketoconazole. Ketoconazole cream is also effective in the treatment of cutaneous candidiasis[64] and tinea versicolor.[65-69] Ketoconazole cream and 2% shampoo have also been shown to be effective in the treatment of seborrheic dermatitis due to its association with *M. furfur* (also known as *Pityrosporum ovale*).[61,70-78] In one study,[61] 78.9% of patients with infantile seborrheic dermatitis achieved a good-to-excellent response after 10 days of ketoconazole application. Comparable success can be expected in adults. A 1% shampoo formulation was recently approved for over-the-counter (OTC) use in the ongoing management of seborrheic dermatitis. The 2% Nizoral shampoo remains available by prescription.

Adverse Effects. In clinical trials during which 905 patients were treated with ketoconazole 2% cream, 5% of the patients reported adverse effects, including irritation and stinging. One of these patients developed a painful allergic reaction at the site of application. In worldwide postmarketing experience, rare reports of contact dermatitis have been associated with Nizoral (ketoconazole) cream or one of its ingredients, namely sodium sulfite or propylene glycol.[79]

Oxiconazole

First approved for use in the United States in 1989 for the topical treatment of human dermatophyte infections, oxiconazole was the first antimycotic to be approved for once daily application.[80]

PHARMACOLOGY. Oxiconazole nitrate is an acetophenone-oxime derivative of the basic imidazole structural unit (substituted heterocyclic ring with a nitrogen in the 3-position), chemically named Z-(2,4-dichloro-2-imidazol-1-yl)aceto-phone-O-(2,4-dichlorobenzyl)-oxime.

Absorption. Topical oxiconazole is rapidly absorbed into the stratum corneum. Fungicidal concentrations of oxiconazole are found in the epidermis within 5 hours of topical application and reach maximum concentrations as early as 100 minutes after application.[81] In animal studies, Polak[82] demonstrated persistence of the drug in the stratum corneum for up to 96 hours after a single application. Because of the pharmacokinetic properties of oxiconazole, it persists in the epidermis at therapeutic levels for 7 days. This reservoir effect accounts for oxiconazole's efficacy in fungus eradication with once daily dosing.[83-85] Systemic absorption of oxiconazole is negligible; in clinical trials, less than 0.3% was recovered in the urine of volunteer patients after up to 5 days of application of oxiconazole cream, and none was recovered from the feces.[86]

Mechanism of Action. Like other imidazole derivatives, oxiconazole mainly acts to block the synthesis of ergosterol by inhibiting demethylation of lanosterol, a cytochrome P-450–dependent step in the ergosterol biosynthesis pathway.[87,88]

CLINICAL USE

Indications. In clinical trials, oxiconazole lotion applied topically once daily was safe and significantly superior to the vehicle when used in the treatment of tinea pedis, including the hyperkeratotic plantar and interdigital subtypes of the disease.[84] In a multicenter, double-blind, parallel-group study, Ellis and co-workers[85] treated 153 patients with mycologically confirmed tinea pedis with either once or twice daily applications of either oxiconazole cream or an inactive vehicle cream. At the 2-week follow-up visit, a mycologic cure was achieved in 80% of the once daily and 75% of patients treated twice daily with oxiconazole cream compared with 34% of those receiving inactive vehicle cream. In clinical trials in Europe,[83,88-95] the United States,[85,86,96,97] Latin America,[98,99] and Japan,[100-103] oxiconazole proved to be highly efficacious in the treatment of superficial fungal infections.[80] Oxiconazole is commercially available in 1% cream and 1% lotion formulations, the latter being useful for large or hairy areas (e.g., the trunk and back)

Adverse Effects. Topical application of oxiconazole is well tolerated, with few side effects. Of 955 patients treated in U.S. clinical trials,[85,86,97] 41 experienced drug-related adverse effects, including pruritus (1.6%), burning (1.4%), irritation (0.4%), erythema (0.2%), maceration (0.1%), and fissuring (0.1%). In a large multicenter trial reported by Meinhof and

associates,[88] only 2.8% of 1759 patients treated with topical oxiconazole cream experienced adverse effects. No adverse effects were reported in several Japanese clinical studies.[102,103]

Econazole

PHARMACOLOGY.   First synthesized in 1969, econazole is a deschloro derivative of miconazole with the chemical name 1-[2-{(4-chlorophenyl) methoxy}-2-(2,4-dichlorophenyl)ethyl]-1H-imidazole mononitrate.

Absorption. Absolute concentrations of econazole in the human stratum corneum after local application far exceed the minimal inhibitory concentrations (MIC) for dermatophytes, and inhibitory concentrations are detected as deep as the middermis.[104,105] Systemic absorption after topical application of econazole is low, with less than 1% recovered in the urine and feces.[106]

Mechanism of Action. Econazole is an imidazole derivative that interferes with ergosterol synthesis by blocking 14α-demethylation of lanosterol, a P-450–dependent step. This in turn leads to an increase in fungal cell membrane permeability associated with the drug's antifungal effect.[22,23]

CLINICAL USE

Indications. In vitro, econazole inhibits most strains of *Trichophyton* organisms, *Microsporum* organisms, *Epidermophyton* organisms, *C. albicans*, and *M. furfur*.[104] Topical econazole is effective in the treatment of tinea pedis, tinea cruris, and tinea corporis caused by dermatophytes, as well as tinea versicolor caused by *Malassezia* organisms and cutaneous candidiasis due to *C. albicans*.[104,107-116] Econazole 1% cream has been shown to be as effective as clotrimazole 1% cream in the treatment of tinea infections and cutaneous candidiasis, but with a more rapid onset of activity in patients treated with econazole.[116] Econazole has also shown activity against some gram-positive and gram-negative bacterial organisms.[104,117] Kates and colleagues[117] treated patients with severe interdigital bacterial toe web infections with no fungi demonstrable by KOH or culture examination with topical econazole. The investigators reported good-to-excellent improvement in 88% of patients treated with topical econazole, whereas no patients treated with the vehicle showed improvement.

Adverse Effects. Topical application of econazole is well tolerated, with rare side effects; in clinical trials, some 3% of the patients treated with econazole experienced adverse effects, including erythema, burning, stinging, and pruritus.[106]

Sulconazole

PHARMACOLOGY. Sulconazole is similar to other azole compounds previously discussed. It has a chemical name of (±)-1-[2,4-dichloro-β-[(p-chlorobenzyl)-thiol]-penethyl imidazole mononitrate.[118] Sulconazole differs from the other azole compounds by having a sulfide (thiol) bond between constituent rings.

Absorption. Sulconazole may be detected in the stratum corneum for up to 96 hours after application. Human percutaneous absorption of sulconazole exceeds that of other azole compounds, being on the order of 8% to 11%.[119] The clinical significance, if any, of this phenomenon is unknown.

Mechanism of Action. As is true of other azoles, sulconazole interferes with ergosterol synthesis by blocking 14α-demethylation of lanosterol. This leads to an increase in fungal cell membrane permeability associated with the drug's antifungal effect.[118,120] Sulconazole also demonstrates some antibacterial activity against gram-positive bacteria.[120]

CLINICAL USE

Indications. Sulconazole offers little advantage over azole compounds previously discussed. It proved effective in the treatment of dermatophytosis due to common organisms,[120-125] tinea versicolor,[126] and cutaneous candidiasis.[127] Sulconazole is available as 1% cream and 1% solution formulations. Sulconazole is applied one to two times daily until clinical resolution, which is generally 2 to 4 weeks. Clinical responses are equivalent to other azoles, although some reports suggest more rapid response when sulconazole is compared with miconazole or clotrimazole.[120] Sulconazole has been reported an effective therapy for impetigo and ecthyma due to Group A β-hemolytic streptococci and staphylococci when applied twice daily for 14 days.[128] However, it is not the preferred drug for these indications.

Adverse Effects. Sulconazole is well tolerated, although there have been a few reports of allergic contact dermatitis.[129]

ALLYLAMINES AND BENZYLAMINES

The allylamines represent a newer class of antimycotic agents. The introduction of allylamines in the 1980s presented a broader spectrum of antimycotic coverage with a new advantage—fungicidal activity. The allylamines were inadvertently discovered during efforts to synthesize an active central nervous system compound.[130] The resulting compound, naftifine, was found to have antimycotic activity during routine laboratory screening tests performed on newly developed compounds.[131] Allylamines are broad-spectrum antimycotics with both fungistatic and fungicidal activity (depending on the organism being tested) that act by inhibiting the synthesis of ergosterol, an essential component of the fungal cell membrane (see Table 24-2). Such inhibition leads to cell membrane fragility, increased membrane permeability, and intracellular accumulation of sterol precursors. The allylamines act at an earlier step in the ergosterol biosynthesis pathway than the azole class of antifungal drugs, and their inhibition is cytochrome P-450–independent.[132-135] Naftifine and terbinafine are the two primary antimycotics of the class of allylamines. Butenafine is the first and only representative of the benzylamine class, a group similar in structure and action to the allylamines.

Naftifine

PHARMACOLOGY. Naftifine is a synthetic allylamine antifungal with the chemical structure (E)-N-methyl-N-(1-naphthylmethyl)-3-phenyl-2-propen-1-amine-hydrochloride.

Absorption. The highly lipophilic nature of this compound allows for efficient penetration and high concentrations in the stratum corneum and hair follicles.[136-138] The tertiary allylamine is the structural element of naftifine with strong antifungal activity.[139-141]

Mechanism of Action. The action of naftifine is both fungicidal and fungistatic.[131,142] Naftifine inhibits squalene epoxidase, the enzyme responsible for the conversion of squalene to squalene oxide in the ergosterol biosynthesis pathway. With this interruption, there is decreased ergosterol production and increased accumulation of the sterol precursor squalene.[139,143-145] Ergosterol is an essential component of the fungal cell membrane and necessary for fungal growth and survival.[146] Studies show that the fungicidal activity of naftifine results from interference with ergosterol synthesis, accumulation of squalene, and consequent disruption of fungal cell membranes. The inhibitory action of naftifine differs from the action of azole antifungals, with its inhibitory effect being independent of the cytochrome P-450–dependent synthesis of steroidal hormones.[134,139,143-145]

CLINICAL USE

Indications. Naftifine's spectrum of in vitro activity includes a broad range of dermatophytes, yeasts, and saprophytes, including *Sporothrix schenckii*.[131,147] It exhibited strong in vivo activity against *T. mentagrophytes* in animal studies.[142,148] Naftifine demonstrated therapeutic efficacy against several dermatomycoses in clinical trials in Europe[54,149-166] and the United States.[167-170] In a controlled double-blind comparison study,[169] investigators found naftifine cream 1% to be as effective as econazole 1% cream in the treatment of tinea cruris and tinea corporis, with an earlier onset of action demonstrated by naftifine. Comparison studies of econazole and naftifine in animal studies produced similar results.[142,148] In comparison with clotrimazole, naftifine was as effective in the treatment of tinea pedis,[156,170-173] tinea cruris,[156] tinea corporis,[156] and candidiasis,[152,162] with a notably earlier onset of symptomatic relief. Naftifine is available in both cream and gel formulations, and is applied once to twice daily. In mild infections (e.g., tinea pedis confined to the toe webs), once daily application is sufficient.

Adverse Effects. Naftifine is well tolerated, with less than 5% of patients experiencing adverse effects, including mild burning/stinging, itching, erythema, irritation, and rarely, allergic reactions.[174]

Terbinafine

PHARMACOLOGY. Terbinafine [(E)-*N*-(6,6-dimethyl-2-hepten-4-ynyl)-N-methyl-1-naphthalena-methanamine] is a broad-spectrum synthetic antimycotic agent of the allylamine chemical family with both fungistatic and fungicidal properties.[131,141,175]

Absorption. Terbinafine is highly lipophilic, resulting in high concentration in and efficient binding to the stratum corneum, sebum, and hair follicles, thus reducing the probability of reinfection. Pharmacokinetic studies demonstrated persistent concentrations well above the MICs for the common dermatophytes 7 days after topical application.[137,176]

Terbinafine is an allylamine derivative similar to naftifine but 10 to 100 times more potent in vitro. After the introduction of naftifine, intense chemical and biologic analysis to identify structure-activity relationships led to the synthesis of a compound with significantly improved antifungal activity. The ultimate result was the compound terbinafine. The key structural modifications to the allylamine group plus the benzene ring, an additional triple bond (the acetylene group), and the addition of a branched side chain led to significantly increased antifungal activity in vitro and in vivo.[134,140-141]

After topical application, 3% to 5% of terbinafine 1% cream is absorbed into the systemic circulation. This amount of absorption is biologically and clinically insignificant. This absorption occurs slowly, with the peak amount of substance appearing as metabolites in the urine 2 to 3 days after the application. This slow absorption is believed to reflect the rate of entry of the drug in the epidermis and dermis.[138,176]

Mechanism of Action. Terbinafine exhibits a broad antifungal spectrum that interferes with the ability of squalene epoxidase to catalyze the conversion of squalene to ergosterol. The suppression of biosynthesis of ergosterol, a sterol critical to cellular integrity, and the intracellular squalene accumulation result in cell death. Terbinafine inhibits ergosterol biosynthesis at an earlier stage than the azole antifungals, without affecting cytochrome P-450–related steroidogenesis. This earlier mode of action may account for its fungicidal rather than fungistatic activity.[133-135,177,178]

CLINICAL USE

Indications. In vitro susceptibility tests showed that terbinafine has fungicidal activity against a wide variety of dermatophytes; certain dimorphic fungi, including *S. schenckii, Blasto-*

myces dermatitidis, and *Histoplasma capsulatum*; and *C. albicans*.[175,179,180] In clinical trials, Savin and co-workers[181] found terbinafine cream applied topically twice daily to be safe and significantly superior to the vehicle when used in the treatment of chronic tinea pedis. Eighty-nine percent of patients treated with terbinafine were clinically and mycologically clear, whereas none of the patients treated with the placebo group cleared. Randomized double-blind, vehicle-controlled parallel group studies were designed to evaluate the safety and efficacy of terbinafine in the treatment of tinea corporis and tinea cruris. In this study, 76% of patients receiving topical terbinafine achieved mycologic cure and clinical improvement, with only 17% of the placebo group achieving similar results. In a large multicenter study in Japan of 629 patients, investigators found terbinafine 1% cream to be both safe and effective in the treatment of tinea pedis, tinea corporis, tinea cruris, tinea versicolor, and intertriginous candidiasis.[182] In a review of clinical experience from 27 studies in which 1258 patients with various dermatomycoses were treated with terbinafine cream, Villars and Jones[183] found the overall efficacy rate of topical terbinafine to range from 70% to 90% for all tinea infections treated and 80% to 90% for the treatment of tinea corporis or tinea cruris.

Adverse Effects. Topical terbinafine is well tolerated, with few reported adverse effects. In a Japanese trial consisting of 629 patients treated with topical terbinafine, only 6 individuals experienced adverse effects, including allergic and acute irritant contact dermatitis.[182] In U.S. clinical trials, 2.2% of the patients experienced mild local side effects, including irritation, burning/tingling sensation, pruritus, and dryness at the site of application.[183]

Butenafine

PHARMACOLOGY. Butenafine, recently approved for use in the United States, is the first and only of the benzylamine class of antifungals. Butenafine hydrochloride (*N*-4-tert-butylbenzyl-*N*-methyl-1-naphthalenemethylamine hydrochloride) is structurally similar to the various allylamines, although there is a butylbenzyl group in the place of the allylamine group.[184,185]

Absorption. Pharmacokinetic studies demonstrated fungicidal concentrations in the skin, particularly the stratum corneum, for at least 72 hours after application.[186,187]

Mechanism of Action. Like the allylamines, butenafine acts by inhibiting the epoxidation of squalene, thus blocking the biosynthesis of ergosterol, an essential component of the fungal cell membrane. The inhibition of sterol synthesis by butenafine is independent of cytochrome P-450. With the inhibition of squalene epoxidase, there is also an accumulation of intracellular squalene leading to disruption of the fungal cell membrane.*

CLINICAL USE

Indications. Recent investigations presented the efficacy of butenafine. Butenafine demonstrated fungicidal activity in vitro and in animal models against dermatophytes, aspergilli, and dimorphic fungi, including *S. schenckii*, with inhibitory activity equal to or greater than that of naftifine and terbinafine.[184,185] Butenafine cream has been the treatment of choice for tinea pedis, tinea corporis, tinea cruris, tinea versicolor, and cutaneous candidal infections in Japan since its introduction in 1992. Clinical trials conducted in Japan revealed 84% to 100% cure rates in tinea cruris, with only 2% to 3% of patients experiencing adverse effects, including erythema and irritation.[189]

Controlled clinical trials indicated butenafine to be a well-tolerated and effective short-term therapy for interdigital tinea pedis, tinea corporis, and tinea cruris.[190-197] Lesher and associates[196] reported 2-week, once daily applications of butenafine to be safe, effective treatment of tinea cruris; in the same study, statistically significant mycologic cure and clinical improvement were also noted after only 1 week of treatment with butenafine. In addition, cure rates continued to increase 2 weeks after the end of treatment, suggesting that butenafine may possess residual therapeutic activity. Savin and co-workers[197] reported short-term, twice daily application of topical butenafine to be clinically and mycologically effective in the treatment of tinea pedis. In a double-blind, placebo-controlled

---

*References 141, 177, 178, 184, 187, 188.

trial,[195] investigators found that a 2-week once daily application of butenafine cream was safe and effective in the treatment of tinea corporis. Several clinical trials of butenafine also demonstrated continued mycologic and clinical improvement after completion of therapy, suggesting a continued benefit after dose completion related to strong keratin binding.

Adverse Effects. The topical allylamine and benzylamine medications are well tolerated, with 2% to 3% of patients experiencing mild adverse effects, including burning, itching, and redness at application sites.[183,188] Lesher and associates[196] noted only one case of burning on topical application of butenafine in a controlled study of 76 patients treated with butenafine cream.

OTHER TOPICAL ANTIFUNGALS
Ciclopirox Olamine
Ciclopirox olamine (6-cyclohexyl-1-hydroxy-4-methyl-2[1H]-pyridone ethanolamine) is a hydroxypyridone antifungal agent with a unique structure and a mode of action unrelated to the other available antifungals. Unlike most antimycotic agents, ciclopirox does not appear to affect sterol biosynthesis but acts by interfering with active membrane transport of essential macromolecular precursors, cell membrane integrity, and cell respiratory processes.[198-202] In vitro, ciclopirox olamine exhibits high inhibitory activity against dermatophytes, yeasts, and fungal saprophytes.[203,204] In one study,[205] ciclopirox olamine demonstrated considerably better in vitro activity against *T. mentagrophytes* and *C. albicans* than oxiconazole, miconazole, clotrimazole, and naftifine. In clinical trials, ciclopirox 1% cream was significantly more effective than its vehicle and clotrimazole 1% cream in the treatment of tinea pedis.[205,206] In clinical trials,[207] ciclopirox 1% cream was also effective in the treatment of tinea corporis, tinea cruris, tinea versicolor,[208,209] and cutaneous candidiasis.[210] Ciclopirox exhibited strong activity in vitro and in vivo against gram-positive and gram-negative bacteria.[201,203,211] Ciclopirox also demonstrated inherent antiinflammatory activity. This compound has been shown to inhibit prostaglandin and leukotriene synthesis in human polymorphonuclear cells.[212] In a comparison study, ciclopirox olamine 1% cream was shown to be as effective as the ciclopirox 1%-hydrocortisone acetate 1% combination in the treatment of inflamed superficial mycoses.[213]

Ciclopirox nail lacquer 8% also demonstrated potential to penetrate the nail plate[214] and clinically and mycologically cleared 40% of patients with fingernail and toenail onychomycosis in one study.[215] Nail penetration studies with ciclopirox nail lacquer varied among volunteers, as have clinical results.[214,216-218] This product was approved for use in the United States in December of 1999 and became commercially available in 2000.

Selenium Sulfide
Selenium sulfide is a liquid antiseborrheic, antifungal preparation for topical application only. It is available in a prescription only 2.5% lotion and in a 1% lotion (Selsun Blue), which is available over the counter. It is currently indicated for the treatment of tinea versicolor and seborrheic dermatitis of the scalp.[69,219-223] In addition, some reports show that selenium sulfide is effective in the treatment of confluent and reticulated papillomatosis of Gougerot-Carteaud syndrome.[224,225] Selenium sulfide has also been shown to be an effective adjuvant to griseofulvin in the treatment of tinea capitis.[226] Selenium sulfide seems to possess a cytostatic effect on cells of the epidermis and follicular epithelium. This allows for the shedding of fungi in the stratum corneum via a reduction in corneocyte adhesion.[227] Selenium sulfide has also shown some fungicidal activity against *P. ovale* in vitro and in vivo.[228] In the past, selenium sulfide was considered by some to be a possible carcinogen, but studies have not confirmed this.[229,230] However, animal reproductive studies have not been performed, and topical selenium is classified as pregnancy category C. Blood and urine levels of selenium have not been found to be increased by the topical courses recommended for the treatment of tinea versicolor.[231,232] Selenium sulfide 2.5% is effective in the treatment of tinea versicolor[219,221-223] and has shown efficacy similar to bifonazole in the treatment of this condition.[220]

Tolnaftate
Tolnaftate is a thiocarbamate antifungal that inhibits sterol biosynthesis of fungal cells by in-

hibiting squalene epoxidase. It is successful in the treatment of the majority of cutaneous mycoses but ineffective against bacteria and *Candida* organisms.[29]

Undecylenic Acid

Undecylenic acid preparations consist of the compound undecylenic acid and its zinc, calcium, or sodium salt in a powder, aerosol, cream, or solution. It is used in the treatment of various dermatomycoses, including tinea pedis, tinea cruris, and diaper dermatitis.[29] With the advent of the previously discussed topical antimycotics, undecylenic acid products are apparently now used.

COMPARATIVE STUDIES

Several laboratory, animal, and clinical investigations have been conducted to compare the safety and efficacy of the various antimycotic agents in the treatment of cutaneous fungal infections. These agents were primarily tested against the most common pathogens responsible for dermatomycosis such as *Trichophyton, Epidermophyton,* and *Microsporum* species.

In Vitro Studies

Results of in vitro susceptibility tests have shown the allylamine- and benzylamine-type drugs to have greater activity against the common dermatophytes than the azole derivatives. For example, Meade and colleagues[195] (Table 24-3) reported butenafine to be 10 to 35 times more potent than clotrimazole against the common dermatophytes. Arika and co-workers[186] reported butenafine to possess 10 to 100 times more antidermatophyte activity than the azoles clotrimazole and bifonazole, and 4 times greater activity than naftifine in vitro. Shadomy and associates[180] (Table 24-4) reported terbinafine to be 2 to 30 times more potent than ketoconazole and 10 times more potent than miconazole against common dermatophytes in vitro. In addition, the MICs of the allylamine and benzylamine groups are equal to or are near the value of their minimal fungicidal concentrations

■ Table 24-3   MICs of Antifungal Agents' Activity Against Dermatophytes (Mean MIC μg/ml)*

Fungus (No. of Strains)	Butenafine	Naftifine	Clotrimazole
Trichophyton rubrum (41)	0.007	0.031	0.267
Trichophyton mentagrophytes (22)	0.012	0.035	0.266
Microsporum canis (14)	0.024	0.100	0.266

Data from Maeda T, Takase M, Ishibashi A, et al: *Yakugaku Zasshi* 111:126-137, 1991.
*Lower MICs indicate stronger inhibition of dermatophytes by allylamines/benzylamines relative to the azole agents.

■ Table 24-4   MICs of Antifungal Agents' Activity Against Dermatophytes (Mean MIC μg/ml)*

Fungus (No. of Strains)	Terbinafine	Naftifine	Ketoconazole
Trichophyton species (13)	≤0.06	0.07	0.21
Microsporum species (6)	≤0.06	0.07	0.35
Epidermophyton floccosum (5)	≤0.06	≤0.06	0.11

Data from Shadomy S, Espinel-Ingroff A, Gebhart RJ: *Sabouraudia* 23:125-132, 1985.
*Lower MICs indicate stronger inhibition of dermatophytes by allylamines/benzylamines relative to the azole agents.

(MFCs) against the dermatophytes, indicating primarily fungicidal activity. This is in contrast to the azole antimycotics that exhibit fungistatic inhibition.

The in vitro dermatophyte potency against can be summarized as follows*:

butenafine = terbinafine > ciclopirox =

naftifine > azoles

In Vivo Studies

Animal study results paralleled the in vitro findings of the various antimycotic efficacies previously reported. In one study, infected guinea pigs with *T. mentagrophytes* and *M. canis* and the resulting dermatophytoses were treated with allylamine/benzylamine and azole antimycotics.[186] After 10 days of treatment, pigs treated with 1.0% topical butenafine achieved a 94% mycologic cure, whereas only 28% of those treated with clotrimazole achieved mycologic cure. In addition, when the same investigators applied butenafine once 24 or 48 hours before infection, no lesions developed, and mycologic cultures of the lesions performed on day 17 after infection were negative for fungi. In contrast, when bifonazole (an azole derivative not approved in the United States) was applied to the skin at 24 hours before infection, lesions developed in four of five animals on day 17 after infection. Hare and Loebener[236] performed a similar investigation on guinea pigs infected with the common pathogenic fungus *T. mentagrophytes*. They ranked common azoles and allylamines according to their efficacy in the treatment of the induced dermatophytoses. Naftifine and terbinafine showed excellent efficacy, with 74% to 100% dermatophyte inhibition, and the azole derivatives clotrimazole, econazole, and oxiconazole showed only 54% to 73% inhibition. Ketoconazole, miconazole, and sulconazole exhibited the least activity, with only 34% to 53% dermatophyte inhibition. In a trial designed to evaluate the relapse rates of tinea pedis in butenafine-treated animals, other investigators[237] reported mycologic clearing in 91.6% of the butenafine-treated animals but only 55.8% of the bifonazole-treated animals. Moreover, at

the 30-day posttreatment follow-up evaluation, the relapse rates were higher in the bifonazole-treated feet (11 of 12 relapsed) than in the butenafine-treated feet (3 of 12 relapsed). The investigators attributed this high efficacy and low relapse rate of butenafine-treated animals to the drug's fungicidal activity (rather than fungistatic) and long cutaneous drug retention after topical application.

Clinical Trials

Controlled clinical trials compared the efficacy of the various allylamine and benzylamine type drugs with the azole antimycotics. In a multicenter, double-blind parallel group study of 256 patients with mycologically confirmed tinea, Evans and colleagues[238] found that a 1-week course of terbinafine 1% cream was more effective than a 4-week course of clotrimazole 1% cream in the treatment of tinea pedis. By week four, mycologic cure was achieved in 93.5% of patients treated with terbinafine compared with only 73.1% of patients treated with clotrimazole. In a multicenter comparison trial by Bergstresser and associates,[239] results of mycologic tests and clinical findings showed topical terbinafine to be significantly more effective than clotrimazole in the treatment of tinea pedis. Patients with mycologically proven tinea pedis were treated with either 1 or 4 weeks of topical terbinafine or 1 or 4 weeks of topical clotrimazole. At the end of week 12, 81% of the patients who received 1 week of terbinafine were mycologically clear, whereas only 30% of the patients who received 1 week of clotrimazole cleared. Sixty-eight percent of those patients who received 4 weeks of clotrimazole had negative fungal cultures at week 12, whereas 85% of the patients treated for 4 weeks with terbinafine were mycologically clear. In addition, overall efficacy at follow-up (combined mycologic and clinical findings) was also significantly greater in the terbinafine group; only 9.3% of patients mycologically cured with terbinafine relapsed. Forty-seven percent of the patients who cleared with 1 week of clotrimazole relapsed, and 30% of the mycologically cleared patients who received a 4-week clotrimazole regimen relapsed.

Ablon, Spedale, and Rosen[240] reported results from a comparative study in which ter-

---

*References 131, 147, 175, 179, 180, 185-187, 233-235.

binafine cream 1%, naftifine gel 1%, and oxiconazole lotion 1% were each applied daily for only 2 weeks in the treatment of chronic tinea pedis. Terbinafine, naftifine, and oxiconazole provided mycologic cure rates of 33.3%, 34.5%, and 21.4%, respectively, at the end of treatment. Although there was no statistically significant difference at the end of treatment, 4-week follow-up mycologic cure rates were significantly superior in the terbinafine and naftifine groups. One month after the cessation of therapy, mycologic cure rates for terbinafine and naftifine had risen to 84.8% and 69.0%, respectively, whereas the oxiconazole cure rate remained low (32.1%). In a comparison of patients with interdigital tinea pedis treated with either 4 weeks of butenafine cream 1% once daily or clotrimazole 1% cream twice daily, Tsuyuki and co-workers[241] found that mycologic cure was achieved in 95% of the patients who received butenafine but in only 88% of the patients treated with clotrimazole. Investigators compared the efficacy of naftifine cream with clotrimazole/betamethasone dipropionate cream in the treatment of tinea pedis.[173] After 4 weeks of twice daily applications, 97% of naftifine-treated patients were mycologically clear, whereas only 70% of the clotrimazole/betamethasone dipropionate group cleared. Two-week posttreatment follow-up examinations revealed negative fungal cultures in 92% of the naftifine-treated group as compared with 55% of the clotrimazole-treated group.

Posttreatment Follow-up Studies

Allylamines and benzylamines produce a significantly lower posttreatment relapse rate compared with the azole antimycotic agents. For example, Bergstresser and colleagues[239] reported that 28% of patients who received a 4-week course of clotrimazole cream for the treatment of tinea pedis had a relapse within 8 weeks of treatment. In contrast, fewer than 10% of patients who received topical terbinafine for only 1 week relapsed within 11 weeks after treatment. Smith and co-workers[173] reported a 9% relapse rate in naftifine-treated patients versus a 29% relapse rate in clotrimazole/betamethasone dipropionate–treated patients. In a long-term follow-up study of patients treated with 1 week of topical terbinafine or 1 week of topical clotrimazole for tinea pedis, Elewski and associates[242] found that 42% of the

terbinafine group reported no new episodes of tinea pedis; however, only 23% of patients treated with 1 week of clotrimazole and only 31% of patients treated with a full 4 weeks of clotrimazole reported no new episodes. In a comparison of oxiconazole, naftifine, and terbinafine in the short-term treatment of tinea pedis, 2 months after cessation of therapy, terbinafine and naftifine provided mycologic cure rates of 80.6% and 75%, respectively, whereas oxiconazole provided only a 26.9% cure rate.[240]

Summary

CLINICAL EFFICACY. In summary, while all the agents mentioned in this chapter may be effective, the allylamine and benzylamine type drugs are more potent in vitro and have a higher efficacy in vivo than the azole type antimycotics in the treatment of dermatophytoses. Allylamines and benzylamines are fungicidal, whereas the azoles are primarily fungistatic against the common dermatophytes. Although there is no conclusive evidence that fungicidal antifungals are more effective than fungistatic antifungals, the higher efficacy and lower relapse rates of the allylamines/benzylamines (which are fungicidal) relative to the azoles (which are fungistatic) might be attributed to the fungicidal action of these drugs. From this evidence, some might conclude that a fungicidal drug is preferable to a fungistatic one. In addition, the highly lipophilic allylamines and benzylamines exhibit a "reservoir" effect and patients continue to improve after cessation of therapy. This retention effect, together with a fungicidal activity, results in shorter duration of therapy and lower relapse rates.

Though not as prevalent as dermatomycoses, cutaneous candidal infections do commonly occur, especially in the immunocompromised patient. Cutaneous candidal infections are amenable to treatment by the azole, allylamine/benzylamine, and hydroxypyridone antifungals, though the efficacy of these agents is not equal among all classes (Table 24-5).

The relative efficacy of the following agents against *Candida* organisms (based on MIC in vitro studies)[201,243,245]:

ciclopirox > azoles >> butenafine > naftifine = terbinafine

■ **Table 24-5**   MICs of Antifungal Agents' Activity Against *Candida albicans* (Mean MIC μg/ml)*

Study (No. of Strains)	Butenafine	Terbinafine	Naftifine	Ketoconazole	Clotrimazole
Maeda et al[185] (57)	>100	—	>100	—	6.4
Shadomy et al[180] (10)	—	128	>128	0.51	—
Georgopapakakou[244] (1)	—	8	64	16	—

*Lower MICs indicate stronger inhibition of *Candida* organisms by azole agents relative to the allylamines/benzylamines.

Despite being the weakest anticandidal agents in vitro, the allylamines are effective in the treatment of cutaneous candidal infections. Butenafine exhibits overall efficacy rates of 81% for intertriginous candidiasis, 73% for interdigital candidiasis, and 83% for paronychial candidiasis.[188] Villars and Jones[183] report that terbinafine was roughly equivalent to its benzylamine relative, as eight studies of cutaneous candidiasis showed terbinafine achieving either a complete clinical cure or a mycologic cure in 75% to 85% of the study population. Nonetheless, in cutaneous candidiasis, both ciclopirox and the various azole compounds are more optimal and are more appropriate therapeutic choices than the allylamine and benzylamine drugs.

Special Properties

ANTIINFLAMMATORY EFFECTS.   Several topical antimycotic agents demonstrated inherent antiinflammatory properties. These properties are not only beneficial in reducing the inflammation associated with dermatomycoses, they have also proved useful in the treatment of other inflammatory skin disorders. These antiinflammatory properties have been demonstrated in a number of in vitro[245-252] and in vivo[201,245,246,253-255] studies.

Certain representative drugs of the azole and allylamine/benzylamine groups possess antiinflammatory properties. However, allylamine and benzylamine agents have been found to possess a greater degree of antiinflammatory action in direct comparison studies.[256] Most of the azoles (e.g., clotrimazole, econazole, ketoconazole, and miconazole) demonstrated an ability to inhibit the chemotaxis of polymorphonuclear cells (PMNs).[249] Bifonazole, in addition to the afore-

mentioned azoles, has also been shown to inhibit calmodulin,[250] a protein that is integral to prostaglandin synthesis and histamine release from mast cells.[256] Elevated levels of calmodulin have been demonstrated in psoriatic plaques.[258-260]

From the azole group, bifonazole and ketoconazole demonstrated utility in a number of inflammatory skin conditions. Bifonazole has been of use in sebopsoriasis[261,262] and seborrheic dermatitis.[263] Leukotriene production by PMNs, an essential step in the inflammatory process, is decreased by bifonazole.[247] Ketoconazole exhibited antiinflammatory effects in the treatment of seborrheic dermatitis.[61,74,75,264] Ketoconazole is able to inhibit 5-lipoxygenase in a dose-dependent fashion, which decreases the production of 5-HETE (5-hydroxyeicosatetraenoic) and leukotriene B$_4$. This action may be related to the inhibition of cytochrome P-450, which may play a role in arachidonic acid metabolism.[246] Ketoconazole possesses antiinflammatory abilities comparable with hydrocortisone when used to combat the inflammation induced by a skin inoculum of both live and killed *Staphylococcus aureus.*[255]

The antiinflammatory action of the allylamines has been inferred by head-to-head clinical outcome comparisons between naftifine and clotrimazole 1%–hydrocortisone 1% combination, where naftifine was found to be equally effective in reducing the clinical erythema associated with inflammatory fungal infections.[265] Whether this was due to naftifine antifungal or antiinflammatory activity is unknown. Nevertheless, the inhibition of inflammation offered by the allylamine class has been borne out in other ways. Naftifine has a dose-dependent inhibitory effect on PMN chemotaxis, which is mediated by interference with leukocyte pseudopod formation. It also impedes the production of reactive oxygen intermediates by PMNs, and its inhibition of 5-lipoxygenase has also been verified.[265]

Naftifine also suppresses ultraviolet B (UVB)–induced erythema, which shares a number of common inflammatory mediators with the inflammatory pathways induced by fungal infections.[256,266-269] Moreover, the structurally similar benzylamine derivative butenafine demonstrates similar prevention of UVB-induced erythema. It has been postulated that this effect is mediated by the same antiinflammatory mechanisms possessed by naftifine.[245]

Ciclopirox olamine also has antiinflammatory properties. Ciclopirox and rilopirox (an experimental hydroxypyridone) were compared with ketoconazole, miconazole, fluconazole, and naftifine in both an in vitro and an in vivo model. In vitro, all agents tested inhibited 5-lipoxygenase, but only ciclopirox olamine inhibited both 5-lipoxygenase and cyclooxygenase. In an in vivo model of arachidonic acid–induced inflammation, only ciclopirox olamine (from the agents previously listed) demonstrated a significant suppression of inflammation.[270] In a double-blind study, ciclopirox olamine 1% cream was compared with a ciclopirox olamine 1%-hydrocortisone acetate 1% combination for 21 days in patients with inflammatory superficial dermatophyte infections. No significant differences (at baseline or at the subsequent weekly evaluations) in the scored clinical assessments of inflammation were noted. This finding suggests that ciclopirox olamine possesses significant antiinflammatory capacity.[213]

ANTIBACTERIAL EFFECTS.　The inherent antibacterial activity of some topical antifungals serves as an adjuvant in the treatment of dermatomycoses where a complex mixed fungal-bacterial infection can be present. Clotrimazole, econazole, miconazole, and oxiconazole demonstrate inhibitory activity in vitro and in vivo against some gram-positive and gram-negative bacteria.* Miconazole inhibits the growth against some gram-positive bacteria and is effective in the treatment of erythrasma, impetigo, or ecthyma caused by Group A β-hemolytic streptococci or pathogenic staphylococci.[39,40,271]

---

*References 29, 36, 39, 40, 83, 104, 117.

▪ Table 24-6　Topical Antifungal Agents—Propylene Glycol Content of Cream Formulations

Generic Name	Trade Name	Contains Propylene Glycol
Nystatin	Various	Yes
Amphotericin B	Various	Yes
Miconazole	Micatin, Monistat Derm	No
Clotrimazole	Lotrimin, Mycelex	No
Ketoconazole	Nizoral	Yes
Oxiconazole	Oxistat	Yes
Econazole	Spectazole	No
Sulconazole	Exelderm	Yes
Naftifine	Naftin	No
Terbinafine	Lamisil	Yes
Butenafine	Mentax	Yes
Ciclopirox	Loprox	No
Selenium	Selsun, Exsel	No
Tolnafate	Tinactin	Yes

The antibacterial activity of econazole accounts for its efficacy in the treatment of interdigital toe web infection uncomplicated by fungi.[117] In vitro, terbinafine exhibits inhibitory activity against both gram-negative and gram-positive bacteria, including *S. aureus, S. faecalis, Propionibacterium acnes*, and *Pseudomonas aeruginosa*.[272]

The in vitro gram-negative antibacterial activity of ciclopirox olamine is seemingly superior to that of other antimycotic drugs. Ciclopirox also demonstrated antibacterial inhibition against gram-positive bacteria, *Mycoplasma* organisms, and *Trichomonas vaginalis*.[201,203,211]

The ancillary antibacterial and antiinflammatory activities of these antimycotics augment the antifungal therapy of inflamed or superinfected dermatomycoses. None of these drugs should be considered agents of choice when treating uncomplicated bacterial pyodermas.

PROPYLENE GLYCOL–INDUCED IRRITANCY.　Propylene glycol as a vehicle ingredient is figuratively a "two-edged sword." This chemical is commonly used in the vehicle by pharmaceutical companies to enhance the percutaneous penetration of various topical medications. In contrast, propylene glycol can be a significant cutaneous irritant in a small percentage of patients, particularly when applied to inflamed, fissured, or ulcerated skin. A list of topical antifungal agents and whether these products contain propylene glycol is found in Table 24-6. If a given patient fails to improve with a topical antifungal medication, the clinician should at least consider whether or not propylene glycol (if present) might be serving as an irritant.

Bibliography

Brennan B, Leyden JJ: Overview of topical therapy for common superficial fungal infections and the role of new topical agents. *J Am Acad Dermatol* 36:S3-S8, 1997.

Espinel-Ingroff A: History of medical mycology in the US. *Clin Microbiol Rev* 9:235-272, 1996.

Gupta AK, Einarson TR, Summerbell RC, et al: An overview of topical antifungal therapy in dermatomycoses: a North American perspective. *Drugs* 55:645-674, 1998.

Lesher JL Jr: Recent developments in antifungal therapy. *Dermatol Clin* 14:163-169, 1996.

References

1. Weitzman I, Summerbell RC: The dermatophytes. *Clin Microbiol Rev* 8:240-259, 1995.
2. Espinel-Ingroff A: History of medical mycology in the US. *Clin Microbiol Rev* 9:235-272, 1996.
3. Smith EB: Topical antifungal drugs in the treatment of tinea pedis, tinea cruris, and tinea corporis. *J Am Acad Dermatol* 28(Suppl):S24-28, 1993.
4. Smith EB: History of antifungals. *J Am Acad Dermatol* 23:776-778, 1990.
5. Medoff G, Kobayashi G: The polyenes. In Speller DCE, editor: *Antifungal chemotherapy*, London, 1980, John Wiley & Sons.

Polyenes—Nystatin
6. Gupta AK, Sauder DN, Shear NH: Antifungal agents: an overview. Part I. *J Am Acad Dermatol* 30:677-698, 1994.
7. Korzybski T, Kowszk-Gindifer Z, et al: *Antifungal antibiotics*, vol I, Oxford, 1967, Pergamon Press, pp 769-845.
8. Hazen EL, Brown R: Nystatin. *Ann NY Acad Sci* 89:258-266, 1960.
9. Hazen EL, Brown R: Fungicidin, an antibiotic produced by a soil actinomycete. *Proc Soc Esptl Biol Med* 76:93-97, 1951.
10. Hazen EL, Brown R: Two antifungal agents produced by a soil actinomycete. *Science* 112:423, 1950.
11. Bennett JE: Antimicrobial agents: antifungal agents. In Gilman AG, Rall TW, Nies AS, editors: *The pharmacological basis of therapeutics*, New York, 1993, McGraw-Hill, pp 1165-1181.
12. Fitzpatrick J: Topical antifungal agents. In Freedberg I, Eisen A, Wolff K, editors: *Dermatology in general medicine*, New York, 1999, McGraw-Hill, pp 2737-2741.
13. Data on file: Westwood-Squibb Inc., Buffalo, NY, 1997.
14. Dixon PN, Warin RP, English MP: Alimentary *Candida albicans* and napkin rashes. *Br J Dermatol* 86:458-462, 1972.
15. Wasilewski C, Jr: Allergic contact dermatitis from nystatin. *Arch Dermatol* 102:216-217, 1970.
16. Coskey RJ: Contact dermatitis due to nystatin. *Arch Dermatol* 103:228, 1971.
17. de Groot AC, Conemans JM: Nystatin allergy. Petrolatum is not the optimal vehicle for patch testing. *Dermatol Clin* 8:153-155, 1990.
18. Cronin E: *Contact Dermatitis*, Edinburgh, 1980, Churchill Livingstone.
19. Lang E, Goos M: Combined allergy to tolnaftate and nystatin. *Contact Dermatitis* 12:182, 1985.
20. Lechner T, Grytzmann B, Baurle G: Hematogenous allergic contact dermatitis after oral administration of nystatin. *Mykosen* 30:143-146, 1987.

21. Wasilewski C, Jr: Allergic contact dermatitis from nystatin. *Arch Dermatol* 104:437, 1971.

Azole Antifungals—General

22. Vanden Bossche H: Mode of action of pyridine, pyrimidine and azole antifungals. In Berg G, Plempel M, editors: *Sterol biosynthesis inhibitors,* Chichester, England, 1988, Ellis Horwood Ltd, p 79.
23. Vanden Bossche H, Marichal P: Mode of action of anti-Candida drugs: focus on terconazole and other ergosterol biosynthesis inhibitors. *Am J Obstet Gynecol* 165:1193-1199, 1991.
24. Vanden Bossche H, Lauwers W, Willemsens G, et al: Molecular basis for the antimycotic and antibacterial activity of N-substituted imidazoles and triazoles: the inhibition of isoprenoid biosynthesis. *Pestic Sci* 15:188-198, 1984.
25. Vanden Bossche H: Cytochrome P450: target for itraconazole. *Drug Dev Res* 8:287-298, 1986.
26. Vanden Bossche H: Biochemical targets for antifungal azole derivatives: hypothesis on the mode of action. In Mcginnis MK, editor: *Current topics in medical mycology,* vol 1, New York, 1985, Springer-Verlag.
27. Ritter W: Pharmacokinetics of azole compounds. In Berg D, Plempel D, editors: *Sterol biosynthesis inhibitors,* Chichester, England, 1988, Ellis Horwood Ltd, pp 398-429.

Miconazole

28. Van Cutsem JM, Thienpont D: Miconazole, a broad-spectrum antimycotic agent with antibacterial activity. *Chemotherapy* 17:392-404, 1972.
29. Gupta AK, Einarson TR, Summerbell RC, et al: An overview of topical antifungal therapy in dermatomycoses: a North American perspective. *Drugs* 55:645-674, 1998.
30. Odds FC, Abbott AB, Pye G, et al: Improved method for estimation of azole antifungal inhibitory concentrations against Candida species, based on azole/antibiotic interactions. *J Med Vet Mycol* 24:305-311, 1986.
31. Yamaguchi H, Hiratani T, Plempel M: In vitro studies of a new imidazole antimycotic, bifonazole, in comparison with clotrimazole and miconazole. *Arzneimittelforschung* 33:546-551, 1983.

32. Botter AA: Topical treatment of nail and skin infections with miconazole, a new broad spectrum antimycotic. *Mykosen* 14:187-191, 1971.
33. Brugmans J, Van Cutsem J, Thienpont D: Treatment of long term tinea pedis with miconazole. *Arch Dermatol* 102:428-432, 1970.
34. Fulton JE Jr: Miconazole therapy for endemic fungal disease. *Arch Dermatol* 111:596-598, 1975.
35. Gip L, Forstrom S: A double-blind parallel study of sulconazole nitrate 1% cream compared with miconazole 2% cream in dermatophytoses. *Mykosen* 26:231-241, 1983.
36. Mandy SJ, Garrott TC: Miconazole treatment for severe dermatophytoses. *JAMA* 230:72-75, 1974.
37. Ongley RC: Efficacy of topical miconazole treatment of tinea pedis. *Can Med Assoc J* 119:353-354, 1978.
38. Tanenbaum L, Anderson C, Rosenberg MJ, et al: 1% sulconazole cream vs 2% miconazole cream in the treatment of tinea versicolor. A double-blind, multicenter study. *Arch Dermatol* 120:216-219, 1984.
39. Pitcher DG, Noble WC, Seville RH: Treatment of erythrasma with miconazole. *Clin Exp Dermatol* 4:453-456, 1979.
40. Nolting S, Strauss WB: Treatment of impetigo and ecthyma. A comparison of sulconazole with miconazole. *Int J Dermatol* 27:716-719, 1988.
41. Mesquita-Guimaraes J, Ramos S, Tavares M, et al: A double-blind clinical trial with a lotion containing 5% benzoyl peroxide and 2% miconazole in patients with acne vulgaris. *Clin Exp Dermatol* 14:357-360, 1989.

Clotrimazole

42. Plempel M, Bartmann K, Buchel KH, et al: BAY b-5097, a new orally applicable antifungal substance with broad-spectrum activity. *Antimicrob Agents Chemother* 9:271-274, 1969.
43. Data on file: Schering Corporation, Kenilworth, NJ, 1993.
44. Holt RJ, Newman RL: Laboratory assessment of the antimycotic drug clotrimazole. *J Clin Pathol* 25:1089-1097, 1972.
45. Clayton YM, Connor BL: Comparison of clotrimazole cream, Whitfield's ointment and nystatin ointment for the topical treatment of ringworm infections, pityriasis versicolor, erythrasma and candidiasis. *Br J Dermatol* 89:297-303, 1973.

46. Clayton R, Du Vivier A, Savage M: Double-blind trial of 1% clotrimazole cream and Whitfield ointment in the treatment of pityriasis versicolor (letter). *Arch Dermatol* 113:849-850, 1977.

47. Clayton YM, Connor BL: Clinical trial of clotrimazole in the treatment of superficial fungal infections. *Postgrad Med J* 50(Suppl 1):66-69, 1974.

48. Fredriksson T: Topical treatment of superficial mycoses with clotrimazole. *Postgrad Med J* 50(Suppl 1):62-64, 1974.

49. Gip L: The topical therapy of pityriasis versicolor with clotrimazole. *Postgrad Med J* 50 (Suppl 1):59-60, 1974.

50. Ipp MM, Boxall L, Gelfand EW: Clotrimazole: intermittent therapy in chronic mucocutaneous candidiasis. *Am J Dis Child* 131:305-307, 1977.

51. Male O: A double-blind comparison of clotrimazole and tolnaftate therapy of superficial dermatophytoses. *Postgrad Med J* 50(Suppl 1):75-76, 1974.

52. Oberste-Lehn H: Ideal properties of a modern antifungal agent—the therapy of mycoses with clotrimazole. *Postgrad Med J* 50(Suppl 1):51-53, 1974.

53. Plempel M, Buchel KH, Bartmann K, et al: Antimycotic properties of clotrimazole. *Postgrad Med J* 50(Suppl 1):11-12, 1974.

54. Polemann G: Clinical experience in the local treatment of dermatomycoses with clotrimazole. *Postgrad Med J* 50(Suppl 1):54-56, 1974.

55. Zaias N, Battistini F: Superficial mycoses: treatment with a new, broad-spectrum antifungal agent: 1% clotrimazole solution. *Arch Dermatol* 113:307-308, 1977.

56. Rajan VS, Thirumoorthy T: Treatment of cutaneous candidiasis: a double blind, parallel comparison of sulconazole nitrate 1% cream and clotrimazole 1% cream. *Australas J Dermatol* 24:33-36, 1983.

Ketoconazole

57. Odds F, Webster C, Abbott A: Antifungal relative inhibition factors: BAY 9139, bifonazole, butoconazole, isoconazole, itraconazole (R51211), oxiconazole, Ro 14-4767/002, sulconazole, terconazole and vibunazole (BAY 7133) compared in vitro with nine established antifungal agents. *J Antimicrob Chemother* 14:105-114, 1984.

58. Odds F, Milne L, Gentles J, et al: The activity in vitro and in vivo of a new imidazole antifungal ketoconazole. *J Antimicrob Chemother* 6:97-104, 1980.

59. Thienpont D, Van Custem J, Van Gervan F, et al: Ketoconazole—a new broad spectrum orally active antimycotic. *Experientia* 35:606-607, 1979.

60. Heeres J, Backx L, Mostmans J, et al: Antimycotic imidazoles: synthesis and antifungal activity of ketoconazole, a new potent orally active broad-spectrum antifungal agent. *J Med Chem* 22:1003-1005, 1983.

61. Taieb A, Legrain V, Palmier C, et al: Topical ketoconazole for infantile seborrhoeic dermatitis. *Dermatologica* 181:26-32, 1990.

62. Borgers M, Van den Bossche H, De Brander M: The mechanism of action of the new antimycotic ketoconazole. *Am J Med* 74:2-8, 1983.

63. Lester M: Ketoconazole 2% cream in the treatment of tinea pedis, tinea cruris, and tinea corporis. *Cutis* 55:181-183, 1995.

64. Greer D, Jolly H: Topical ketoconazole treatment of cutaneous candidiasis. *J Am Acad Dermatol* 18:748-749, 1988.

65. Savin RC, Horwitz SN: Double-blind comparison of 2% ketoconazole cream and placebo in the treatment of tinea versicolor. *J Am Acad Dermatol* 15:500-503, 1986.

66. el Euch D, Riahi I, Mokni M, et al: Ketoconazole 2% foaming gel in tinea versicolor. Report of 60 cases. *Tunis Med* 77:38-40, 1999.

67. Rekacewicz I, Guillaume JC, Benkhraba F, et al: A double-blind placebo-controlled study of a 2 percent foaming lotion of ketoconazole in a single application in the treatment of pityriasis versicolor. *Ann Dermatol Venereol* 117:709-711, 1990.

68. Caterall MD: Ketoconazole therapy for pityriasis versicolor (letter). *Clin Exp Dermatol* 7:679, 1982.

69. Danby FW, Maddin WS, Margesson LJ, et al: A randomized, double-blind, placebo-controlled trial of ketoconazole 2% shampoo versus selenium sulfide 2.5% shampoo in the treatment of moderate to severe dandruff. *J Am Acad Dermatol* 29:1008-1012, 1993.

70. Carr MM, Pryce DM, Ive FA: Treatment of seborrhoeic dermatitis with ketoconazole: I. Response of seborrhoeic dermatitis of the scalp to topical ketoconazole. *Br J Dermatol* 116:213-216, 1987.

71. Ive FA: An overview of experience with ketoconazole shampoo. *Br J Clin Pract* 45:279-284, 1991.

72. Katsambas A, Antoniou C, Frangouli E, et al: A double-blind trial of treatment of seborrhoeic dermatitis with 2% ketoconazole cream compared with 1% hydrocortisone cream. *Br J Dermatol* 121:353-357, 1989.

73. Peter RU, Richarz-Barthauer U: Successful treatment and prophylaxis of scalp seborrhoeic dermatitis and dandruff with 2% ketoconazole shampoo: results of a multicentre, double-blind, placebo-controlled trial. *Br J Dermatol* 132:441-445, 1995.

74. Stratigos JD, Antoniou C, Katsambas A, et al: Ketoconazole 2% cream versus hydrocortisone 1% cream in the treatment of seborrheic dermatitis. A double-blind comparative study. *J Am Acad Dermatol* 19:850-853, 1988.

75. Green CA, Farr PM, Shuster S: Treatment of seborrhoeic dermatitis with ketoconazole: II. Response of seborrhoeic dermatitis of the face, scalp and trunk to topical ketoconazole. *Br J Dermatol* 116:217-221, 1987.

76. McGrath J, Murphy GM: The control of seborrhoeic dermatitis and dandruff by antipityrosporal drugs. *Drugs* 41:178-184, 1991.

77. Cauwenbergh G, De Doncker P, Schrooten P, et al: Treatment of dandruff with a 2% ketoconazole scalp gel. A double-blind placebo-controlled study. *Int J Dermatol* 25:541, 1986.

78. Farr P, Shuster S: Treatment of seborrheic dermatitis with topical ketoconazole. *Lancet* 2:1271-1272, 1984.

79. Data on file: Janssen Pharmaceutica, Titusville, NJ, 1995.

Oxiconazole

80. Jegasothy BV, Pakes GE: Oxiconazole nitrate: pharmacology, efficacy, and safety of a new imidazole antifungal agent. *Clin Ther* 13:126-141, 1991.

81. Stuttgen G, Bauer E: Permeation of labeled oxiconazole. *Mykosen* 28:138-147, 1985.

82. Polak A: Antifungal activity of four antifungal drugs in the cutaneous retention time test. *Sabouraudia* 22:501-503, 1984.

83. Ramelet AA, Walker-Nasir E: One daily application of oxiconazole cream is sufficient for treating dermatomycoses. *Dermatologica* 175:293-295, 1987.

84. Pariser DM, Pariser RJ: Oxiconazole nitrate lotion, 1 percent: an effective treatment for tinea pedis. *Cutis* 54:43-44, 1994.

85. Ellis CN, Gammon WR, Goldfarb MT, et al: A placebo controlled evaluation of once-daily versus twice-daily oxiconazole nitrate 1% cream in the treatment of tinea pedis. *Curr Ther Res* 46:269-276, 1989.

86. Data on file: Glaxo Dermatology, Research Triangle Park, NC, 1996.

87. Hiratani T, Yamaguchi H: Mode of antifungal action of oxiconazole nitrate toward *Candida albicans*. *Chemotherapy* 33:215-226, 1985.

88. Meinhof W, Fischer M, Durand R: Studies on antimycotic action of oxiconazole. *Therapiewoche* 35:4580-4585, 1985.

89. Beierodorffer H, Picolin K, Herbold D: Oxiconazole, a new antimycotic for the topical treatment of dermatomycoses. *Acta Therapeutica* 9:147-155, 1983.

90. Kastellitz G: Experiences with single daily application of the new antimycotic oxiconazole. *Z Allgemeinmed* 61:611-613, 1985.

91. Wagner W: Comparison of clinical efficacy and tolerance of oxiconazole administered once daily or twice daily. *Mykosen* 29:280-284, 1986.

92. Parissis N, Noutsis C, Koumantaki E, et al: Comparative clinical studies with imidazolyl derivative Ro 13-8996, tolnaftate and miconazole. In Periti P, Grassi G, editors: *Current chemotherapy and immunotherapy*, Washington, DC, 1982, American Society for Microbiology, pp 1025-1027.

93. Gip L: Comparison of oxiconazole (13-8996) and econazole in dermatomycoses. *Mykosen* 27:295-302, 1984.

94. Wagner W, Reckers-Czaschka R: Oxiconazole in dermatomycosis—a double-blind, randomized therapy compared with bifonazole. *Mykosen* 30:484-492, 1987.

95. Gall H: Pityriasis versicolor: treatment with the broad range antimycotic oxiconazole. *Der Kassenarzt* 10:41-48, 1986.

96. Elewski B, Jones T, Zaias N: Comparison of an antifungal agent used alone with an antifungal used with a topical steroid in inflammatory tinea pedis. *Cutis* 58:305-307, 1996.

97. Lebwohl M, Rex I, Tschen E, et al: Oxiconazole nitrate cream 1%, once or twice daily in the treatment of tinea pedis. *Clin Res J* 92:468, 1989.

98. Arreaza de Arreaza F, Diaz de Torres E, Briceno Maaz T: Double-blind comparison of oxiconazole with miconazole for efficacy and local tolerance in patients with cutaneous mycoses. *Med Cutanea Ibero-Lat-Am* 12:57-61, 1984.

99. Machado-Pinto J, Laborne M: The use of 1% oxiconazole cream in the treatment of dermatophytoses. *Folha Med* 95:381-384, 1987.
100. Clinical Research Group for Oxiconazole Cream: Oxiconazole cream for dermatomycoses. *Skin Res* 29:318-325, 1987.
101. Oxiconazole Study Group: Clinical evaluation of oxiconazole in dermatomycosis: comparison with clotrimazole cream in a well-controlled comparative study. *Nishi Nihon* 47:89-100, 1985.
102. Hishikawa J, Higashida T, Asada Y: Clinical effects of oxiconazole nitrate on dermatomycosis. *Skin Res* 26:706-710, 1984.
103. Kawaguchi T, Shimao S: Clinical effects of oxiconazole cream studied in 100 patients with mycoses. *Acta Ther* 8:361-365, 1982.

Econazole
104. Heel RC, Brogden RN, Speight TM, et al: Econazole: a review of its antifungal activity and therapeutic efficacy. *Drugs* 16:177-201, 1978.
105. Schaefer H, Stuttgen G: Absolute concentrations of an antimycotic agent, econazole, in the human skin after local application. *Arzneimittelforschung* 26:432-435, 1976.
106. Data on file: Ortho Pharmaceuticals Inc, Raritan, NJ, 1996.
107. Brenner M: Efficacy of twice-daily dosing of econazole nitrate 1% cream for tinea pedis. *J Am Podiatr Med Assoc* 80:583-587, 1990.
108. Cullen S, Millikan L, Mullen R: Treatment of tinea pedis with econazole nitrate cream. *Cutis* 7:388-389, 1986.
109. Daily A, Kramer S, Rex I, et al: Econazole nitrate (Spectazole) cream, 1 percent: a topical agent for the treatment of tinea pedis. *Cutis* 35:278-279, 1985.
110. Grigoriu D, Pallares J: Follow-up study after more than one year including 100 patients treated for superficial mycoses. *Dermatologica* 160:62-68, 1980.
111. Cullen S, Rex I, Thorne E: A comparison of a new antifungal agent, 1% econazole nitrate (Spectazole) cream versus 1% clotrimazole cream in the treatment of intertriginous candidosis. *Curr Ther Res* 35:606-609, 1984.
112. Wong E, Hay R, Clayton Y, et al: Comparison of the therapeutic effect of ketoconazole tablets and econazole lotion in the treatment of chronic paronychia. *Clin Exp Dermatol* 9:489-496, 1984.

113. Hira S, Din S, Patel J: Econazole 1% in the treatment of pityriasis versicolor in Zambia. *J Am Acad Dermatol* 12:580-581, 1985.
114. Vicik G, Mendiones M, Qinones C, et al: A new treatment for tinea versicolor using econazole nitrate 1.0 percent cream once a day. *Cutis* 33:570-571, 1984.
115. Lassus A, Forstrom S: A double-blind parallel study comparing sulconazole and econazole in the treatment of dermatophytoses. *Mykosen* 27:592-598, 1984.
116. Fredriksson T: Treatment of dermatomycoses with topical econazole and clotrimazole. *Curr Ther Res* 25:590-594, 1979.
117. Kates S, Myung K, McGinley K, et al: The antibacterial efficacy of econazole nitrate in interdigital toe web infections. *J Am Acad Dermatol* 22:583-586, 1990.

Sulconazole
118. Anonymous: Sulconazole—a new antifungal for the skin. *Drug Ther Bull* 24:67-68, 1986.
119. Franz TJ, Lehman P: Percutaneous absorption of sulconazole nitrate in humans. *J Pharm Sci* 77:489-491, 1988.
120. Benfield P, Clissold SP: Sulconazole: a review of its antimicrobial activity and therapeutic use in superficial dermatomycoses. *Drugs* 35:143-153, 1988.
121. Lassus A, Forstrom S, Salo O: A double-blind comparison of sulconazole nitrate 1% cream with clotrimazole cream in the treatment of dermatophytoses. *Br J Dermatol* 108:195-198, 1983.
122. McVie DH, Littlewood S, Allen BR, et al: Sulconazole versus clotrimazole in the treatment of dermatophytosis. *Clin Exp Dermatol* 11:613-618, 1986.
123. Akers WA, Lane A, Lynfield Y, et al: Sulconazole nitrate 1% cream in the treatment of chronic moccasin-type tinea pedis caused by Trichophyton rubrum. *J Am Acad Dermatol* 21:686-689, 1989.
124. Tanenbaum L, Taplin D, Lavelle C, et al: Sulconazole nitrate 1 percent for treating tinea cruris and corporis. *Cutis* 44:344-347, 1989.
125. Gugnani HC, Gugnani A, Malachy O: Sulconazole in the therapy of dermatomycoses in Nigeria. *Mycoses* 40:139-141, 1997.
126. Tham SN: Treatment of pityriasis versicolor: Comparison of sulconazole nitrate 1% solution and clotrimazole 1% solution. *Australas J Dermatol* 28:123-125, 1987.
127. Tanenbaum L, Anderson C, Rosenberg M, et al: A new treatment for cutaneous candidiasis: sulconazole nitrate cream 1%. *Int J Dermatol* 22:318-320, 1983.

128. Nolting S, Strauss WB: Treatment of impetigo and ecthyma. A comparison of sulconazole with miconazole. *Int J Dermatol* 27:716-719, 1988.

129. Bigardi AS, Pigatto PD, Altomare G: Allergic contact dermatitis to sulconazole. *Contact Dermatitis* 26:281-282, 1992.

Allylamines—General

130. Berney D, Schuh K: Heterocyclic spiro-naphthalenones. Part I: Synthesis and reactions of some Spiro [(1H-naphthalenone)]-1,3',-piperidines. *Helv Chim Acta* 61: 1262-1273, 1978.

131. Georgopoulos A, Petranyi G, Mieth H, et al: In vitro activity of naftifine, a new antifungal agent. *Antimicrob Agents Chemother* 19:386-389, 1981.

132. Ryder N, Dupont M: Inhibition of squalene epoxidase by allylamine antimycotic compounds: a comparative study of the fungal and mammalian enzymes. *Biochem J* 230: 765-770, 1985.

133. Ryder N: Specific inhibition of fungal sterol biosynthesis by SF 86-327, a new orally active allylamine derivative. *Antimicrob Agents Chemother* 27:252-256, 1985.

134. Ryder N: Mode of action of allylamines. In Berg D, Plempel M, editors: *Sterol biosynthesis inhibitors*, Chichester, England, 1988, Ellis Horwood, Ltd.

135. Ryder N: The mechanism of action of terbinafine. *Clin Exp Dermatol* 14:98-100, 1989.

Naftifine

136. Grassberger M, Mieth M, Petranyi G, et al: Aspects of antimycotic research exemplified by the allylamines. *Triangle* 25:711-784, 1986.

137. Schuster I, Schaude M, Schatz F, et al: Preclinical characteristics of allylamines. In Berg D, Plempel M, editors: *Sterol biosynthesis inhibitors*, Chichester, England, 1988, Ellis Horwood, Ltd, pp 449-470.

138. Jones TC: Treatment of dermatomycoses with topically applied allylamines: naftifine and terbinafine. *J Dermatol Treat* 1(Suppl 2):29-32, 1990.

139. Petranyi G, Ryder N, Stutz A: Allylamine derivatives: new class of synthetic antifungal agents inhibiting fungal squalene epoxidase. *Science* 224:1239-1241, 1984.

140. Stutz A: Synthesis and structure-activity correlations within allylamine antimycotics. *Ann N Y Acad Sci* 544:46-62, 1988.

141. Stutz A: Allylamine derivatives—a new class of active substances in antifungal chemotherapy. *Angew Chemie* (International Edition: England) 26:320-328, 1987.

142. Petranyi G, Georgopoulos A, Mieth H: In vivo antimycotic activity of naftifine. *Antimicrob Agents Chemother* 19:390-392, 1981.

143. Paltauf F, Daum G, Zuder G, et al: Squalene and ergosterol biosynthesis in fungi treated with naftifine, a new antimycotic agent. *Biochim Biophys Acta* 712:267-273, 1982.

144. Ryder NS, Seidl G, Troke PF: Effect of the antimycotic drug naftifine on growth of and sterol biosynthesis in *Candida albicans*. *Antimicrob Agents Chemother* 25:483-487, 1984.

145. Ryder N, Troke P: The activity of naftifine as a sterol synthesis inhibitor in *Candida albicans*. In Periti P, Grassi G, editors: *Current chemotherapy and immunotherapy*, Proceedings of the 12th International Congress of Chemotherapy. Washington, D.C., 1981, American Society of Microbiology, pp 1016-1017.

146. Vanden Bossche H: Importance and role of sterols in fungal membranes. In Kuhn PJ, Trinci APJ, Jung MJ, et al, editors: *Biochemistry of cell walls and membranes in fungi*, Berlin, 1990, Springer-Verlag, p 135.

147. Faruqi A, Khan K, Qazi A, et al: In vitro antifungal activity of naftifine (SN 105-843 GEL) against dermatophytes. *J Pakistani Med Assoc* 31:279-282, 1981.

148. Petranyi G, Leitner I, Mieth H: The "hair root invasion test," a semi-quantitative method for experimental evaluation of antimycotics in guinea-pigs. *Sabouraudia* 20:101-108, 1982.

149. Hantschke D, Reichenberger M: Double blind, randomized in vivo investigations comparing the antifungals clotrimazole, tolnaftate and naftifine (author's translation). *Mykosen* 23:657-668, 1980.

150. Klaschka F, Gartmann H, Weidinger G: The antifungal agent naftifin. Placebo-controlled therapeutic comparison in tinea pedis. *Z Hautkr* 59:1218-1226, 1984.

151. Meinicke K, Striegel C, Weidinger G: Treatment of dermatomycosis with naftifine. Therapeutic effectiveness following once and twice daily administration. *Mykosen* 27:608-614, 1984.

152. Zaun H, Luszpinski P: Multicenter double-blind contralateral comparison of naftifine and clotrimazole cream in patients with dermatophytosis and candidiasis. *Z Hautkr* 59:1209-1217, 1984.

153. Bojanovsky A, Haas P: Antimycotic effect of naftifine in tinea pedis. Comparative double-blind study with bifonazole. *Fortschr Med* 103:677-679, 1985.

154. Effendy I, Friedrich HC: Double-blind, comparative trial of naftifine solution (once-a-day) and clotrimazole solution (twice-a-day) in the treatment of dermatomycoses. *Mykosen* 28(Suppl 1):126-134, 1985.

155. Haas PJ, Tronnier H, Weidinger G: Naftifine in tinea pedis: Double-blind comparison with clotrimazole. *Mykosen* 30(Suppl 1):50-56, 1987.

156. Kagawa S: Comparative clinical trial of naftifine and clotrimazole in tinea pedis, tinea cruris, and tinea corporis. *Mykosen* 30(Suppl 1):63-69, 1987.

157. Nolting S, Weidinger G: Naftifine in severe dermatomycosis—controlled comparison of efficacy with econazole. *Mykosen* 28:69-76, 1985.

158. Tronnier H: Inflammatory dermatomycoses: comparison of naftifine and a corticosteroid/imidazole compound preparation. *Mykosen* 28(Suppl 1):98-108, 1985.

159. Ganzinger U, Stutz A, Petranyi G, et al: Allylamines: topical and oral treatment of dermatomycoses with a new class of antifungal agents. *Acta Derm Venereol Suppl (Stockh)* 121:155-60, 1986.

160. Male O: Comparison of naftifine with clotrimazole and tolnaftate in patients with superficial dermatophytoses. In Periti P, Grassi G, editors: *Current chemotherapy and immunotherapy,* Proceedings of the 12th International Congress of Chemotherapy. Washington, D.C., 1981, American Society of Microbiology, pp 1019-1021.

161. Ganzinger U, Stephen A, Moritz A: Open systematic clinical evaluation of naftifine in patients with dermatomycosis. In Periti P, Grassi G, editors: *Current chemotherapy and immunotherapy,* Proceedings of the 12th International Congress of Chemotherapy. Washington, D.C., 1981, American Society of Microbiology, pp 1018-1019.

162. Zaun H, Luszpinski P: Antimycotic treatment of in-patients—contralateral comparison of naftifine and clotrimazole. *Mykosen* 28(Suppl 1):59-65, 1985.

163. Weidinger G, Striegel C, Meinicke K: Validation of the "once-a-day principle" by a controlled trial. *Mykosen* 28(Suppl 1):119-125, 1985.

164. Paetzold O, Engst R, Kneist W, et al: Yeast infections of the skin—double-blind therapeutic comparison of naftifine and clotrimazole. *Mykosen* 28(Suppl 1):135-141, 1985.

165. Klaschka F: Therapy of onychomycosis with naftifine gel. *Mykosen* 28(Suppl 1):142-146, 1985.

166. Gip L, Brundin G: A double-blind, two group multicenter study, comparing naftifine 1% cream with placebo cream in the treatment of tinea cruris. *Mykosen* 28(Suppl 1):55-58, 1985.

167. Naftifine Podiatric Study Group: Naftifine cream 1% versus clotrimazole cream 1% in the treatment of tinea pedis. *J Am Podiatr Med Assoc* 80:314-318, 1990.

168. Naftifine Study Group: Naftifine gel in the treatment of tinea pedis: two double-blind, multicenter studies. *Cutis* 48:85-88, 1991.

169. Millikan LE, Galen WK, Gewirtzman GB, et al: Naftifine cream 1% versus econazole cream 1% in the treatment of tinea cruris and tinea corporis. *J Am Acad Dermatol* 18:52-56, 1988.

170. Maibach H: Naftifine. Dermatotoxicology and clinical efficacy. *Mykosen* 28(Suppl 1):75-81, 1985.

171. Haas PJ, Tronnier H, Weidinger G: Naftifine in foot mycoses. Double-blind therapeutic comparison with clotrimazole. *Mykosen* 28:33-40, 1985.

172. Smith EB, Wiss K, Hanifin JM, et al: Comparison of once- and twice-daily naftifine cream regimens with twice-daily clotrimazole in the treatment of tinea pedis. *J Am Acad Dermatol* 22:1116-1117, 1990.

173. Smith EB, Breneman DL, Griffith RF, et al: Double-blind comparison of naftifine cream and clotrimazole/betamethasone dipropionate cream in the treatment of tinea pedis. *J Am Acad Dermatol* 26:125-127, 1992.

174. Data on file: Herbert Laboratories, Irvine, CA, 1985.

Terbinafine

175. Petranyi G, Meingassner JG, Mieth H: Antifungal activity of the allylamine derivative terbinafine in vitro. *Antimicrob Agents Chemother* 31:1365-1368, 1987.

176. Hill S, Thomas R, Smith SG, et al: An investigation of the pharmacokinetics of topical terbinafine (Lamisil) 1% cream. *Br J Dermatol* 127:396-400, 1992.

177. Elewski B: Mechanisms of action of systemic antifungal agents. *J Am Acad Dermatol* 28(Suppl):S28-34, 1993.

178. Ryder NS: Terbinafine: mode of action and properties of the squalene epoxidase inhibition. *Br J Dermatol* 126(Suppl 39):S2-S7, 1992.

179. Clayton YM: In vitro activity of terbinafine. *Clin Exp Dermatol* 14:101-103, 1989.

180. Shadomy S, Espinel-Ingroff A, Gebhart RJ: In-vitro studies with SF 86-327, a new orally active allylamine derivative. *Sabouraudia* 23:125-132, 1985.

181. Savin R: Treatment of chronic tinea pedis (athlete's foot type) with topical terbinafine. *J Am Acad Dermatol* 23:786-789, 1990.

182. Kagawa S: Clinical efficacy of terbinafine in 629 Japanese patients with dermatomycosis. *Clin Exp Dermatol* 14:116-119, 1989.

183. Villars V, Jones TC: Clinical efficacy and tolerability of terbinafine (Lamisil)—a new topical and systemic fungicidal drug for treatment of dermatomycoses. *Clin Exp Dermatol* 14:124-127, 1989.

Butenafine

184. Nussbaumer P, Dorfsatter G, Grassberger M, et al: Synthesis and structure-activity relationships of phenyl-substituted benzylamine antimycotics: a novel benzylamine antifungal agent for systemic treatment. *J Med Chem* 36:2115-2120, 1993.

185. Maeda T, Takase M, Ishibashi A, et al: Synthesis and antifungal activity of butenafine hydrochloride (KP- 363), a new benzylamine antifungal agent. *Yakugaku Zasshi* 111:126-137, 1991.

186. Arika T, Yokoo M, Hase T, et al: Effects of butenafine hydrochloride, a new benzylamine derivative, on experimental dermatophytosis in guinea pigs. *Antimicrob Agents Chemother* 34:2250-2253, 1990.

187. Arika T, Hase T, Yokoo M: Anti-*Trichophyton mentagrophytes* activity and percutaneous permeation of butenafine in guinea pigs. *Antimicrob Agents Chemother* 37:363-365, 1993.

188. Fukushiro R: Butenafine hydrochloride, a new antifungal agent: clinical and experimental study. In Kabayashi HY, editor: *Recent progress in antifungal therapy,* New York, 1992, Marcel Dekker.

189. Data on File: Penederm Inc, Foster City, CA, 1996.

190. Reyes BA, Beutner KR, Cukllen SI, et al: Butenafine, a fungicidal benzylamine derivative, used once daily for the treatment of interdigital tinea pedis. *Int J Dermatol* 37:450-453, 1998.

191. Tschen E, Elewski B, Gorsulowsky DC, et al: Treatment of interdigital tinea pedis with a 4-week once-daily regimen of butenafine hydrochloride 1% cream. *J Am Acad Dermatol* 36:S9-S14, 1997.

192. Savin R, Lucky A, Brennan B: One-week treatment of tinea pedis with butenafine HCl 1%: A multi-center, double-blind, randomized trial. 55th Annual American Academy of Dermatology Meeting; March, 1997.

193. Lesher J, Babel D, Stewart D, et al: Butenafine HCl 1% cream in the treatment of tinea cruris: A multicenter, vehicle controlled, double-blind trial. 55th Annual American Academy of Dermatology Meeting; March, 1997.

194. Greer D, Weiss J, Rodriguez D, et al: Treatment of tinea corporis with topical once-daily butenafine HCl 1%: A double-blind, placebo controlled trial. 55th Annual American Academy of Dermatology Meeting; March, 1997.

195. Greer DL, Weiss J, Rodriguez DA, et al: A randomized trial to assess once-daily topical treatment of tinea corporis with butenafine, a new antifungal agent. *J Am Acad Dermatol* 37:231-235, 1997.

196. Lesher JL Jr, Babel DE, Stewart DM, et al: Butenafine 1% cream in the treatment of tinea cruris: a multicenter, vehicle-controlled, double-blind trial. *J Am Acad Dermatol* 36:S20-24, 1997.

197. Savin R, De Villez RL, Elewski B, et al: One-week therapy with twice-daily butenafine 1% cream versus vehicle in the treatment of tinea pedis: a multicenter, double-blind trial. *J Am Acad Dermatol* 36:S15-S19, 1997.

Other Topical Antifungals—Ciclopirox

198. Sakurai K, Sakaguchi T, Yamaguchi H, et al: Mode of action of 6-cyclohexyl-1-hydroxy-4-methyl-2(1H)-pyridone ethanolamine salt (Hoe 296). *Chemotherapy* 24:68-76, 1978.

199. Gasparini G, Contini D, Torti A, et al: The effect of ciclopirox olamine investigated by means of the freeze- fracture technique. *Mykosen* 29:539-544, 1986.

200. del Palacio-Hernanz A, Guarro-Artigas J, Figueras-Salvat MJ, et al: Changes in fungal ultrastructure after short-course ciclopirox olamine therapy in pityriasis versicolor. *Clin Exp Dermatol* 15:95-100, 1990.
201. Abrams B, Heinz H, Hoehler T: Ciclopirox olamine: A hydroxypyridone antifungal agent. *Clin Dermatol* 9:471-477, 1992.
202. Kruse R: La ciclopirox olamine, inhibiteur energetique fongique. *JAMA* (French edition), Suppl(Sept):7-10, 1991.
203. Dittmar W, Lohaus G: HOE 296, a new antimycotic compound with a broad antimicrobial spectrum. Laboratory results. *Arzneimittelforschung* 23:670-674, 1973.
204. Riviera L, Bellotti M: Laboratory evaluation of ciclopirox olamine: In vitro and in vivo studies on its antimicrobial activity. *Chemotherapia* 2:97-102, 1983.
205. Aly R, Bagatell F, Dittmar W, et al: Ciclopirox olamine lotion 1%: bioequivalence to ciclopirox olamine cream 1% and clinical efficacy in tinea pedis. *Clin Ther* 11:290-303, 1989.
206. Kligman AM BH, Cordero C: Evaluation of ciclopirox olamine cream for the treatment of tinea pedis: multicenter, double-blind comparative studies. *Clin Ther* 7:409-417, 1985.
207. Bogaert H, Cordero C, Ollague W, et al: Multicentre double-blind clinical trials of ciclopirox olamine cream 1% in the treatment of tinea corporis and tinea cruris. *J Int Med Res* 14:210-216, 1986.
208. Corte M, Jung K, Linker U, et al: Topical application of a 0.1% ciclopirox olamine solution for the treatment of pityriasis versicolor. *Mycoses* 32:200-203, 1989.
209. Cullen SI, Frost P, Jacobson C, et al: Treatment of tinea versicolor with a new antifungal agent, ciclopirox olamine cream 1%. *Clin Ther* 7:574-583, 1985.
210. Bagatell F, Bogaert H, Cullen S, et al: Evaluation of a new antifungal cream, ciclopirox olamine 1% in the treatment of cutaneous candidosis. *Clin Ther* 8:41-48, 1985.
211. Kellner H, Arnold C, Christ O, et al: Untersuchungen kotkums Ciclopirox olamin bei Tieren und beim Menschen nach topischer und systemischer Anwendung. *Arzneimittel-Forschung* 31:1338, 1981.
212. Data on file: Hoechst-Marion Roussel, Kansas City, MO, 1991.
213. Lassus A, Nolting KS, Savopoulos C: Comparison of ciclopirox 1% cream with ciclopirox 1%-hydrocortisone acetate 1% cream in the treatment of inflamed superficial mycoses. *Clin Ther* 10:594-599, 1988.
214. Ceschin-Roques CG, Hanel H, Pruja-Bougaret SM, et al: Ciclopirox nail lacquer 8%: in vivo penetration into and through nails and in vitro effect on pig skin. *Skin Pharmacol* 4:89-94, 1991.
215. Baran R, Viraben R, Bougaret S, et al: Effect of an 8% ciclopirox antifungal lacquer in onychomycosis: a multicenter, double-blind clinical trial versus systemic ketoconazole (abstract). Second Congress of the European Academy of Dermatology and Venereology. Athens:182, 1991.
216. Wu T, Chuan MT, Lu YC: Efficacy of ciclopirox olamine 1% cream in onychomycosis and tinea pedis. *Mycoses* 34:93-95, 1991.
217. Qadriput S, Horn G, Hohler T: Zur Lokalwirksamkeit von Ciclopiroxamin bei Nagelmykosen. *Arzneim-Forsch* 31:1369, 1981.
218. Qadriput S, Hochler T: Initial results on the topical effectiveness of ciclopirox olamine in onychomycosis. Proceedings of the 8th Congress of the International Society for Human and Animal Mycology. Feb 8-12, 1982.

Selenium Sulfide
219. Albright SD, Hitch JM: Rapid treatment of tinea versicolor with selenium sulfide. *Arch Dermatol* 93:460-462, 1966.
220. Chu AC: Comparative clinical trial of bifonazole solution versus selenium sulfide shampoo in the treatment of pityriasis versicolor. *Dermatologica* 169(Suppl 1):81-86, 1984.
221. Hersle K: Selenium sulphide treatment of tinea versicolor. *Acta Derm Venereol* 51:476-478, 1971.
222. Hernanz ADP, Vicente SD, Ramos FM, et al: Randomized comparative clinical trial of itraconazole and selenium sulfide shampoo for the treatment of pityriasis versicolor. *Rev Infect Dis* 9:121-127, 1987.
223. Sanchez JL, Torres VM: Double-blind efficacy study of selenium sulfide in tinea versicolor. *J Am Acad Dermatol* 11:235-238, 1984.

224. Friedman SJ, Albert HL: Confluent and reticulated papillomatosis of Gougerot and Carteaud: Treatment with selenium sulfide lotion (letter). *J Am Acad Dermatol* 14:280-282, 1986.

225. Nordby CA, Mitchell AJ: Confluent and reticulated papillomatosis responsive to selenium sulfide. *Int J Dermatol* 25:194-199, 1986.

226. Allen HB, Honig PJ, Leyden JJ, et al: Selenium sulfide: adjunctive therapy for tinea capitis. *Pediatrics* 69:81-83, 1982.

227. Rezabek GH, Friedman AD: Superficial fungal infections of the skin. Diagnosis and current treatment recommendations. *Drugs* 43:674-682, 1992.

228. Van Cutsem J, Van Gerven F, Fransen J, et al: The in-vitro antifungal activity of ketoconazole, zinc pyrithione, and selenium sulfide against Pityrosporum and their efficacy as a shampoo in the treatment of experimental pityrosporosis in guinea pigs. *J Am Acad Dermatol* 22:993-998, 1990.

229. Millikan LE: The safety of selenium sulfide, and other news from Washington [editorial]. *J Am Acad Dermatol* 3:430-431, 1980.

230. Cummins LM, Kimura ET: Safety evaluation of selenium sulfide antidandruff shampoos. *Toxicol Appl Pharmacol* 20:89-96, 1971.

231. Kalivas J: Lack of serum selenium rise after overnight application of selenium sulfide (letter). *Arch Dermatol* 129:646-648, 1993.

232. Sanchez JL, Torres VM: Selenium sulfide in tinea versicolor: blood and urine levels. *J Am Acad Dermatol* 11:238-241, 1984.

Comparative Studies—Various Antifungal Agents

233. Shadomy S, Wang H, Shadomy H: Further in vitro studies with oxiconazole nitrate. *Diagn Microbiol Infect Dis* 9:231-237, 1988.

234. Grant SM, Clissold SP: Itraconazole. A review of its pharmacodynamic and pharmacokinetic properties, and therapeutic use in superficial and systemic mycoses. *Drugs* 37:310-344, 1989.

235. Gebhart R, Espinel-Ingroff A, Shadomy S: In vitro susceptibility studies with oxiconazole (Ro 13-8996). *Chemotherapy* 30:244-247, 1984.

236. Hare R, Loebenberg D: Animal models in the search for antifungal agents. *Amer Soc Microbiol New* 54:235-239, 1988.

237. Arika T, Yokoo M, Yamaguchi H: Topical treatment with butenafine significantly lowers relapse rate in an interdigital tinea pedis model in guinea pigs. *Antimicrob Agents Chemother* 36:2523-2525, 1992.

238. Evans EG: A comparison of terbinafine (Lamisil) 1% cream given for one week with clotrimazole (Canesten) 1% cream given for four weeks, in the treatment of tinea pedis. *Br J Dermatol* 130(Suppl 43):1-4, 1994.

239. Bergstresser PR, Elewski B, Hanifin J, et al: Topical terbinafine and clotrimazole in interdigital tinea pedis: a multicenter comparison of cure and relapse rates with 1- and 4-week treatment regimens. *J Am Acad Dermatol* 28:648-651, 1993.

240. Ablon G, Rosen T, Spedale J: Comparative efficacy of naftifine, oxiconazole, and terbinafine in short-term treatment of tinea pedis. *Int J Dermatol* 35:591-593, 1996.

241. Tsuyuki S, Ito M, Unno T, et al: Clinical usefulness of butenafine hydrochloride on tinea pedis: comparative study with clotrimazole. *Acta Dermatol* 85:299-306, 1990.

242. Elewski B, Bergstresser PR, Hanifin J, et al: Long-term outcome of patients with interdigital tinea pedis treated with terbinafine or clotrimazole. *J Am Acad Dermatol* 32:290-292, 1995.

243. Vanden Bossche H, Willemsens G, Cools W, et al: Biochemical effects of miconazole on fungi. II. Inhibition of ergosterol biosynthesis in *Candida albicans*. *Chem Biol Interact* 21:59-78, 1978.

244. Georgopapadakou NH, Bertasso A: Effects of squalene epoxidase inhibitors on *Candida albicans*. *Antimicrob Agents Chemother* 36:1779-1781, 1992.

245. Nahm WK, Orengo I, Rosen T: The antifungal agent butenafine manifests anti-inflammatory activity in vivo. *J Am Acad Dermatol* 41:203-206, 1999.

246. Beetens JR, Loots W, Somers Y, et al: Ketoconazole inhibits the biosynthesis of leukotrienes in vitro and in vivo. *Biochem Pharmacol* 35:883-891, 1986.

247. Bremm KD, Plempel M: Modulation of leukotriene metabolism from human polymorphonuclear granulocytes by bifonazole. *Mycoses* 34:41-45, 1991.

248. Choi TS, Solomon B, Nowakowski M, et al: Effect of naftifine on neutrophil adhesion. *Skin Pharmacol* 9:190-196, 1996.

249. Davies RR, Zaini F: Antifungal drugs affecting the chemotaxis of polymorphonuclear neutrophils. *Sabouraudia* 23:119-123, 1985.

250. Hegemann L, Toso SM, Lahijani KI, et al: Direct interaction of antifungal azole-derivatives with calmodulin: a possible mechanism for their therapeutic activity. *J Invest Dermatol* 100:343-346, 1993.

251. Solomon B, Lee WL, Geen SC, et al: Modifications of neutrophil functions by naftifine. *Br J Dermatol* 128:393-398, 1994.

252. Steinhilber, Jaschonek K, Knopse J, et al: Effects of novel antifungal azole derivatives on the 5-lipoxygenase and cyclooxygenase pathways. *Drug Res* 40:1260-1263, 1990.

253. Agut J, Tarrida N, Sacristan A, Ortiz JA: Antiinflammatory activity of topically applied sertaconazole nitrate. *Methods Find Exp Clin Pharmacol* 18:233-234, 1996.

254. Uzunoglu S, Tosun AU, Ozden T, et al: Synthesis and activities of 5-substituted-2-(p-substituted phenyl)-1-dialkylaminomethyl benzimidazole derivatives. *Farmaco* 52:619-623, 1997.

255. Van Cutsem J, Van Gerven F, Cauwenbergh G, et al: The antiinflammatory effects of ketoconazole. A comparative study with hydrocortisone acetate in a model using living and killed *Staphylococcus aureus* on the skin of guinea-pigs (see comments). *J Am Acad Dermatol* 25:257-261, 1991.

256. Rosen T, Schell BJ, Orengo I: Anti-inflammatory activity of antifungal preparations. *Int J Dermatol* 36:788-792, 1997.

257. Tomlinson S, MacNeil S, Walker SW, et al: Calmodulin and cell function. *Clin Sci* 66:497-507, 1984.

258. van de Kerkhof PC, van Erp PE: Calmodulin levels are grossly elevated in the psoriatic lesion. *Br J Dermatol* 108:217-218, 1983.

259. Tucker WF, MacNeil S, Dawson RA, et al: Calmodulin levels in psoriasis: the effect of treatment. *Acta Derm Venereol* 66:2412-2414, 1986.

260. Tucker WF, MacNeil S, Dawson RA, et al: An investigation of the ability of antipsoriatic drugs to inhibit calmodulin activity: a possible mode of action of dithranol (anthralin). *J Invest Dermatol* 87:232-235, 1986.

261. Doring HF: Experience gained with topical therapy with bifonazole in unusual indications. In Hay RJ, editor: *Advances in topical antifungal therapy,* Berlin, 1986, Springer Verlag, pp 26-31.

262. Faergemann J: Treatment of seborrhoeic dermatitis with bifonazole. *Mycoses* 32:309-311, 1989.

263. Massone L, Borghi S, Pestarino A, et al: Seborrheic dermatitis in otherwise healthy patients and in patients with lymphadenopathy syndrome/AIDS-related complex: treatment with 1% bifonazole cream. *Chemioterapia* 7:109-112, 1988.

264. Faergemann J: Treatment of seborrhoeic dermatitis of the scalp with ketoconazole shampoo. A double-blind study. *Acta Derm Venereol* 70:171-172, 1990.

265. Evans EG, James IG, Seaman RA, et al: Does naftifine have anti-inflammatory properties? A double-blind comparative study with 1% clotrimazole/1% hydrocortisone in clinically diagnosed fungal infection of the skin. *Br J Dermatol* 129:437-442, 1993.

266. Swan JW, Dahl MV, Coppo PA, et al: Complement activation by *Trichophyton rubrum*. *J Invest Dermatol* 80:156-158, 1983.

267. Calderon RA: Immunoregulation of dermatophytosis. *Crit Rev Microbiol* 16:339-368, 1989.

268. Dahl MV: Immunological resistance to dermatophyte infections. *Adv Dermatol* 2:305-320, 1987.

269. Dahl MV: Host defense: fungus. In Dahl MV, editor: *Clinical immunodermatology,* St Louis, 1996, Mosby, pp 201-213.

270. Hanel H, Smith-Kurtz E, Pastowsky S: Therapy of seborrheic eczema with an antifungal agent with an antiphlogistic effect. *Mycoses* 34(Suppl 1):91-93, 1991.

271. Heel RC, Brogden RN, Pakes GE, et al: Miconazole: a preliminary review of its therapeutic efficacy in systemic fungal infections. *Drugs* 19:7-30, 1980.

272. Nolting S, Brautigam M: Clinical relevance of the antibacterial activity of terbinafine: a contralateral comparison between 1% terbinafine cream and 0.1% gentamicin sulphate cream in pyoderma. *Br J Dermatol* 126(Suppl 39):56-60, 1992.

Jennifer L. Baumbach
Pranav B. Sheth

Topical and Intralesional Antiviral Agents

The subject of topical and intralesional antiviral agents encompasses a wide variety of pharmacologic agents. The three broad categories forming the basis and sequence of discussion in this chapter are the viricidal drugs, the immunoenhancing drugs, and the cytodestructive drugs (Table 25-1). The drugs in these categories that have a proprietary formulation available in the United States are listed in Table 25-2. These drugs are primarily used for various manifestations of human papillomavirus (HPV) infections and herpes simplex virus (HSV) infections, with imiquimod and topical formulations of cidofovir being investigated for molluscum contagiosum.

VIRICIDAL DRUGS
Acyclovir
Acyclovir was discovered in 1974. The first formulation of the drug was the topical form, which became available in 1982.[1] Numerous concentrations and preparations have been studied; however, the 5% ointment is the only Food and Drug Administration (FDA)–approved topical preparation.

PHARMACOLOGY
Structure. Acyclovir (9-[2-hydroxyethoxymethyl] guanine) is an acyclic analog of guanosine (Figure 25-1).

Absorption. Even when applied topically to damaged skin, systemic absorption of acyclovir is limited. In patients treated for genital herpes with 5% acyclovir in polyethylene glycol 4 to 6 times a day for 5 to 7 days, plasma acyclovir levels are undetectable.[2,3]

Mechanism of Action. Acyclovir is specific for certain herpes virus (HSV-1, HSV-2, varicella-zoster virus [VZV]) infected cells because the drug requires phosphorylation by viral thymidine kinase. Phosphorylation of acyclovir leads to acyclovir monophosphate. The acyclovir monophosphate is then further metabolized to acyclovir triphosphate by human cellular guanylate kinase. Acyclovir triphosphate then inhibits viral deoxyribonucleic acid (DNA) polymerase. In addition, acyclovir triphosphate is mistaken for deoxyguanosine triphosphate and becomes incorporated irreversibly into newly synthesized viral DNA. Because acyclovir lacks a 3' hydroxyl-group for DNA elongation to continue, incor-

◼ Table 25-1   Drug Categories—Topical and Intralesional Antiviral Agents*

Viricidal	Immunoenhancing	Cytodestructive
Acyclovir	Imiquimod	Bleomycin
Penciclovir	Interferon-α†	Podophyllin/podofilox
Cidofovir		Trichloroacetic acid
Foscarnet		Cantharidin
Idoxuridine		Salicylic acid
		5-Fluorouracil

*Drugs follow the sequence of discussion in this chapter.
†Systemic forms of various interferons are discussed in Chapter 16.

◼ Table 25-2   Topical Antiviral Agents*

Generic Name	Trade Name	Manufacturer	Generic	Cream	Ointment	Special Formulations	PPS
VIRICIDAL DRUGS							
Acyclovir	Zovirax	Glaxo-Wellcome	No	No	Yes	Oral, injectable	C
Penciclovir	Denavir	SmithKline Beecham	No	Yes	No		B
Cidofovir	Forvade	Gilead Sciences	No	No	No	Only in injectable forms	C†
Foscarnet	Foscavir	Astra	No	No	No	Only in injectable forms	C†
Idoxuridine	Stoxil/ Dendrid	SmithKline Beecham/Alcon	No	No	No	Ophthalmic ointment and solution	C
IMMUNOENHANCING DRUG							
Imiquimod	Aldara	3M Pharmaceuticals	No	Yes	No		B
CYTODESTRUCTIVE DRUGS							
Bleomycin	Blenoxane	Bristol-Myers Squibb	No	No	No	Injectable	D†
Podofilox	Condylox	Oclassen	No	No	No	Solution	C
Cantharidin	Canthacur, Canthacur PS	Pharmascience	No	No	No	Colloidal solution	NR
Salicylic acid	Multiple	Multiple	Yes	Yes	Yes	Solution, gel, film, plaster, patch, spray	C
5-fluorouracil	Efudex, Fluoroplex	Roche, Allergan	No	Yes	No	Solution, injectable	X

PPS, Pregnancy prescribing status—U.S. FDA (NR, not rated).
*Only listing drugs with proprietary formulations that are currently available in United States—trichloroacetic acid is excluded.
†The PPS listed is for the injectable formulation of this drug.

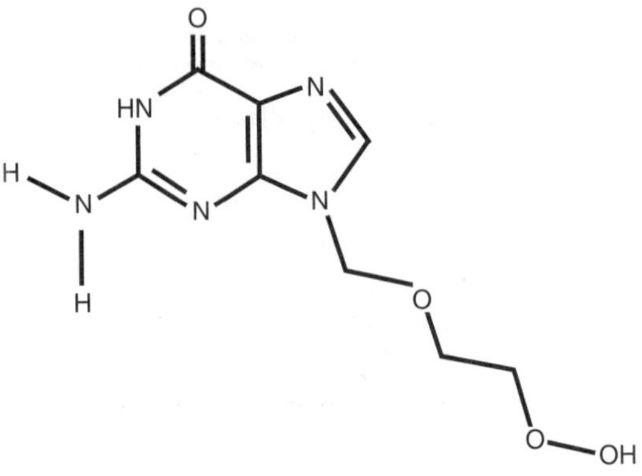

Acyclovir

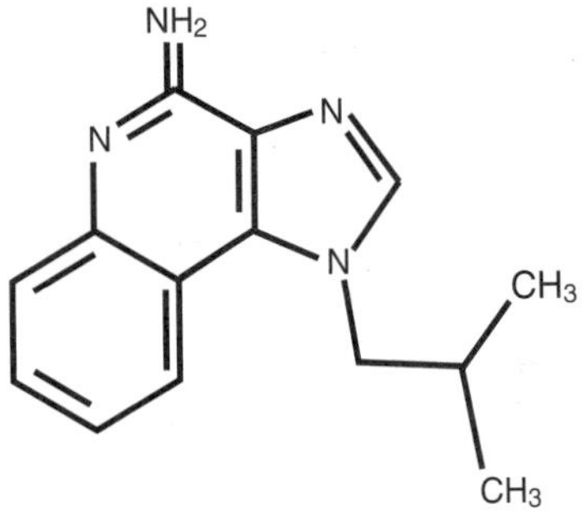

Imiquimod

Figure 25-1 Topical antiviral agents.

poration of acyclovir triphosphate into viral DNA leads to chain termination.[3]

Spectrum of Activity. Acyclovir is effective against HSV-1, HSV-2, and VZV but not cytomegalovirus (CMV) because CMV does not encode thymidine kinase.

CLINICAL USES

Genital Herpes Simplex Infections. Acyclovir 5% ointment is approved for the treatment of initial genital herpes infections. In the largest double-blind, placebo-controlled trial, acyclovir 5% ointment applied four times daily to lesions of an initial or first episode of genital herpes decreased the duration of viral shedding from 7 days (placebo) to 4.1 days, and the time to complete crusting from 10 days (placebo) to 7.1 days. No statistically significant difference

was seen in duration of pain, time to healing, frequency of new lesion formation, or recurrence of blisters after cessation of therapy from the placebo group. In the treatment of recurrent genital HSV, there was no significant clinical improvement in symptoms or duration of disease, although there was a significant decrease in viral shedding (1.90 days for placebo to 0.90 days with the active drug).[4] Smaller European studies with the 5% ointment (polyethylene glycol base) and 5% cream base (not proprietary in United States) reveal more statistically significant improvements in viral shedding, new lesion formation, time to complete healing, duration of pain, and itching in both initial genital herpes[5,6] and recurrent genital HSV.[5,7] Early application (within 24 hours of onset of prodrome) and patient training are important for maximal benefit from the topical form of acyclovir.

Given these data, topical acyclovir has limited use. Oral acyclovir remains the treatment of choice over topical acyclovir for recurrent genital herpes because of its greater efficacy in decreasing the duration of viral shedding and the time to crusting and healing of lesions.[8] Oral acyclovir is also believed to be more efficacious and convenient in the treatment of initial genital HSV.[9,10]

Herpes Labialis. Acyclovir 5% ointment also has FDA approval for use in "limited non-life threatening mucocutaneous herpes simplex virus infections in immunocompromised patients." In studies in immunocompromised patients with mainly herpes labialis, there was a decrease in duration of viral shedding and a slight decrease in duration of pain. There was no clinical benefit in nonimmunocompromised patients.[11]

Dosing. Application is recommended every 3 hours, 6 times per day for 7 days. A finger cot or rubber glove should be used when applying the medication to prevent autoinoculation or transmission to other persons. Therapy should be initiated as early as possible after onset of signs or symptoms.[11]

Adverse Effects. The common adverse effects have been shown to be mild pain, burning, and stinging. Rash, pruritus, and vulvitis have also been reported. However, placebo patients experienced similar side effects with an overall similar frequency.[4,5]

Pregnancy Prescribing Status. The pregnancy prescribing category for acyclovir is listed in Table 25-2. For all other antiviral agents discussed in this chapter that have an established pregnancy prescribing category the pregnancy rating is listed in this table as well.

Penciclovir

The limited bioavailability of oral acyclovir and the limited efficacy of topical acyclovir led to the discovery of penciclovir. This drug was approved by the FDA in 1996.

PHARMACOLOGY

Structure. Penciclovir (9-(4-hydroxy-3-hydroxymethylbut-1-yl) guanine is an acyclic purine nucleoside analog of guanine and is structurally related to ganciclovir. Penciclovir is available only in a topical preparation because of poor oral bioavailability. Famciclovir, a prodrug of penciclovir, is available in oral form.[12]

Mechanism of Action. The mechanism of action of penciclovir is similar to that of acyclovir in that the drug is selectively phosphorylated to the monophosphate form by viral thymidine kinase. Penciclovir monophosphate is further phosphorylated by cellular enzymes to the active penciclovir triphosphate form. This triphosphate form subsequently interferes with viral DNA synthesis and inhibits viral replication by competing with deoxyguanosine triphosphate for viral DNA polymerase and inhibiting viral DNA chain elongation. Even though acyclovir and penciclovir are qualitatively similar, penciclovir does have certain advantages over acyclovir. Penciclovir exhibits more efficient phosphorylation, a higher affinity of viral DNA polymerases for the triphosphate form, and increased stability of the triphosphate form leading to a longer duration of activity.[13]

Spectrum of Activity. Penciclovir exhibits inhibitory activity against several of the herpes viruses including HSV-1, HSV-2, VZV, and Epstein-Barr virus (EBV). It has limited in vitro activity against CMV.

CLINICAL USES

Herpes Labialis. Penciclovir 1% cream is indicated for the treatment of recurrent herpes labialis in immunocompetent patients. In a randomized, double-blind, placebo-controlled study, penciclovir 1% cream was found to speed healing of classic lesions and decrease pain and viral shedding from 5.5 days (placebo) to 4.8 days. The efficacy was similar whether the medication was started in the early prodromal phase or whether it was started in the later papule/vesicular phase.[12]

Dosage. Penciclovir 1% cream should be applied at the earliest sign or symptom to all lesions every 2 hours (or at least six times a day) for 4 days.

Adverse Effects. The incidence of local irritation, hyperesthesia, and paresthesia is similar for placebo and penciclovir cream.

Contraindications. Topical penciclovir is contraindicated in patients hypersensitive to the drug or any of the components of the formulation.

Summary. Given the inconvenience of frequent application, the expense of penciclovir, and the reduction of symptoms and viral shedding by only half a day, the clinical benefit of topical penciclovir over oral antiviral therapy is limited.

Cidofovir

Cidofovir is an acyclic nucleotide that exhibits antiviral activity against a broad range of DNA viruses. Currently, cidofovir is available in an intravenous (IV) form for treating CMV retinitis in patients with acquired immunodeficiency syndrome (AIDS). No oral preparations are currently available; however, cidofovir has been compounded in topical formulations and is currently under investigation for several potential indications.

PHARMACOLOGY

Structure. Cidofovir (1-[{S}-3-hydroxy-2-{phosphonomethoxy}propyl] cytosine) is a nucleoside analog of deoxycytidine monophosphate.

Mechanism of Action. After incorporation into virally infected cells, cidofovir requires two stages of phosphorylation to form the active metabolite cidofovir diphosphate. Unlike acyclovir and penciclovir, however, cidofovir does not depend on viral thymidine kinase for its phosphorylation. Cidofovir diphosphate then acts as a competitive inhibitor of deoxycytosine-5'-triphosphate for incorporation into viral DNA by viral DNA polymerases. After incorporation, cidofovir blocks further viral DNA synthesis.[14]

CLINICAL USES—UNDER INVESTIGATION

Molluscum Contagiosum. Three cases of human immunodeficiency virus (HIV)–positive men with recalcitrant molluscum were reported to have clearance of their lesions with either IV or topical cidofovir. Only one of the three had topical cidofovir compounded in a 3% cream. After application of the 3% cream daily Monday through Friday for 2 weeks, the patient had 70% clearance of lesions. By 1 month of therapy the patient had complete resolution of lesions without inflammation or sequelae.[15]

Condyloma Acuminatum. Three patients with AIDS with relapsing anogenital HPV lesions were treated with a 1% cidofovir topical preparation. Patients were treated daily for 5 days to 5 weeks, with complete resolution of all lesions and no recurrence at 6-month follow-up.[16] Further clinical trials are currently underway.

Verruca Vulgaris. Two cases of children being treated with 3% cidofovir cream for recalcitrant verruca have been reported. The first, a 7-year-old, was treated twice daily for 10 days with complete clearance and maintained a remission for greater than 40 weeks. The second, a girl 13 years of age with verruca on her hands, responded completely to 3% cidofovir cream daily for 10 weeks with continued clearance at 12 months.[17]

Herpes Simplex. A randomized, double-blind, placebo-controlled study of cidofovir gel in patients with AIDS with acyclovir-resistant HSV was performed to compare 0.3% gel versus 1.0% gel versus placebo. In cidofovir-treated patients, 50% had greater than 50% improvement compared with 0% improvement in the placebo group. Overall, 30% of cidofovir patients had complete healing.[18]

Another report of two immunocompromised patients with acyclovir-resistant HSV infections experienced clearance of their HSV with topical 3% cidofovir gel. When the HSV reemerged, it was paradoxically resensitized to acyclovir.[19]

In healthy patients with recurrent HSV, cidofovir gel (i.e., 1%, 3%, or 5%) used within 12 hours of an outbreak decreased the number of days to complete healing and duration of viral shedding from 3 days (placebo) to 1 to 2 days.[20]

Adverse Effects. Complaints of systemic adverse effects, such as headache, nausea, and pharyngitis, occurred in 6% to 11% of patients receiving topical cidofovir, which was comparable in frequency with patients receiving placebo.[20] Local adverse effects reported included itching, rash, pain, paresthesia, and ulceration and appeared to be increased in patients receiving higher concentrations of topical cidofovir. Placebo application site reactions occurred in 3% of patients compared with 5%, 19%, and 22% of patients receiving 1%, 3%, or 5% topical cidofovir, respectively.[20]

Foscarnet

Foscarnet exhibits in vitro activity against all herpes viruses and currently is used in the treatment of CMV infection in immunocompromised patients. It is also the drug of choice for acyclovir-resistant herpes virus infections.[21] Topical preparations are currently under investigation.

PHARMACOLOGY

Structure. Foscarnet (trisodium phosphonoformic acid) is a pyrophosphate analog.

Mechanism of Action. Foscarnet does not require activation by either cellular or viral enzymes. In addition, because the drug is not a nucleoside analog, nucleoside-resistant viral polymerases are susceptible to foscarnet. Foscarnet acts by competitively blocking pyrophosphate-binding sites on viral polymerases, which leads to interference with the cleavage of pyrophosphate from deoxyadenosine triphosphate.[22,23]

CLINICAL USES—UNDER INVESTIGATION

Herpes Labialis. A 3% foscarnet cream was evaluated in ultraviolet (UV) radiation–induced herpes labialis. The subjects applied either placebo or 3% foscarnet cream eight times a day immediately after exposure to UV. There was no significant difference between the two groups in the number of lesions developed or the duration of lesions. However, there was a statistically significant decrease in the mean lesion area and the maximum lesion area in foscarnet-treated patients.[21]

Genital Herpes.   In general, studies evaluating topical foscarnet cream have not shown a significant benefit over placebo for genital HSV infections.[22,23] One double-blind trial suggested some decrease in redness, swelling, and blisters with 0.3% foscarnet cream.[23] Overall, although the drug appears to be safe, the clinical response rate in studies has been disappointing and appears to not warrant the drug's expense.

Idoxuridine

Idoxuridine (5-iodo-2'-deoxyuridine) is a thymidine analog, which was synthesized in 1959 and was the first FDA-approved antiviral medication.[24] Idoxuridine has in vitro activity against HSV and VZV. Topical idoxuridine 5% to 15% in dimethyl sulfoxide has been evaluated in the treatment of genital herpes, herpes labialis, and herpes zoster. In genital HSV infections, idoxuridine was not found to be effective.[25] However, some studies did show some decrease in duration of pain and in mean healing time by approximately 1.7 days in both herpes zoster and herpes labialis. In herpes zoster and herpes labialis, idoxuridine needed to be applied every 4 hours for 4 consecutive days.[26,27] Idoxuridine has since been replaced by newer antiviral therapies. Currently, idoxuridine is only available as an ophthalmic solution (Stoxil) for the treatment of herpes keratitis.

IMMUNOENHANCING DRUGS
Imiquimod

Imiquimod is an immunomodulating agent that was approved by the FDA in 1997 for use in genital HPV infections.

PHARMACOLOGY

Structure.   Imiquimod 1-(2-2-methyl-propyl)-1*H*-imidazo[4,5-c] quinolin-4-amine is a non-nucleoside heterocyclic amine (see Figure 25-1).

Mechanism of Action.   The exact mechanism of action for imiquimod has not been fully elucidated; however, it is thought to be related to the drug's immunomodulating properties. In vitro, imiquimod does not exhibit direct antiviral activity; however, in vivo, imiquimod has been demonstrated to be a potent inducer of several cytokines including tumor necrosis factor (TNF)-α, interferon (IFN)-γ, IFN-α, interleukin (IL)-6, IL-1α, IL-1β, IL-8, IL-12, granulocyte-macrophage colony–stimulating factor (GM-CSF), and granulocyte colony–stimulating factor (G-CSF). Through these immunomodulating properties, imiquimod has potent antiviral and antitumor activity.[28,29] In the treatment of genital warts with topical 5% imiquimod cream, the mechanism of action may be attributed to the stimulation primarily of IFN-α, IFN-γ, TNF-α, IL-12, and a cell-mediated immune response.[29]

Absorption.   When applied topically, systemic absorption of imiquimod appears to be minimal.

CLINICAL USES

External Genital and Perianal Warts.
The only current FDA-approved indication for imiquimod 5% cream is in the treatment of external genital and perianal warts/condyloma acuminatum in adults. Fifty percent of patients had complete clearance of warts in a 12-week, double-blind, placebo-controlled trial.[28] These clearance results compared favorably with the 1% imiquimod cream, which demonstrated a 21% clearance rate versus the 11% clearance rate with placebo. Clearance of lesions generally occurred within 8 to 12 weeks. Median time to complete wart clearance was 10 weeks. In addition, 81% of patients experienced a 50% or greater reduction in wart area. Women were found to have a higher clearance rate of 77% compared with just 40% clearance in men. Recurrence rate at 12 weeks posttreatment of patients who experienced complete resolution was 13% with no gender differences.[28,30-32]

Molluscum Contagiosum.   Imiquimod is currently not approved for the treatment of molluscum. However, double-blind, placebo-controlled studies evaluating imiquimod 1% cream in treating molluscum demonstrated a clearance rate of 82% when it was applied to lesions three times a day for 5 days for 4 weeks. Clearance with placebo occurred in just 16% of patients.[33]

Herpes Simplex Virus.   Imiquimod has been shown to have activity against HSV in a guinea pig model.[34,35] If applied within 72 hours of inoculation (intravaginally) in the guinea pig, imiquimod reduced primary lesions, viral shedding, and viral content of spinal cords. If applied once lesions began to appear, imiquimod treatment was not able to stop lesion development. Imiquimod is currently in clinical trials for treating human HSV infections.[35]

Adverse Effects.   Imiquimod is generally well tolerated, with the most frequent adverse reactions being mild-to-moderate inflammation with erythema, erosion, excoriation, flaking, and edema. Erythema is the most common adverse reaction, occurring in approximately 33% to 80% of patients receiving 5% imiquimod cream. Pruritus, burning, tenderness, stinging, rash, and hypopigmentation occur in 10% to 35% of patients. Serious systemic effects have not been reported. The incidence of flulike symptoms was equivalent for 5% imiquimod cream and placebo-treated patients. Other reported adverse effects include fatigue, diarrhea, and fever.[28,30,32]

Dosage.   Imiquimod 5% cream should be applied to the affected area at bedtime and left in place for 6 to 10 hours before washing it off. Recommended dosing is three times a week on nonconsecutive days (e.g., Monday, Wednesday, and Friday) until complete clearance for a maximum of 16 weeks. Occlusive dressings or wrappings are not recommended because of an increased risk of irritation.

Contraindications.   Contraindications to imiquimod use are hypersensitivity to any of the formulation's components.

Interferon-α

Topical IFN-α preparations have been formulated and evaluated in the treatment of condyloma acuminatum and recurrent genital herpes. Overall, the topical formulations have not proved to be efficacious over placebo.[36-38] Intralesional IFN is discussed in detail in Chapter 16.

CYTODESTRUCTIVE DRUGS
Bleomycin (Intralesional)

Bleomycin, initially discovered in 1996, is the generic name for a group of sulfur-containing glycopeptide cytotoxic antibiotics derived from *Streptomyces verticillus* and found to have antitumor, antibacterial, and antiviral activity.[39,40] Un-

like other medications in this chapter, bleomycin is not applied topically in the treatment of viral infections. Bleomycin has been shown to be effective against HPV infections only with intralesional administration.

PHARMACOLOGY

Mechanism of Action.   The exact mechanism against HPV infection is unclear; however, bleomycin selectively inhibits DNA by binding to DNA, leading to single strand scission in DNA and elimination of pyrimidine and purine bases, as well as altering DNA metabolism.[41] Bleomycin is most effective at DNA damage in the M and G2 phase of the cell cycle. Bleomycin is also believed to have an effect on protein synthesis, which is thought to cause biochemical changes leading to apoptosis and necrosis of keratinocytes. It is unlikely that bleomycin binds specifically to HPV,[42] and therefore effectiveness is through cytotoxicity to infected keratinocytes.

Systemic Absorption.   In one study, plasma concentrations of bleomycin after injection of 1 mg/1 ml (1 mg/ml = 1 U/ml) intralesionally showed levels as high as 113 ng/ml in one patient, which is similar to patients receiving slow subcutaneous infusion for cancer chemotherapy.[42] However, no clinical evidence of systemic toxicity had been noted.

CLINICAL USES

Verruca Vulgaris.   Intralesional bleomycin has been investigated in the treatment of recalcitrant warts. Studies demonstrate that the efficacy of intralesional bleomycin 0.1% aqueous solution (1 mg/1 ml) at 2-week intervals is variable depending on the location of the warts. Overall, 47% to 67% of plantar warts, 71% to 94% of periungual warts, and 77% to 95% of warts in other locations responded favorably. The overall complete cure rate was 68% to 81% with one or two injections.[39,40,43,44]

Adverse Effects.   The most common adverse effect is local pain and burning at the injection site. Within the first 24 to 72 hours there may be erythema, swelling, and pain before a blackened thrombotic eschar forms. Scarring is uncommon. Although uncommon, Raynaud's phenomenon after treatment of both periungual and plantar warts has been described.[40,43,45] Reports indicate that the Raynaud's remains localized to only the digits that receive intralesional bleomycin.[46-48] There are also case reports of loss of the nail plate with no subsequent regrowth, as well as a report of persistent nail dystrophy after treatment with intralesional bleomycin.[49,50] Avoidance of injection into the nail matrix may decrease the risk of nail dystrophy.

Contraindications.   Because bleomycin is not currently FDA approved for the treatment of warts and there are case reports of significant side effects, recommendations have been made to limit the use of bleomycin. It is recommended that intralesional bleomycin not be used in pregnant women, children, immunosuppressed patients, or patients with possible vascular compromise.[46]

Dosage.   Each individual lesion receives 0.1 ml of 1 U/ml bleomycin in a 0.1% solution with normal saline. No more than a total of 2 ml of bleomycin (approximately 10 to 20 small warts) should be administered per session to any patient. Treatments are performed every 2 to 3 weeks until resolution. Due to the pain of injecting bleomycin, many clinicians anesthetize the treatment site before the bleomycin injection. Other methods to reduce the pain of injection include reconstituting bleomycin with injectable anesthetic (e.g., Marcaine) without epinephrine instead of normal saline. Topical anesthetics (e.g., EMLA, Frigiderm) or placing the wart-infected site on ice packs for 10 to 15 minutes (until numb) may be used before injection. Local nerve blocks may be indicated in some patients. After bleomycin injection, ice water soaks for 10 to 15 minutes two times per day for 4 days may decrease the pain during the postbleomycin swelling phase.[51]

Because of the rapid deterioration of reconstituted bleomycin (24 hours) at room temperature and the high cost of the medication, bleomycin 0.1% aqueous solution should be stored at −20° C freezing temperature. If stored in glass (rather than plastic) at freezing temperatures, it keeps its immunoreactivity for at least 27 months.[42]

Podophyllin and Podofilox

Podophyllin, which has been in use since the 1940s to treat condyloma, is a crude extract of cytotoxic material from the May apple plant (either *Podophyllum peltatum* or *Podophyllum emodi*). The most active ingredient and the cytodestructive agent in podophyllin is podophyllotoxin. One difficulty in using podophyllin is that the concentration of podophyllotoxin in office-based podophyllin is not standardized. However, the commercial product podofilox (Condylox), prepared in a solution or gel, has a stable concentration of 0.5% podophyllotoxin.[52] Although, in general, this is a lower concentration than found in office-based podophyllin, podofilox does not contain quercetin or kaempherol (known mutagens), and it can to be used on an outpatient basis.[53]

PHARMACOLOGY

Mechanism of Action.   Podophyllotoxin is an antimitotic agent and exerts its effect by arresting cells in metaphase by binding reversibly to tubulin.[53]

CLINICAL USES

Condyloma   Acuminatum.   Podofilox 0.5% was found to have better clearance rates when compared with podophyllin 20% in the treatment of penile warts.[52] Podofilox solution and gel have both been found to be safe and effective in the treatment of genital warts. Clearance rates have been reported to be from 37% to as high as 71%, particularly when used on mucosal surfaces.[53-55] Recurrence rates are typically in the 20% to 30% range.

Adverse Effects.   The most common side effects are inflammation, burning, erythema, and erosions, which occurred in up to 75% of patients treated with 0.5% podofilox gel.[53,54]

Contraindications.   Podophyllin is contraindicated in pregnancy secondary to its mutagenic properties. Birth defects, fetal death, and stillbirth have been reported. In contrast, podofilox is a pregnancy prescribing status category C medication. Embryotoxicity in rats has been reported when administered intraperitoneally; however, no teratogenicity was noted during topical application in rabbits.[53]

Trichloroacetic Acid

Trichloroacetic acid (TCAA) works through the destruction of tissue by causing hydrolysis of cellular proteins, leading to inflammation and cell death.[56] Because the drug is nonspecific regarding effect on virus-infected cells, care must be taken when applying TCAA so that surrounding tissue is not destroyed. TCAA is advantageous over podophyllin because it can be used in treating genital warts in pregnant patients. Adequate application is achieved when the wart and surrounding area turn white.[57]

CLINICAL USES

External Genital Warts.   In studies comparing TCAA with cryotherapy, TCAA has been found to have similar efficacy with response rates between 70% and 81%. The average number of treatments required for clearance was between four and six. The recurrence rate for TCAA is around 39%.[58,59]

Cervical Human Papillomavirus Infection. Variable results have been obtained for the effectiveness of TCAA in treating cervical HPV. One study showed no significant difference between TCAA and placebo.[56] However, another study revealed an 81% clearance rate of cervical HPV infection (measured by koilocytes on Papanicolaou smears) with 85% TCAA to the entire cervix (1 to 4 applications).[60]

Nongenital Warts.   TCAA is generally thought to be more effective on smaller, less keratotic warts. There are no good studies to support this opinion.

Adverse Effects.   The major adverse effects following treatment with TCAA are local pain and ulceration. Ulceration was found to be somewhat more common with TCAA than with cryotherapy for genital warts.[58]

Cantharidin

Cantharidin is a vesiculating agent derived from the "blister beetle" *Lytta vesicatoria*, also known as the "Spanish fly." Cantharidin acts by interfering with mitochondria, leading to epidermal cell death, acantholysis, and clinical blister formation.[61] It has no direct antiviral effect.

Cantharidin's use is limited to in-office treatment for verruca vulgaris applied by a physician. Initially a "grandfather drug," the FDA changed its requirements in 1992 and required a new drug application for cantharidin. Cantharone and Cantharone Plus were pulled off the market in the United States.[62] Cantharidin is now available from compounding pharmacists or from Pharmscience (Canada)/

Omniderm as Canthacur solution (active ingredient cantharidin 0.7%) or Canthacur PS (cantharidin 1%, podophyllin 2%, salicylic acid 30%).

The colloidion solution can be applied with the wooden end of an applicator stick or a toothpick directly to the wart. After application, the lesion should be occluded for 24 hours with adhesive tape. A blister usually forms within 24 to 48 hours and often heals within 1 week. Retreatment is recommended on a 1- to 3-week interval. The cure rate is reported to be as high as 80% for common, plantar, and periungual warts.[61,63]

Some benefits of cantharidin are that the application itself is painless (an advantage in children) and there is no scarring. The major adverse side effect is pain from the blister. Less common, but quite frustrating for the patient and physician, is the formation of a ring wart (annular wart formed at the periphery of a resolving blister induced by cantharidin and less frequently cryotherapy). Cantharidin has also been used in the treatment of molluscum contagiosum in a similar fashion. The main difference is that occlusion is not used, except for large papules or persistent lesions.[63]

Salicylic Acid

Salicylic acid is a keratolytic agent that is a common component of over-the-counter verruca vulgaris treatments ranging in concentrations between 10% and 60%. Salicylic acid is available in both liquid and plaster preparations and is recommended for use in the treatment of warts located on the hands and feet. For best results, the wart can be soaked in warm water for 5 minutes and the dead tissue removed with an emery board or pumice stone. The salicylic acid–containing medication is applied. The lesions can be subsequently occluded for enhanced penetration of the active ingredient. Cure rates vary depending on the lesion location. After 3 months of treatment, 67% of hand, 84% of simple plantar, and 45% of mosaic warts completely resolve.[64] (See Chapter 34 for further details on salicylic acid.)

5-Fluorouracil

5-Fluorouracil (5-FU) is a fluorinated pyrimidine analog with cytotoxic effects that has been found to penetrate abnormal skin to a greater extent than normal skin. The FDA-approved indications for topical 5-FU (Efudex/Fluoroplex) are for multiple actinic keratoses and superficial basal cell carcinomas; however, the drug demonstrated some degree of efficacy in the treatment of resistant genital condylomata, verruca plana, and verruca vulgaris.[65] Application of 5% 5-FU on a once weekly basis has been found to be as effective as daily treatment, albeit with fewer adverse effects.[66,67] The main adverse effect is discomfort at the application site, manifested clinically by erythema and edema. If the patient continues to apply 5-FU after significant inflammation develops, erosive dermatitis and mucositis may occur.[65] (See Chapter 29 for further details on 5-fluorouracil.)

Bibliography

Goldfarb MT, Gupta MA, Sawchuk WS: Office therapy for human papillomavirus infection in non-genital sites. *Dermatol Clin* 9:287-296, 1991.

Lea AP, Bryson HM: Cidofovir. *Drugs* 52:225-230, 1996.

Memar O, Tyring S: Antiviral agents in dermatology: current status and future prospects. *Int J Dermatol* 34:597-606, 1995.

Moscicki AB: Human papillomavirus infections in adolescents. *Pediatr Clin North Am* 46:783-807, 1999.

Mroczkowski TF, McEwen C: Warts and other human papillomavirus infections. *Postgrad Med* 78:91-98, 1985.

O'Brien JJ, Campoli-Richards DM: Acyclovir: an updated review of its antiviral activity, pharmacokinetic properties and therapeutic efficacy. *Drugs* 37:233-309, 1989.

Reusser P: Herpesvirus resistance to antiviral drugs: a review of the mechanism, clinical importance and therapeutic options. *J Hosp Infect* 33:235-248, 1996.

References

Acyclovir

1. King DH: History, pharmacokinetics, and pharmacology of acyclovir. *J Am Acad Dermatol* 18:176-179, 1988.
2. O'Brien JJ, Campoli-Richards DM: Acyclovir: an updated review of its antiviral activity, pharmacokinetic properties and therapeutic efficacy. *Drugs* 37:233-309, 1989.
3. Balfour HH: Acyclovir and other chemotherapy for herpes group viral infections. *Annu Rev Med* 35:279-291, 1984.
4. Corey L, Nahmias AJ, Guinan ME: A trial of topical acyclovir in genital herpes simplex virus infections. *N Engl J Med* 306:1313-1319, 1982.
5. Kinghorn GR, Turner EB, Barton IG: Efficacy of topical acyclovir cream in first and recurrent episodes of genital herpes. *Antiviral Res* 3:291-301, 1983.
6. Thin RN, Nabarro JM, Parker JD, et al: Topical acyclovir in the treatment of initial genital herpes. *Br J Vener Dis* 59:116-119, 1983.
7. Fiddian AP, Kinghorn GR, Goldmeier D, et al: Topical acyclovir in the treatment of genital herpes: a comparison with systemic therapy. *J Antimicrob Chemother* 12(Suppl B):67-77, 1983.
8. Reichman RC, Badger GJ, Mertz GJ, et al: Treatment of recurrent genital herpes simplex infections with oral acyclovir. *JAMA* 251:2103-2107, 1984.
9. Bryson VJ, Dillon M, Lovett M, et al: Treatment of first episodes of genital herpes simplex virus infection with oral acyclovir. *N Engl J Med* 308:916-921, 1983.
10. Spruance SL, Freeman DJ: Topical treatment of cutaneous herpes simplex virus infections. *Antiviral Res* 14:305-321, 1990.
11. *Physicians' desk reference*, ed 54, Montvale, NJ, 2000, Medical Economics Company.

Penciclovir

12. Spruance SL, Rea TL, Thoming C, et al: Penciclovir cream for the treatment of herpes simplex labialis. A randomized multicenter, double-blind, placebo-controlled trial. *JAMA* 277:1374-1379, 1997.
13. Bacon TH, Howard BA, Spender LC, et al: Activity of penciclovir in antiviral assays against herpes simplex virus. *J Antimicrob Chemother* 37:303-313, 1996.

Cidofovir

14. Lea AP, Bryson HM: Cidofovir. *Drugs* 52:225-230, 1996.
15. Meadows KP, Tyring SK, Pavia AT, et al: Resolution of recalcitrant molluscum contagiosum virus lesions in human immunodeficiency virus-infected patients treated with cidofovir. *Arch Dermatol* 133:987-990, 1997.
16. Snoeck R, van Ranst M, Andrei G, et al: Treatment of anogenital papillomavirus infections with an acyclic nucleoside phosphonate analogue (letter). *N Engl J Med* 333:943-944, 1995.
17. Zabawski EJ, Sands B, Goetz D, et al: Treatment of verruca vulgaris with topical cidofovir (letter). *JAMA* 278:1236, 1997.
18. Lalezari J, Schacker T, Feinberg J: A randomized, double-blind, placebo-controlled trial of cidofovir gel for the treatment of acyclovir-unresponsive mucocutaneous herpes simplex virus infection in patients with AIDS. *J Infect Dis* 176:892-898, 1997.
19. Snoeck R, Andrei G, Gerard M: Successful treatment of progressive mucocutaneous infection due to acyclovir- and foscarnet-resistant herpes simplex virus with (S)-l-(3-hydroxy-2-phosphonylmethoxypropyl) cytosine (HPMPC). *Clin Infect Dis* 18:570-578, 1994.
20. Sacks SL, Shafrun SD, Diaz-Mitoma F: A multicenter phase I/II dose escalation study of single-dose cidofovir gel treatment of recurrent genital herpes. *Antimicrob Agents Chemother* 42:2996-2999, 1998.

Foscarnet

21. Bernstein DI, Schleupner CJ, Evans TG: Effect of foscarnet cream on experimental UV radiation-induced herpes labialis. *Antimicrob Agents Chemother* 41:1961-1964, 1997.
22. Barton SE, Munday PE, Kinghorn GR: Topical treatment of recurrent genital herpes simplex virus infections with trisodium phosphonoformate (foscarnet): double blind, placebo controlled, multicenter study. *Genitourin Med* 62:247-250, 1986.

23. Wallin JN, Lernestedt J, Ogenstad S, et al: Topical treatment of recurrent genital herpes infections with foscarnet. *Scand J Infect Dis* 17:165-172, 1985.

Idoxuridine

24. Memar O, Tyring S: Antiviral agents in dermatology: current status and future prospects. *Int J Dermatol* 34:597-606, 1995.
25. Silvestri DL, Corey L, Holmes KK: Ineffectiveness of topical idoxuridine in dimethyl sulfoxide for therapy for genital herpes. *JAMA* 248:953-959, 1982.
26. Spruance SL, Stewart JC, Freeman DJ, et al: Early application of topical 15% idoxuridine in dimethyl sulfoxide shortens the course of herpes simplex labialis: a multicenter placebo-controlled trial. *J Infect Dis* 161:191-197, 1990.
27. Dawber R: Idoxuridine in herpes zoster: further evaluation of intermittent topical therapy. *BMJ* 2:526-527, 1974.

Imiquimod

28. Beutner KR, Tyring SK, Trofatter KF Jr: Imiquimod, a patient-applied immune-response modifier for treatment of external genital warts. *Antimicrob Agents Chemother* 42:789-794, 1998.
29. Arany I, Tyring SK, Stanley MA, et al: Enhancement of the innate and cellular immune response in patients with genital warts treated with topical imiquimod cream 5%. *Antiviral Res* 43:55-63, 1999.
30. Edwards L, Ferenczy A, Eron L, et al: Self-administered topical 5% imiquimod cream for external anogenital warts. *Arch Dermatol* 134:25-30, 1998.
31. Syed TA, Ahmadpour OA, Ahmad SA, et al: Management of female genital warts with an analog of imiquimod 2% in cream: a randomized, double-blind, placebo-controlled study. *J Dermatol* 25:429-433, 1998.
32. Beutner KR, Spruance SL, Hougham AJ: Treatment of genital warts with an immune-response modifier (imiquimod). *J Am Acad Dermatol* 38:230-239, 1998.
33. Syed TA, Goswami J, Ahmadpour OA, et al: Treatment of molluscum contagiosum in males with an analog of imiquimod 1% in cream: a placebo-controlled, double-blind study. *J Dermatol* 25:309-313, 1998.

34. Bernstein DI, Miller RL, Harrison CJ: Effects of therapy with an immunomodulator (imiquimod, R-837) alone with acyclovir on genital HSV-2 infection in guinea pigs when begun after lesion development. *Antiviral Res* 20:45-55, 1993.

35. Miller RL, Imbertson LM, Reiter MJ, et al: Treatment of primary herpes simplex virus infection in guinea pigs by imiquimod. *Antiviral Res* 44:31-42, 1999.

Interferon-alpha

36. Shupack J, Stiller M, Knobler E, et al: Topical alpha-interferon in recurrent genital herpes simplex infection. *Dermatologica* 181:134-138, 1990.

37. Keay S, Teng N, Eisenberg M, et al: Topical interferon for treating condyloma acuminata in women. *J Infect Dis* 158:934-939, 1988.

38. Lebwohl M, Sacks S, Conant M: Recombinant alpha-2 interferon gel treatment of recurrent herpes genitalis. *Antiviral Res* 17:235-243, 1992.

Bleomycin

39. Bremner RM: Warts: treatment with intralesional bleomycin. *Cutis* 18:264-266, 1976.

40. Shumer SM, O'Keefe EJ: Bleomycin in the treatment of recalcitrant warts. *J Am Acad Dermatol* 9:91-96, 1983.

41. Munkvad M, Genner J, Staberg B, et al: Locally injected bleomycin in the treatment of warts. *Dermatologica* 167:86-89, 1983.

42. James MP, Collier PM, Aherne W, et al: Histologic, pharmacologic and immunocytochemical effects of injection of bleomycin into viral warts. *J Am Acad Dermatol* 28:933-937, 1993.

43. Amer M, Diab N, Ramadan A, et al: Therapeutic evaluation for intralesional injection of bleomycin sulfate in 143 resistant warts. *J Am Acad Dermatol* 18:1313-1316, 1988.

44. Cordero AA, Guglielmi HA, Woscoff A: The common wart: intralesional treatment with bleomycin sulfate. *Cutis* 26:319-324, 1980.

45. Munn SE, Higgins E, Marshall M, et al: A new method of intralesional bleomycin therapy in the treatment of recalcitrant warts. *Br J Dermatol* 135:969-971, 1996.

46. Epstein E: Persisting Raynaud's phenomenon following intralesional bleomycin treatment of finger warts. *J Am Acad Dermatol* 13:468-469, 1985.

47. Epstein E: Intralesional bleomycin and Raynaud's phenomenon. *J Am Acad Dermatol* 24:785-786, 1991.

48. Gregg L: Intralesional bleomycin and Raynaud's phenomenon. *J Am Acad Dermatol* 26:279-280, 1992.

49. Miller R: Nail dystrophy following intralesional injection of bleomycin for a periungual wart. *Arch Dermatol* 120:963-964, 1984.

50. Gonzalez FU, Gil M, Martinez AA: Cutaneous toxicity of intralesional bleomycin administration in the treatment of periungual warts. *Arch Dermatol* 122:974-975, 1986.

51. Estes SA: Personal communication, 2000.

Podophyllin

52. Edwards A, Atma-Ram A, Thin RN: Podophyllotoxin 0.5% v podophyllin 20% to treat penile warts. *Genitourin Med* 64:263-265, 1988.

53. Tyring S, Edwards C, Cherry LK: Safety and efficacy of 0.5% podofilox gel in the treatment of anogenital warts. *Arch Dermatol* 134:33-38, 1998.

54. Baker DA, Douglas JM Jr, Buntin DM: Topical podofilox for the treatment of condyloma acuminata in women. *Obstet Gynecol* 76:656-659, 1990.

55. Petersen CS, Weismann K: Quercetin and kaempherol: an argument against the use of podophyllin? *Genitourin Med* 71:92-93, 1995.

Trichloroacetic Acid

56. Boothby RA, Carlson JA, Rubin M, et al: Single application treatment of human papillomavirus infection of the cervix and vagina with trichloroacetic acid: a randomized trial. *Obstet Gynecol* 70:278-280, 1990.

57. Baker GE, Tyring SK: Therapeutic approaches to papillomavirus infections. *Dermatol Clin* 15:331-340, 1997.

58. Godley MJ, Bradbeer CS, Gellan M, et al: Cryotherapy compared with trichloroacetic acid in treating genital warts. *Genitourin Med* 63:390-392, 1987.

59. Abdullah AN, Walzman M, Wade A: Treatment of external genital warts comparing cryotherapy (liquid nitrogen) and trichloroacetic acid. *Sex Trans Dis* 20:344-345, 1993.

60. Malviya VK, Deppe G, Pluszczynski R, et al: Trichloroacetic acid in the treatment of human papillomavirus infection of the cervix without associated dysplasia. *Obstet Gynecol* 70:72-74, 1987.

Cantharidin

61. Epstein WL, Kingman AM: Treatment of warts with cantharidin. *Arch Dermatol* 77:508, 1958.
62. Seres Laboratories: Personal communication, 2000.
63. Funt TR, Mehr KA: Cantharidin: a valuable office treatment of molluscum contagiosum. *South Med J* 72:1019, 1979.

Salicylic Acid

64. Mroczkowski TF, McEwen C: Warts and other human papillomavirus infections. *Postgrad Med* 78:91-98, 1985.

5-Fluorouracil

65. Krebs HB: Use of topical 5-fluorouracil in the treatment of genital condylomas. *Obstet Gynecol Clin North Am* 14:559-568, 1987.
66. Krebs HB: Treatment of extensive bulbar condylomata acuminata with topical 5-fluorouracil. *South Med J* 83:761-764, 1990.
67. Krebs HB: Treatment of vaginal condylomata acuminata by weekly topical application of 5-fluorouracil. *Obstet Gynecol* 70:68-71, 1987.

James E. Rasmussen

Antiparasitic Agents

SCABIES AND LICE

Table 26-1 lists antiparasitic agents.

Permethrin

PHARMACOLOGY.   Key pharmacologic concepts for permethrin are listed in Table 26-2. Permethrin is a synthetic pyrethroid used as an approximate 1:3 mixture of the *cis-* and *trans-*isomers of (±)-3-phenoxybenzyl 3-(2,2-dichlorovinyl)-2,2-dimethyl cyclopropane-carboxylate (Figure 26-1). It has a molecular formula of $C_{21}H_{20}Cl_2O_3$ and a molecular weight of 391.29.[1] Permethrin is available as a 5% cream (Elimite) for the total body topical treatment of scabies and as a 1% cream rinse (Nix) for the treatment of head lice.

After application of the 5% permethrin cream, mean absorption was less than 1%, with a maximum of 2%.[2] In studies using 5% permethrin lotion (not commercially available), most of the test subjects had undetectable levels of permethrin in plasma samples, and the maximum absorption was .032% of the applied dose. Permethrin is metabolized through ester cleavages, and inactive metabolites are secreted in the urine. These esterases have been identified in the skin.

Mechanism of Action.   Permethrin is reported to act on the cell membrane of arthropods by disabling the sodium transport mechanism, which is responsible for maintenance of polarization of arthropod neuromembranes.[3] Paralysis is the consequence.

CLINICAL USE
Approved Indications
Scabies.   The treatment of choice for scabies is either topical permethrin (Elimite) or systemic ivermectin (Stromectol 200 μg/kg as a single dose). Scabies is an ancient disease, for which the worldwide incidence is unknown. It is probably much more common in conditions of poverty, poor hygiene, and overcrowding. Before the 1940s, the treatment of choice was probably 6% precipitated sulfur in a cream or ointment base applied on multiple consecutive days. This drug appears to have been relatively safe and effective. The 1940s through the 1960s saw the advent of organochloride and organophosphate insecticides, which soon began to have widespread use in the treatment of scabies. During the years 1950 to 1990, 1% lindane was probably the treatment of choice for scabies. In many countries of the world, malathion has been used extensively, although this product was only available for a very short period of time in the United States (circa 1990).

Pyrethrins are organic compounds that were originally derived from a species of the genus *Compositae*, which is related to chrysanthemums. Because of the chemical instability and relative lack of effectiveness, chemists soon developed synthetic pyrethroids such as permethrin, which have a wide range of activity against lice, scabies, ticks, and many other arthropods. Ivermectin (Stromectol) is the most recent addition to the list of drugs used to treat scabies.

Table 26-1 Antiparasitic Agents

Drug	Trade Name	Formulations/Sizes	Clinical Indications
Permethrin	Elimite (Rx)	5% cream—60 g	Scabies
	Nix (OTC)	1% cream rinse—60 ml	Head lice, pubic lice
Ivermectin	Stromectol (Rx)	6 mg tablets	Scabies, head lice
Pyrethrins	Rid, A200 (OTC)	0.3% shampoo, 60 ml	Head lice, pubic lice
	Barc, etc	0.18% lotion, 60, 120 ml	
		0.3% lotion	
Lindane	None (Rx)	1% shampoo—59 ml	Head lice, pubic lice
		1% lotion—59 ml	Scabies
Crotamiton	Eurax (Rx)	10% cream—60 g	Scabies
		10% lotion 60, 465 ml	
Malathion	*	0.5%-1% solution	Head lice, pubic lice
Benzyl benzoate	None (Rx)	20%-25% solution	Scabies
Thiabendazole	Mintezol (Rx)	500 mg tablets	"Creeping eruption"
Precipitated sulfur	6% in cream/ ointment base (Rx)	500 mg per 5 ml suspension, 120 ml	Scabies

Rx, Prescription; *OTC*, over the counter.
*Not commercially available in the United States.

Table 26-2 Key Pharmacologic Concepts—Antiparasitic Agents

	Permethrin	Ivermectin	Lindane	Malathion	Topical Thiabendazole
Absorption	<1%	Not well studied	5%-10%	Unknown	Unknown
Mechanism	Blocks neural transmission	Blocks glutamate-gated chloride	Organochloride, blocks neural transmission	Organophosphate; cholinesterase inhibitor, blocks neural transmission	May inhibit fumarate reductase
Metabolism	Ester cleavage	Hepatic	Stored in fat	Hepatic	Liver going to the glucuronide
Excretion	Urine	Feces	Urine, stool	Unknown	Urine
Toxicity	None	None	Central nervous system, primarily seizures	Seizures and paralysis, respiratory distress	None serious

THERAPEUTIC GUIDELINES. The cream should be applied from neck to toes and not just to visibly affected body sites. Particular care should be paid to the hands and fingernail areas because these sites harbor the greatest concentration of mites. In addition, intertriginous sites (including between digits) need careful application. Infants and young children who exhibit visible disease on the head and neck should have the cream applied to these areas as well. Permethrin cream is approved for use in patients 2 months of age and older. It has no recognized toxicity in infants younger than this and is commonly used in young patients of any age.

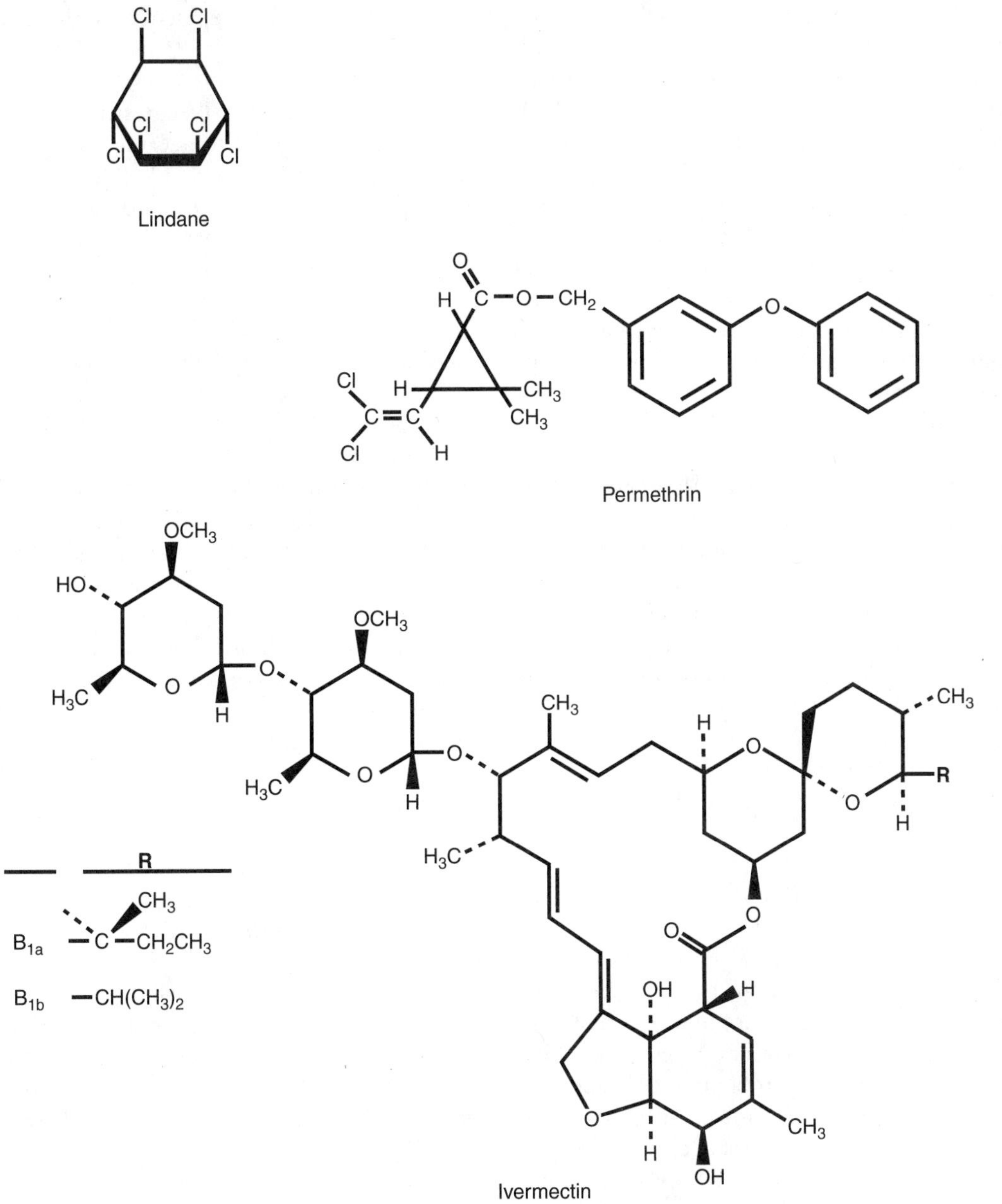

Lindane

Permethrin

Ivermectin

Figure 26-1   Antiparasitic agents.

HEAD LICE
Permethrin

The drug of choice for head lice is permethrin 1% cream rinse (Nix). Other drugs are pyrethrins with piperonyl butoxide (Rid, A-200, and others), malathion, lindane, and ivermectin.

PHARMACOLOGY.   The pharmacology of permethrin is discussed in the previous section on scabies.

CLINICAL USE
Approved Indications

Head Lice.   Pyrethrins with piperonyl butoxide (Rid, A-200, others) and permethrin (Nix) are approved by the FDA for the treatment of head lice. These compounds are available as over-the-counter agents. Some authors[4] consider 5% permethrin cream (Elimite) to be a more effective agent for the treatment of head lice than either of these two compounds.

Permethrin 5% cream (Elimite) is approved by the FDA for the treatment of infestation with *Sarcoptes scabiei*. It can also be used in the treatment of head and pubic lice, particularly when resistance to the 1% cream rinse (Nix) currently available is thought to be a problem.

Although 1% permethrin (Nix) and pyrethroids (Rid, etc) are marketed as a single application treatment for head lice, all products should be reapplied at the end of a week. Resistance to these agents has been reported to be common,[5] although "resistance" sometimes represents improper application technique or incorrect diagnosis.

ADVERSE EFFECTS. There have been no serious reported adverse reactions other than local irritation, which is common to all topical applications on inflamed skin.

It is not known if permethrin is secreted in human milk; however, the manufacturers suggest that nursing be discontinued or withheld if the drug is used in a nursing mother.

PREGNANCY PRESCRIBING STATUS. The pregnancy prescribing status of these drugs is category B.

CLINICAL COMPARISONS. To date, there have been no side-by-side clinical comparisons in which naive populations have been studied. Permethrin will probably be more effective when introduced into populations that had long-term exposure to other scabeticides, which is due to the theoretic problem of resistance developing with prior exposure. Although there are anecdotal reports of resistance developing to permethrin,[6-8] it is rare. In fact, most of the patients who are referred to clinicians with "resistant scabies" either do not have scabies or have been treated improperly.

Ivermectin

Ivermectin (Stromectol) is an anti-helminthic agent approved by the FDA for the treatment of strongyloidiasis and onchocerciasis.[9] Published reports on the efficacy of this drug in the treatment of scabies and head lice are few but impressive.[10] Several authors and publications consider it to be the treatment of choice in part because of its effectiveness and ease of administration, particularly in epidemics of these parasitic infestations.

PHARMACOLOGY. Ivermectin is 5-O-demethyl-22,23-dihydroavermectin A_{1A}. The empiric formula is $C_{48}H_{74}O_{14}$. As used commercially, the drug also contains less than 10% ivermectin A_{1B} 5-O-demethyl-25-de(1-methylpropyl)-22,23-dihydro-25-(1-methylethyl), which is sometimes referred to as ivermectin B.[9] Ivermectin is available in 6 mg tablets and is used at a dose of 200 μg/kg. The final dose is usually about 12 to 18 mg per adult administered as a single dose.

After a single dose, mean peak plasma concentration peaks at 4 hours. The drug is extensively metabolized in the liver, with the excretion primarily in the feces over the next 10 to 14 days. Plasma half-life is approximately 16 hours.

Mechanism of Action. Ivermectin blocks glutamate-gated, chloride ion channels, with adverse effects on nerve and muscle resulting in paralysis and death of the helminth.[10] The drug has a very low affinity for mammalian chloride channels. Although it has not been well studied in scabies and head lice, it is presumed that its mechanism of action for ivermectin is similar.

CLINICAL USES
Approved Indications
Onchocerciasis and Strongyloidiasis. Ivermectin is approved by the FDA for the treatment of onchocerciasis and strongyloidiasis. Its clinical use in scabies has been described in only a few publications, one of which reported it as effective when used in a 1% cream base.[5,10,11]
Other Indications
Scabies. Meinking and colleagues[10] reported that a single dose of ivermectin produced 100% cures in 11 patients with scabies. In 11 human immunodeficiency virus (HIV)–positive patients, the authors' reported clinical effectiveness rate was about 70% with a single ivermectin dose and greater than 90% efficacy with two doses.[10] Two of the HIV-positive patients had "crusted scabies." Only a few other reports described the use of ivermectin for scabies.[12-14]

ADVERSE EFFECTS. Adverse effects of ivermectin used in a single oral dose are reported to be very infrequent.[10] Because of the ease of administration, high rate of effectiveness, and low rate of adverse effects, some authors consider ivermectin to be the treatment of choice for scabies and head lice. Most of the reported adverse effects[12,13] in the treatment of onchocerciasis and strongyloidiasis have been noted with accidental intoxication from veterinary formulations and include headache, dizziness, nausea, vomiting, ataxia, and seizures. In one epidemiologic study done by Barkwell and Shields,[15] an increased death rate was thought to be due to this drug when used in a nursing home setting. Other authors scrutinized the Barkwell report and presented additional data, casting significant doubt regarding the true causal relationship of ivermectin with these nursing home deaths.[16,17]

PREGNANCY PRESCRIBING STATUS.   The pregnancy prescribing status of ivermectin is category C.

DRUG INTERACTIONS.   There are no drug interactions known involving oral ivermectin therapy.

Lindane
PHARMACOLOGY.   Lindane is the gamma isomer of 1,2,3,4,5,6 hexachlorocyclohexane with a formula of $C_6H_6Cl_6$ and a molecular weight of 290.83. It is currently available as a prescription only in 1% lotion for the treatment of scabies and 1% shampoo for the treatment of head lice. The familiar brand Kwell is no longer manufactured. After topical application in infants and children, peak serum half-life is observed at 18 hours, with a mean peak blood level of 28 ng/ml 6 hours after total body application.[18] Lindane is widely distributed throughout the body and slowly metabolized. It has a predilection for storage in fatty tissues as well as the brain. Minute amounts of lindane can be detected for months after application.

Franz and associates[2] estimated lindane absorption at 10 times that of permethrin, with serum levels about 40 times higher because of differences in metabolism. Lindane levels rise rapidly with repeated frequent application. Levels are reported to be higher in infants, in young children, and in those with reduced body fat levels such as premature infants.[19]

Mechanism of Action.   Lindane is an organochlorine insecticide that inhibits neurotransmission, inducing respiratory and muscular paralysis in parasitic arthropods.

CLINICAL USE
Approved Indications
Scabies.   Lindane 1% lotion is approved by the FDA "only for the treatment of patients infested with *Sarcoptes scabiei* (scabies) who have either failed to respond to adequate doses or are intolerant of other approved therapies."[18] Lindane cream is no longer available for use in scabies.

Lindane 1% shampoo is indicated "only for the treatment of patients with pediculosis capitis (head lice) and pediculosis pubis (crab lice) who have either failed to respond to adequate doses or are intolerant of other approved therapies."[18]

All readers should appreciate that this is a substantial change from earlier FDA approval, in which lindane was considered first-line therapy (at times the drug of choice) for the treatment of pediculosis and scabies. The reasons for these changes are clear, and lindane must now be considered more toxic than other choices.

Lindane lotion 1% should be applied to all affected areas for the treatment of scabies, which usually means from the neck to the toes. Particular attention should be given to the fingernail areas. It should be left on 8 to 12 hours (usually overnight) and then rinsed off. Shorter periods of exposure (up to 4 hours) have not been well studied but are probably effective. The drug should never be given on a daily basis, although some clinicians use two treatments separated by a 1-week interval.

ADVERSE EFFECTS.   Toxicity with proper use of lindane is rare. With ingestion of or repeated exposure to lindane, adverse effects seem to center around the central nervous system with multiple reports of seizures due to this drug.[20-23] Other concerns have been about reported emergence of resistant scabies and lice.

In laboratory animals the drug is rated as a possible hepatic carcinogen, although this statement is based on long-term, high-dose feeding studies.[18] It is difficult to extrapolate these animal studies to a single lifetime exposure given in a clinical setting.

Other infrequently reported adverse effects include hematologic disorders such as aplastic anemia.[18]

Medical and consumer opinion has swung solidly against lindane. A leading consumer magazine lists lindane as a remedy "which should not be used."[24] For a variety of reasons stated in this section, lindane is no longer indicated for the treatment of scabies or lice in any patient.

PREGNANCY PRESCRIBING STATUS. The pregnancy prescribing status of lindane is category B.

CLINICAL COMPARISONS. Some studies indicate that permethrin products used for the treatment of head lice have a repository effect and are therefore more effective against hatching nits. In some clinical populations frequently exposed to lindane, resistance developed, and in these areas, recently introduced products are more effective. In the United States, however, reports of lindane resistance are anecdotal and may represent inadequate treatment methods rather than true resistance.[25-29] However, it is quite logical to assume that arthropods could eventually develop resistance to any antiparasitic agent in use.

Malathion

PHARMACOLOGY. Malathion is available as a 0.5% solution for the treatment of head lice. The chemical formula is $C_{10}H_{19}O_6PS_2$, with a molecular weight of 330.36. Malathion is an organophosphate cholinesterase inhibitor, which produces neuromuscular paralysis in arthropods.

CLINICAL USE

Head Lice. Malathion is used throughout the world as a very effective treatment for head lice[30] and scabies. Like almost all the other described agents, it is extensively used as a pesticide in agriculture. The product was marketed in the United States for only a few years around 1990 and then withdrawn. Malathion is no longer available in the United States.

ADVERSE EFFECTS. Percutaneous absorption of malathion in vivo has not been well studied, although toxicity from topical application is extremely rare.[31] The drug is rapidly inactivated. It is widely used on commercial crops meant for human consumption.

The solution marketed in the United States was odoriferous and flammable. Systemic toxicity has only been reported with oral ingestion where the symptoms are similar to those of other organophosphate poisonings with cholinesterase depletion. Severe respiratory distress is the most serious toxicity of organophosphate poisoning. Malathion is not known to be a carcinogen.

Nonpharmacologic Therapy for Head Lice

Many authorities believe that removing nits from the scalp hair is essential in the treatment of head lice. There are several products and home remedies (such as vinegar) that are reported to help loosen the nits from the hair, although published data on their effectiveness are sparse. Many authorities and patient advocacy groups promote the concept of a no-nit policy, such as the policy that children are allowed to return to school only when free from carrying any nits in their scalp hair. Whether this is effective in assisting the pharmacologic therapy of head lice is logical, yet unproved. There are no published studies that document the effectiveness of nit combing. Many of the nit combs may be inadequate for the job and can impose a significant temporal and psychologic burden on both the patient and the parent. A recent consumer publication promotes the use of a redesigned metal comb called the "Lice Meister," which is available from the National Pediculosis Association (781-449-NITS).[24] Adequate nit combing can be time consuming and must be repeated every few nights for a couple of weeks.

Less Frequently Used Drugs

Table 26-3 lists indications and contraindications for antiparasitic agents.

CROTAMITON. Crotamiton (Eurax) is available as a 10% cream or lotion that is FDA approved for the eradication of scabies. Thirty grams should be applied from neck to toes on 2 consecutive days. In published studies,[30] this drug is only minimally effective for the treatment of scabies. There are no significant adverse

■ **Table 26-3**   Indications and Contraindications

	FDA-Approved Indications	Off-Label Uses	Contraindications
Permethrin	Scabies, lice (as primary therapy)		Children less than 2 months of age
Ivermectin	Strongyloidiasis, onchocerciasis	Scabies, head lice	None
Lindane	Scabies, lice (only if unresponsive to other therapy)	None	Premature children, patients with history of seizures, Norwegian scabies
Crotamiton	Scabies	None	None
Malathion	None	Head lice, pubic lice	None
Benzyl benzoate	None	Scabies	None
Precipitated sulfur	None	Scabies, head lice	None
Thiabendazole	Cutaneous larva migrans	None	None

reactions to crotamiton. The pregnancy prescribing status is category C.

BENZYL BENZOATE.   Benzyl benzoate can be made in 20% to 25% solutions for the topical treatment of scabies. There are no commercially available preparations, although this drug is often used in veterinary medicine. There are few published studies on its use in scabies in humans.[32] It is commonly used in many countries outside of the United States where it is reported to be a very inexpensive and effective compound. Adverse reactions are usually limited to skin irritation. Safety in pregnancy has not been established.

PRECIPITATED SULFUR.   A compound containing 6% precipitated sulfur is a time-honored and accepted therapy for the treatment of scabies. Although no commercial preparation exists, it can be compounded in a 6% cream or ointment vehicle and is usually prescribed daily until the patient has improved. Many authors consider it to be the drug of choice for the treatment of scabies in pregnant women, although there are no published studies for this indication. In addition, reports that precipitated sulfur is safer in this patient group cannot be substantiated. The only well-documented adverse effect is the drug's obnoxious odor.

LARVA MIGRANS AND LARVA CURRENS

This section discusses drugs used for larva migrans and larva currens. Larva migrans is also referred to as cutaneous larva migrans, creeping eruption, and sandworm disease.

Thiabendazole
PHARMACOLOGY.   Thiabendazole is 2-(4-thiazoly)-1H-benzimidazole.[33] The empiric formula is $C_{10}H_7N_2S$. The drug has a molecular weight of 201.26.

After oral administration the drug is rapidly absorbed with peak blood concentration seen at about 1 to 2 hours.[33] It is metabolized extensively in the liver and excreted in the urine as glucuronide or sulfate conjugates. The pharmacology of topical applications has not been well studied.

Mechanism of Action.   Thiabendazole probably acts via inhibition of the helminth-specific enzyme fumarate reductase.

CLINICAL USE
Approved Indications.   Common causes of larva migrans are dog and cat hookworms (e.g., *Ancylostoma braziliense, Ancylostoma caninum*). Larva currens is caused by *Strongyloides stercoralis*.

These round worms characteristically parasitize the intestines of their natural hosts (e.g., dogs, cats, and others). Eggs are deposited in the feces and incubate in the soil. Humans are exposed in temperate or tropical areas, such as the beaches of tropical islands, as well as relatively sandy soil in southern portions of the United States. The eruption usually begins on exposed areas such as the feet, buttocks, or back.

The extremely pruritic cutaneous eruption is characteristic, consisting of numerous inflammatory threadlike serpiginous tracks. An observant patient is able to recognize in which direction the larva is headed. Larva currens is usually noted around the buttocks, thighs, and upper back. The affected patient usually carries the *Strongyloides* organisms in the intestine, with the eggs frequently hatching before they are deposited outside the body. The hatched nematodes then crawl out the anal opening and infest the surrounding skin. Lesions of larva currens are noted to migrate at a faster rate, hence the Latin terminology "running larva."

In the past treatment has been limited to locally destructive applications of liquid nitrogen; however, this requires an appreciation of which direction the parasite is headed because the organism is several mm to 1 cm ahead of the visible inflammatory trail. Even without therapy, the lesions are self-limited, usually resolving spontaneously in 1 to 3 weeks. Topical steroids may be somewhat effective in providing symptomatic relief during this phase.

More effective therapy involves the topical or systemic use of thiabendazole. Other agents used include oral albendazole and ivermectin.

THERAPEUTIC GUIDELINES. Thiabendazole (Mintezol) is available as 500 mg chewable tablets and as a suspension containing 500 mg per 5 ml.[33] Thiabendazole has FDA approval for the treatment of *Strongyloides* organisms, cutaneous larva migrans, visceral larva migrans, and trichinosis. The standard dose for cutaneous larva migrans is 1.5 g (3 tablets) for 2 successive days.[33] The tablet should be chewed before swallowing.

Thiabendazole can also be used topically by applying the suspension to the lesions three or four times daily for 3 to 4 days.[34]

ADVERSE EFFECTS. Gastrointestinal symptoms, such as nausea, vomiting, and diarrhea, are common when the drug is used orally. Aside from local irritation, adverse effects from topical thiabendazole are rare.

DRUG INTERACTIONS. Oral thiabendazole may elevate levels of theophylline.[33]

PREGNANCY PRESCRIBING STATUS. The pregnancy prescribing status of thiabendazole is category C.

Bibliography

Medical Reviews

Anonymous: Drugs for head lice. *Med Lett Drugs Ther* 39:6-7, 1997.

Anonymous: Drugs for parasitic infections. *Med Lett Drugs Ther* 40:1-12, 1998.

Burkhart CG, Burkhart CN, Burkhart KM: An assessment of topical and oral prescription and over-the-counter treatments for head lice. *J Am Acad Dermatol* 38:979-982, 1998.

Elgart M: A risk-benefit assessment of agents used in the treatment of scabies. *Drug Saf* 14:386-393, 1996.

Liu LX, Weller PF: Antiparasitic drugs. *N Engl J Med* 334:1178-1184, 1996.

Meinking TL, Taplin D: Safety of permethrin vs lindane for the treatment of scabies. *Arch Dermatol* 132:959-962, 1996.

Taplin D, Meinking TL: Permethrin. *Curr Probl Dermatol* 24:255-260, 1996.

Consumer Oriented Articles

Consumer Reports Cray D, Ghosh C, King W, et al: A lousy nit-picking epidemic. February:62-63, 1998.

Time January 12:73-74, 1998.

References

Permethrin

1. Elimite Cream. Allergan, Inc. *Physicians' desk reference,* Montvale, NJ, 2000, p 497.
2. Franz TJ, Lehman PA, Franz SF, et al: Comparative percutaneous absorption of lindane and permethrin. *Arch Dermatol* 132:901-905, 1996.
3. Narahashi T: Nerve membrane Na+ channels as targets of insecticides. *Trends Pharmacol Sci* 13:236-241, 1992.
4. Meinking TL, Taplin D: Safety of permethrin vs lindane for the treatment of scabies. *Arch Dermatol* 132:959-962, 1996.
5. Drugs for head lice. *Med Lett Drugs Ther* 39:6-7, 1997.
6. Burgess IF, Peock S, Brown CM, et al: Head lice resistant to pyrethroid insecticides in Britain. *BMJ* 311:752, 1995.
7. Mumcuoglu KY, Hemingway J, Miller J, et al: Permethrin resistance in the head louse *Pediculus capitis* from Israel. *Med Vet Entomol* 9:427-432, pp 447, 1995.
8. Rupes V, Moravec J, Chmela J, et al: A resistance of head lice *(Pediculus capitis)* to permethrin in Czech Republic. *Centr Europ J Public Health* 3:30-32, 1995.

Ivermectin

9. Stromectol Tablets, Merck & Co, Inc: *Physicians' desk reference,* Montvale, NJ, 2000, pp 1886-1887.
10. Meinking TL, Taplin D, Hermida JL, et al: Treatment of scabies with ivermectin. *N Engl J Med* 333:26-30, 1995.
11. Drugs for parasitic infections. *Med Lett Drugs Ther* 40:1-12, 1998.
12. Gardon J, Gardon-Wendel N, Demanga-Ngangue, et al: Serious reactions after mass treatment of onchocerciasis with ivermectin in an area endemic for Loa loa infection. *Lancet* 350:18-22, 1997.
13. Cook GC: Adverse effects of chemotherapeutic agents used in tropical medicine. *Drug Saf* 13:31-45, 1995.
14. Corbett EL, Crossley I, Holton J, et al: Crusted ("Norwegian") scabies in a specialist HIV unit: successful use of ivermectin and failure to prevent nosocomial transmission. *Genitourin Med* 72:115-117, 1996.
15. Barkwell R, Shields S: Deaths associated with ivermectin treatment of scabies (letter). *Lancet* 349:1144-1145, 1997.

16. Coyne PE, Addiss DG: Deaths associated with ivermectin for scabies (letter). *Lancet* 350:215-216, 1997.
17. Diazgranados JA, Costa JL: Deaths after ivermectin treatment (letter). *Lancet* 349:1698, 1997.

Lindane

18. Lindane lotion USP, 1%. Alpharma U.S. Pharmaceuticals Division: *Physicians' desk reference,* Montvale NJ, 1998, pp 497-498.
19. Ginsburg CM, Loury W, Reisett JS: Absorption of lindane in infants and children. *J Pediatric* 91:353-357, 1997.
20. Solomon BA, Haut SR, Carr EM, et al: Neurotoxic reaction to lindane in an HIV-seropositive patient. An old medication's new problem. *J Fam Pract* 40:291-296, 1995.
21. Boffa MJ, Brough PA, Ead RD: Lindane neurotoxicity. *Br J Dermatol* 133:1013, 1995.
22. Sunder Ram Rao CV, Shreenivas R, Singh V, et al: Disseminated intravascular coagulation in a case of fatal lindane poisoning. *Vet Hum Toxicol* 30:132-134, 1988.
23. Davies JE, Dedhia HV, Morgade C, et al: Lindane poisonings. *Arch Dermatol* 119:142-144, 1983.
24. *Consumer Reports* February:62-63, 1998.
25. Hernandez-Perez E: Resistance to antiscabetic drugs. *J Am Acad Dermatol* 8:121-123, 1983.
26. Boix V, Sanchez-Paya J, Portilla J, et al: Nosocomial outbreak of scabies clinically resistant to lindane. *Infect Control Hosp Epidemiol* 18:677, 1997.
27. Brown S, Becher J, Brady W: Treatment of ectoparasitic infections: review of the English-language literature, 1982-1992. *Clin Infect Dis* 20(Suppl 1):S104-109, 1995.
28. Purvis RS, Tyring SK: An outbreak of lindane-resistant scabies treated successfully with permethrin 5% cream. *J Am Acad Dermatol* 25:1015-1016, 1991.

Malathion

29. Burgess I, Robinson RJF, Robinson J, et al: Aqueous malathion 0.5% as a scabicide: clinical trial. *BMJ* 292:1172, 1986.
30. Moeller HC, Rider JA: Plasma and red blood cell cholinesterase activity as indications of the threshold of incipient toxicity of EPN and malathion in human beings. *Toxicol Appl Pharmacol* 4:123-130, 1962.

31. Cubela V, Yawalkar SJ: Clinical experience with crotamiton cream and lotion in the treatment of infants with scabies. *Br J Clin Pract* 32:229-231, 1978.

Other Antiparasitic Agents

32. Haustein UF, Hlawa B: Treatment of scabies with permethrin versus lindane and benzyl benzoate. *Acta Derm Venereol* 69:348-351, 1989.

33. Mintezol, Merck & Co: *Physicians' desk reference,* Montvale, NJ, 2000, pp 1838-1839.

34. Jelinek T, Maiwald H, Nothdruft HD, et al: Cutaneous larva migrans in travelers: synopsis of histories, symptoms, and treatment of 98 patients. *Clin Infect Dis* 19:1062-1066, 1994.

PART VI

Topical Immunomodulatory and Antiproliferative Drugs

CHAPTER 27

Michael Warner
Charles Camisa

Topical Corticosteroids

The human body regulates inflammatory immunoreactions via endogenous glucocorticoids such as cortisol (hydrocortisone). In the early 1950s, physicians began using systemically administered cortisol to treat inflammatory dermatoses. Unfortunately, corticosteroids with a ketone group at C 11 (e.g., cortisone) must be reduced to their corresponding 11-hydroxyl analogs (e.g., hydrocortisone) to be active—a reduction that does not occur effectively in the skin. Thus early attempts to use topical cortisone failed until 1952, when Sulzberger and Witten successfully treated eczematous dermatitis with topical hydrocortisone. Their success marked a cornerstone in dermatology and the birth of a major new market for pharmaceutical companies. The next 5 decades of research, experience, and marketing led to the development of an ever-growing list of topical corticosteroid preparations and an array of interrelated facts attempting to explain their clinical effects. The pertinent points of topical corticosteroid (TCS) pharmacology and the appropriate use of TCS in dermatology are summarized in this chapter.

PHARMACOLOGY

To understand the pharmacology and pharmacokinetics of TCS, one must first understand how their clinical effect is measured and compared.

Estimating Potency

The term *potency* is used to describe the intensity of a TCS's clinical effect. To estimate clinical effect, assays measure aspects of the antiinflammatory and/or the antiproliferative properties of TCS (see Mechanisms of Action section) using laboratory animals or human volunteers (Box 27-1). The vasoconstrictor assay is the most commonly used test. In fact, the term *potency* is often misused to describe the vasoconstrictor rating of a TCS, which does not always correlate with clinical efficacy.

The actual vasoconstrictor assay usually involves the following[1]:

1. Preparing the test corticosteroid in 95% alcohol
2. Applying it to the volar surface of a normal volunteer's forearm
3. Allowing the alcohol to evaporate, then covering the test area with an occlusive dressing for 16 hours
4. Washing off the area
5. Assessing vasoconstriction (0 = none, 1 = mild, 2 = moderate, and 3 = intense) 2 hours later on a blind basis by an experienced investigator
6. Using statistical analysis mostly with the Wilcoxson's rank sum test based on the sum of signed ranks of difference

For more precise evaluation of the vasoconstrictive potential, one can use tenfold serial

Box 27-1

Examples of Commonly Used Glucocorticoid Assays

ASSAYS OF ANTIINFLAMMATORY POTENCY	ASSAYS OF ATROPHOGENICITY
Studies Using Laboratory Animals	**_Studies Using Cell Cultures_**
• Mitotic index suppression—hairless mouse	**_or Laboratory Animals_**
• Antigranuloma assay—rat	• Inhibition of fibroblast growth in vitro
• Croton oil inflammation assay—rat	• Neutral red release assay[†]
• 6-chloro-2-4-dinitrobenzene inflammation—	• Mouse tail epidermis
guinea pig	• Transgenic mouse model expressing human
	elastin promoter/chloramphenicol
Studies Using Human Volunteers	acetyltransferase[‡]
• Vasoconstrictor assay	• Guinea pig epidermis
• Artificially induced inflammation	
Tape stripping	**_Studies Using Human Volunteers_**
Ultraviolet light	• Micrometer calipers
Mustard oil	• Histopathologic examination of skin biopsies
Nitric acid	• X-ray radiography
Tetrahydrofurfuryl alcohol	• Pulsed ultrasound
Nickel-induced positive patch tests[*]	
• Spontaneously occurring skin disease (psoriasis)	

Adapted from Yohn JJ, Weston WL: *Curr Probl Dermatol* 2:40, 1990.
*Seidenari S, Di Nardo A, Mantovani L, et al: *Exp Dermatol* 6:75-80, 1997.
†Korting HC, Hulsebus E, Kerscher M, et al: *Br J Dermatol* 133:54-59, 1995.
‡Katchman SD, Del Monaco M, Wu M, et al: *Arch Dermatol* 131:1274-1278, 1995.

dilutions from 10^{-2} to 10^{-7} g/dl of TCS in ethanol and then plot dose-response curves for comparison.[2]

The vasoconstrictor assay is the assay of choice because it usually correlates well with clinical efficacy and is reproducible. In patients with psoriasis, for example, the vasoconstrictor assay demonstrated excellent correlation in bilateral, symmetric-paired comparisons of psoriatic target lesions treated one to three times daily for 2 to 3 weeks with 30 of 32 different TCS compounds.[3] The two exceptions were aclometasone ointment and hydrocortisone valerate cream, which both demonstrated greater vasoconstrictive activities than clinical efficacy. The vasoconstrictor assay proved to be reproducible by the same and other observers in completely different settings, locations, climates, and subjects.[4] The disadvantages are that the test is subjective, only measures one aspect of TCS effects, and produces no "hard copy" such as with an electrocardiogram or chest x-ray for subsequent comparisons, analysis, and validation. TCS preparations are best evaluated

with the vasoconstrictor assay and a second assay on spontaneously occurring skin diseases in human volunteers (e.g., psoriasis).

Pharmacokinetics

The pharmacokinetics and resultant clinical potency of a TCS preparation depend on three interrelated factors—the structure of the corticosteroid molecule, the vehicle, and skin onto which it is applied. The exact relationship between these factors is neither clear nor predictable; however, certain aspects have been elucidated.

STRUCTURE OF THE TCS MOLECULE. Hydrocortisone is considered the backbone of most TCS molecules (Figure 27-1 and Table 27-1). These molecules are formed by placing hydroxyl groups into the 11-β, 17-α, and 21 positions; ketone groups into the 3 and 20 positions; and a double bond into the 4 position of the glucocorticoid nucleus. The further addition or alteration of functional groups (e.g., hydroxy, hydrocarbon, ester, fluoro, chloro, acetonide, ketone) at certain positions can greatly

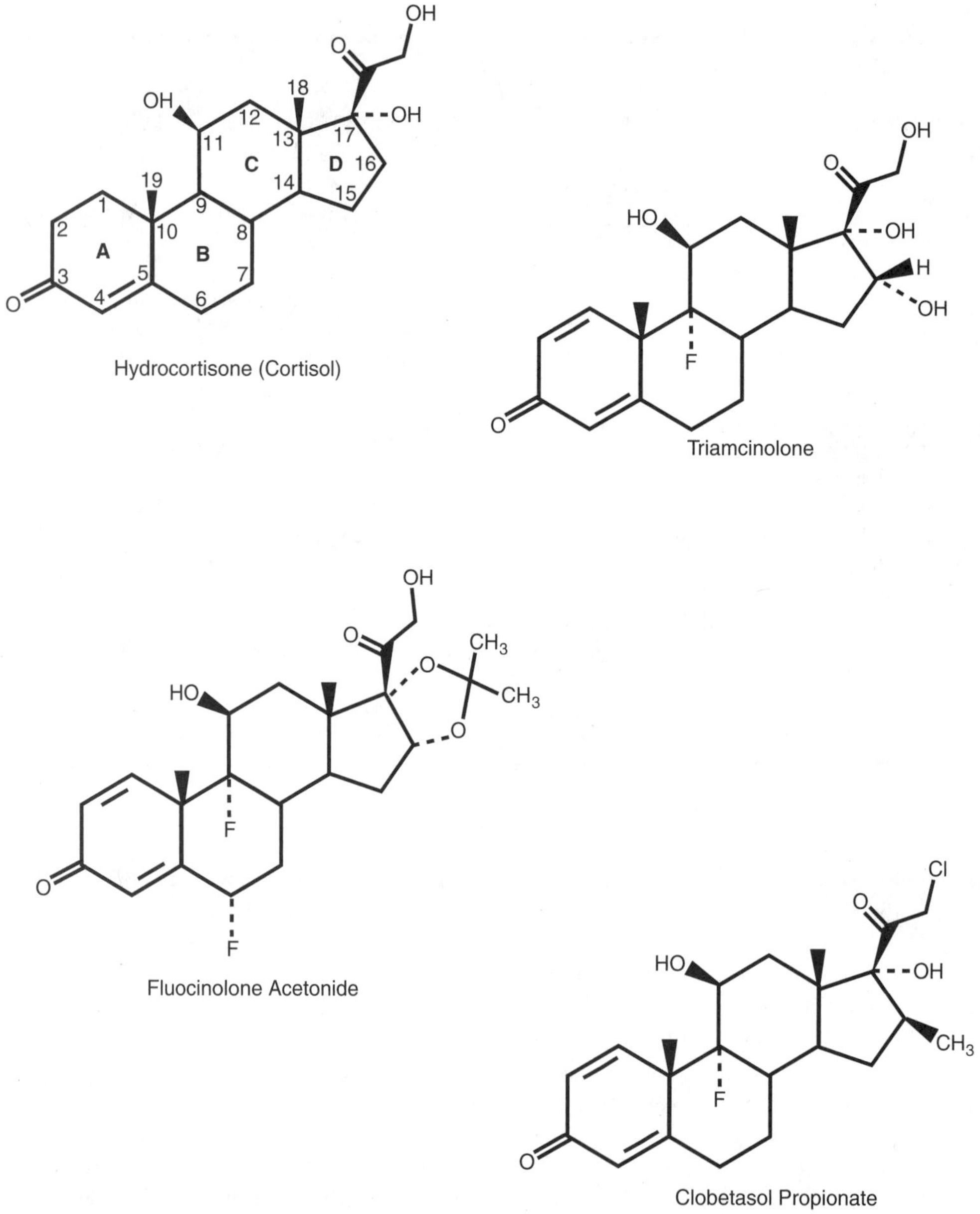

Figure 27-1   Topical corticosteroids.

affect the molecule's pharmacokinetics (see Table 27-1).

The removal, replacement, or masking of hydroxyl groups changes a molecule's lipophilicity, solubility, percutaneous absorption, and glucocorticoid receptor (GCR)-binding activity. Replacement of the 21-hydroxy group in betamethasone with a chloro moiety creates clotamethasone with a chloro moiety creates clo-

betasol, which binds much more tightly to the GCR.[5] Esterification or addition of acetonide groups masks hydroxyl groups. Esterification at the 17 position of betamethasone creates betamethasone-17-valerate, which binds much more tightly to GCR[5] and is approximately 125 times more potent than betamethasone in the vasoconstrictor assay.[1] Esterification at the 21

■ **Table 27-1** Structural Comparisons with Potency—Selected Topical Corticosteroids

Name	Relevant Functional Groups	Vasoconstrictor Potency Rating*
Hydrocortisone	C11: beta-hydroxyl C17: hydroxyl C20: ketone C21: hydroxyl	Class VII Low potency (1.0, 2.5%) Generic ointment
Triamcinolone acetonide	C1,2: double bond C9: fluorine C11: hydroxyl C16: hydroxyl	Class V Moderate (0.1%) Generic ointment
Fluocinolone acetonide acetate (fluocinonide)	C1,2: double bond C6: fluorine C9: fluorine C16,17: acetonide C21: ester (acetate)	Class II High potency (0.05%) Generic ointment
Clobetasol propionate	C1,2: double bond C9: fluorine C16: methyl C17: ester C21: chlorine	Class I Superpotent (0.05%) Generic ointment

*Vasoconstrictor potency of selected ointment for the TCS listed.

position of betamethasone creates betamethasone-21-valerate, which binds less tightly to the GCR[1] but significantly increases percutaneous absorption (and potency) by increasing the molecule's lipophilicity. Acetonide groups are formed from the 16-α, 17-α dihydroxy groups of triamcinolone and fluocinolone. Triamcinolone acetonide binds much more tightly to GCR than triamcinolone,[6] and fluocinolone acetonide penetrates human skin and hairless mouse skin 14 to 23 times faster than fluocinolone.[1] Fluocinolone acetonide can be further esterified at the 21 position to create fluocinolone acetonide acetate (fluocinonide), which is even more potent.

A double bond in the 1 position increases glucocorticoid activity. Halogenation at the 6-α or 9-α position increases GCR-binding activity, augmenting both glucocorticoid and mineralocorticoid activity. An additional fluorination (e.g., difluorisone diacetate-6-α) or chlorination further enhances the potency.[7] Addition of a 16-α methyl, 16-β methyl, or 16-α hydroxy group decreases mineralocorticoid activity; thus these functional groups are often incorporated into molecules containing 9-α or 6-α halogens such as dexamethasone, betamethasone, and triamcinolone.

Structural modifications also affect biotransformation. Enzymes in the epidermis cause deesterification of TCS into inactive metabolites. Halogenation at the 21 position (e.g., clobetasol propionate) inhibits deesterification at the 17 position and significantly increases potency.[8] Halogenation at the 9-α position also decreases biotransformation.

VEHICLE.   The vehicle is a highly engineered balance of numerous chemicals, each serving a separate or overlapping purpose (Box 27-2). Emollients are incorporated to retard transepidermal water loss, occlude the corticosteroid molecule, and increase flexibility of the skin. Emulsifying agents are required to create oil-in-water preparations such as creams and lotions. Other chemicals act to stabilize emulsions and thicken the final preparation. Solvents are used in lotions,

Box 27-2

Selected Vehicle Ingredients by Function

EMOLLIENTS
Butyl stearate
Caprylic/capric triglyceride
Castor oil
Cetearyl alcohol
Cetyl alcohol
Diisopropyl adipate
Glycerin
Glyceryl monostearate
Isopropyl myristate
Isopropyl palmitate
Lanolin
Lanolin alcohol
Lanolin, hydrogenated
Mineral oil
Petrolatum
Polyethylene glycols
Polyoxypropylene 15-stearyl ether
Propylene glycol stearate
Squalene
Stearic acid
Stearyl alcohol

EMULSIFYING AGENTS
Amphoteric-9
Carbomer
Cetearyl alcohol (and) ceteareth-20
Cholesterol
Disodium monooleamideosulfosuccinate
Emulsifying wax, NF
Lanolin
Lanolin alcohol
Lanolin, hydrogenated
Polyethylene glycol 1000 monocetyl ether
Polyoxyl 40 stearate
Polysorbates
Sodium laureth sulfate
Sodium lauryl sulfate
Sorbitan esters
Stearic acid
Triethanol amine stearate
Trolamine

HUMECTANTS
Glycerin
Propylene glycol
Sorbitol solution

EMULSION STABILIZERS AND VISCOSITY BUILDERS
Carbomer
Cetearyl alcohol
Cetyl alcohol

EMULSION STABILIZERS AND VISCOSITY BUILDERS—cont'd
Glyceryl monostearate
Polyethylene glycols
Propylene glycol stearate
Stearyl alcohol

THICKENING, STIFFENING SUSPENDING AGENTS
Beeswax (white wax or yellow wax)
Canthum gum
Carbomer
Cetyl esters wax
Dextrin
Polyethylene

SOLVENTS
Alcohol
Diisopropyl adipate
Glycerin
1,2,6-hexanetriol
Isopropyl myristate
Polyoxypropylene 15 stearyl ether
Propylene carbonate
Propylene glycol

PRESERVATIVES, ANTIOXIDANTS, AND CHEMICAL STABILIZERS
Alcohol
Benzyl alcohol
2-Bromo-2-nitropropane-1,3,-diol
Butylated hydroxyanisole (BHA)
Butylated hydroxytoluene (BHT)
Chlorocresol (P-chloro-m-cresol)
Citric acid
Diazolidinyl urea
Dimethyloldimethyl (DMDM) hydantoin
Edetate disodium
Glutaraldehyde
Methylchlororisothiazoline/methyliso-
    thiazolinone (Kathon CG)
Parabens
Potassium sorbate
Propyl gallate
Propylene glycol
Quaternium-15
Sodium bisulfite
Sorbic acid
Thimerosal

Adapted from *The base book,* Syntex Laboratories, Inc. USA, 1982.

solutions, gels, and sprays to create a less viscous product. Humectants are necessary in all oil-in-water preparations to maintain the required water content.

The vehicle can indirectly alter a given preparation's therapeutic and adverse actions by altering the pharmacokinetics of the TCS molecule.[9] Solvents like propylene glycol and ethanol, for example, affect the TCS molecule's solubility in the vehicle and skin by affecting its percutaneous absorption.[10] Very occlusive vehicles also enhance a TCS molecule's percutaneous absorption probably by increasing the hydration of the stratum corneum.[11] For this reason, a TCS molecule in an ointment vehicle tends to be more potent than the same concentration of the molecule in a cream or lotion. Emulsifiers help to distribute the drug evenly on the skin surface. The vehicle can also directly contribute to a preparation's therapeutic and adverse effects (see Adverse Effects and Therapeutic Guidelines sections) and ultimately determine a given TCS preparation's acceptance by the patient.

CONDITION OF THE SKIN.   The condition of the skin also affects bioavailability. Penetration of the applied drug correlates inversely with the thickness of the stratum corneum.[11] Penetration increases with inflamed or diseased skin[9] and increases with increased hydration of the stratum corneum, relative humidity, and temperature.[11] The stratum corneum may also act as a reservoir for TCS for up to 5 days; this retention is TCS concentration- and formulation-dependent.[12]

MECHANISMS OF ACTION

The list of available TCS preparations can only be matched by the list of possible mechanisms of action (Boxes 27-3 and 27-4). An understanding of the mechanisms helps direct research toward more effective TCS derivatives.

TCS exert their effects through both direct and indirect mechanisms, which are mediated via the GCR as follows:

1. The corticosteroid diffuses into the target cell and binds to the GCR in the cytoplasm.[13]

2. The corticosteroid-GCR complex undergoes necessary conformational changes.[14]
3. The resulting active complex traverses the nuclear envelope and binds to "acceptor sites" on DNA.[15]
4. Gene regulation and transcription of various specific messenger ribonucleic acid (mRNA) occur.[16,17]

GCR can be found in almost all types of cells in the human body, accounting for the long list of GCR-mediated effects.

Antiinflammatory Effects

TCS seem to affect every aspect of cutaneous inflammation—inflammatory cells, chemical mediators, and tissue responses. All cells involved with inflammation are affected. Epidermal Langerhans' cells, the antigen-presenting cell responsible for initiation of both nonspecific and acquired immune responses, are reduced in number and demonstrate decreased cellular receptors, indicating decreased antigen-presenting function. Polymorphonuclear leukocytes have less ability to adhere to vascular endothelium and are reduced in number at sites of inflammation.[18-20] Their phagocytic and antibacterial capabilities are diminished.[21] Monocytes are also decreased in number at sites of inflammation and show decreased fungicidal activity and clearance of opsonized particles.[22-24] Lymphocytes demonstrate decreased antibody-dependent cellular cytotoxicity[25] and decreased natural killer cell activity.[26] Mast cell sensitization and mediator release induced by immunoglobulin E (IgE) are inhibited.[27,28] TCS also reduce the synthesis and secretion of cytokines and inflammatory proteins necessary to initiate and sustain an immune response. Production of interleukin (IL)-1, IL-2, interferon (IFN)- γ, tumor necrosis factor, and granulocyte-monocyte-stimulating factor is reduced.[29] TCS induce lipocortins,[30] which inhibit phospholipase A_2 and subsequent cell surface liberation of platelet-activating factor (PAF) and arachidonic acid as well as associated potent inflammatory mediators. TCS even affect the vascular component of inflammation by augmenting the vasoconstrictive response to epinephrine and norepinephrine[31-34] and reducing the responses to histamine and bradykinin.[35] To-

Box 27-3

Corticosteroid Mechanisms of Action—Antiinflammatory Effects

DIRECT EFFECTS (IMMEDIATE)
- Stabilize cell and lysosomal membranes, prevent release of lysosomal contents and phospholipid precursors for synthesis of prostaglandins and PAF
- Potentiate vascular response to catecholamines
- Reduce vascular smooth muscle sensitivity to histamine and bradykinin
- Inhibit mast cell sensitization induced by IgE
- Inhibit release of histamine and other mast cell mediators

GCR-MEDIATED EFFECTS (DELAYED)
- Induction of antiinflammatory proteins— lipocortins, vasocortin, and vasoregulin
- Lipocortins inhibit phospholipase A_2 and block release of arachidonic acid and PAF from cell membranes; therefore prevent formation of potent inflammatory mediators including prostaglandins, leukotrienes, 12-HETE, and 15-HETE
- Lipocortins also prevent PAF-induced wheal and flare reactions and leukocyte chemotaxis
- Vasocortin and vasoregulin decrease vascular permeability

ANTIINFLAMMATORY ACTIONS ON SPECIFIC CELLS (PROBABLY BOTH DIRECT AND GCR-MEDIATED EFFECTS)
Polymorphonuclear Leukocytes
- Decrease ability to adhere to vascular endothelium
- Decrease migration to sites of inflammation
- Reduce number at sites of inflammation
- Reduce phagocytosis, bactericidal activity, release of acid hydrolases and pyrogens

Polymorphonuclear Leukocytes—cont'd
- Cause abnormal nitroblue tetrazolium test in vitro

Monocytes
- Reduce number at sites of inflammation
- Decrease fungicidal activity and clearance of opsonized particles
- Decrease response to macrophage activating factor and decreased chemotaxis
- Decrease response to mixed leukocyte reaction

Lymphocytes
- Decrease response to concanavalin A–induced T-cell blastogenesis
- Decrease response to tetanus toxoid and streptodornase-streptokinase
- Suppress response to mixed lymphocyte reaction
- Decrease antibody-dependent cell-mediated cytotoxicity
- Decrease natural killer cell activity

Langerhans' Cells
- Moderate-potency TCS cause decreased expression of Fc receptor, C3b receptor, and HLA DR positivity, but no alteration in CD1a antigen expression
- Superpotent TCS cause loss of all cells expressing Langerhans' cell markers

EFFECTS ON IMMUNE CYTOKINE PRODUCTION
- Decrease production of IL-1 (both IL-1α and IL-1β), IFN-γ, tumor necrosis factor, IL-2, and granulocyte-monocyte colony-stimulating factor

Adapted from Yohn JJ, Weston WL: *Curr Probl Dermatol* 2:42, 1990.

gether, the antiinflammatory properties of TCS are useful for dermatoses in which inflammation is a problem like atopic dermatitis and contact dermatitis but can be deleterious for dermatoses in which inflammation is a useful host response, like dermatophyte infections.

Antiproliferative and Atrophogenic Effects

TCS reduce mitotic activity in the epidermis,[36,37] leading to flattening of the basal cell layer and thinning of the stratum corneum and stratum granulosum.[38] Keratinocyte ultrastructure and the basement membrane[39] are not affected. TCS promote atrophy of the dermis mostly through inhibition of fibroblast proliferation, migration, chemotaxis, and protein synthesis.[40] Fibroblast synthesis of both glycosaminoglycans (GAGs)[41,42] and collagen[43-47] is inhibited. The loss of GAGs occurs early because their normal turnover rate in the skin is 2 to 18 days.[48] Their loss combined with TCS-induced vasoconstriction leads to the reduced dermal volume (water) observed after just 3 weeks

Box 27-4

Corticosteroid Mechanisms of Action—Antiproliferative Actions*

EPIDERMIS
- Number of keratinocyte mitoses is diminished
- Stratum corneum thickness reduced
- Granular layer reduced or absent
- Basal layer of keratinocytes flattened
- Keratinocyte growth factors suppressed†
- Keratinocyte ultrastructure (keratin filaments, keratohyalin granules, membrane-coating granules) normal
- Basement membrane unaffected
- Melanocyte pigment production inhibited

DERMIS
Early Atrophy
- Dermal volume reduced—decreased water content, loss of glycosaminoglycans

Early Atrophy—cont'd
- Hypoactive fibroblasts—suppression of procollagen I mRNA transcription, reduced activity of prolyl 4-hydroxylase and lysyl oxidase, collagenase activity reduced, hyaluronate synthetase activity suppressed
- Collagen and elastic fibers unchanged

Late Atrophy (Continuation of the Atrophogenic Process)
- Dermal volume reduced
- Collagen and elastic fibers diminished and abnormally aggregated
- Hypoactive fibroblasts (as above)
- Dermal vessels fragile, due to loss of fibrous and ground substance support

Adapted from Yohn JJ, Weston WL: *Curr Probl Dermatol* 2:42, 1990.
*Probably both direct and GCR-mediated effects.
†Brauchle M, Fassler R, Werner S: *J Invest Dermatol* 105:579-584, 1995.

of superpotent (also called "ultrapotent" or "megapotent") TCS application. Late dermal atrophy results from continuation of the early processes and reduction of elastin and collagen fibers, which also become abnormally aggregated.[49] Together, the antiproliferative and atrophogenic effects of TCS are helpful in proliferative dermatoses such as psoriasis; however, these effects are injurious when TCS are used in the wrong disease, location, or potency or used in excessive quantities.

Systemic Effects
The mechanisms of systemic actions of percutaneously absorbed TCS are the same as those of systemically administered corticosteroids (see Chapter 6).

CLINICAL USE
Indications
Table 27-2 lists the indications and contraindications for TCS, some of which are discussed here.

ATOPIC DERMATITIS. Moderate-potency TCS are frequently successful treatments for flares of atopic dermatitis on the trunk and extremities. Usually, control of the disease occurs after 2 to 3 weeks of twice daily therapy, and

then a lower potency of the TCS can be used twice daily to finish treatment or for early signs of recurrence (see Therapeutic Guidelines section). Fluticasone propionate 0.05% cream applied once daily was as effective as twice daily treatment in a multicenter, randomized study.[50] Fluticasone propionate 0.05% cream once daily was equal in safety and efficacy to clobetasone butyrate 0.05% cream twice daily in a randomized, double-blind clinical trial with 22 children having moderately active atopic dermatitis.[51]

Generally, only low-potency TCS are recommended for atopic dermatitis in children (see Therapeutic Guidelines section). Occasionally, intermediate-potency TCS are necessary for very short courses. Four weeks of twice daily desonide 0.05% ointment or hydrocortisone 2.5% ointment did not affect morning serum cortisol levels or adrenocorticotropic hormone (ACTH) stimulation tests in children with atopic dermatitis of 20% to 70% of total body surface area in a randomized, parallel, open-label study.[52] Mometasone furoate 0.1% cream once daily was significantly more effective than twice daily hydrocortisone valerate 0.2% cream in a 3-week, multicenter, randomized, evaluator-blinded, parallel group study with 219 children ages 2 to 12 years who had failed to respond to

Table 27-2	Selected Indications and Contraindications of Topical Corticosteroids

DERMATOLOGIC USES

Dermatitis/Papulosquamous
Atopic dermatitis*
Diaper dermatitis*
Dyshidrotic eczema
Erythroderma
Lichen planus
Lichen simplex chronicus
Nummular dermatitis*
Pityriasis rosea
Psoriasis—intertriginous*
Psoriasis—plaque or palmoplantar
Seborrheic dermatitis*

Bullous Dermatoses
Bullous pemphigoid
Cicatricial pemphigoid
Epidermolysis bullosa acquisita
Herpes gestationis (pemphigoid gestationis)
Pemphigus foliaceus

Connective Tissue Diseases
Dermatomyositis
Lupus erythematous spectrum

Neutrophilic Dermatoses
Beçhet's disease
Pyoderma gangrenosum

Other Dermatologic Uses
Alopecia areata
Acne keloidalis nuchae
Chondrodermatitis nodularis helicis
Cutaneous T-cell lymphoma, patch-stage
Granuloma annulare
Jessner's lymphocytic infiltrate
Lichen planopilaris
Lichen sclerosis et atrophicus
Morphea
Pruritic urticarial papules and plaques of pregnancy (PUPPP)
Pruritus—perianal, vulvar, scrotal
Sarcoidosis
Vitiligo
Well's syndrome

CONTRAINDICATIONS TO TOPICAL CORTICOSTEROIDS

Absolute
Known hypersensitivity to the topical corticosteroid
Known hypersensitivity to a component of the vehicle

Relative
Bacterial, mycobacterial, fungal, viral infection
Infestation
Ulceration

USAGE IN PREGNANCY—only when potential benefits justify possible risk to the fetus

USAGE IN LACTATION—used with caution at sites other than the breast or nipple (Not known if TCS are distributed into the breast milk)

*Conditions typically very sensitive to TCS.

at least 7 consecutive days of a topical hydrocortisone preparation. No treatment-related atrophy was seen in either group.[53]

CHONDRODERMATITIS NODULARIS. When betamethasone valerate cream is applied for more than 8 weeks in combination with triamcinolone 0.2 ml to 0.5 ml; a 10 mg/ml concentration injected into the skin around the ulcer is effective in about 25% of cases.[54,55]

GRANULOMA ANNULARE. Superpotent TCS alone or high-potency corticosteroids under occlusion are effective treatments for localized granuloma annulare. Occlusive TCS preparations such as Cordran tape and intralesional TCS treatment such as 5 to 10 mg/ml triamcinolone acetonide are also effective.[56]

LICHEN PLANUS. Localized cutaneous lichen planus (LP) generally responds to TCS. TCS in double-blind comparative trials were better than the other vehicles at treating LP.[57,58] Clobetasol propionate 0.05% ointment was superior to fluocinonide 0.05% ointment in a placebo-controlled, comparative study for treatment of atrophic-erosive oral lichen planus.[59]

LICHEN SCLEROSUS ET ATROPHICUS. Clobetasol propionate twice daily for 45 days and then once daily for an additional 45 days was successful at improving the subjective and objective components of lichen sclerosus et atrophicus (LS et A) in an open, uncontrolled clinical trial with 10 patients.[60] A regimen of high-potency or superpotent TCS followed by maintenance with low-potency TCS was safe and effective for treating LS et A in children.[61,62] In a prospective, observational study of vulvar LS et A in 54 patients of various ages, 94% responded to a diminishing regimen of TCS.[63] Similarly, a retrospective clinical and histopathologic study of penile LS et A in 22 patients showed clobetasol dipropionate 0.05% cream to be safe and effective; however, there seemed to be some potential for triggering latent human papillomavirus infections.[64]

PSORIASIS.   TCS are most useful for localized psoriasis or psoriasis of the scalp. Localized plaque psoriasis generally requires a high-potency or superpotent TCS twice daily followed by a maintenance regimen to obtain and preserve remission. Katz and associates[65] obtained 75% to 100% clearance in 28 of 59 and 26 of 59 patients with psoriasis via twice daily application of clobetasol ointment or betamethasone dipropionate in optimized vehicle (BDOV, Diprolene), respectively. In a parallel design study for 3 weeks, 15 of 18 and 17 of 19 patients showed similar results.[66] The majority (60% to 74%) of patients who cleared or almost cleared by twice daily BDOV could be maintained in remission status for up to 6 months by applying three consecutive doses of 3.5 g at 12-hour intervals each week (Saturday AM, PM, and Sunday AM). Other studies showed the success of clobetasol propionate 0.05% ointment twice daily for 14 days separated by at least 1 week according to the rate of relapse.[67] Many physicians treat thick psoriatic plaques on the scalp with a high-potency or superpotent TCS solution

nightly to twice daily 2 weeks on and 1 week off combined with the daily AM use of a therapeutic shampoo containing coal tar or salicylic acid. Augmented betamethasone dipropionate lotion was as effective as and more rapid acting than clobetasol propionate solution in a 2-week, randomized, multicenter, investigator-blinded, parallel-group study.[68] Betamethasone valerate foam (0.12%) was more effective than betamethasone valerate lotion in a randomized, multicenter, double-blind, active- and placebo-controlled trial in adult patients with moderate-to-severe scalp psoriasis; 72% were clear or almost clear after 28 days of treatment.[69]

Because the long-term efficacy of TCS for psoriasis is controversial and not well studied, many physicians' treatment of choice for localized plaque psoriasis is topical calcipotriene (previously named calcipotriol), which generally has less adverse effects than TCS. Topical calcipotriene treatment of plaque psoriasis compares favorably to mid- and high-potency TCS[70-72] but was less effective than superpotent TCS in 2-week, multicenter studies.[73,74] In the latter study, a regimen of calcipotriene ointment in the morning and halobetasol ointment in the evening produced better clinical results and less local adverse effects than either ointment alone. Similarly, calcipotriene in the morning and betamethasone dipropionate in the evening were superior to calcipotriene alone.[75] Clobetasol propionate ointment twice daily for 2 weeks followed by calcipotriol ointment twice daily for 4 weeks was superior to calcipotriol ointment alone in a randomized, double-blind, right-side versus left-side comparison.[76]

TCS have been tested for patients with psoriasis in combination with various other therapies such as phototherapy, systemic therapy, and other topical therapies. At least five clinical studies showed more rapid clearing rates of psoriasis using psoralen plus ultraviolet A (PUVA) plus TCS compared with PUVA alone.[4] An intermediate-to high-potency TCS may be used concurrently during PUVA photochemotherapy to achieve a faster clearing, lower total UVA dose at clearing, and lower final UVA dose. The combination of TCS with UVB phototherapy appears to have no substantial effect on the time to clearing or the percentage of responders. TCS have been associated with an increased risk of earlier relapse after the Goeckerman regimen. Triamcinolone cream 0.1% compounded with 5% salicylic acid allowed low-dose oral etretinate to be as effective as higher doses in a double-blind trial.[77] The addition of TCS leads to more rapid clearing of psoriatic plaques with short-course cyclosporine therapy, although relapse rates remained unchanged.[78] Combining fluocinonide 0.01% ointment with increasing concentrations of anthralin did not change the final time to clearance in a bilateral comparison study.[79] Tazarotene 0.1% gel once daily in the evening with mometasone furoate once daily in the morning was superior to tazarotene 0.1% gel alone in an open-label study with 20 patients.[80] Other studies showed that triamcinolone acetonide ointment 0.1% is more effective under occlusion than either clobetasol propionate cream 0.05% twice daily or triamcinolone acetonide ointment 0.1% alone.[81,82] Similarly, once-daily flurandrenolide tape was superior to twice-daily diflorasone diacetate ointment in an investigator-blinded, randomized, bilateral comparison study on psoriatic plaques.[83] Weekly clobetasol lotion applied under occlusion with a hydrocolloid dressing demonstrated excellent results in chronic plaque psoriasis, psoriasis of the palms and soles, palmoplantar pustulosis, and in skin lesions of Reiter's disease.[84] Hydrocolloid occluded clobetasol propionate lotion once weekly induced a faster remission of localized psoriasis than did unoccluded clobetasol propionate ointment twice daily; relapse and safety characteristics were comparable.[85]

SEBORRHEIC DERMATITIS. Only low-potency TCS creams are necessary for control of seborrheic dermatitis on the face. If traditional antidandruff shampoos fail, moderate- to high-potency TCS lotions or solutions may be used on the scalp. Physicians frequently use Vytone (iodoquinol and 1% hydrocortisone) cream twice daily 2 weeks on and 1 week off as needed for the face and 0.01% fluocinolone acetonide solution nightly for the scalp.

Treatments for seborrheic dermatitis are many, but comparative trials are few. Ketoconazole 2% foaming gel was significantly more effective at reducing *Pityrosporum ovale* counts, erythema, and scale than 0.05% betamethasone

dipropionate lotion in a 4-month single-blind comparative study.[86]

WELL'S SYNDROME. TCS successfully treat initial or subsequent episodes of eosinophilic cellulitis.[87-90]

BULLOUS DERMATOSES. The mucous membrane lesions of vesiculobullous disorders, such as pemphigus vulgaris (PV), can often be treated with TCS preparations.[91] For mild oral PV with no cutaneous involvement, a fluorinated TCS, such as fluocinonide 0.05%, in a dental paste, such as Orabase, can be applied four times daily (after meals and at bedtime). For moderate oral PV, physicians frequently use Decadron elixir 0.5 mg/5 ml 1 teaspoon swish, held in the mouth for a few minutes, and spit four times daily. After the initial lesions respond, a less potent 0.1% triamcinolone acetonide in a dental paste can be substituted.[92] Epidermal atrophy from TCS is not cosmetically or functionally significant on the oral mucous membranes. Similarly, treatment of mucosal lesions of cicatricial pemphigoid, bullous pemphigoid, or pemphigus foliaceus might respond to just TCS prescribed as previously described. Paraneoplastic pemphigus lesions are typically refractory to TCS.

Treatment of cutaneous bullous pemphigoid (BP) with TCS has been successful for limited skin involvement.[93,94] A trial of superpotent TCS ointment or cream twice daily, 2 weeks on and 1 week off, is recommended for limited BP. There are also reports of generalized BP successfully treated with TCS alone[95] or in combination with oral tetracycline with[96] or without[97] niacinamide.

BEHÇET'S DISEASE. Treatment of Behçet's disease with TCS is based on anecdotal or open clinical trials.[98] A high-potency or superpotent TCS in an ointment or vehicle like Orabase should be applied directly to the oral or genital erosions four times daily for 1 to 2 weeks until resolved.

PYODERMA GANGRENOSUM. Application of a superpotent TCS might halt the progression of a very early papular or pustular lesion, but intralesional or systemic corticosteroids are usually required for more advanced lesions of pyoderma gangrenosum (PG).[99] Potent TCS sped the resolution of PG on the scrotum of a patient with dermatomyositis already on oral prednisolone and azathioprine.[100]

ACNE KELOIDALIS NUCHAE. Superpotent TCS may help reduce the inflammation associated with acne keloidalis nuchae but may aggravate the acneiform condition.[101]

ALOPECIA AREATA. Treatment of alopecia areata (AA) with TCS is based mostly on anecdotal experience. High-potency or superpotent TCS preparations can improve hairless patches.[102] Application of a superpotent TCS preparation in a gel, lotion, or solution base to the patch and 1 cm of adjacent skin twice daily for 2 weeks on and 1 week off is recommended. If there is a progressive response after a period of 2 to 3 months, we continue the product until an arbitrary amount of hair has regrown, usually a few months longer.

PATCH-STAGE CUTANEOUS T-CELL LYMPHOMA. Prospective reviews demonstrate that TCS, especially ultrapotent compounds, are an effective treatment for patch-stage cutaneous T-cell lymphoma (CTCL).[103]

VITILIGO. TCS can be effective repigmenting agents.[104] The recommendations are a mid-to-lower potency TCS cream daily for a 3- to 4-month trial.[105] Therapy is continued if repigmentation occurs but stopped if it does not. A Wood's lamp is useful for monitoring progress at 6-week intervals. Metaanalysis showed medium-potency TCS to have success rates of approximately 55%.[106]

Adverse Effects

The adverse effects from TCS preparations (Box 27-5) are mostly from the TCS molecule. The vehicle, however, can potentiate these adverse effects and cause additional problems.

SYSTEMIC EFFECTS. TCS molecules can be absorbed percutaneously in significant quantities to cause systemic adverse effects identical to systemically administered corticosteroids—suppression of hypothalamic-pituitary-adrenal axis, iatrogenic Cushing's syndrome, and growth retardation in infants and children.

The actual number of reports of such adverse effects is small and seems to involve gross misuse of a TCS preparation. For example, growth impairment was reported in an infant who had received an estimated 30 g of Betnovate ointment (0.1% betamethasone 17-valerate) weekly over 3 years.[107] Cushing's syndrome was reported in a patient who had been using an estimated 38 g daily of 0.1% triamcinolone acetonide under polyethylene film for 4 years; adrenal insufficiency occurred on withdrawal.[108] Cushing's syndrome was also reported in a pa-

Box 27-5

Adverse Effects of Topical Corticosteroids

SYSTEMIC
- Suppression of hypothalamic-pituitary-adrenal axis
- Iatrogenic Cushing's syndrome
- Growth retardation in infants and children

LOCAL
- Epidermal atrophy—shiny, wrinkled, fragile skin with hypopigmentation, prominent vasculature, stellate pseudoscars, striae, or purpura
- Steroid addiction/rebound
- Glaucoma/cataracts

LOCAL—cont'd
- Allergic or irritant contact dermatitis
- Tachyphylaxis
- Facial hypertrichosis
- Folliculitis, miliaria
- Genital ulceration
- Granuloma gluteale infantum
- Crusted (Norwegian) scabies
- Exacerbation or increased susceptibility to bacterial, fungal, and viral infections
- Reactivation of Kaposi's sarcoma
- Perioral dermatitis, rosacea, acne
- Delayed wound healing

tient who applied an estimated 30 g daily of 0.25% dexamethasone cream without occlusion over a 5-year period; adrenal insufficiency occurred on withdrawal.[109] Clinical and laboratory evidence of Cushing's syndrome was reported in two Hispanic adults after using up to 100 g/week of clobetasol propionate 0.05% ointment and approximately 80 g/week of betamethasone dipropionate 0.05% in an augmented base presumably for many months to years.[110] Cushing's syndrome was reported during TCS treatment for nonbullous ichthyosiform erythroderma.[111] Betamethasone valerate also caused iatrogenic Cushing's syndrome.[112] Dwarfism has been reported after long-term TCS treatment.[113]

Laboratory evidence strongly suggests that systemic adverse effects from TCS preparations are a definite risk. Desoximetasone cream applied to 80% of the body area in amounts of 50 to 60 g/24 hours caused fasting hyperglycemia and increased insulin-glucose ratios within 24 hours; the increases in carbohydrate metabolism paralleled increases in circulating leukocytes.[114] Normal and psoriatic or eczematous adult volunteers applying over 50 g of Dermovate (0.05% clobetasol propionate) cream or ointment weekly showed either depressed 9 AM serum cortisol levels or decreased peak insulin stress tests by 1 week. Over 100 g caused profound AM cortisol suppression.[115] Betnovate ointment, applied in amounts of 30 g under occlusion by polyethylene for 20 out of 24 hours daily in hospital, depressed 9 AM plasma cortisol levels after 1 week.[107] Dermovate ointment 15 g twice daily without occlusion caused complete suppression of 7:30 AM plasma cortisol as early as 9.5 hours later.[116] Clobetasol or betamethasone dipropionate in optimized vehicle 3.5 g twice daily dramatically suppressed AM plasma cortisol and urinary free cortisol in 8 of 40 psoriatic patients (20%) by 3 to 8 days; the suppression was sustained for 24 and 10 days after withdrawal, respectively.[66]

Risk factors for systemic adverse effects (Box 27-6) are thought to include young age, liver and renal disease, amount of corticosteroid applied, extent of skin surface treated, frequency of application, length of treatment, potency of drug, and the use of occlusion. Children and infants have a greater skin surface-to-body volume ratio and may be less able to quickly metabolize glucocorticoids.[117] In infants and young children, catch-up growth is expected when TCS are discontinued. Continuous long-term treatment with a TCS preparation near puberty should also be avoided because growth suppression may cause premature epiphyseal closure before catch-up growth can occur.[118] The liver is the main organ for systemic corticosteroid metabolism, and the kidneys excrete metabolized and unmetabolized corticosteroid.[119]

The test of choice for screening and monitoring adrenal suppression is the 8 AM plasma cortisol; definitive diagnosis requires the metyrapone test (see Systemic Corticosteroids—Chapter 6). Treatment of TCS-induced adrenal suppression involves treatment with an oral corticosteroid while reducing the potency and amount of TCS. There are no formal practice guidelines; the length and rate of corticosteroid taper depend on the degree of adrenal suppression and the potency, amount, and duration of TCS treatment. Consultation with a specialist in endocrinology is recommended.

In pregnancy, TCS preparations may cause fetal abnormalities in animals if used in large amounts, with occlusive dressing, for prolonged periods of time, or if the more potent agents are used. Fetal abnormalities due to TCS have not been documented in human beings.[105] It is not known whether TCS molecules are excreted in breast milk, but no adverse effects on lactation from the use of TCS preparations have been

---

Box 27-6

Risk Factors for Systemic Effects and Local Atrophy

SYSTEMIC EFFECTS
- Young age (infancy/childhood)
- Liver disease
- Renal disease
- Amount of TCS applied
- Potency of TCS
- Use of occlusion

LOCAL ATROPHY
- Young age (infancy/childhood)
- Potency of TCS
- Use of occlusion
- Location (face, neck, axilla, groin, and upper inner thighs)

documented in humans. TCS products should not be applied to the nipples before nursing.[105]

LOCAL EFFECTS—GENERAL. Local adverse effects occur more frequently than systemic adverse effects but are generally uncommon. In a study of 2349 patients, the incidence of local adverse effects with unoccluded corticosteroids was low and about equal to the vehicle alone.[120]

ATROPHY. The most common local adverse effect is atrophy.[121] Cutaneous atrophy is characterized clinically by lax, wrinkled, shiny skin with telangiectasias, purpura, striae, stellate pseudoscars, hypopigmentation, or prominent deep vessels. Microscopic features are discussed in the Mechanisms of Action section. Atrophy of the epidermis may be seen within the first 7 days of daily superpotent TCS application under occlusion[49] and within 2 weeks of daily use of less potent TCS or superpotent TCS without occlusion.[122,123] Significant atrophy and striae are generally seen after many weeks or months of application, but striae have been observed on a man's medial thighs after 2 weeks of a proprietary combination of betamethasone dipropionate 0.05% and clotrimazole 1% cream. Risk factors for atrophy (see Box 27-6) include corticosteroid potency, occlusion, infancy/childhood, and location of TCS use. High-risk locations are the face, neck, axilla, groin, and upper inner thighs. Corticosteroid absorption by the genitalia can be over 40 times greater than that of glabrous skin.[124] Atrophy of the fat and muscle in the diaper area has occurred with fluorinated TCS.[125] Most signs of cutaneous atrophy resolve by 1 to 4 weeks after discontinuation of the TCS; however, striae are permanent. Most published studies involving humans are only 4 to 6 weeks in duration; therefore there are very few data on the long-term use of TCS.[9]

ADDICTION/REBOUND SYNDROME AND PERIORAL DERMATITIS. The addiction/rebound syndrome is characterized by initial improvement with a TCS, followed by lack of response after continued application, followed by a flare after TCS withdrawal. The treated skin might appear atrophic and erythematous, and the patient might report a burning sensation. The syndrome frequently occurs on facial, genital, or perianal skin. The classic example of the addiction/rebound syndrome is perioral dermatitis. Perioral dermatitis usually occurs after chronic or potent TCS exposure on the face. The exposure may be intentional or occult (e.g., dripped from the hairline or rubbed there unknowingly from the hands). The dermatitis is characterized by both eczema and acne in a perioral and sometimes periocular distribution. Treatment involves tetracycline 500 to 1000 mg daily followed by a slow taper to 250 mg daily for several weeks. The corticosteroid can be tapered by the use of a nonfluorinated TCS such as 1% hydrocortisone acetate cream.[126] Similarly, TCS initially improve but eventually exacerbate inflammatory conditions, such as acne,[127] rosacea,[128] and infections, such as scabies[129] and the dermatophytoses (a condition named "tinea incognito").[130]

OCULAR EFFECTS. Penetration around the eyelid skin can be 36 to 40 times that of thicker skin such as the palm or sole.[4] Although reports of ocular side effects from TCS applied to the eyelid skin are rare, studies with ophthalmologic preparations indicate that prolonged use on conjunctival tissue can lead to glaucoma, cataracts, decreased healing of traumatic ulcers, exacerbation of herpetic ulcers, and increased susceptibility to fungal and bacterial infections.[131] Glaucoma and blindness have occurred after 12 years intermittent use of 1% hydrocortisone cream for periorbital involvement of atopic dermatitis.[132] Glaucoma also occurred in a patient with a history of hand eczema, for which he had been using 0.1% betamethasone-17-valerate cream at bedtime for the previous 7 years in varying frequency.[133]

ALLERGIC CONTACT DERMATITIS. Only 7 years after the successful use of hydrocortisone was reported, the first case of allergic contact dermatitis (ACD) appeared in the literature.[134] Currently, more than 50 different TCS products have been reported to cause positive patch-test reactions.[135] In patient populations undergoing standard patch-test series (i.e., those suspected of ACD to the full spectrum of potential allergens), prevalence ranges from 0.2% to 4.8%.

ACD to a TCS is suspected when a corticosteroid-sensitive dermatitis fails to respond readily to TCS therapy[136] or if the dermatitis worsens with TCS therapy.[137] Predisposing factors for

TCS allergy are a history of numerous positive patch tests to non-TCS allergens, treatment-resistant eczema, leg ulcers, stasis dermatitis, perineal dermatitis, and chronic actinic dermatitis.[138,139] Budesonide has been reported to cause an erythema multiforme (EM)–like contact dermatitis,[140] and desoximetasone has been reported to cause a morbilliform, EM-like eruption.[141]

ACD to a TCS product may involve allergy to either a component of the vehicle (see below) or the actual TCS molecule. Confirmation of ACD to a TCS requires patch testing and occasionally prick and intradermal testing. Usage tests on normal skin produce too many false-negative results, possibly because of insufficient TCS absorption.[142] Patch testing to TCS is an evolving science. Problems exist with choosing a suitable agent at a suitable concentration in a suitable vehicle. TCS have been classified into four groups based on cross-reactivity elucidated by patch testing (Box 27-7)—hydrocortisone type, triamcinolone acetonide type, betamethasone type, and hydrocortisone-17-butyrate type.[143,144] Tixocortol pivolate, hydrocortisone-17-butyrate, and budesonide are usually the screening agents of choice, but most patch-test experts utilize a larger TCS "allergen" series. The accepted vehicle is ethanol, despite problems with irritation and degradation. The irritation lasts for only 24 to 48 hours, whereas patch-test reactions to TCS generally persist for at least 96 hours.[145] One month of storage in ethanol lowers the chromatographic purity of triamcinolone acetonide, fluocinolone acetonide, and betamethasone-17-valerate from 95% to 75%.[146] In general, the complexity and uncertainty of patch testing with TCS necessitates referral to a patch-test expert. The exact antigenic determinants have yet to be resolved.

Treatment of a TCS-induced ACD involves choosing a TCS from a different cross-reactivity group. A patient with a delayed-type hypersensitivity to a TCS should be warned that there is a small but definite risk of a generalized reaction to systemic administration of that corticosteroid.[147]

TACHYPHYLAXIS. Tachyphylaxis is the acute development of tolerance to the action of a drug after repeated doses. Loss of clinical effect is a well-known problem with chronic TCS application, particularly with higher potency TCS. Studies demonstrate tachyphylaxis to occur both to the

Box 27-7

Topical Corticosteroid Allergic Contact Dermatitis Cross-Reaction Groups

GROUP A
Hydrocortisone*
Hydrocortisone acetate
Cortisone acetate
Tixocortol pivalate†
Prednisolone
Methylprednisolone
Prednisone

GROUP B
Triamcinolone acetonide*
Triamcinolone alcohol
Amcinonide
Budesonide†
Desonide
Fluocinonide
Fluocinolone acetonide
Halcinonide

GROUP C
Betamethasone*
Betamethasone sodium phosphate
Dexamethasone
Dexamethasone sodium phosphate
Fluocortolone

GROUP D
Hydrocortisone-17-butyrate*†
Hydrocortisone-17-valerate
Aclometasone dipropionate
Betamethasone valerate
Betamethasone dipropionate
Prednicarbate
Clobetasone-17-butyrate
Clobetasol-17-propionate
Fluocortolone caproate
Fluocortolone pivalate
Fluprednidene acetate

Adapted from Coopman S, Degreef H, Dooms-Goossens A: *Br J Dermatol* 121:27-34, 1989.
*Prototype for this group of TCS—contact allergy.
†Common screening TCS for this group (see text).

vasoconstrictive effects on human skin[148] and to the antiproliferative effects in hairless mouse skin.[149-151] In the vasoconstrictor assay studies, significant tachyphylaxis occurred by day 4 of three times daily application of 0.5% or 0.1% triamcinolone acetonide in N,N-dimethylacetamide and twice daily or alternate-day application of Lidex cream. Recovery generally occurred after a 3- to 4-day rest period. Complete tolerance to histamine-induced wheal suppression by occluded topical 0.05% clobetasol propionate has been shown to occur earlier in croton oil–induced dermatitic skin than in normal controls.[152] A proven regimen to prevent tachyphylaxis does not exist. Twice daily application for 2 weeks on, then 1 week off is recommended because it seems easier for patients to remember.

OTHER LOCAL ADVERSE EFFECTS.   These local effects of TCS include facial hypertrichosis, folliculitis, miliaria, genital ulceration, and granuloma gluteale infantum.[9] The latter condition results from treatment of diaper dermatitis with potent TCS, and is characterized by reddish-purple plaques and nodules in the groin, inner thigh, and buttocks, which show syphilis-like plasma cell infiltrates on light microscopy. This has been seen to develop around an intergluteal fissure in an adult patient with systemic lupus erythematosus receiving a potent TCS preparation for severe inverse psoriasis. Long-term application of a TCS resulted in a case of crusted (Norwegian) scabies requiring treatment with ivermectin.[153] New lesions of Kaposi's sarcoma (KS) developed at the site of TCS application for erosive LP in a patient with known erythroblastopenia, thymoma, and KS.[154]

VEHICLE-RELATED ADVERSE EFFECTS. The vehicle of a TCS preparation can potentiate the adverse effects of the TCS or cause local adverse effects of its own.

Components of the vehicle can cause itching, burning, stinging, urticaria, and irritant contact dermatitis. Frequent causes of stinging include benzoic acid, cinnamic acid compound, lactic acid, urea, emulsifiers, formaldehyde, and sorbic acid. Propylene glycol, alcohol, and acetone can be very irritating. TCS preparations that do not contain propylene glycol are listed in Table 27-3. TCS preparations can contain agents

■ **Table 27-3**   Selected Topical Corticosteroids Without Propylene Glycol in the Vehicle

Generic Name	Trade Name	Formulation	Manufacturer
LOW-POTENCY PRODUCTS			
Desonide	DesOwen	Ointment 0.05%	Galderma
Desonide	Tridesilon	Cream 0.05%, ointment 0.05%	Bayer
Hydrocortisone	Hytone	Ointment 1.0%, 2.5%	Dermik
MEDIUM-POTENCY PRODUCTS			
Clocortolone pivalate	Cloderm	Cream 0.1%	Healthpoint
Fluocinolone	Synalar	Ointment 0.025%	Pantheon
Flurandrenolide	Cordran	Lotion 0.05%, tape	Occlassen
Hydrocortisone butyrate	Locoid	Cream 0.1%, ointment 0.1%, solution 0.1%	Hamanouchi Europe
Triamcinolone acetonide	Aristocort A	Cream 0.025%, 0.1%, 0.5%	Fujisawa
HIGH-POTENCY PRODUCTS			
Amcinonide	Cyclocort	Cream 0.1%, lotion 0.1%	Lederle
Desoximetasone	Topicort	Emollient cream 0.25%, LP emollient cream 0.05%	Hoechst-Roussel
Diflorasone	Florone	Ointment 0.05%	Dermik
Diflorasone	Maxiflor	Ointment 0.05%	Allergan
Halcinonide	Halog	Ointment 0.1%, solution 0.1%	Westwood-Squibb
SUPERPOTENT PRODUCTS			
Clobetasol	Temovate	Scalp application 0.05%	GlaxoWellcome
Halobetasol	Ultravate	Cream 0.05%	Westwood-Squibb

Table 27-4 Considerations for Choosing a Topical Corticosteroid Product

Potency (Class)*	Type of Dermatoses	Extent of Dermatoses	Duration of TCS Usage	Location of Dermatoses	Usage in Infants and Children	State of the Epidermis
Superpotent (I)	Dermatoses resistant to intermediate- or high-potency TCS	Avoid extensive application (>50 g weekly)	For short-term use only, ideally 2-3 weeks at a time	Do not use on the face, axillae, submammary area, or groin	Avoid use in infants and children under 12 years of age	Best for thick, lichenified, or hypertrophic skin; avoid with thin skin
High (II & III)	Severe	Avoid extensive application (>50 g weekly)	For short-term use if extensive application to atrophy-prone areas	Do not use on the face, axillae, submammary area, or groin	Avoid use in infants and children under 12 years of age	Best for thick, lichenified, or hypertrophic skin; avoid with thin skin
Intermediate (IV & V)	Moderate	Best for short-term treatment of extensive dermatoses	Avoid extended use (>1-2 weeks) in infants and children	Best on trunk and extremities	Avoid extended use (>1-2 weeks) in infants and children	Safer for short-term use on thin skin; less effective on thicker skin
Low (VI & VII)	Steroid sensitive	Preferred for treatment of large areas	Best if long-term treatment is required	Best choice for face, axilla, groin, and other moist, occluded areas	Infants and children	Best for thin skin; not effective on thick skin

*Potency class based on the Stoughton vasoconstrictor assay (see text).

that cause Type I nonimmunologic contact urticaria including acetic acid, alcohols, balsam of Peru, benzoic acid, cinnamic acid, formaldehyde, sodium benzoate, and sorbic acid. Immunologic causes include acrylic monomer, alcohols, ammonia, benzoic acid, benzophenone, diethyl toluamide, formaldehyde, henna, menthol, parabens, polyethylene glycol, polysorbate 60, salicylic acid, and sodium sulfide.[155] Very occlusive vehicles can cause folliculitis, miliaria, and exacerbation of acne and rosacea.

Vehicle ingredients can be the cause of ACD to a TCS preparation. Certain preservatives[156] have been implicated. Propyl gallate in a desonide preparation (Locapred) caused ACD.[157] Sorbic acid, a common preservative in TCS preparations, can potentially cause ACD.[158] Certain TCS preparations (e.g., Ultravate cream and Cutivate cream) contain formaldehyde-releasing preservatives (diazolidinyl urea and imidazolidinyl urea, respectively), which could cause ACD in formaldehyde-sensitive patients. Other common preservatives like parabens, BHA, BHT, and p-chloro-m-cresol seem to have very low potential for ACD. The perfume in the original Mycolog cream has caused ACD.[159] ACD from vehicle ingredients is much less common than irritant contact dermatitis from the preparation.

THERAPEUTIC GUIDELINES

The proper administration of TCS involves choosing a TCS preparation, estimating the necessary amount, and then supervising the therapy.

Choosing a TCS Preparation

The list of available TCS preparations is large and growing. The physician should become familiar with a few TCS preparations in each class, so that their clinical effects are known and predictable.

First, one must choose the desired potency. This decision is based on the patient's age and the type, severity, extent, location, and expected duration of the dermatoses. Table 27-4 illustrates the complexity of these considerations (see Indications section). In general, choose the least potent TCS necessary to achieve a response, and then taper the potency as quickly as possible.

After choosing the potency, one must select the proper vehicle. Table 27-5 displays the various considerations in choosing a vehicle for the topical corticosteroid. The most important factors in selecting a vehicle are location of use, potential for irritation, and past allergic reactions. Ultimately, patient compliance and clinical response determine the best vehicle. Table 27-6 displays selected TCS with unique vehicles/bases.

Supplementation of brand name TCS with generic products is not straightforward. Table 27-7 lists selected brand name TCS and their respective generic names. *First*, no comparative potency labeling exists to ensure equal efficacy between generic and brand name products. *Second*, studies confirm that the potency of generic products is not always equivalent to the brand name preparation and vice versa.[160,161] Valisone 0.1% cream (Schering) and Kenalog 0.1% cream (Westwood-Squibb) demonstrate significantly better vasoconstriction than some generics. Similarly, Synalar 0.025% cream is more potent than generic fluocinolone acetonide 0.025% cream (Fougera and Company), but Aristocort 0.025% cream and Aristocort 0.05% cream (Lederle Laboratories) are significantly less potent than generic triamcinolone 0.025% and 0.05% cream (Fougera and Company), respectively. As a general rule, ointments score closer to brand names than creams on vasoconstrictor assays, but there are exceptions. *Third*, studies show that variability exists between the different generic preparations,[162] emphasizing the effect of vehicle on a preparation's potency. Similarly, studies demonstrate different vasoconstrictor potency between brand name preparations of the same TCS.[163] *Fourth*, substitution of a brand name product with a generic does not always ensure a better price for the patient. The pharmacist wants to fill prescriptions correctly according to the law while receiving a legitimate profit. The cost of the generic product to the pharmacist is usually much less than the brand name, but the pharmacist can mark up the retail price of the generic product to nearly equal the price of the brand name product and therefore realize a larger profit. The cost to the pharmacist, for example, is much higher for 30 g of brand name Kenalog

■ **Table 27-5** Considerations for Choosing a Vehicle for the Topical Corticosteroid

Prepa-ration	Compo-sition	Moistur-izing Versus Drying	Preferred Dermatoses or Site of Use	Preferred Location of Use	Cosmesis	Potential for Irritation
Ointment	Water in oil	Very moisturizing	Best for thick, lichenified, or scaly dermatoses	Best for thick palmar or plantar skin; avoid occluded areas	Very greasy	Generally low
Cream	Oil in water emulsion	Moderate in moisturizing tendency	Best for acute, subacute, or weeping dermatoses	Good for moist skin and inter-triginous areas	Elegant	Variable; re-quire pre-servatives
Gel	Cellulose cut with alcohol or acetone	Drying	Scalp or derma-toses in dense hair areas	Best for oc-cluded areas, scalp, and mucosa	Elegant	High
Lotion	Oil in water	Drying	Scalp or derma-toses in dense hair areas	Best for oc-cluded areas, scalp, and mucosa	Elegant	High
Solution	Alcohol	Drying	Scalp or derma-toses in dense hair areas	Best for oc-cluded areas, scalp, and mucosa	Elegant	High

ointment (e.g., $18.95) than for the generic (e.g., $3.09), but the subsequent markup may be much higher, resulting in a very similar price to the customer. In general, substitution of a brand name product with a generic requires knowledge of the specific generic product available and its price at a given pharmacy.

With regard to price, increasing concentration of TCS in a product correlates with increasing price but not always increasing efficacy. Table 27-8 lists TCS preparations with more than one concentration (strength) available. Aristocort 0.5% cream costs almost three times more than Aristocort 0.025% cream, yet the preparations are equivalent on vasoconstriction assays.[163] The following preparations also show equivalent potency between different concentrations of the brand name product: Kenalog 0.025%, 0.1%, and 0.5% ointments; Aristocort

0.1% and 0.5% ointments; Topicort 0.05% and 0.25% cream; and Hytone 1.0% and 2.5% cream. Aristocort A 0.1% cream is more potent than the 0.05% and 0.025% creams, which are equal. Both Synalar and Valisone creams show dose-response relationships with increasing concentrations of the TCS.

Determining the Necessary Amount

Prescribing the proper amount of a TCS preparation requires estimating the body surface area involved and converting that measurement into grams supplied. A fingertip unit (FTU)[164] is the amount of ointment expressed from a tube with a 5-mm diameter nozzle, applied from the distal skin crease to the tip of the palmar aspect of the index finger. One FTU weighs 0.49 g and covers 312 cm^2 in adult males, and weighs 0.43 g and covers 257 cm^2 in adult females. Tables

Table 27-6   Topical Corticosteroids in Unique Bases/Vehicles

Base/Vehicle	Potency	Brand Name
Gels	Superpotent	Diprolene
		Temovate
	High potency	Lidex
		Topicort
Lotions	High potency	Cyclocort
		Diprolene
		Maxivate
	Medium potency	Cordran
		Diprosone
		Elocon
		Kenalog (0.01%, 0.025%)
	Low potency	Betatrex
		DesOwen
Solutions	Superpotent	Cormax Scalp Application
		Temovate Scalp Application
	High potency	Halog
		Lidex
	Medium potency	Locoid
	Low potency	Fluonid
		Synalar (0.01%)
Oils	Low potency	Derma-Smoothe/FS
Sprays	Low potency	Diprosone
		Kenalog
Other	Superpotent	Cordran Tape
		Cordran Tape Patch
	Medium potency	Kenalog in Orabase paste
		Luxiq foam

Table 27-7   Generic and Trade Names of Commonly Used Topical Corticosteroids

Superpotent/High Potency		Medium/Low Potency	
Trade Name	Generic Name	Trade Name	Generic Name
Cyclocort	Amcinonide	Aclovate	Alclometasone dipropionate
Dermacin	Fluocinonide	Alphatrex	Betamethasone dipropionate
Diprolene AF	Betamethasone dipropionate*	Aristocort	Triamcinolone acetonide
Diprosone	Betamethasone dipropionate	Betatrex	Betamethasone valerate
Flurone	Diflorasone diacetate	Cloderm	Clocortolone pivalate
Halog	Halcinonide	Cordran	Flurandrenolide
Lidex	Fluocinonide	Cutivate	Fluticasone propionate
Maxiflor	Diflorasone diacetate	Dermatop	Prednicarbate
Maxivate	Betamethasone dipropionate	Dermasmoothe	Fluocinolone acetonide
Psorcon	Diflorasone diacetate	DesOwen	Desonide
Temovate	Clobetasol propionate	Elocon	Mometasone furoate
Topicort	Desoximetasone	Hytone	Hydrocortisone acetate
Ultravate	Halobetasol propionate	Kenalog	Triamcinolone acetonide
		Locoid	Hydrocortisone butyrate
		Penecort	Hydrocortisone acetate
		Pandel	Hydrocortisone buteprate
		Synalar	Fluocinolone acetonide
		Tridesilon	Desonide
		Uticort	Betamethasone benzoate
		Westcort	Hydrocortisone valerate

*Augmented-base version of betamethasone dipropionate.
AF, Advanced formula

■ **Table 27-8** Topical Corticosteroid Products with Multiple Concentrations Available

Vehicle	Potency	Product (concentration)
Cream	Medium	Aristocort cream (0.5%)
		Aristocort A cream (0.5%)
		Kenalog cream (0.5%)
	Low	Aristocort cream (0.1%, 0.025%)
		Aristocort A cream (0.1%, 0.025%)
		Kenalog cream (0.1%, 0.025%)
		Synalar cream (0.025%, 0.01%)
		Hytone cream (0.5%, 1.0%, 2.5%)
Ointment	Medium	Aristocort ointment (0.5%, 0.1%)
		Aristocort A ointment (0.1%)
		Cordran ointment (0.05%)
	Low	Cordran ointment (0.025%)
Lotion	Low	Kenalog lotion (0.1%, 0.025%)

■ **Table 27-9** Estimating the Necessary Amount of Topical Corticosteroid for Adults

Anatomic Area	FTU Required to Cover	Amount for bid Application (g)	Amount for 1 Week of bid Application (g)	Amount for 4 Weeks of bid Application (g)
Face and neck	2.5	2.5	17.5	70
Anterior or posterior trunk	7	7	49	196
Arm	3	3	21	84
Hand (both sides)	1	1	7	28
Leg	6	6	42	168
Foot	2	2	14	56

Adapted from Long CC, Finlay AY: *Clin Exp Dermatol* 16:444-447, 1991.

27-9 and 27-10 are conversion tables for 1 month, twice daily application in adults and children, respectively.

Compounding

Compounding TCS with certain salicylates, tar, antibiotics, and antifungals may alter the stability[165] or solubility of the corticosteroid or cause contact allergy. Urea 10% has been shown to cause significant degradation of the TCS in Topicort, Kenalog, and Westcort creams.[166] No degradation of TCS occurred with 0.25% menthol, camphor, or phenol; 2% salicylic acid; or 5% LCD.

Supervising the Therapy

Like most prescription drugs, TCS therapy requires supervision to optimize benefits and minimize adverse effects. The most effective form of supervision is the follow-up visit. Unfortunately, recent health care trends move toward allowing less frequent office visits, which typically means less opportunity for careful follow-up. More emphasis must be placed on educating the patient at the first visit. From our experience, even the more intelligent patients cannot remember more than two or three instructions from a given visit; thus handouts are helpful. Box 27-8 lists a sample patient instructions sheet.

Table 27-10   Estimating the Necessary Amount of Topical Corticosteroid for Children

Anatomic Area	FTU Required to Cover				Amount for bid Application (g)				Amount for 1 Week of bid Application (g)				Amount for 4 Weeks of bid Application (g)			
	3-6 mos	1-2 yrs	3-5 yrs	6-10 yrs	3-6 mos	1-2 yrs	3-5 yrs	6-10 yrs	3-6 mos	1-2 yrs	3-5 yrs	6-10 yrs	3-6 mos	1-2 yrs	3-5 yrs	6-10 yrs
Face and neck	1	1.5	1.5	2	1	1.5	1.5	2	7	10.5	10.5	14	28	42	42	56
Arm and hand	1	1.5	2	2.5	1	1.5	2	2.5	7	10.5	14	17.5	28	42	56	70
Leg and foot	1.5	2	3	4.5	1.5	2	3	4.5	10.5	14	21	31.5	42	56	84	126
Anterior trunk	1	2	3	3.5	1	2	3	3.5	7	14	21	24.5	28	56	84	98
Posterior trunk and buttocks	1.5	3	3.5	5	1.5	3	3.5	5	10.5	21	24.5	35	42	84	98	140

Patient Age Range

Adapted from Long CC, Mills CM, Finlay AY: *Br J Dermatol* 138:293-296, 1998.

Box 27-8

Sample Patient Instructions Sheet—Topical Corticosteroids

MEDICATION: _____

DIRECTIONS: _____
- This information summary is applicable to most topical corticosteroid preparations.
- There is a large list of potential side effects from topical corticosteroids. Although patients' awareness of these side effects is important, overconcern and overattention to these possible side effects is potentially disruptive and best avoided.

CONTRAINDICATIONS
- Absolute contraindications to the use of a topical corticosteroid include known hypersensitivity (allergy) to the topical corticosteroid or a component of the vehicle.
- Other possible contraindications include ulceration, scabies infestation, and bacterial, viral, mycobacterial, or fungal infection.

SIDE EFFECTS
Minor Effects from Short-Term Therapy
(2 to 3 weeks or less)
- In the absence of any of the aforementioned contraindications, topical corticosteroid therapy is rarely associated with serious side effects.
- The most common side effects include mild irritation such as redness, burning, stinging, or itching.

Potential Effects from Long-Term Therapy
- Important side effects from long-term therapy include skin atrophy (thinning) characterized by shiny, wrinkled, easily bruised skin; pigment changes; prominent small blood vessels; and ulceration.
- Long-term therapy with certain topical corticosteroids can lead to absorption into the blood

Potential Effects from Long-Term Therapy—cont'd
stream and can cause weight gain and fluid retention, blood pressure elevation, mood alterations, significant fever or chills, excessive thirst and urinary frequency or volume, or severe or persistent bone, joint, or muscle pain.
- Long-term therapy can cause worsening of scabies, fungal, and yeast infections; extension of herpetic ulcers; increased susceptibility to fungal and bacterial infections; inflammation of hair follicles or sweat ducts; exacerbation of acne or rosacea; and glaucoma.
- Local side effects generally occur at the site of application and are not common.

SPECIAL CIRCUMSTANCES
- Usage in pregnancy should be restricted to times when the potential benefits justify possible risk to the fetus.
- Use with caution when breast-feeding. Avoid application to the breast or nipple. It is not known if topical corticosteroids are distributed into the breast milk.

SUMMARY
- The vast majority of patients receiving short- or long-term topical corticosteroids do not experience important or serious side effects; however, early reporting to your physician of the more serious side effects listed earlier is important.
- Apply the topical corticosteroid according to directions from your physician. Incorrect usage of topical steroids can greatly increase the risk of local and systemic side effects.
- Do not share your product with other people.

Bibliography

Ahluwalia A: Topical glucocorticoids and the skin—mechanisms of action: an update. *Mediators Inflammation* 7:183-193, 1998.

Camisa C: Corticosteroids: In Camisa C, editor: *Psoriasis*, Boston, 1994, Blackwell Scientific Publications, pp 177-196.

Chaffman MO: Topical corticosteroids: a review of properties and principles in therapeutic use. *Nurse Practitioner Forum* 10:95-105, 1999.

Drake LA, Dinehart SM, Farmer ER, et al: Guidelines of care for the use of topical glucocorticosteroids. *J Am Acad Dermatol* 35:615-619, 1996.

Katz HI: Topical corticosteroids. *Dermatol Clin* 13:805-815, 1995.

Schafer-Korting M, Schmid MH, Korting HC: Topical glucocorticoids with improved risk-benefit ratios. Rationale of a new concept. *Drug Saf* 14:375-385, 1996.

Sloan KB, Araujo OE, Flowers FP: Topical corticosteroid therapy. In Arndt KA, Leboit PE, Robinson JK, et al, editors: *Cutaneous medicine and surgery*, Philadelphia, 1996, WB Saunders, pp 160-166.

Yohn JJ, Weston WL: Topical Glucocorticosteroids. *Curr Probl Dermatol* 2:38-63, 1990.

References

Pharmacology

1. Stoughton RB: Vasoconstrictor activity and percutaneous absorption of glucocorticosteroids. *Arch Dermatol* 99:753-756, 1969.

2. Place VA, Velazquez JG, Burdick KH: Precise evaluation of topically applied corticosteroid potency. *Arch Dermatol* 101:531-537, 1970.

3. Cornell RC, Stoughton RB: Correlation of the vasoconstrictor assay and clinical activity in psoriasis. *Arch Dermatol* 121:63-67, 1985.

4. Camisa C: Corticosteroids. In Camisa C, editor: *Psoriasis*, Boston, 1994, Blackwell Scientific Publications, pp 177-196.

5. Ponec M: Glucocorticoids and cultured human skin cells: specific intracellular binding and structure-activity relationships. *Br J Dermatol* 107(Suppl 23):24-29, 1982.

6. Ponec M, Kenpenaar J, Shroot B, et al: Glucocorticoids: binding affinity and lipophilicity. *J Pharm Sci* 75:973-975, 1986.

7. Phillips GH: Locally active corticosteroids: structure-activity relationships. In Wilson L, Marks R, editors: *Mechanisms of topical corticosteroid activity*, Edinburgh, 1976, Churchill Livingstone, p 1.

8. Kamm A: The pharmacologic profile of clobetasol propionate: a new high potency steroid. In *Clobetasol: an investigator's report*, Philadelphia, 1986, Glaxo Monograph, pp 10-18.

9. Yohn JJ, Weston WL: Topical glucocorticosteroids. *Curr Probl Dermatol* 2:38-63, 1990.

10. Stoughton RB, Cornell RC: Topical steroids in dermatology. In Christophers E, Schopf E, Kligman AM, et al, editors: *Topical corticosteroid therapy: a novel approach to safer drugs*, New York, 1988, Raven Press, pp 1-12.

11. Vickers CFH: Existence of a reservoir in the stratum corneum. *Arch Dermatol* 88:20-23, 1963.

12. Clarys P, Gabard B, Barel AO: A qualitative estimate of the influence of halcinonide concentration and urea on the reservoir formation in the stratum corneum. *Skin Pharmacol Appl Skin Physiol* 12:85-89, 1999.

Mechanisms of Action

13. Catt KJ, Dufau ML: Hormone action: Control of target cell function by peptide, thyroid and steroid hormones. In Felig P, Baxter JD, Broadus AE, et al, editors: *Endocrinology and metabolism*, New York, 1981, McGraw-Hill Book Co, pp 61-105.

14. Thompson EB: The structure of the human glucocorticoid receptor and its gene. *J Steroid Biochem* 27:105-108, 1987.

15. Lan NC, Karin M, Nguyen T, et al: Mechanisms of glucocorticoid hormone action. *J Steroid Biochem* 20:77-88, 1984.

16. Spindler SR, Mellon-Nussbaum S, Baxter JD: Growth hormone gene transcription is regulated by thyroid and glucocorticoid hormones in cultured rat pituitary tumor cells. *J Biol Chem* 257:11627-11632, 1982.

17. Evans RM, Birnberg NC, Rosenfeld MG: Glucocorticoid and thyroid hormones transcriptionally regulate growth hormone gene expression. *Proc Natl Acad Sci USA* 79:7659-7663, 1982.

18. MacGregor RR: Inhibition of granulocyte adherence: potential mechanism of action of anti-inflammatory drugs. *Clin Res* 22:423A, 1974.

19. Dale DC, Rauci AS, Wolff SM: Alternate-day prednisone. Leukocyte kinetics and susceptibility to infections. *N Engl J Med* 291:1154-1158, 1974.

20. Dale DC, Fauci AS, Guerry DIV, et al: Comparison of agents producing a neutrophilic leukocytosis in man. Hydrocortisone, prednisone, endotoxin, and etiocholanolone. *J Clin Invest* 56:808-813, 1975.

21. Rebuck JW, Mellinger RC: Interruption by topical cortisone of leukocyte cycles in acute inflammation in man. *Ann NY Acad Sci* 56:715-732, 1953.

22. Balow JE, Rosenthal AS: Glucocorticoid suppression of macrophage inhibitory factor. *J Exp Med* 137:1031-1041, 1973.

23. Weston WL, Claman HN, Krueger CG: Site of action of cortisol in cellular immunity. *J Immunol* 110:880-883, 1973.

24. Rinehart JJ, Balcerzak SP, Sagone AL, et al: Effects of corticosteroids on human monocyte function. *J Clin Invest* 54:1337-1343, 1974.

25. Hattori T, Hirata F, Hoffman T, et al: Inhibition of human natural killer (NK) activity and antibody-dependent cellular cytotoxicity (ADCC) by lipomodulin, a phospholipase inhibitory protein. *J Immunol* 131:662-665, 1983.

26. Hoffman T, Hirata F, Bougnouz P, et al: Phospholipid methylation and phospholipase A2 activation in cytotocixity by human natural killer cells. *Proc Natl Acad Sci USA* 78:3839-3843, 1981.

27. Hellewell PG, Williams TJL: An anti-inflammatory steroid inhibits tissue sensitization by IgE in vivo. *Br J Pharmacol* 96:5-7, 1989.

28. Altura BM: Role of glucocorticoids in local regulation of blood flow. *Am J Physiol* 211:1393-1397, 1966.

29. Guyre PM, Bodwell JE, Hollbrook NJ, et al: Glucocorticoids and the immune system: activation of glucocorticoid-receptor complexes in thymus cells; modulation of Fc receptors of phagocytic cells. In Lee HJ, Walker CA, editors: *Progress in research and clinical applications of corticosteroids,* Philadelphia, 1981, Heyden and Son, pp 14-27.

30. DiRosa M, Flower RJ, Hirata F, et al: Antiphospholipase proteins. *Prostaglandins* 28:441-442, 1984.

31. Ramey ER, Goldstein MS: The adrenal cortex and the sympathetic nervous system. *Physiol Rev* 37:155-195, 1957.

32. Fritz I, Levine R: Action of adrenal cortical steroids and norepinephrine on vascular responses of stress in adrenalectomized rats. *Am J Physiol* 165:456-465, 1951.

33. Besse JC, Bass AD: Potentiation by hydrocortisone of responses to catecholamines in vascular smooth muscle. *J Pharmacol Exp Ther* 154:224-238, 1966.

34. Kalsner S: Steroid potentiation of responses to sympathomimetic amines in aortic strips. *Br J Pharmacol* 36:582-593, 1969.

35. Altura BM: Role of glucocorticoids in local regulation of blood flow. *Am J Physiol* 211:1393-1397, 1966.

36. Marks R, Williams K: The action of topical steroids on the epidermal cell cycle. In Wilson L, Marks R, editors: *Mechanisms of topical corticosteroid activity,* Edinburgh, 1976, Churchill Livingstone, p 39.

37. Fisher LB, Maibach HI: The effect of corticosteroids on epidermal mitotic activity. *Arch Dermatol* 103:39-44, 1971.

38. Lehman P, Zheng P, Lavker RM, et al: Corticosteroid atrophy in human skin. A study by light, scanning and transmission elecron microscopy. *J Invest Dermatol* 81:169-176, 1983.

39. Oikarinen A, Peltonen L, Hintikka J, et al: A local potent glucocorticosteroid decreases the induction of galactosylhydroxylysl glucosyltransferase in suction blisters but has no effect on basement membrane structures. *Br J Dermatol* 108:171-178, 1983.

40. Hein R, Krieg T: Effects of corticosteroids on human fibroblasts in vitro. In Christophers E, Schopf E, Kligman AM, et al, editors: *Topical corticosteroid therapy: a novel approach to safer drugs,* New York, 1988, Raven Press, pp 57-65.

41. Saarni H: Cortisol effects on the gly-cosaminoglycan synthesis and molecular weight distribution in vitro. *Biochem Pharmacol* 27:1029-1032, 1978.

42. Smith TJ: Dexamethasone regulation of glycosaminoglycan synthesis in cultured human skin fibroblasts. Similar effects of glucocorticoid and thyroid hormones. *J Clin Invest* 74:2157-2163, 1984.

43. Rokowski RJ, Sheehy J, Cutroneo KR: Glucocorticoid selective reduction of functioning collagen messenger ribonucleic acid. *Arch Biochem Biophys* 210:74-81, 1981.

44. Oikarinen J, Pihlajaniemi T, Hamalainen L, et al: Cortisol decreases the cellular concentration of translatable type-I procollagen mRNA species in cultured human skin fibroblasts. *Biochem Biophys Acta* 741:297-302, 1983.

45. Oikarinen A, Hannuksela M: Effect of hydro-cortisone-17-butyrate, hydrocortisone and clobetasol-17-propionate on prolyl hydroxy-lase activity in human skin. *Arch Dermatol Res* 267:79-82, 1980.

46. Benson SC, Lu Valle PA: Inhibition of lysyl oxidase and prolyl hydroxylase activity in glucocorticoid treated rats. *Biochem Bio-phys Res Commun* 99:557-562, 1981.

47. Jeffrey JJ, Coffey RJ, Eisen AZ: Studies on uterine collagenase in tissue culture, II: effect of steroid hormones on enzyme production. *Biochem Biophys Acta* 252:143-149, 1971.

48. Silbert JE: Proteoglycans and glycosamino-glycans. In Goldsmith LA, editor: *Biochem-istry and physiology of the skin*, New York, 1983, Oxford University Press, pp 448-461.

49. Marks R: Survey of methods for assessment of corticosteroid atrophogenicity. In Christophers E, Schopf E, Kligman AM, et al, editors: *Topical corticosteroid therapy: a novel approach to safer drugs*, New York, 1988, Raven Press, pp 105-110.

Atopic Dermatitis

50. Bleehan SS, Chu AC, Hamann I, et al: Fluti-casone propionate 0.05% cream in the treatment of atopic eczema: a multicentre study comparing once-daily treatment and once-daily vehicle cream application versus twice-daily treatment. *Br J Dermatol* 133:592-597, 1995.

51. Wolkerstorfer A, Strobos MA, Glazenburg EJ, et al: Fluticasone propionate 0.05% cream once daily versus clobetasone bu-tyrate 0.05% cream twice daily in children with atopic dermatitis. *J Am Acad Dermatol* 39:226-231, 1998.

52. Lucky AW, Grote GD, Williams JL, et al: Effect of desonide ointment, 0.05%, on the hypothalamic-pituitary-adrenal axis of children with atopic dermatitis. *Cutis* 59:151-153, 1997.

53. Lebwohl M: A comparison of once-daily application of mometasone furoate 0.1% cream compared with twice-daily hydrocor-tisone valerate 0.2% cream in pediatric atopic dermatitis patients who failed to respond to hydrocortisone. *Int J Dermatol* 38:604-606, 1999.

Miscellaneous Dermatoses

54. Beck MH: Treatment of chondrodermatitis nodularis helicis and conventional wisdom. *Br J Dermatol* 113:504-505, 1985.

55. Lawrence CM: The treatment of chondro-dermatitis nodularis with cartilage removal alone. *Arch Dermatol* 127:530-535, 1991.

56. Muhlbauer JE: Granuloma annulare. *J Am Acad Dermatol* 3:217, 1980.

57. Garretts M: Controlled double-blind comparative trial with fluprednylidene acetate cream and its base. *Archiv fur Dermatolo-gische Forschung* 251:165-168, 1975.

58. Beylot C, Babin MB: Clinical trial of Top-ifram. *Bordeaux Medical* 5:1091-1100, 1972.

59. Carbone M, Conrotto D, Carrozzo M, et al: Topical corticosteroids in association with miconazole and chlorhexidine in the long-term management of atrophic-erosive lichen planus: a placebo-controlled and comparative study between clobetasol and fluocinonide. *Oral Diseases* 5:44-49, 1999.

60. Cattani P, Manfrin E, Presti F, et al: Our experience in treating lichen sclerosus. *Mi-nerva Ginecologica* 49:207-212, 1997.

61. Fischer GO: Lichen sclerosus in childhood. *Aust J Dermatol* 36:166-167, 1995.

62. Garzon MC, Paller AS: Ultrapotent topical corticosteroid treatment of childhood genital lichen sclerosus. *Arch Dermatol* 135:525-528, 1999.

63. Sinha P, Sorinola O, Luesley DM: Lichen sclerosus of the vulva. Long-term steroid maintenance therapy. *J Reprod Med* 44:621-624, 1999.

64. Dahlman-Ghozlan K, Hedblad MA, von Krogh G: Penile lichen sclerosus et atrophicus treated with clobetasol dipropionate 0.05% cream: a retrospective clinical and histopathological study. *J Am Acad Dermatol* 40:451-457, 1999.

Psoriasis

65. Katz HI, Prawer WE, Medansky RS, et al: Intermittent corticosteroid maintenance treatment of psoriasis: a double blind, multicenter trial of augmented betamethasone dipropionate ointment in a pulse dose treatment regimen. *Dermatologica* 183:269-274, 1991.
66. Katz HI, Hien NT, Prauer SE, et al: Superpotent topical steroid treatment of psoriasis vulgaris—clinical efficacy and adrenal function. *J Am Acad Dermatol* 16:804-811, 1987.
67. Gammon WR, Krueger GG, Van Scott EJ, et al: Intermittent short courses of clobetasol propionate ointment 0.05% in the treatment of psoriasis. *Curr Ther Res* 42:419-427, 1987.
68. Katz HI, Lindholm JS, Weiss JS, et al: Efficacy and safety of twice-daily augmented betamethasone dipropionate lotion versus clobetasol propionate solution in patients with moderate-to-severe scalp psoriasis. *Clin Therapeutics* 17:390-401, 1995.
69. Franz TJ, Parsell DA, Halualani RM, et al: Betamethasone valerate foam 0.12%: a novel vehicle with enhanced delivery and efficacy. *Int J Dermatol* 38:628-632, 1999.
70. Kragballe K, Gjertsen BT, de Hoop D, et al: Calcipotriol, a novel principle in the treatment of psoriasis vulgaris: results of a double-blind, multicenter, right-left comparison with betamethasone 17-valerate. *Lancet* 1:193-196, 1991.
71. Bruce S, Epinette WW, Funicella T, et al: Comparative study of calcipotriene (MC 903) ointment and fluocinonide ointment in the treatment of psoriasis. *J Am Acad Dermatol* 31:755-759, 1994.
72. Molin L, Cutler TP, Helander I, et al: Comparative efficacy of calcipotriol (MC903) cream and betamethasone 17-valerate cream in the treatment of chronic plaque psoriasis. A randomized, double-blind, parallel group, multicenter study. Calcipotriol Study Group. *Br J Dermatol* 136:89-93, 1997.
73. Lebwohl M, Siskin S, Pharm D, et al: A multicenter trial of calcipotriene ointment and halobetasol ointment compared to either agent alone for the treatment of psoriasis. *J Am Acad Dermatol* 35:268-269, 1996.
74. Lebwohl M: Topical application of calcipotriene and corticosteroids: combination regimens. *J Am Acad Dermatol* 37:S55-58, 1997.
75. Ortonne JP: Psoriasis: nouvelle modalite therapeutique par le calcipotriol plus le dipropionate de betamethasone. *Nouv Dermatol* 13:746-751, 1994.
76. Austad J, Bjerke JR, Gjertsen BT, et al: Clobetasol propionate followed by calcipotriol is superior to calcipotriol alone in topical treatment of psoriasis. *J Eur Acad Dermatol Venereol* 11:19-24, 1998.
77. Van Der Rhee JH, Tijssen JGP, Herrmann WA, et al: Combined treatment of psoriasis with a new aromatic retinoid (Tigason) in low dosage orally and triamcinolone cream topically: a double blind trial. *Br J Dermatol* 102:203-212, 1980.
78. Finzi AF: Individualized short-course cyclosporin therapy in psoriasis. *Br J Dermatol* 135(Suppl 48):31-34, 1996.
79. Gratten CEH, Christopher AP, Robinson M, et al: Double-blind comparison of a dithranol and steroid mixture with a conventional dithranol regimen for chronic psoriasis. *Br J Dermatol* 119:623-626, 1988.
80. Poulin YP: Tazarotene 0.1% gel in combination with mometasone furoate cream in plaque psoriasis: a photographic tracking study. *Cutis* 63:41-48, 1999.
81. Kragballe K, Larsen FG: A hydrocolloid occlusive dressing and triamcinolone acetonide cream is superior to clobetasol cream and in palmo-plantar psoriasis. *Acta Derm Venereol* 71:540-542, 1991.
82. David M, Lowe NJ: Psoriasis therapy: comparative studies with a hydrocolloid dressing, plastic film occlusion, and triamcinolone acetonide cream. *J Am Acad Dermatol* 21:511-512, 1989.
83. Krueger GG, O'Reilly MA, Weidner M, et al: Comparative efficacy of once-daily flurandrenolide tape versus twice-daily diflorasone diacetate ointment in the treatment of psoriasis. *J Am Acad Dermatol* 38:186-190, 1998.

84. Volden G: Successful treatment of chronic skin disease with clobetasol propionate and a hydrocolloid occlusive dressing. *Acta Derm Venereol* 72:69-71, 1992.

85. Van der Vleuten CJ, van Vlijmen-Willems IM, de Jong EM, et al: Clobetasol-17-propionate lotion under hydrocolloid dressing (Duoderm ET) once weekly versus unoccluded clobetasol-17-propionate ointment twice daily in psoriasis: an immunohistochemical study on remission and relapse. *Arch Dermatol Res* 291:390-395, 1999.

Other Dermatoses

86. Ortonne JP, Lacous JP, Vitetta A, et al: Comparative study of ketoconazole 2% foaming gel and betamethasone dipropionate lotion in the treatment of seborrheic dermatitis in adults. *Dermatology* 184:275-280, 1992.

87. Wells GC, Smith NP: Eosinophilic cellulitis. *Br J Dermatol* 100:101-109, 1979.

88. Andreano JM, Kantor GR, Bergfeld WF, et al: Eosinophilic cellulitis and eosinophilic pustular folliculitis. *J Am Acad Dermatol* 20:934-936, 1989.

89. Mitchell AJ, Anderson TF, Headington JT, et al: Recurrent granulomatous dermatitis with eosinophilia: Well's syndrome. *Int J Dermatol* 23:198-202, 1984.

90. Schorr WF, Tauscheck AL, Dickson KB, et al: Eosinophilic cellulitis (Well's syndrome): histologic and clinical features in arthropod bites. *J Am Acad Dermatol* 11:1043-1049, 1984.

91. Camisa C, Rindler J: Diseases of the oral mucous membranes. *Curr Probl Dermatol* 8:41-96, 1996.

92. Camisa C, Warner M: Treatment of pemphigus. *Dermatol Nursing* 10:115-131, 1998.

93. Muramatsu T, Iida T, Shirai T: et al: Foliaceus successfully treated with topical corticosteroids. *J Dermatol* 23:683-688, 1996.

94. Zimmermann R, Faure M, Claudy A: Prospective study of treatment of bullous pemphigoid by a class I topical corticosteroid. *Ann Dermatol Venereol* 126:13-16, 1999.

95. Spuls PI, Brakman M, Westerhof W, et al: Treatment of generalized bullous pemphigoid with topical corticosteroids (letter). *Acta Derm Venereol* 75:89, 1995.

96. Hornschuh B, Hamin H, Wever S, et al: Treatment of 16 patients with bullous pemphigoid with oral tetracycline and niacinamide and topical clobetasol. *J Am Acad Dermatol* 36:101-103, 1997.

97. Thomas I, Khorenian S, Arbesfeld DM: Treatment of generalized bullous pemphigoid with oral tetracycline. *J Am Acad Dermatol* 28:74-77, 1993.

98. Mangelsdorf HC, White WL, Jorizza JL: Behçet's disease. Report of 25 patients from the United States with prominent mucocutaneous involvement. *J Am Acad Dermatol* 34:745-750, 1996.

99. Chow RK. Ho VC: Treatment of pyoderma gangrenosum. *J Am Acad Dermatol* 34:1047-1060, 1996.

100. Shah M, Lewis FM, Harrington CTR: Scrotal pyoderma gangrenosum associated with dermatomyositis. *Clin Exp Dermatol* 21:151-153, 1996.

101. Halder RM: Hair and scalp disorders in blacks. *Cutis* 32:378-380, 1988.

102. Leydon JL, Kligman A: Treatment of alopecia areata with a steroid solution. *Arch Dermatol* 106:924, 1972.

103. Zackheim HS, Kashani-Sabet M, Amin S: Topical corticosteroids for mycosis fungoides. Experience in 79 patients. *Arch Dermatol* 134:949-954, 1998.

104. Kumari J: Vitiligo treated with topical clobetasol propionate. *Arch Dermatol* 120:631-635, 1984.

105. Drake LA, Dinehart SM, Farmer ER, et al: Guidelines for care for vitiligo. *J Am Acad Dermatol* 35:620-626, 1996.

106. Njoo MD, Westerhof W, Bos JD, et al: Development of guidelines for the treatment of vitiligo. *Arch Dermatol* 135:1514-1521, 1999.

Systemic Adverse Effects

107. Munro DD: Percutaneous absorption in humans with particular reference to topical steroids and their systemic influence, thesis for doctorate in medicine, University of London, 1975.

108. May P, Stein EJ, Ryter RJ, et al: Cushing syndrome from percutaneous absorption of triamcinolone cream. *Arch Intern Med* 136:612-613, 1976.

109. Himathongkam T, Dasanabhairochana P, Pitchayayothin N, et al: Florid Cushing's syndrome and hirsutism induced by desoximetasone. *JAMA* 239:430-431, 1978.

110. Gilbertson EO, Spellman MC, Piacquadio DJ, et al: Super potent topical corticosteroid use associated with adrenal suppression: clinical considerations. *J Am Acad Dermatol* 38:318-321, 1998.

111. Brozyskowski M, Grant DB, Wells RS: Cushing's syndrome induced by topical steroids used for the treatment of nonbullous icthyosiform erythroderma. *Clin Exp Dermatol* 1:337-342, 1976.

112. Keipert JA, Kelly R: Temporary Cushing's syndrome from percutaneous absorption of betamethasone valerate. *Med J Aust* 1:542-544, 1971.

113. Bode HH: Dwarfism following long-term topical corticosteroid treatment. *JAMA* 244:813-814, 1980.

114. Cook LJ, Freinkel RK, Zugerman C, et al: Iatrogenic hyperadrenocorticism during topical steroid therapy: assessment of systemic effects by metabolic criteria. *J Am Acad Dermatol* 6:1054-1060, 1982.

115. Carruthers JA, August PJ, Staughton RCD: Observations on the systemic effect of topical clobetasol propionate (Dermovate). *BMJ* 4:203-204, 1975.

116. Ortega E, Burdick KH, Segre EJ: Adrenal suppression by clobetasol propionate. *Lancet* 1:1200, 1975.

117. West DP, Worobec S, Solomon LM: Pharmacology and toxicology of infant skin. *J Invest Dermatol* 76:147-150, 1981.

118. Drake LA, Dinehart SM, Farmer ER, et al: Guidelines of care for the use of topical glucocorticosteroids. *J Am Acad Dermatol* 35:615-619, 1996.

119. Cunliffe WJ, Burton JL, Holti G, et al: Hazards of steroid therapy in hepatic failure. *Br J Dermatol* 93:183-185, 1975.

Local Adverse Effects

120. Akers WA: Risks of unoccluded topical steroids in clinical trials. *Arch Dermatol* 116:786-788, 1980.

121. Kligman AM: Adverse effects of topical corticosteroids. In Christophers E, Schopf E, Kligman AM, et al, editors: *Topical corticosteroid therapy: a novel approach to safer drugs*, New York, 1988, Raven Press, pp 181-187.

122. Kirby JD, Munro DD: Steroid-induced atrophy in an animal and human model. *Br J Dermatol* 94(Suppl 12):111-119, 1976.

123. Katz HI, Prawer SE, Mooney JJ, et al: Preatrophy: covert sign of thinned skin. *J Am Acad Dermatol* 20:731-735, 1989.

124. Feldman RJ, Maibach HI: Regional variation in percutaneous penetration of 14C cortisol in man. *J Invest Dermatol* 48:181-183, 1967.

125. Johns AM, Bower BD: Wasting of the napkin area after repeated use of fluorinated steroid ointment. *BMJ* 1:347-348, 1970.

126. O'Donoghue MN: Perioral dermatitis. In Arndt KA, Leboit PE, Robinson JK, et al, editors: *Cutaneous medicine and surgery,* Philadelphia, 1996, WB Saunders, pp 497-502.

127. Fulton JE, Kligman AM: Aggravation of acne vulgaris by topical application of corticosteroids under occlusion. *Cutis* 4:1106-1109, 1968.

128. Leyden JJ, Thew M, Kligman AM: Steroid rosacea. *Arch Dermatol* 110:619-622, 1974.

129. MacMillan AL: Unusual features of scabies associated with topical fluorinated steroids. *Br J Dermatol* 87:497, 1972.

130. Ive FA, Marks R: Tinea incognito. *BMJ* 3:149-152, 1968.

131. Wilson FM: Adverse external ocular effects of topical ophthalmic medications. *Surg Ophthalmol* 24:57-88, 1979.

132. Aggarwa RK, Potamitis T, Chong NHV, et al: Extensive visual loss with topical facial steroids. *Eye* 7:664-666, 1993.

133. Schwartzenberg GWS, Buys Y: Glaucoma secondary to topical use of steroid cream. *Can J Ophthalmol* 34:222-225, 1999.

134. Burckhardt W: Kontaktekzem durch Hydrocortison. *Hautarzt* 10:42-43, 1959.

135. Lauerma AI: Contact hypersensitivity to glucocorticosteroids. *Am J Cont Derm* 3:112-132, 1992.

136. Guin JD: Contact sensitivity to topical corticosteroids. *J Am Acad Dermatol* 10:773-782, 1984.

137. Tegner E: Contact allergy to corticosteroids. *Int J Dermatol* 15:520-523, 1976.

138. Wilkinson SM, English JS: Hydrocortisone sensitivity: clinical features of fifty-nine cases. *J Am Acad Dermatol* 27:683-687, 1992.

139. Marks JG, Belsito DV, DeLeo VA, et al: North American Contact Dermatitis Group patch test results for the detection of delayed-type hypersensitivity to topical allergens. *J Am Acad Dermatol* 38:911-918, 1998.

140. Stingeni L, Caraffin S, Assalve D, et al: EM-like contact dermatitis from budesonide. *Contact Dermatitis* 34:154-155, 1996.

141. Stingeni L, Hansel K, Lisi P: Morbilliform EM-like eruption from desoximetasone. *Contact Dermatitis* 35:363-364, 1996.

142. Lauerma AI, Reitamo S: Contact allergy to corticosteroids. *J Am Acad Dermatol* 28:618-622, 1993.

143. Coopman S, Degreef H, Dooms-Goossens A: Identification of cross-reaction patterns in allergic contact dermatitis from topical corticosteroids. *Br J Dermatol* 121:27-34, 1989.

144. Goossens A, Matura M, Degreef H: Reactions to corticosteroids: some new aspects regarding cross-sensitivity. *Cutis* 65:43-45, 1999.

145. Lauerma AI: Contact hypersensitivity to glucocorticosteroids. *Am J Contact Dermat* 3:112-132, 1992.

146. Förström L, Lassus A, Salde L, et al: Allergic contact eczema from topical corticosteroids. *Contact Dermatitis* 8:128-133, 1982.

147. Bircher AJ, Levy F, Langauer S, et al: Contact allergy to topical corticosteroids and systemic contact dermatitis from prednisolone with tolerance of triamcinolone. *Acta Derm Venereol* 75:490-493, 1995.

148. Du Vivier A, Stoughton RB: Tachyphylaxis to the action of topically applied corticosteroids. *Arch Dermatol* 3:581-583, 1975.

149. Du Vivier A: Tachyphylaxis to topically applied steroids. *Arch Dermatol* 112:1245-1248, 1976.

150. Du Vivier A, Stoughton RB: Acute tolerance to effects of topical glucocorticosteroids. *Br J Dermatol* 94(Suppl 12):25-32, 1976.

151. Du Vivier A, Phillips H, Hehir M: Applications of glucocorticosteroids. *Arch Dermatol* 118:305-308, 1982.

152. Singh G, Gupta A, Pandey SS, et al: Tachyphylaxis to histamine-induced wheal suppression by topical 0.05% clobetasol propionate in normal versus croton oil-induced dermatitic skin. *Dermatology* 193:121-123, 1996.

153. Marliere V, Roul S, Labreze C, et al: Crusted (Norwegian) scabies induced by use of topical corticosteroids and treated successfully with ivermectin. *J Pediatrics* 135:122-124, 1999.

154. Perez E, Barnadas MA, Garcia-Patos V, et al: Kaposi's sarcoma in a patient with erythroblastopenia and thymoma: reactivation after topical corticosteroids. *Dermatology* 197:264-267, 1998.

155. Warner M, Taylor J: Agents causing contact urticaria. *Clin Dermatol* 15:623-635, 1997.

156. Fisher AA, Pascher F, Kanoff NB: Allergic contact dermatitis due to ingredients of vehicles. *Arch Dermatol* 104:286-290, 1971.

157. Hernandez N, Assier-Bonnet H, Terki N, et al: Allergic contact dermatitis from propyl gallate in desonide cream (Locapred). *Contact Dermatitis* 36:111, 1997.

158. Ramsing DW, Menne T: Contact sensitivity to sorbic acid. *Contact Dermatitis* 28:124-125, 1993.

159. Goldberg HS: Allergic contact dermatitis from the perfume in Mycolog cream. *Arch Dermatol* 105:896-897, 1972.

Therapeutic Guidelines

160. Stoughton RB: Are generic formulations equivalent to trade name topical glucocorticoids? *Arch Dermatol* 123:1312-1314, 1987.

161. Olsen EA: A double blind controlled comparison of generic and trade name topical steroids using the vasoconstriction assay. *Arch Dermatol* 127:197-201, 1991.

162. Jackson DB, Thompson C, McCormack JR, et al: Bioequivalence (bioavailability) of generic topical corticosteroids. *J Am Acad Dermatol* 20:791-796, 1989.

163. Stoughton TB, Wullich K: The same glucocorticoid in brand-name products. *Arch Dermatol* 125:1509-1511, 1989.

164. Long CC, Finlay AY: The fingertip unit—a new practical measure. *Clin Exp Dermatol* 16:444-447, 1991.

165. Timmins P Gray EA: Degradation of hydrocortisone in a zinc oxide lotion. *J Clin Hosp Pharm* 8:79-85, 1983.

166. Krochmal L, Wang JCT, Patel B, et al: Topical corticosteroid compounding: effects on physiochemical stability and skin penetration rate. *J Am Acad Dermatol* 21:979-984, 1989.

Janet Hill Prystowsky

Topical Retinoids

Topical forms of vitamin A (retinoids) have been utilized widely in the United States for nearly 30 years. The first retinoid to be used topically, all-*trans* retinoic acid, dominated treatment with this class of compounds. In the last 5 years the number of choices available in topical vitamin A therapy has increased from a variety of prescription choices to the seemingly effective over-the-counter (OTC) formulations. Continued research into the area of topical retinoids is likely to bring additional formulations of existing compounds, possible combination drug products, and new derivatives.

The major drugs and compounds discussed in this chapter include all-*trans* retinoic acid (tretinoin), all-*trans* retinol, adapalene, and tazarotene (Table 28-1). Other drugs, such as azelaic acid, possess some retinoid-like activity but are not considered chemically to be retinoids and are not included in this chapter.

DRUG DEVELOPMENT
All-*trans* Retinoic Acid (Tretinoin)
Dr. Albert Kligman developed tretinoin for topical use at the University of Pennsylvania.[1] The drug loosened comedones and thus was developed as an acne drug. It was brought to market in the 1970s by Ortho Pharmaceuticals as Retin-A. Approximately 10 years later, Dr. Kligman and colleagues noted that middle-aged female patients with acne were reluctant to stop the Retin-A therapy even when their acne was under good control because they perceived an improvement in fine lines and general skin appearance while using Retin-A. The first report on the use of Retin-A for photoaging was published in 1986,[2] leading to a succession of clinical and basic studies to more firmly define the efficacy of the product in correcting photoaging changes of facial skin and to define possible mechanisms at the cellular level.[3-9] In addition, the safety of topical applications of the drug was studied to assess the potential for teratogenicity when women of childbearing potential used the drug.[10-15]

Finally, in the early 1990s, a new vehicle for tretinoin was developed. This product was introduced as Renova, with photoaging of the skin as a Food and Drug Administration (FDA) approved indication. Because of the drying nature of the vehicles (in addition to the innate drying tendency of tretinoin) used in Retin-A and the resultant dryness of the skin found in adult patients undergoing treatment for photoaging, the new vehicle in Renova had a moisturizing quality appropriate for dry, photoaged skin.[16] In the mid1990s other formulations of tretinoin entered the marketplace, including Avita and Retin-A Micro. Avita is a tretinoin formulation that complexes with a unique polymer, polyoprepolymer-2, to slow percutaneous absorption and reduce irritation.[17-20] The vehicle in Retin-A Micro incorporates microsponge technology to deliver the tretinoin in a more controlled manner, also decreasing irritating side effects.[21-23]

■ Table 28-1   Topical Retinoids

Generic Name	Trade Name	Date Released	Formulations Available	Natural or Synthetic
All-*trans* retinol*	Avon Bioadvance	1984	Cream	Natural
	Avon Anew Retinol PM	1998	0.15% retinol	
	Avon Anew Retinol Hand Cream	1998	0.3% retinol microsponge carrier in creams	
All-*trans* retinoic acid	Retin-A	1971	0.01% to 0.1% cream	Natural
	Renova	1996	0.05% moisturizing cream	
	Avita	1996	0.025% polyoprepolymer 2 in cream vehicle	
	Retin-A Micro	1996	0.05% microsponge carrier in cream	
Tazarotene	Tazorac	1997	0.05% and 0.1% gel, cream	Synthetic
Adapalene	Differin	1996	0.1% gel 0.1% lotion	Synthetic

*All-*trans* retinol is present in over-the-counter formulations by Avon, Neutrogena, and others.

In addition to acne and photoaging, topical tretinoin was studied during the past 25 years for a large number of other conditions. It was found to have significant beneficial effects in the skin for pigmentation, prevention of steroid atrophy, improved wound healing, treatment of actinic keratoses, and treatment of skin ailments characterized by altered keratinization such as ichthyosis.[24,25]

All-*trans* Retinol

Avon initially introduced all-*trans* retinol in cosmetic products in 1984 in a product that was difficult for consumers to use because of irritation. However, after additional development, Avon and others incorporated all-*trans* retinol into effective OTC products to help counteract photoaging. The newest Avon formulations deliver all-*trans* retinol to the skin in a microsponge carrier, which allows for a slower, more controlled delivery of all-*trans* retinol into the skin. Because all-*trans* retinol represents the parent form of vitamin A, the addition of this compound in various products is not considered a drug. However, in vitro evidence suggests that after absorption into skin cells, all-*trans* retinol is oxidized to form tretinoin and therefore causes many of the changes that occur with tretinoin treatment.[26,27] Clinical evidence suggests beneficial changes in pigmentation and fine lines in women who used topical all-*trans* retinol in OTC formulations.[28]

Adapalene

Due to the irritation from topical tretinoin that often limits the acceptance of the treatment by patients, the search for a retinoid with more selective antiacne effects and less skin irritation led to the development of adapalene. Adapalene was found to be selective in its interaction with retinoid receptors. In comparisons with tretinoin, adapalene was found to be less irritating and at least as efficacious in the treatment of acne.[29-31] Galderma launched this drug in the mid1990s as Differin.

Tazarotene

Tazarotene represents a retinoid with benefits for the topical treatment of both acne and psoriasis. The 0.1% tazarotene gel is approved for both acne and psoriasis whereas the 0.05% tazarotene gel is only approved for psoriasis.[32] A majority of the clinical application of this drug focuses on its role as a drug for mild-to-moderate psoriasis.[33-35] Although its usefulness is limited by its irritating tendency and possible adverse koebnerization potential, the drug is very effective in reducing plaque thickness and clearing psoriatic plaques. These clinical benefits are most significant when tazarotene is combined with mid- to high-potency topical corticosteroids[36] or phototherapy. An additional benefit of tazarotene is that healed psoriatic plaques are less likely to rebound flare when compared with plaques treated with topical steroids alone.[37] Also, because tazarotene is a retinoid, prevention of topical corticosteroid atrophy is less likely when used in combination with topical corticosteroids. Tazarotene was launched in the mid1990s by Allergan under the brand name Tazorac.

PHARMACOLOGY

Table 28-2 lists key pharmacologic concepts for topical retinoids. The structures of the three retinoids discussed in this chapter are shown in Figure 28-1. Note that tretinoin represents an oxidized form of all-*trans* retinol and is endogenously synthesized in the skin from all-*trans* retinol after delivery of all-*trans* retinol via the bloodstream to basal keratinocytes.[38] Thus both all-*trans* retinoic acid (tretinoin) and all-*trans* retinol are naturally occurring retinoids, which means that the human body has the binding proteins and enzymatic machinery in place to properly metabolize these retinoids. In comparison, significant structural differences are evident for adapalene and tazarotene, which are not naturally occurring retinoids, making metabolic pathways more challenging to predict.[39,40] The structure of the different retinoids is important because it determines how they are transported in the bloodstream and within cells. Affinity to binding proteins, both cytoplasmic and nuclear,

■ Table 28-2   Key Pharmacologic Concepts—Topical Retinoids

Drug	All-*trans* Retinol	All-*trans* Retinoic Acid	Adapalene	Tazarotene
Systemic absorption	NA	1%-2% in normal skin; up to 31% in dermatitic skin	Trace	Up to 5% topically applied to normal skin; up to 15% in psoriatic skin
Onset of action	NA	NA	NA	2 wks
Timing of improvement	8-12 wks	8-12 wks; peak effect may be as long as 6 mos	8-12 wks	8-12 wks
Plasma half-life	Normally present in plasma	Normally present in plasma	NA	18 hrs for tazarotenic acid
Distribution	Keratinocytes; unknown dermal uptake	Keratinocytes; minimal uptake in dermis	Follicular penetration 5 min after topical application	Keratinocytes, with dermal penetration and uptake into bloodstream
Metabolism	All-*trans* retinoic acid becomes the active metabolite	No conversion required because it is an active metabolite	Active without metabolic transformation	Rapid (<20 min) metabolism to tazarotenic acid
Excretion	Hepatobiliary and skin desquamation	Hepatobiliary and skin desquamation	Hepatobiliary and skin desquamation	Urine, feces, and skin desquamation
Teratogenicity	Excessive oral vitamin A is teratogenic; no data available on topical all-*trans* retinol	Category C	Category C	Category X

NA, Not available.

is critical for retinoid effects on gene transcription and resultant biologic activity.

Teratogenicity

Vitamin A is required for normal growth and differentiation of many tissues. Excessive quantities adversely affect the developing embryo and fetus of a number of animal species.[10,11] Thus while topical absorption of retinoids is generally slight, there is a concern when large surface areas are treated. For example, patients with psoriasis potentially have large surface areas involved with disruption of the epidermal barrier; therefore the rate of retinoid absorption is likely to be significantly increased. A pregnancy test is recommended before the use of tazarotene in women of childbearing potential, and appropriate birth control measures should be in place for the duration of treatment.[37] Topical retinoids should be avoided during pregnancy.

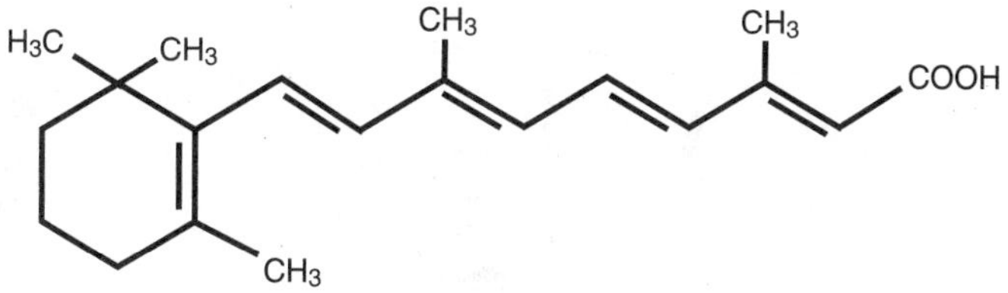

Tretinoin

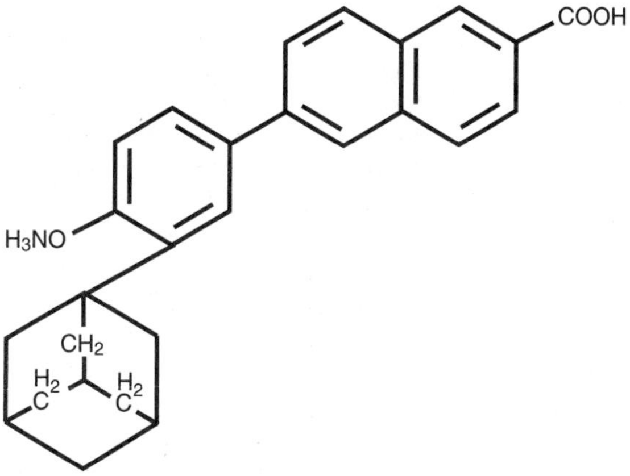

Adapalene

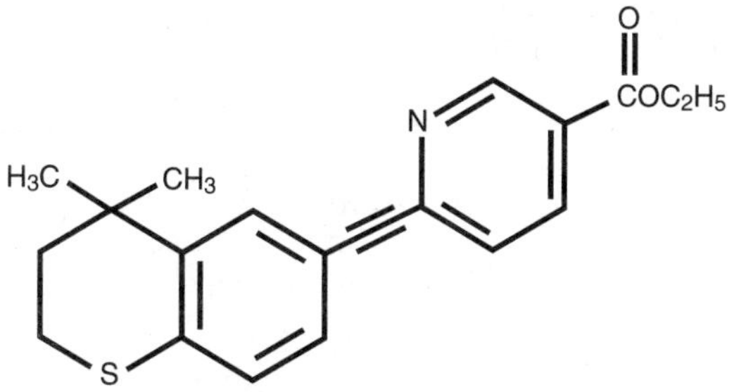

Tazarotene

Figure 28-1 Topical retinoids.

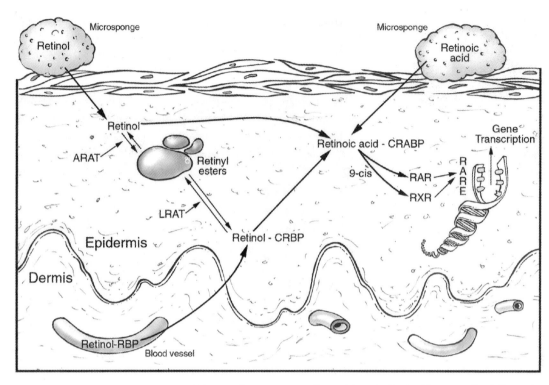

Figure 28-2 Topical and systemic delivery of vitamin A to the epidermis. Retinol is normally delivered to the skin via the dermal vasculature bound to retinol-binding protein. It is taken up into the keratinocyte where it then binds to cellular (or cytosolic) retinol-binding protein (CRBP). Excess retinol in the lower layers of the epidermis is stored as retinyl esters by esterification to long-chain fatty acids through the action of lecithin:retinol acyl transferase (LRAT). Topically applied retinol and retinoic acid are taken up as indicated. Retinol, when in excess in the outer layers of the epidermis, is stored through conversion by acyl CoA:retinol acyl transferase to retinyl esters. Topically applied retinoic acid immediately expands the intracellular pool of retinoic acid because it cannot be reduced to retinol and stored. Thus direct delivery of retinoic acid has the potential, in theory, to overwhelm cellular processes leading to side effects. In contrast, retinol is less irritating when applied topically, presumably because it is stored when plenty of retinoic acid is available. When retinoic acid levels in the epidermis are low, retinol is mobilized from stores of retinyl esters and is oxidized to form all-*trans* retinoic acid, as well as other isomers (e.g., 9-*cis* retinoic acid). These latter two active metabolites bind to the nuclear retinoic acid receptors, RAR and RXR, respectively. These receptors complex to form homodimers and heterodimers that function as transcription factors, binding to retinoic acid response elements (RARE) in deoxyribonucleic acid (DNA) to influence gene transcription. The genes affected are known to influence cell differentiation and proliferation. Modifications of the expression of these genes are associated with improvement of acne, psoriasis, photoaging, hyperpigmentation, and keratinization disorders.

All-*trans* Retinol and All-*trans* Retinoic Acid

The pathway of metabolism for all-*trans* retinol and all-*trans* retinoic acid is illustrated in a summary manner in Figure 28-2. All-*trans* retinol is the natural alcohol form of vitamin A that is transported in the bloodstream from storage in the liver to peripheral target tissues bound to the serum transport protein, retinol-binding protein (RBP) (Table 28-3). All-*trans* retinol then traverses the interstitial spaces in the papillary dermis and is taken up by basal keratinocytes. As these cells divide and move up through the epidermis, vitamin A is distributed across the epidermis.[38] When all-*trans* retinol is topically applied to the skin, this drug is taken up by the keratinocytes in the outer epidermis and diffuses through the skin as a fat-soluble

◼ Table 28-3   Topical Retinoids—Abbreviations and Definitions

Abbreviation	Full Name	Comments
BINDING PROTEINS		
RBP	Retinol-binding protein	Serum transport protein
CRBP	Cytoplasmic retinol-binding protein	Binds all-*trans* retinol in cell
CRABP	Cellular retinoic acid–binding protein	Binds all-*trans* retinoic acid in cell
RECEPTORS AND DNA RESPONSE ELEMENTS		
RAR	Retinoic acid receptor (nuclear)	Three types—RAR-α, RAR-β, RAR-γ
RXR	Retinoid X receptor (nuclear)	Three types—RXR-α, RXR-β, RXR-γ
RARE	Retinoic acid response elements	Enhancing elements—retinoid gene transcription
TIG	Tazarotene inducible gene	Three types—TIG-1, TIG-2, TIG-3
KERATINOCYTE METABOLIC ENZYME SYSTEM		
ARAT	Acyl CoA:retinol acyltransferase	Important for topical retinol
LRAT	Lecithin:retinol acyltransferase	For endogenous all-*trans* retinol
OTHER ABBREVIATIONS		
K6, K16	Keratin 6, keratin 16	Hyperproliferative keratins
MRP-8	Migration inhibition factor related protein	Marker of inflammation, inhibited by tazarotene
Tgase I	Transglutaminase I	Enzyme downregulated by tazarotenic acid

◼ Table 28-4   Binding of Retinoids to Cytoplasmic-Binding Proteins and Nuclear Receptors

Retinoid	CRBP	CRABP	RAR-α	RAR-β	RAR-γ
All-*trans* retinol	++	(−)	(−)	(−)	(−)
All-*trans* retinoic acid	(−)	++	++	++	++
Adapalene	NA	(−)	Weak	++	++
Tazarotenic acid*	NA	NA	+	+++	++

+, minimal binding; ++, moderate binding; +++, relatively strong binding; (−), no binding of the specific retinoid to this binding protein or nuclear receptor; *NA*, not available.
*Tazarotenic acid is the active metabolite of tazarotene.

drug. Within keratinocytes, excess all-*trans* retinol is esterified to long-chain fatty acids to form retinyl esters, which form lipid droplets; this is similar to how vitamin A is stored in the liver.[27]

There are two different enzyme systems in keratinocytes that direct esterification and hydrolysis of retinyl esters—acyl CoA: retinol acyltransferase (ARAT), which is more important for topically applied retinol, and lecithin:retinol acyltransferase (LRAT), which is dominant for endogenously supplied all-*trans* retinol. When all-*trans* retinol exists free within the cell, it binds to the cytoplasmic RBP (CRBP) (Table 28-4). All-*trans* retinol is oxidized to form all-*trans* retinoic acid when needed by the cell.[27,38] All-*trans* retinoic acid formed by this mechanism binds to cellular all-*trans* retinoic acid–binding protein CRABP. From this pool, all-*trans* retinoic acid is transported to the nucleus where it binds to nuclear retinoic acid receptors (RARs). These drug-RAR complexes subsequently bind to retinoic acid response elements (RAREs), which are enhancing elements for gene transcription (Table 28-5). All-*trans* retinoic acid isomerizes to form 9-*cis* retinoic acid, which binds to retinoid X receptors (RXRs). RARs and RXRs bind together as heterodimers to function as transcription factors. Further details on the resultant gene transcription are beyond the scope of this chapter[24,25,41] (see Chapter 13).

A number of all-*trans* retinoic acid responsive genes have been identified. Examples of retinoic acid–influenced genes include the following: (1) Type I epidermal transglutaminase, (2) CRBP, (3) CRABP, and (4) RARs. One of the most pronounced effects of either all-*trans* retinol or all-*trans* retinoic acid treatment of the skin is on epidermal hyperplasia. For thin or atrophic, photoaged epidermis, the effect of topical retinoids is to cause epidermal thickening, or hyperplasia. In hypertrophic skin, such as that found in actinic keratoses or psoriasis, the net effect is normalization of the epidermal thickness.* It should be noted that a number of other retinoid intermediary forms and metabolites are formed through enzymatic reactions in the epidermis. This discussion represents a simplification of the key processes as they are currently understood.

---

*References, 2, 24, 25, 35, 41, 42.

Table 28-5 Topical Retinoid Drug Mechanisms

Retinoid	Mechanism of Action	Resultant Therapeutic Effects	Resultant Adverse Effects
All-*trans* retinol	Gene transcription after conversion to all-*trans* retinoic acid	Comedolysis, epidermal thickening, dermal regeneration, pigment lightening	Irritation, erythema, desquamation
All-*trans* retinoic acid	Gene transcription affects growth and differentiation of cells in the skin; also normalizes follicular epithelial differentiation	Comedolysis; palliative effects on fine wrinkling, mottled hyperpigmentation, and tactile roughness of facial skin	Irritation, erythema, desquamation
Adapalene	Normalizes the differentiation of follicular epithelial cells resulting in decreased microcomedone formation	Comedolysis	Irritation, erythema, desquamation, pruritus, burning
Tazarotene	Blocks induction of ornithine decarboxylase activity, which is associated with cell proliferation and hyperplasia Suppresses MRP8, a marker of inflammation in psoriasis Also inhibits cornified envelope formation and corneocyte accumulation in Rhino mouse skin Inhibits cross-linked envelope formation	Normalization of differentiation and proliferation of the epidermal keratinocytes in psoriasis Also comedolysis in acne	Irritation, erythema, desquamation, pruritus, burning, worsening of psoriasis, photosensitivity, dry skin, fissuring, bleeding Also teratogenic precautions

Adapalene

Adapalene is a derivative of naphthoic acid. It is available as a 0.1% gel or lotion for the treatment of acne. When adapalene 0.1% gel is applied to skin, a comedolytic reaction is seen utilizing the Rhino mouse in vivo model.[39] Fluorescence microscopy shows that adapalene microcrystals penetrate follicular openings to the level of the sebaceous gland within 5 minutes after topical application.[43] The selective uptake by follicles is thought to be due to its lipophilicity and may contribute to adapalene's success in the treatment of acne. It is theorized that after follicular penetration, the lipophilicity of adapalene will result in dissolution within sebum, thus preventing appreciable systemic exposure. Only trace amounts of adapalene are systemically absorbed.

Systemically absorbed adapalene is excreted through the hepatobiliary route. Although adapalene is similar to all-*trans* retinoic acid in its effects on acne, it is more stable chemically, less photolabile, and more lipophilic, which enables it to penetrate follicles quickly. It has selective affinity for RAR-β and RAR-γ. Adapalene does not bind to the CRABP but induces CRABP-II messenger ribonucleic acid (mRNA) when applied under occlusion for 4 days to human skin.[39,44] There is less production of erythema, spongiosis, and hyperplasia of the epidermis by adapalene when compared with all-*trans* retinoic acid.[29-31,39,45,46]

Tazarotene

Tazarotene is a prodrug that is hydrolyzed rapidly in tissues to the active metabolite termed *tazarotenic acid*. Tazarotenic acid has a high affinity to the RAR-γ nuclear receptor that is the predominant receptor present in the epidermis. Tazarotenic acid also binds to RAR-α and RAR-β (see Table 28-2) but not to RXRs. By binding to the various RARs, tazarotenic acid modulates the expression of retinoid responsive genes, including those that regulate cell proliferation, cell differentiation, and inflammation.[32,35,40,42] Modulation of these genes occurs in psoriasis, a disease characterized by increased epidermal proliferation and inflammation. Tazarotene downregulates the abnormal expression of keratinocyte transglutaminase I (Tgase I), epidermal growth factor receptor, and hyperproliferative keratins K6 and K16.[34,47] Tazarotene induces tazarotene inducible gene (TIG-1, TIG-2, and TIG-3) in patients with psoriasis; these are proteins whose role in psoriasis pathophysiology remains to be determined. Migration inhibitory factor–related protein (MRP-8), a marker of inflammation, is decreased by tazarotene treatment.[42,47]

Tazarotene gel produces high cutaneous concentrations, but the systemic absorption of the prodrug is practically nonexistent because of its rapid metabolism to tazarotenic acid. Total systemic absorption is up to 5% of the drug applied in normal skin and 15% of the amount applied in psoriatic skin.[33,48,49] The maximal concentration of tazarotenic acid in the blood occurs 9 hours after tazarotene application. The half-life of tazarotene is less than 20 minutes. Small amounts of tazarotene, which are absorbed systemically and not degraded, are excreted in both the urine and feces. The degradation of tazarotenic acid is via oxidation to inactive sulfoxide and sulfone derivatives that are excreted in the urine. The terminal half-life of tazarotenic acid is approximately 18 hours.[49]

Tazarotene was determined to be nonmutagenic and had no chromosomal effects in a series of in vitro mutagenicity tests. No carcinogenicity was found with topical administration; however, in the hairless mouse model, tazarotene was found to produce increased photocarcinogenicity associated with ultraviolet (UV) radiation.[40,42,48] Not unlike other retinoids, oral administration of tazarotene at high doses was found to be teratogenic in rats and rabbits. However, no teratogenicity was seen in either species with topical application at high doses (limited only by topical irritation).[40,42,48]

Adverse effects observed are those typical for topical retinoids and are discussed in the next section. These include erythema, pruritus, and burning. Six women have become pregnant while using tazarotene, but all had normal births. Nevertheless, the product carries a Category X warning such that tazarotene therapy should be avoided during pregnancy.[32,50] Chronic administration of topically applied tazarotene in animal studies and human studies was found to be safe from a systemic standpoint otherwise. This safety record includes no clinically significant systemic, ophthalmologic, hematologic, or clinical chemistry abnormalities.[48]

CLINICAL USE
Indications

The indications for the topical retinoids are shown in Table 28-6. The contraindications, adverse effects, and drug interactions are summarized in Table 28-7.

ACNE VULGARIS. The systemic retinoid 13-*cis* retinoic acid (isotretinoin) is known to decrease sebum production, and this activity is thought to significantly contribute to its efficacy in treating severe acne vulgaris.[51,52] In contrast, the clinical experience with topical retinoids sug-

---

■ **Table 28-6**   Indications for the Clinical Use of Topical Retinoids

Retinoid	FDA-Approved Indications	Off-Label Uses	Under Investigation
All-*trans* retinol	NA	Photoaging Hyperpigmentation	
All-*trans* retinoic acid	Acne vulgaris Fine wrinkling, mottled hyperpigmentation, tactile roughness of facial skin	Actinic keratoses Hyperpigmentation (e.g., melasma, solar lentigines) Hyperkeratotic disorders Pretreatment of skin to augment wound healing	Prevent atrophy from use of topical steroids
Adapalene	Acne vulgaris		
Tazarotene	Acne vulgaris Psoriasis (<20% of body surface area)		Prevent atrophy from use of topical steroids

---

■ **Table 28-7**   Precautions for Topical Retinoid Clinical Use

Retinoid	Contraindications	Adverse Effects	Drug Interactions
All-*trans* retinol	Hypersensitivity to the vehicle	Irritation of the skin	
All-*trans* retinoic acid	Nursing Pregnancy (relative) Hypersensitivity to the vehicle Caution for eczematous skin, sunburn, permanent wave solutions, electrolysis, hair depilatories or waxes	Irritation, erythema, peeling, temporary worsening of acne Photosensitivity	Photosensitizing drugs (e.g., thiazides, tetracyclines, fluoroquinolones, phenothiazines, sulfonamides) Skin irritants (topical medications or cosmetic products that are abrasive or drying) Possible "neutralization" with simultaneous benzoyl peroxide application
Adapalene	Pregnancy (relative) Hypersensitivity to adapalene or the vehicle	Skin irritation, erythema, peeling, burning, pruritus	Topical sulfur, resorcinol, salicylic acid, alcohol, astringents
Tazarotene	Pregnancy (absolute) Hypersensitivity to tazarotene or the vehicle Eczematous skin, sunburn, exposure to weather extremes	Skin irritation, erythema, peeling Koebnerization of psoriasis	Dermatologic medications and cosmetics that have a strong drying effect should be avoided Photosensitizing medications

gests that their primary mode of action in improving acne is through normalization of the follicular epithelium, which leads to loosening of comedones, thereby allowing sebum to reach the surface of the epidermis more easily.[21,22,51,53-55] Thus preventing sebum buildup, and not sebum production, in follicles is the major therapeutic action for topical retinoid treatment of acne. Although studies using topical isotretinoin have been performed,[51] the mechanism of topical isotretinoin is largely similar to topical tretinoin because of intraepithelial isomerization of isotretinoin to tretinoin.[40] The development of topical isotretinoin has lagged and has not received FDA approval for use in the United States.

Another important difference in topical therapy of acne with retinoids compared with systemic isotretinoin is the duration of remission of acne after discontinuing the retinoid. Although long-term remissions (months to years) are routinely observed after systemic isotretinoin therapy,[52] treatment with topical retinoids needs to be continuous to maintain its comedolytic effects.[54,56] Although numerous studies demonstrated in vitro antiinflammatory effects for retinoids, it is difficult to clinically appreciate the antiinflammatory action of topical retinoids because of the erythema that occurs as a consequence of epidermal irritation.[21,56] Finally, because topical therapy of acne with retinoids is less durable than systemic therapy, it is typically reserved for milder cases of acne. This typically includes cases that are nonscarring and characterized by open and closed comedones with moderate pustule formation. Cystic acne responds poorly to topical retinoid therapy and is better approached systemically with isotretinoin.[52]

Topical retinoid therapy of acne consists of application of the retinoid cream, gel, or lotion to the entire region of the face that is prone to develop acne lesions. Specifically, topical retinoids are not used as a spot treatment for individual lesions. The skin is cleaned with a mild cleansing agent and is left to dry, preferably for up to 30 minutes. A thin film of the topical retinoid is applied once daily, typically at nighttime to avoid photodestruction of the light-sensitive retinoid molecules. This photodestruction theoretically could occur if application were to occur just before sun exposure.

Combination therapy with topical antimicrobial agents is frequently utilized to enhance the therapeutic outcome in acne vulgaris patients. A mild topical vehicle for the antimicrobial agent is advisable, however, to avoid exacerbation of the typical retinoid cutaneous irritation. For more severe cases of acne or where retinoid dermatitis is problematic, oral antibiotic therapy is frequently a better way to deliver antimicrobial action for the treatment of acne.[53,56]

Acne therapy with topical retinoids is a relatively slow process, with worsening of the disease activity commonly occurring in the first 2 to 4 weeks of treatment as the follicular epithelium is loosening. However, by the end of 2 months of treatment, a significant improvement is typically noted with continuing improvement over the months that follow with long-term topical retinoid use. Prevention of new comedones becomes the maintenance therapeutic goal. During topical retinoid therapy, patients must be counseled to avoid astringents, harsh soaps, buff puffs, and other potentially irritating agents (including some benzoyl peroxide products) that traumatize the epidermis to minimize the retinoid dermatitis that accompanies treatment.[56]

ACTINIC KERATOSES.

Rhytides, blotchy pigmentation, telangiectasias, solar comedones, and actinic keratoses (AKs) characterize photodamaged skin. All-*trans* retinoic acid (tretinoin) is the only topical retinoid that has been thoroughly studied for treatment of photodamage and found to be definitively beneficial.[2] AKs are precancerous lesions consisting of dysplastic epithelium that over time may develop into squamous cell carcinomas. Topical tretinoin has been found to decrease the number of AKs on the face by about 50% when used as a monotherapy over a prolonged period of time (minimum of 6 months).[57,58] However, no significant drug effect has been seen on the scalp and extremities.[59] A different approach for treatment of AKs with tretinoin is to use it adjunctively in the treatment of actinic keratoses with topical 5-fluorouracil (5-FU).[60,61] Topical tretinoin, when utilized in this manner, probably leads to enhanced penetration of the 5-FU cream and enhanced efficacy. Thus combination therapy with retinoic acid and topical 5-FU leads to an enhanced therapeutic effect for AKs.[60,61] Because topical tretinoin has been determined to normalize the differentiation of dysplastic epithelium in AKs, it has been considered as a potentially useful agent for chemoprevention in patients at high risk of basal or squamous cell carcinomas of the skin.[58,62,63] In this application, tretinoin is considered a relatively weak agent, and no studies proved it to prevent skin cancer. A limited number of animal studies suggest that topical tretinoin enhanced UV-induced skin tumor production under laboratory-defined conditions.[40,42,48] Caution should be exercised in using the product in patients who continue to have significant sun exposure. In contrast, systemic retinoid therapy in several patient populations has been demonstrated to be efficacious in chemoprevention of keratinocyte malignancies of the skin.[64-69]

PHOTOAGING.   Photoaging is a consequence of UV-induced damage to the skin. This topic is discussed therapeutically in this section separately from AKs because the goal in treating photoaging is to improve the appearance of the skin from a cosmetic point of view. While in the process of treating photoaging changes of the skin, precancerous lesions may simultaneously be treated. Patients who seek medical attention for treatment of photodamage come from a different perspective. A patient with AKs may be concerned about the potential for developing skin cancer but may not care about looking old. Likewise, a patient may have many changes from photodamage, with or without AKs, but may be concerned only with how he or she looks. Although both of these groups benefit from topical tretinoin treatment, the approach to the patient differs. In the case of patients seeking improvement of their appearance in the absence of precancerous lesions, therapy is often considered to be elective. This lack of medical necessity reduces the likelihood of insurance reimbursement for treatment.

The only retinoid that has been proven to decrease fine wrinkling, increase dermal collagen, and repair elastin fiber formation is tretinoin.[2,7-9] Because topical all-*trans* retinol is converted into tretinoin (all-*trans* retinoic acid), it is reasonable to presume that similar effects from its use would also occur. For the other topical retinoids discussed in this chapter, definitive studies to look at their effects on photoaging are necessary to determine their efficacy.

Photoaging is typically treated with a once nightly application of tretinoin in an emollient cream, using a product such as Renova. It gen-

erally takes 3 to 6 months of continuous use to note significant clinical improvement. Just as acne patients need to be counseled regarding gentle skin care while under therapy, so must patients using the product for photoaging. Sunscreen use is particularly stressed because topical tretinoin can increase sensitivity to sunlight due to reduced stratum corneum thickness. In addition, continued sunlight exposure works against the topical retinoid-induced repair processes. Typical instructions include the daily application of a moisturizer that contains sunscreen. Moisturizers that contain alpha-hydroxy acids are often used to get additional improvement of the photoaging changes; however, combination studies have not been done proving an added benefit. Also, high alpha-hydroxy acid concentrations in moisturizers may lead to stinging and burning sensations because of enhanced penetration through the topical retinoid–treated epidermis.

The histologic changes noted with prolonged tretinoin therapy are (1) epidermal hyperplasia of atrophic skin, (2) elimination of dysplastic keratinocytes, including AKs, (3) dispersion of melanin granules, (4) new collagen formation, (5) angiogenesis, and (6) comedolysis.[2,7-9,70] Clinically these changes are seen as smoother skin, a rosy glow, decreased blotchy pigmentation, and diminished fine lines and wrinkles.

PIGMENTARY DISORDERS.   Hyperpigmentation of the skin can be successfully treated with topical retinoids when caused by postinflammatory hyperpigmentation, melasma, or photoaging (lentigines). When the pigmentation problem is mild, topical retinoids are often effective as a solo therapy. However, more significant pigmentary problems are typically treated with tretinoin used in combination with hydroquinone, topical steroids, or alpha-hydroxy acids. As previously noted the retinoid causes melanin granule dispersion, which allows light to pass through the skin more readily, yielding a less pigmented appearance.[71-73]

DYSPLASTIC NEVI.   Another application of topical tretinoin has been to dysplastic nevi with potential utility as a chemopreventive strategy for malignant melanoma. Less melanocytic atypia was noted in treated dysplastic nevi.[74,75] It is unclear as to whether the effects are long lasting, however, as dysplasia recurred 6 months after cessation of therapy in at least one study.[75] Additional studies to clarify the effects of long-term topical retinoids on melanocytic atypia are indicated. It is cumbersome to apply a cream to numerous dysplastic nevi throughout the body. In addition, irritation and photosensitivity secondary to the retinoid therapy may occur, making this treatment approach impractical at the present time.

PLAQUE-TYPE PSORIASIS. When topical tretinoin was introduced for acne in the 1970s, dermatologists also used it to treat psoriasis. The results demonstrated that the irritation from the topical retinoids was unacceptable.[76,77] Thus use of topical retinoids in this setting was never popularized. It was reported that topical tretinoin helped prevent topical corticosteroid atrophy in laboratory animals.[78] Subsequently, topical retinoids were used to prevent topical corticosteroid atrophy in patients who are dependent on topical steroids for their psoriasis treatment.

The development of tazarotene led to a renewed evaluation of topical retinoid therapy for psoriasis. Tazarotene was developed as an antipsoriatic drug due to the therapeutic results of decreasing scaling and decreasing plaque thickness.[33,34,79-81] Tazarotene therapy in psoriasis remains limited somewhat by its tendency for cutaneous irritation requiring combination therapy with medium-to-high potency topical corticosteroids to achieve optimal results and improved patient tolerance of this product.[82] Typically, the tazarotene is applied thinly to the plaques at bedtime and allowed to dry. The following morning, a mid-to-high potency topical corticosteroid is used. Because significant amounts of the active metabolite, tazarotenic acid, are systemically absorbed, it is recommended that tazarotene not be used in pregnant women and that pregnancy be excluded before therapy (Category X). It is useful for mild-to-moderate psoriasis but can rarely be utilized as a monotherapy. Aside from the discomfort from retinoid dermatitis forming at the periphery of psoriatic plaques, tazarotene has on occasion been so irritating that koebnerization reactions

have been observed. The argument can be made that only physicians very familiar with the use of topical retinoids should attempt to treat patients with psoriasis with this product to minimize complications.

WOUND HEALING. Application of tretinoin to the skin for approximately 2 weeks or more before wounding has been demonstrated to enhance the wound healing process and speed the healing time. Studies show that pretreatment with topical retinoids before dermabrasion, medium depth chemical peels, and CO_2 resurfacing results in decreased healing time, as well as overall improvement in cosmetic outcome.[83-87]

Studies also show that pretreatment with topical retinoids can accelerate the healing of full thickness punch biopsy–induced wounds.[88] However, continued application of tretinoin after wounding occurs may stimulate granulation tissue formation but appears to slow reepithelialization. Treatment to stimulate granulation tissue has been frequently tried for stasis ulcers, but no definitive studies have been reported.

Moreover, *early* topical application of retinoids has also been shown to improve the appearance of striae distensae, a type of closed dermal wound.[89,90]

OTHER DERMATOSES. Because retinoids normalize the proliferation and differentiation of keratinocytes, topical retinoids can be used to treat a variety of disorders characterized by abnormal keratinization. In addition to the disorders discussed in detail in this chapter, topical retinoids have been successfully used to treat Darier's disease, ichthyosis, and flat warts.[63,91-93] Other possible clinical uses may include molluscum, oral lichen planus, pityriasis rubra pilaris, palmoplantar hyperkeratosis, vellus hair cysts, pearly penile papules, lichen nitidus, hyperkeratotic epidermal nevi, lichen simplex chronicus, Grover's disease, and more. However, clinical studies and even individual successes (case reports) need to be evaluated more formally to advocate the use of topical retinoids in the aforementioned disease states. Moreover, the practicality of their topical use in the treatment of such disorders may be limited by the extent of the disease. Patients with widespread involvement may be better served with use of an oral retinoid or another systemic therapy to more efficiently treat widespread lesions.

Adverse Effects

See Table 28-7 for a list of the adverse effects of topical retinoids. All topical retinoids produce similar reactions in the skin. Although the pharmaceutical companies focus on big differences between the products regarding irritation, the clinically observed differences are often greater between patients using the same product than between products. The local adverse effects observed include erythema, scaling, pruritus, burn-ing, stinging, dryness, and irritation. Patients also note a decreased tolerance to UV radiation leading to phototoxicity reactions. Because these side effects are not well tolerated, they can lead to a discontinuation of therapy or noncompliance. It is helpful for patients to avoid concomitant use of irritating topical products such as medicated or abrasive soaps and cosmetics, and products with high concentrations of alcohol, astringents, spices, or lime. Also, topical products containing sulfur, resorcinol, or salicylic acid should be avoided while using topical retinoids to minimize irritancy.

Bibliography

Drug Development

Kligman AM, Grove GL, Hirose R, et al: Topical tretinoin for photoaged skin. *J Am Acad Dermatol* 15:836-859, 1986.

Special Issue: Emerging topical retinoid therapies. *J Am Acad Dermatol* 38:S1-30, 1998.

Special Issue: The evolving role of retinoids in the management of cutaneous conditions. *J Am Acad Dermatol* 39:S1-122, 1998.

Special Issue: Topical tretinoin: photodamage treatment overview and developmental toxicology studies. *J Am Acad Dermatol* 36:S25-90, 1997.

Special Issue: Adapalene: a novel topical retinoid receptor agonist for acne. *J Am Acad Dermatol* 36:S91-134, 1997.

Special Issue: Tazarotene: a new generation of receptor-selective retinoids. *J Am Acad Dermatol* 37:S1-40, 1997.

Special Issue: Tazarotene: optimizing the therapeutic benefits of a new topical receptor-selective retinoid. Proceedings of a symposium held during the 19th World Congress of Dermatology. *J Am Acad Dermatol* 39:S123-152, 1998.

References

Drug Development

1. Kligman AM, Fulton JE, Plewig G: Topical vitamin A acid in acne vulgaris. *Arch Dermatol* 99:469-476, 1969.
2. Kligman AM, Grove GL, Hirose R, et al: Topical tretinoin for photoaged skin. *J Am Acad Dermatol* 15:836-859, 1986.
3. Weiss JS, Ellis CN, Headington JT, et al: Topical tretinoin improves photoaged skin; a double blind vehicle controlled study. *JAMA* 259:527-532, 1988.
4. Leyden JJ, Grove GL, Grove MJ, et al: Treatment of photodamaged facial skin with topical tretinoin. *J Am Acad Dermatol* 21:638-644, 1989.
5. Angeles AM, Kahari VM, Chen YQ, et al: Enhanced collagen gene expression in fibroblast cultures treated with all trans retinoic acid: evidence for up-regulation of the alpha 2-promoter activity. *J Invest Dermatol* 94:504A, 1990.
6. Lever L, Kumar P, Marks R: Topical retinoic acid for treatment of solar damage. *Br J Dermatol* 122:91-98, 1990.
7. Olsen EA, Katz HI, Levine N, et al: Tretinoin emollient cream: a new therapy for photodamaged skin. *J Am Acad Dermatol* 26:215-224, 1992.
8. Gilchrest BA: Retinoids and photodamage. *Br J Dermatol* 127(Suppl 41):14-20, 1992.

9. Griffiths CEM, Russman AN, Majmudar G, et al: Restoration of collagen formation in 9 photodamaged human skin by tretinoin (retinoic acid). *N Engl J Med* 329:530-535, 1993.

10. Latriano L, Tzimas G, Wong F, et al: The percutaneous absorption of topically applied tretinoin and its effect on endogenous concentrations of tretinoin and its metabolites after single doses or long-term use. *J Am Acad Dermatol* 36:S37-S46, 1997.

11. Kochhar DM, Christain MS: Tretinoin; a review of the nonclinical developmental toxicology experience. *J Am Acad Dermatol* 36:S47-S59, 1997.

12. Seegmiller RE, Ford WH, Carter MW, et al: A developmental toxicity study of tretinoin administered topically and orally to pregnant Wistar rats. *J Am Acad Dermatol* 36:S60-S66, 1997.

13. Christian MS, Mitala JJ, Powers WJ, et al: A developmental toxicity study of tretinoin emollient cream (Renova) applied topically to New Zealand white rabbits. *J Am Acad Dermatol* 36:S67-S76, 1997.

14. Clewell HJ, Andersen ME, Wills RJ, et al: A physiologically based pharmacokinetic model for retinoic acid and its metabolites. *J Am Acad Dermatol* 36:S77-S85, 1997.

15. Johnson EM: A risk assessment of topical tretinoin as a potential human developmental toxin based on animal and comparative human data. *J Am Acad Dermatol* 36:S86-S90, 1997.

16. Kligman AM: Topical retinoic acid (tretinoin) for photoaging: conceptions and misperceptions. *Cutis* 57:142-144, 1996.

17. Quigley JW, Bucks DAW: Reduced skin irritation with tretinoin containing polyoprepolymer-2, a new topical tretinoin delivery system: a summary of preclinical and clinical investigations. *J Am Acad Dermatol* 38:S1-5, 1998.

18. Mills OH, Berger RS: Irritation potential of a new topical tretinoin formulation and a commercially available tretinoin formulation as measured by patch testing in human subjects. *J Am Acad Dermatol* 38:S11-16, 1998.

19. Lucky AW, Cullen SI, Jarratt MT, et al: Comparative efficacy and safety of two 0.025% tretinoin gels: results from a multicenter, double blind, parallel study. *J Am Acad Dermatol* 38:S17-23, 1998.

20. Lucky AW, Cullen SI, Finicella T, et al: Double-blind vehicle-controlled, multicenter comparison of two 0.025% tretinoin creams in patients with acne vulgaris. *J Am Acad Dermatol* 38:S24-30, 1998.

21. Leyden JJ: Topical treatment of acne vulgaris: retinoids and cutaneous irritation. *J Am Acad Dermatol* 38:S1-4, 1998.

22. Gibson JR: Rationale for the development of new topical treatments for acne vulgaris. *Cutis* 57(1S):13-19, 1996.

23. *Physicians' desk reference,* Montvale, NJ, 1999, Medical Economics Co, Inc.

24. Craven NM, Griffiths CEM: Topical retinoids and cutaneous biology. *Clin Exper Dermatol* 21:1-10, 1996.

25. Orfanos CE, Zouboulis CC, Almond-Roesler B, et al: Current use and future potential role of retinoids in dermatology. *Drugs* 53:358-388, 1997.

26. Kang S, Duell EA, Datta SC, et al: Application of retinol to human skin in vivo induces epidermal hyperplasia and cellular retinoid binding proteins characteristic of but without measurable retinoic acid levels of irritation. *J Invest Dermatol* 105:549-556, 1995.

27. Kurlandsky SB, Xiao J-H, Duell EA, et al: Biological activity of all-*trans* retinol requires metabolic conversion to all-*trans* retinoic acid and is mediated through activation of nuclear retinoid receptors in human keratinocytes. *J Biol Chem* 269:32821-32827, 1994.

28. Kligman AM: Topical treatments for photoaged skin: Separating the reality from the hype. *Postgraduate Med* 102:115-126, 1997.

29. Shalita A, Weiss JS, Chalker DK, et al: A comparison of the efficacy and safety of adapalene gel 0.1% and tretinoin 0.025% gel in the treatment of acne vulgaris: a multicenter trial. *J Am Acad Dermatol* 34:482-485, 1996.

30. Cunliffe WJ, Caputo R, Dreno B, et al: Clinical efficacy and safety comparison of adapalene gel and tretinoin gel in the treatment of acne vulgaris: Europe and US multicenter trials. *J Am Acad Dermatol* 36:S126-134, 1997.

31. Verschoore M, Poncet M, Czernielewski J, et al: Adapalene 0.1% gel has low skin-irritation potential. *J Am Acad Dermatol* 36:S104-109, 1997.

32. Foster RH, Brogden RN, Benfield P: Tazarotene. *Drugs* 55:705-711, 1998.

33. Weinstein GD, Krueger GG, Lowe NJ, et al: Tazarotene Gel, a new retinoid, for topical therapy of psoriasis: vehicle-controlled study of safety, efficacy and duration of therapeutic effect. *J Am Acad Dermatol* 37:85-92, 1997.

34. Esgleyes-Ribot T, Chandraratna RA, Lew-Kaya DA, et al: Response of psoriasis to a new topical retinoid, AGN 190168. *J Am Acad Dermatol* 30:581-590, 1994.

35. Duvic M, Nagpal S, Asano AT, et al: Molecular mechanisms of tazarotene action in psoriasis. *J Am Acad Dermatol* 37:S18-S24, 1997.

36. Lebwohl M, Poulin Y: Tazarotene in combination with topical corticosteroids. *J Am Acad Dermatol* 39:S139-143, 1998.

37. Weinstein GD: Tazarotene gel: efficacy and safety in plaque psoriasis. *J Am Acad Dermatol* 37:S33-38, 1997.

Pharmacology

38. Kurlandsky SB, Duell EA, Kang S, et al: Autoregulation of retinoic acid biosynthesis through regulation of retinol esterification in human keratinocytes. *J Biol Chem* 271:15346-15352, 1996.

39. Shroot B, Michel S: Pharmacology and chemistry of adapalene. *J Am Acad Dermatol* 36:S96-103, 1997.

40. Chandraratna RAS: Tazarotene: the first receptor-selective topical retinoid for the treatment of psoriasis. *J Am Acad Dermatol* 37:S12-17, 1997.

41. Fisher GJ, Voorhees JJ: Molecular mechanisms of retinoid actions in skin. *FASEB J* 10:1002-1013, 1996.

42. Chandraratna RAS: Tazarotene—first of a new generation of receptor-selective retinoids. *Br J Dermatol* 135(S49):18-25, 1996.

43. Allec J, Chatelus A, Wagner N: Skin distribution and pharmaceutical aspects of adapalene gel. *J Am Acad Dermatol* 36:S199-205, 1997.

44. Shroot B: Pharmacodynamics and pharmacokinetics of topical adapalene. *J Am Acad Dermatol* 39:S17-24, 1998.

45. Clucas A, Verschoore M, Sorba V, et al: Adapalene 0.1% gel is better tolerated than tretinoin 0.025% gel in acne patients. *J Am Acad Dermatol* 36:S116-118, 1997.

46. Caron D, Sorba V, Kerrouche N, et al: Split-face comparison of adapalene 0.1% gel and tretinoin 0.025% gel in acne patients. *J Am Acad Dermatol* 36:S110-112, 1997.

47. Duvic M, Asano AT, Hager C, et al: The pathogenesis of psoriasis and the mechanism of action of tazarotene. *J Am Acad Dermatol* 39:S129-133, 1998.

48. Marks R: Clinical safety of tazarotene in the treatment of plaque psoriasis. *J Am Acad Dermatol* 37:S25-32, 1997.

49. Marks R: Pharmacokinetics and safety review of tazarotene. *J Am Acad Dermatol* 39:S134-138, 1998.

50. Allergan: Tazorac 12-week post-maintenance of therapeutic benefit data is from one study. Explicit maintenance claim denied. FDC Reports Pharmaceutical Approvals Monthly 2(12):36-41, 1997.

Clinical Use—Acne

51. Chalker DK, Lasher JL, Smith JG, et al: Efficacy of topical isotretinoin 0.05% gel in acne vulgaris; results of a multicenter, double blind investigation. *J Am Acad Dermatol* 17:251-254, 1987.

52. Leyden JJ: The role of isotretinoin in the treatment of acne: personal observations. *J Am Acad Dermatol* 39:S45-49, 1998.

53. Leyden JJ, Shalita AR: Rational therapy for acne vulgaris: an update on topical treatment. *J Am Acad Dermatol* 15:907-914, 1986.

54. Webster GF: Topical tretinoin in acne therapy. *J Am Acad Dermatol* 39:S38-44, 1998.

55. Lavker RM, Leyden JJ, Thorne EG: An ultrastructural study of the effects of topical tretinoin on microcomedones. *Clin Therap* 14:773-779, 1992.

56. Kligman AM: The treatment of acne with topical retinoids: One man's opinions. *J Am Acad Dermatol* 36:S92-95, 1997.

Clinical Use—Actinic Keratoses

57. Thorne EG: Long-term clinical experience with a topical retinoid. *Br J Dermatol* 127S:31-36, 1992.

58. Lotan R: Retinoids in cancer chemoprevention. *FASEB J* 10:1031-1039, 1996.

59. Alirezai M, Dupuy P, Amblard P, et al: Clinical evaluation of topical isotretinoin in the treatment of actinic keratoses. *J Am Acad Dermatol* 30:447-451, 1994.

60. Robinson TA, Kligman AM: Treatment of solar keratoses of the extremities with retinoic acid and 5 fluorouracil. *Br J Dermatol* 92:703-706, 1975.

61. Bercovitch L: Topical chemotherapy of actinic keratoses of the upper extremity with tretinoin and 5-fluorouracil: a double blind controlled study. *Br J Dermatol* 116:549-552, 1987.
62. Peck GL: Topical tretinoin in actinic keratosis and basal cell carcinoma. *J Am Acad Dermatol* 15:829-835, 1986.
63. Euvrard S, Verschoore M, Touraine JL, et al: Topical retinoids for warts and keratoses in transplant recipients. *Lancet* 340:48-49, 1992.
64. Rook A, Jaworsky C, Nguyen T, et al: Beneficial effect of low dose systemic retinoid in combination with topical tretinoin for the treatment and prophylaxis of premalignant and malignant skin lesions in renal transplant recipients. *Transplantation* 59:714-719, 1995.
65. Kelly JW, Sabbto J, Gurr FW, et al: Retinoids to prevent skin cancer in organ transplant recipients. *Lancet* 338:1407, 1991.
66. Bavinckk JN, Tieben LM, Van der Woude FJ, et al: Prevention of skin cancer and reduction of keratotic skin lesions during acitretin therapy in renal transplant recipients: a double blind, placebo-controlled study. *J Clin Oncol* 13:1933-1938, 1995.
67. Lippman S, Meyskens F: Treatment of advanced squamous cell carcinoma of the skin with isotretinoin. *Ann Intern Med* 107:499, 1987.
68. Peck GL, Digiovanna JJ, Sarnoff DS, et al: Treatment and prevention of basal cell carcinoma with oral isotretinoin. *J Am Acad Dermatol* 19:176, 1988.
69. Kraemer KH, Digiovanna JJ, Moshell AN, et al: Prevention of skin cancer in xeroderma pigmentosum with the use of oral isotretinoin. *N Engl J Med* 318:1633, 1988.

Clinical Use—Photoaging and Pigmentary Disorders

70. Gilchrest BA: Treatment of photodamage with topical tretinoin: an overview. *J Am Acad Dermatol* 36:S27-36, 1997.
71. Kligman AM, Willis I: A new formula for depigmenting human skin. *Arch Dermatol* 111:40-48, 1975.
72. Pathak MA, Fitzpatrick TB, Kraus EW: Usefulness of retinoic acid in treatment of melasma. *J Am Acad Dermatol* 15:894-899, 1986.
73. Griffiths CEM, Finkel LJ, Ditre CM, et al: Topical tretinoin (retinoic acid) improves melasma: a vehicle controlled clinical trial. *Br J Dermatol* 129:415-421, 1993.

Clinical Use—Dysplastic Nevi

74. Halpern A, Schuchter LM, Elder DE, et al: Effects of topical tretinoin on dysplastic nevi. *J Clin Oncol* 12(5):1028-1035, 1994.
75. Edwards L, Jaffe P: The effect of topical tretinoin on dysplastic nevi: a preliminary trial. *Arch Dermatol* 126:494-499, 1990.

Clinical Use—Psoriasis

76. Frost P, Weinstein GD: Topical administration of vitamin A acid for ichthyosiform dermatoses and psoriasis. *JAMA* 207:1863-1868, 1969.
77. Orfanos CE, Schmidt HW, Mahrle G, et al: Retinoic acid in psoriasis: its value for topical therapy with and without corticosteroids. Clinical, histological, and electron microscopic studies on forty-four hospitalized patients with extensive psoriasis. *Br J Dermatol* 88:167-182, 1973.
78. Schwartz E, Mezick JA, Gendimenico GJ, et al: In vivo prevention of corticosteroid-induced skin atrophy by tretinoin in the hairless mouse is accompanied by modulation of collagen, glycosaminoglycans, and fibronectin. *J Invest Dermatol* 102:241-246, 1994.
79. Asano AT, Nagpal S, Chandraratna RAS, et al: Tazarotene (AGN 190168), a topical retinoid, improves psoriasis and alters epidermal gene expression in vivo. *J Invest Dermatol* 194:694, 1995.
80. Krueger GG, Drake LA, Elias PM, et al: The safety and efficacy of topical tazarotene gel, a topical acetylenic retinoid, in the treatment of psoriasis. *Arch Dermatol* 134:57-60, 1998.
81. Weinstein GD: Safety, efficacy, and duration of therapeutic effect of tazarotene used in the treatment of plaque psoriasis. *Br J Dermatol* S49:32-36, 135, 1995.
82. Lebwohl MG, Breneman DL, Goffe BS, et al: Tazarotene 0.1% gel plus corticosteroid cream in the treatment of plaque psoriasis. *J Am Acad Dermatol* 39:590-596, 1998.

Wound Healing and Other Dermatoses

83. Vagotis FI, Brundage SR: Histologic study of dermabrasion and chemical peel in an animal model after pretreatment with Retin A. *Aesthetic Plast Surg* 19:243-246, 1995.
84. Kim IH, Kim HK, Kye YC: Effects of tretinoin pretreatment on TCA chemical peel in guinea pig skin. J Korean Med Sci 11:335-341, 1996.
85. Mandy S: Tretinoin in the preoperative and postoperative management of dermabrasion. *J Am Acad Dermatol* 15:848, 1986.

86. Hevia O, Nemeth AJ, Taylor JR: Tretinoin accelerates healing after trichloroacetic acid chemical peel. *Arch Dermatol* 127:678, 1991.

87. Apfelberg DB: Ultrapulse carbon dioxide laser with CPG scanner for full face resurfacing for rhytids, photoaging, and acne scars. *Plast Reconstr Surg* 99:1817-1825, 1997.

88. Popp C, Kligman AM, Stoudemayer TJ: Pretreatment of photodamaged forearm skin with topical tretinoin accelerates healing of full-thickness wounds. *Br J Dermatol* 132:46-53, 1995.

89. Kang S, Kim KJ, Griffiths CEM, et al: Topical tretinoin (retinoic acid) improves early stretch marks. *Arch Dermatol* 132:519-526, 1996.

90. Elson ML: Treatment of striae distensae with topical tretinoin. *J Dermatol Surg Oncol* 16:3, 1990.

91. Burkhart CG, Burkhart CN: Tazarotene gel for Darier's disease. *J Am Acad Dermatol* 38:1001, 1998.

92. Burge SM, Buxton PK: Topical isotretinoin in Darier's disease. *Br J Dermatol* 133:924-928, 1995.

93. Steijlen PM, Reifenschweiler DO, Ramaekers FC, et al: Topical treatment of ichthyoses and Darier's disease with 13-*cis*-retinoic acid. A clinical and immunohistochemical study. *Arch Dermatol* Res 285:221-226, 1993.

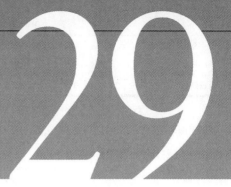
Herschel S. Zackheim

Topical and Intralesional Chemotherapeutic Agents

This chapter discusses the rationale for and experience with topical 5-fluorouracil (5-FU), mechlorethamine, and carmustine, as well as intralesional vinblastine in the management of a number of premalignant, malignant, and various benign dermatoses (Table 29-1).

5-FLUOROURACIL (TOPICAL)

5-FU was synthesized by Heidelberger and co-workers in 1957 and was established as an anticancer agent in 1963.[1] It is a structural analog of thymine in which the 5-methyl group is replaced by fluorine. 5-FU competes for enzymes with normal metabolites such as uracil. It is eventually incorporated into ribonucleic acid (RNA), and inhibits deoxyribonucleic acid (DNA) formation by blocking thymidylate synthetase. This ultimately results in cell death.

Falkson and Schulz[2] in 1962 reported inflammation and clearing of actinic keratoses in a patient treated systemically with 5-FU for cancer. Soon thereafter Klein[3] and Dillaha[4] described destruction of a keratoacanthoma, superficial cutaneous carcinomas, and actinic keratoses with topical 5-FU.

Clinical Use
INDICATIONS
Actinic Keratoses and Related Disorders. The principal indication for topical 5-FU is actinic keratoses. Pearlman[5] reported favorable results in 10 patients treated with pulse therapy (1 to 2 days per week) for a mean of 6.7 weeks rather than a daily schedule. Six patients remained 86% clear at 9 months. Local irritation was limited to erythema. Thus with this regimen, irritation was reduced to an acceptable level while maintaining efficacy. However, Epstein[6] was unable to confirm the efficacy of the pulse regimen. Eight of 13 patients failed to show discernible improvement, and efficacy was linked to the degree of skin irritation. Unis[7] used a short-term intensive 5-FU schedule. Applications were 4 times daily for 7 to 21 days. The same brisk reactions and therapeutic response as achieved with the standard regimen were obtained, with greater patient acceptability.

Bercovitch[8] compared 5% 5-FU cream applied to one arm followed by 0.05% tretinoin cream with 5-FU followed by a control cream to the other arm. The combination of 5-FU with tretinoin appeared to enhance the efficacy of 5-FU. Sander and associates[9] used a combina-

▆ Table 29-1 Topical and Intralesional Chemotherapeutic Agents

Generic Name	Synonym	Trade Name	Manu-facturer	Standard Concentrations	Vial Size
TOPICAL ADMINISTRATION					
5-fluorouracil	5-FU	Efudex*	Roche	5% cream, 2% and 5% solutions*	N/A
		Fluoroplex*	Allergan	1% cream, 1% solution*	
Mechlorethamine	Nitrogen mustard	Mustargen	Merck	10-mg % ointment† 10 mg in 60 ml water	10 mg vials
Carmustine	BCNU	BiCNU	Bristol-Myers Squibb	300 mg in 150 ml stock solution‡	100 mg vial
INTRALESIONAL ADMINISTRATION					
Vinblastine	N/A	Velban	Lilly	0.5 mg/ml	10 mg vials

*Proprietary formulations exist—all other products in this table must be compounded.
†Ointment compounded 10 mg Mustargen in 10 ml absolute alcohol; subsequently compounded in 100 g of petrolatum or Aquaphor. (For total body use 90 mg Mustargen in 10 ml absolute alcohol, then 900 g same bases, lasts 1 month.)
‡Stock solution adequate for 1 month—daily use takes 2.5 ml stock solution in 30 ml water.

tion of topical 5-FU and oral isotretinoin daily for disseminated actinic keratoses for a median treatment time of 21 days. Actinic keratoses disappeared, and photodamaged skin improved in all patients. Adverse effects included burning, itching, and painful erosions. The authors conclude that the combination is highly effective for widespread actinic keratoses on photodamaged skin.

Lawrence and co-workers[10] evaluated a medium depth chemical peel versus 5-FU for facial actinic keratoses. A single application of Jessner's solution (resorcinol, lactic acid, and salicylic acid) and 35% trichloroacetic acid was applied to one side of the face, and 5% 5-FU cream was applied twice daily to the other side for 3 weeks. The authors conclude that the chemical peel is particularly valuable for poorly compliant patients because it is as effective as 5-FU with little morbidity and has the convenience of a single application. The same group reported the long-term results (32 months) of the comparative study of the chemical peel versus 5-FU.[11] There was little difference in the rate of recurrences or improvement of actinically damaged skin as between the two treatments.

Kurwa and colleagues[12] compared a single treatment of photodynamic therapy (PDT) versus 5-FU for 3 weeks for actinic keratoses on the back of the hands. There was no significant difference between the two treatments with regard to efficacy or adverse effects.

Jansen[13] states that actinic cheilitis responds well to 5-FU. Although the response may be more erosive and painful compared with that seen with actinic keratoses, the end result justifies the discomfort.

Keratoacanthomas. In one study, 14 patients were treated with 20% 5-FU ointment for 2 to 4 weeks by Goette and coauthors.[14] All lesions cleared in a mean period of 3.4 weeks. Allergic contact dermatitis occurred in 2 patients. Jansen[13] noted that even giant keratoacanthomas respond to 5% 5-FU under occlusion.

Verruca. Hursthouse[15] evaluated 5% 5-FU cream versus the placebo cream base in a randomized, double-blind study involving 64 patients with verruca. Comparisons were made as to the response of verruca on the right side versus the left side of the body, with one side receiving just a placebo cream. Results were significantly better with 5-FU than with the placebo cream ($p < 0.001$). However, the overall cure rate was only about 60%. Bunney[16] found no advantage of 5-FU over salicylic acid in the treatment of mosaic plantar warts.

Krebs[17] treated 49 nonpregnant women

with extensive condylomata acuminata of the vulva with 5% 5-FU cream. The overall response rate was 71%. Periodic treatment, consisting of twice weekly applications for 10 weeks, was as effective as a continuous daily regimen for 6 weeks with fewer side effects. Rosemberg[18] found that topical 5-FU was an excellent modality in the management, prophylaxis, and treatment of men with recurrent genital human papillomavirus infections.

Other Cutaneous Disorders. Complete clearing was obtained in 2 patients with resistant Darier's disease treated with topical 5-FU by Knulstand and associates.[19] There were no significant adverse effects. One patient with porokeratosis treated by McDonald and Peterka[20] cleared with topical 5-FU. However, results with 5-FU for carcinoma in situ of the vulva are unimpressive.[21]

Therapeutic Guidelines

5-FU is commercially available as 1%, 2%, and 5% solutions and 1% and 5% creams. Applications are made twice daily to the involved areas including normal skin with care not to allow accumulation of excessive amounts about the nose, nasolabial folds, or eyes. A brisk inflammatory reaction is desired and expected; this may include edema, oozing, and crusting. The usual treatment period for the face is 2 weeks. If a minimal reaction occurs, treatment is continued for another 1 to 2 weeks. Topical corticosteroids may be used to relieve the inflammatory reaction. Lesions on the hands and arms may require 4 to 6 weeks treatment to achieve the desired reaction. In addition to inflammation, patients may experience pain, pruritus, hypopigmentation or hyperpigmentation, and burning at the site of application.

MECHLORETHAMINE/NITROGEN MUSTARD (TOPICAL)

Although mechlorethamine (MCH) is commonly referred to as "nitrogen mustard," MCH is but one of a number of nitrogen mustard compounds used in cancer chemotherapy (Figure 29-1). These other nitrogen mustards include melphalan, cyclophosphamide, ifosfamide, and chlorambucil. Nitrogen mustards exert their antineoplastic effect by means of

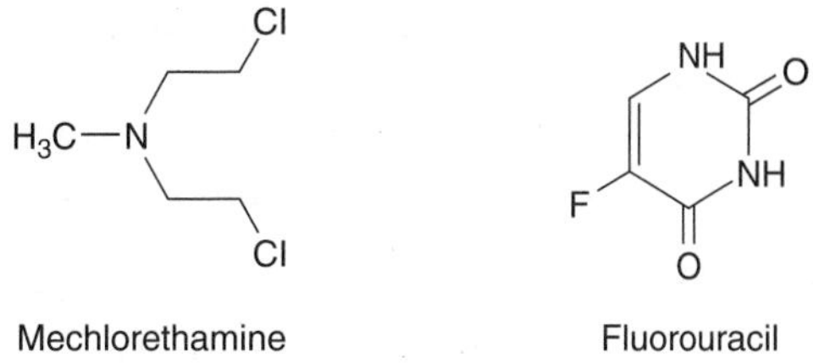

Figure 29-1 Topical and intralesional chemotherapy agents.

alkylation, in which an alkyl or substituted alkyl group becomes covalently linked to cellular constituents, most importantly DNA. The net result is inhibition of DNA replication. All alkylating agents are potentially mutagenic and carcinogenic, as well as cytotoxic. MCH is currently used mostly as part of combination chemotherapy for Hodgkin's disease.[22]

Clinical Use
INDICATIONS

Treatment of Cutaneous T-Cell Lymphoma. Topical MCH has been used predominantly for mycosis fungoides (MF), the most common form of cutaneous T-cell lymphoma (CTCL). The first report of this use, which was published in Hungarian in 1956, was by Sipos, who referenced it in his 1965 report.[23] The first English language report was by Haserick in 1959.[24] Since then, numerous studies documented the efficacy of topical MCH for MF.[25]

MCH is available as Mustargen (Merck), which comes as a vial containing 10 mg MCH hydrochloride and 90 mg sodium chloride. Topical MCH is used either as an aqueous solution or as an ointment. The aqueous solution is prepared by dissolving the MCH powder (and sodium chloride) in tap water in the desired concentration. The initial concentration is usually 10 mg MCH in 60 ml. If this is ineffective, then the concentration may be increased to 20 mg or even 40 mg per 60 ml. Treatments are usually applied daily to the entire cutaneous surface, although intertriginous areas are treated lightly, and the face and genitals are spared unless they have active lesions. Some investigators treat only the involved areas. Treatments are generally continued until a maximum response is obtained, which usually occurs within 3 to 6 months. After clearing, maintenance therapy is often continued daily for varying periods of time and followed by tapering schedules, according to the preference of the investigator (see later discussion).[25]

MCH ointment is prepared by dissolving one 10 mg vial of MCH in 10 ml of 95% (absolute) alcohol, subsequently mixing this solution with an anhydrous ointment base such as Aquaphor or white petrolatum USP. The usual initial concentration is 10 mg/100 g ointment base (10 mg %). If total body MCH therapy is desired, then mixing 90 mg of MCH in 900 g of petrolatum or Aquaphor would give a full month's supply of the compound. Proportionately smaller amounts can be compounded if "spot treatment" is utilized. If this initial concentration is ineffective, then concentrations of 20 mg or 40 mg/100 g base are often used. Applications are made daily similarly to the technique described for MCH solution. Time to clearing (6 to 12 months) with the ointment formulation is usually longer than the time required for clearing with the MCH solution.

It should be noted, however, that for both MCH solution and ointment there have been no prospective, randomized studies comparing total body treatment, regardless of extent of involvement, with treatment to just the involved areas. Neither have there been randomized studies comparing the long-term results of postclearing maintenance therapy versus retreatment only in the event of relapse. Therefore the rationale for postclearing maintenance therapy and for total skin treatment for all patients has not been confirmed.

In this regard the report of Volden[26] is relevant. Two patients developed infiltrated plaques during the period of weekly maintenance therapy after complete clearing. They were then resistant to topical MCH. However, after rest periods of 4 and 6 months, they again became responsive. The investigators favor intermittent therapy to be used only in the event of a relapse.

The Stanford University Experience. Hoppe and co-workers[27] reported combined results in 123 patients treated with either MCH aqueous solution or MCH in Aquaphor ointment base. Applications were made to the entire cutaneous surface. From 1968 to 1980, patients were treated with the solution and, since 1980, with the ointment. The solution was used in 53% of the patients and the ointment in 42%. A polyethylene glycol lotion base was used in 5%. In patients with less than 10% skin involvement, 51% achieved complete remission (CR) and 37% achieved partial remission (PR) (50% or more improvement) for a total response rate (TR) of 88%. For those with 10% or more skin involvement the comparable response rates were CR 26%, PR 43%, TR 69%.

Response rates for the two vehicles were similar—76% for the solution and 79% for the ointment. Time to clearing ranged from 1 to 51 months (median 7.9 months). Duration of maintenance therapy after clearing was from 0 to 57 months (median 8.2 months). Total follow-up was from 6 months to 16 years (median 5.2 years). Relapse occurred in 56% of the patients who achieved CR. When a second course of MCH was used the CR rate was 54%.

In addition, 13 patients with tumor stage disease were treated with topical MCH. None achieved CR, and all subsequently developed progressive skin disease. Nine patients with generalized erythroderma were treated. Two patients cleared but later relapsed. Seven other patients failed to clear, including two who were unable to tolerate concentrations of greater than 2 mg/100 ml because of contact hypersensitivity.

Allergic contact dermatitis occurred in two thirds of the patients treated with the aqueous solution, but in less than 5% of the patients treated with the ointment-based preparation. In addition, 11% of the patients developed squamous cell or basal cell carcinomas; however, all but one received additional therapy including electron beam, psoralen plus ultraviolet A (PUVA), and systemic chemotherapy. Two of the four patients who developed squamous cell cancers died of metastatic disease.

The authors conclude that ointment-based preparations of MCH have the advantage of fewer cutaneous reactions than the aqueous solution while providing equally good control.

The Stanford University group recently reported a retrospective analysis of 148 patients with either generalized patch/plaque MF or tumor stage disease treated with total skin electron beam (TSEB) therapy with or without adjuvant topical MCH.[28] The adjuvant MCH therapy was administered 4 to 8 weeks after completion of TSEB in patients who had achieved CR, and was continued for 1 to 40 months (median 16.5 months). TSEB therapy with or without MCH gave significantly higher response rates as compared with MCH alone. Treatment with adjuvant MCH after TSEB provided an improvement in freedom from relapse as compared with TSEB alone; however, the difference was not quite statistically significant ($p = 0.068$). Additionally, survival was not improved in the group receiving adjuvant therapy as compared with TSEB alone. Nevertheless, the investigators recommend adjuvant MCH therapy because it provides a longer disease-free interval. In addition to the well-recognized adverse effects of TSEB, 21 patients (14%) developed skin cancer, including basal and squamous cell carcinoma and melanoma (3 cases).

The New York University Experience. Ramsay and coauthors[29] reported results with topical MCH aqueous solution in 107 patients with patch/plaque stage MF and in 10 patients with tumor stage MF. However, patients with tumor stage MF also received local radiation and therefore cannot be evaluated with regard to MCH. A solution with a concentration of 10 mg/60 ml was used. Applications were made daily to the "cutaneous surface" with the precaution to apply sparingly to intertriginous sites.

CRs were obtained in 67% of patients with less than 10% skin involvement at the end of 1 year of treatment and in 77% at the end of 2 years. The corresponding CRs for those with over 10% involvement were 40% and 52%, respectively. When classified according to depth of infiltrate (based on clinical judgment), 59% of patients with patch stage disease (stage I) achieved CR after 1 year of treatment, and 76% achieved CR after 2 years. The corresponding CRs for plaque stage (stage II) were 41% and 45% after 1 and 2 years, respectively.

The median time to achieve CR was 4.4 months for those with less than 10% involvement, and 20 months for those with over 10% involvement. The median time to relapse was 66 months for stage I patients and 44 months for stage II patients. Of 29 patients who relapsed, 21 achieved a second CR after retreatment.

Delayed hypersensitivity reactions occurred in 58% of the patients. However, because of successful topical desensitization with dilute solutions, treatment had to be discontinued in only one patient. Twelve (10%) of the patients developed an immediate-type urticarial reaction and had to discontinue MCH due to the possibility

of anaphylaxis. No increase in secondary cutaneous malignancies after topical MCH was seen, with a median follow-up duration of 3.3 years.

The Temple University Experience. Vonderheid and associates at Temple University[30] treated 331 patients with CTCL using topical MCH over a period of 14 years. An aqueous solution of MCH 10 to 20 mg in 40 to 60 ml water was applied once daily to "the entire skin surface except for the genital skin."[30] Patients who achieved CR were treated daily or every other day for at least 3 years after clearing.

Because "many patients with slowly responsive disease, extensive skin or extracutaneous involvement, or otherwise problematic disease were often treated with other modalities,"[30] the effectiveness of MCH as a single agent cannot be evaluated in this study. The other modalities included local radiotherapy, TSEB, ultraviolet light, or systemic drugs such as methotrexate or alkylating agents. Nevertheless, this large study is noteworthy in a number of respects.

CRs were obtained in 80% of CTCL patients with less than 10% skin involvement by patch/plaque disease and in 68% of those with 10% or more involvement. Allergic contact dermatitis occurred in 35% of the patients; all patients used the aqueous solution of MCH.

The frequency of secondary primary cancers was determined. A highly significant relative risk (RR) of 7.8 ($p < 0.001$) for cutaneous squamous cell carcinomas and a significant RR of 1.8 ($p < 0.01$) for basal cell carcinomas were found. Additionally, a highly significant RR of 58.9 ($p < 0.001$) for Hodgkin's disease and a significant RR of 2.6 ($p < 0.005$) for colon cancer were noted. Metastases occurred in 4 of 31 (13%) patients who developed cutaneous squamous cell carcinomas.

Although the authors' original protocol called for maintenance therapy after CR for at least 3 years, they conclude with the recommendation for maintenance therapy for only 6 months. This may reflect concern over the increased risk of secondary skin cancers observed during the study period.

Other Studies Using Topical Mechlorethamine for CTCL. Breneman and coworkers[31] studied the adequacy of skin coverage from a single application of the aqueous solution or ointment vehicle in 6 patients who had been self-treating (or with the help of an assistant) their MF with MCH. A fluorescent dye was added to the solution or ointment vehicle. Approximately 1 hour after application the skin surface and immediate environment, including other persons present, were examined with a Wood's light. Results revealed that an average of 78% of the skin surface was covered by the liquid, compared with 55% coverage for the ointment. Only minimal environmental contamination was found. However, the authors comment that it is likely that more contamination would occur after multiple applications.

Esteve and colleagues[32] recently performed a multicenter study to determine the frequency and histologic features of cutaneous intolerance to MCH in patients treated predominantly for CTCL with an aqueous solution. (MCH ointment cannot be used in France.) Cutaneous intolerance developed in 23 of 43 patients (53%); 21 patients developed intolerance within 3 months. Biopsy specimens showed histologic features of spongiotic dermatitis in nine patients, irritant dermatitis in two, and insignificant changes or normal in three patients. All nine patients with spongiotic dermatitis discontinued MCH, but all five patients who did not show such features were able to resume therapy.

SEVERE COMPLICATIONS
AFTER TOPICAL MCH

Hypersensitivity Reactions. Daughters[33] reported the first case of urticaria and anaphylactoid reaction after topical MCH, which occurred in a woman 68 years of age with MF. Grunnet[34] reported two additional patients with MF who developed urticaria and anaphylactoid reaction after topical MCH. Newman and coauthors[35] reported a woman who developed Stevens-Johnson syndrome after a 1-month treatment course with MCH ointment for CTCL.

Carcinogenic Potential of Topical MCH. Smith and Konnikov[36] described a man who developed four cutaneous squamous cell carcinomas after 2 to 3 years treatment with topical MCH for CTCL. MCH was stopped, and he was then treated with PUVA for 5 months. During the next year he developed a total of 25 squamous cell carcinomas, in addition to multiple

eruptive epidermoid cysts. Death resulted from metastatic disease 1 year later.

Studstrup[37] measured sister chromatid exchanges (SCEs) in lymphocytes of MF patients before and 2 hours and 24 hours after topical application of MCH. No increase in SCEs was found. However, Reddy[38] studied biopsy specimens of MF lesions treated with topical MCH for 10 to 76 months and found atypical histologic changes not present before treatment. These included atypical keratinocytes with large nuclei, suprabasal mitotic figures, increased number of slightly enlarged junctional melanocytes, atypical endothelial cells, and large fibroblasts with atypical nuclei.

Zackheim and Smuckler[39] found topical MCH to be a strong carcinogen in mice. Squamous cell carcinomas developed in 9 of 36 (27%) Swiss mice painted three times weekly on the back for 23 weeks with 0.1 ml MCH 0.2 ml in 95% ethanol. An additional mouse developed a premalignant papilloma. No tumors occurred in control mice painted with ethanol.

As is evident from the preceding review of experience with topical MCH for CTCL, there appears to be a difference regarding the relative hazard of secondary cutaneous malignancies as observed by different investigators.

Thus 11% of patients reported by Hoppe[27] developed squamous or basal cell carcinomas; however, all but one received additional therapy, which could have contributed to the development of malignancy. Ramsay and colleagues[29] found no increase in secondary cutaneous malignancies related to topical MCH. Only two of their patients received additional therapy. However, the median follow-up period of 3.3 years in that study was considerably shorter than the median follow-up of 5.2 years in the Hoppe study. Vonderheid[30] reported in the largest series a highly significant relative risk of 7.8 for cutaneous squamous cell carcinoma and a statistically significant relative risk of 1.8 for basal cell carcinomas in MCH-treated patients. Once again, many patients were treated with other modalities, which could have facilitated the development of malignancy. The median period of follow-up was not stated.

DuVivier and associates[40] analyzed the frequency and etiology of skin cancer in 202 patients with MF treated with topical MCH. (This cohort was later incorporated in the study of Vonderheid.[30]) Two patients who had no prior skin cancers developed squamous cell skin cancers after topical MCH without other therapy.

Lee and co-workers[41] reported a man 58 years of age who developed a squamous cell carcinoma of the scrotum 4 years after starting daily total body treatments with MCH. No other treatment had been given. Additionally, they reported an invasive squamous cell carcinoma of the vulva in a woman who had total body treatments with topical MCH for 2 years. She had also received 25 local ultraviolet B (UVB) treatments to the inner thighs but with shielding of the adjacent genital skin.

Halprin and colleagues[42] studied the frequency of skin cancer in 150 psoriasis patients who had not received PUVA phototherapy. Squamous cell carcinomas occurred in nonsun-exposed areas in six patients who had been treated with MCH in addition to other therapies. Ganor[43] analyzed the data of Halprin[42] and found that skin cancers in nonsun-exposed areas occurred in 6 of 44 patients treated with MCH as compared with only 2 of 106 patients not so treated. The difference was statistically significant ($p < 0.02$). In their reply, Halprin and coauthors[44] concur that MCH is acting as a carcinogen or cocarcinogen and caution against its use in psoriasis.

OTHER INDICATIONS FOR TOPICAL NITROGEN MUSTARD

Langerhans' Cell Histiocytosis. Sheehan[45] treated 16 children with multisystem Langerhans' cell histiocytosis (LCH) and severe skin involvement with topical MCH. Rapid clinical improvement was seen; subsequent healing occurred in 14 patients and partial healing in two others. Mean duration of treatment was 3.5 months (range 2 to 6 months). Adverse effects were minimal. Successful use of topical MCH solution in LCH otitis externa in five children was described by Hadfield and associates.[46] Berman and co-workers[47] produced clearing of cutaneous LCH with topical MCH within 2 to 3 weeks in two elderly patients. Remission was maintained with daily treatment. Nethercott[48] obtained sustained remission in one adult with

LCH whose disease was limited to the skin, but only short-term remission was achieved in an adult with extensive systemic disease and cutaneous involvement.

Psoriasis. In 1959, Van Scott and Reinertson[49] noted involutionary effects of MCH under occlusion on lesions of psoriasis in three patients. This was followed by a clinical report by Epstein and Ugel in 1970[50] and several other series in the 1970s[51,52] demonstrating the efficacy of topical MCH for psoriasis. However, interest soon waned with the development of more potent topical corticosteroids, and there appears to be little current use of topical MCH for psoriasis, at least in the United States. The carcinogenic effect of topical MCH in psoriasis was noted earlier in this chapter.

Other Dermatoses. Arrazola[53] treated 11 patients with severe alopecia areata with topical MCH. Seven had cosmetically acceptable terminal hair growth. Only two patients had a recurrence during a follow-up period of 12 months.

Tsesle and colleagues[54] obtained complete healing of new lesions of pyoderma gangrenosum with topical MCH in a man 69 years of age. Ulcerating skin lesions of chronic granulocytic leukemia improved in a patient treated with topical MCH.[55]

CARMUSTINE/BCNU (TOPICAL)

Carmustine (also named "BCNU" for bischloroethylnitrosourea) is one of several nitrosourea compounds currently used in cancer chemotherapy. Its principal indications are for central nervous system malignancies, lymphomas, melanoma, and gastrointestinal tumors. The principal mechanism of action is by alkylation.[56]

Zackheim[57] first reported the topical use of several nitrosoureas for CTCL in 1972, and since then there have been a number of studies by Zackheim and co-workers on the use of topical BCNU for CTCL.[25,58,59]

Clinical Use

BCNU is marketed as BiCNU (Bristol-Myers Squibb) as a 100-mg powder in a rubber-stoppered, dark-glass vial.

BCNU Solution

BCNU is not directly soluble in water; it must first be dissolved in 95% (or absolute) ethanol and then diluted with tap water. The alcoholic solution is stable at refrigerator temperature for at least 3 months[60] and, based on clinical experience, probably longer. The aqueous solution ideally should be used soon after preparation.

MYCOSIS FUNGOIDES—TOTAL BODY VERSUS LOCALIZED APPLICATION.

A vial of BCNU (100 mg) is dissolved in 50 ml of 95% ethanol, yielding a concentration of 2 mg/ml (the stock solution). Then 5 ml of this solution (10 mg BCNU) is diluted with 60 ml water for total skin coverage. As a rule, 300 mg BCNU in 150 ml ethanol is prescribed; this gives enough stock solution for 1 month. Because only the involved areas are treated, the patient is often instructed to use smaller amounts, such as 2.5 ml stock solution in 30 ml water, as needed. The face, genitals, and intertriginous areas are not treated unless involved. The solution is best applied with a 2-inch nylon brush. Plastic or latex gloves should be worn.

Relatively limited areas (less than 3% of skin involved) can be treated with the undiluted alcoholic stock solution (2 mg/ml) by cautious applications using a cotton-tipped applicator once daily.

STUDY RESULTS—BCNU SOLUTION.

Zackheim[59] reported response rates in 109 patients with patch/plaque MF treated with BCNU solution. In patients with less than 10% skin involvement (T1), CRs were obtained in 86% and PRs in 12%, for a TR of 98%. For those with 10% or more involvement (T2), the corresponding responses were CR 47%, PR 37%, TR 84%.

Zackheim[25] subsequently reported results in 188 patients with patch/plaque MF treated with BCNU solution. Because of the long-term nature of the study, responses were reported in terms of freedom from treatment failure (FFTF). Patients were followed for up to 218 days. The median FFTF for T1 patients was not reached; for T2 patients the median FFTF was 86 months. At 36 months, 91% of T1 patients and 62% of T2 patients had not failed treatment.

The great majority of patients experienced some degree of erythema.[25] This was almost always macular, simulating a sunburn. Body folds were most often involved. Severe reactions were commonly accompanied by skin tenderness, which tended to persist for some months after the erythema subsided. Severe reactions were also often followed some months later by telangiectasia. Varying with the severity, the telangiectasia lasted from several months to as long as 11 years. However, the telangiectasia was benign; biopsies for up to 11 years showed no premalignant changes.

Mild leukopenia (lowest WBC 2700/mm^3) occurred in 3.7% of the patients.[25] Allergic reactions occurred in less than 10% of the patients, were limited to the skin, and were not severe. No skin cancers related to treatment were noted. This is in accord with experiments in mice in which BCNU was found to be a weak topical carcinogen in contrast to MCH, which was a strong topical carcinogen.[26]

BCNU Ointment Preparation

The ointment containing BCNU is prepared by mixing an alcoholic solution of BCNU with white petrolatum USP. The ointment appears to be stable (judged by clinical efficacy) at refrigerator temperature for at least 1 year. Brownish discoloration indicates oxidation and loss of activity.

Concentrations most often used are 20 mg/100 g ointment base (20-mg % concentration) or 40 mg/100 g ointment base (40-mg % concentration). The 20-mg % strength is usually used initially; if response is inadequate, the 40-mg % strength preparation is used. However, the 40-mg % ointment should not be used to over 10% of the skin because of the hazard of bone marrow suppression. Applications are once daily to involved areas only, using protective gloves, with precautions similar to those for BCNU solution.

STUDY RESULTS—BCNU OINTMENT.

Experience with BCNU ointment is considerably less than with the solution. A report of a series of patients has not been published. It is our impression that the ointment causes milder cutaneous reactions than the solution but is less effective. It is easier to use than the solution but is messier. At about the time BCNU ointment was evaluated, it was noted in one study that results with topical corticosteroids, especially the class I compounds, were as good as, or even better than, those with BCNU ointment, with fewer adverse effects. Trials were therefore abandoned with BCNU ointment.

Monitoring Guidelines

Complete blood counts should be obtained at the beginning and once monthly during treatment for both the BCNU solution and the ointment. Treatment must be stopped if erythema, pruritus, or other symptoms develop during treatment. Topical corticosteroids or other antiinflammatory measures should be used.

VINBLASTINE (INTRALESIONAL)

Although intralesional (IL) injection of vinblastine (VBL) has been used with some success in the treatment of cutaneous Kaposi's sarcoma associated with the acquired immunodeficiency syndrome (AIDS-KS), documentation of response rates is limited. Injections are often painful. Boudreaux and coauthors[61] evaluated the efficacy and associated pain of IL VBL 0.5 mg/ml

in 11 homosexual men when administered with or without 1% bicarbonate-buffered lidocaine (BBL). There was a complete or partial clinical response in 88% of the VBL-treated lesions. The addition of BBL did not reduce the efficacy but neither did it reduce the pain of the injections.

Smith[62] treated six patients with multiple cutaneous plaques and tumors of KS with IL VBL, VBL preceded by IL hyaluronidase, or IL hyaluronidase alone. Both IL VBL and IL VBL preceded by IL hyaluronidase caused regression of KS lesions. However, the combination of hyaluronidase and VBL was more effective for tumor nodules. Additionally, lesions treated with hyaluronidase and VBL recurred less often than those treated with VBL alone and showed no evidence of residual KS in two patients biopsied 4 and 6 months after therapy.

Smith and co-workers[63] also treated KS lesions in human immunodeficiency virus (HIV) patients with VBL using iontophoresis. Thirty-one lesions were treated with partial-to-complete clearing and symptomatic improvement. Iontophoresis was well tolerated in contrast to the pain sometimes associated with IL injections.

Bibliography

Chabner BA, Allegra CJ, Curt GA, et al: Antineoplastic agents. In Hardman JG, Limbird LE, Molinoff PB, et al, editors: *Goodman & Gilman's the pharmacological basis of therapeutics,* ed 9, New York, 1996, McGraw-Hill, pp 1233-1287.

Hoppe RT, Abel EA, Deneau DG, et al: Mycosis fungoides: management with topical nitrogen mustard. *J Clin Oncol* 5:1796-1803, 1987.

Jansen T: Topical chemotherapy. *Clin Dermatol* 10:305-307, 1992.

Ramsay DL, Meller JA, Zackheim HS: Topical treatment of early cutaneous T-cell lymphoma. *Hematol Oncol Clin North Am* 9:1031-1056, 1995.

Zackheim HS: Treatment of cutaneous T-cell lymphoma. *Semin Dermatol* 13:207-215, 1994.

References

5-Fluorouracil

1. Heidelberger C, Ausfield FJ: Experimental and clinical use of fluorinated pyrimidines in cancer chemotherapy. *Cancer Res* 23:1226-1243, 1963.

2. Falkson G, Schultz EJ: Skin changes in patients treated with 5-fluorouracil. *Br J Dermatol* 74:229-236, 1962.

3. Klein E, Milgrom H, Helm F, et al: Tumors of the skin. I. Effects of local use of cytostatic agents. *Skin* 1:81-87, 1962.

4. Dillaha CJ, Jansen GT, Honeycutt WM, et al: Selective effect of topical 5-fluorouracil. *Arch Dermatol* 88:247-256, 1963.

5. Pearlman DL: Weekly pulse dosing: effective and comfortable topical 5-fluorouracil treatment of multiple facial actinic keratoses. *J Am Acad Dermatol* 25:665-667, 1991.

6. Epstein E: Does intermittent "pulse" topical 5-fluorouracil therapy allow destruction of actinic keratoses without significant inflammation? *J Acad Dermatol* 38:77-80, 1998.

7. Unis ME: Short-term intensive 5-fluorouracil treatment of actinic keratoses. *Dermatol Surg* 21:162-163, 1995.

8. Bercovitch L: Topical chemotherapy of actinic keratoses of the upper extremity with tretinoin and 5-fluorouracil: a double-blind controlled study. *Br J Dermatol* 116:549-552, 1987.

9. Sander CA, Pfeiffer C, Kligman AM, et al: Chemotherapy for disseminated actinic keratoses with 5-fluorouracil and isotretinoin. *J Am Acad Dermatol* 36:236-238, 1997.

10. Lawrence N, Cox SE, Cockerell CJ, et al: A comparison of the efficacy and safety of Jessner's solution and 35% trichloroacetic acid vs fluorouracil in the treatment of widespread facial actinic keratoses. *Arch Dermatol* 131:176-181, 1995.

11. Witheiler DD, Lawrence N, Cox SE, et al: Long-term efficacy and safety of Jessner's solution and 35% trichloroacetic acid vs 5% 5-fluorouracil in the treatment of widespread facial actinic keratoses. *Dermatol Surg* 23:191-196, 1997.

12. Kurwa HA, Yong-Gee SA, Seed PT, et al: A randomized paired comparison of photodynamic therapy and topical 5-fluorouracil in the treatment of actinic keratoses. *J Am Acad Dermatol* 41:414-418, 1999.

13. Jansen T: Topical chemotherapy. *Clin Dermatol* 10:305-307, 1992.

14. Goette DK, Odom RB, Arrott JW, et al: Treatment of keratoacanthoma with topical application of fluorouracil. *Arch Dermatol* 118:309-311, 1982.

15. Hursthouse MW: A controlled trial on the use of 5-fluorouracil on viral warts. *Br J Dermatol* 92:93-96, 1975.

16. Bunney M: The treatment of plantar warts with 5-fluorouracil. *Br J Dermatol* 89:96-97, 1973.

17. Krebs HB: Treatment of extensive vulvar condylomata acuminata with topical 5-fluorouracil. *South Med J* 83:761-764, 1990.

18. Rosemberg SK: Sexually transmitted papillomaviral infections: V. Prophylactic use of topical 5-fluorouracil in refractory infection in the male. *Urology* 34:86-88, 1989.

19. Knulst AC, De La Faille HB, Van Vloten WA: Topical 5-fluorouracil in the treatment of Darier's disease. *Br J Dermatol* 133:463-466, 1995.

20. McDonald SG, Peterka ES: Porokeratosis (Mibelli): treatment with topical 5-fluorouracil. *J Am Acad Dermatol* 8:107-110, 1983.

21. Lifshitz S, Roberts JA: Treatment of carcinoma in situ of the vulva with topical 5-fluorouracil. *Obstet Gynecol* 56:242-244, 1980.

Mechlorethamine/Nitrogen Mustard

22. Pratt WB, Ruddon RW, Ensminger WD, et al: *The anticancer drugs,* New York, 1994, Oxford University Press, pp 108-154.

23. Sipos K: Painting treatment of nitrogen mustard in mycosis fungoides. *Dermatologica* 130:3-11, 1965.

24. Haserick JR, Richardson JH, Grant DJ: Remission of lesions in mycosis fungoides following topical application of nitrogen mustard. *Cleve Clin Q* 26:144-147, 1959.

25. Ramsay DL, Meller JA, Zackheim HS: Topical treatment of early cutaneous T-cell lymphoma. *Hematol Oncol Clin NA* 9:1031-1056, 1995.

26. Volden G, Molin L, Thomsen K: Topical mechlorethamine therapy for mycosis fungoides. Proposed schedule to overcome drug resistance. *Arch Dermatol* 118:138-139, 1982.

27. Hoppe RT, Abel EA, Deneau DG, et al: Mycosis fungoides: management with topical nitrogen mustard. *J Clin Oncol* 5:1796-1803, 1987.

28. Chinn DM, Chow S, Kim TH, et al: Total skin electron beam therapy with or without adjuvant topical nitrogen mustard or nitrogen mustard alone as initial treatment of T2 and T3 mycosis fungoides. *Int J Rad Oncol Biol Phys* 43:951-958, 1999.

29. Ramsay DL, Halperin PS, Zeleniuch-Jacquotte A: Topical mechlorethamine therapy for early stage mycosis fungoides. *J Am Acad Dermatol* 19:684-691, 1988.

30. Vonderheid EC, Tan ET, Kantor AF, et al: Long-term efficacy, curative potential, and carcinogenicity of topical mechlorethamine chemotherapy in cutaneous T cell lymphoma. *J Am Acad Dermatol* 20:416-428, 1989.

31. Breneman DL, Nartker AL, Ballman EA, et al: Topical mechlorethamine in the treatment of mycosis fungoides. Uniformity of application and potential for environmental contamination. *J Am Acad Dermatol* 25:1059-1064, 1991.

32. Esteve E, Bagot M, Joly P, et al: A prospective study of cutaneous intolerance to topical mechlorethamine therapy in patients with cutaneous T-cell lymphomas. *Arch Dermatol* 135:1349-1353, 1999.

33. Daughters D, Zackheim H, Maibach HI: Urticaria and anaphylactoid reactions after topical application of mechlorethamine. *Arch Dermatol* 107:429-430, 1973.

34. Grunnet E: Contact urticaria and anaphylactoid reaction induced by topical application of nitrogen mustard. *Br J Dermatol* 94:101-103, 1976.

35. Newman JM, Rindler JM, Bergfeld WF, et al: Stevens-Johnson syndrome associated with topical nitrogen mustard therapy. *J Am Acad Dermatol* 36:112-114, 1997.

36. Smith SP, Konnikov N: Eruptive epidermal cysts and multiple squamous cell carcinomas after therapy for cutaneous T-cell lymphoma. *J Am Acad Dermatol* 25:940-943, 1991.

37. Studstrup L, Beck HI, Bjerring P, et al: No detectable increase in sister chromatid exchanges in lymphocytes from mycosis fungoides patients after topical treatment with nitrogen mustard. *Br J Dermatol* 119:711-715, 1988.

38. Reddy VB, Ramsay D, Garcia JA, et al: Atypical cutaneous changes after topical treatment with nitrogen mustard in patients with mycosis fungoides. *Am J Dermatopathol* 18:19-23, 1996.

39. Zackheim HS, Smuckler EA: Tumorigenic effect of topical mechlorethamine, BCNU and CCNU in mice. *Experientia* 36:1211-1212, 1980.

40. Du Vivier A, Vonderheid EC, Van Scott EF, et al: Mycosis fungoides, nitrogen mustard and skin cancer. *Br J Dermatol* 99:61-63, 1978.

41. Lee LA, Fritz KA, Golitz L, et al: Second cutaneous malignancies in patients with mycosis fungoides treated with topical nitrogen mustard. *J Am Acad Dermatol* 7:590-598, 1982.

42. Halprin KM, Comerford M, Taylor JR: Cancer in patients with psoriasis. *J Am Acad Dermatol* 7:633-638, 1982.

43. Ganor S: Skin cancer in psoriatics treated with nitrogen mustard. *J Am Acad Dermatol* 9:164, 1983.

44. Halprin KM, Comerford M, Taylor JR: Reply. *J Am Acad Dermatol* 9:164-165, 1983.

45. Sheehan MP, Atherton DJ, Broadbent V, et al: Topical nitrogen mustard: an effective treatment for cutaneous Langerhans cell histiocytosis. *J Pediatr* 119:317-321, 1991.

46. Hadfield PJ, Birchall MA, Albert DM: Otitis externa in Langerhans' cell histiocytosis—the successful use of topical nitrogen mustards. *Int J Ped Otorhinolaryngol* 30:143-149, 1994.

47. Berman B, Chang DL, Shupack JL, et al: Histiocytosis X: treatment with topical nitrogen mustard. *J Am Acad Dermatol* 3:23-29, 1980.

48. Nethercott JR, Murray AH, Melwidsky W, et al: Histiocytosis X in two adults. Treatment with topical mechlorethamine. *Arch Dermatol* 119:157-161, 1983.

49. Van Scott EJ, Reinertson RP: Morphologic and physiologic effects of chemotherapeutic agents in psoriasis. *J Invest Dermatol* 33:357-362, 1959.

50. Epstein EH, Ugel AR: Effects of topical mechlorethamine on skin lesions of psoriasis. *Arch Dermatol* 102:504-506, 1970.

51. Zackheim HS, Arnold JE, Farber EM, et al: Topical therapy of psoriasis with mechlorethamine. *Arch Dermatol* 105:702-706, 1972.

52. Taylor JR, Halprin KM: Topical use of mechlorethamine in the treatment of psoriasis. *Arch Dermatol* 106:362-364, 1972.

53. Arrazola JM, Sendagorta E, Harto A, et al: Treatment of alopecia areata with topical nitrogen mustard. *Int J Dermatol* 24:608-610, 1985.

54. Tsele E, Yu RC, Chu AC: Pyoderma gangrenosum—response to topical nitrogen mustard. *Clin Exp Dermatol* 17:437-440, 1992.

55. Murphy WG, Fotheringham GH, Busuttil A, et al: Skin lesions in chronic granulocytic leukemia. Treatment of a patient with topical nitrogen mustard. *Cancer* 55:2630-2633, 1985.

Carmustine/BCNU

56. Chabner BA, Allegra CJ, Curt GA, et al: Antineoplastic agents. In Hardman JG, Limbird LE, Molinoff PB, et al, editors. *Goodman & Gilman's the pharmacological basis of therapeutics*, ed 9, New York, 1996, McGraw-Hill, pp 1233-1287.

57. Zackheim HS: Treatment of mycosis fungoides with topical nitrosourea compounds. *Arch Dermatol* 106:177-182, 1972.

58. Zackheim HS, Epstein EH Jr, McNutt NS, et al: Topical carmustine (BCNU) for mycosis fungoides and related disorders: a 10-year experience. *J Am Acad Dermatol* 9:363-374, 1983.

59. Zackheim HS, Epstein EH Jr, Crain WR: Topical carmustine (BCNU) for cutaneous T cell lymphoma: a 15 year experience in 143 patients. *J Am Acad Dermatol* 22:802-810, 1990.

60. Chan KK, Zackheim HS: Stability of nitrosourea solutions. *Arch Dermatol* 107:298, 1973; (correction *Arch Dermatol* 107:782, 1973).

Vinblastine

61. Boudreaux AA, Smith LL, Cosby CD, et al: Intralesional vinblastine for cutaneous Kaposi' sarcoma associated with acquired immunodeficiency syndrome. A clinical trial to evaluate efficacy and discomfort associated with infection. *J Am Acad Dermatol* 28:61-65, 1993.

62. Smith KJ, Skelton HG, Turiansky G, et al: Hyaluronidase enhances the therapeutic effect of vinblastine in intralesional treatment of Kaposi's sarcoma. Military Medical Consortium for the Advancement of Retroviral Research (MMCARR). *J Am Acad Dermatol* 36:239-242, 1997.

63. Smith KJ, Konzelman JL, Lombardo FA, et al: Iontophoresis of vinblastine into normal skin and for treatment of Kaposi's sarcoma in human immunodeficiency virus-positive patients. The Military Medical Consortium for Applied Retroviral Research. *Arch Dermatol* 128:1365-1370, 1992.

Andrew N. Lin

Topical Immunotherapy

Topical immunotherapy can be used to describe any topical agent with immunomodulatory properties. This phrase most often refers to a class of compounds that treat various dermatoses by inducing an allergic contact dermatitis in a previously unsensitized host and maintaining the dermatitis at the site of the skin disease being treated. Three such agents have been extensively studied, mainly in the treatment of alopecia areata and warts—diphenylcyclopropenone (DPC, diphencyprone), squaric acid dibutyl ester (SADBE), and dinitrochlorobenzene (DNCB). In this chapter, these three agents are referred to as *contact allergens*.

More recently, topical formulations of a different class of compounds with direct immunosuppressive actions have been tested in diseases believed to have an immunologic basis, especially atopic dermatitis and psoriasis. These *topical immunosuppressive agents* include tacrolimus (FK 506) and the structurally related ascomycin derivatives (SDZ ASM 981, ABT-281 and SDZ 281-240, all still experimental).

This chapter reviews the pharmacology, clinical efficacy, and adverse effects of these two categories of topical immunotherapy in dermatology (Box 30-1).

CONTACT ALLERGENS

The ideal contact allergen with therapeutic potential fulfills the following criteria: (1) it is a potent topical sensitizer; (2) it is not widely found in the environment; (3) it does not cause significant side effects; and (4) it does not cross sensitize with other substances. DNCB was the first agent to be studied extensively but was found to be mutagenic in the Ames test and has been largely replaced by DPC and SADBE (Figure 30-1). All three agents show favorable results in treatment of alopecia areata and warts. However, many studies are uncontrolled, and the data may be influenced by "publication bias," where positive results are reported more readily than negative ones.[1] Furthermore, alopecia areata and warts are clinically heterogeneous diseases, making it difficult to establish clearly defined, consistently used criteria concerning patient selection and treatment.[1,2] Also, the variable natural course of these conditions can sometimes make it difficult to correlate outcome with treatment.[2]

These agents are *not approved* by the Food and Drug Administration (FDA), and treatment should be initiated only after approval by the appropriate ethics/institutional review board and after obtaining informed consent from the patient[3,4] (Box 30-2). Women of childbearing potential should take contraceptive measures, and in case of pregnancy, treatment should be immediately stopped.[4,5] For DPC and SADBE, some investigators suggest that complete blood count and liver and kidney function should be monitored before treatment and every 3 to 6 months.[4,5] Although children with alopecia

Box 30-1

Topical Immunotherapy Agents

CONTACT ALLERGENS	TOPICAL IMMUNOSUPPRESSANTS
Diphencyclopropenone (diphencyprone, DPC)*	Tacrolimus†
Squaric acid dibutyl ester (SADBE)*	SDZ ASM 981‡
Dinitrochlorobenzene (DNCB)*	ABT-281§
	SDZ 281-240§

*None of these contact allergens has FDA approval for any indication—the uses discussed in this chapter should be considered investigational.
†FDA approval expected in 2001 for tacrolimus use in atopic dermatitis.
‡This drug is currently under investigation for dermatologic use.
§Currently, clinical research on these two drugs has been suspended.

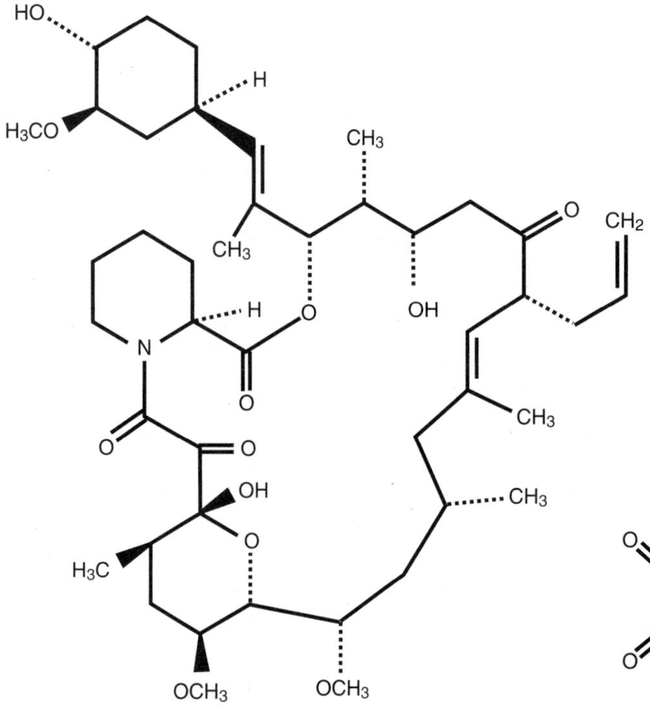

Tacrolimus

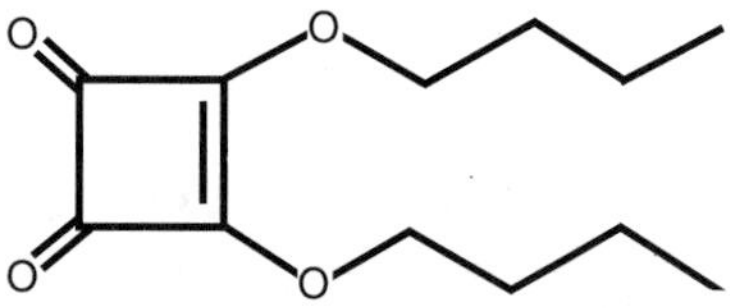

Squaric acid
dibutyl ester (SADBE)

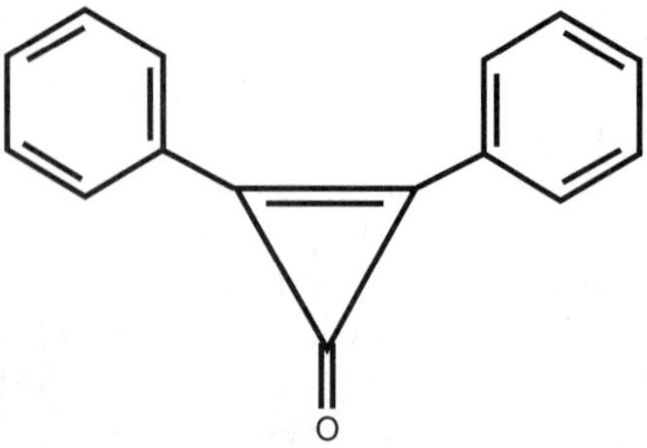

Diphenylcyclopropenone (DPC)

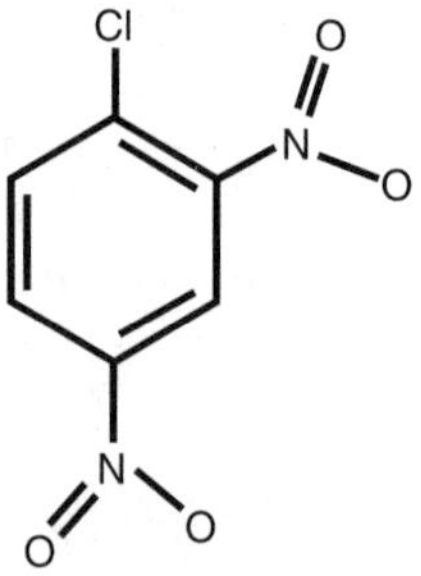

Dinitrochlorobenzene
(DNCB)

Figure 30-1 Topical immunotherapeutic agents.

Box 30-2

Contact Allergens—Clinical Uses Reported in Human Subjects*

DIPHENCYCLOPROPENONE (DPC)
Alopecia areata
Warts
Melanoma (one reported case)

SQUARIC ACID DIBUTYL ESTER (SADBE)
Alopecia areata
Warts

DINITROCHLOROBENZENE (DNCB)
Alopecia areata
Warts
Skin cancers (including melanoma)
HIV infection
Atopic dermatitis
Systemic lupus erythematosus
Lichen nitidus
Chronic nodular prurigo

*All of these uses are investigational—none of the contact allergens currently have FDA approval for any indication. (See text for details and references.)

areata have been treated in several studies, some investigators do not treat children because of the experimental nature of these agents.[4]

Mechanism of Action in Alopecia Areata

It is not known how topical immunotherapy may improve alopecia areata. The "antigenic competition" theory proposes that an immunoreaction to one antigen may inhibit the development of the immune response to another unrelated antigen.[6] In untreated alopecia areata, the peribulbar infiltrate consists predominantly of CD4+ T cells, with a CD4:CD8 ratio of approximately 4:1.[7] With successful treatment with DPC, this ratio changes to 1:1, reflecting a relative increase in peribulbar CD8+ T cells. It is possible that the suppressor T cells may nonspecifically inhibit the immunoreaction to an unidentified hair-associated antigen that is assumed to be the main target in the pathogenesis of alopecia areata.[8] Also, long-term treatment of alopecia areata with DPC or SADBE potentially leads to significant nonspecific systemic suppression of delayed hypersensitivity reactions.[9] In alopecia areata,

DPC treatment also reduces the abnormal expression of human leukocyte antigen (HLA)-A, HLA-B, HLA-C and HLA-DR in the epithelium of lower hair follicles.[10] Investigators reported successful treatment of alopecia areata–like hair loss in mice and rats using topical DPC[10a] and in mice using topical SADBE.[10b]

Mechanism of Action in Warts

The mechanism of action of topical immunotherapy in warts is unknown. It may result from a nonspecific cell–mediated immune response, triggering virus-infected cell lysis and death.[11] Treatment with DNCB increases the incidence of complement-binding wart virus antibodies from 15% to 48%, suggesting a role for humoral factors.[12]

Diphenylcylopropenone

PHARMACOLOGY. Since the 1980s, DPC has been the preferred topical immunotherapeutic agent for alopecia areata. It is not mutagenic in the Ames test, but its synthetic precursor (α,α'-dibromodibenzylketone) is a potential contaminant of commercially obtained samples and is a potent mutagen.[13] Some investigators routinely screen for its presence before use and periodically thereafter with high-performance liquid chromatography.[14,15] DPC is extremely light sensitive, and its photolysis product (diphenylacetylene) is not mutagenic.[13] There are data suggesting the existence of a short-lived, photochemically produced, high-energy mutagenic intermediate, for which the significance is unclear.[13] There is no teratogenicity or organ toxicity in the hen's egg test or in the mouse teratogenicity assay.[16,17] DPC was not detected in serum or urine of 18 human subjects after a minimum of 0.5 ml of 1% DPC solution was applied to the scalp.[18] DPC is stable for at least 4 weeks if stored in a dark container and shielded from light,[19] but some investigators believe its stability can last 3 months[4] and even up to 6 months.[17]

Acetone is a standard solvent because it is a strong ultraviolet (UV) light absorber[3] and because it dries rapidly and allows patients to put on a wig immediately after application.[4] Female patients with childbearing potential should have a negative pregnancy test before being starting DPC treatment and should use reliable birth control during treatment.[20,21] Five women became accidentally pregnant while undergoing DPC treatment for alopecia areata, but all delivered healthy babies.[21] Because the adverse effects are not fully understood, some investigators do not treat children under 10 years of age.[4] DPC costs $87.20 for 5 g, whereas the same amount of SADBE costs $149.50.[2]

CLINICAL USE.   See Box 30-2 for clinical uses of DPC.

Alopecia Areata—Treatment Protocol.   A protocol for treating alopecia areata with DPC has been published in several reviews.* Most patients studied had alopecia totalis, alopecia universalis, or severe alopecia areata. Patients should be sensitized by applying 2% solution in acetone to a 5 × 5 cm area of the scalp with a cotton swab. Some investigators attempt sensitization on the forearm, but this may cause flare-up reactions on the forearm during treatment.[4] Often, an eczematous response is seen 5 to 7 days after initial sensitization.[5,22] Failure to sensitize is observed in 1% to 2% of cases.[5] Elicitation of allergic contact dermatitis can begin as early as 2 weeks after sensitization. This should be done with 0.001% solution if response to sensitization has faded or has not been visible.[5] If eczema is still visible, then elicitation should wait until the eczematous changes disappear. The longer the initial response persists, the lower the initial elicitation concentration should be. In either case, in clinical studies it is important to perform elicitation on one side of the scalp, or one half of a hairless patch, to rule out a possible spontaneous remission. After this, DPC is applied weekly, using the lowest concentration (e.g., 0.0000001%, 0.000001%, 0.00001%, 0.0001%, 0.001%, 0.01%, 0.05%, 0.1%, 0.5%, 1%, or 2%) that maintains erythema, itching, and scaling for 2 to 3 days. In a few patients, 2% concentration does not result in eczema, and a second or third application with the 2% solution is then necessary. It is generally believed that an allergic reaction is an integral part of successful treatment[23] and that some degree of itching, erythema, desquamation, and even adenopathy should be considered desirable side effects.[22] However, some authors believe

discomfort is not required for satisfying and long-lasting therapeutic results.[24] Some patients are exquisitely sensitive, requiring only 0.0001% solution to maintain reaction.[25] On the other hand, some patients who experience regrowth can develop tolerance, which is defined as "continuous increase in DPC concentration until 2.0% was reached without producing an adequate dermatitis, resulting in loss of all regrowth hair."[26,27] In one study, 15 such patients were subsequently treated with topical SADBE, and 3 achieved complete regrowth.[26] Exceeding a 2% concentration is not recommended[4] (Box 30-3).

Box 30-3

Contact Allergens—Topical Preparations

DIPHENCYCLOPROPENONE (DPC)
Sensitization
2% acetone solution for alopecia areata
1% to 3% acetone solution for warts

Elicitation
0.0000001% to 2% acetone solution for
   alopecia areata
0.001% to 2% acetone solution for warts

Comments
Negative Ames test
Store in dark container, shield from light
Screen for potential mutagenic contaminants
   with high pressure liquid chromatography

SQUARIC ACID DIBUTYL ESTER (SADBE)
Sensitization
2% solution in acetone for alopecia areata
   or warts

Elicitation
0.0000001% to 2% acetone solution for
   alopecia areata
0.01% to 1% acetone solution for warts

Comments
Negative Ames test
Should be refrigerated

DINITROCHLOROBENZENE (DNCB)
Comments
Positive Ames test
Seldom used currently for alopecia areata and
   warts

---

*References 4, 5, 15, 16, 21, 22.

To prevent photolysis, the patient's head should be covered with a hair piece or scarf [21] for at least 6 hours, but preferably 48 hours, when the DPC should be washed off.[15] In successful cases, vellus-like hairs usually appear within 8 to 12 weeks, and these become thicker and darker with continued treatment.[4] When unilateral regrowth is noted, DPC should be applied to the entire scalp. Some authors consider the treatment has failed if no regrowth is seen after 20 weeks.[15] Treatment should be stopped after 30 weeks of uninterrupted treatment after the first successful elicitation because a good response later is unlikely.[17] Other investigators, however, empirically continue treatment for up to 3 years.[28] In one study of 26 children, it was shown that continued treatment beyond 1 year in nonresponders was unlikely to promote further hair growth.[29] Eyebrows should be treated with extreme caution, and it has been suggested that the concentration applied to this site should be one-tenth of that used for the scalp.[16] The patient should lie flat and the eyes should be shielded with gauze.[21] Eyelashes should not be treated.[4,16]

Alopecia Areata—Response Rates. The English language literature contains at least 18 studies evaluating DPC as an individual treatment in alopecia areata.* Two additional studies exclusively evaluated children,[14,29] and three others evaluated DPC in combination with other agents.[25,41,42] Overall, there was considerable variation in the response rate, ranging from "whole scalp regrowth" in only 1 of 26 patients (4%),[31] to "excellent or satisfactory" regrowth in 70 of 139 patients (50.4%).[17] In 1998, Rokhsar and colleagues[2] reviewed 17 studies in the English language literature and reclassified all reported treatment outcomes as follows: *complete response* was defined as hair growth described by different authors as excellent; cosmetically acceptable (wig no longer required), or hair growth greater than 90%; *partial response* denoted hair growth referred to as moderate-to-good, or growth between 30% and 90% (wig may be required); *inadequate response* denoted the growth of vellus hair, sparse pigmented or nonpigmented terminal hair, or poor. With these definitions, they determined that the total response

rate (complete plus partial responses) for all 17 DPC studies ranged from 29% to 87%, with a weighted average response rate of 59%.

In 14 studies, DPC was applied only to one side of the scalp and the other half served as control.* Sometimes, hair growth occurred only on the treated side, but subsequent bilateral treatment resulted in growth over the entire scalp.† These observations support a direct therapeutic effect of DPC, rather than just placebo effect or spontaneous remission.[2,4] On the other hand, bilateral regrowth in spite of unilateral treatment may reflect spontaneous remission, and treatment can be stopped.[2,22]

Some patients with good results suffer relapses after stopping treatment. Macdonald Hull and Cunliffe examined 19 patients who were successfully treated (14 had complete regrowth, 5 had almost complete regrowth) after these patients stopped all therapy for 6 months.[33] Two (10%) had lost all the regrown hair, 10 (53%) had patchy alopecia, and 7 (37%) had no hair loss. Van der Steen and associates[26] followed 54 patients who had total regrowth for a mean of 15 months after stopping DPC and found 25 (46%) had not relapsed. Gordon and co-workers[28] followed a cohort of 47 patients for 18 to 36 months. Of the 32 patients who originally responded to DPC treatment, 9 (28%) had maintained cosmetically acceptable regrowth without continuing application of DPC, another 9 (28%) maintained the same regrowth with continued DPC application, and a further 9 (28%) had poor hair regrowth despite continued DPC use. The remaining 5 patients (16%) had to discontinue DPC because of adverse effects.

In two studies, the following factors were associated with a poor response to treatment: extent of hair loss, duration of alopecia before treatment, nail involvement, early age of alopecia onset, and personal history of atopic eczema.[39,40] In another study, nonresponders tended to have rather pronounced inflammatory reactions with dense perifollicular lymphocytic infiltrates.[42a]

Addition of 5% minoxidil had no significant clinical benefit in 13 patients treated with DPC, 5 of whom showed marked regrowth of coarse terminal hair after 24 weeks of DPC treat-

---

ment.[42] Similarly, oral administration of the immunomodulatory agent inosine pranobex did not enhance the efficacy of topical DPC in 33 patients with alopecia totalis.[41] Good response occurred in only 1 of 11 patients receiving DPC only, 1 of 11 receiving both, and none of 10 receiving only inosine pranobex.[41] In a study of 119 patients, Tosti and colleagues[32] found the following rates of complete hair regrowth in response to 4 different treatments were not statistically significant: 28 of 44 (64%) patients treated with SADBE, 27 of 35 (77%) with DPC, 12 of 20 (60%) with topical minoxidil, and 12 of 20 (60%) with placebo.

Alopecia Areata—Adverse Effects. Regional adenopathy is a common adverse effect, occurring in "virtually all" of 139 patients in one study[18] (see Box 30-4). Eczema at the treated site is also common, and this can be quite intense,[34] sometimes causing blisters[14,17,20,37] and sleep impairment.[17,28] The eczema can spread to different sites[17,20,29,34] and even become generalized.[28,34] Less common effects include fever and chills,[34] fainting,[34] and flu-like symptoms.[36]

Vitiligo is a rare event and has been reported at treated sites in seven patients,[28,34,41,43,44] but it extended to distant sites in two of them.[34,44] In one patient, electron microscopy confirmed absence of melanocytes and melanosomes.[43] It is unclear if this reflects koebnerization caused by DPC-induced eczema, a direct chemical effect of DPC, or the higher incidence of vitiligo in patients with alopecia areata when compared with the general population.[35] Because of this rare but disfiguring occurrence, dark-skinned individuals should be treated with extreme caution.[15] A pattern of hyperpigmentation and hypopigmentation, termed *dyschromia in confetti*, occurred in 4 of 243 patients undergoing DPC treatment.[45] This can occur in areas where DPC was applied and can appear in nontreated sites as well. It is unclear if this pigmentary abnormality is a toxic or allergic reaction to the DPC.[45] Three of the four patients had a "rather dark complexion," raising additional caution about DPC use in such individuals.[45]

Erythema multiforme occurred in one patient,[28] two others developed "erythema multiforme–like eruption,"[17] and two other patients who were treated with topical DPC for warts developed "erythema-like" reactions.[46,47] Other adverse effects include urticaria and contact urticaria.[17,48,49] The wife of a patient who was undergoing DPC treatment for alopecia universalis developed vitiligo, presumably due to inadvertent exposure to DPC that the husband was using.[50] Occupational exposure to DPC also resulted in sensitization,[51-55] and staff involved in administering DPC treatment must be protected with gloves, gowns, and barrier creams to avoid accidental exposure.[21]

No significant abnormalities have been noted in blood count, liver function, renal function, electrolytes, ferritin, thyroid function, autoantibody profile, immunoglobulins, and uric acid.[17,20,28,30]

Biopsy of the scalp during or after treatment shows variable results. In children, these results include downward migration of hair follicles to the subcutis, change in follicles from miniature to normal size, reduction of perifollicular fibrosis, and lymphocytic infiltrate.[29]

Warts. Four large studies involving 44 to 134 patients have been reported concerning the use of DPC in treating resistant warts.[11,55-57]

In three of these studies, patients were sensitized on the forearm with 1% to 3% DPC solution in acetone. Starting in 2 to 3 weeks, the lowest concentration (0.001% to 2%) was applied to the warts once a week to produce mild inflammation. Buckley and associates[57] used DPC 0.1% for digital warts and 2% for plantar warts and found clearance of all warts in 42 of 48 patients who persisted with treatment. The median number of treatments to clear was five (range 1 to 22), and median time to clear was 5 months (range 0.5 to 14). Rampen and Steijlen[11] found "complete remission" in 9 of 134 patients after 8 weeks, but a 4-month follow-up showed 49 patients had complete remission. Orrechia and colleagues[55] achieved "complete cure" in 20 of 44 patients.

Naylor and co-workers used a somewhat different approach and were able to sensitize 60 of 62 patients using only 0.1% solution applied to the forearm; they initiated treatment with 0.01% solution applied daily to the warts, except for those lesions on the face or groin, where 0.004% to 0.1% solution was used.[56] "Cure" occurred in 62% of 45 patients, and the majority resolved within 3 to 4 months.[56] The highest cure rate was seen in plantar warts (12 of 16 patients) and periungual warts (9 of 14 patients). In contrast, only 1 of 6 patients with palmar warts achieved cure, and either of 2 patients with genital warts.[56]

Adverse effects included contact dermatitis at distant sites,[56] pigmentation,[55] and severe reactions at treated sites.[11] In one additional report, one patient developed extrasystole during treatment and another experienced generalized urticaria.[58] One technician preparing the solution was inadvertently sensitized to DPC.[55] As with alopecia areata, the long-term effects of DPC treatment for warts are unknown, and it has been suggested that it should be used only as a last resort for treating relapsing multiple warts that resist several other treatments.[55] In one additional case report, a girl 14 years of age with disseminated facial warts experienced clearance after 8 weeks of treatment with DPC.[58a]

Melanoma. A woman 76 years of age with about 400 cutaneous lesions of metastatic melanoma was considered to be too old for aggressive surgical or medical treatment and was treated with oral cimetidine and topical immunotherapy with DPC.[59] After about 66 weeks of treatment, there was "complete histologic resolution."[59] The remission persisted 70 weeks without evidence of distal spread. A delayed hypersensitivity reaction induced by DPC was postulated to augment T-lymphocyte and macrophage response to melanoma cells.

Squaric Acid Dibutyl Ester
PHARMACOLOGY. Like DPC, SADBE is not mutagenic.[60,61] Lifetime subcutaneous injection of squaric acid into ICR/Ha Swiss mice resulted in a low incidence of tumors at the injection site, equal to that observed with saline.[62] No contaminants were found by gas chromatography–mass spectroscopy.[63]

SADBE should not be compounded in absorbent ointment because in this medium it undergoes 41.4% hydrolysis.[63] In one study, investigators found that SADBE in hydrophilic petrolatum or isopropyl alcohol was unsuccessful in producing a dermatitis, and all patients had to eventually switch to SADBE in acetone.[64] SADBE is prone to hydrolysis, but this can be decreased by adding molecular sieves (i.e., molecules that trap and remove water from organic solvents)

to the solution.[63] This chemical is not as stable in acetone as DPC, and requires refrigeration.[3]

CLINICAL USE. See Box 30-2 for clinical uses of SADBE.

Alopecia Areata—Clinical Studies. The treatment protocol for SADBE is identical to that for DPC.[5] The English language literature contains 14 studies evaluating its use in alopecia areata,[60,64-76] with two studies involving children exclusively.[73,74] In seven of these studies,* one part of the scalp was treated, and the untreated part served as control. One study compared SADBE with sodium lauryl sulfate,[68] and another study compared SADBE with DPC, topical minoxidil, and placebo.[34] As with DPC, results varied widely. The largest study involved 144 patients.[75] Of 129 patients with alopecia areata, the following results were obtained: regrowth in 81 patients (63%), no regrowth in 23 patients (17%), and initial regrowth followed by hair loss in 6 patients (5%). Overall, 19 patients (15%) discontinued the study. Of 13 patients with alopecia totalis, 11 patients experienced regrowth, whereas 2 patients had no regrowth. Two patients had alopecia universalis, and one showed regrowth, whereas the other had no regrowth. However, in another series of 17 patients (11 with alopecia areata and 6 with alopecia totalis), terminal hair growth was detected in none of 15 patients who completed 1 month, and only 3 of 6 who completed 3 months of therapy. The study was prematurely terminated because of severe adverse effects such as eczema.[67] One study of 20 patients did show statistically significant improvement in the treated side compared with the untreated side.[72] In 1998, Rokhsar and co-workers reviewed 13 studies in the English language literature and reclassified all reported treatment outcomes as complete, partial, or inadequate response, using the same definitions for their analysis of DPC treatment studies.[2] They found that the total response rate (complete plus partial responses) for all 13 SADBE studies ranged from 9% to 85%, with a weighted average of 58%, almost identical to the figures for DPC.

As with DPC, relapses after successful treatment can occur. Tosti and co-workers reported

---

*References 60, 66, 67, 69, 72, 75, 76.

complete hair regrowth in 10 of 33 children (30.3%), but relapse occurred in 7 of those 10 during follow-up of 1 month to 3 years, while all were still being treated.[74] Similarly, Orrechia's series[73] of pediatric subjects reported a relapse rate of 87%, even 2 to 6 months after treatment.

Some patients were noted to show regrowth at sites distant from the site of SADBE application,[75,77] or showed denser and faster growth on the untreated site compared with the treated site.[60] This is termed the *castling phenomenon*, in reference to the chess maneuver where the rook jumps over the king to the other side of the board. The mechanism is unclear, but a systemic effect of localized application has been proposed.[78] It has been observed also with DPC treatment of alopecia areata[17,79] and is estimated to occur in 1% to 2% of cases treated with DPC.[79]

In one study, early age of onset (before 15 years) was associated with poor treatment outcome with SADBE.[76] Orrechia and associates,[73] however, found no relation between response and age of onset, sex, extent, duration, or clinical type of disease. Combination of PUVA and SADBE was not better than either alone.[80] Tolerance developed in five patients[64,69] and was restored by cimetidine in one.[64] One study found no difference in efficacy between DNCB and SADBE.[71]

During treatment, no abnormalities were detected in blood count, reticulocyte count, liver and kidney function, urinalysis, erythrocyte sedimentation rate, blood sugar, serum protein electrophoresis, uric acid, toxic granules, and Heinz bodies.[60,64,72,75]

In one study, histologic examination of the treated side of the head in 10 patients showed changes of chronic dermatitis in the epidermis.[60] In one study of 19 patients, immunohistologic evaluation of biopsy specimens showed no specific alterations in lymphocyte subclasses and macrophages in relation to the hair growth response.[68] In another study, one patient showed mild granulomatous infiltrate in the area of the hair papillae (significance of this histologic finding is unclear), whereas two others showed chronic dermatitis.[66]

Alopecia Areata—Adverse Effects. Adverse effects observed have been similar to those seen during DPC treatment (Box 30-4). The

Box 30-4

Adverse Effects of Contact Allergens (DPC, SADBE, DNCB)

COMMON
Localized contact eczema (erythema, blistering)
Spread of contact eczema to distant sites
Regional lymphadenopathy
Mutagenicity (positive Ames test only for DNCB)

UNCOMMON
Vitiligo
Dyschromia in confetti
Leukoderma
Erythema multiforme
Erythema multiforme–like reaction
Urticaria
Contact urticaria

most common adverse effects were local and distant eczema, local lymphadenopathy, and pruritus. In one study of 14 patients sensitized with 2% SADBE over a large 9-cm^2 area of the forearms, severe local eczematous reactions occurred in 10 patients, and 9 subjects developed disseminated eczematous reactions.[81] If sensitization is done on the forearm, flexion of the elbow can result in unintentional transfer of the chemical to the biceps area, leading to a spread of the eczematous reaction.[82,83] Uncommon adverse effects include persistence of eczematous reactions,[84] sometimes up to 18 months after only one sensitizing application,[82] benign lymphoplasia at treated site,[85] and development of contact allergy to the acetone vehicle.[86] One patient developed nickel contact allergy, but the relation to SADBE treatment was unclear.[87] In one patient with preexisting vitiligo, SADBE therapy for alopecia areata resulted in leukoderma over the whole scalp.[88] A girl 16 years of age with no history of vitiligo was treated with SADBE for alopecia areata of the scalp and developed transient leukoderma on the untreated forehead, but it faded as soon as treatment was discontinued.[89] Another patient had leukoderma that disappeared at the end of treatment.[75]

Warts. The English language literature contains three large studies of SADBE in treatment of warts. One study involved 20 subjects aged 5 to 50 years; 14 had plantar warts, four had warts around fingernails, and one had warts on the hand and another on the leg.[90] The warts were present for a mean of 15.3 months. Patients were sensitized with 2% SADBE in acetone on the arm and were treated with 0.1% or 0.01% solution once weekly or every other week to maintain mild contact dermatitis. Twelve patients were "cured" after an average of six applications (range 2 to 12), five patients showed either poor or no response after 9 to 18 applications, and three patients developed contact dermatitis and presumably did not respond to therapy.[90]

The second study involved 29 patients (ages 22 months to 40 years) with warts mainly on the hands and feet.[91] Patients were sensitized with 1% or 2% solution in acetone under overnight occlusion on the upper arm, then washed off. Treatment was done by applying 0.5% to 1% solution directly to the warts every 2 to 4 weeks. The 0.5% solution was used in the perianal region and on warts of patients with exuberant contact dermatitis. The face was not treated. Twelve patients received adjunctive therapy such as cryotherapy, salicylic acid, soaking, and cimetidine. Clearing of all warts (for at least 1 month) occurred in 20 of 29 patients, with a mean duration of treatment of 4.2 months. Six patients developed blisters on treated sites.

The third study was an open-label, retrospective study of 59 children.[91a] Sensitization with 2% SADBE on the forearm was followed with home treatment of 0.2% SADBE to the warts 3 to 7 nights per week for at least 3 months. Complete clearing occurred in 34 patients (58%) with mean duration of therapy of 7 weeks, partial clearing in 11 (18%), and no response in 14 (24%). Clearance coordinated with plantar distribution, wart duration under 2 years, and first-line therapy with SADBE. One third of patients had mild adverse effects mainly limited to mild erythema at the site of sensitization.

Dinitrochlorobenzene

PHARMACOLOGY.   DNCB was the first topical sensitizer to be extensively studied for the treatment of alopecia areata and warts. However, this chemical is mutagenic in the Ames test[61,92,93] and is genotoxic by sister chromatid exchange in

human fibroblasts.[94] One study found that commercial grades of DNCB contain contaminants that are mutagenic and carcinogenic in animals.[95] Toxicity or carcinogenicity, however, did not occur in rats and mice who orally ingested DNCB.[96] When applied topically to human skin, greater than 40% of the drug is absorbed systemically.[97] Because of these concerns about safety, DPC and SADBE largely replaced DNCB in treatment of alopecia areata and warts. Topical DNCB has also been studied as an immunologic adjuvant in skin cancers, and its immunomodulatory effects have been studied in human immunodeficiency virus (HIV) disease.

CLINICAL USE.   See Box 30-2 for clinical uses of DNCB.

Alopecia Areata.   The use of DNCB in alopecia areata is very similar to the use of DPC or SADBE. One double-blind study found that DNCB is more effective than croton oil,[98] whereas open studies showed that it can be effective in some patients.[99-105] In one study of 905 patients, DNCB or DPC treatment showed better results than intralesional injection of triamcinolone acetonide but only for patients with bald areas exceeding 50 cm^2 (including alopecia totalis and universalis).[106]

Warts.   The treatment protocol is very similar to that for DPC and SADBE. Patients are usually sensitized on the forearm, although this sensitization can be done on a wart as well.[107] Open studies[12,107-112] showed a cure rate of up to 80%.[12] In one study, 8 of 10 patients who treated the warts on only one side of the body noted healing of warts on the untreated side as well.[113]

Skin Cancers.   DNCB has been used as an immunologic adjuvant in treatment of various types of cancers, meaning that this contact allergen increases host responsiveness to antigenic challenge and potentiates any preexisting antitumor response.[114]

Nonmelanoma Skin Cancers.   Topical DNCB has been found useful in some patients with cutaneous cancers. The mechanism leading to improvement is unclear. It is possible that the sensitizing agent acts as a hapten and interacts with weak tumor antigens that by themselves are not sufficiently immunogenic to evoke an effective immune response.[115]

A man 54 years of age treated about 60 lesions of Bowen's disease with topical DNCB; all except one large lesion resolved after 15 months, and the resistant lesion responded to additional treatment with topical 5-fluorouracil (5-FU).[115] In one study, 36 of 113 basal cell carcinomas in five patients showed complete clinical regression after topical DNCB treatment.[116] In another study of actinic keratoses in 10 patients, 5-FU with DNCB gave only slightly better results than 5-FU alone.[117]

In one study, DNCB resulted in "total eradication" of resistant vulvar carcinoma in situ in four of six patients.[118] However, another study found that DNCB cannot be recommended in the routine management of patients with positive cervical smears.[119] Similarly, one patient with conjunctival squamous cell tumor experienced rapid regression after DNCB treatment,[114] whereas another with conjunctival squamous papilloma did not respond.[120]

Melanoma.   In one randomized prospective study, intralesional DNCB was just as effective as intralesional bacillus Calmette-Guérin in treating recurrent metastatic cutaneous malignant melanoma. Both treatments resulted in 90% regression of lesions.[121] In a woman 71 years of age who was considered unsuitable for surgical treatment of a 1.91 mm Breslow depth acral lentiginous melanoma on the heel, application of DNCB to the lesion resulted in a "severe toxic-allergic reaction," but continued treatment resulted in disappearance of the lesion after 5 months. Ten months later and again 36 months after the initial treatment, local recurrence was similarly treated successfully.[122] Topical DNCB combined with systemic dacarbazine showed promising results in treating 59 patients with recurrent melanoma.[123] Fifteen patients demonstrated a complete response, seven had partial response, and no response was seen in the remaining 37 patients. In another study, 19 patients with melanoma metastatic to the skin were "not amenable to any other form of treatment."[124] Topical DNCB resulted in complete remission in three patients, partial remission in three others, "stabilization" in one, and no improvement in 12 patients.[124]

HIV Infection.   Because DNCB modulates the function of Langerhans' cells, which play an important role in HIV infection, investigators studied the use of topical DNCB sensitization in patients with HIV infection.[125-128] This treatment was associated with improved cellular immune function[129-132] and decreased viral load.[133] More extensive studies are required to better define the role of topical DNCB in HIV infection.

Atopic Dermatitis.   In one open study, six of eight patients (ages 15 to 48 years) with refractory atopic dermatitis treated with topical DNCB showed clinical improvement, and this improvement correlated with eosinophil counts, immunoglobulin E (IgE) levels, and serum soluble interleukin-2 (IL-2) receptor levels. One patient did not show clear improvement, and another showed deterioration.[134] In another open study of nine adults with atopic dermatitis, DNCB treatment led to significant decrease in the total body surface area of involved skin.[134a]

Other Dermatoses.   A woman 71 years of age with systemic lupus erythematosus experienced decreased joint pains and drop in antinuclear antibody (ANA) titer after DNCB treatment.[135] DNCB improved lichen nitidus in a man 40 years of age,[136,137] as well as chronic prurigo nodularis in a woman 50 years of age.[138]

TOPICAL IMMUNOSUPPRESSIVE AGENTS
Topical Tacrolimus
PHARMACOLOGY.   Tacrolimus is a macrolide lactone produced by the soil fungus *Streptomyces tsukubaensis*[139] (see Figure 30-1). It is available in both intravenous and oral formulation for the prevention of organ rejection after allogeneic liver or kidney transplantation. Oral tacrolimus has been found useful in treatment of psoriasis,[140] but potentially serious adverse effects, such as nephrotoxicity and hypertension, limit its use for dermatologic indications. Topical formulations have been extensively studied and show promise in the treatment of inflammatory skin diseases such as atopic dermatitis and psoriasis.[139,141-143]

Cyclosporine lacks topical activity presumably because its large molecular weight (1202.635) results in poor epidermal penetration.[139] In contrast, topical tacrolimus (molecular weight 822.05) can better permeate intact human skin.[144,145] Topically applied tacrolimus is considered to be safe and effective in treatment of skin diseases.[139] Whole blood levels should be monitored to ensure that drug levels do not exceed or even enter the higher end of the range (5 to 20 ng/ml) considered acceptable for transplant recipients.[139]

Topical tacrolimus did not cause atrophy when used to treat an inflammatory reaction in pigskin at a concentration that had efficacy similar to that of 0.13% clobetasol.[146] In atopic patients and normal human volunteers, tacrolimus does not alter collagen synthesis (even under occlusion) and is not atrophogenic.[147] It may therefore have a special role in treating dermatitis of the face and neck, where topical corticosteroids are prone to cause atrophy.[139] A 0.1% ointment can be made by incorporating tacrolimus powder (obtained from 1-mg capsules, Prograf) into hydrophilic petrolatum.[148] This "hydrophilic petrolatum" is composed of white petrolatum containing 8% bleached beeswax, 3% stearyl alcohol, and 3% cholesterol.[148] FDA approval of topical tacrolimus for treatment of atopic dermatitis is expected in 2001.

MECHANISM OF ACTION.

Tacrolimus exerts 10 to 100 times higher immunosuppressive activity than cyclosporine in vitro.[142] This is mediated by a direct effect on T lymphocytes to inhibit IL-2 transcription, which decreases responsiveness of T lymphocytes to foreign antigens.[139] Its action in atopic dermatitis may be related to alteration of the antigen-presenting cells,[149] suppression of IL-2 and costimulatory molecule expression,[150] impairment of phenotypic and functional differentiation of epidermal Langerhans' cells,[151] and suppression of Th1 and Th2 cytokine induction in lymph node cells.[152] The effect of tacrolimus on pruritus may be related to inhibition of histamine release from skin mast cells and impairment of de novo mast cell prostaglandin D_2 synthesis[153] along with diminished release of histamine from basophils.[154] In NC/Nga mice, tacrolimus ointment suppresses development of "spontaneous dermatitis," which normally appears about 8 weeks after birth in untreated animals, and whose pathogenesis is believed to involve immunologic factors.[155] In mouse skin, topical tacrolimus markedly inhibits tumor promotion induced by 12-O-tetradecanoyl phorbol-13-acetate (TPA).[156]

CLINICAL USE

Box 30-5 lists clinical uses of topical immunosuppressants reported in human subjects.

Alopecia Areata. In a vehicle-controlled study,[157] investigators showed that topical tacrolimus causes hair regrowth in an animal model of alopecia areata (the Dundee experimental bald rat model). Topical tacrolimus stimulates hair growth in severe combined immunodeficiency (SCID) mice that lack B- and T-cell immunity, suggesting that this effect is not mediated through immunosuppression.[158] The drug stimulates hair growth also in CD1 mice, rats, and Syrian golden hamsters.[158,159] In mice, topical tacrolimus causes induction of anagen hair, inhibition of massive catagen development, and relative protection from chemotherapy-induced alopecia.[160,161] In a boy 9 years of age with alopecia areata, application of 0.3% tacrolimus ointment twice daily to an approximately 8 × 8 cm hairless patch on the scalp did not result in regrowth, and the patient progressed to alopecia totalis.[162]

Atopic Dermatitis. Topical tacrolimus has been shown to be effective and safe in treatment of atopic dermatitis in several open stud-

Box 30-5

Clinical Uses of Topical Immunosuppressants Reported in Human Subjects*

TACROLIMUS†
Atopic dermatitis
   (0.03%, 0.1%, or 0.3% ointment)
Psoriasis
Contact hypersensitivity
Pyoderma gangrenosum
Lichen planus

SDZ ASM 981‡
Psoriasis
Atopic dermatitis
Allergic contact dermatitis

SDZ 281-240‡
Psoriasis

*See text for details and references.
†FDA approval for tacrolimus use in atopic dermatitis is expected in 2001.
‡These drugs are not currently approved by the FDA for any indication.

ies,[148,163-166] in one double-blind study of 213 patients (ages 13 to 60 years),[167] and in another double-blind study of 180 children.[168]

In 1994, Nakagawa and co-workers[163] reported an open study of 50 patients with recalcitrant facial atopic dermatitis who were treated twice daily with 0.03%, 0.1%, or 0.3% ointment. Improvement was noted within 3 days for those without lichenification and within 7 days for those with lichenification. One third of the patients had detectable whole blood tacrolimus concentration, which ranged from 0.4 to 0.9 ng/ml for those patients without lichenification and from 0.09 to 0.7 ng/ml for those patients with lichenification. Mild skin irritation occurred in one third of patients, but no systemic adverse effects were noted. Histologic findings at days 3 to 7 showed that T-cell and eosinophil infiltrates were markedly diminished.

In 1998, Alaiti and associates reported another open study of 39 patients (31 adults and 8 children) treated with 0.3% ointment for 8 days. Overall, 95% of patients showed at least good improvement.[165] Burning (15%) was the most common application site adverse event. Vasodilation was the only drug-related nonapplication site adverse event experienced by more than one patient and occurred in four patients. No clinically significant changes in laboratory profile were associated with tacrolimus ointment administration, and trough (predose) blood levels were well below those associated with adverse events in transplant recipients. Comparison with historic intravenous data indicates that absolute bioavailability of topical tacrolimus was less than 0.5%.

Aoyama and colleagues[148] reported in 1995 that three patients (17 to 25 years of age) showed marked improvement within 1 to 2 weeks of using 0.1% ointment. Slight stinging occurred in one patient, and none showed evidence of systemic adverse effects. Kawashina[166] reported that a patient with erythroderma treated with 20 g daily of 1 mg/g tacrolimus ointment had a blood level of 20 ng/ml on day 2, which decreased after 1 week with clinical improvement. These data highlight the need for monitoring blood levels because the normal range for transplant recipients is considered to be 5 to 20 ng/ml.[139]

Ruzicka and fellow investigators reported a randomized, double-blind study of 213 patients (13 to 60 years of age).[167] Tacrolimus ointment was applied twice daily for 3 weeks. Median percentage decrease in the summary score for dermatitis for trunk and extremities was 66.7% (0.03% ointment), 83.3% (0.1% ointment), 75.0% (0.3% ointment), and 22.5% (vehicle), with the p value <0.001. There was no statistically significant difference among the active treatments, but there was a trend toward an advantage for the 0.1% concentration over 0.03%. Sensation of burning at the site of application was the only adverse event that was significantly more frequent with tacrolimus than with vehicle alone. Most patients had blood levels below 0.25 ng/ml; the highest blood level was 4.9 ng/ml, which occurred in the group receiving the 0.3% ointment.

Boguniewicz and co-workers[168] reported a randomized, double-blind, vehicle-controlled multicenter study of 180 children (7 to 16 years of age) treated for up to 22 days with 0.03%, 0.1%, or 0.3% tacrolimus ointment. Treated patients showed significantly better results than vehicle in all parameters (i.e., Physician's Global Evaluation of clinical response, modified Eczema Area and Severity Index, patient's assessment of pruritus, Head and Neck total score), although there was no statistically significant difference among the three groups treated with tacrolimus. Blood tacrolimus levels were all substantially below 20 ng/ml, which is the concentration associated with increased risk of toxicity in transplant patients. Mean and median hematology and chemistry parameters (including renal and hepatic function testing) remained within normal range. The most common reported adverse events were local increased pruritus and burning during the first 4 days of the study.

Psoriasis. Oral tacrolimus is effective in treatment of psoriasis, but its use is limited by potentially serious adverse effects such as nephrotoxicity and hypertension.[140] Studies of topical tacrolimus in psoriasis yielded conflicting results. In 1998, a double-blind pilot study showed no statistically significant difference between topical tacrolimus and placebo in chronic plaque psoriasis.[169] The next year a double-blind, randomized study showed that topical tacrolimus applied under occlusion to descaled psoriatic microplaques induced a statistically significant decrease in (1) erythema and infiltration, (2) superficial blood flow, and (3) epidermal thickness.[170]

Contact Hypersensitivity. Topical tacrolimus suppresses allergic and irritant contact dermatitis in guinea pigs[145,171] and mice.[172] In addition, the drug profoundly inhibits dinitrofluorobenzene-induced inflammation in pigskin with a potency similar to that of 0.13% clobetasol[146] and suppresses oxazolone-induced lymph node cell proliferation in mice.[173] In an animal model of delayed allergic cutaneous reactions, its suppressive effects may be due to inhibition of activation of sensitized T lymphocytes already accumulated in the dermis.[174] In five male human subjects, pretreatment of each subject with 100 μl of 1%, 0.1%, or 0.01% tacrolimus in ethanol suppressed DNCB-induced contact allergy.[175]

Pyoderma Gangrenosum. A woman 32 years of age with a 10-cm calf ulcer with "typical features" of pyoderma gangrenosum was initially treated with oral prednisolone.[176] The addition of topical 0.5% tacrolimus solution under hydrocolloid dressing resulted in complete healing after 12 weeks. The only adverse effect was burning on application of the solution. A man 48 years of age with recurrent pyoderma gangrenosum developed a 2.5 cm inflammatory supraclavicular skin nodule with early ulceration. This ulcer cleared with 0.1% tacrolimus ointment applied twice daily for 3 weeks.[177] A woman 27 years of age was receiving oral cyclosporine for recurrent pyoderma gangrenosum.[177] One large malleolar ulcer was also treated with 0.1% tacrolimus ointment applied once daily under occlusion with a hydrocolloid dressing, and this was thought to accelerate healing. In the latter two patients, side effects were not noted, and serum levels remained below 5 to 15 ng/ml. A woman 30 years of age with Crohn's disease had pyoderma gangrenosum that did not respond to oral prednisolone, azathioprine, doxycycline, clofazimine, dapsone, and intravenous granulocyte-macrophage colony–stimulating factor.[177a] Oral cyclosporine improved the ulcers, but the disease progressed within months. Oral tacrolimus resulted in improvement in 2 months, but the ulcers later recurred. She then responded slowly to oral

tacrolimus, azathioprine, prednisolone, and intravenous immunoglobulin. Addition of 0.1% tacrolimus ointment under occlusion resulted in healing over 3 months.[177a]

Lichen Planus. Six patients with erosive mucosal lichen planus were treated with 0.1% tacrolimus in hydrophilic ointment.[178] All reported rapid relief from pain and burning. Complete resolution occurred in three patients (within 4 weeks), with two others showing "good improvement" and with one showing "little improvement."[178] In five patients, no systemic blood levels could be measured, but one patient had blood levels between 9 and 15 ng/ml, presumably because of frequent application and extensive disease. The only adverse effect was slight burning immediately after application. None showed systemic adverse effects attributable to tacrolimus ointment.

Ichthyosis Linearis Circumflexa. A man 20 years of age with ichthyosis linearis circumflexa showed marked improvement after applying 0.1% tacrolimus ointment to the back for 4 weeks.[179] During a follow-up of more than 1 year, he continued to be free of erythema, but intermittent scaling on the body occurred when tacrolimus was applied to the whole body. There was no hypertension or renal dysfunction.

Ascomycin Derivatives

Several other macrolide immunosuppressants have been evaluated for topical treatment of inflammatory skin diseases. These drugs are all analogs of ascomycin, which is isolated from the fermentation product of *Streptomyces hygroscopicus* var. *ascomyceticus* for its antifungal activity. The best studied of these drugs is SDZ ASM 981. Others are ABT-281 and SDZ 281-240. Their structures are closely related to tacrolimus (see Figure 30-1).

SDZ ASM 981

SDZ ASM 981 is the best studied topical ascomycin derivative currently under development.[180,181] This drug down regulates production of Th1 (IL-2, interferon-γ [IFN-γ]) and Th2 (IL-4, IL-10) type cytokines after antigen-specific stimulation of a human helper T-cell clone isolated from the skin of an atopic dermatitis patient.[182] It also inhibits production of proinflammatory cytokines from mast cells.[182,183]

Topical SDZ ASM 981 showed antiinflammatory activity in treating allergic contact dermatitis in mouse, rat, and pig models and did not cause skin atrophy in pigs.[18]

CLINICAL USE

Psoriasis. Ten patients with plaque type psoriasis were treated with SDZ ASM 981 ointment under occlusion (0.3 and 1.0%), placebo (ointment base), or clobetasol-17-propionate ointment (0.05%) in a randomized, double-blind, within-subject comparison for 2 weeks, using the microplaque assay.[185] Clinical scores for erythema and induration decreased by 92% for clobetasol, by 82% for 1% SDZ ASM 981, by 63% for 0.3% SDZ ASM 981, and by 18% for the placebo.[185] No adverse drug effects were seen.

Atopic Dermatitis. A randomized, double-blind, placebo-controlled, right-left comparison study was done to assess SDZ ASM 981 in treatment of atopic dermatitis in 38 adults (28 patients completed the study).[186] Within 3 weeks of therapy with 1% SDZ ASM 981 cream twice daily, a mean reduction of 71.9% in the Atopic Dermatitis Severity Index (ADSI) score was observed at the actively treated test sites, compared with a mean reduction of 10.3% at the placebo-treated sites ($p < 0.001$). Greater improvement occurred in those patients treated twice daily compared with once daily application. There were no clinically relevant drug-related adverse effects. Only 2 of 121 whole blood samples obtained from patients treated twice daily were above the limit of quantification (0.1 ng/ml), and these were considered to

be due to contamination of the blood sample during blood draw.

In another study, blood levels of 12 adult patients with atopic dermatitis were collected during treatment with 1% SDZ ASM 981 cream applied up to 59% of the total body surface area twice daily for 3 weeks. The investigators found that 99% of the 444 blood samples had concentrations of SDZ ASM 981 below 1 ng/ml, and 72% were below the limit of quantitation of the assay (0.4 ng/ml).[187]

Allergic Contact Dermatitis. In a multicenter, randomized, within-patient controlled study of nickel allergic contact dermatitis involving 66 patients, SDZ ASM 981 cream was significantly more effective than placebo.[188]

ABT-281

ABT-281 potently inhibits production of both human Th1 cytokines (IL-2 and IFN-γ), and Th2 cytokines (IL-4 and IL-5).[189,190] It also has potent topical activity in a swine model of allergic contact hypersensitivity, and topical application over 25% of the body surface of swine resulted in undetectable blood levels.[189] Abbott Laboratories has suspended further investigation and development for this compound.

SDZ 281-240

SDZ 281-240 is an ascomycin analog with immunosuppressive mechanisms similar to tacrolimus.[191] In a randomized, double-blind, placebo-controlled study, all 15 patients with psoriasis showed significant improvement with SDZ 281-240 but not with placebo.[191] However, further development of SDZ 281-240 was curtailed because of technical difficulties.[180]

Bibliography

Buckley DA, Keane FM, Munn SE, et al: Recalcitrant viral warts treated by diphencyprone immunotherapy. *Br J Dermatol* 141:292-296, 1999.

Epstein WL, Stricker RB: Immunomodulation by allergic contact sensitization: the dinitrochlorobenzene story. *Am J Contact Dermatitis* 6:117-121, 1995.

Hoffmann R, Happle R: Topical immunotherapy in alopecia areata: what, how and why? *Dermatol Clin* 14:739-744, 1996.

Lee AN, Mallory SB: Contact immunotherapy with squaric acid dibutylester for the treatment of recalcitrant warts. *J Am Acad Dermatol* 41:595-599, 1999.

Paul C, Ho V: Ascomycins in dermatology. *Semin Cutan Med Surg* 17:256-259, 1998.

Rokhsar CK, Shupack JL, Vafai JJ, et al: Efficacy of topical sensitizers in the treatment of alopecia areata. *J Am Acad Dermatol* 39:751-761, 1998.

Ruzicka T, Assmann T, Homey B: Tacrolimus: the drug for the turn of the millennium? *Arch Dermatol* 135:574-580, 1999.

Ruzicka, T, Bieber T, Schopf E, et al: European Tacrolimus Multicenter Atopic Dermatitis Study Group. A short-term trial of tacrolimus ointment for atopic dermatitis. *N Engl J Med* 337:816-821, 1997.

References

Contact Allergens—Introduction and Mechanism of Action

1. Naldi L, Parazzini F, Cainelli T, et al: Role of topical immunotherapy in the treatment of alopecia areata. Quality analysis of articles published between January 1977 and January 1988 about three treatments. *J Am Acad Dermatol* 22:654-656, 1990.

2. Rokhsar CK, Shupack JL, Vafai JJ, et al: Efficacy of topical sensitizers in the treatment of alopecia areata. *J Am Acad Dermatol* 39:751-761, 1998.

3. Buckley DA, Du Vivier AWP: Topical immunotherapy in dermatology. *Int J Clin Pract* 53:130-137, 1999.

4. Hoffmann R, Happle R: Topical immunotherapy in alopecia areata. What, how and why? *Dermatol Clin* 14:739-744, 1996.

5. van der Steen PHM, Happle R: Topical immunotherapy of alopecia areata. *Dermatol Clin* 11:619-622, 1993.

6. Happle R: Antigenic competition as a therapeutic concept for alopecia areata. *Arch Dermatol Res* 267:109-114, 1980.

7. Happle R, Klein HM, Macher E: Topical immunotherapy changes the composition of the peribulbar infiltrate in alopecia areata. *Arch Dermatol Res* 278:214-218, 1986.

8. Happle R: Topical immunotherapy in alopecia areata. *J Invest Dermatol* 96:71S, 1991.

9. Brocker E-B, John SM, Steinhausen D, et al: Topical immunotherapy with contact allergens in alopecia areata: evidence for nonspecific systemic suppression of cellular immune reactions. *Arch Dermatol Res* 283:133-134, 1991.

10. Brocker E-B, Echternacht-Happle K, Hamm H, et al: Abnormal expression of class I and class II major histocompatibility antigens in alopecia areata: modulation by topical immunotherapy. *J Invest Dermatol* 88:564-568, 1987.

10a. Shapiro J, Sundberg JP, Bissonnette R, et al: Alopecia areata-like hair loss in C3H/HeJ mice and DEBR rats can be reversed using topical diphencyprone. *J Invest Dermatol Symp Proc* 4:239, 1999.

10b. Freyschmidt-Paul P, Sundberg JP, Happle R, et al: Successful treatment of alopecia areata-like hair loss with the contact sensitizer squaric acid dibutylester (SADBE) in C3H/HeJ mice. *J Invest Dermatol* 113:61-68, 1999.

11. Rampen FHJ, Steijlen PM: Diphencyprone in the management of refractory palmoplantar and periungual warts: an open study. *Dermatology* 193:236-238, 1996.

12. Eriksen K: Treatment of the common wart by induced allergic inflammation. *Dermatologica* 160:161-166, 1980.

DPC Pharmacology

13. Wilkerson MG, Connor TH, Henkin J, et al: Assessment of diphencyclopropenone for photochemically induced mutagenicity in the Ames assay. *J Am Acad Dermatol* 17:606-611, 1987.

14. MacDonald Hull S, Pepall L, Cunliffe WJ: Alopecia areata in children: response to treatment with diphencyprone. *Br J Dermatol* 125:164-168, 1991.

15. Shapiro J: Topical immunotherapy in the treatment of chronic severe alopecia areata. *Dermatol Clin* 11:611-617, 1993.

16. Perret CM, Steijlen PM, Happle R: Alopecia areata: pathogenesis and topical immunotherapy. *Int J Dermatol* 29:83-88, 1990.

17. van der Steen PHM, van Baar MJ, Perret CM, et al: Treatment of alopecia areata with diphencyclopropenone. *J Am Acad Dermatol* 24:253-257, 1991.

18. Berth-Jones J, McBurney A, Hutchinson PE: Diphencyprone is not detected in serum or urine following topical application. *Acta Derm Venereol* 74:312-313, 1994.

19. Wilkerson MG, Henkin J, Wilkin JK: Diphencyclopropenone: examination for potential contaminants, mechanisms of sensitization, and photochemical stability. *J Am Acad Dermatol* 11:802-807, 1984.

DPC—Alopecia Areata

20. MacDonald Hull DS, Norris JF: Diphencyprone in treatment of long-standing alopecia areata. *Br J Dermatol* 119:367-374, 1988.

21. MacDonald N, Wiseman MC, Shapiro J: Alopecia areata: topical immunotherapy— application and practical problems. *J Cutan Med Surg* 3(Suppl 3):S3-36-S3-40, 1999.

22. Happle R: Alopecia areata—principles of treatment. In Burgdorf WHC, Katz SI, editors: *Dermatology: progress and perspectives*, The Proceedings of the 18th World Congress of Dermatology, New York, June 12-18, 1992. New York, 1993, The Parthenon Publishing Group, pp 207-210.

23. MacDonald Hull S, Cunliffe WJ: Alopecia areata treated with diphencyprone: is an allergic response necessary? *Br J Dermatol* 122:716-717, 1990.

24. Orrechia G, Rabbiosi G: Squaric acid dibutyl ester in alopecia areata: is discomfort really necessary? *J Am Acad Dermatol* 16:876, 1987.

25. Ashworth J, Tuyp E, Mackie RM: Allergic and irritant contact dermatitis compared in the treatment of alopecia totalis and universalis. A comparison of the value of topical diphencyprone and tretinoin gel. *Br J Dermatol* 120:397-401, 1989.

26. van der Steen PHM, Boezeman JBM, Happle R: Topical immunotherapy for alopecia areata: re-evaluation of 139 cases after an additional follow-up period of 19 months. *Dermatology* 184:198-201, 1992.

27. van der Steen PHM, Happle R: Immunological treatment of alopecia areata including the use of diphencyprone. *J Dermatol Treat* 3:35-40, 1992.

28. Gordon PM, Aldridge RD, McVittie E, et al: Topical diphencyprone for alopecia areata: evaluation of 48 cases after 30 months' follow up. *Br J Dermatol* 134:869-871, 1996.

29. Schuttelaar M-LA, Hamstra JJ, Plinck EPB, et al: Alopecia areata in children: treatment with diphencyprone. *Br J Dermatol* 135:581-585, 1996.

30. Happle R, Hausen BM, Wiesner-Menzel L: Diphencyprone in the treatment of alopecia areata. *Acta Derm Venereol* 63:49-52, 1983.

31. Orrechia G, Rabbiosi G: Treatment of alopecia areata with diphencyprone. *Dermatologica* 171:193-196, 1985.

32. Tosti A, Padova MP, Minghetti G, et al: Therapies versus placebo in the treatment of patchy alopecia areata. *J Am Acad Dermatol* 15:209-210, 1986.

33. MacDonald Hull DS, Cunliffe WJ: Posttherapy relapse rate in alopecia areata after successful treatment with diphencyprone. *J Dermatol Treat* 1:71-74, 1989.

34. Hatzis J, Georgiotouo K, Kostakis P, et al: Treatment of alopecia areata with diphencyprone. *Austral J Dermatol* 29:33-36, 1988.

35. Hatzis J, Gourgiotou K, Tosca A, et al: Vitiligo as a reaction to topical treatment with diphencyprone. *Dermatologica* 177:146-148, 1988.

36. Monk B: Induction of hair growth in alopecia totalis with diphencyprone sensitization. *Clin Exp Dermatol* 14:154-157, 1989.

37. MacDonald Hull S, Cunliffe WJ: Successful treatment of alopecia areata using the contact allergen diphencyprone. *Br J Dermatol* 124:212-213, 1991.

38. Hoting E, Boehm A: Therapy of alopecia areata with diphencyprone. *Br J Dermatol* 127:625-629, 1992.

39. van der Steen PHM, van Baar HMJ, Happle R, et al: Prognostic factors in the treatment of alopecia areata with diphencyclopropenone. *J Am Acad Dermatol* 24:227-230, 1991.

40. Weise K, Kretzschmar L, John SM, et al: Topical immunotherapy in alopecia areata: anamnestic and clinical criteria of prognostic significance. *Dermatology* 192:129-133, 1996.

40a. Pericin M, Trueb RM: Topical immunotherapy with diphencyprone in Indians with alopecia areata with diphencyclopropenone: evaluation of 68 cases. *Dermatology* 196:418-421, 1998.

40b. Sharma VK, Muralidhar S: Topical immunotherapy with diphencyprone in Indians with alopecia areata. *Clin Exp Dermatol* 23:291-292, 1998.

41. Berth-Jones J, Hutchinson PE: Treatment of alopecia totalis with a combination of inosine pranobex and diphencyprone compared to each treatment alone. *Clin Exp Dermatol* 16:172-175, 1991.

42. Shapiro J, Tan J, Ho V, et al: Treatment of severe alopecia areata with topical diphencyclopropenone and 5% minoxidil: a clinical and immunopathological evaluation. *J Invest Dermatol* 104(Suppl):36S, 1995.

42a. Freyschmidt-Paul P, Hamm H, Happle R, et al: Pronounced perifollicular lymphocytic infiltrates in alopecia areata are associated with poor treatment response to diphencyprone. *Eur J Dermatol* 9:111-114, 1999.

DPC—Adverse Effects

43. Duhra P, Foulds IS: Persistent vitiligo induced by diphencyprone. *Br J Dermatol* 123:415-416, 1990.

44. Henderson CA, Ilchyshyn A: Vitiligo complicating diphencyprone sensitization therapy for alopecia universalis. *Br J Dermatol* 133:496-497, 1995.

45. van der Steen P, Happle R: "Dyschromia in confetti" as a side effect of topical immunotherapy with diphenylcyclopropenone. *Arch Dermatol* 128:518-520, 1992.

46. Perret CM, Steijlen PM, Zaun H, et al: Erythema multiforme-like eruptions: a rare side effect of topical immunotherapy with diphencyclopropenone. *Dermatologica* 180:5-7, 1990.

47. Puig L, Alegre M: Erythema multiforme-like reaction following diphencyprone treatment of plane warts. *Int J Dermatol* 33:201-203, 1994.

48. Alam M, Gross EA, Savin RC: Severe urticarial reaction to diphencyclopropenone therapy for alopecia areata. *J Am Acad Dermatol* 40:110-112, 1999.

49. Tosti A, Guerra L, Bardazzi F: Contact urticaria during topical immunotherapy. *Contact Dermatitis* 21:196-197, 1989.

50. MacDonald-Hull SP, Cotterill JAC, Norris JFB: Vitiligo following diphencyprone dermatitis. *Br J Dermatol* 120:323, 1989.

51. Sansom JE, Molloy KC, Lovell CR: Occupational sensitization to diphencyprone in a chemist. *Contact Dermatitis* 32:363, 1995.

52. Whittaker M: Severe dermatitis caused by diphencyclopropenone. *Contact Dermatitis Newsletter* 11:264-265, 1972.

53. Adisesh A, Beck M, Cherry NM: Hazards in the use of diphencyprone. *Br J Dermatol* 136:470, 1997.

54. Shah M, Lewis FM, Messenger AG: Hazards in the use of diphencyprone. *Br J Dermatol* 134:1153, 1996.

DPC—Warts and Melanoma

55. Orrechia G, Douville H, Santagostino L, et al: Treatment of multiple relapsing warts with diphencyprone. *Dermatologica* 177:225-231, 1988.

56. Naylor MF, Nelder KH, Yarbrough GK, et al: Contact immunotherapy of resistant warts. *J Am Acad Dermatol* 19:679-683, 1988.

57. Buckley DA, Keane FM, Munn SE, et al: Recalcitrant viral warts treated with diphencyprone immunotherapy. *Br J Dermatol* 141:292-296, 1999.

58. Lane PR, Hogan DJ: Diphencyprone. *J Am Acad Dermatol* 19:364-365, 1988.

58a. Weisshaar E, Neumann H-J, Gollnick H: Successful treatment of disseminated facial verrucae with contact immunotherapy. *Eur J Dermatol* 8:488-491, 1998.

59. Harland CC, Saihan EM: Regression of metastatic malignant melanoma with topical diphencyprone and oral cimetidine. *Lancet* 2:445, 1989.

SADBE—Pharmacology

60. Happle R, Kalveram KJ, Buchner U, et al: Contact allergy as a therapeutic tool for alopecia areata. *Dermatologica* 161:289-297, 1980.

61. Strobel R, Rohrborn G: Mutagenic and cell transforming activities of 1-chlor-2, 4-dinitrobenzene (DNCB) and squaric-acid-dibutylester (SADBE). *Arch Toxicol* 45:307-314, 1980.

62. van Duuren B, Melchionne S, Blair R, et al: Carcinogenicity of isoesters of epoxides and lactones: aziridine ethanol, propane sulfone, and related compounds. *J Natl Cancer Inst* 46:143-149, 1971.

63. Wilkerson MG, Henkin J, Wilkin JK, et al: Squaric acid and esters: analysis for contaminants and stability in solvents. *J Am Acad Dermatol* 13:229-234, 1985.

SADBE—Alopecia Areata

64. Case PC, Mitchell AJ, Swanson NA, et al: Topical therapy of alopecia areata with squaric acid dibutyl ester. *J Am Acad Dermatol* 10:447-451, 1984.

65. Giannetti A, Orrechia G: Clinical experience on the treatment of alopecia areata with squaric acid dibutyl ester. *Dermatologica* 167:280-282, 1983.

66. Flowers FP, Slazinski L, Fenske NA, et al: Topical squaric dibutyl ester therapy for alopecia areata. *Cutis* 30:733-736, 1982.

67. Barth JH, Darley CR, Gibson JR: Squaric acid dibutyl ester in the treatment of alopecia areata. *Dermatologica* 170:40-42, 1985.

68. Johansson E, Ranki A, Reunala T, et al: Immunohistological evaluation of alopecia areata treated with squaric acid dibutyl ester (SADBE). *Acta Derm Venereol* 66:485-490, 1986.

69. Caserio RJ: Treatment of alopecia areata with squaric acid dibutyl ester. *Arch Dermatol* 123:1036-1041, 1987.

70. Valsecchi R, Cainelli T, Tornaghi A, et al: Squaric acid dibutyl ester treatment of alopecia areata. *Clin Exper Dermatol* 10:233-238, 1985.

71. Valsecchi R, Cainelli T, Foiadelli L, et al: Topical immunotherapy of alopecia areata. A follow-up study. *Acta Derm Venereol* 66:269-272, 1986.

72. Chua SH, Goh CL, Ang CB: Topical squaric dibutyl ester therapy for alopecia areata: a double-sided patient-controlled study. *Ann Acad Med Singapore* 25:842-847, 1996.

73. Orrechia G, Malagoli P, Santagostino L: Treatment of severe alopecia areata with squaric acid dibutyl ester in pediatric patients. *Pediatr Dermatol* 11:65-68, 1994.

74. Tosti A, Guidetti MS, Bardazzi F, et al: Long-term results of topical immunotherapy in children with alopecia areata or alopecia universalis. *J Am Acad Dermatol* 35:199-201, 1996.

75. Micali G, Cicero RL, Nasca MR, et al: Treatment of alopecia areata with squaric acid dibutyl ester. *Int J Dermatol* 35:52-56, 1996.

76. Iijima S: Prognostic factors for clinical response of alopecia areata to topical immunotherapy with squaric acid dibutyl ester. *Arch Dermatol* 133:539-540, 1997.

77. Cicero RL, Micali G, Sapuppo A: A paradoxical hair regrowth during the treatment of severe alopecia areata with squaric acid dibutyl ester (SADBE). *Eur J Dermatol* 3:321, 1993.

78. Orecchia G: The "castling" phenomenon: a possible explanation. *Eur J Dermatol* 4:161-162, 1994.

79. Van der Steen PHM, Happle R: The "castling" phenomenon in topical immunotherapy of alopecia areata. *Eur J Dermatol* 2:151-153, 1992.

80. Orrechia G, Perfetti L, Borroni G, et al: Photochemotherapy plus squaric acid dibutyl ester in alopecia areata treatment. *Dermatologica* 181:167-169, 1990.

SADBE—Adverse Effects

81. Foley S, Blattel SA, Martin AG: Clinical sequelae associated with squaric acid dibutyl ester topical sensitization. *Am J Contact Dermat* 7:104-108, 1996.

82. Fowler JF, Hodge SF, Tobin GR: Persistent allergic contact dermatitis from squaric acid dibutyl ester. *J Am Acad Dermatol* 28:259-260, 1993.

83. Frattasio A, Germino M, Cargnello S, et al: Side effects during treatment with SADBE. *Contact Dermatitis* 36:118-119, 1997.

84. Nasca MR, Cicero RL, Innocenzi D, et al: Persistent allergic contact dermatitis at the site of primary sensitization with squaric acid dibutyl ester. *Contact Dermatitis* 33:438, 1995.

85. Nishioka K, Ogasawara M, Kurata K, et al: Iatrogenic benign lymphoplasia induced by allergic contact dermatitis from squaric acid dibutyl ester: immunohistologic study of cellular infiltrates. *Contact Dermatitis* 28:3-5, 1993.

86. Tosti A, Bardazzi F, Ghetti P: Unusual complication of sensitizing therapy for alopecia areata. *Contact Dermatitis* 18:322, 1988.

87. Valsecchi R, Cainelli T: Nickel sensitivity as a complication of squaric acid dibutyl ester treatment of alopecia areata. *Contact Dermatitis* 12:234, 1985.

88. Valsecchi R, Cainelli T: Depigmentation from squaric acid dibutyl ester. *Contact Dermatitis* 10:109, 1984.

89. Nasca MR, Micali G, Pulvirenti N, et al: Transient leukoderma appearing in an untreated area following contact immunotherapy for alopecia areata. *Eur J Dermatol* 8:125-126, 1998.

SADBE—Warts

90. Iijima S, Otsuka F: Contact immunotherapy with squaric acid dibutyl ester for warts. *Dermatology* 187:115-118, 1993.

91. Lee AN, Mallory SB: Contact immunotherapy with squaric acid dibutyl ester for the treatment of recalcitrant warts. *J Am Acad Dermatol* 41:595-599, 1999.

91a. Silverberg NB, Lim JK, Paller AS, et al: Squaric acid immunotherapy for warts in children. *J Am Acad Dermatol* 42:803-808, 2000.

DNCB—Pharmacology

92. Kratka J, Goerz G, Vizethum W, et al: Dinitrochlorobenzene: influence on the cytochrome P-450 system and mutagenic effects. *Arch Dermatol Res* 266:315-318, 1979.

93. Summer K-H, Goggelmann W: 1-chloro-2,4-dinitrobenzene depletes glutathione in rat skin and is mutagenic in *Salmonella typhimurium. Mutation Res* 77:91-93, 1980.

94. DeLeve LD: Dinitrochlorobenzene is genotoxic by sister chromatid exchange in human skin fibroblasts. *Mutation Res* 371:105-108, 1996.

95. Wilkerson MG, Wilkin JK, Smith RG: Contaminants of dinitrochlorobenzene. *J Am Acad Dermatol* 9:554-557, 1983.

96. Weisburger EK, Russfield AB, Homburger F, et al: Testing of twenty-one environmental aromatic amines or derivatives for long-term toxicity or carcinogenicity. *J Environ Pathol Toxicol* 2:325-356, 1978.

97. Feldmann RJ, Maibach HI: Absorption of some organic compounds through the skin in man. *J Invest Dermatol* 54:399-404, 1970.

DNCB—Alopecia Areata

98. Swanson NA, Mitchell AJ, Leahy MS, et al: Topical treatment of alopecia areata: Contact allergen vs primary irritant therapy. *Arch Dermatol* 117:384-387, 1981.

99. Frentz G, Eriksen K: Treatment of alopecia areata with DNCB—an immunostimulation? *Acta Derm Venereol* 57:370-371, 1977.

100. Happle R, Echternacht K: Induction of hair growth in alopecia areata with DNCB. *Lancet* 2:1102-1103, 1977.

101. Happle R, Cebulla K, Echternacht-Happle K: Dinitrochlorobenzene therapy for alopecia areata. *Arch Dermatol* 114:1629-1631, 1978.

102. Daman L, Rosenberg W, Drake L: Treatment of alopecia areata with dinitrochlorobenzene. *Arch Dermatol* 114:1036-1038, 1978.

103. Breuillard F, Szapiro E: Dinitrochlorobenzene in alopecia areata. *Lancet* 2:1304, 1978.

104. Warin AP: Dinitrochlorobenzene in alopecia areata. *Lancet* 1:927, 1979.

105. de Prost Y, Paquez F, Rouraine R: Dinitrochlorobenzene treatment of alopecia areata. *Arch Dermatol* 118:542-545, 1982.

106. Ro BI: Alopecia areata in Korea. *J Dermatol* 22:858-864, 1995.

DNCB—Warts

107. Sanders BB, Smith KW: Dinitrochlorobenzene immunotherapy of human warts. *Cutis* 27:389-392, 1981.

108. Greenberg JH, Smith L, Katz R: Verrucae vulgaris rejection: a preliminary study of contact dermatitis and cellular immunity response. *Arch Dermatol* 107:580-582, 1973.

109. Lewis HM: Topical immunotherapy of refractory warts. *Cutis* 12:863-867, 1973.

110. Bruckner D, Price NM: Immunotherapy of verrucae vulgaris with dinitrochlorobenzene. *Br J Dermatol* 98:451-455, 1978.

111. Dunagin WG, Millikan LE: Dinitrochlorobenzene immunotherapy for verrucae resistant to standard treatment modalities. *J Am Acad Dermatol* 6:40-45, 1982.

112. Lee S, Cho CK, Kim JG, et al: Therapeutic effect of dinitrochlorobenzene (DNCB) on verruca plana and verruca vulgaris. *Int J Dermatol* 23:624-626, 1984.

113. Goihman-Yahr M, Fernandez J, Boatswain A, et al: Unilateral dinitrochlorobenzene immunopathy of recalcitrant warts. *Lancet* 1:447-448, 1978.

DNCB—Various Malignancies

114. Ferry AP, Meltzer MA, Taub RN: Immunotherapy with dinitrochlorobenzene (DNCB) for recurrent squamous cell tumor of the conjunctiva. *Trans Am Ophthalmol Soc* 74:154-171, 1977.

115. Raaf JH, Krown SE, Pinsky CM, et al: Treatment of Bowen's disease with topical dinitrochlorobenzene and 5-fluorouracil. *Cancer* 37:1633-1642, 1976.

116. Levis WR, Kramer KH, Klingler WG, et al: Topical immunotherapy of basal cell carcinomas with dinitrochlorobenzene. *Cancer Res* 33:3036-3042, 1973.

117. Price NM: Actinic keratoses treated with a combination of topical 5-fluorouracil and dinitrochlorobenzene. *Dermatologica* 158:279-286, 1979.

118. Foster DC, Woodruff D: The use of dinitrochlorobenzene in the treatment of vulvar carcinoma in situ. *Gynecol Oncol* 11:330-339, 1981.

119. Guthrie D, Way S: Failure of topical DNCB immunotherapy in most patients with non-clinical carcinoma of the cervix. *Br J Cancer* 39:445-448, 1979.

120. Novick NL, Bosniak SL: The failure of immunotherapy with dinitrochlorobenzene and Rhus extract for recurrent conjunctival squamous papillomas. *J Dermatol Surg Oncol* 12:602-605, 1986.

121. Cohen MH, Jessup M, Felix M, et al: Intralesional treatment of recurrent metastatic
cutaneous malignant melanoma: a randomized prospective study of intralesional bacillus Calmette-Guerin versus intralesional
dinitrochlorobenzene. *Cancer* 41:2456-
2463, 1978.

122. Sigg C, Schnyder UW: Successful immunotherapy by dinitrochlorobenzene in a
case of recurrent acrolentiginous melanoma. *Dermatologica* 181:250-251, 1990.

123. Strobbe LJ, Hart AA, Rumke P, et al: Topical
dinitrochlorobenzene combined with systemic dacarbazine in the treatment of recurrent melanoma. *Melanoma Res* 7:507-512,
1997.

124. Budzanowska E, Pawlicki M: An attempt at
topical DNCB immunomodulation in advanced malignant melanoma. *Tumori*
74:519-522, 1988.

DNCB—HIV Infections

125. Epstein WL, Stricker RB: Immunomodulation by allergic contact sensitization: the
dinitrochlorobenzene story. *Am J Contact
Dermatitis* 6:117, 1995.

126. Mills LB: Stimulation of T-cell immunity by
cutaneous application of dinitrochlorobenzene. *J Am Acad Dermatol* 14:1089-1090,
1986.

127. Stricker RB, Elswood BF, Abrams DI: Den-
dritic cells and dinitrochlorobenzene
(DNCB): a new treatment approach to
AIDS. *Immunol Lett* 29:191-196, 1991.

128. Stricker RB, Zhu YS, Elswood BF, et al: Pilot
study of topical dinitrochlorobenzene
(DNCB) in human immunodeficiency virus
infection. *Immunol Lett* 36:1-6, 1993.

129. Stricker RB, Elswood BF: Topical dinitrochlorobenzene in HIV disease. *J Am
Acad Dermatol* 28:796-797, 1993.

130. Stricker RB, Elswood BF, Goldberg B, et al:
Clinical and immunologic evaluation of
HIV-infected patients treated with dinitrochlorobenzene. *J Am Acad Dermatol*
31:462-466, 1994.

131. Stricker RB, Goldberg B, Mills BL, et al: Improved results of delayed-type hypersensitivity skin testing in HIV-infected patients
treated with topical dinitrochlorobenzene.
J Am Acad Dermatol 33:608-611, 1995.

132. Traub A, Margulis SB, Stricker RB: Topical
immune modulation with dinitrochlorobenzene in HIV disease: a controlled trial from
Brazil. *Dermatology* 195:369-373, 1997.

133. Stricker RB, Goldberg B, Mills LB, et al: Decrease in viral load associated with topical
dinitrochlorobenzene therapy in HIV disease. *Res Virol* 148:343-348, 1997.

DNCB—Other Dermatoses

134. Yoshizawa Y, Matsui H, Izaki S, et al: Topical
dinitrochlorobenzene therapy in the treatment of refractory atopic dermatitis: systemic immunotherapy. *J Am Acad Dermatol*
42:258-262, 2000.

134a. Mills LB, Mordan LJ, Roth HL, et al: Treatment of severe atopic dermatitis by topical
immune modulation using dinitrochlorobenzene. *J Am Acad Dermatol*
42:687-689, 2000.

135. Stricker RB, Goldberg B, Epstein WL: Immunologic changes in patients with systemic lupus erythematosus treated with
topical dinitrochlorobenzene. *Lancet*
345:1505-1506, 1995.

136. Kano Y, Otake Y, Shiohara T: Improvement
of lichen nitidus after topical dinitrochlorobenzene application. *J Am Acad Dermatol* 39:305-308, 1998.

137. Stricker RB, Goldberg B: Lichen nitidus and
dinitrochlorobenzene. *J Am Acad Dermatol*
40:647-648, 1999.

138. Yoshizawa Y, Kitamura K, Maibach HI: Successful immunotherapy of chronic nodular
prurigo with topical dinitrochlorobenzene.
Br J Dermatol 141:387-389, 1999.

Topical Tacrolimus—Pharmacology

139. Lawrence ID: Tacrolimus (FK 506): experience in dermatology. *Dermatol Ther*
5:74-84, 1998.

140. Jegasothy B, Ackerman CD, Todo S, et al:
Tacrolimus (FK506)—a new therapeutic
agent for severe recalcitrant psoriasis. *Arch
Dermatol* 128:781-785, 1992.

141. Lauerma AI, Maibach H: Topical FK506:
clinical potential or laboratory curiosity?
Dermatology 188:173-176, 1994.

142. Ruzicka T, Assmann T, Homey B: Tacrolimus:
the drug for the turn of the millenium? *Arch
Dermatol* 135:574-580, 1999.

143. Fleischer AB Jr: Treatment of atopic dermatitis: role of tacrolimus ointment as a
topical noncorticosteroid therapy. *J Allergy
Clin Immunol* 104:S126-130, 1999.

144. Lauerma AI, Surber C, Maibach HI: Absorption of topical tacrolimus (FK506) in vitro
through human skin: comparison with cyclosporin A. *Skin Pharmacol* 10:230-234,
1997.

145. Lauerma AI, Stein B, Homey B, et al: Topical FK506 (tacrolimus): Percutaneous absorption and effect on allergic and irritant contact dermatitis (abstract). *J Invest Dermatol* 100:491, 1993.
146. Meingassner JG, Stutz A: Immunosuppressive macrolides of the type FK-506: A novel class of topical agents for treatment of skin diseases? *J Invest Dermatol* 98:851-855, 1992.
147. Reitamo S, Rissanen J, Remitz A, et al: Tacrolimus ointment does not affect collagen synthesis: results of a single-center randomized trial. *J Invest Dermatol* 111:396-398, 1998.
148. Aoyama H, Tabata N, Tanaka M, et al: Successful treatment of residual facial lesions of atopic dermatitis with 0.1% FK506 ointment. *Br J Dermatol* 133:494-496, 1995.

Topical Tacrolimus—Mechanism of Action

149. Wollenberg A, Regele D, Sharma S, et al: Topical tacrolimus (FK506) treatment leads to profound alterations of the antigen presenting cells in lesional atopic dermatitis skin (abstract). *J Invest Dermatol* 107:468, 1996.
150. Homey B, Assmann T, Vohr H-W, et al: Topical FK506 suppresses interleukin-12 and costimulatory molecule expression in vivo (abstract). *J Invest Dermatol* 109:454, 1997.
151. Panhans A, Bieber T: FK506 (tacrolimus) impairs the phenotypic and functional differentiation of human epidermal Langerhans cells (abstract). *J Invest Dermatol* 107:485, 1996.
152. Homey B, Assmann T, Vohr H-W, et al: Topical FK506: suppression of TH1 and TH2 cytokine induction in lymph node cells in vivo (abstract). *J Invest Dermatol* 107:476, 1996.
153. de Paulis A, Stellato C, Cirillo R, et al: Anti-inflammatory effect of FK-506 on human skin mast cells. *J Invest Dermatol* 99:723-728, 1992.
154. Eberlein-Konig B, Michel G, Ruzicka T, et al: Modulation of histamine release in vitro by FK506 and interleukin-3 is determined by sequence of incubation. *Arch Dermatol Res* 289:606-608, 1997.
155. Hiroi J, Sengoku T, Morita K, et al: Effect of tacrolimus hydrate (FK506) ointment on spontaneous dermatitis in NC/Nga mice. *Japan J Pharmacol* 76:175-183, 1998.

156. Jiang H, Yamamoto S, Nishikawa K, et al: Anti-tumor-promoting action of FK506, a potent immunosuppressive agent. *Carcinogenesis* 14:67-71, 1993.

Topical Tacrolimus—Alopecia Areata

157. McElwee KJ, Rushton DH, Trachy R, et al: Topical FK506: a potent immunotherapy for alopecia areata? Studies using the Dundee experimental bald rat model. *Br J Dermatol* 137:491-497, 1997.
158. Yamamoto S, Jiang H, Kato R: Stimulation of hair growth by topical application of FK506, a potent immunosuppressive agent. *J Invest Dermatol* 102:160-164, 1994.
159. Yamamoto S, Kato R: Hair growth stimulating effects of cyclosporin A and FK 506, potent immunosuppressants. *J Dermatol Sci* 7(Suppl):S47-54, 1994.
160. Maurer M, Handjuski B, Paus R: Hair growth modulation by topical immunophilin ligands: Induction of anagen, inhibition of massive catagen development, and relative protection from chemotherapy-induced alopecia. *Am J Pathol* 150:1433-1441, 1997.
161. Jiang H, Yamamoto S, Kato R: Induction of anagen in telogen mouse skin by topical application of FK506, a potent immunosuppressant. *J Invest Dermatol* 104:523-525, 1995.
162. Thiers BH: Topical tacrolimus: treatment failure in a patient with alopecia areata. *Arch Dermatol* 136:124, 2000.

Topical Tacrolimus—Atopic Dermatitis

163. Nakagawa H, Etoh T, Ishibashi Y, et al: Tacrolimus ointment for atopic dermatitis. *Lancet* 344:883, 1994.
164. Nakagawa H, Etoh T, Ishibashi Y, et al: Effects of tacrolimus (FK506) ointment for facial atopic dermatitis (abstract). *Allergy* 50(Suppl 26):368, 1995.
165. Alaiti S, Kang S, Fiedler VC, et al: Tacrolimus (FK506) ointment for atopic dermatitis: a phase I study in adults and children. *J Am Acad Dermatol* 38:69-76, 1998.
166. Kawashima M, Nakagawa H, Ohtuski M, et al: Tacrolimus concentrations in blood during topical treatment of atopic dermatitis. *Lancet* 348:1240-1241, 1996.
167. Ruzicka T, Bieber T, Schopf E, et al: A short-term trial of tacrolimus ointment for atopic dermatitis. *N Engl J Med* 337:816-821, 1997.

168. Boguniewicz M, Fiedler VC, Raimer S, et al: A randomized, vehicle-controlled trial of tacrolimus ointment for treatment of atopic dermatitis in children. *J Allergy Clin Immunol* 102:637-644, 1998.

Topical Tacrolimus—Psoriasis
169. Zonneveld IM, Rubins A, Jablonska S, et al: Topical tacrolimus is not effective in chronic plaque psoriasis: a pilot study. *Arch Dermatol* 134:1101-1102, 1998.
170. Remitz A, Reitamo S, Erkko P, et al: Tacrolimus ointment improves psoriasis in microplaque assay. *Br J Dermatol* 141:103-107, 1999.

Topical Tacrolimus—Contact Dermatitis
171. Lauerma AI, Homey B, Lee CH, et al: Topical FK506: suppression of allergic and irritant contact dermatitis in the guinea pig. *Arch Dermatol Res* 286:337-340, 1994.
172. Meingassner JG, Stutz A: Anti-inflammatory effects of macrophilin-interacting drugs in animal models of irritant and allergic contact dermatitis. *Int Arch Allergy Immunol* 99:486-489, 1992.
173. Homey B, Assmann T, Vohr H-W, et al: Topical FK506 suppresses cytokine and costimulatory molecule expression in epidermal and local draining lymph node cells during primary skin immune responses. *J Immunol* 160:5331-5340, 1998.
174. Sengoku T, Morita K, Sakuma S, et al: Possible inhibitory mechanism of FK506 (tacrolimus hydrate) ointment for atopic dermatitis based on animal models. *Eur J Pharmacol* 379:183-189, 1999.
175. Lauerma A, Maibach HI, Granlund H, et al: Inhibition contact allergy reactions by topical FK506. *Lancet* 340:556, 1992.

Topical Tacrolimus—Other Indications
176. Schuppe H-C, Homey B, Assmann T, et al: Topical tacrolimus for pyoderma gangrenosum. *Lancet* 351:832, 1998.
177. Reich K, Vente C, Neumann C: Topical tacrolimus for pyoderma gangrenosum. *Br J Dermatol* 139:755-757, 1998.
177a. Jolles S, Niclasse S, Benson E: Combination oral and topical tacrolimus in therapy-resistant pyoderma gangrenosum. *Br J Dermatol* 140:564-565, 1999.
178. Vente C, Reich K, Rupprecht R, et al: Erosive mucosal lichen planus: response to topical treatment with tacrolimus. *Br J Dermatol* 140:338-342, 1999.

179. Suga Y, Tsuboi R, Hashimoto Y, et al: A case of ichthyosis linearis circumflexa successfully treated with topical tacrolimus. *J Am Acad Dermatol* 42:520-522, 2000.

Ascomycin Derivatives
180. Paul C, Ho V: Ascomycins in dermatology. *Semin Cutan Med Surg* 17:256-259, 1998.
181. Mrowietz U: Macrolide immunosuppressants. *Eur J Dermatol* 9:346-351, 1999.
182. Grassberger M, Baumruker T, Enz A, et al: A novel anti-inflammatory drug, SDZ ASM 981, for the treatment of skin diseases: in vitro pharmacology. *Br J Dermatol* 141:264-273, 1999.
183. Hultsch T, Muller KD, Meingassner JG, et al: Ascomycin macrolactam derivative SDZ ASM 981 inhibits the release of granule-associated mediators and of newly synthesized cytokines in RBL 2H3 mast cells in an immunophilin-dependent manner. *Arch Dermatol Res* 290:501-507, 1998.
184. Meingassner JG, Grassberger M, Fahrngruber H, et al: A novel anti-inflammatory drug, SDZ ASM 981, for the topical and oral treatment of skin diseases: in vivo pharmacology. *Br J Dermatol* 137:568-576, 1997.
185. Mrowietz U, Graeber M, Brautigam M, et al: The novel ascomycin derivative SDZ ASM 981 is effective for psoriasis when used topically under occlusion. *Br J Dermatol* 139:992-996, 1998.
186. van Leent EJM, Graber M, Thurston M, et al: Effectiveness of the ascomycin macrolactam SCZ ASM 981 in the topical treatment of atopic dermatitis. *Arch Dermatol* 134:805-809, 1998.
187. Graber M, van Leent EJM, Burtin P, et al: Profiling SDZ ASM 981: Evaluation of local tolerability and safety in the treatment of atopic dermatitis. *Ann Dermatol Venereol* 125(Suppl 1):S214-S215, 1998.
188. Queille-Roussel C, Graber M, Thurston M, et al: Topical treatment with the anti-inflammatory macrolactam SDZ ASM 981 inhibits established nickel contact dermatitis. *Austral J Dermatol* 38(Suppl 2):234, 1997.
189. Mollison KW, Fey TA, Gauvin DM, et al: A macrolactam inhibitor of T helper type 1 and T helper type 2 cytokine biosynthesis for topical treatment of inflammatory skin diseases. *J Invest Dermatol* 112:729-738, 1999.

190. Mollison KW, Fey TA, Gauvin DM, et al: Discovery of ascomycin analogs with potent topical but weak systemic activity for treatment of inflammatory skin diseases. *Curr Pharmaceut Design* 4:367-379, 1998.

191. Rappersberger K, Meingrassner JG, Fialla R, et al: Clearing of psoriasis by a novel immunosuppressive macrolide. *J Invest Dermatol* 106:701-710, 1996.

PART VII

Miscellaneous Topical Drugs

Stanley B. Levy

Sunscreens

Encouraging photoprotection is the leading preventive health strategy employed by physicians involved in the care of the skin. Although it is becoming increasingly clear that sun avoidance is most desirable, outdoor occupations and lifestyles make total avoidance impossible for most individuals. The regular use of sunscreens represents a practical compromise in this regard. Sunscreens prevent the formation of squamous cell carcinomas in animals.[1] In humans, the regular use of sunscreens has been shown to reduce actinic keratoses[2] and solar elastosis.[3] Sunscreens also prevent immunosuppression.[4] Drug photosensitization and photo-induced or photo-aggravated dermatoses can be avoided with sunscreen use. Understanding available sunscreen products allows selection of the most appropriate one for a given patient (Box 31-1). Familiarity with not only active sunscreen ingredients, but also their vehicles, increases the likelihood that patients will comply with specific recommendations.

DEFINITIONS

Table 31-1 lists UV spectrum wavelengths. Table 31-2 lists definitions and labels of sunscreens. Ultraviolet radiation (UVR) reaching the Earth's surface can be divided into UVB (290 to 320 nm) and UVA (320 to 400 nm). UVA can be further subdivided into UVA I (340 to 400 nm) or far UVA and UVA II (320 to 340 nm) or near UVA.

Sunscreen products are regulated by the U.S.

Food and Drug Administration (FDA) as over-the-counter (OTC) drugs. The Final Monograph for Sunscreen Drug Products for Over-the-Counter Use was recently issued (Federal Register 64:27666-27693, 1999) established the conditions for safety, efficacy, and labeling of these products. The sun-protection factor (SPF) is defined as the dose of UVR required to produce 1 minimal erythema dose (MED) on protected skin after application of 2 mg/cm² of product divided by the UVR to produce 1 MED on unprotected skin. A "water-resistant" product maintains the SPF level after 40 minutes of water immer-

Box 31-1

Common Sunscreen Components

UVB BLOCKERS
Padimate O
Octyl methoxycinnamate (Octinoxate)
Octyl salicylate (Octisalate)
Octocrylene
Phenylbenzimidazole sulfonic acid

UVA BLOCKERS
Oxybenzone
Methyl anthranilate
Avobenzone (Parsol 1789)

PHYSICAL BLOCKERS
Titanium dioxide
Zinc oxide

sion. A "very water-resistant" (formerly water-proof) product is tested after 80 minutes of water immersion.

A "broad-spectrum" or "full-spectrum" sunscreen provides protection through the entire spectrum of both UVB and UVA. Until recently, products claiming this protection relied on ingredients absorbing in the UVA II region. Despite the availability of newer ingredients, which also protect against UVA I, some manufacturers continue to make this claim without effective UVA I protection.

SUNSCREEN OPTIONS
Active Sunscreen Ingredients
Sunscreens have been traditionally divided into chemical absorbers and physical blockers based on their mechanism of action. Chemical sunscreens are generally aromatic compounds conjugated with a carbonyl group.[5] These chemicals absorb high intensity UV rays, producing

excitation to a higher energy state. With return to the ground state, the result is conversion of the absorbed energy into longer lower energy wavelengths. Physical blockers reflect or scatter UVR. Recent research indicates that the newer microsized forms of physical blockers may also function in part by absorption.[6] Sometimes referred to as "nonchemical" sunscreens, they may be more appropriately designated as inorganic particulate sunscreen ingredients.

The most commonly used active sunscreen ingredients are listed in Table 31-3 by their generic drug name. Allowable ingredients are listed in the FDA monograph, as are appropriate concentrations. The lower limits apply only to sunscreens used in combination with others, except for the UVA I blockers, which are also assigned minimum concentrations, even when used as the single active ingredient. Sunscreen nomenclature can be quite confusing. They may

■ Table 31-1   UV Spectrum Wavelengths

UV Spectrum	Wavelengths
UVC	200-290 nm
UVB	290-320 nm
UVA	320-400 nm
UVA I	340-400 nm
UVA II	320-340 nm

■ Table 31-2   Sunscreen Labeling Definitions

Terminology	Definition
SPF	MED-protected skin/MED-unprotected skin
Broad-spectrum protection	Full-spectrum UVB/UVA Protection
Water-resistant	SPF maintained after 40 minutes of water immersion
Very water-resistant (waterproof)	SPF maintained after 80 minutes of water immersion

■ Table 31-3   FDA Final Monograph Sunscreen Ingredients

Drug Name	Concentration	Absorbance
Aminobenzoic acid (PABA)	Up to 15%	UVB
Avobenzone (Parsol 1789)	2%-3%	UVA I
Cinoxate	Up to 3%	UVB
Dioxybenzone	Up to 3%	UVB, UVA II
Homosalate	Up to 15%	UVB
Menthyl anthranilate	Up to 5%	UVA II
Octocrylene	Up to 10%	UVB
Octyl methoxycinnamate	Up to 7.5%	UVB
Octyl salicylate	Up to 5%	UVB
Oxybenzone	Up to 6%	UVB, UVA II
Padimate O	Up to 8%	UVB
Phenylbenzimidazole sulfonic acid	Up to 4%	UVB
Sulisobenzone	5%-10%	UVB, UVA II
Titanium dioxide	2%-25%	Physical
Trolamine salicylate	5%-12%	UVB
Zinc oxide	2%-25%	Physical

■ **Table 31-4**   Sunscreen Nomenclature

OTC Drug*	INCI Terminology†	Trade Name
Avobenzone	Butyl methoxydibenzoylmethane	Parsol 1789
Octinoxate	Octyl methoxycinnamate	Parsol MCX
Oxybenzone	Benzophenone-3	Eusolex 4360
		Uvinul M-40
Padimate O	Octyldimethyl PABA	Escalol 507

*Final Over-the-Counter Drug Products Monograph on Sunscreens (Federal Register 64:27666-27798, 1999).
†International Cosmetic Ingredient (INCI) Dictionary and Handbook , ed 7, Washington, DC, 1997, The Cosmetic, Toiletry, and Fragrance Association.

also be referred to by their chemical INCI (cosmetic ingredient) name or by their trade name (Table 31-4). Representative chemical structures are shown in Figure 31-1.

Sunscreen ingredients can also be classified by which portion of the UV spectrum they effectively absorb, as well as their role in a particular formulation with a combination of ingredients. The absorption spectrum of the most commonly used sunscreens is shown in Figure 31-2. The sunscreen ingredients are discussed individually.

UVB Sunscreens

PADIMATE O.   Paraaminobenzoic acid (PABA) was one of the first chemical sunscreens to be widely available. Several problems limited the use of PABA. It required an alcoholic vehicle, stained clothing, and was associated with a number of adverse reactions including subjective stinging and contact dermatitis. Ester derivatives, mainly Padimate O (octyl dimethyl PABA), became more popular with greater compatibility in a variety of cosmetic vehicles and a lower potential for staining or adverse reactions. Because of problems with PABA formulations, manufacturers emphasized the "PABA-free" claim, so that these derivatives are now less frequently used.

Padimate O is the most potent UVB absorber. The decline in PABA use along with the demand for higher SPF products led to the incorporation of multiple active ingredients in a single product to achieve the desired SPF. Products utilizing just PABA esters are very uncommon.

OCTYL METHOXYCINNAMATE (OCTINOXATE).   The cinnamates largely replaced PABA

derivatives as the next most potent UVB absorbers. Octyl methoxycinnamate is the most frequently used sunscreen ingredient.[7] As shown in Figure 31-2, demonstrating absorbance curves on a logarithmic scale, octyl methoxycinnamate is an order of magnitude less potent than Padimate O. Diethanolamine methoxycinnamate is a water-soluble cinnamate derivative that is less commonly utilized in sunscreens.

OCTYL SALICYLATE (OCTISALATE).   Octyl salicylate is used to augment the UVB protection in a sunscreen. Salicylates are weak UVB absorbers and are generally used in combination with other UV sunscreens. Other salicylates need to be used in higher concentrations. They all share a good safety profile.

OCTOCRYLENE.   Octocrylene may also be used in combination with other UV absorbers to achieve higher SPF formulas. Difficulties in formulating with this ingredient and its expense to manufacturers limit its use.

PHENYLBENZIMIDAZOLE SULFONIC ACID. Most chemical sunscreen ingredients are oils soluble in the oil phase of emulsion systems, accounting in part for the heavy, greasy aesthetics of many of these products. Phenylbenzimidazole sulfonic acid is water-soluble and used in products formulated to feel lighter and less oily such as daily use cosmetic moisturizers. This chemical is a very selective UVB filter, allowing almost complete UVA transmission. Diethanolamine methoxycinnamate is also water-soluble and may be used in these lighter, more aesthetic sunscreen products.

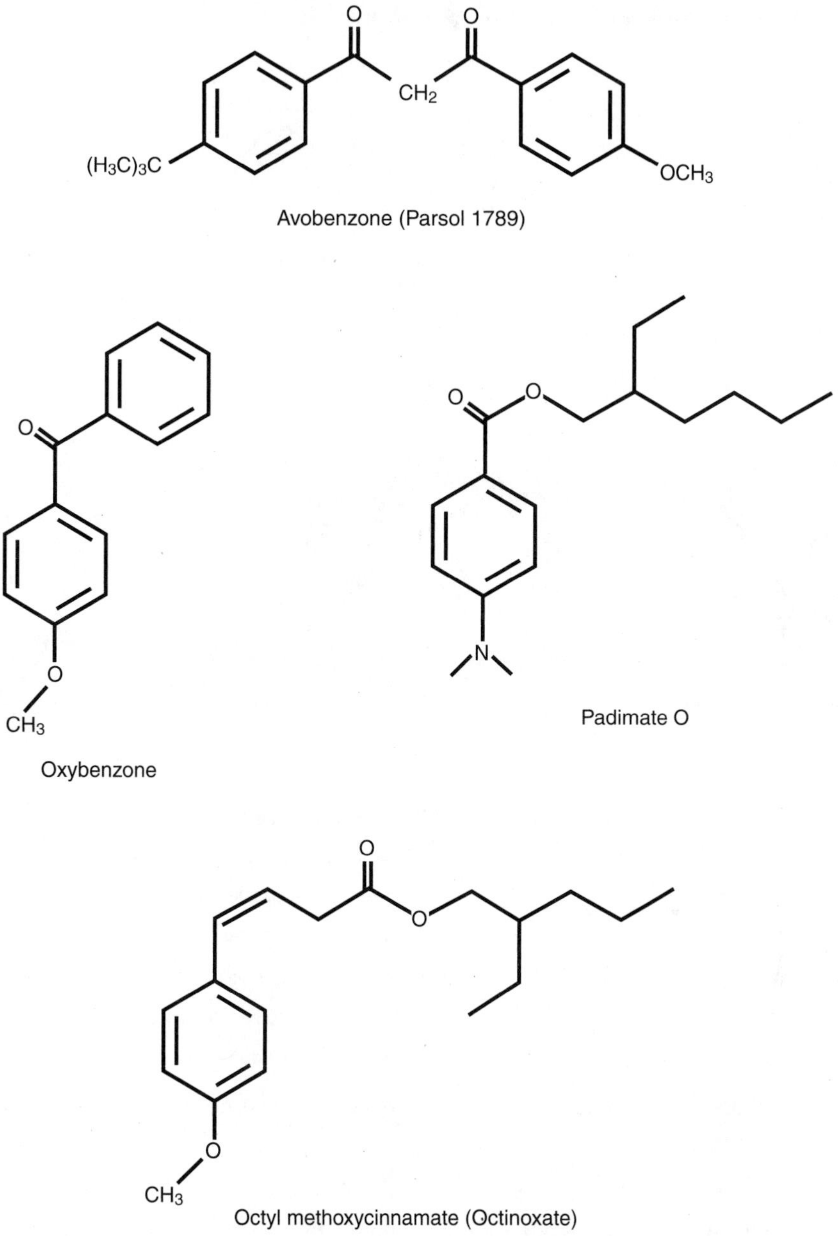

Avobenzone (Parsol 1789)

Oxybenzone

Padimate O

Octyl methoxycinnamate (Octinoxate)

Figure 31-1 Sunscreens.

UVA Sunscreens

OXYBENZONE. Although benzophenones are primarily UVB absorbers (as shown in Figure 31-2), oxybenzone absorbs well through UVA II. It can be considered a broad-spectrum UVR absorber. Benzophenones significantly augment the UVB protection of a sunscreen product when employed in a given formula.

MENTHYL ANTHRANILATE. Menthyl anthranilate is a weak UVB filter that absorbs mainly in the near UVA (UVA II) portion of the spectrum. This suncreen ingredient is less effective in this UVA II range than benzophenones and is less widely used.

AVOBENZONE. Often referred to by its trade name, Parsol 1789, avobenzonel provides

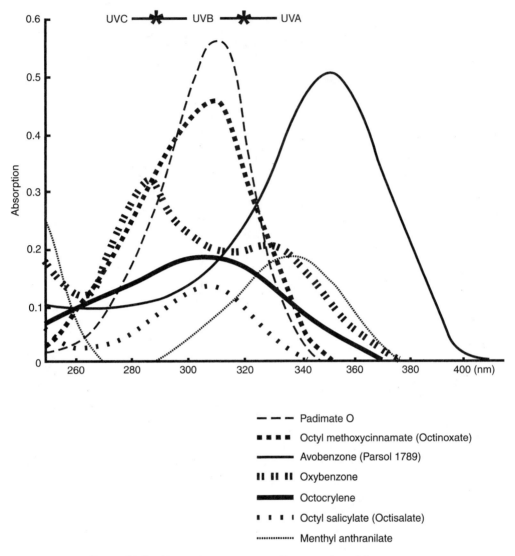

Figure 31-2   Absorption spectrum of commonly used sunscreens.

superior protection through a large portion of the UVA range (see Figure 31-2), including the majority of the UVA I spectrum. It has been widely used in Europe for the last decade. Avobenzone, recently approved by the FDA for use in the United States, is a significant addition to sunscreen products for true broad-spectrum UV protection. Concerns have been raised regarding its photostability and potential to degrade other sunscreen ingredients in products where it is used.[8] Further studies with standardized protocols need to be done to answer formulation stability issues with avobenzone. For

now clinicians need to rely on the integrity of the sunscreen manufacturer who uses this ingredient. Clinicians are again reminded as to the limitations of sunscreen products and the need to counsel patients in total sun protection.

Physical Blockers

Some of the original sunblocks were opaque formulations reflecting or scattering UVR. During World War II, red petrolatum was extensively used by the military. Titanium dioxide and zinc oxide also functioned in this fashion. Poor cosmetic acceptance limited the widespread use of the latter two ingredients until recently, when microsized forms became available.

TITANIUM DIOXIDE.   The ideal sunscreening agent would be chemically inert, safe, and absorb or reflect through the full UV spectrum. Titanium dioxide meets these criteria limited only by aesthetics. By decreasing the particle size of this pigment to a microsize or ultrafine grade and making it less visible on the skin surface, some of these advantages could be utilized. This ingredient can be classified as a broad-spectrum agent.

Despite advances in the technology, it is difficult to formulate products with titanium dioxide that do not whiten the skin secondary to pigment residue. Adding other pigments simulating fleshtones may partially camouflage this effect. The net effect may be that the user is inclined to make a less heavy application of the product, effectively lowering the SPF.[9] "Hybrid" products employing a combination of chemical UV absorbers with inorganic particulate sunscreens may represent a practical compromise.

ZINC OXIDE.   Zinc oxide has recently been approved as an allowable active ingredient in sunscreen products by the FDA, having been used for many years in opaque blocks. Like titanium dioxide, microsized grades of this ingredient have been developed, offering the same advantages and disadvantages previously described and including the ability to provide more full-spectrum protection.

CLINICAL USE
Indications
Table 31-5 lists indications and contraindications for sunscreens. Sunscreens were originally developed for the prevention of acute sunburn. The SPF designation directly addresses this indication. Theoretically, an SPF 15 product allows an individual to remain in the sun up to 15 times longer without sunburning than what that individual's intrinsic unprotected skin would allow. SPF 15 products block 93.3% of UVR from penetrating the skin.[10] A fair-complected individual who sunburns in 10 minutes would have more than 2.5 hours of protection from SPF 15.

Most dermatologists recommend the regu-

Table 31-5	Sunscreen Indications and Contraindications

INDICATIONS
Protection from ultraviolet radiation to
   prevent the following:
Sunburn—FDA approved
Skin or lip damage, freckling, skin
   discoloration—FDA approved
Skin aging—FDA approved
Skin cancer—FDA approved
Phototoxic or photoallergic drug reactions
Photosensitivity diseases

CONTRAINDICATIONS
Known sensitivity to any active sunscreen
   ingredient or vehicle ingredient contained
   in product
Infants less than 6 months of age
As the sole component of an overall program of photoprotection*

---

*A complete program of sun protection includes protective clothing, shade, and sun avoidance (see Box 31-3).

lar use of sunscreens for a broader range of indications, including prevention of photoaging and carcinogenesis. UVR exposure causes chronic changes in the skin by direct tissue and cellular damage, where the principal target is DNA.[11] Indirectly, it is likely that UV-induced immunosuppression plays a permissive role in the development of skin cancers. Prevention of UV-induced immunosuppression by sunscreens has been demonstrated in humans.[4,12]

A large number of medications increase sun sensitivity, requiring patient compliance with photoprotection. Phototoxicity by direct light-mediated damage to the skin, either from ingested or topically applied compounds, is much more common than immunomediated photoallergic reactions. Many skin diseases are photoinduced or aggravated by UVR. These processes can be prevented or attenuated by proper sunscreen selection and usage.

SPF Level
The FDA sunscreen monograph provides qualitative definitions of sun protection products for

product labeling and consumer guidance based on SPF ranges recommended for specific skin phototypes (Table 31-6). Most dermatologists recommend SPF 15 or greater to all their patients regardless of their skin type and would question the use of lower SPF products.

An argument can be made that an SPF 15 sunscreen theoretically provides full protection for normal individuals.[13] The SPF number is correlated with the proportion of UVR that is filtered out. An SPF 2 product prevents 50% of the incident radiation from penetrating. An SPF 50 allows 2% penetration and blocks 98% of UVR. As shown in Table 31-7, the difference in UVR penetration between an SPF 15 and SPF 30 product of about 4% would not seem significant for most individuals or clinical situations.

Product application technique alters SPF. The FDA SPF testing standard provides for product thickness application of 2 mg/cm². Outside the laboratory under real world conditions, most individuals approximate a thickness application closer to 1 mg/cm².[14] Additionally, when SPF testing is performed outdoors, lower SPF levels are obtained than in the laboratory.[15]

Erythema, the key measurement in the SPF assay, is a crude biologic endpoint. Comparison of an SPF 15 with an SPF 30 sunscreen showed subclinical damage with the formation of sunburn cells in the former without visible erythema. The SPF 30 product provided significantly greater protection, with respect to sunburn cell production.[16] It also appears that the higher the SPF the greater the UVA II protection.[17]

Concerns that higher SPF products would be associated with a greater incidence of side effects do not appear to be well founded. Objective irritation appears unrelated to sunscreen levels in formulations.[18] Therefore a strong case can be made for the use of higher SPF products, at least up to the proposed upper limit designation of SPF 30 as recommended in the most recent FDA monograph. The current monograph allows products with SPF values above 30; however, the SPF declaration for sunscreens with SPF values above 30 is limited to "SPF 30 plus" or "+."

UVA Protection

SPF is primarily a measure of UVB protection. Some correlation is present with near UVA or UVA II protection. With the availability of higher SPF products allowing individuals to spend greater amounts of time in the sun without burning, concerns have been raised as to the adequacy of UVA protection in these products.[11] Individuals relying on conventional sunscreens as their sole form of photoprotection may in fact now be subject to greater cumulative UVA exposure. Patients with photosensitivity conditions or who take certain drugs may be particularly at risk, given the role of UVA in many of these conditions.

Although UVA has lower energy than UVB, UVA penetrates more deeply into the dermis and is more constant in intensity throughout the day and year-round. UVA is additive to UVB erythema[19] and is carcinogenic by itself.[20] Recent studies document that multiple low-dose UVA exposures in humans are associated with significant dermal and epidermal histologic changes,[21,22] with the action spectrum for dermal damage particularly broad, extending through 400 nm.[23]

■ **Table 31-6**   FDA Monograph Sunscreen Product Guide

Sunburn Protection	SPF
Minimal	2 to 12
Moderate	12 to under 30
High	30 or above

■ **Table 31-7**   Percent Reduction of UVB Penetration Based on SPF

SPF	UVB Absorption*
2	50%
4	75%
8	87.5%
15	93.3%
20	95%
30	96.7%
45	97.8%
50	98%

*UVB absorption (as a percent = $100 - 100/SPF$).

There is no consensus as to the best method for measuring UVA protection. A variety of methods have been proposed. Available methods have been reviewed in detail and summarized by Lowe[24] as shown in Table 31-8. A detailed discussion is beyond the scope of this chapter. At best, each method has its limitations and indications for a particular clinical situation or skin type. Physicians generally want to recommend to their patients a truly broad- or full-spectrum sunscreen. If protection from UVR through 400 nm is indicated, then the formula should contain either avobenzone or an inorganic particulate sunscreen as an active ingredient.

Sunscreen Vehicles

Vehicle type is critical for determining sunscreen efficacy and aesthetics. Ingredients such as solvents and emollients can have a profound effect on the strength of UV absorbance because of the active ingredients and wavelengths the ingredients absorb.[25] Film formers and emulsifiers determine the nature of film formed on the skin surface. Higher SPF products require a formula that provides a uniform and thick sunscreen film with minimum interaction of inert ingredients with active ingredients.[26] Durability and water resistance are obviously vehicle-dependent. Lastly, product aesthetics play a large role in patient compliance with specific sunscreen recommendations.

EMULSIONS.   The most commonly used sunscreens are lotions and creams. Oil-in-water and water-in-oil emulsion systems allow for the greatest variety of formulations. Because the most effective UV absorbers are oils, by necessity they are incorporated into the oil phase of the emulsion. Higher SPF products may therefore contain 20% to 40% sunscreen oils, accounting for the heavy, greasy feel of many of these products. So-called dry lotions, often labeled as "sport lotions," are an attempt to formulate a less oily product utilizing newer polymeric film formers and less greasy silicone oils.

GELS.   Water-based gels rely on the limited number of water-soluble active sunscreen ingredients, such as phenylbenzimidazole sulfonic acid or trolamine salicylate. Alcohol or hydroalcoholic vehicles have similar limitations. Gels are easily removed by swimming or perspiration. They tend to more readily cause facial or eye stinging. They may, however, be favored by individuals with oily skin or who are acne-prone. They are also easier to use for individuals with thinning scalp hair or abundant body hair.

SPRAYS.   For convenience of application, some individuals prefer sprays. Sprays may be difficult to apply evenly and can produce a discontinuous film, resulting in a less effective sunscreen product. They also share some of the disadvantages of gels previously mentioned. Sprays are also useful for thinning scalp hair.

STICKS.   Thickened with waxes and petrolatum, most lipid-soluble sunscreens can be readily incorporated into sticks. Sticks are helpful for protecting limited areas of the body, such as the lips, nose, or around the eyes. They may not

■ Table 31-8   Various Measures of UVA Protection Methods

Method	Endpoint	Indication
SPF	Erythema	UVA II
UVA protection factor	Erythema	UVA II—skin phototypes I and II
Persistent pigment darkening	Delayed pigment darkening	Full UVA—skin phototypes III and IV
Phototoxic protection factor	Erythema with topical photosensitizer	Full UVA photosensitivity
Photosensitivity disease study	Flare in disease process	Specific photosensitivity diseases
In vitro	Transmittance through substrate (such as thin film)	Screening materials—convenient and practical

be practical for application to large areas of the body.

COSMETICS.　Cosmetic and skin care products containing sunscreen are increasingly available to consumers. The FDA monograph recognizes this category and distinguishes between beach and nonbeach products. These cosmetic sunscreen products offer several advantages. Daily protection is facilitated for a large segment of the population. They provide superior aesthetics, facilitating compliance with their use. Perhaps most importantly, these products are available to consumers year-round as opposed to seasonally available beach products.

Foundation makeup, even without sunscreen, may provide some protection (generally around SPF 4) due to its pigment content. By raising the level of pigments (including titanium dioxide), or by adding a chemical sunscreen, a higher SPF can easily be achieved. By virtue of its opacity, foundation makeup also provides the benefit of some UVA protection.

Adverse Reactions

A major factor accounting for failed compliance with sunscreen recommendations is adverse reactions to these products (Box 31-2). In a longitudinal prospective study of 603 subjects applying sunscreen daily (applying either an SPF 15+ broad-spectrum sunscreen containing octyl methoxycinnamate and avobenzone or a vehicle cream), 19% developed an adverse reaction.[27] Interestingly, the rates of reactions to both the

---

Box 31-2

Adverse Reactions to Sunscreens

Subjective irritation—stinging, burning, itching
Contact urticaria—immunologic, nonimmunologic
Irritant contact dermatitis
Allergic contact dermatitis
Photosensitivity
Acnegenicity (induce or exacerbate acne)
　Comedogenicity
　Folliculitis
Exacerbation of preexisting acne

---

active and vehicle cream were similar, emphasizing the importance of excipient ingredients. The majority of reactions were irritant in nature. A disproportionate 50% of the reacting subjects were atopic. Less than 10% of the reactions were labeled allergic, with none of the subjects (who were labeled as allergic) patch tested proving to be allergic to an individual sunscreen ingredient.

SUBJECTIVE IRRITATION.　The most common complaint associated with sunscreen use is immediate stinging or burning on application without associated visible erythema. This is most frequently experienced in the eye area. Even sunscreen applied away from the eye may migrate, particularly with perspiration, causing stinging of the eyes. This stinging sensation can occur even if several hours have elapsed since sunscreen application. Patients often interpret these symptoms as true allergy.

CONTACT URTICARIA.　Erythema occurring immediately on contact with sunscreen may represent contact urticaria. Urticaria occurring from topically applied substances may be either immunologic (immunoglobulin E [IgE]-mediated Type I allergy) or nonimmunologic (toxic or due to direct mast cell degeneration). Nonimmunologic contact urticaria may be part of the spectrum of subjective irritation. Sunscreens do not appear to be associated with a higher incidence of contact urticaria than other toiletries or cosmetics.

IRRITANT CONTACT DERMATITIS.　Longerlasting irritation may be difficult to distinguish from true allergic contact dermatitis without patch testing. In a postmarket survey of sunscreen complaints in 57 individuals, 20 users had relatively brief symptoms, lasting minutes to hours. Overall, 26 individuals had intermediateduration symptoms of 1 to 3 days.[28] Half of the study participants were patch and photopatch tested, and only three showed positive reactions to sunscreen ingredients.

ALLERGIC CONTACT DERMATITIS.　Irritation is clearly a more prevalent problem than true Type IV delayed hypersensitivity reactions. Considering their widespread use, the number of documented allergic reactions to individual sunscreen ingredients is not high.[29] PABA and PABA esters historically accounted for many reported reactions to sunscreens. With a decrease in their use, the relative frequency of reactions to benzophenones appears to be increasing.[30] Fragrances, preservatives, and other excipients account for a large number of the allergic reactions seen.[31]

PHOTOSENSITIVITY.   Virtually all sunscreen ingredients reported to cause allergy may also be photoallergens. Although still relatively uncommon, sunscreen active ingredients seem to have become the leading cause of photocontact allergic reactions.[32,33] There have been increasing reports of photocontact allergy to benzophenones[34] as the use of PABA and its derivatives has decreased. In Europe, avobenzone is a significant cause of photoallergy in patients suspected of photosensitivity.[31,35] Individuals with eczematous conditions have a significant predisposition to sensitization (contact or photocontact dermatitis) due to an impaired cutaneous barrier. This seems particularly true of patients with photosensitivity dermatoses who develop the majority of photocontact dermatitis to sunscreens.[31] Allergic and photoallergic contact dermatitis should be considered in patients with a photosensitivity condition that suddenly changes or worsens.

ACNE INDUCTION AND EXACERBATION. As with many of the previously described adverse reactions, aggravation of acne by sunscreens appears more related to vehicle than to sunscreen ingredients. Sunscreen vehicle ingredients may be comedogenic, while individual sunscreen oils are not.[36] Comedone formation leading to acne is a very gradual process. More commonly, physicians see aggravation of acne in an acne-prone individual. Relating this solely to sunscreens is problematic because acne may be aggravated by UV exposure, as in patients with acne aestivale.[37] Contact folliculitis, the rapid onset of small follicular papules and pustules shortly after product application, represents another form of irritation. Lack of reproducibility of reactions makes this problem difficult to study systematically. Gel or spray formulation may reduce the frequency of this adverse effect.

General Photoprotection Instructions to Patients

Presenting patients with clear instructions on the proper use of sunscreens (Box 31-3) and guidelines for choosing the appropriate products specific for their needs enhances compliance.

Latitude determines the need for sunscreen at a given time of year. In the northern part of the United States, sunscreens are most important from April to October, but arguably should

Box 31-3

Instructions to Patients Regarding Sun Protection Measures

- Depending on latitude and climate, sunscreens may be needed year-round, including on cloudy days, when up to 80% of UV rays may still reach the earth's surface.
- Sunscreens are most important from 10 AM to 4 PM (Daylight Savings Time) when the sun's rays are strongest. If possible, try to avoid significant sun exposure during these peak hours by staying in the shade or indoors.
- For intermittent, casual daily use, an SPF 15 is sufficient. For prolonged recreational exposures, an SPF 30 is more desirable, particularly for fair-skinned individuals.
- Sunscreen should be applied 15 to 30 minutes before sun exposure to allow sufficient time for the protective film to develop.

- Sunscreen should be reapplied after prolonged swimming or vigorous activity. If swimming or perspiring heavily, a water-resistant or waterproof product should be used.
- Sunscreen needs to be applied liberally. Up to 1 oz (about 30 g) of the product may be needed to cover the whole body. Remember to apply to all areas including the back of the neck, ears, and areas of the scalp with thin hair.
- Clothing is an excellent form of sun protection provided it is tightly woven. Check by seeing if light comes through when held up to visible light. Otherwise, sunscreen may be needed under clothing or hats.
- A 4-inch wide, broad brimmed hat is required to cover the entire face and neck.

be used year-round when outdoors for any sufficient period of time. In the southern part of the United States, sunscreens should be used year-round. Patients need to be reminded that on cloudy days, depending on density of the cloud cover, up to 80% of UVR is still transmitted to the Earth's surface.[38]At higher altitudes, more UVR is transmitted.

Sunscreens are most important 3 hours before and 3 hours after the sun is at its daytime apogee. As a rough guide, this would be 3 hours before and 3 hours after noon, although logically this time frame shifts in the setting of "daylight savings time." Application 15 to 30 minutes before sun exposure allows sufficient time for the sunscreen film to set on the skin surface. This is particularly important for water-resistant sunscreens. Individuals who are outdoors regularly (even intermittently outdoors) may do best with daily morning applications of sunscreen. This morning application can be in the form of a moisturizer, makeup base, or after-shave. UVA varies much less in intensity throughout the day than UVB. Patients specifically requiring UVA protection should wear their sunscreen for more extended daylight hours.

Sunscreens needs to be applied liberally and evenly all over exposed areas. Most people probably apply sunscreens in a patchy distribution and in an insufficient amount to achieve the labeled SPF.[39] Up to 1 oz (about 30 g) of sunscreen may be needed to cover the entire body. Roughly 3 to 5 g are needed to cover the head and neck. Individuals are particularly disinclined to apply product in the periorbital and ear areas.[40] Patients also need to be reminded to protect the lower lip and areas of thinning hair in the scalp.

Special Patient Group Instructions

Based on the previous discussion on SPF level and the realities of product application, it would seem prudent to recommend to lighter-complected individuals, subject to prolonged sun exposure, the use of at least an SPF 30 product. Some patients require more detailed instructions to ensure appropriate use (Table 31-9).

PHOTOSENSITIVE PATIENTS.   Patients subject to a variety of photodermatoses need to take particular care with the selection and application of their sunscreen. Frequently, individuals with polymorphous light eruption, taking photosensitizing drugs, or in whom melasma or lentigines darken despite the use of sunscreens need better UVA protection through the entire spectrum, including UVA I protection. Therefore these groups of patients may benefit from a higher SPF product that contains avobenzone, titanium dioxide, or zinc oxide.

PATIENTS WITH SENSITIVE SKIN.   A careful history of previous sunscreen use can be quite helpful in dealing with the patient who complains of sunscreen intolerance. Patients should be informed that subjective stinging in or near the eyes should not be interpreted as a sign of true allergy. Recommending a PABA-free sunscreen is only helpful to the patient still using the less widely available PABA-containing sunscreens. The patient can be instructed to perform a limited usage or repeat open application test with a previously used or recommended sunscreen product. If true allergy is suspected, consider patch testing the patient with the product as is. Sunscreen products have individual sunscreen ingredients at concentration levels comparable with the concentration used in diagnostic patch testing.[10] Chronically photosensitive patients with eczematous changes who flare despite the use of a broad-spectrum product may need patch tests or photopatch tests with a complete sunscreen series.

The availability of sunscreens with the chemically inert inorganic particulate materials (e.g., titanium dioxide or zinc oxide) as the only active ingredients provides a suitable alternative to patients, regardless of what kind of sunscreen intolerance they experience.

ACNE-PRONE PATIENTS.   Individuals with oily complexions may prefer an oil-free, alcohol-based gel or a lighter feeling cosmetic sunscreen moisturizer. Even an oil-free product may feel somewhat oily because the active sunscreen ingredients are themselves oils. The oil-free claim merely refers to the vehicle. Although, as stated previously, sunscreen oils and most film-forming vehicular ingredients are noncomedogenic, their occlusivity may be an issue for some acne patients. Sunscreen products intended for oily skin types can be recommended in these patients.

■ **Table 31-9   Some Commercially Available Sunscreens***

Product Type	Indications/Advantages	Commercial Products (Noninclusive)
Waterproof	Recreational Occupational All-day exposure	Bain de Soleil All Day 15 or 30 BioSun 15, 30, or 45 Coppertone Sunblock Lotion 15, 30, or 45 Neutrogena 15 or 30 Shade Sunblock Lotion 30 or 45 Solbar 50
Daily use moisturizer	Casual exposure Lighter feel on application Under makeup Aftershave	Almay Moisture Balance Lotion SPF 15 Eucerin Daily Facial Lotion SPF 25 Lubriderm Daily UV Lotion SPF 15 Neutrogena Moisture SPF 15 Oil of Olay UV Complete UV Protective Moisture Lotion SPF 15 (contains zinc oxide) Purpose Dual Moisturizer SPF 15
Full spectrum (contain avobenzone)	Drug photosensitivity Photodermatoses Dyspigmentations	Almay Lasting Moisture SPF 25 BioSun Sunblock Oil Free Gel SPF 30 Ombrelle Lotion SPF 15 or 30 Pre Sun Ultra Lotion or Gel SPF 30 Shade UVA Guard SPF 30
Dry lotion	Avoiding eye stinging Less heavy application	Coppertone Sport SPF 15 or 30 Neutrogena No Stick SPF 30
Inorganic particulate	Skin sensitivity	Clinique City Block SPF 15 Estee Lauder Advanced Sunblock for Face Neutrogena Sensitive Skin Sunblock SPF 17 PreSun Block SPF 28
Oil-free gel	Oily skin type Acne-prone Thin hair	Bull Frog Quickgel SPF 36 PreSun Clear Gel SPF 30 Shade Sunblock Oil-Free Gel SPF 30
Oil-free lotion	Oily skin type Less heavy feel Acne-prone	Clinique Oil-Free Sunblock SPF 15 Coppertone Oil-Free SPF 30 Neutrogena Oil-Free Sunblock SPF 30
Spray	Ease of application Thin hair	Neutrogena Sunblock Spray SPF 20 Ombrelle Spray Mist SPF 15 PreSun Mist Sunscreen SPF 23
Stick	Lips Eye area	Almay Stay Smooth Lipcolor SPF 25 Blistex Ultra Protection SPF 30 Neutrogena Sunblock Stick SPF 30 Shade SPF 30 UVA/UVB Stick
Foundation makeup	Daily use Convenience	Almay Amazing Sheer SPF 12 Clinique Almost Make-up SPF 15 Clinique Sensitive Skin Foundation SPF 15 Estee Lauder Futurist Age Resisting SPF 15 Estee Lauder Double Matte SPF 15 Revlon ColorStay Lite SPF 15 Revlon New Complexion One-Step SPF 15 Revlon New Complexion Even Out SPF 20

*This list is not meant to be inclusive. Mass market, relatively cost-effective, and readily available brands have been emphasized. Product listings quickly become outdated as manufacturers are constantly redesigning their product presentation and, to a lesser degree, their formulas.

CHILDREN. The importance of sun protection for children cannot be overstated.[41] Parents who regularly apply sunscreen to their children at an early age typically find that as adolescents they are more likely to continue this practice.[42] Sunscreen products specifically marketed for children are essentially no different than adult products. The FDA monograph states that the use of sunscreens is not recommended for infants under 6 months of age. Although these products are not hazardous per se, sun avoidance is most appropriate for very young infants.

Theoretic Inhibition of Vitamin D Synthesis

Regular sunscreen use can diminish UVR-dependent cutaneous synthesis of vitamin D. The elderly are particularly susceptible to the consequences of vitamin D deficiency, including osteopenia and bone fractures.[43] An Australian study showed that under real world conditions, patients instructed in the regular use of sunscreens still received enough sunlight to support vitamin D metabolism[44] probably through lack of total skin coverage. Despite rigorous photoprotection, patients with xeroderma pigmentosum still maintain normal vitamin D levels.[45] Patients compliant with sunscreen use probably get enough UVR through their sunscreen and non-covered areas to maintain adequate vitamin D levels. It would still seem prudent to recommend to older individuals daily supplementation consistent with current recommendations of 400 IU of vitamin D. This amount of vitamin D is found in most general multivitamins.

Sunless Tanners—Dihydroxyacetone

The notion that a suntanned appearance is desirable and healthy remains prevalent in our culture, despite greater general awareness of the hazards of sun exposure. Self-tanning or sunless tanning products can be recommended as a safe option, provided that the user is aware of the limited true sunscreen potential of these products. These products contain dihydroxyacetone (DHA) as the active ingredient[46] (see Chapter 36). DHA is a three-carbon sugar that reacts with the amino group of amino acids, peptides, or proteins found in the keratin and epidermis. Melanoidins are formed as a result of the Maillard or "browning reaction" in the stratum corneum. DHA has at most a modest effect on SPF,[47] providing perhaps SPF 3 or 4 protection. The brown color obtained on the skin does absorb in the low end of the visible spectrum with overlap into the long UVA and may provide some UVA I protection.[48] Patients need to be informed that, although their skin has a tanned appearance with products containing DHA, they provide only minimal sun protection. Many sunless tanning products also contain sunscreen and a have labeled SPF. Because the resultant color from these products can last up to several days, patients also need to be reminded that the duration for UV protection is more short-lived than that of the skin color change.

SUMMARY

Despite recent controversy regarding sunscreen efficacy,[11] sunscreens represent a key component in any overall program for photoprotection. A thorough understanding of active sunscreen ingredients and their vehicles ensures that sunscreen recommendations are appropriate for specific indications and helps to assure adequate patient compliance.

Bibliography

Gasparro FP, Metchnik M, Nash JF: A review of sunscreen safety and efficacy. *Photochem Photobiol* 68:243-256, 1998.

Gonzalez E, Gonzalez S: Drug photosensitivity, idiopathic photodermatoses, and sunscreens. *J Am Acad Dermatol* 35:871-885, 1996.

Lowe NJ, Shaath NA, Pathak MA, editors: *Sunscreens: development, evaluation, and regulatory aspects,* ed 2, New York, 1997, Marcel Dekker.

McLean DI, Gallagher R: Sunscreens, use and misuse. *Dermatol Ther* 16:219-226, 1998.

Naylor MF, Farmer KC: The case for sunscreens: a review of their use in preventing actinic damage and neoplasia. *Arch Dermatol* 133:1146-1154, 1997.

Taylor CR, Stern RS, Leyden JJ, et al: Photoaging/photodamage and photoprotection. *J Am Acad Dermatol* 22:1-15, 1990.

References

Definitions and Sunscreen Options

1. Gurish MF, Roberts LK, Krueger GG, et al: The effect of various sunscreen agents on skin damage and the induction of tumor susceptibility in mice subjected to ultraviolet irradiation. *J Invest Dermatol* 65:543-546, 1975.
2. Thompson SC, Jolley D, Marks R: Reduction of solar keratoses by regular sunscreen use. *N Engl J Med* 329:1147-1151, 1993.
3. Boyd AS, Naylor M, Cameron GS, et al: The effects of chronic sunscreen use on the histologic changes of dermatoheliosis. *J Am Acad Dermatol* 33:941-946, 1995.
4. Roberts LK, Beasley DG: Commercial sunscreen lotions prevent ultraviolet-radiation-induced immune suppression of contact hypersensitivity. *J Invest Dermatol* 105:339-344, 1995.
5. Shaath NA: The chemistry of sunscreens. *Cosmet Toilet* 101:55-70, 1986.
6. Sayre RM, Killias N, Roberts RL, et al: Physical sunscreens. *J Soc Cosmet Chem* 41:103-109, 1990.
7. Steinberg DC: Sunscreen encyclopedia regulatory update. *Cosmet Toilet* 111:77-86, 1996.
8. Sayre RM, Dowdy JC: Avobenzone and the photostability of sunscreen products. Presented at the 7th Annual Meeting of the Photomedicine Society. Orlando, Florida: February 26, 1998.
9. Diffey BL, Grice J: The influence of sunscreen type on photoprotection. *Br J Dermatol* 137:103-105, 1977.

Clinical Use

10. Levy SB: Sunscreens for photoprotection. *Dermatol Ther* 4:59-71, 1997.
11. Naylor MF, Farmer KC: The case for sunscreens: a review of their use in preventing actinic damage and neoplasia. *Arch Dermatol* 133:1146-1154, 1997.
12. Whitmore SD, Morison WL: Prevention of UVB-induced immunosuppression in humans by a high sun protection factor sunscreen. *Arch Dermatol* 131:1128-1133, 1995.
13. Marks R: Summer in Australia: skin cancer and the great SPF debate. *Arch Dermatol* 131:462-464, 1995.
14. Bech-Thomsen N, Wulf HC: Sunbather's application of sunscreen is probably inadequate to obtain the sun protection factor assigned to the preparation. *Photodermatol Photoimmunol Photomed* 9:242-244, 1992/1993.
15. Toda K, Pathak MA: Determination of sun protection values of three test products under indoor and outdoor test conditions using Japanese volunteers. *J Jpn Cosmet Sci Soc* 12:139-144, 1988.
16. Kaidbey KH: The photoprotective potential of the new superpotent sunscreens. *J Am Acad Dermatol* 22:449-452, 1990.
17. Urbach F: Ultraviolet A transmission by modern sunscreens: is there a real risk? *Photodermatol Photoimmunol Photomed* 9:237-241, 1992/1993.
18. Silber PM, Mills OH Jr, Dammers KS, et al: Comparative skin irritation of high and low SPF sunscreen products. *J Toxicol—Cutan Ocular Toxicol* 9(2):555-563, 1989/1990.
19. Ying CY, Parris JA, Pathak MA, et al: Additive erythemogenic effects of middle (280-320 nm) and longwave (320-400 nm) ultraviolet light. *J Invest Dermatol* 63:273-278, 1974.
20. Sterenborg HJCM, van der Leun JC: Tumorigenesis by a long wavelength UVA source. *Photochem Photobiol* 51:325-330, 1990.
21. Lavker RM, Gerberick GF, Veres D, et al: Cumulative effects from repeated exposures to suberythemal doses of UVB and UVA in human skin. *J Am Acad Dermatol* 32:53-62, 1995.
22. Lowe NJ, Meyers DP, Wieder JM, et al: Low doses of repetitive ultraviolet A include morphologic changes in human skin. *J Invest Dermatol* 105:739-743, 1995.

23. Lavker RM, Kaidbey K: The spectral dependence for UVA-induced cumulative damage in human skin. *J Invest Dermatol* 108:17-21, 1997.

24. Lowe NJ: Ultraviolet A claims and testing procedures for OTC sunscreens: a summary and review. In Lowe NJ, Shaath NA, Pathak MA, editors: *Sunscreens: development, evaluation, and regulatory aspects,* ed 2, New York, 1997, Marcel Dekker, pp 499-512.

25. Agrapidis-Paloympis LE, Nash RA, Shaath NA: The effect of solvents on the ultraviolet absorbance of sunscreens. *J Soc Cosmet Chem* 38:209-221, 1987.

26. Klein K: Formulating sunscreen products. In Lowe NJ, Shaath NA, editors: *Sunscreens: development, evaluation, and regulatory aspects,* New York, 1990, Marcel Dekker, pp 235-266.

Adverse Reactions

27. Foley P, Nixon R, Marks R, et al: The frequency of reactions to sunscreens: results of a longitudinal population-based study on the regular use of sunscreens in Australia. *Br J Dermatol* 128:512-518, 1993.

28. Fischer T, Bergstrom K: Evaluation of customers' complaints about sunscreen cosmetics sold by the Swedish pharmaceutical company. *Contact Dermatitis* 25:319-322, 1991.

29. Dromgoole SH, Maibach HI: Sunscreening agent intolerance: contact and photocontact sensitization and contact urticaria. *J Am Acad Dermatol* 22:1068-1078, 1990.

30. Lenique P, Machet L, Vaillant L, et al: Contact and photocontact allergy to oxybenzone. *Contact Dermatitis* 26:177-181, 1992.

31. Schauder S, Ippen H: Contact and photocontact sensitivity to sunscreens. Review of a 15-year experience and of the literature. *Contact Dermatitis* 37(5):221-232, 1997.

32. Fotiades J, Soter NA, Lim HW: Results of evaluation of 203 patients for photosensitivity in a 7.3-year period. *J Am Acad Dermatol* 33(4):597-602, 1995.

33. Trevisi P, Vincenzi C, Chieregato C, et al: Sunscreen sensitization: a three-year study. *Dermatology* 189:55-57, 1994.

34. Szczurko C, Dompmartin A, Michel M, et al: Photocontact allergy to oxybenzone: ten years of experience. *Photodermatol Photoimmunol Photomed* 10:144-147, 1994.

35. Berne B, Ros AM: 7 years experience of photopatch testing with sunscreen allergens in Sweden. *Contact Dermatitis* 38(2):61-64, 1998.

36. Mills OH, Porte M, Kligman AM: Enhancement of comedogenic substances by ultraviolet radiation. *Br J Dermatol* 100:699-702, 1979.

37. Mills OH, Kligman AM: Acne aestivalis. *Arch Dermatol* 111:891-892, 1975.

Patient Instructions

38. Smith RC, Tyler JE: Transmission of solar radiation into natural waters. In Smith RC, editor: *Photochemical and photobiological reviews,* New York, 1976, Plenum Press, p 117.

39. Gaughan MD, Padilla RS: Use of a topical fluorescent dye to evaluate effectiveness of sunscreen application. *Arch Dermatol* 134:515-517, 1998.

40. Loesch H, Kaplan DL: Pitfalls in sunscreen application. *Arch Dermatol* 130:665-666, 1994.

41. Stern RS, Weinstein MC, Baker SG: Risk reduction for nonmelanoma skin cancer with childhood sunscreen use. *Arch Dermatol* 122:537-545, 1986.

42. Banks BA, Silverman RA, Schwartz RM, et al: Attitudes of teenagers toward sun exposure and sunscreen use. *Pediatrics* 89:40-42, 1992.

43. Gloth M, Gundberg CM, Hollis BW, et al: Vitamin D deficiency in homebound elderly persons. *JAMA* 274:1683-1686, 1995.

44. Marks R, Foley PA, Jolley D, et al: The effect of regular sunscreen use on vitamin D levels in an Australian population. *Arch Dermatol* 131:415-421, 1995.

45. Sollitto RB, Kraemer KH, DiGiovanna JJ: Normal vitamin D levels can be maintained despite rigorous photoprotection: six years' experience with xeroderma pigmentosum. *J Am Acad Dermatol* 37(6):942-947, 1997.

46. Levy SB: Dihydroxyacetone-containing sunless or self-tanning lotions. *J Am Acad Dermatol* 27:989-993, 1992.

47. Muizzuddin N, Marenus KD, Maes DH: UV-A and UV-B protective effect of melanoids formed with dehydroxyacetone and skin. Poster 360 presented at the 55th Annual Meeting of the American Academy of Dermatology, San Francisco, 1997.

48. Johnson JA, Fusaro RM: Protection against long ultraviolet radiation: topical browning agents and a new outlook. *Dermatologica* 175:53-57, 1987.

CHAPTER 32

Robert T. Brodell
Kevin D. Cooper

Therapeutic Shampoos

Therapeutic shampoos are widely available dermatologic products that commonly are used for scaling and pruritus of the scalp. Because scalp hair covers the affected area in the majority of patients, the chief complaint may be embarrassing flakes in the hair and on the clothing. All of these shampoos perform cleansing actions through the emulsification of oily secretions and can be substituted for standard (salon) shampoos. Therefore they are very convenient to use on a regular basis. The additional active ingredients provide the basis for categorization of these agents (Table 32-1).

VARIOUS DERMATOSES INVOLVING THE SCALP

Clinically, the scaling conditions of the scalp can be categorized as dandruff, cradle cap, seborrheic dermatitis, psoriasis, atopic dermatitis, or irritant contact dermatitis. Dandruff is a condition that causes dry, grayish-white scales scattered over the scalp. In contrast with psoriasis, there is no underlying plaque and the lesions show indistinct borders. The earliest onset of dandruff is at puberty. Itching is inconsistently present. Dandruff can persist through life but tends to diminish with age. This may represent a variant of seborrheic dermatitis.

Cradle cap is often seen 1 to 2 weeks after birth but can occur at any time through infancy.

Children with cradle cap have yellowish-brown, greasy scales on the scalp with indistinct borders associated with underlying erythema and pruritus. It can also involve the retroauricular skin, nasolabial folds, and skin folds of the neck, axillae, and diaper area. This condition usually clears in 2 to 8 weeks. Cradle cap also appears to be a variant of seborrheic dermatitis.

Seborrheic dermatitis shows white-to-yellow scales on an erythematous base and involves the scalp, eyebrows, postauricular area, nasolabial folds, body folds, and central chest and back. When the scaling is dry, it can be referred to as *seborrhea capitis sicca* (dandruff).[1] When scaling is accompanied by excessive sebum production of the scalp, the condition is also called *seborrhea capitis oleosa*.[1] Seborrheic dermatitis occurs after puberty. This condition occurs more frequently in patients with neurologic diseases or human immunodeficiency virus (HIV) infection, where it can be a marker for early disease.[2-4] Pruritus is commonly present. Though it can persist for life, seborrheic dermatitis is characterized by remissions and exacerbations. Vitamin deficiencies have not been tied to this condition.

Psoriasis shows thick, well-demarcated purple-red plaques with white micaceous scaling on the scalp. Other sites of involvement particularly include the knees, elbows, and sacral area. The nails often show pitting, dystrophy, and onycholysis. Psoriasis often appears in young

■ Table 32-1   Therapeutic Shampoos Used in Dermatology

Generic Name	Trade Name	Active Ingredient	Size	AWP
KERATOLYTIC SHAMPOOS				
Salicylic acid (salacid)	T-sal	Salacid 3%	4.5 oz	$5.35
	Baker's P & S	Salacid 2%	4 oz	$8.95
	Ionil	Salacid 2%	8 oz	$12.08
	Ionil Plus	Salacid 2%	8 oz	$12.46
Salicylic acid and sulfur	MG 217 Tar-free Shampoo	Salacid 3%, sulfur 5%	4 oz	$3.96
	Sebulex	Salacid 2%, sulfur 2%	4 oz	$5.58
CYTOSTATIC SHAMPOOS				
Selenium sulfide	Selsun Blue	Selenium sulfide 1%	4 oz	$3.34
	Head & Shoulders Intensive Treatment	Selenium sulfide 1%	15.2 oz	$3.51
	Selenium sulfide 1%	Selenium sulfide 1%	4 oz	$3.25
	Selsun 2.5%*	Selenium sulfide 2.5%	4 oz	$6.73
	Exsel 2.5%*	Selenium sulfide 2.5%	4 oz	$15.46
	Selenium sulfide 2.5%*	Selenium sulfide 2.5%	4 oz	$6.95
Zinc pyrithione	Head & Shoulders	Zinc pyrithione 1%	7 oz	$2.59
	Zincon	Zinc pyrithione 1%	4 oz	$2.59
	Sebulon	Zinc pyrithione 2%	??	??
	DHS Zinc	Zinc pyrithione 2%	8 oz	$6.65
ANTIMITOTIC SHAMPOOS				
Tar	Pentrax	CTE 7%	4 oz	$6.74
	T-Gel XS	Solubilized CTE 4%	4.4 oz	$7.09
	T-gel	Solubilized CTE 2%	4.4 oz	$4.45
	Ionil T	Coal tar solution 2%; Benzalkonium chloride; Salacid 2%	4 oz	$8.08
	Ionil T plus	Coal tar solution 2%	8 oz	$12.46
	Zetar	Whole coal tar 1%	6 oz	$14.21
	DHS Tar	Coal tar 0.5%	4 oz	$4.57
	Tegrin	Coal tar solution 7%	7 oz	$4.96
	Polytar	"Polytar" 4.5%	5.9 oz	$7.41
	Reme'T	Coal tar 5%	8 oz	$9.49
ANTIMICROBIAL SHAMPOOS				
Ketoconazole	Nizoral	Ketoconazole 1%	4 oz	$8.99
	Nizoral*	Ketoconazole 2%	4 oz	$20.74
Chloroxine	Capitrol*	Chloroxine 2%	4 oz	$19.57
Iodophors	Betadine Surgical Scrub	Povidone-iodine 7.5%	4 oz	$9.64
ANTIINFLAMMATORY SHAMPOOS				
Fluocinolone	Derma-Smoothe/FS*	Fluocinolone 0.01%	4 oz	$14.62

Price index adapted from *Drug topics*. The Red Book, 1999.
AWP, Average wholesale price; *CTE*, coal tar extract.
*Available only by prescription.

adulthood but can occur at any age. Half of patients with psoriasis experience pruritus. This condition is also characterized by remissions and exacerbations. Environmental stimuli are thought to explain exacerbations and include streptococcal infection, medications, fever, and a variety of emotional and physical stressors. Psoriatic arthritis, which occurs in 10% of patients with psoriasis, represents the only systemic complication.

Irritant contact dermatitis and atopic dermatitis are often termed *lichen simplex chronicus* when they occur on the scalp. These patients have extreme itching. Rubbing and scratching is a central part of the disease process. Dermatitis can occur anywhere on the body, but the occipital scalp is commonly involved. This condition will last until the "itch-scratch cycle" is broken.

Many of these conditions can result in severe accumulation of adherent scale, resulting in matted hair in the scalp. This is referred to as tinea amiantacea, although the condition is not itself a tinea infection. Scalp infections with dermatophytes (tinea capitis) such as *Trichophyton tonsurans* must be ruled out in all scaling scalp conditions, particularly in children. Scalp conditions can be signs of serious disease elsewhere (e.g., pityriasis rubra pilaris, lupus erythematosus, cutaneous T-cell lymphoma) or can result in permanent scarring alopecia of the scalp (e.g., lichen planopilaris, lupus erythematosus, folliculitis, and perifolliculitis capitis abscedens et suffodiens) must also be ruled out on clinical or histologic grounds before using the therapeutic shampoos discussed in this chapter.

HISTORICAL PERSPECTIVE

In 1874, Malassez[5] implicated yeast organisms as the cause of seborrheic dermatitis. Sabouraud[6] supported this observation in 1904. For over 100 years most experts believed these yeast forms were secondary invaders of diseased skin. The response of seborrheic dermatitis to oral ketoconazole rejuvenated the view that yeast organisms may be an important etiology of this condition. Oral ketoconazole does not have a cytostatic effect, although metabolic effects (e.g., inhibition of cytochrome P-450 enzymes)

that may alter the pathogenesis of seborrheic dermatitis have not been ruled out.[7-9] *Staphylococcus aureus* colonization may also contribute to the disease process.

The use of topical medications to treat scaling scalp conditions dates to 1876 when Duhring wrote, "Among external remedies which are of the greatest service and should be employed in all cases, baths of various kinds, simple or medicated, the preparations of tar, the mercurial ointments, sulphur, sapo viridis, and solutions of caustic potassa, will be found most useful."[10] A number of scalp medicaments have been available for many years, several of which have not been through the rigorous testing of modern clinical trials. Available for over 20 years are numerous tar solutions and shampoos, salicylic acid preparations, phenol and saline solutions, and selenium sulfide.

PHARMACOLOGY
Mechanism of Action

Most of the shampoos discussed in this chapter contain "wetting agents," also known as surfactants, which have hydrophilic and hydrophobic portions on each molecule. These shampoos degrease the skin of the scalp through emulsification of sebum, promoting "wetting" of the scalp, which enhances the effect of the "active" ingredients. The end result is washing away flakes of scale and facilitating separation of scale into smaller, less visible flakes. Improvement of seborrheic dermatitis by decreasing high skin surface lipid levels, when compared with controls, may also result in therapeutic benefit.[11,12] Perhaps the high surface lipid levels provide the substrate required for growth of *Pityrosporum* yeast. Alternatively, they may provide substrates for inflammatory prostaglandins and cell signaling. Interestingly, previous studies found that sebaceous output was not elevated in patients with seborrheic dermatitis.[13-16] Cationic wetting agents include quaternary ammonium compounds such as benzalkonium chloride and cetyl trimethyl ammonium bromide. Anionic wetting agents include the sulfates, sulfonates, and soaps such as sodium lauryl sulfate and dioctyl sodium sulfosuccinate. Nonionic wetting agents include propylene glycol, spans, and tweens.[17]

KERATOLYTIC EFFECTS. The mechanism by which keratolytic agents (e.g., salicylic acid and sulfur) soften, dissolve, or release the adherent scale of psoriasis, lichen simplex chronicus, and seborrheic dermatitis is not well understood, although these chemicals became an important component of standard scalp care in these scaling conditions. The stratum corneum is the outermost layer of the skin and is composed of an aggregation of flattened keratinocytes forming a relatively impermeable barrier. This serves to limit water loss, protect against environmental chemicals, and provide protection from mechanical forces. In normal skin, corneocytes (dead flattened epidermal cells) are shed from the outer layers of the stratum corneum in concert with the production of new cells at the basal layer, which differentiate and continually replace the lost cells. This slough is continuous and imperceptible. In psoriasis and to a lesser extent in seborrheic dermatitis, hyperproliferation is associated with a decreased transit time from the basal layer to the outer stratum corneum, leading to imperfect keratinization and faulty desquamation of the cornified layer.[18] A basal cell may reach the stratum corneum in 3 days rather than the usual 25 to 30 days. Corneocytes remain tightly adherent, creating large flakes of scale that are visible to the naked eye when they break away in an irregular fashion. Eczemas, including lichen simplex chronicus and atopic dermatitis, also show hyperkeratosis. Keratolytic agents in selected therapeutic shampoos loosen the "cement" between corneocytes, allowing them to release from the scalp and to be washed away during subsequent shampooing. The thinner stratum corneum induced by these keratolytic agents leads to less dandruff and permits better contact with active therapeutic agents in topical shampoo preparations. No studies have proven the effectiveness of salicylic acid or sulfur as a monotherapy in psoriasis or eczema, although scaling is clearly reduced in seborrheic dermatitis.[19]

Alternative abrasive approaches to dandruff control using fingernails, combs, or brushes to remove scales are rarely helpful. Vigorous scrubbing can lead to bleeding (Auspitz sign in psoriasis), crusting, increasing pruritus, and worsening of the underlying disease. This process is known as Koebner's phenomenon or "isomorphic effect" in psoriasis.[20] In addition, the itch-scratch cycle is the underlying cause of lichen simplex chronicus and also can exacerbate atopic dermatitis. Thus keratolytic agents in therapeutic shampoos may improve papulosquamous diseases of the scalp by eliminating the symptoms of dandruff, which provoke patients to traumatize their scalps.

ANTIINFLAMMATORY EFFECTS. Many shampoos and scalp lotions or sprays contain topical corticosteroids, which have potent antiinflammatory and antipruritic effects. A scalp-directed, corticosteroid-containing foaming mousse that penetrates scales is now available (betamethasone valerate foam 0.12%—Luxiq). A fluocinolone-containing scalp application (Derma-Smoothe/FS) is formulated in peanut oil, which helps this mid-strength topical corticosteroid penetrate through the scale and deliver the active drug to the underlying epidermis. The exact mode of action is likely complex and multifactorial. Inhibitions of immunologic factors, such as induction of inflammatory cascades by cytokines from T cells, keratinocytes, and macrophages, and inflammatory mediators, such as histamines, proteases, and leukotrienes, may be central to the mechanism of action for corticosteroid-containing shampoos. In addition, decreasing pruritus reduces scratching and thereby decreases Koebner's phenomenon in psoriasis and irritation and excoriation of seborrheic dermatitis, atopic dermatitis, and lichen simplex chronicus. Perhaps because the underlying *Pityrosporum* infection is not being directly treated, recurrence is prompt and relapse rates are high.[21]

A new scalp treatment involves the incorporation of a retinoid (tazarotene) into a gel that can be worked into the base of the scalp of patients with psoriasis or lichen simplex chronicus.[22,23] The mechanism may be either epidermal differentiation or immunologic but is unlikely to be antimicrobial. Tazarotene shampoos are not yet available.

ANTIPROLIFERATIVE EFFECTS. Tar shampoos most probably work through antimitotic (antiproliferative) and cytostatic effects, although the huge number of biologically active components in coal tar products complicates analysis of the mechanism.[24] Specifically, coal tar suppresses epidermal cell deoxyribonucleic acid (DNA) synthesis, which may normalize the increased DNA synthesis that characterizes psoriasis and in addition may be immunosuppressive.[25] Antibacterial and antimycotic activity of tars is likely but is poorly studied. In addition, tar products disperse scales, which in and of itself may reduce *Pityrosporum* colonization.[26]

Selenium sulfide also has significant cytostatic effects that may play a key role in this drug's action in scaling scalp diseases.[17] Selenium sulfide and zinc pyrithione reduce cell turnover rate significantly. It is possible that selenium sulfide has a direct antimitotic effect. Zinc pyrithione mechanism of action is unknown but may be due to a mild nonspecific toxicity for epidermal cells.[26]

ANTIPITYROSPORUM EFFECTS.   A favored proposed mechanism of action of ketoconazole shampoo, zinc pyrithione, and perhaps selenium sulfide shampoo is that they suppress superficial fungal infection of the scalp.[22,27-32] Specifically, in seborrheic dermatitis, the hyperproliferative and inflammatory pathways may be reactive effects caused by superficial *Pityrosporum* infection. The central role of *Pityrosporum* infection is supported by studies showing that the density of *Pityrosporum* is correlated with the severity of seborrheic dermatitis.[33] In addition, *Pityrosporum* is cultured much more frequently in seborrheic dermatitis than in other papulosquamous diseases.[34] The efficacy of antifungal therapy in seborrheic dermatitis is paralleled by the reduction in the number of *P. ovale* cells.[35-37] In addition, topical ketoconazole has also been shown to have antiinflammatory effects.[38] Patients with HIV and other immunodeficiency states commonly develop seborrheic dermatitis, perhaps because the immunodeficiency is directly related to overgrowth of *Pityrosporum* yeast, although unregulated inflammatory processes during HIV infection may also play a role. In patients with psoriasis, yeast organisms may colonize the abnormal scaling scalp and subsequently koebnerize the scalp skin, triggering the inflammatory cascade.

Lithium succinate ointment has been shown to be effective in the treatment of seborrheic dermatitis. It blocks the release of free fatty acids from tissues and is postulated to reduce the substrate needed for *Pityrosporum* growth.[39] In the future, lithium base shampoos may become available. However, lithium effects on neutrophil and leukocyte activation must also be taken into account in seborrhea, which has an active neutrophilic inflammatory component.

EFFECTS IN INFANTILE SEBORRHEIC DERMATITIS.   Altered essential fatty acid production caused by transient impaired enzyme function may play a role in infantile seborrheic dermatitis.[40] Specific treatments to normalize essential fatty acid enzyme pathways have not been developed.

Systemic Absorption

The potential for significant absorption of tar compounds is worrisome because the mutagenic effects of crude coal tar and its components have been well documented.[41] Significant absorption of tar occurs when the normal scalp is shampooed with tar shampoo. In one study, polycyclic aromatic hydrocarbons (which are present in coal tar shampoos) were detected in the urine of patients using tar shampoos in amounts equivalent to levels detected in coke-oven workers. These workers have a documented increased incidence of cancer due to polycyclic aromatic hydrocarbons.[42] It would be expected that diseased skin in psoriasis and seborrheic dermatitis would lead to even more systemic absorption. However, the use of tar products in shampoos for decades has not been shown to induce localized or systemic tumor formation.[43] Metabolic conjugation of tars occurs in the liver with excretion in the urine.

Absorption of salicylic acid leading to salicylate intoxication has been reported when patients use concentrations greater than 10% over more than 50% of their body surface in ointment forms.[44] This systemic absorption has not been reported from available salicylic acid shampoos. Small amounts of salicylic acid that are absorbed are metabolized in the liver and excreted by the kidneys.

Selenium sulfide and zinc pyrithione absorption must occur to some extent when these products are used in shampoos but generally have a high safety margin with minor skin irritation reported infrequently.[45-47] An isolated report documented that a patient with damaged scalp skin using selenium sulfide shampoo 2 to 3 times per week developed selenium intoxication. Elevated selenium levels as high as 32 μg/ml were documented in this case. This systemic absorption was evidenced by tremors, perspiration, garlicky breath, weakness, vomiting, and abdominal pain.[48] Rarely, contact dermatitis to zinc pyrithione has been reported.[26]

Percutaneous corticosteroid absorption occurs with topical use of shampoos containing corticosteroids. Factors such as relatively decreased absorption of topical corticosteroids through scalp skin, relatively infrequent use of shampoos (daily at most), and the relatively small percentage of body surface area treated limit the potential for systemic corticosteroid levels that could suppress the hypothalamus-pituitary-adrenal axis. Scalp skin thinning and telangiectasias can occur with repeated heavy use due to corticosteroid atrophy.

Only small amounts of ketoconazole are absorbed when this agent is used in shampoo form.[49] Metabolism of this small quantity of absorbed ketoconazole by the liver ensures that significant serum levels are not achieved. Ketoconazole persists in hair keratin for up to 72 hours after shampoo application. No systemic adverse effects have been reported in patients using ketoconazole shampoo.

CLINICAL USE

Indications

All of the shampoos described are useful in the treatment of scaling inflammatory skin diseases of the scalp. They are used to control scaling scalp conditions rather than cure these conditions. Prolonged or intermittent use is the rule rather than the exception. Because there is relatively little published scientific information regarding these therapeutic shampoos, art must be combined with science as treatment is tailored for each patient. Physically washing the scalp on a regular basis with even nonmedicated (salon) shampoos may be an important factor in dandruff control.[1,50] Specific Food and Drug Administration (FDA)–approved indications are listed in Table 32-2 (see Therapeutic Guidelines section).

Table 32-2	Indications for Therapeutic Shampoos

FDA-APPROVED INDICATIONS
Scaling Scalp and Dandruff
Salicylic acid
Selenium sulfide 1% and 2.5%
Zinc pyrithione
Tar
Ketoconazole

Seborrheic Dermatitis
Ketoconazole
Tar
Topical steroids
Selenium sulfide 2.5%

Psoriasis
Tar

OFF-LABEL USES
Adjunctive Treatment of Tinea Capitis
Selenium sulfide
Ketoconazole

Adverse Effects

Each of the therapeutic shampoos is contraindicated in individuals shown to be allergic to the active ingredients, preservatives, stabilizers, fragrances, and other ingredients. None of the products have been adequately tested in pregnancy, although they would not appear to present a significant risk to the fetus.

SAFETY IN CHILDREN.   Similarly, many of these products have not been tested in children. Except with products labeled for use in "cradle cap," use of these products in infants is not recommended. This is because the amount of skin surface in proportion to body weight is greater in very young children than in adults. Furthermore, hepatic enzyme systems are not fully developed in neonates and infants for handling toxic substances that might be absorbed.

Preliminary information suggests that ketoconazole shampoo is safe and effective in infants with cradle cap.[49,51] The rare occurrence of idiosyncratic hepatotoxicity due to this drug with systemic use must be kept in mind if significant and prolonged exposure to ketoconazole is contemplated in this age group.

ALLERGIC AND IRRITANT CONTACT DERMATITIS.

Drying, burning, stinging, irritation, and discomfort have been reported with each of the products and are most commonly irritant in nature. Irritation commonly occurs with keratolytic agents present in therapeutic shampoos.[26] The short contact time, dilution with water, and quick rinse reduce the sensitizing potential of these products. However, allergic contact dermatitis is possible either to the active ingredients, such as topical steroids, or to other contents of the products, including anionic detergents, amphoteric detergents, fatty acid amides, fragrance, formaldehyde, and other preservatives that are formaldehyde releasers.[52] Patch-testing to individual ingredients is necessary to incriminate allergens in shampoos.

OTHER ADVERSE EFFECTS.

There are few adverse effects from the use of these shampoos. Topical corticosteroid shampoos could induce the same local adverse effects reported for the use of other topical corticosteroids. These potential adverse effects include folliculitis, skin atrophy, telangiectasia, hypertrichosis, hypopigmentation, secondary infection, and striae. Specific case reports of adverse effects from corticosteroid shampoos could not be identified in the literature. In addition, tachyphylaxis has been reported with the use of topical corticosteroids, though not specifically with corticosteroid shampoos.[53]

Avoiding eye contact is recommended in the cases of tars, salicylic acid, selenium sulfide, and topical corticosteroids.[26] Tar shampoos can stain blonde or dyed hair a greenish or brown color. Selenium sulfide may leave a residual smell, discolor hair, and make hair more oily.[26,50] Staining of clothing by tar products seems to be less common with newer tar shampoos. In addition, tar shampoos should be avoided in patients receiving psoralen plus ultraviolet A (PUVA) therapy to avoid "tar smarts" that have been associated with other topical tar preparations. Objectionable features of early tar shampoos, such as unpleasant odor, staining of blonde or white hair,

and difficulty removing the tar, have been largely overcome with modern formulations.[26,54]

Therapeutic Guidelines

Generally, any of the shampoos discussed in this chapter is applied to the scalp after wetting the hair and massaged vigorously, allowing the shampoo to contact the scalp for 5 minutes.[26] After rinsing the shampoo, the product may be applied a second time. These products are safe with daily use, although they may also be effective by shampooing as little as once or twice weekly in patients with dandruff, seborrheic dermatitis, or cradle cap. Whereas the benefits of Nizoral shampoo plateau at 2 to 3 times per week, selenium sulfide and other medicated shampoos continue to improve scalp scaling with increased use up to daily.[55,56] Ad lib use to maintain adequate control is often recommended.

Many clinical studies support the clinical efficacy of ketoconazole shampoo for seborrheic dermatitis or dandruff.[29,57-66] Similarly, ketoconazole cream can be used effectively for seborrheic dermatitis of the face.[67,68] In comparative studies, ketoconazole shampoo suppresses *Pityrosporum* organisms more effectively than either zinc pyrithione or selenium sulfide shampoo.[69] Among the imidazoles, both MICs in vitro and clinical experience suggest that ketoconazole is highly effective in seborrheic dermatitis.[70] Selenium sulfide also demonstrated efficacy in clinical studies.[60,63] Relapse may be delayed in patients using ketoconazole 2% shampoo when compared with placebo[71] and when compared with selenium sulfide 2.5% shampoo as well.[63] Zinc pyrithione has also been shown to be efficacious in a shampoo formulation.[72] Selenium sulfide may be somewhat more efficacious than zinc pyrithione.[72,73] The clinical effectiveness of tar shampoos has also been demonstrated.[74] Patients should be educated to anticipate using the shampoos for long periods of time to "control" seborrhea and psoriasis rather than expect a "cure."[75] Chronic use of 2% ketoconazole shampoo has been shown to be safe.[76] Remission of scalp psoriasis can occur with the use of various therapeutic shampoos but is unpredictable.

Many patients with scaling scalp diseases benefit from rotational therapy.[56] A specific shampoo is used for 3 to 4 weeks, then rotated to another shampoo from a different class.[77] In another commonly used approach, two products are used on alternate days, with less frequent application as the condition improves. Some patients find that salicylic acid and tar products can be mixed together before shampooing for maximum effectiveness.

Salicylic acid lotions (e.g., 5% to 10% salicylic acid in a cream base, Bakers P&S Solution, Epilyt, or 5% salicylic acid plus 5% liquor carbonis detergens [LCD] in Ponds Softening Lotion) may be applied to the scalp 2 to 8 hours before shampooing with a tar shampoo. If irritation occurs, the patient should avoid shampooing with the responsible product for a few days, then resume shampooing less frequently.

Finally, topical corticosteroid lotions, tazarotene gel, or anthralin scalp solution can be used in conjunction with therapeutic shampoos. None of these products stands out as clearly superior in controlling scalp psoriasis. In contrast, topical corticosteroid solutions or lotions are an appropriate adjunctive therapy if scalp pruritus is not adequately controlled by the shampoo alone. Physicians must rely on feedback from the patient to select the approach that is most effective and best tolerated for these chronic scalp conditions.

This chapter considers therapeutic shampoos separately from other treatment modalities. In the case of psoriasis, many different treatment modalities, including systemic approaches and phototherapy, may be utilized in the same patient. Systemic therapies, which produce general improvement of the burden of psoriasis over the entire cutaneous surface, may assist the therapeutic shampoos in achieving or maintaining remission.[78] It is interesting that scalp psoriasis, even under a full head of hair, can improve with phototherapy (e.g., PUVA) that is delivered to remaining areas of the body.

Both selenium sulfide shampoo and ketoconazole shampoo have been shown to decrease dermatophyte fungus in scale and may decrease infectivity in patients who have tinea capitis.[79,80] Neither of these adjunctive shampoo treatments eradicates the disease, and therefore these shampoos should be used in conjunction with systemic antifungal agents to eradicate tinea capitis and to reduce contagion.

All of the products discussed in this chapter are available over-the-counter with the exception of ketoconazole 2% shampoo, selenium sulfide 2.5% shampoo, betamethasone valerate foam 0.12% (Luxiq), and fluocinolone acetonide 0.01% (Derma-Smoothe/FS Shampoo).

Drug Interactions

There are no known drug interactions of these agents in routine use. If systemic levels of ketoconazole were achieved through misuse, a variety of drug interactions mediated by the cytochrome P-450 enzyme system would require consideration. There are no requirements for monitoring of therapy with ketoconazole shampoo.

SUMMARY

Therapeutic shampoos are widely used in a variety of conditions associated with scaling of the scalp. Their usefulness has met the test of time, but comparative outcome studies are required to document the most cost-effective uses of these products in the future.

Bibliography

Chesterman KW: An evaluation of O-T-C dandruff and seborrhea products. *J Am Pharm Assoc* 12:578-581, 1972.

Faergemann J: Pityrosporum infections. *J Am Acad Dermatol* 31:S18-S20, 1994.

Greaves MW, Weinstein GD: Treatment of psoriasis. *N Engl J Med* 332:581-587, 1995.

Jacobs PH: Seborrheic dermatitis: causes and management. *Cutis* 41:182-186, 1988.

Leyden JJ: Overview: *Pityrosporum* and scaling disorders of the scalp. *J Int Postgrad Med* 2:5-9, 1990.

McGrath J, Murphy GM: The control of seborrhoeic dermatitis and dandruff by antipityrosporal drugs. *Drugs* 41:178-184, 1991.

Robinson JR, Gauger LJ: Dermatitis, dry skin, dandruff, seborrheic dermatitis and psoriasis products. In: Nonprescription products, formulations and features. Washington, DC. *American Pharmaceutical Association* 30:597-623, 1986.

Webster G: Seborrheic dermatitis. *Int J Dermatol* 30:843-844, 1991.

References

Introduction

1. Chesterman KW: An evaluation of O-T-C dandruff and seborrhea products. *J Am Pharm Assoc* 12:578-581, 1972.
2. Binder RL, Jonelis FJ: Seborrheic dermatitis in neuroleptic-induced parkinsonism. *Arch Dermatol* 119:473-475, 1983.
3. Groisser D, Bottone EJ, Lebwohl M: Association of *Pityrosporum orbiculare (Malassezia furfur)* with seborrheic dermatitis in patients with acquired immunodeficiency syndrome (AIDS). *J Am Acad Dermatol* 20:770-773, 1989.
4. Wishner AJ, Teplitz ED, Goodman DS: Pityrosporum, ketoconazole, and seborrheic dermatitis. *J Am Acad Dermatol* 17:140-141, 1987.
5. Malassez L: Note sur le champignon de la pelade. *Arch Physiol Norm Pathol II* I:203, 1874.
6. Sabouraud R: *Pityriasis et alopecies peculaires: les maladies desquamatives,* ed 1, Paris, 1904, Masson et cie, pp 295-374.
7. Farr PM: Initial studies on the treatment of seborrheic dermatitis with oral ketoconazole. Seborrhoeic dermatitis and dandruff—a fungal disease. Royal Society of Medicine Services Limited. International Congress and Symposium Series. 132:5-11, 1988.
8. Ford GP, Farr PM, Ive FA, et al: The response of seborrheic dermatitis to ketoconazole. *Br J Dermatol* 3(Suppl 26):603-607, 1984.
9. Jacobs PH: Seborrheic dermatitis: causes and management. *Cutis* 41:182-186, 1988.
10. Duhring LA: *Atlas of skin diseases,* Philadelphia, 1876, JB Lippincott.

Mechanism of Action

11. Bergbrant IM: Seborrhoeic dermatitis and *Pityrosporum ovale:* cultural, immunological and clinical studies. *Acta Derm Venereol* 167(Suppl):7-36, 1991.

12. Leyden JJ: Overview: *Pityrosporum* and scaling disorders of the scalp. *J Int Postgrad Med* 2:5-9, 1990.
13. Federal Register 47(238), Friday December 3, 1982/ Proposed Rules, pp 54646-54684.
14. Webster G: Seborrheic dermatitis. *Int J Dermatol* 30:843-844, 1991.
15. Kligman AM, Leyden JJ: Seborrheic dermatitis. *Semin Dermatol* 2:57-59, 1983.
16. Pye RJ, Meyrich G, Burton JL: Skin surface lipids in seborrheic dermatitis. *Br J Dermatol* 97(Suppl):12-15, 1977.
17. Plewig G, Kligman AM: The effect of selenium sulfide on epidermal turnover of normal and dandruff scalps. *J Soc Cosmet Chem* 20:767-775, 1969.
18. Ackerman AB, Kligman AM: Some observations on dandruff. *J Soc Cosmet Chem* 20: 81-101, 1969.
19. Greaves MW, Weinstein GD: Treatment of psoriasis. *N Engl J Med* 332:581-587, 1995.
20. Jablonska S, Chowaniec, O, Beutner EH, et al: Stripping of the stratum corneum in patients with psoriasis. *Arch Dermatol* 118:652-657, 1982.
21. McGrath J, Murphy GM: The control of seborrhoeic dermatitis and dandruff by antipityrosporal drugs. *Drugs* 41:178-184, 1991.
22. Weinstein GD, Krueger GG, Lowe NJ, et al: Tazarotene gel, a new retinoid, for topical therapy of psoriasis: vehicle-controlled study of safety, efficacy, and duration of therapeutic effect. *J Am Acad Dermatol* 37:85-92, 1997.
23. Lebwohl MG, Breneman DL, Goffe BS, et al: Tazarotene 0.1% gel plus corticosteroid cream in the treatment of plaque psoriasis. *J Am Acad Dermatol* 39:590-596, 1998.
24. Wortzman M, Breeding J, Lowe N: Efficacy of a new coal tar extract and four coal tar shampoos by DNA synthesis suppression assay (abstract). *J Invest Dermatol* 77:315, 1981.

25. Lowe NJ, Breeding JH, Wortzman MS: New coal tar extract and coal tar shampoos. *Arch Dermatol* 118:487-489, 1982.

26. Robinson JR, Gauger LJ: Dermatitis, dry skin, dandruff, seborrheic dermatitis and psoriasis products. In Nonprescription products, formulations and features. Washington, DC, *American Pharmaceutical Association* 30:597-623, 1986.

27. Spoor HJ: A study of anti-dandruff agents, *Drug and Cosmetic Industry* 77:44-45, 134-137, 1955.

28. Schmidt A: *Malassezia furfur:* a fungus belonging to the physiological skin flora and its relevance in skin disorders. *Cutis* 59:21-24, 1997.

29. Degreef H: World wide experiences with ketoconazole shampoo in seborrhoeic dermatitis and dandruff.. Satellite Symposium to the 2nd International Skin Therapy Symposium, Antwerp, Belgium, May 5, 1988, 32-37.

30. Richardson MD, Shankland GS: Enhanced phagocytosis and intracellular killing of *Pityrosporum ovale* by human neutrophils after exposure to ketoconazole is correlated to changes of the yeast cell surface. *Mycoses* 34:29-33, 1991.

31. Segal R, David M, Ingber A, et al: Treatment of bifonazole shampoo for seborrhea and seborrheic dermatitis: a randomized, double-blind study. *Acta Derm Venereol (Stockh)* 72:454-455, 1992.

32. Thulliez M, Cornelis H, Schiettekatte L, et al: Ketoconazole shampoo in dandruff and/or seborrhoeic dermatitis. In Janssen in touch with the skin Abstract of the Satellite Symposium to the 17th World Congress of Dermatology, Berlin, May 1987, p 47.

33. Heng MCY, Henderson CL, Barker DC, et al: Correlation of *Pityrosporum ovale* density with clinical severity of seborrheic dermatitis as assessed by a simplified technique. *J Am Acad Dermatol* 23:82-86, 1990.

34. Ruiz-Maldonado R, López-Martínez R, Pérez Chavarría EL, et al: *Pityrosporum ovale* in infantile seborrheic dermatitis. *Pediatr Dermatol* 6:16-20, 1989.

35. Faergemann J: Seborrheic dermatitis and *Pityrosporum orbiculare:* treatment of seborrheic dermatitis of the scalp with miconazole-hydrocortisone (Daktacort), miconazole and hydrocortisone. *Br J Dermatol* 114:695-700, 1986.

36. Sei Y, Hamaguchi T, Ninomiya J, et al: Seborrhoeic dermatitis: treatment of anti-mycotic agents. *J Dermatol* 21:334-340, 1994.

37. Groisser D, Bottone EJ, Lebwohl M: Association of *Pityrosporum orbiculare (Malassezia furfur)* with seborrheic dermatitis in patients with acquired immunodeficiency syndrome (AIDS). *J Am Acad Dermatol* 20:770, 1989.

38. Van Cutsem J, Van Gerven F, Cauwenbergh G, et al: The antiinflammatory effects of ketoconazole. *J Am Acad Dermatol* 25:257-261, 1991.

39. Efalith Multicenter Trial Group: A double-blind, placebo-controlled, multicenter trial of lithium succinate ointment in the treatment of seborrheic dermatitis. *J Am Acad Dermatol* 26:452-457, 1992.

40. Tollesson A, Frithz A, Berg A, et al: Essential fatty acids in infantile seborrheic dermatitis. *J Am Acad Dermatol* 28:957-961, 1993.

Systemic Absorption

41. Storer JS, DeLeon I, Millikan LE, et al: Human absorption of crude coal tar products. *Arch Dermatol* 120:874-877, 1984.

42. van Schooten FJ, Moonen EJ, Rhijnsburger E, et al: Dermal uptake of polycyclic aromatic hydrocarbons after hairwash with coal-tar shampoo (letter). *Lancet* 344:1505-1506, 1994.

43. Jemec GBE, Osterlind A: Cancer in patients treated with coal tar: a long-term follow up study. *J Eur Acad Dermatol Venereol* 3:153-156, 1994.

44. Pec J, Strmenova M, Palencarova E, et al: Salicylate intoxication after use of topical salicylic acid ointment by a patient with psoriasis. *Cutis* 50:307-309, 1992.

45. Opdyke D: Antiseborrheic qualities of zinc pyrithione in a cream vehicle. II. Safety evaluation. *Food Cosmet Toxicol* 5:321, 1967.

46. Snyder F: Safety evaluation of zinc 2-pyridinethiol 1-oxide in a shampoo formulation. *Toxicol Appl Pharmacol* 7:425, 1965.

47. Matson E: Selenium sulfide as an antidandruff agent. *J Soc Cosmet Chem* 7:459, 1956.

48. Ransone JW, Scott NM, Knoblock EC: Selenium sulfide intoxication. *N Engl J Med* 264:384-385, 1961.

49. Brodell RT, Patel S, Venglarcyk J, et al: The safety of ketoconazole shampoo for infantile seborrheic dermatitis (letter). *Pediatr Dermatol* 15:406-407, 1998.

Adverse Effects

50. Treatment of dandruff. *Med Lett Drugs Ther* 19:63-64, 1977.

51. Janniger CK: Infantile seborrheic dermatitis: an approach to cradle cap. *Pediatr Dermatol* 51:233-235, 1993.

52. Maibach HI, Engasser PG: Dermatitis due to cosmetics. In AA Fisher, editor: *Contact dermatitis*, ed 3, Philadelphia, 1986, Lea & Feibiger, p 380.

53. DuVivier A, Stoughton RB: Tachyphylaxis to the action of topically applied corticosteroids. *Arch Dermatol* 111:581-583, 1975.

54. Olansky S: Whole coal tar shampoo: a therapeutic hair repair system. *Cutis* 25:99-104, 1980.

Therapeutic Guidelines

55. Neumann PB, Coffindaffer TW, Cothran PD, et al: Clinical investigation comparing 1% selenium sulfide and 2% ketoconazole shampoos for dandruff control. *Cosmetic Dermatol* 9:20-26, 1996.

56. Luppino M, Burkhart CG: Seborrheic dermatitis. *Dermatology* July:28-29, 1982.

57. Arlette J, Giroux JM, Maddin SW, et al: Ketoconazole shampoo in seborrheic dermatitis. *Can J Dermatol* 3:175-180, 1991.

58. Berger R, Mills OH, Jones EL, et al: Double-blind, placebo-controlled trial of ketoconazole 2% shampoo in the treatment of moderate to severe dandruff. *Adv Ther* 7:247-256, 1990.

59. Carr MM, Pyrce DM, Ive FA: Treatment of seborrhoeic dermatitis with ketoconazole: I. Response of seborrhoeic dermatitis of the scalp to topical ketoconazole. *Br J Dermatol* 116:213-216, 1987.

60. Danby FW, Maddin WS, Margesson LJ, et al: A randomized, double-blind, placebo-controlled trial of ketoconazole 2% shampoo versus selenium sulfide 2.5% shampoo in the treatment of moderate to severe dandruff. *J Am Acad Dermatol* 29:1008-1012, 1993.

61. Dobrev H, Zissova L: Effect of ketoconazole 2% shampoo on scalp sebum level in patients with seborrhoeic dermatitis. *Acta Derm Venereol (Stockh)* 77:132-134, 1997.

62. Peter RU, Richarz-Barthauer U: Successful treatment and prophylaxis of scalp seborrhoeic dermatitis and dandruff with 2% ketoconazole shampoo: results of a multicentre, double-blind, placebo-controlled trial. *Br J Dermatol* 132:441-445, 1995.

63. Tanew A: A randomized study with ketoconazole shampoo 2% or Selsun (selenium sulfide 2.5%) in the treatment of seborrheic dermatitis and/or dandruff. Satellite Symposium to the 2nd International Skin Therapy Symposium, Antwerp, Belgium, May 5, 1988.

64. Cauwenbergh G: International experience with ketoconazole shampoo in the treatment of seborrhoeic dermatitis and dandruff. In Shuster S, Blatchford N, editors: Seborrhoeic dermatitis and dandruff—a fungal disease. International Congress and Symposium Series of the Royal Society of Medicine. 132:35-45, 1988.

65. Rigopoulos D, Katsambas A, Antoniou C, et al: Facial seborrheic dermatitis treated with fluconazole 2% shampoo. *Int J Dermatol* 33:136-137, 1994.

66. Arrese JE, Piérard-Franchimont C, Doncker PD, et al: Effect of ketoconazole-medicated shampoos on squamometry and *Malassezia ovalis* load in pityriasis capitis. *Cutis* 58:235-236, 1996.

67. Kousidou T, Panagiotidou D, Boutli F, et al: A double-blind comparison of 2% ketoconazole cream and 1% hydrocortisone cream in the treatment of seborrheic dermatitis. *Curr Ther Res* 51:723-728, 1992.

68. Skinner RB, Noah PW, Taylor RM, et al: Double-blind treatment of seborrheic dermatitis with 2% ketoconazole cream. *J Am Acad Dermatol* 12:852-856, 1985.

69. Van Cutsem J, Van Gerven F, Fransen J, et al: The in vitro antifungal activity of ketoconazole, zinc pyrithione, and selenium sulfide against *Pityrosporum* and their efficacy as a shampoo in the treatment of experimental pityrosporosis in guinea pigs. *J Am Acad Dermatol* 22:993-998, 1990.

70. Faergemann J: Severe seborrheic dermatitis. *J Int Postgrad Med* 2:10-13, 1990.

71. Brown M, Evans TW, Poyner T, et al: The role of ketoconazole 2% shampoo in the treatment and prophylactic management of dandruff. *J Dermatol Treat* 1:177-179, 1990.

72. Kligman AM, Marples RR, Lantis LR, et al: Appraisal of efficacy of antidandruff formulations. *J Soc Cosmet Chem* 25:73-91, 1974.

73. Rapaport M: A randomized controlled clinical trial of four anti-dandruff shampoos. *J Int Med Res* 9:152-156, 1981.

74. Amos HE, MacLennan AI, Boorman GC: Clinical efficacy of Polytar AF (Fongitar) and Nizoral scalp treatments in patients with dandruff/seborrhoeic dermatitis. *J Dermatol Treat* 5:127-130, 1994.

75. Klauder JV: Modern concept and treatment of dandruff and seborrheic eruptions. *J Soc Cosmetic Chem* 6:443-459, 1955.

76. Van Lint J, DeDoncker P, Woestenborghs R:
    Chronic use of 2% ketoconazole shampoo in
    patients with seborrheic dermatitis and dan-
    druff: ketoconazole plasma levels and safety.
    Curr Ther Res 43:43-47, 1988.

77. Fishman HC: Seborrheic dermatitis: practical
    therapy. *Cutis* 20:724-726, 1977.

78. Langner A, Wolska H, Hebborn P: Treatment
    of psoriasis of the scalp with coal tar gel and
    shampoo preparations, *Cutis* 32:290-296,
    1983.

79. Allen HB, Honig PJ, Leyden JJ, et al: Sele-
    nium sulfide: adjunctive therapy for tinea
    capitis. *Pediatrics* 69:81-83, 1982.

80. Silverman RA: Pedatric mycoses in topics in
    clinical dermatology: cutaneous fungal infec-
    tions. In Elewski BE, editor: *Cutaneous fun-
    gal infections*, New York, 1992, Igaku-Shoin
    Medical Publishers Inc., p 218.

Amy B. Lewis

Alpha-Hydroxy Acids

Alpha-hydroxy acids (AHAs) are a class of compounds that continue to generate extensive media attention and consumer interest for the treatment of aging skin. As the search for eternal youth continues, this old family of carboxylic acids has been rediscovered to add to the armamentarium for rejuvenation. The most commonly used are lactic acid and glycolic acid. For years before, these were used to acidify products with a high pH that were unacceptable for skin application. Other AHAs, such as malic acid, citric acid, mandelic acid, and tartaric acid, have not been as extensively studied as lactic and glycolic acids and therefore are not as widely used. They are also called "fruit acids" because they are derived from various fruits, although they are also derived from sugar cane and milk. Because they are derived from organic products, patients often think this represents a natural form of treatment. However, the products used in practice are chemically synthesized.

PHARMACOLOGY

Structure

The smallest of the AHAs is the 2-carbon molecule, glycolic acid. It conforms to the formula $HOCH_2COOH$ (Figure 33-1). The advantages of glycolic acid are that it is stable, colorless, odorless, water-soluble, and nontoxic if ingested.

Next in size is lactic acid with a 3-carbon chain. The formula is diagrammed in Table 33-1. Lactic acid can exist in several isomeric forms; the L-lactic acid (dextro-rotatory), the D-lactic acid (levo-rotatory), or the DL racemic mixture. This terminology is sometimes confusing. The L-lactic acid, with a capital L, is synonymous in the literature with d-lactic acid (with a small case d), whereas the D-isomer (capital D) is also referred to as l-lactic acid (small case l). These forms are enantiomorphic isomers (mirror images). The DL or L forms are more likely to be used in cosmetic formulations. Ammonium lactate is prepared by neutralizing DL-lactic acid with ammonium hydroxide. This is commercially available under the name Lac-Hydrin 12% lotion or cream (Bristol-Myers Squibb). This drug is approved by the Food and Drug Administration (FDA) for the treatment of ichthyosis vulgaris and xerosis. Lactic acid is converted to another AHA, pyruvic acid, by lactic acid dehydrogenase.

The other AHAs are larger with longer carbon chains (Table 33-1). Mandelic acid is named after the German word for almond, *mandel*, because it is derived from bitter almond extract. It is an 8-carbon AHA, much larger than the glycolic acid molecule (chemical formula = $HOCH(C_6H_5)COOH$). It is also available in two enantiomeric and pharmacologically distinct forms.

Mechanism of Action

All AHAs cause detachment of keratinocytes in low concentrations. When applied consistently to rough dry skin, normalization of keratiniza-

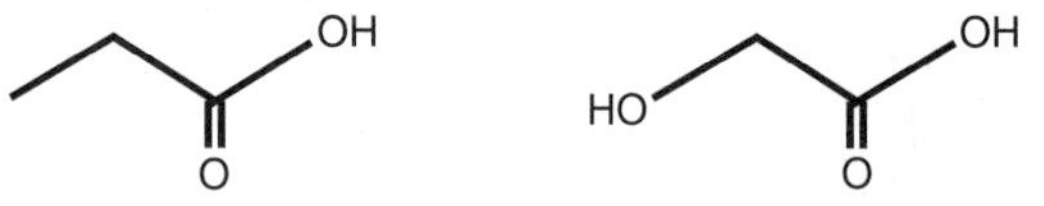

Lactic Acid   Glycolic Acid

Figure 33-1 Alpha-hydroxy acids.

Box 33-1

Epidermolysis—Order of Rapidity

Pyruvic acid
Glycolic acid
Lactic acid

■ **Table 33-1** Alpha-Hydroxy Acids of Varying Carbon Chain Length

2 Carbons	3 Carbons	4 Carbons	6 Carbons	6 Carbon ring†	8 Carbons
Glycolic acid	Lactic acid Pyruvic acid*	Malic acid Tartaric acid Alpha methyl lactic acid	Citric acid Gluconic acid Glucuronic acid	Monophenyl glycolic acid Diphenyl glycolic acid	Mandelic acid

*Pyruvic acid is the keto form of lactic acid.
†Both of these compounds are glycolic acid derivatives.

■ **Table 33-2** Biologic Responses to Varying Alpha-Hydroxy Concentrations and pH*

Stratum Corneum Response	Epidermal and Dermal Response
Less than 10% AHA application daily with pH greater than 3.0 Low pH with high AHA concentration in short exposure times (i.e., office peels)	Single exposure to high-concentration, unneutralized glycolic or lactic acid Repeated exposures to low AHA concentrations with pH less than 3.0 Repeated exposures to high AHA concentrations, pH greater than 3.0 but less than neutral

*Adapted from Van Scott EJ, Yu RJ: *J Geriatr Dermatol* 3(Suppl 3):19A-25A, 1995.

tion yields a smoother, less scaly surface.[1] Desquamation from follicular orifices cleanses the pores and prevents follicular occlusion. These superficial follicular effects are readily seen, thus making these products popular with those seeking a quick fix for mild aging of the skin. Patients note control of dry skin, ichthyosis, and acne, and a disappearance of solar lentigines.[1] Higher concentrations of some of these products effect not only diminished corneocyte cohesion but can cause complete epidermolysis (Box 33-1). This makes the higher concentration AHAs potentially useful for treating seborrheic keratoses, actinic keratoses, verrucae, and facial rhytides.[2]

With long-term use, the AHAs produce measurable dermal changes (Table 33-2). Some think that the increase in collagen, elastin, and glycosaminoglycan (GAG) synthesis in the dermis occurs due to regeneration of protein,[3] whereas others claim that the increase in protein synthesis is mediated by the functional activation of fibroblasts.[4,5] The increase in intercellular ground substances, namely, GAGs and especially hyaluronic acid, leads to increased dermal hydration and thickness.[6] AHAs also cause a decrease in oxidative damage after ultraviolet radiation.[7] As opposed to the topical retinoids, there is no increase in vasculature.[8] In addition, there is a reversal of the atrophic

■ **Table 33-3**   Effects of Preparations Applied Twice Daily on Ichthyosiform Dermatoses—Response of Selected Patients with Various Ichthyosis Subsets

Chemical	L1	L2	L3	L4	L5	L6	X1	X2	X3	IV1	IV2	EH1	U1	U2
Citric acid	Ex	VG	Ex	Ex	Ex	—	VG	Ex	Ex	Ex	Ex	Gd	—	—
Ethyl pyruvate	Ex	—	VG	Ex	VG	Ex	VG	Ex	Ex	Ex	Ex	No	Fr	—
Glycolic acid	Ex	VG	Ex	Ex	Ex	—	Ex	Ex	Ex	Ex	Ex	Fr	—	—
Glucuronic acid	Ex	—	VG	Ex	Gd	—	—	—	—	Ex	Ex	Gd	—	—
Lactic acid	Ex	—	Ex	Ex	Ex	VG	Ex	Ex	Ex	Ex	Ex	No	VG	—
Malic acid	VG	VG	VG	Ex	Ex	—	Ex	Ex	—	Ex	Ex	No	—	—
Pyruvic acid	Ex	—	Ex	Ex	Ex	Ex	Ex	Ex	Ex	Ex	Ex	Ex	Ex	Ex
Tartaric acid	Ex	—	Ex	Ex	VG	—	Gd	Ex	—	Ex	Ex	Fr	—	—
Tartonic acid	Ex	—	VG	Ex	Ex	—	—	—	—	Ex	Ex	No	—	—

Adapted from Van Scott EJ, Yu RJ: *Arch Dermatol* 110:586-590, 1974.
Note: Number following these ichthyoses represents patient number.
L, Lamellar ichthyosis; *X*, X-linked ichthyosis; *IV*, ichthyosis vulgaris; *EH*, epidermolytic hyperkeratosis; *U*, uncertain type; *Ex*, excellent with restoration to normal-looking skin; *VG*, very good with disappearance of scale from lesions; —, not done; *Gd*, good with substantial improvement of the lesions; *Fr*, fair with slight improvement over that provided by vehicle alone; *No*, no improvement.

changes on the epidermis that are associated with corticosteroid treatment.[9]

CLINICAL USE
Indications
XEROSIS AND ICHTHYOSIS. Ammonium lactate has been used for over two decades for dry skin therapy. This and other AHAs are useful as moisturizing agents. This effect is mediated by their bonding to molecules in the stratum corneum and making that layer more flexible and less susceptible to cracking. The use of occlusive materials in the base may also add to the hydration. Some formulations have small amounts of petrolatum in the lotions or creams for this reason. Leyden and colleagues[8] studied the effects of 12% ammonium lactate (Lac-Hydrin) on severely dry skin. Besides the expected reversal of abnormal hyperkeratosis in xerotic or ichthyotic skin, there were measurable changes in the epidermis and the dermis. There was a 20% increase in the viable epidermis thickness and a 50% increase in the dermal GAGs, particularly hyaluronic acid. These results have been confirmed by other investigators.[10] Because hyaluronic acid can bind water up to 10,000 times its weight, it

may cause significant clinical improvement in fine lines and wrinkles due to photoaging.

It was thought that thinning of the stratum corneum in normal skin may result in more skin sensitivity to potentially irritating chemicals. This is an important issue in treating patients with dry or eczematous skin, which can often have a tendency to be easily irritated or sensitive. However, with prolonged use, some formulations of AHA actually make the stratum corneum more resistant to potentially irritating substances such as detergents.[8] Takahashi and colleagues[11] reported that AHAs were more effective than β-hydroxy acids (such as salicylic acid) for skin plasticization (skin smoothing), and that the flexibility increased with increasing AHA chain length to 4 carbons.

Lactic acid, partially neutralized with ammonium hydroxide in 8% to 12% concentrations, is also indicated for treating severe cases of lamellar ichthyosis and X-linked ichthyosis.[12] As early as 1974, Van Scott demonstrated the effect of lactic and other AHAs in the improvement of epidermal keratinization in ichthyosis (Table 33-3). In particular, Van Scott reported a patient with lamellar ichthyosis in whom topical treatment three times daily for 4 days with

5% glycolic acid caused an "abrupt loss of the entire abnormal stratum corneum and a greatly diminished epidermal thickness."[1]

DERMATOHELIOSIS (PHOTOAGED SKIN).

A controlled study using 25% glycolic, lactic, or citric acid to the forearm for 6 months showed an approximately 25% increase in skin thickness. Both the epidermis and papillary dermis were thicker, with increased GAGs, increased collagen density, disbursement of melanin, and an increase in elastic fibers, without causing inflammation. These correlated with a reversal of the epidermal and dermal markers of photoaging.[4]

However, most available daily use AHAs contain much less than the above 25% concentration. There are many companies that market AHAs to the physician. The most common brands and their leading products are listed in Table 33-4. A study was designed to evaluate the cosmetic and histologic effects of a commercially available 5% and 12% lactic acid formulation. Treatment with 12% lactic acid resulted clinically in increased epidermal and dermal firmness and histologically in thickness along with clinical improvement in skin smoothness and a decrease in lines and wrinkles. In contrast, no dermal changes were observed with 5% lac-

■ **Table 33-4**   Common Alpha-Hydroxy Acid Formulations for Glycolic Acid

Pharmaceutical Company	Product Name and Labeled Acid Value	Free Acid Value (Bioavailability)
GLYCOLIC ACID PRODUCTS		
MD Formulations	MD Forte I facial cream 15%	4.68%
	MD Forte II facial cream 20%	5.76%
	MD Forte I facial lotion 15%	4.68%
	MD Forte II facial lotion 20%	6.84%
	MD Forte I body cream 20%	9%
Glytone	Day cream for dry skin 12%	9.70%
	Day cream for normal skin 10%	8.00%
	Day cream for oily skin 16%	14.00%
	Body lotion 20%	17.5%
	Ultra heel & elbow cream 30%	29.5%
Neostrata	AHA skin smoothing cream 8%	4.80%
	AHA Neo-15 face cream 15%	9.75%
	AHA skin smoothing lotion 10%	6.30%
	AHA Neo-15 face lotion 15%	8.5%
	AHA Neo-15 foot gel 15%	5.5%
Glyderm	Cream 5%	2.5%
	Cream Plus 10%	5.00%
	Cream Plus 12%	6.0%
	Lotion Lite 5%	2.5%
	Lotion Lite Plus	5.00%
	Lotion Plus 12%	6.00%
	Body lotion 10%	4.8%
MIXED PRODUCTS		
Therapeutics	AHA Revitalizing cream 8%	4.56%
	AHA Revitalizing cream HP 20%	13.00%
	AHA Revitalizing lotion 10%	6.4%
	AHA Revitalizing lotion HP 20%	12.8%

Adapted from Genesis Pharmaceuticals, Inc, Hazel Park, Minn.
Free acid value (FAV) is determined by applying both the pH of each product and the percentage of AHA in the product to and Henderson-Hasselbalch equation (per Van Scott).

tic acid; however, similar clinical and epidermal changes were seen.[13] Two of the most widely used AHAs, 8% glycolic acid and 12% lactic acid (L-isoform), were studied in the treatment of photodamaged skin on the face and the arms. Compared with vehicle cream alone, the glycolic acid preparation was significantly superior in improving the overall photodamage score and degree of sallowness. The L-lactic acid was much better than vehicle in reducing overall photodamage, sallowness, mottled pigmentation, and roughness on the forearms.[14] A controlled study of 20% citric acid lotion versus vehicle alone showed changes similar to those observed with the more commonly used glycolic or lactic acids. Biopsy specimens after 3 months of treatment showed increase in epidermal and dermal GAGs along with viable epidermal thickness.[15] High doses of lactic acid at 85% can be used to rapidly remove solar lentigines by causing epidermolysis within several minutes.[16] These concentrated products are not readily available.

The clinical improvement in photoaging from glycolic acids is well documented, but the reasons for these changes are not completely understood. One reason that has been suggested is that glycolic acid products produce a functional activation of fibroblasts. A recent study was designed to evaluate the effect of glycolic and malic acids on cultured dermal fibroblasts. Results showed an increase in cell proliferation and collagen production in response to glycolic acid in a dose-dependent manner but showed minimal change with malic acid or control.[17]

For deeper or faster remodeling, higher concentrations of glycolic acid can be applied in sequential peels. They usually range from 20% to 70% glycolic acid (Table 33-5). Various techniques are used, but all aim to increase either the concentration or duration of application with each treatment. A double-blind study examined the effect of unneutralized 50% glycolic acid on photoaged skin on the face, forearms, and hands. The peels were applied in gel form on one side for 5 minutes for a total of four applications. A control gel was applied to the contralateral side concomitantly. Statistically significant improvements were observed in rough texture, the number of solar keratoses, darkness of solar lentigines, and amount of fine wrinkling. On light microscopy, there was a 53% decrease in stratum corneum thickness and a 19% increase in overall epidermal thickness, with a 50% increase in the stratum granulosum. These changes were not seen in the control specimens. There was transient erythema, scaling, and irritant dermatitis postpeel, along with mild stinging on application of the acid.[18]

Glycolic acid peels can be administered in many ways. There are multiple products available in differing pH values and concentrations. It is important to always start on a low percentage of glycolic acid for a short amount of time and increase both parameters only as tolerated. Patients with oily skin are usually less reactive, whereas those with excessive sun-induced or environmental damage are more sensitive.

Peels should be tailored to the individual patient depending on condition, skin type, and tolerance. The patient should be watched carefully during each peel and should be encouraged to verbalize any discomfort. A hand-held fan is often given to the patient to decrease discomfort. A bicarbonate or water neutralizer is sometimes applied to the entire treated area at the

■ **Table 33-5**   Common Office Glycolic Acid Peel Regimens*

Regimen #1	Regimen #2
Month 1: 20% glycolic acid for 5 min	Month 1: 20% glycolic acid for 4 min
Month 2: 35% glycolic acid for 5 min	Month 2: 30% glycolic acid for 4 min
Month 3: 50% glycolic acid for 5 min	Month 3: 40% glycolic acid for 4 min
Month 4: 70% glycolic acid for 4 min	Month 4: 50% glycolic acid for 4 min
Month 5: 70% glycolic acid for 5 min	Month 5: 60% glycolic acid for 4 min
Month 6: 70% glycolic acid for 7 min	Month 6: 70% glycolic acid for 4 min

*Regimen based on experience and personal communications with many cosmetic dermatologists.

end of the peel. Immediately afterwards, an emollient cream is applied. The patient is instructed to avoid the sun, use the appropriate sunscreens, and not use any AHA- or retinoid-containing creams for 24 to 48 hours. Two of the most widely used peel regimens are outlined in Table 33-3. Variations on either regimen can be used, and patients are encouraged to repeat a previous treatment if they experienced excessive irritation or peeling.

Kligman[19] reported on the concomitant use of AHAs and tretinoin at different times of the day, in terms of compatibility and efficacy, compared with tretinoin alone at night. Furthermore, use of both agents provided greater benefit than tretinoin alone with regard to early signs of aging such as fine lines and dyspigmentation.[19] It is common practice to prescribe a tretinoin-based medication in the evening along with a glycolic acid product once or twice daily. The appropriate base should be chosen for the patient's skin condition. Because most aging skin is often dry, an emollient-based cream is usually preferred. All patients are started on a low concentration of AHA, such as 5%, which is increased to 10% when tolerated. Patients are instructed to use a broad-spectrum sunscreen in the morning as part of their daily regimen. The superficial peels are often recommended on a monthly basis as described. They have earned the title "lunchtime peels" because they can be performed during a quick break from work and the patient can return to work without any signs of the "escapade."

NAIL DISORDERS. The AHAs can also be used to reverse the changes seen in brittle, aged nails. These include longitudinal ridging, splitting, and delamination of the nail plate. Application of 8% glycolic acid or 12% lactic acid 3 to 4 times daily was helpful in reversing these processes.[8]

ACNE VULGARIS AND RELATED CONDITIONS. Aside from an increase in *Propionibacterium acnes* and excessive sebum production, the third pathophysiologic cause of acne is the abnormal desquamation of the sebaceous epithelium in the pilosebaceous unit.

Because of their unique effect on the stratum corneum, the AHAs can produce superfi-

cial and controlled desquamation, making them useful in the treatment of acne. The corneocyte cohesion is diminished, normalizing follicular keratinization. Low concentrations of glycolic acid (5% to 10%) can be applied once or twice daily as a home regimen. In the office setting, higher concentrations of AHA, usually 35% to 70%, can be administered for short exposure times, creating a superficial chemical peel. These can augment the healing response by causing subcorneal epidermolysis, opening of comedones, and unroofing of pustules.[20]

In 1989, Van Scott and Yu[2] reported on the use of topical applications of 70% glycolic acid alone as a treatment for acne in 28 patients. The duration of exposure of the skin to the acid solutions was "gauged to provoke minimal erythema," which was claimed to fade after a few hours and was sometimes followed by mild desquamation for a few days. The authors concluded that this treatment leads to a precipitous improvement of acne, adding a "distinct benefit to the standard acne treatment regimens."[2] However, this solitary regimen has been disputed by other authors. Kligman,[21] for instance, believes the consensus that glycolic acid as a single therapy for acne is less effective than tretinoin. However, he concedes that it has a synergistic effect when combined with tretinoin—an opinion also shared by Elson,[22] who reported a synergistic behavior with topical tretinoin and glycolic acids in the treatment of acne vulgaris without significant problems with irritancy.

A treatment plan commonly used by dermatologists for acne vulgaris is to prescribe a tretinoin nightly, along with an appropriate AHA for the morning. Patients with acne and increased oil production are most likely to be given glycolic acid in an alcohol solution or water-based lotion as a base. The superficial peels are often added to the regimen on a monthly basis.

Glycolic acid is also reported to be effective in treating pseudofolliculitis barbae, with an 8% lotion resulting in a reduction of lesions with little irritation.[23]

ROSACEA. Briden and colleagues[24] report on patients with chronic acne rosacea recalcitrant to conventional therapies. Glycolic acid peels were added to their regimen, resulting in a dramatic decrease in the inflammatory process. There was a marked reduction in the papules, pustules, and erythematous components.[24] The etiology of rosacea is unclear, but theories include hypersensitivity to *Demodex folliculorum* or an underlying vascular disorder.[25] Topical retinoids have been used for rosacea, but they can produce excessive irritation and can exacerbate the telangiectatic component. AHAs, however, do not promote angiogenesis.[4] AHAs may prevent attachment of the *Demodex* mite in the follicle through their effect on corneocyte adhesion. In addition, the low pH of the glycolic acids may deplete bacterial nutrients and therefore reduce the presence of viable pathogens. Glycolic acids are used on a daily basis and, as in office peels, similar to that described for acne vulgaris.

MELASMA.   Glycolic acid may be used in combination with other bleaching agents, such as hydroquinones, for the amelioration of melasma, probably promoting normal epidermal cell growth and down regulating melanocyte activity.[26] In addition, the glycolic acid may enhance the penetration of the hydroquinone, yielding a better response. Glycolic acid peels are effective and safe in medium- to dark-skinned individuals. The concentration of glycolic acid and the peeling time must be increased with caution in these darker skin types. Risks include more chemical irritancy, and possible postinflammatory hyperpigmentation. Peels should be initiated at 20% glycolic acid for 2 minutes and increased as tolerated.[27]

ACTINIC KERATOSES.   In 1995, the status of AHAs in the treatment of actinic keratoses was still investigational according to the guidelines of the American Academy of Dermatology.[28] However, in 1997, the use of chemical peels utilizing AHAs became acceptable by the Academy as a method of destruction of actinic keratoses.[29]

Formulations

Dermatologists are formulating or dispensing AHA-containing products through their offices in increasing amounts. Pharmaceutical companies and major cosmetic lines are incorporating AHAs into their products. These include cleansers, shampoos, toners, cuticle softeners, lotions, creams, gels, masks, sprays, peeling agents, and sunscreens. These products range from less than 1% in skin fresheners to 20% AHA (usually glycolic acid) in creams and lotions and as peeling agents used in physicians' offices at concentrations of AHA from 20% to 70%.

BIOAVAILABILITY.   The topical efficacy of an AHA formulation depends on the bioavailable concentration and the vehicle used.[30] The bioavailability depends on the fraction of free AHA present in the formulation. Many of the current products on the market claim to be neutralized or buffered to create less irritation. These terms are not synonymous. AHAs can be neutralized with an inorganic alkali or organic base (sodium hydroxide or ammonium hydroxide) to raise the pH. The closer the pH is to neutral, the less irritation to the skin. This principle was utilized by Westwood-Squibb Pharmaceuticals in developing Lac-Hydrin lotion, which contains 12% ammonium lactate. The AHAs can also be buffered to create a compound that resists pH changes when an acid or alkali is added. For example, glycolic acid can be buffered with sodium glycolate and monosodium phosphate to maintain a pH between 2.8 and 4.8. These manipulations, however, decrease the free acid levels.

Many currently available AHA preparations are partially neutralized. A base has been added to the glycolic acid, which allows for formation of ammonium glycolate salt, resulting in a higher pH and lower free acid levels. AHAs in free acid form are bioavailable, but the metallic salt dissociates into the AHA ion and the metallic ion. These ions cannot permeate the stratum corneum of intact human skin nearly as well as the free acid form. Because it is assumed that free acid concentration in the preparation produces the antiphotoaging effect, one would expect a partially neutralized product to be less effective. The glycolic acid dissociates into the glycolate ion and the hydrogen ion, whereas the lactic acid becomes a lactate ion and hydrogen ion mix.[25] Interestingly, both clinical and in vitro studies show partially neutralized glycolic acid and other AHA preparations to be somewhat beneficial with regard to skin rejuvenation or remodeling. Some studies show that higher concentrations of AHAs work better than lower concentrations.[13,31,32] However, those products that are partially neutralized to maintain a higher pH (approaching 4.4) have been shown to be better moisturizers by maintaining a higher water content in the skin.[13]

The bioavailability of AHAs at room temperature (25° C) can be calculated from both the pH of the preparation and the concentration of the AHA. In most circumstances, this can be plugged into the Henderson-Hasselbalch equation and the free acid value and bioavailability can be determined. This becomes extremely important for the clinician in the real world. If a specific brand of AHA claims to have 10% AHA, many physicians and patients believe that the product delivers nearly that amount. They strive to use a stronger concentration in the future. However, changing brands may completely throw the best laid plans off track. Comparing two major brands of glycolic acid, one 15% formula yields less than 5% free acid, whereas in the other, a 10% preparation, actually has 8% free acid (see Table 33-3). When switching to another brand of AHA it is important to compare free acid values. Patients often feel they are doing more for their skin if they use an AHA with a high concentration on the label. What is written on the bottle is definitely not what the patient is getting. Most companies label only the AHA concentration before neutralization. Patient education regarding what the numbers really mean and a chart of free acid values are often helpful.

VEHICLE ISSUES.   The vehicle used for formulation also plays a role in absorption.[30] For example, because glycolic acid is water-soluble, most glycolic acid in the water phase is in direct contact with the stratum corneum when topically applied. Certain components may interfere with or enhance these pharmacologic effects. Glycerin has a strong affinity for the AHAs, and because glycerin cannot substantially penetrate the stratum corneum, it decreases the AHA absorption. In contrast, propylene glycol can enhance the penetration of AHA by modifying the permeability of the stratum corneum.[33]

There is clearly an inverse relationship between the pH of AHA preparations and their potential for skin irritation. The concentration of AHA seems to be independent of irritation when the pH is constant. As the pH is lowered, the potential for irritation is increased. A 10% glycolic acid–based product was tested at six pH levels ranging from 2.0 to 4.4. In addition, identical 10%, 15%, and 20% glycolic acid preparations at pH 3.0 were tested in the same manner. Subjects were patch-tested on the back to each of these products. Results showed that regardless of glycolic concentration (from 10% to 20%), irritation did not change as long as the pH was maintained. The group of preparations with varying pH showed that the lower the pH, the higher the irritation. As the pH increased nearer to neutrality at 4.4, the cutaneous irritation dropped off markedly.[34]

With regard to the stimulation of collagen and GAGs for dermal thickening and removal of rhytides, varying the concentration of AHA at a standard pH of 3.8 gave different results. Even though a 20% concentration of AHA resulted in more collagen production, a 5%, 10%, and 15% concentration still resulted in a significant amount of collagen deposition. All concentrations increase collagen deposition; however, higher percentages give more significant amounts of new collagen deposition. There are more superficial changes, with thinning of the stratum corneum and thickening of the epidermis, when patients are treated with a high pH product such as 3.8. However, when the pH is pushed higher to 4.4, the effects on the stratum corneum decline. A pH of 3.8 seems to be a threshold above which skin irritation potential begins to decrease markedly.[35]

PRESCRIPTION   VERSUS   OVER-THE-COUNTER STATUS.   Most AHAs are available without prescription; one such product is Am-Lactin (12% ammonium lactate). In contrast, Lac-Hydrin 12% lotion and cream are available only by prescription. Stronger concentrations, such as the 20% glycolic acid (Glytone) body lotion, can be obtained only through a physician's office. The FDA has received adverse reaction reports regarding AHAs, including redness, swelling, burning, itching, blistering, and skin discoloration. However, in spite of the wide use of various AHA products, the number of complaints is relatively small. Larger molecular weight (MW) chemically synthesized AHAs tend to remain on the skin surface longer, producing more of an epidermal effect. The stratum corneum resists penetration of the higher MW AHAs such as citric, gluconic, and mandelic acids.[30] This also eliminates some of the stinging and burning associated with the smaller MW AHAs such as glycolic acid. Therefore some cosmetic companies are using larger AHA molecules in their sensitive skin products.

COSMECEUTICAL USES

AHAs bridge the gap from cosmetics, which are formulated to deliver an aesthetic effect, to products that are made to deliver a pharmacologic effect on the structure and function of the skin. Many contend that by altering the physiologic processes of the skin, the AHAs should be classified as drugs. The term *cosmeceutical* was introduced to better define a product that combines the beneficial effects of a cosmetic product with those of a pharmaceutical agent. It is very difficult to delineate the difference between the pharmacologic and cosmetic uses of AHAs because of the wide variety in formulations and differing effects. Many dermatologists feel that the benefits of low concentrations of AHAs are focused on the superficial layers of the skin and therefore could easily be classified as cosmetic.[32] A preparation with a free acid concentration under 10% is considered to be relatively low. However, the FDA adamantly responds that it does not officially recognize a hybrid category such as cosmeceutical. Cosmetics do not require premarket approval for both safety and efficacy as necessitated with drugs. Therefore there is concern that these products may be marketed freely as cosmetics but may truly be functioning as drugs.[36,37]

The Cosmetic Ingredient Review (CIR) panel was given the task of analyzing the data available on the AHAs. It was predicted that there would be a recommendation of a three-tiered system; home, professional, and medical uses. On June 24, 1997 the Cosmetic, Fragrance and Toiletry Association (CFTA) and the FDA Office of Cosmetics met in Washington, DC to formally present the CIR panel findings. They reaffirmed the safety of glycolic and lactic acids in retail formulations at a concentration of 10% or less with a pH of 3.5 or higher. It was shown

conclusively that more rapid absorption and subsequent irritation occurred at lower pH levels.[38] Professional products formulated at a concentration of 30% or less with a pH of 3.0 or higher were approved as long as each is accompanied with instructions for daily use of an adequate sunscreen. This sunscreen should protect against any potential increase in sun sensitivity from the AHA products. Formulations containing stronger concentrations of AHA (over 30%) or with a lower pH than these thresholds would be recommended only for medical use supervised by a physician. It was felt that additional studies were needed to answer two safety concerns. First, there is concern whether the use of AHAs makes the user more sensitive to sunlight and, consequently, more at risk for photodamage and photocarcinogenicity. Secondly, the chemical irritation over a long period of time may cause chronic irritation and potential adverse effects.

ADVERSE EFFECTS

The most common adverse effect is an irritant contact dermatitis. This problem can generally be managed by decreasing the AHA concentration, altering the application schedule, or increasing the pH of the product. After a superficial peel, most patients experience mild erythema with burning or stinging for several minutes to hours.[39] If the reaction is more severe or prolonged with scaling, crusting, or blistering, a topical corticosteroid can be helpful. Rarely, hyperpigmentation or hypopigmentation may result with a deeper peel, which can necessitate additional treatment. Pigmentary problems are more often encountered in dark-skinned patients.[40]

Very rarely, a herpes infection can be triggered with a glycolic acid peel due to the fact that the peel is an acid burn on the face. Thus prophylactic acyclovir (Zovirax) or similar antiviral medications might be warranted in patients prone to such outbreaks.[41]

There is conflicting evidence regarding the AHAs and photosensitivity. The short-term effects of the dermal application of glycolic acid on the sensitivity of skin to ultraviolet B (UVB) light were determined by assessing the effect on sunburn cell (SBC) production. Ten percent glycolic acid with a pH of 3.5 was compared with vehicle cream. Each site was exposed to one minimal erythema dose (MED) of UVB, and the number of SBC was determined from biopsy specimens 24 hours postirradiation. The glycolic acid formula did not increase the amount of SBC compared with control.[42]

Another study, using the same design, evaluated the effect of 10% glycolic acid, with pH of 3.5 and 4.0, after 12-week application. Both glycolic acid products resulted in a statistically increased number of SBC as compared with untreated or moisturized skin. Others added methoxycinnamate with an SPF of 3 to 4 to 8% glycolic acid mixtures. With a similar study protocol as above, there was no increase in SBC in the glycolic acid–treated sites after direct irradiation.[43] A large study using 8% glycolic acid or lactic acid at a pH of 3.8 examined patients after 22 weeks during normal incidental sun exposure. There was no increase in SBC in any of the treated sites.[44] More UV is transmitted through normally moisturized skin than through dry skin because dry skin scatters or reflects ultraviolet radiation. Typical cosmetic moisturizers decrease the MED approximately 5% to 7.5%.[45]

Perricone and associates evaluated areas of skin pretreated with daily application of glycolic acid, with and without superimposed peels, versus untreated skin. An SPF of 2.4 was achieved by pretreating the skin with glycolic acid prior to UVB. The addition of glycolic acid peels reduced the sun-protection factor (SPF) by 50%, but the SPF was still 1.7 compared with untreated skin. It was determined that pretreatment with glycolic acid increased the skin's natural protection from UVB and minimized the additional UVB damage before chemical peeling.[46]

With their diverse properties and adaptability to many clinical scenarios, it is no wonder the AHAs became one of the most popular classes of dermatologic agents of the last few years. Interestingly, however, although they are often touted as a beneficial treatment for a host of skin conditions, some of the data supporting this generalization are conflicting. The clinician needs to use sound medical judgment when determining whether the AHAs are appropriate for individual patients. It is probably accurate to say that the full story on AHAs in clinical practice is not yet in. It remains to be seen whether this category of dermatologic agents will be an increasingly important tool in the dermatologic armamentarium of the new millennium.

Bibliography

Bergfeld W: Improving the cosmetic appearance of photoaged skin with glycolic acid. *J Am Acad Dermatol* 36:1011-1013, 1997.

Ditre CM: Effects of alpha-hydroxy acids on photoaged skin: a pilot clinical, histologic, and ultrastructural study. *J Am Acad Dermatol* 34:187-195, 1996.

Kempers S: An evaluation of the effect of an alpha hydroxy acid-blend skin cream in the cosmetic improvement of symptoms of moderate to severe xerosis, epidermolytic hyperkeratosis, and ichthyosis. *Cutis* 61:347-350, 1998.

Kneedler JA: Understanding alpha-hydroxy acids. *Dermatol Nurs* 10:247-254, 259-262, 1998.

Lewis AB: Resurfacing with topical agents. *Semin Cutan Med Surg* 15:139-144, 1996.

Smith WP: Epidermal and dermal effects of topical lactic acid. *J Am Acad Dermatol* 35:388-391, 1996.

Vidt DG: Cosmetic use of alpha-hydroxy acids. *Cleve Clin J Med* 64:327-329, 1997.

References

Pharmacology

1. Van Scott EJ, Yu RJ: Control of keratinization with the alpha hydroxy acids and related compounds. *Arch Dermatol* 110:586-590, 1974.
2. Van Scott EJ, Yu RJ: Alpha hydroxy acids. Procedures for use in clinical practice. *Cutis* 43:222-228, 1989.
3. Lewis AB: Resurfacing with topical agents. *Semin Cutan Med Surg* 15:139-144, 1996.
4. Ditre CM: Effects of alpha-hydroxy acids on photoaged skin: a pilot clinical, histologic, and ultrastructural study. *J Am Acad Dermatol* 34:187-195, 1996.
5. Kim SJ, Park JH, Kim DH, et al: Increased in vivo collagen synthesis and in vitro cell proliferative effect of glycolic acid. *Dermatol Surg* 24:1054-1058, 1998.
6. Van Scott EJ, Yu RJ: Actions of alpha hydroxy acids on skin compartments. *J Ger Dermatol* 3(Suppl 3):19A-25A, 1995.
7. Perricone NV: An alpha hydroxy acid acts as an antioxidant. *J Ger Dermatol* 1:101-104, 1993.
8. Leyden J, Lavker RM, Groove G, et al: Alpha hydroxy acids are more than moisturizers. *J Ger Dermatol* 3(Suppl 3):33A-37A, 1995.
9. Lanker RM, Kaidby K, Leyden J: Effects of topical ammonium lactate on cutaneous atrophy from a potent topical steroid. *J Am Acad Dermatol* 26:535-544, 1992.

Clinical Use

10. Bernstein EF, Uitto J: Connective tissue alterations in photodamaged skin and the effects of alpha hydroxy acids. *J Ger Dermatol* Suppl A(3):7A-18A, 1995.
11. Takahashi M, Machida Y, Tsuda Y: The influence of hydroxy acids on the rheological properties of the stratum corneum. *J Soc Cosmet Chem* 36:177-187, 1985.
12. Van Scott EJ, Yu RJ: Hyperkeratinization, corneocyte adhesion, and hydroxy acids. *J Am Acad Dermatol* 111:867-879, 1984.
13. Smith WP: Epidermal and dermal effects of topical lactic acid. *J Am Acad Dermatol* 35:388-391, 1996.
14. Stiller MJ, Bartolone J, Stern R, et al: Topical 8% glycolic acid and 12% L-lactic acid creams for the treatment of photodamaged skin. A double blind vehicle-controlled clinical trial. *Arch Dermatol* 132:631-636, 1996.
15. Bernstein EF, Underhill CB, Lakkaakorpi J, et al: Citric acid increases viable epidermal thickness and glycosaminoglycan content of sun-damaged skin. *Dermatol Surg* 23:689-694, 1997.
16. Van Scott EJ, Yu RJ: Alpha hydroxy acids. Therapeutic potentials. *Can J Dermatol* 1:108-112, 1989.
17. Kim SJ, Won YH: The effect of glycolic acid on cultured human skin fibroblasts: cell proliferative effect and increased collagen synthesis. *J Dermatol* 25:85-89, 1998.
18. Newman N, Newman A, Moy LS, et al: Clinical improvement of photodamaged skin with 50% glycolic acid. A double blind vehicle-controlled study. *Dermatol Surg* 22:455-460, 1996.
19. Kligman AM: The compatibility of combinations of glycolic acid and tretinoin in acne and in photoaged skin. *J Ger Dermatol* 3(Suppl A):25A-28A, 1995.
20. Briden ME, Cacatua LS, Patriots MA, et al: Treatment of acne with glycolic acid. *J Ger Dermatol* 4(SB):22B-27B, 1996.
21. Kligman A: Result of a pilot study evaluating the compatibility of topical tretinoin in combination with glycolic acid. *Cosmet Dermatol* 6:28-32, 1993.
22. Elson ML: Differential effects of glycolic acid and tretinoin in acne vulgaris. *Cosmet Dermatol* 5:36-40, 1992.
23. Perricone NV: Treatment of pseudofolliculitis barbae with topical glycolic acid: A report of two studies. *Cutis* 52:232-235, 1993.
24. Briden ME, Rent-Pellerano MI: Treatment of rosacea with glycolic acid. *J Ger Dermatol* 4(SB):17B-21B, 1996.
25. Wilken J: Rosacea: pathophysiology and treatment. *Arch Dermatol* 130:359-362, 1987.
26. Dial WF: Use of AHAs add new dimensions to chemical peeling. *Cosmet Dermatol* 3:32-34, 1990.
27. Kakita LS, Petratos MA: The use of glycolic acid in Asian and darker skin types. *J Ger Dermatol* 4(SB):8B-11B, 1996.
28. Report of the Committee on Guidelines of care. *J Am Acad Dermatol* 32:95-98, 1995.
29. Callen JP, Bickers DR, Moy RL: From the Academy. *J Am Acad Dermatol* 36:650-653, 1997.

Formulations—Cosmeceutical Uses

30. Yu EJ, Van Scott EJ: Bioavailability of alpha-hydroxy acids in topical formulations. *Cosmet Dermatol* 9:954-962, 1996.
31. Meszaros L, editor: What to consider when choosing an alpha-hydroxy acid. *Dermatol Times*, January:34, 1996.
32. Rubin M: pH is an important element in determining the safety and efficacy of AHAs. *Cosmet Dermatol* 9(Suppl 5):14-15, 1996
33. Smith WP: Comparative effectiveness of α-hydroxy acids on skin properties. *Intl J Cosmet Sci* 18:75-83, 1996.
34. Scientific Literature Review: On glycolic and lactic acids, their common salts, and their simple esters. Final Report. April 7, 1995. Cosmetic Ingredient Review. Wash, D.C.
35. Dinardo JC: Studies show cumulative irritation potential based on pH. *Cosmet Dermatol* 9(Suppl 5):12-13, 1996.
36. Schwartz RM: Why AHAs have FDA's attention. *Cosmet Dermatol* 7:40-42, 1994.
37. McEwen G, Milstein SR: The safety and beneficial effects of AHAs. *Cosmet Dermatol* 9(Suppl 5):19, 1996.
38. Schwartz RM: News and information from our nation's capital. *Cosmet Dermatol* 10:18-20, 22, 1997.

Adverse Effects

39. Piacquadio D, Dobry J, Hunt S, et al: Short contact 70% glycolic acid peels as a treatment for photodamaged skin: a pilot study. *Dermatol Surg* 22:449-452, 1996.

40. Scheinberg RS: Alpha-hydroxy acids for skin rejuvenation. *West J Med* 160:366-367, 1994.
41. Rubin MG: *Manual of chemical peels superficial and medium depth*, Philadelphia, 1995, Lippincott Williams & Wilkins.
42. KGL, Inc. (1996a): An investigation of the short-term effects of topical treatments on the sensitivity of human skin to UVR. KGL Protocol #3800. Final report dated Dec 11. Unpublished data submitted by CTFA, 34 pp.
43. KGL, Inc. (1996b): A study to investigate the effects of several topical treatments on the sensitivity of human skin to UVR. Protocol #3813. Final report dated Dec 11. Unpublished data submitted by CTFA, 42 pp.
44. Unilever research U.S. (1996): A double-blind, vehicle controlled, randomized study to evaluate the efficacy and safety of 8% L-Lactic Acid and 8% Glycolic acid in the cosmetic improvement of the signs of photo-damaged skin. (URUS-93-MG-1) Part 7: Evaluation of sunburn cell formation. Unpublished data submitted by CTFA, 21 pp.
45. TKL Research (1995): Effect of emollients on the minimal erythema dose (MED) response. Unpublished data submitted by industry, 8 pp.
46. Perricone NV, DiNardo JC: Photoprotective and anti-inflammatory effects of topical glycolic acid. *Dermatol Surg* 22:435-437, 1996.

Adam B. Hessel
Julio C. Cruz-Ramon
Andrew N. Lin

Agents Used for Treatment of Hyperkeratosis

Substances used to treat hyperkeratosis are frequently referred to as *keratolytic* agents. These agents significantly decrease the clinical extent of hyperkeratosis. However, some of these keratolytic agents may not be truly "lysing" keratin at the molecular level. In this chapter, the most commonly used topical agents to treat hyperkeratosis are reviewed (Box 34-1). See Chapter 33 for a complete discussion of alpha-hydroxy acids such as lactic acid and glycolic acid.

SALICYLIC ACID

For over 2000 years, salicylic acid has been used as a topical agent to treat skin disorders.[1] Willow bark, which contains salicylic acid, was used to treat corns and calluses by Pliny in the first century AD Leerovx, in 1829, isolated salicylic acid from willow bark. In the 1860s, with the newfound chemical synthesis of salicylic acid, the ability of salicylic acid to soften and exfoliate the stratum corneum was discovered.[2]

Pharmacology
CHEMISTRY. Figure 34-1 lists agents for the treatment of hyperkeratosis. Salicylic acid, also known as 2-hydroxybenzoic acid or orthohydrobenzoic acid, is a white, crystalline powder. Salicylic acid and salicylates (which are easily converted to salicylic acid) are present in willow bark, wintergreen leaves, and sweet birch. Salicylic acid can be synthesized as well.[1,3]

Whereas salicylic acid has been described as a beta-hydroxy acid by Kligman,[4] Yu and Van Scott classify salicylic acid as a phenolic aromatic acid.[5] Yu and Van Scott refute the concept of salicylic acid being a beta-hydroxy acid because, unlike a true beta-hydroxy acid, salicylic acid has both the hydroxyl and the carboxyl groups directly attached to an aromatic benzene ring. In addition, unlike true beta-hydroxy acids, the hydroxyl group of salicylic acid exhibits acid properties. The hydroxyl group of true β-hydroxy acids is neutral and not acidic.

In contrast to the alpha-hydroxy acids (such as lactic acid and glycolic acid), salicylic acid is lipid-soluble and therefore is miscible with epidermal lipids and sebaceous gland lipids in hair follicles. Thus salicylic acid can interact with the lipids that surround keratinized cells. Salicylic acid is able to interact with multilamellar structures surrounding keratinocytes in the stratum corneum and in hair follicles. In addition, due

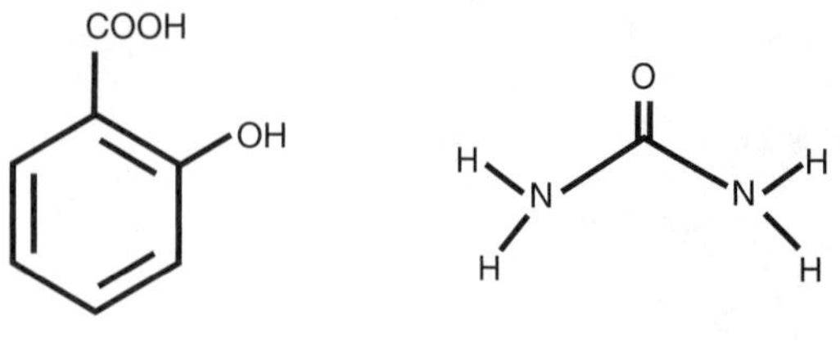

Figure 34-1 Agents used for treatment of hyperkeratosis.

Box 34-1

Agents Used for Treatment of Hyperkeratosis

Salicylic acid	Tar
Sulfur	Urea

to the greater lipophilic qualities (as compared with alpha-hydroxy acids), the clinical effect of salicylic acid may be limited to the superficial epidermis. In contrast, the alpha-hydroxy acids may penetrate deeper into the epidermis and probably the dermis.[3]

Salicylic acid has a pKa of 2.98. To obtain a significant exfoliative effect, salicylic acid must be formulated at a proper pH to allow enough free acid to be present compared with the salt form of this drug. Thus various formulations with concentrations of salicylic acid at a pH close to the pKa give significantly more exfoliation than formulations at any pH significantly greater than the pKa.[6]

MECHANISM OF ACTION.   The mechanism of salicylic acid as a keratolytic and comedolytic agent is not exactly known.[7] Proposed mechanisms include reduction of corneocyte adhesion,[8] solubilizing effect on intercellular cement,[9] and loosening and detachment of corneocytes. Human upper arm skin stratum corneum treated with 2% salicylic acid is significantly more easily removed by tape stripping than control sites treated with only the vehicle.[11] The increased removal of scale from human skin may be due to reduced cohesion between corneocytes. Al-

though salicylic acid appears to have no effect on the mitotic activity of the normal human epidermis,[8] studies of pathologic epithelial proliferation in guinea pigs demonstrated a reduction in hyperplasia in viable keratinocyte.[12] Salicylic acid causes an irregular and thinner stratum corneum without altering epidermal thickness.[11]

Salicylic acid and its derivatives can be used as sunscreens.[13,14] The mechanism of the sunscreen effect is due to the benzene ring's transformation of ultraviolet radiation (UVR) into longer wave radiation that is emitted from the skin as heat.[15]

Salicylates are also known to possess antiinflammatory properties. Acetylsalicylic acid, commonly known as aspirin, is well known as an analgesic, antipyretic, and antiinflammatory agent. Acetylsalicylic acid inhibits prostaglandin biosynthesis.[16] Salicylic acid shares some of the antiinflammatory effects of acetylsalicylic acid.[17] The antiinflammatory effect of salicylic acid is most pronounced at concentrations between 0.5% and 5% (w/w).[7]

Clinical Use

INDICATIONS.   Box 34-2 lists clinical uses for salicylic acid. Salicylic acid is found in numerous topical preparations. Many of these preparations do not require a prescription.[18] Salicylic acid is present in a wide variety of wart and callus topical treatments and is often compounded with other keratolytic agents such as lactic acid. Salicylic acid, 2% to 20%, is available in collodion-based paints and gels,[18] which dry and form a film from which salicylic acid is absorbed into the skin. In higher concentrations (10% to 50%), salicylic acid is used as a plaster that can be cut to fit a wart, corn, or callus.[18] Many shampoos contain 2% salicylic acid, often with tar and sulfur[1] (see Chapter 32). These shampoos are useful in treating psoriasis, seborrheic dermatitis, and cradle cap of the scalp.[7] Salicylic acid in ointments and oils, which are usually applied under occlusion, is a useful treatment for thick plaques of scalp psoriasis.[19]

A proprietary compound (Keralyt gel) 6% salicylic acid, 60% propylene glycol, and 20% ethanol, formulated as a gel, is useful in removing thick scales of ichthyosis vulgaris, sex-linked ichthyosis, lamellar ichthyosis, and epidermolytic hyperkeratosis, especially under occlu-

Box 34-2

Salicylic Acid Clinical Uses

HYPERKERATOTIC DISORDERS
Calluses
Corns
Ichthyosis
Keratoderma
Hyperkeratosis

COSMETIC/AESTHETIC USES
Hyperpigmentation
Rejuvenation/Peeling

PAPULOSQUAMOUS DERMATOSES
Psoriasis

CUTANEOUS INFECTIONS
Dermatophyte infections
Verruca

DERMATITIS
Seborrheic dermatitis
Cradle cap

OTHER USES
Acne
Photoprotection (salicylates)

sion.[20] This gel is also useful in plantar keratoderma climactericum, hyperkeratosis palmaris and plantaris of Unna, pityriasis rubra pilaris, and psoriasis. The keratolytic effect of this gel has been credited with clearing three patients with *Trichophyton rubrum* infection of the sole.[20] Whitfield's ointment, a time honored remedy for tinea infection, contains 6% salicylic acid and 12% benzoic acid in wool fat and petrolatum.[1,7] The concentrations of salicylic and benzoic acids can be used at half-strength to reduce irritation. Whitfield's ointment has been largely replaced by more effective and elegant preparations. A compound of 10% salicylic acid and 20% urea has been useful as a means of avulsing toenails nonsurgically.[21] Salicylic acid is believed to have a mild comedolytic effect and is thus used in acne preparations, including creams, liquid cleansers, astringents, medicated pads, and bar soaps.[22] Salicylic acid is added into topical preparations containing an-

thralin to prevent its oxidation.[23] The original Lassar's paste contained 2% salicylic acid, 24% zinc oxide, 24% starch, and 50% white soft paraffin.[7] Compounds duplicating the formulation of the original Lassar's paste should always be freshly prepared because, on standing, the ingredients combine to form zinc salicylate.[24] Modern formulations of Lassar's paste do not contain salicylic acid due to the interaction of salicylic acid and zinc oxide.[25]

Salicylic acid and related salicylates can be used as sunscreen ingredients (see Chapter 31). Salicylates absorb ultraviolet B (UVB) in the range of 300 to 310 nm.[14] Topical salicylic acid, which is frequently used in psoriasis, can interfere with UVB phototherapy for psoriasis.[26] Octyl salicylate (2-ethyl hexyl salicylate) and homomenthyl salicylate are used as sunscreen agents in many cosmetic products.[14] Salicylic acid cannot be incorporated into vanishing creams because salicylic acid "cracks" the cream by decomposing the soap that is needed to form the appropriate emulsion.[26] Although in vitro data suggest that salicylic acid enhances absorption of topical corticosteroids, this was not confirmed by in vivo studies in animals[27] and human subjects.[28] However, a study comparing the efficacy of mometasone furoate 0.1% combined with salicylic acid 5% in an ointment versus a stronger corticosteroid, fluocinonide 0.05% ointment, in the treatment of psoriasis showed that the mometasone furoate–salicylic acid was more effective.[29]

Salicylic acid is used in antipruritic formulations at a concentration of 1% to 2%.[7] Choline salicylate is used as a topical anesthetic for aphthous ulcers.[30] Methyl salicylate, found in oil of wintergreen, is used for topical musculoskeletal symptomatic pain relief.[31]

Salicylic acid has been used as a peeling agent.[32,33] Jessner's solution, which consists of 14% salicylic acid, 14% resorcinol, and 14% lactic acid, has been used as a superficial peeling agent. More recently, salicylic acid in concentrations of 20% to 30% in a hydroethanolic vehicle (5% water) gained popularity as a superficial chemical peeling agent for the treatment of acne, photodamage, and hyperpigmentation.[32,33]

A 50% salicylic acid ointment has been used to treat severely photodamaged hands and forearms.[34] At lower concentrations, 1% to 2%, salicylic acid is used as an exfoliant to increase corneocyte shedding and improve the appearance of aged skin.[35] In a controlled study, a 1.5% to 2% salicylic acid proprietary formulation in a moisturizing vehicle resulted in greater improved facial skin appearance, exfoliation of follicular contents, and increased stratum corneum turnover compared with a bland moisturizer and glycolic acid formulations.[36]

ADVERSE EFFECTS. When topically applied to the skin, salicylic acid is readily absorbed.[37] If salicylic acid is applied onto erythrodermic skin, it can be detected in the urine in 24 hours.[38] Percutaneous absorption of salicylic acid is enhanced by incorporation into a hydrophilic ointment,[39] tape stripping of the stratum corneum,[40] or application under occlusion.[41]

Systemic toxicity from percutaneous absorption of salicylic acid is a rare but potentially serious event (Box 34-3). Salicylates in high concentrations are toxic to the central nervous system. Clinical manifestations of salicylate toxicity include nausea, vomiting, confusion, dizziness, delirium, psychosis, stupor, coma, and death.[37,42] Tinnitus due to salicylate toxicity is caused by increased labyrinthine pressure and effects on cochlear hair cells, perhaps secondary to vasoconstriction in the auditory microvasculature.[37] With salicylate toxicity there is stimulation of the medullary respiratory center that causes marked hyperventilation and respiratory alkalosis; in infants and children, metabolic acidosis may also occur.[37] Signs of salicylate toxicity generally occur when blood concentrations exceed 35 mg/dl.

In a recent review of the English literature, 32 cases of salicylate toxicity from topical application were found.[1] Most of the patients were being treated for psoriasis and ichthyosis. Symptoms of salicylate toxicity appeared early in the course of treatment, frequently within 2 to 3 days of initiating therapy. Topical application of salicylic acid with concentrations as low as 3%, applied three times daily for 5 days to the entire skin below the neck in an adult, resulted in toxicity.[43] In one case of salicylate-induced tinnitus, naproxen was proposed to increase unbound (free) serum salicylic acid by competing for protein binding and hepatic metabolism.[37] In two patients, death occurred with topical application of 20.7% salicylic acid to "over 50%" of the body.[42] These patients had symptoms of salicylism, although blood salicylate levels were not reported.

In addition, salicylates affect glucose utilization. This can lead to hypoglycemia, especially in patients with uremia, in whom there is reduced protein binding of salicylates.[44]

Salicylic acid is considered a weak contact sensitizer,[45] with only a few reports of contact sensitization to salicylates having been recorded.[1] Patients with presumed allergic contact dermatitis to salicylic acid preparations may not be allergic to salicylic acid. The patients may be reacting to other components of the preparation. Two patients who had an allergic contact dermatitis to a salicylic acid wart remedy had negative patch-test results to salicylic acid and positive patch-test results to colophony contained in the same preparation.[46]

Box 34-3

Salicylic Acid Systemic Toxicity

GASTROINTESTINAL
Nausea
Vomiting

NEUROLOGIC
Confusion
Dizziness
Delirium
Psychosis
Stupor
Coma
Death

METABOLIC
Respiratory alkalosis
Metabolic acidosis (infants and children)
Hypoglycemia

MISCELLANEOUS
Tinnitus
Hyperventilation

SULFUR

Sulfur has been used for medicinal purposes since the time of Hippocrates for the treatment of plague.[47] For centuries, sulfur has been used in dermatologic treatment. Mild antiseptic, antiparasitic, antiacne, and antiseborrheic properties have been attributed to sulfur. The uses of sulfur include treatment of acne, seborrheic dermatitis, rosacea, scabies, and tinea versicolor.

Pharmacology

CHEMISTRY.　Sulfur is a yellow nonmetallic element. Various preparations of sulfur (Table 34-1) are produced as follows:

1. *Sublimed* sulfur—This form of sulfur is produced by direct conversion of crude sulfur from solid phase to gas. Then the vapor is condensed to yield a fine yellow powder.[48]
2. *Precipitated* sulfur—This form of sulfur is produced by boiling sublimed sulfur with lime and water and then adding hydrochloric acid, which then results in very fine particles. These particles are significantly smaller than the particles of sublimed sulfur. The smaller particle size allows for greater sulfur-cutaneous interaction, thereby enhancing the therapeutic effect.[49]
3. *Colloidal* sulfur—This form of sulfur has even smaller particles than precipitated sulfur. This form of sulfur is considered to be the most active form of sulfur.[47]
4. Sulfurated *potash*—This form of sulfur is produced by heating sublimed sulfur with potassium carbonate.
5. Sulfurated *lime*—This form of sulfur is formed by boiling a suspension of sublimed sulfur, calcium carbonate, and water. This re-

sults in formation of calcium pentasulfide and calcium thiosulfate.[50]
6. *Washed* sulfur—This form of sulfur is prepared when sublimed sulfur is treated with ammonia and washed with water to remove impurities such as arsenic.[48]

The various preparations of sulfur lend themselves to various dermatologic therapeutic uses based on the properties of the form of sulfur. Smaller particle sizes are thought to have greater pharmacologic effect due to greater area available for sulfur-cutaneous interactions. In addition, water and alcohol solubility, as well as particle size, determine the preferred vehicles for the various sulfur preparations.

Both sublimed and precipitated sulfur have United States Pharmacopeia official formulations. Precipitated sulfur is the most common form of sulfur used in dermatology.[50]

MECHANISM OF ACTION.　The precise mechanism of sulfur's keratolytic effects is unknown.[51] The interaction of sulfur with cysteine within keratinocytes probably accounts for the keratolytic effect.[47,49] In low concentrations, sulfur has keratoplastic effects.[52] At higher concentrations, sulfur is thought to induce a keratolytic effect. Cysteine combines with sulfur to form cystine and release hydrogen sulfide (2 cysteine + sulfur → cystine + H_2S).[49]

Due to cystine being a normal constituent of the stratum corneum at low concentrations, sul-

■ Table 34-1　Various Forms of Sulfur

Form	Color/Consistency	Particle Size	Solubility	Clinical Use
Sublimed sulfur (flower of sulfur)	Yellow powder	Relatively large	Insoluble in water, alcohol	In ointments
Precipitated sulfur (milk of sulfur)	Yellow-white powder	Relatively small	Insoluble in water, slightly soluble in alcohol	In ointments
Colloidal sulfur		Relatively small		Suspended in colloidal solution
Sulfurated potash	Yellow-brown to brown lumps		Soluble in water	In lotions
Sulfurated lime	Clear to orange-colored solution	May be particles of polysulfides of calcium	In a solution of polysulfides of calcium	In lotions or solutions

fur is believed to promote normal keratinization, giving a keratoplastic effect.[52] A keratoplastic effect represents a slowing of the desquamation of keratin, thus leading to hyperkeratosis at the treated site. However, hydrogen sulfide can break down keratin; higher concentrations of sulfur presumably lead to greater amounts of hydrogen sulfide, which causes dissolution of the stratum corneum.[48] The antifungal properties of sulfur are related to formation of pentathionic acid ($H_2S_5O_6$) by cutaneous bacteria and keratinocytes. Further antifungal activity may also be related to sulfur's keratolytic action, which causes shedding of infected stratum corneum.[53,54]

In regard to scabies, the action of sulfur is poorly understood. Formation of hydrogen sulfide and polythionic acid, which are toxic to the mite, in addition to shedding of the stratum corneum from the mite's burrow, may be the mechanism of action in the treatment of scabies.[48,55]

Clinical Uses

INDICATIONS.   The therapeutic uses of sulfur in dermatology are summarized in Box 34-4. Various over-the-counter (OTC) preparations contain sulfur, frequently in combination with other agents such as tar and salicylic acid. The keratolytic effect of sulfur may be enhanced by concomitant use with other agents such as salicylic acid.[63]

Box 34-4

Sulfur Clinical Uses

ACNE AND RELATED DERMATOSES
Acne
Rosacea
Perioral dermatitis

DERMATITIS
Seborrheic dermatitis

CUTANEOUS INFECTIONS
Scabies
Tinea versicolor
Dermatophyte infections
Demodex-induced eruptions
Verruca

The therapeutic effect of sulfur in acne may not be related to keratolytic effect but may instead be related to nonspecific "irritant" effect, which leads to peeling. Sulfur may not be comedolytic and may even be comedogenic[56,64]; however, comedogenicity was not found by Strauss.[65]

Before the availability of permethrin for the treatment of scabies, 5% to 10% sulfur preparations had been used to treat scabies in pregnant and lactating women, as well as infants. However, there are no well-designed studies regarding the efficacy and toxicity of sulfur in the therapy of scabies.[51]

ADVERSE EFFECTS.   Fatal toxicity after sulfur was applied to large areas of the skin of infants has been reported rarely.[66] In addition, allergic contact dermatitis to sulfur has been described.[67,68] The limiting factor of the use of sulfur is its offensive odor, which is similar to the odor of rotten eggs.[50]

TAR

The use of tar to treat skin diseases dates back nearly 2000 years. The Greek physician Pedanius Dioscorides (circa 20 AD) used tar preparations in the form of asphalt to treat cutaneous afflictions.[69] In 1925, Goeckerman[70] introduced the use of crude coal tar and UV light for the treatment of psoriasis.

Pharmacology

CHEMISTRY.   Tar is the dry distillation product of organic matter heated in the absence of oxygen. Tar preparations of dermatologic importance are derived from three main organic sources—bituminous coal, wood, and marine fossils.

Crude coal tar, the most widely used tar in dermatology, is produced from gases obtained during the distillation of coal at temperatures ranging from about 900° C to 1200° C. The solid distillation byproduct of this chemical process is coke, used to manufacture steel. Condensation of these gases to liquid and subsequent ammonia extraction produces crude coal tar—a dark, odorous, and thick liquid. Crude coal tar is composed of a complex mixture of thousands of individual organic components, which include polycyclic aromatic hydrocarbons (PAHs), phenols, and nitrogen bases. Fractional distillates obtained at different temperatures produce coal tar of different color, smell, consistency, and organic composition. Also, an alcohol extract of coal tar emulsified with polysorbate (Tween 80) yields a more cosmetically acceptable product known as liquor carbonis detergens (LCD).[71]

Wood tar preparations are derived from distillation of trees, such as birch *(Oleum rusci)*, beech, juniper (Cade oil) or pine, at temperatures not exceeding 700° C. They have fewer carcinogenic agents, such as pyridines and anthracene, but are more irritating and toxic than coal tar because of higher phenol absorption properties.

Bituminous tar, also known as sulfonated shale oils (ichthyol), is derived from distillation of marine fossil sediments and natural rock, at temperatures ranging from 150° C to 500° C. Subsequent chemical degradation of byproducts is accomplished using ammonia and sulfuric acid. Bituminous tar preparations can be of light or dark color, depending on the manufacturing temperature.

MECHANISM OF ACTION.   The mode of action of tar is not understood. Because of its inherent chemical complexity, tar is not pharmacologically standardized, and the specific therapeutic activity of the components is not known. Nonetheless, tar has conclusive antiproliferative effects on the epidermis. Studies by Lavker and colleagues[72] demonstrated a progressive thinning of the epidermis that follows a transient epidermal hyperplasia attributed to primary irritation. Tar appears to exert its actions through suppression of deoxyribonucleic acid (DNA) synthesis and consequent reduction of mitotic activity in the basal layer of the epidermis.[73-75] In combination with UV light, coal tar reduces epidermal proliferation more effectively than either treatment modality alone.[76] In addition to antiproliferative action, shale tar (bituminous tar) has antiinflammatory activity caused by inhibition of chemotaxis of neutrophils due to leukotriene B_4 and C5a.[77,78] Listermann[79] also demonstrated fungicidal properties of shale tar, but the antifungal mechanism of action is not known.

Clinical Uses
Table 34-2 lists clinical uses of tar.

INDICATIONS.   Tar preparations are a useful topical therapy in the management of inflammatory skin diseases, especially psoriasis vulgaris, atopic dermatitis, seborrheic dermatitis, and eczematous dermatitides. Coal tar in combination with UVR for psoriasis (known as the "Goeckerman regimen") has been diversified and customized according to institutional experiences. The use of modified regimens using LCD or other tars is generally thought to be beneficial. The original regimen was based on topical daily use of crude coal tar followed by gradually increasing doses of UV light.[70]

Sulfonated shale oils is of interest for their use in seborrheic dermatitis and other inflammatory dermatoses. In addition, these shale oils have antifungal properties against yeast, dermatophytes, and hyphomycetes.[79]

Coal tar, in concentrations up to 20% (usually in range of 5% to 20%), can be compounded in creams, ointments, and pastes. Coal tar is frequently compounded with salicylic acid. In addition, tar preparations are available as bath soaks.

ADVERSE EFFECTS.   The safety of tar, especially coal tar, has been a matter of debate for decades. In the United States, the Food and Drug Administration (FDA) scrutinized topical tar use because of concerns regarding carcinogenic potential but declared tar effective and safe.[80] Skin

■ **Table 34-2**   Tar Clinical Uses

Dermatosis	Coal Tar	Wood Tar*	Shale Tar*
Psoriasis	x	x	x
Atopic dermatitis	x		
Seborrheic dermatitis	x		x
Tinea versicolor	x		
Yeast/dermatophyte infections			x
Vitiligo	x		
Pruritus	x		

*Both wood tar and shale tar are useful for other inflammatory dermatoses (see text).

cancer has been induced in mice exposed to coal tar preparations.[81] However, clinical studies done with numerous patients who have chronically used topical tar preparations demonstrated that skin cancer incidence in these patients was not different than the skin cancer incidence in the general population.[82-85] In contrast, other, mostly anecdotal studies reported skin cancer occurrence in patients who used tar preparations.[86-88] However, in patients with psoriasis who received extensive treatment with tar or UVR, the incidence of skin cancer was increased.[89]

Scrotal squamous cell carcinoma in association with tar exposure is a well-known, occupationally induced cancer. However, the use of protective clothing, better hygiene, and less scrotal exposure to carcinogens made tar-induced scrotal squamous cell carcinoma primarily of historical significance only.[90] Nonetheless, there are numerous reports in the urology literature referring to the use of tar in the genital area and the occurrence of scrotal carcinoma.[91-93]

The cancer potential of tar has been linked to its carcinogen content. The major carcinogenic agents in tar are PAHs, anthracene derivatives, and pyridines. Coal tar is rich in all of these carcinogenic agents; wood tar is rich in PAHs. Bituminous tar (shale oil) has comparatively low levels of these carcinogenic agents.[94]

A major disadvantage of the use of coal tar is poor compliance. Crude coal tar is unattractive to use because of its unwelcome smell, appearance, and capacity to stain clothing and other items. Consequently, crude coal tar has been modified in several ways such as fractional distillates and LCD. LCD appears more therapeutically effective than fractional distillates but is therapeutically inferior to crude coal tar.[94] Patient acceptance of LCD tends to exceed other forms of tar.

Phototoxicity is an adverse effect of coal tar that is also responsible (at least in part) for the therapeutic effect of the Goeckerman regimen. There are several phototoxic components in coal tar that include anthracene, fluoranthene, phenanthrene, benzpyrene, and acridine.[95] In addition, wood tar and bituminous tar do not photosensitize and are more cosmetically attractive than coal tar.

The acute toxic potential of tar, particularly wood tar, has been linked to phenol content. But newer tar products have been manufactured with reduced phenol content, minimizing the risk for phenol toxicity.[94]

In addition, tar products can induce different types of contact allergy. Phototoxic and photoallergic reactions to coal tar products have been reported.[96] The phototoxic dermatitis can result in a poikiloderma.[97] More often, contact dermatitis appears to occur with wood tar, which may cross-react with colophony, balsam of Peru, and turpentine.[97,98] Irritant reactions to tar can occur as well. Tar can also produce pruritus, folliculitis, comedones, acneiform eruptions, keratoses (tar warts), and keratoacanthomas.[97]

UREA

In 1828, the German chemist Frederich Wohler was the first to synthesize an organic compound and, as a result, originated the discipline of organic chemistry. This compound was urea.[99] Urea is found in urine. Ancient Babylonians instilled urine into wounds. This unusual practice by the ancient Babylonians may have had some utility due to the antimicrobial properties of urea.[100] For many years, urea has been used effectively in topical preparations as a moisturizing, hygroscopic (the ability to attract water), antimicrobial, and keratolytic agent.

Pharmacology
CHEMISTRY. Urea is produced by dehydration of ammonium carbamate ($NH_2CO_2NH_4$) at high temperatures and pressure. Ammonium carbamate is obtained by reaction of ammonia and carbon dioxide.

The molecule of urea is bipolar, rendering the molecule highly water-soluble and capable of ionic interactions with salt solutions. This latter property causes an increase in the water-binding capacity of urea when mixed with sodium chloride.[101]

The ability of urea to retain water is especially illustrated by sharks. Sharks generate and preserve high concentrations of urea in their tissues. These levels of urea slightly surpass seawater's salt concentration, preventing dehydration by osmosis and eliminating the need for sharks to swallow seawater.[102]

Urea is the end product of the catabolism of animal proteins. Hence urea is not an energy source for most pathogenic bacteria and does not promote bacterial growth. Urea is present in urine.

MECHANISM OF ACTION.   Urea has various pharmacologic and chemical actions relevant to the skin. Urea is an antimicrobial agent, protein solvent and denaturant, and enhancer of protein water-binding capacity. In addition, urea enhances percutaneous absorption of various chemicals and pharmaceutical agents.[103]

Topically applied urea is capable of incorporating itself into the cornified layer of the epidermis by breaking hydrogen bonds and reaching the interior of epidermal keratins.[104] Because of urea's properties of high water solubility and low water vapor pressure, urea is capable of absorbing water from the atmosphere in a high humidity environment. With urea, the hydrated stratum corneum preserves its flexibility and softness.[105] Loden[106] demonstrated that urea-containing moisturizers decrease transepidermal water loss and increase skin hydration. Urea also enhances penetration of various topically administered drugs, including some topical steroids.[107]

High concentrations of urea dissolve proteins and can be used as a denaturant.[103] The ability of urea to macerate dystrophic nails has been attributed to a "proteolytic effect,"[100] but other authors attributed the maceration to the hydrating properties of urea.[108] Maceration of full thickness dermatitic skin occurs at greater than 20% concentration of urea in water.[103] A dead frog immersed in a saturated solution of urea becomes macerated and disintegrated in a few hours. Urea has been shown to inhibit the growth of some microorganisms.[103]

The keratolytic mechanism of urea is not known. However, the bipolar molecular structure gives the urea molecule keratin dispersing and denaturing capabilities without disrupting the epidermal water barrier.[109] Some authors dispute the categorization of urea as a keratolytic agent because urea does not cause direct metabolic or enzymatic alterations of the epidermis. However, urea promotes keratolysis by exerting physical alterations such as improved hydration in the horny layer.[11,104,105] Urea's water solubility and binding capacity give the emollient and hygroscopic characteristics, leading to increased desquamation of corneocytes.

Clinical Uses

INDICATIONS.   Table 34-3 lists clinical uses of urea. Topical urea in concentrations of 10% and 20% can be used as an emollient and mild keratolytic agent.[110] There is also one double-blind study showing antipruritic qualities of urea.[111] Urea is effective for conditions associated with dry skin, including atopic dermatitis, xerotic eczema, keratosis pilaris, ichthyosiform dermatoses, and keratodermas.[110] There are numerous OTC topical preparations of urea, typically with urea concentrations from 10% to 25%. Recently an OTC product with 40% urea (Carmol 40) was released.

Preparations containing 40% urea can be used topically for treatment of calluses. A compound of 40% urea, 20% anhydrous lanolin, 5% white wax, and 35% white petrolatum, under occlusion, can be used for chemical avulsion of dystrophic nails.[100,112] The compound was subsequently modified to 40% urea, 5% white beeswax (or paraffin), 20% anhydous lanolin,

■ **Table 34-3**   Urea Clinical Uses

Concentration	Pharmacologic Properties	Dermatoses Treated
Urea 10%-25%	Moisturizing Hydroscopic Antipruritic Keratolytic (mild)	Xerosis Atopic dermatitis Xerotic dermatitis Keratosis pilaris Keratodermas Ichthyosis
Urea 40%	Chemical hygroscopic keratolysis	Calluses Chemical avulsion of dystrophic nails

25% white petrolatum, and 10% silica gel type H with very specific compounding instructions.[113] However, a similar rate of success was found in the chemical avulsion of dystrophic nails when an emollient cream under occlusion was compared with a 40% urea compound under occlusion.[108] Although 40% urea compounds are not effective for the avulsion of normal nails (i.e., nondystrophic nails), 10% salicylic acid with 20% urea in a topical compound can be effective to avulse symptomatic nondystrophic nails,[114] but the efficacy of the urea and salicylic acid combination for normal nail avulsion has been disputed.[113]

Unusual uses of urea include intralesional injection for treatment of basal cell and squamous cell carcinoma, as well as topical application for superficial basal cell carcinoma and actinic keratosis[115] and as an adjunct to wound healing.[116]

ADVERSE EFFECTS.   Topical urea preparations can cause irritant reactions, which is more likely with the higher concentration products. Use of urea in excoriated or fissured skin can produce stinging and irritation. These adverse effects are related to the high acidity of many preparations (usually pH 3.0 or less).[110] However, new stabilized preparations claim less acidity and consequently less skin irritation.

Bibliography

Banerjee PK, Choudhury AK, Panja SK: Topical urea in dermatology. *Indian J Dermatol* 36:17-25, 1990.

Kligman AM: Salicylic acid: an alternative to alpha-hydroxy acids. *J Geriatr Dermatol* 5:128-131, 1997.

Lin AN, Nakatsui T: Salicylic acid revisited. *Int J Dermatol* 37:335-342, 1998.

Lin AN, Moses K: Tar revisited. *Int J Dermatol* 24:216-219, 1985.

Lin AN, Reimer RJ, Carter DM: Sulfur revisited. *J Am Acad Dermatol* 18:553-558, 1988.

References

Salicylic Acid

1. Lin AN, Nakatsui T: Salicylic acid revisited. *Int J Dermatol* 37:335-342, 1998.
2. Draelos ZD: Rediscovering the cutaneous benefits of salicylic acid. *Cosmet Derm* 10(Suppl 4):4, 1997.
3. Brackett W: The chemistry of salicylic acid. *Cosmet Derm* September 10(Suppl 4):5-6, 1997.
4. Kligman AM: Salicylic acid: an alternative to alpha-hydroxy acids. *J Geriatr Dermatol* 5:128-131, 1997.
5. Yu RJ, Van Scott EJ: Salicylic acid: not a beta-hydroxy acid. *Cosmet Derm* 10:27, 1997.
6. Smith WP: Hydroxy acids and skin aging. *Soap/Cosmetics/Chemical Specialties* 69:54-76, 1993.
7. Draelos ZD: Salicylic acid in the dermatologic armamentarium. *Cosmet Derm* September 10(Suppl 4):7-8, 1997.
8. Roberts DL, Marshall R, Marks R: Detection of the action of salicylic acid on the normal stratum corneum. *Br J Dermatol* 102:191-196, 1980.
9. Marks R, Davies M, Cattell A: An explanation for the keratolytic effect of salicylic acid. *J Invest Dermatol* 64:283, 1975.
10. Davies M, Marks RL: Studies on the effect of salicylic acid on normal skin. *Br J Dermatol* 95:187, 1976.
11. Loden M, Bostrom P, Kneczke M: Distribution and keratolytic effect of salicylic acid and urea in human skin. *Skin Pharmacol* 8:173-178, 1995.
12. Weirich EG, Longauer JK, Kirkwood AH: Dermatopharmacology of salicylic acid. II. Epidermal anti-hyperplastic effect of salicylic acid in animals. *Dermatologica* 151:321-332, 1975.

13. Sunscreen drug products for over-the-counter human drugs; proposed safety, efficacy and labeling conditions. Federal register: August 25, 1978, p 38206.

14. Shaath NA: Evolution of modern chemical sunscreens. In Lowe NJ, Shaath NA, editors: *Sunscreens development, evaluation and regulatory aspects,* New York, 1990, Marcel Dekker, pp 3-35.

15. Lowe NJ: Sun protection factors: comparative techniques and selection of ultraviolet sources. In Lowe NJ, editor: *Physicians guide to sunscreens,* New York, 1991, Marcel Dekker, pp 161-165.

16. Insel PA: Analgesic-antipyretics and anti-inflammatory agents: drugs employed in the treatment of rheumatoid arthritis and gout. In Gilman AG, Rall TW, Nies AS, et al, editors: *Goodman and Gilman's the pharmacological basis of therapeutics,* New York, 1990, Pergamon Press, pp 644-653.

17. Weirch EG, Longauer JK, Kirkwood AH: Dermatopharmacology of salicylic acid. III. Topical contra-inflammatory effect of salicylic acid and other drugs in animal experiments. *Dermatologica* 152:98, 1976.

18. United States Pharmacopeial Convention I. Salicylic acid: topical. In Drug Information for the Health Care Professional. Rockville: United States Pharmacopeial Convention, Inc, 2607-2611, 1996.

19. Larko O: Problem sites: scalp, palm and sole, and nail. *Dermatol Clin* 13:771-777, 1995.

20. Baden HP, Alper JC: A keratolytic gel containing salicylic acid in propylene glycol. *J Invest Dermatol* 62:330-333, 1973.

21. Buselmeier TJ: Combination urea and salicylic acid ointment nail avulsion in nondystrophic nails: a follow up observation. *Cutis* 25:397-405, 1980.

22. Leyden JL, Shalita AR: Rational therapy for acne vulgaris: an update on topical treatment. *J Am Acad Dermatol* 15:907-914, 1986.

23. Christophers E, Sterry W: Psoriasis. In Fitzpatrick TB, Eisen AZ, Wolff K, et al, editors: *Dermatology in general medicine,* New York, 1993, McGraw-Hill, pp 489-514.

24. Polano MK: *Skin therapeutics: prescription and preparation (materia medica Dermatologica),* Amsterdam, 1952, Elsevier, pp 57-58, 111.

25. Young E, Weiffenbach N: About the conversion of salicylic acid into zinc salicylate in ointment and pastes containing both zinc oxide and salicylic acid. *Dermatologica* 118:74, 1959.

26. Harvey SC: Topical drugs. In Osol A, editor: *Remington's pharmaceutical sciences,* Easton PA, 1975, Mack Publishing, pp 724-725.

27. Wester RC, Noonan PK, Maibach HI: Effect of salicylic acid on the percutaneous absorption of hydrocortisone: in vivo studies in the Rhesus monkey. *Arch Dermatol* 114:1162-1164, 1978.

28. Tauber U, Weiss C, Matthes H: Does salicylic acid increase the percutaneous absorption of diflucortolone-21-valerate? *Skin Pharmacol* 6:276-281, 1993.

29. Medansky RS, Cuffie CA, Tanner DJ: Mometasone furoate 0.1% salicylic acid 5% ointment twice daily versus fluocinonide 0.5% ointment twice daily in the management of patients with psoriasis. *Clin Ther* 19:701-709, 1997.

30. Reedy BLEC: A topical salicylate gel in the treatment of oral aphthous ulceration. *Practitioner* 204:846, 1970.

31. Goldsmith LA: Salicylic acid. *Int J Dermatol* 18:32-36, 1979.

32. Kligman D, Kligman AM: Salicylic acid as a peeling agent for the treatment of acne. *Cosmet Derm* 10:44-47, 1997.

33. Kligman D, Kligman AM: Salicylic acid peels for the treatment of photoaging. *Dermatol Surg* 24:325-328, 1998.

34. Swinehart JM: Salicylic acid ointment peeling of the hands and forearms: effective nonsurgical removal of pigmented lesions and actinic damage. *J Dermatol Surg Oncol* 18:495-498, 1992.

35. Freedburg I, Baden H: Metabolic response to exfoliation. *J Invest Dermatol* 38:277, 1962.

36. Kligman AM: A comparative evaluation of a novel low-strength salicylic acid cream and glycolic acid products on human skin. *Cosmet Derm* 10(Suppl 4):11-15, 1997.

37. Insel PA: Analgesics-antipyretics and anti-inflammatory agents and drugs employed in the treatment of gout. In Hardman JG, Limbard LE, Molinoff PB, et al, editors: *Goodman and Gilman's the pharmacological basis of therapeutics,* New York, 1996, McGraw-Hill, pp 617-657.

38. Kvorning SA: On ointments containing salicylic acid. *Acta Dermatol Venereol (Stockh)* 34:89-91, 1954.

39. Stolar ME, Rossi GV, Barr M: The effect of various ointment bases on the percutaneous absorption of salicylates. I. Effect of type of ointment base. *J Am Pharm Assoc* 49:144-147, 1960.

40. Birmingham BK, Greene DS, Rhodes CT: Systemic absorption of topical salicylic acid. *Int J Dermatol* 18:228-231, 1979.

41. Taylor JR, Halprin KM: Percutaneous absorption of salicylic acid. *Arch Dermatol* 111:740-743, 1975.

42. Lindsey CP: Two cases of fatal salicylate poisoning after topical application of an antifungal solution. *Med J Australia* 1:353-354, 1968.

43. Shupp DL: An unusual case of salicylate toxicity. *J Am Acad Dermatol* 15:300-301, 1986.

44. Raschke R, Arnold-Capell PA, Richeson R, et al: Refractory hypoglycemia secondary to topical salicylate intoxication. *Arch Intern Med* 151:591-593, 1991.

45. Goh CL, Ng SK: Contact allergy to salicylic acid. *Contact Dermatitis* 14:114, 1986.

46. Lachapelle J-M, Leroy B: Allergic contact dermatitis to colophony included in the formulation of flexible collodion BP, the vehicle of a salicylic and lactic acid wart paint. *Dermatol Clin* 8:143-146, 1990.

Sulfur

47. Harvey SC: Antiseptics and disinfectants; fungicides; ectoparasiticides. In Gilman AG, Goodman LS, Rall TW, et al, editors: *The pharmacological basis of therapeutics*, ed 7, New York, 1985, Macmillan, pp 959-979.

48. McMurtry CW: Dermatologic therapeutics: sulfur. *J Cutan Dis* 31:322-328, 399-408, 1913.

49. Combes FC: Colloidal sulfur: some pharmacodynamic considerations and their therapeutic application in seborrheic dermatoses. *NY State J Med* 46:401-406, 1946.

50. McEvoy GK, McQuarrie GM, editors: Drug Information 86, American Hospital Formulary Service, Bethesda, American Society of Hospital Pharmacists, 1800-1802, 1986.

51. Lin AN, Reimer RJ, Carter DM: Sulfur revisited. *J Am Acad Dermatol* 18:553-558, 1988.

52. Strakosch EA: Studies on ointments. *Arch Dermatol Syphilol* 47:216-225, 1943.

53. Salter WT: *A textbook of pharmacology*, Philadelphia, 1952, WB Saunders, p 913.

54. Miller HE: Colloidal sulfur in dermatology. *Arch Dermatol Syphilol* 31:516-525, 1935.

55. Osol A, Pratt R, Gennaro AR: *The United States dispensatory*, ed 27, Philadelphia, 1973, JB Lippincott, pp 1123-1124.

56. Hjorth N: Traditional topical treatment of acne. *Acta Derm Venereol (Stockh)* 89:53-55, 1980.

57. Blom I, Hornmark AM: Topical treatment with sulfur 10 per cent for rosacea. *Acta Derm Venereol (Stockh)* 64:358-359, 1984.

58. Bamford JTM: Treatment of tinea versicolor with sulfur salicylic shampoo. *J Am Acad Dermatol* 8:211-213, 1983.

59. Bendl BJ: Perioral dermatitis: etiology and treatment. *Cutis* 17:903-908, 1976.

60. Hjorth N, Osmundsen P, Rook AJ, et al: Perioral dermatitis. *Br J Dermatol* 80:307-313, 1968.

61. Ayres S Jr, Ayres S III: Demodectic eruptions (demodicoidosis) in the human. *Arch Dermatol* 83:816-827, 1964.

62. Thomas JR III, Daniel Su WP: The treatment of plane warts. *Arch Dermatol* 118:626, 1982.

63. Sheard C: *Treatment of skin diseases: a manual*, Chicago, 1978, Year Book, pp 21-22.

64. Mills OH Jr, Kligman AM: Is sulfur helpful or harmful in acne vulgaris? *Br J Dermatol* 86:620-627, 1972.

65. Strauss JS, Goldman PH, Nacht S, et al: A re-examination of the potential comedogenicity of sulfur. *Arch Dermatol* 114:1340-1342, 1978.

66. Rasmussen JR: Percutaneous absorption in children. In Dobson RL, editor: *Year book of dermatology*, Chicago, 1979, Year Book, pp 15-38.

67. Wilkinson DS: Sulfur sensitivity. *Contact Dermatitis* 1:58, 1975.

68. Schneider HG: Schwereallergie. *Hautarzt* 29:340-342, 1978.

Tar

69. Kinmont PDC: Tar and the skin. *Practitioner* 179:598-601, 1957.

70. Goeckerman WH: Treatment of psoriasis. *Northwest Med* 24:229, 1925.

71. Lin AN, Moses K: Tar revisited. *Int J Dermatol* 24:216-219, 1985.

72. Lavker RM, Grove GL, Kligman AM: The atrophogenic effect of crude coal tar on human epidermis. *Br J Dermatol* 105:77-82, 1981.

73. Lowe NJ, Breeding J, Wortzman MS: The pharmacological variability of crude coal tar. *Br J Dermatol* 107:475-479, 1982.

74. Walter JF, Stoughton RB, DeQuoy PR: Suppression of epidermal proliferation by ultraviolet light, coal tar and anthralin. *Br J Dermatol* 99:89-96, 1978.

75. Gloor M, Dressel M, Schnyder UW: The effect of coal tar distillate, cadmium sulfide, ichthyol sodium and omadine mds on the epidermis of the guinea pig. *Dermatologica* 156:238-243, 1978.

76. Stoughton RB, DeQuoy PR, Walter JF: Crude coal tar plus near ultraviolet light suppresses DNA synthesis in the epidermis. *Arch Dermatol* 114:43-45, 1978.

77. Czarnetzki B: Inhibitory effect of shale oils (ichthyols) on the secretion of chemotactic leukotrienes from human leukocytes and on leukocyte migration. *J Invest Dermatol* 87:694-697, 1986.

78. Kownatzki E, Kapp A, Uhrich S: Inhibitory effect of sulfonated shale oils (ammonium bituminosulfate) on the stimulation of neutrophilic granulocytes by the chemotactic tripeptide f-Met-Leu-Phe. *Arch Dermatol Res* 278:190-193, 1986.

79. Listemann H, Scholermann A, Meigel W: Antifungal activity of sulfonated shale oils. *Arzneimittelforschung* 43:784-788, 1993.

80. Final Rule: Dandruff, seborrheic dermatitis and psoriasis drug products for over-the-counter human use. Federal Register December 4, 1991; 56:63554-63569.

81. Yamaggiwa K, Ichikawa K: Experimental study of the pathogenesis of carcinoma. *J Cancer Res* 3:1-29, 1971.

82. Jemec GBE, Ostelind A: Cancer in patients treated with coal tar: a long-term follow-up study. *J Eur Acad Dermatol Venereol* 3:153-156, 1994.

83. Pittelkow MR, Perry HO, Muller SA, et al: Skin cancer in patients with psoriasis treated with coal tar. *Arch Dermatol* 117:465-468, 1981.

84. Jones SK, Mackie RM, Hole DJ, et al: Further evidence of the safety of tar in management of psoriasis. *Br J Dermatol* 113:97-101, 1985.

85. Maughan WZ, Muller SA, Perry HO, et al: Incidence of skin cancers in patients with atopic dermatitis treated with coal tar. *J Am Acad Dermatol* 3:612-615, 1980.

86. Alexander JO, Macrosson KI: Squamous epithelioma probably due to tar ointment in a case with psoriasis. *BMJ* 2:1089, 1954.

87. Rasmussen JE: The crudeness of coal tar. *Prog Dermatol* 12:23-29, 1978.

88. Rook AJ, Greshman GH, Davis RA: Squamous epithelioma possibly induced by therapeutic application of tar. *Br J Cancer* 10:17-23, 1956.

89. Stern R, Zierler S, Parrish JA: Skin carcinoma in patient with psoriasis treated with topical tar and artificial ultraviolet radiation. *Lancet* 1:732-735, 1980.

90. Lowe FC: Squamous cell carcinoma of the scrotum. *J Urol* 130:423-427, 1983.

91. McGarry GW: Scrotal carcinoma following prolonged use of tar ointment. *Br J Urol* 63:211, 1989.

92. Andrews PE: Squamous cell carcinoma of the scrotum: long-term follow up of 14 patients. *J Urol* 146:1299-1304, 1991.

93. Moy LS: Scrotal squamous cell carcinoma in a psoriatic patient treated with coal tar. *J Am Acad Dermatol* 14:518-519, 1986.

94. Schmid MH, Korting HC: Coal tar, pine tar and sulfonated shale oil preparations: comparative activity, efficacy and safety. *Dermatology* 193:1-5, 1996.

95. Kaidbey KH, Kligman AM: Clinical and histological study of coal tar phototoxicity in humans. *Arch Dermatol* 113:592-595, 1977.

96. Goncalo S, Sousa I, Moreno A: Contact dermatitis to coal tar. *Contact Derm* 10:57-58, 1984.

97. Rietschel RL, Fowler JF, editors: *Fisher's contact dermatitis,* ed 4, Baltimore, 1995, Williams & Wilkins, p 153.

98. Rosyanto ID, van der Akker TW, van Joost TW: Wood tar allergy, cross-sensitization and coal tar. *Contact Dermatitis* 22:95-98, 1990.

Urea

99. Wohler F: On the artificial production of urea. *Annalen der Physik und Chemie* 12:88, 1828.

100. Port M, Sanicola KF: Nonsurgical removal of dystrophic nails utilizing urea ointment occlusion. *J Am Podiatry Assoc* 70:521-523, 1980.

101. Swanbeck G: The effect of urea on the skin with special reference to the treatment of ichthyosis. In Marks R, Dykes PJ, editors: The Ichthyoses. Proc. 2nd Ann Clin Oriented Symp Eur Soc Dermatol. Re Cardiff, 1977, Lancaster 1978, Technical Press, pp 163-166.

102. Alexander MD: Osmotic control and urea biosynthesis in selachians. *Comp Biochem Physiol* 26:971-978, 1968.

103. Ashton H, Frenk E, Stevenson CJ: Urea as a topical agent. *Br J Dermatol* 84:194-196, 1971.

104. Hellgren L, Larsson K: On the effect of urea on human epidermis. *Dermatologica* 49:289-293, 1974.

105. Swanbeck G: Urea in the treatment of dry skin. *Acta Derm Venereol (Stockh)* 177(Suppl):7-8, 1992.

106. Loden M: Urea-containing moisturizers influence barrier properties of normal skin. *Arch Dermatol* Res 288:103-107, 1996.

107. Feldman RJ, Maibach H: Percutaneous penetration of hydrocortisone with urea. *Arch Dermatol* 109:58-59, 1974.

108. Pinner TAF, Jones RH, Bandisode MS: Study of efficacy of urea compound versus emollient cream in avulsive therapy of dystrophic nails. *Cutis* 46:155-157, 1990.

109. Grice K, Sattar H, Baker H: Urea and retinoic acid in ichthyosis and their effect on transepidermal water loss and water holding capacity of stratum corneum. *Acta Derm Venereol* 53:114-118, 1973.

110. Banerjee PK, Choudhury AK, Panja SK: Topical urea in dermatology. *Indian J Dermatol* 36:17-25, 1990.

111. Swanbeck G, Rajka G: Antipruritic effect of urea solutions. An experimental and clinical study. *Acta Derm Venereol (Stockh)* 50:225-227, 1970.

112. Farber EM, South DA: Urea ointment in the nonsurgical avulsion of nail dystrophies. *Cutis* 22:689-692, 1978.

113. South DA, Farber EM: Urea ointment in the nonsurgical avulsion of nail dystrophies—a reappraisal. *Cutis* 25:609-612, 1980.

114. Buselmeier TJ: Combination urea-salicylic acid ointment in nondystrophic nails: a follow-up observation. *Cutis* 25:397, 405, 1980.

115. Danopoulos ED, Danopoulou IE: Urea treatment of skin malignancies. *Lancet* 1:115-118, 1974.

116. Robinson W: Use of urea in stimulating healing in chronic purulent wounds. *Am J Surg* 33:192-197, 1936.

CHAPTER 35

Dana Sachs
Susan Baur
Sewon Kang

Topical Vitamin D$_3$

Vitamin D is both a vitamin and a hormone whose well-known physiologic function is to maintain serum calcium and phosphorus levels within a normal range.[1] Its critical importance in calcium homeostasis was revealed in rickets, a devastating bone disease for which the incidence reached an epidemic level in industrialized cities of northern Europe and the northeastern United States by the turn of the 20th century. Smoke-polluted and sunless alleyways were prevalent in these cities at the time. With the observation that rickets was much less common among children living in rural areas, the cause of rickets was postulated to be from the lack of sun exposure as early as 1882.[2] However, the proof with radiographic documentation that sunlight alone could cure rickets was made about 40 years later.[3] Rickets was also noted to be responsive to ingestion of cod liver oil. Eventually vitamin D was determined to be the nutrient responsible for the clinical improvement. Subsequent elucidation that ultraviolet (UV) radiation is the initiating signal for vitamin D biosynthesis in the skin finally completed the loop linking sun exposure, vitamin D, and rickets.

Dermatologic interest in vitamin D centers on the fact that the skin is both a site of initial vitamin D biosynthesis (where 7-dehydrocholesterol is converted to vitamin D$_3$ in the presence of UV irradiation) and a target organ of vitamin D action. The presence of Vitamin D receptors (VDR), the transducer of 1,25-dihydroxyvitamin D$_3$ effects, has been demonstrated in keratinocytes, Langerhans' cells, melanocytes, fibroblasts, and endothelial cells.[4] The ability of 1,25-dihydroxyvitamin D$_3$ to affect cell proliferation and differentiation, in both in vitro and in vivo conditions, helped initiate its pharmacologic development. More recently, the increased understanding of the immunomodulatory effects of vitamin D and its analogs paralleled the growth in knowledge of the vitamin D mode of action in psoriasis and other inflammatory dermatologic disorders.[5]

PHARMACOLOGY
Structure and Biosynthesis

Provitamin D$_3$ (7-dehydrocholesterol) (Figure 35-1) is found in plants and animals. It is easily detected in human skin. UVB irradiation causes a bond cleavage of *provitamin* D$_3$ to form previtamin D$_3$ (9,10-secosterol precholecalciferol), which is inert. A temperature-dependent isomerization of *previtamin* D$_3$ generates vitamin D$_3$ (cholecalciferol) in the skin. Vitamin D$_3$ is a very labile molecule that may become inactivated if it does not promptly enter into circu-

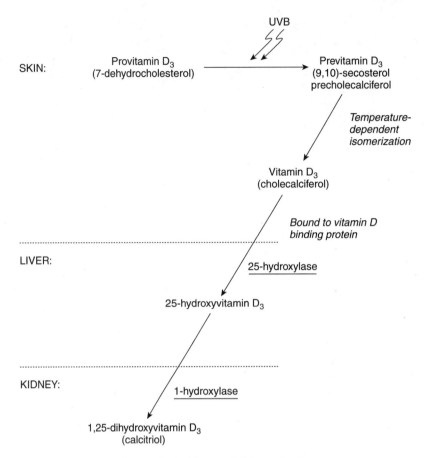

Figure 35-1 Vitamin D biosynthesis.

lation. Once in circulation, vitamin D_3 is transported to the liver where it undergoes hydroxylation by the cytochrome P-450–dependent enzyme 25-hydroxylase to become 25-hydroxyvitamin D_3. In the kidney (as well as in other tissues such as placenta, pulmonary alveolar macrophages, and bone cells), the 25-hydroxyvitamin D_3 is hydroxylated again to form calcitriol (1,25-dihydoxyvitamin D_3), the active hormone.

Metabolism
The active form of vitamin D, 1,25-dihydroxyvitamin D_3 (1,25[OH]$_2$D$_3$), is metabolized by 24-hydroxylase to 1,24,25-trihydroxyvitamin D_3, which has very little biologic activity when compared with the active form. The 24-hydroxylase is expressed both in the kidney and

in human skin. It is an inducible enzyme in that topical application of calcitriol to human skin markedly enhances its activity.[6]

Mechanism of Action
Vitamin D in the form of 1,25-dihydroxyvitamin D_3 acts mainly via the VDR to regulate cell growth, differentiation, and immune function, as well as calcium and phosphorus metabolism. The VDR protein belongs to the family of nuclear receptors that includes the corticosteroid, thyroid hormone, and retinoic acid receptors. When the VDR is activated by its ligand 1,25(OH)$_2$D$_3$ or the synthetic analogs discussed in this chapter, the drug/receptor complex binds to specific deoxyribonucleic acid (DNA) binding sites, known as vitamin D response elements, and regulates the genes that contain

■ Table 35-1   Topical Vitamin D₃

Generic Name	Trade Name	Manufacturer	Generic	Cream	Ointment	Special Formulations
Calcipotriene	Dovonex	Westwood-Squibb	No	.005%	.005%	.005% lotion for scalp use
Tacalcitol*	(Europe, Asia)	(Europe, Asia)	No	No	.0004%† .0002%‡	

Note: Calcitriol is only available in the United States in oral and intravenous formulations (not pertinent to this chapter).
*Not yet released in the United States.
†Formulation available in Japan.
‡Formulation available in the United Kingdom, Germany, Switzerland, and several other European countries.

them. Vitamin D has been shown to inhibit the proliferation of keratinocytes in culture and to modulate epidermal differentiation. In addition, it has a number of effects on inflammation. Vitamin D inhibits production of interleukin (IL)-2 and IL-6 by T cells, blocks transcription of interferon (IFN)-γ and granulocyte-macrophage colony–stimulating factor (GM-CSF) messenger ribonucleic acid (mRNA), and inhibits cytotoxic and natural killer T cell activity.[7]

VITAMIN D ANALOGS

Pharmacologic doses of oral $1,25(OH)_2D_3$ produce substantial hypercalcemia and hypercalciuria, thus limiting its use for dermatologic indications. Many vitamin D analogs have been synthesized in search of those with reduced hypercalcemic activity, without compromising the desired pharmacologic activity. Only three analogs are discussed in this chapter—calcipotriene (originally named *calcipotriol*), calcitriol, and tacalcitol (Table 35-1, Figure 35-2). There are no comparative clinical studies between the vitamin D analogs. However, regarding the pharmacokinetics of these analogs, calcipotriene is much less likely to induce hypercalcemia (with resultant hypercalciuria) as compared with tacalcitol and calcitriol.[7]

Calcipotriene

Calcipotriene (calcipotriol) is a synthetic analog of calcitriol. Calcipotriene binds to the VDR with the same affinity as calcitriol, although it is 100 times less active on calcium metabolism, due to its rapid local metabolism when applied topically.[8] It is available under the trade names Dovonex (USA), Daivonex (Asia), and Psorcutan (Europe). Ointment, cream, and solution (50 μg/g, thus .005%) formulations of Dovonex are available.

Tacalcitol

Tacalcitol is a dihydroxyvitamin D₃ like calcitriol. Tacalcitol differs structurally from calcitriol by the presence of a hydroxyl group at the 24-position, rather than at the 25-position. This drug is available in Japan as 2 μg/g (.0002%) ointment for twice daily application. In the United Kingdom, Germany, Switzerland, and several other European countries, tacalcitol is available as a 4 μg/g (.0004%) ointment for once daily application for the treatment of psoriasis. It is currently not available in the United States.[9]

Calcitriol

Calcitriol is the natural, bioactive, 1,25 dihydroxyvitamin D₃. The drug is available for systemic administration (oral and intravenous routes) strictly for nondermatologic indications.

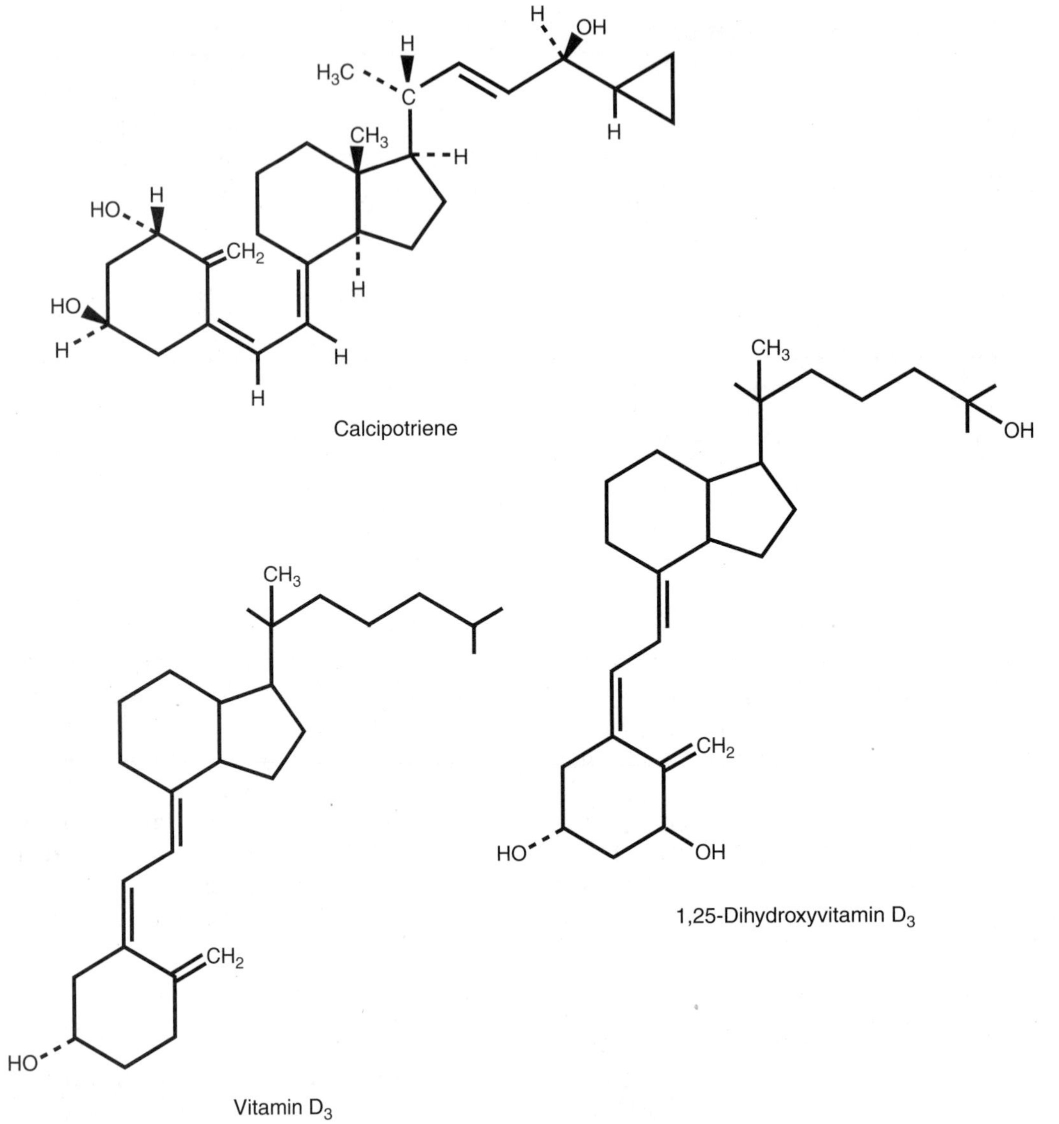

Figure 35-2   Topical vitamin D.

It is not available as a topical preparation and therefore is not further discussed.

CLINICAL USE

Table 35-2 lists indications and contraindications for calcipotriene.

FDA-Approved Indication—Psoriasis

PLAQUE PSORIASIS. Calcipotriene has been approved for the treatment of plaque-type psoriasis in adults. The early studies were all short-term, lasting from 4 to 8 weeks. These studies showed calcipotriene to be superior to vehicle in double-blind controlled studies. In left-right comparison studies and parallel group studies with betamethasone-17-valerate (betamethasone valerate), calcipotriene was as effective or more so in reducing the psoriasis area and severity index (PASI) score.

In short-term studies, class I topical corticosteroids were found to be superior to calcipo-

Table 35-2	Calcipotriene Indications and Contraindications

FDA-APPROVED INDICATION
Psoriasis[10-25]

OFF-LABEL USES

Autoimmune Dermatoses
Morphea[26,27]
Vitiligo[28]

Disorders of Keratinization
X-linked recessive ichthyosis[29]
Lamellar ichthyosis[30]
Epidermolytic hyperkeratosis[30]
Sjögren-Larsson syndrome[31]

Miscellaneous Dermatoses
Acanthosis nigricans[32]
Confluent and reticulated papillomatosis[33]
Grover's disease[34]
Inflammatory linear verrucous epidermal
   nevus[35]

CONTRAINDICATIONS

Absolute
None

Relative
Erythrodermic psoriasis with concurrent renal
   insufficiency

PREGNANCY PRESCRIBING STATUS—CATEGORY C*

*It should be used during pregnancy only if the potential benefit justifies the potential risk to the fetus.

triene. When compared with short-contact anthralin or 15% coal tar, calcipotriene was found to be more effective. The efficacy of calcipotriene is not reduced with long-term treatment, indicating the lack of tachyphylaxis with its continuous use.[10] Calcipotriene applied twice daily is more effective than once daily use. The greater efficacy of a twice daily regimen is not necessarily associated with more frequent occurrence of irritation side-effects as compared with once daily application.[11]

INTERTRIGINOUS PSORIASIS. In an open and uncontrolled study, patients with psoriasis in the axillary, inguinal, and anal regions were treated with calcipotriene. Despite concerns of it causing significant irritation at these sites, calcipotriene was found to be well tolerated and was an effective treatment.[12]

NAIL PSORIASIS. Calcipotriene has been compared with betamethasone dipropionate with salicylic acid in the treatment of nail psoriasis. The two treatment regimens were comparable in reducing subungual hyperkeratosis and in their tolerability.[13]

ACRODERMATITIS CONTINUA OF HALLO-PEAU. Anecdotal reports describe calcipotriene to be an effective treatment for this difficult to manage variant of psoriasis.[14]

SCALP PSORIASIS. The Dovonex solution formulation improves the delivery of calcipotriene to psoriatic plaques in the scalp. It is significantly more effective than the vehicle in reducing scalp psoriasis. However, when compared with betamethasone valerate solution, calcipotriene solution was found to be less effective.[10]

USE IN CHILDREN. Calcipotriene ointment was shown to be effective in children with plaque psoriasis in a prospective, noncontrolled, openlabel trial.[15] Similar to adults, the most common adverse effect observed with its use in children was local skin irritation. There was no evidence of hypercalcemia, as assessed by serum calcium levels, with use of up to 45 g of calcipotriene ointment per week in these children. In a prospective, double-blind, randomized, placebo-controlled, parallel group trial, calcipotriene ointment was shown to be significantly better than vehicle in reducing the redness and scaliness of psoriatic plaques in children.[16]

HIGH-DOSE CALCIPOTRIENE.   Inpatients with psoriasis were treated with 200 g of calcipotriene ointment for 1 week, followed by from 300 g up to 360 g of calcipotriene the second week. This was found to be an effective mode of therapy for patients with extensive psoriasis. Overall, 65% of the patients responded and of those responders, 69% were controlled for 3 months. Five of the 28 patients developed asymptomatic hypercalcemia, which resolved within 3 days after withdrawal of the drug. All of these patients received maximum doses of more than 5 g/kg/week.[17]

Use With Other Antipsoriatic Therapies

UVB AND PSORALEN PLUS ULTRAVIOLET A.
Several studies have examined combination treatment for psoriasis using calcipotriene with UVB or psoralen plus ultraviolet A (PUVA).[18] In one randomized study, psoriasis patients received either UVB phototherapy alone, calcipotriene (100 g/week) alone, or UVB plus calcipotriene. The greatest improvement in the PASI score was achieved in those who received both UVB and calcipotriene.[19] Similarly, an investigator-blinded, right-left comparison study between calcipotriene plus UVB and mineral oil plus UVB revealed that the calcipotriene plus UVB combination was superior to the mineral oil plus UVB regimen.[20] The addition of calcipotriene to PUVA provided greater reduction in the PASI scores and more rapid clearing of skin lesions in patients receiving the combination than either agent alone.[18] Therefore calcipotriene enhances the efficacy of both UVB and PUVA.

When used in combination with UVB or PUVA, calcipotriene should be applied after UV irradiation for several reasons. First, although calcipotriene is stable under UVB, it is significantly photodegraded by UVA.[21] This UVA exposure markedly reduces the bioavailability of calcipotriene. Secondly, applying calcipotriene after phototherapy eliminates the possibility of any attenuation in UV light transmission introduced by the topical ointment. In essence, this combination maximizes the effectiveness of phototherapy. Finally, topical administration of calcipotriene after UV exposure minimizes the discomfort that has been described in some patients when the drug application preceded phototherapy.

CORTICOSTEROIDS.   Topical corticosteroids have been used in combination with calcipotriene to enhance the efficacy and reduce the local irritant reaction. Indeed, a study that compared halobetasol ointment with calcipotriene alone and with calcipotriene plus halobetasol showed that the combination therapy was both more effective in clearing psoriasis plaques and had fewer adverse effects.[22] Another study looked at different potencies of topical corticosteroids in combination with calcipotriene. Twice daily application of calcipotriene was found to be as effective as calcipotriene *plus* clobetasone butyrate but not as effective as calcipotriene *plus* betamethasone valerate.[11] In this study, there was also less irritation in the patients who used a topical corticosteroid in conjunction with calcipotriene, compared with patients who used calcipotriene alone. Another study demonstrated that clobetasol propionate ointment twice daily for 2 weeks followed by calcipotriene twice daily for 4 weeks was superior to calcipotriene alone.[23]

COMPATIBILITY STUDY.   When considering combining calcipotriene with another topical agent, one must consider stability of each active agent in the mixture. For example, calcipotriene is degraded when mixed with hydrocortisone valerate 0.2%, ammonium lactate lotion 12%, or salicylic acid 6%. It is quite stable when mixed with halobetasol propionate and hence is compatible.[24]

CYCLOSPORINE.   In a study evaluating the efficacy and tolerability of calcipotriene plus cyclosporine versus cyclosporine alone, calcipotriene was useful in reducing the total dosage of cyclosporine needed to improve psoriasis.[25]

Off-Label Uses

MORPHEA.   In an open-label study, patients with morphea and linear scleroderma were treated with calcipotriene for 3 months under occlusion. All patients were shown to have statistically significant improvement in their plaques with respect to dyspigmentation, induration, erythema, and telangiectasia.[26] Although randomized, double-blind, placebo-controlled studies have not yet been done, calcipotriene may be a reasonable treatment for this condition. In vitro, calcipotriene has been shown to inhibit the proliferation of fibroblasts cultured from morphea lesions.[27]

VITILIGO.   A placebo-controlled, right-left comparative study was performed to evaluate the efficacy of the combination of psoralens with exposure to solar radiation (PUVAsol) with calcipotriene in the treatment of vitiligo. The onset of repigmentation was faster on the PUVAsol *plus* calcipotriene-treated side as compared with the PUVAsol only side. In addition, patients had better repigmentation of the hands and feet when treated with the combination regimen.[28]

DISORDERS OF KERATINIZATION.   Calcipotriene was applied to patients with congenital ichthyosis (including X-linked, lamellar, and epidermolytic hyperkeratosis subtypes), hereditary palmoplantar keratoderma, keratosis pilaris, and Darier's disease in a randomized, double-blind, placebo-controlled, right-left comparative study. Calcipotriene was found to be effective in X-linked ichthyosis and congenital ichthyosis. It was either not effective or not well tolerated in patients with keratosis pilaris, palmoplantar keratoderma, and Darier's disease.[29] Lamellar ichthyosis and epidermolytic hyperkeratosis had a positive response to calcipotriene in a prospective and double-blind, bilaterally paired, comparative study.[30] The cutaneous manifestations of Sjögren-Larsson syndrome, a genodermatosis characterized by ichthyosis and spastic paralysis, have also reported to improve with calcipotriene.[31]

ACANTHOSIS NIGRICANS.   No randomized controlled studies were found in the literature regarding the use of calcipotriene in acanthosis nigricans. However, a published report describes a patient with mixed-type acanthosis nigricans who after a 3-month treatment with twice daily calcipotriene showed marked improvement.[32] The patient had biopsy-proven acanthosis nigricans and metastatic transitional cell carcinoma of the urinary bladder, as well as insulin-resistant diabetes secondary to obesity.

CONFLUENT AND RETICULATED PAPILLOMATOSIS OF GOUGEROT AND CARTEAUD.   A patient whose skin biopsy was consistent with this diagnosis and who had no evidence of *Pityrosporum orbiculare* infection was treated with twice daily application of calcipotriene. A marked improvement was reported after only 1 month of use.[33]

GROVER'S DISEASE.   Alternating use of calcipotriene ointment and a topical corticosteroid has been a successful treatment regimen for a patient with Grover's disease. The efficacy of calcipotriene was impressive in this patient, considering that previously dapsone, etretinate, and oxytetracycline all failed to be beneficial.[34]

INFLAMMATORY LINEAR VERRUCOUS EPIDERMAL NEVUS (ILVEN).   Calcipotriene has been reported to be effective in the treatment of ILVEN, which is considered by some to be a linear form of psoriasis.[35]

Adverse Effects
HYPERCALCEMIA.   The only major concern with the use of topical vitamin D preparations is the possibility of adverse effects on calcium homeostasis. The risk for the development of hypercalcemia and hypercalciuria in patients using calcipotriene is real, although this risk is a function of the cumulative weekly dose. When the amount used does not exceed the recommended 100 g/week, calcipotriene can be used with a great margin of safety.[36,37] In general, product cost limits use of calcipotriene to quantities much less than 100 g/week.

IRRITATION.   Treatment with calcipotriene may cause lesional, perilesional, and ectopic (inadvertent application) facial irritation.[38] The irritant effects are self-limited and quickly resolve once the drug is discontinued, particularly with adjunctive topical corticosteroids. Concern has been expressed over the use of calcipotriene in intertriginous sites and on the face. However, most patients do not develop irritant dermatitis even at these sites.[39]

PHOTOSENSITIVITY.   There are reports of photosensitivity developing in patients with chronic plaque psoriasis treated with UVB after calcipotriene had been introduced to the treatment regimen. Several mechanisms have been proposed for this, including a phototoxic reaction to calcipotriene or possibly a change in the delayed erythema response induced by calcipotriene.[40] However, such photosensitivity is infrequent and the severity is mild for it to be a significant problem.

ALLERGIC CONTACT DERMATITIS.   There has been debate over whether or not calcipotriene can also cause allergic contact dermatitis. Evidence to date suggests that calcipotriene is at best a weak contact allergen, although the drug can be a contact irritant.[41]

Bibliography

Holick MF: McCollum Award Lecture, 1994: vitamin D—new horizons for the 21st century. *Am J Clin Nutr* 60:619-630, 1994.

Kragballe K: The future of vitamin D in dermatology. *J Am Acad Dermatol* 37:S72-S76, 1997.

Kragballe K, Iversen L: Calcipotriol: a new topical antipsoriatic. *Dermatol Clin* 11:137-141, 1993.

Peters DC, Balfour JA: Tacalcitol. *Drugs* 54:265-271, 1997.

Thiers BH: The use of topical calcipotriene/calcipotriol in conditions other than plaque-type psoriasis. *J Am Acad Dermatol* 37:S69-S71, 1997.

van der Kerkhof PCM: An update on vitamin D_3 analogues in the treatment of psoriasis. *Skin Pharmacol Appl Skin Physiol* 11:2-10, 1998.

References

Introduction

1. Holick MF: McCollum Award Lecture, 1994: vitamin D—new horizons for the 21st century. *Am J Clin Nutr* 60:619-630, 1994.
2. Snaidecki J, Cited by W: Mozolowski, Jerdrzej Snaidecki (1768-1883) on the cure of rickets. *Nature* 143:121, 1939.
3. Hess AF, Unger LF: Cure of infantile rickets by sunlight. *JAMA* 77:39, 1921.
4. Kragballe K: The future of vitamin D in dermatology. *J Am Acad Dermatol* 37:S72-S76, 1997.
5. Kang S, Yi S, Fancher L, et al: Calcipotriene-induced improvement in psoriasis is associated with reduced interleukin-8 and increased interleukin-10 levels within lesions. *Br J Dermatol* 138:77-83, 1998.

Pharmacology

6. Kang S, Li XY, Duell EA, et al: The retinoid-X-receptor agonist 9-*cis* retinoic acid and the 24-hydroxylase inhibitor ketoconazole increase activity of 1,25-dihydroxyvitamin D_3 in human skin *in-vivo*. *J Invest Dermatol* 108:513-518, 1997.
7. van der Kerkhof PCM: An update on vitamin D_3 analogues in the treatment of psoriasis. *Skin Pharmacol Appl Skin Physiol* 11:2-10, 1998.
8. Kragballe K: Calcipotriol: a new drug for topical psoriasis treatment. *Pharmacol Toxicol* 77:241-246, 1995.
9. Peters DC, Balfour JA: Tacalcitol. *Drugs* 54:265-271, 1997.

Clinical Use—Psoriasis

10. Ramsay CA: Management of psoriasis with calcipotriol used as monotherapy. *J Am Acad Dermatol* 37:S53-S54, 1997.
11. Kragballe K, Barnes L, Hamberg KJ, et al: Calcipotriol cream with or without concurrent topical corticosteroid in psoriasis: tolerability and efficacy. *Br J Dermatol* 139:649-654, 1998.
12. Kienbaum S, Lehmann P, Ruzicka T: Topical calcipotriol in the treatment of intertriginous psoriasis. *Br J Dermatol* 135:647-650, 1996.

13. Tosti A, Piraccini BM, Cameli N, et al: Calcipotriol ointment in nail psoriasis: a controlled double-blind comparison with betamethasone dipropionate and salicylic acid. *Br J Dermatol* 139:655-659, 1998.

14. Mozzanica N, Cattaneo A: The clinical effect of topical calcipotriol in acrodermatitis continua of Hallopeau. *Br J Dermatol* 138:556, 1998.

15. Darley CR, Cunliffe WJ, Green CM, et al: Safety and efficacy of calcipotriol ointment (Dovonex®) in treating children with psoriasis vulgaris. *Br J Dermatol* 135:390-393, 1996.

16. Oranje AP, Marcoux D, Svensson A, et al: Topical calcipotriol in childhood psoriasis. *J Am Acad Dermatol* 36:203-208, 1997.

17. Bleiker TO, Bourke JF, Mumford R, et al: Long-term outcome of severe chronic plaque psoriasis following treatment with high-dose topical calcipotriol. *Br J Dermatol* 139:285-286, 1998.

Clinical Use—Combination Therapies

18. Koo J: Calcipotriol/calcipotriene (Dovonex/Daivonex) in combination with phototherapy: a review. *J Am Acad Dermatol* 37:S59-S61, 1997.

19. Bourke JF, Iqbal SJ, Hutchinson PE: The effects of UVB plus calcipotriol on systemic calcium homeostasis in patients with chronic plaque psoriasis. *Clin Exp Dermatol* 22:259-261, 1997.

20. Hecker D, Lebwohl M: Topical calcipotriene in combination with UVB phototherapy for psoriasis. *Int J Dermatol* 36:302-303, 1997.

21. Lebwohl M, Hecker D, Martinez J, et al: Interactions between calcipotriene and ultraviolet light. *J Am Acad Dermatol* 37:93-95, 1997.

22. Lebwohl M, Siskin S, Epinette W, et al: A multicenter trial of calcipotriene ointment and halobetasol ointment compared with either agent alone for the treatment of psoriasis. *J Am Acad Dermatol* 35:268-269, 1996.

23. Austad J, Bjerke JR, Gjertsen BT, et al: Clobetasol propionate followed by calcipotriol is superior to calcipotriol alone in topical treatment of psoriasis. *J Eur Acad Dermatol Venereol* 11:19-24, 1998.

24. Patel B, Siskin S, Krazmien R, Lebwohl M: Compatibility of calcipotriene with other topical medications. *J Am Acad Dermatol* 38:1010-1011, 1998.

25. Kokelj F, Torsello P, Plozzer C: Calcipotriol improves the efficacy of cyclosporine in the treatment of psoriasis vulgaris. *J Eur Acad Dermatol Venereol* 10:143-146, 1998.

Off-Label Uses

26. Cunningham BB, Landells IDR, Langman C, et al: Topical calcipotriene for morphea/linear scleroderma. *J Am Acad Dermatol* 39:211-215, 1998.

27. Bottomley WW, Jutley J, Wood EJ, et al: The effect of calcipotriol on lesional fibroblasts from patients with active morphea. *Acta Derm Venereol* 75:364-366, 1995.

28. Parsad D, Saini R, Verma N: Combination of PUVAsol and topical calcipotriol in vitiligo. *Dermatology* 197:167-170, 1998.

29. Kragballe K, Steijlen PM, Ibsen HH, et al: Efficacy, tolerability, and safety of calcipotriol ointment in disorders of keratinization. *Arch Dermatol* 131:556-560, 1995.

30. Lucker GPH, van de Kerkhof PCM, van Dijk MR, et al: Effect of topical calcipotriol on congenital ichthyoses. *Br J Dermatol* 131:546-550, 1994.

31. Lucker GPH, van de Kerkhof PCM, Cruysberg JRM, et al: Topical treatment of Sjögren-Larsson syndrome with calcipotriol. *Dermatology* 190:292-294, 1995.

32. Bohm M, Luger TA, Metze D: Treatment of mixed-type acanthosis nigricans with topical calcipotriol. *Br J Dermatol* 139:932-933, 1998.

33. Kurkcuoglu N, Celebi CR: Confluent and reticulated papillomatosis: response to topical calcipotriol. *Dermatology* 191:341-342, 1995.

34. Koehane SG, Cork MJ: Treatment of Grover's disease with calcipotriol (Dovonex®). *Br J Dermatol* 132:832-833, 1995.

35. Micali G, Nasca MR, Musumeci ML: Effect of topical calcipotriol on inflammatory linear verrucous epidermal nevus. *Pediatr Dermatol* 12:386-387, 1995.

Adverse Effects

36. Bourke JF, Iqbal SJ, Hutchinson PE: Vitamin D analogues in psoriasis: effects on systemic calcium homeostasis. *Br J Dermatol* 135:347-354, 1996.

37. Bourke JF, Mumford R, Whittaker P, et al: The effects of topical calcipotriol on systemic calcium homeostasis in patients with chronic plaque psoriasis. *J Am Acad Dermatol* 37:929-934, 1997.

38. Fullerton A, Benfeldt E, Petersen JR, et al:
    The calcipotriol dose-irritation relationship:
    48 hour occlusive testing in healthy volun-
    teers using Finn Chambers®. *Br J Dermatol*
    138:259-265, 1998.
39. Lebwohl M: Topical application of cal-
    cipotriene and corticosteroids: combination
    regimens. *J Am Acad Dermatol* 37:S55-S58,
    1997.
40. McKenna KE, Stern RS: Photosensitivity asso-
    ciated with combined UV-B and calcipotriene
    therapy. *Arch Dermatol* 131:1305-1307,
    1995.
41. Frosch PJ, Rustemeyer T: Contact allergy to
    calcipotriol does exist. *Contact Dermatitis*
    40:66-71, 1999.

CHAPTER 36

Zoe Diana Draelos

Cosmetic Therapy

Products designed for cosmetic care are an important part of dermatologic therapy for their ability to maintain the integrity of the skin, hair, and nails, as well as beautify appearance. Historically, cosmetics represent the first dermatologic agents ever used by humans. This chapter discusses methods of chemically altering skin and hair color, physically altering hair shape, and temporarily coloring nails and skin. Cleansing and moisturizing of the hair and skin are also discussed.

HYDROQUINONE

Hydroquinone, also known as 1,4 dihydroxybenzene (Figure 36-1), is utilized in products designed to lighten skin color.[1] This chemical functions as an active agent to decrease melanocyte pigment production through degradation by autooxidation of melanin, tyrosinase, and phenol oxidases into highly reactive oxygen radicals, semiquinones, and quinones.[2,3] These reactive substances prevent melanin production. The reactivity of hydroquinone can be attested to by the fact that it can even oxidize in the tube or bottle, becoming a brown color instead of white. Lightening ("bleaching") products that have undergone this color change are ineffective and should be discarded.

Hydroquinone is present in the United States in over-the-counter skin lightening products in concentrations of 2% and in prescription products of 3% to 5%. Many times hydroquinone is combined with topical skin exfoliants, such as glycolic acid or topical tretinoin, to enhance the absorption and apparent concentration of hydroquinone.

Both allergic and irritant contact dermatitis to hydroquinone have been reported. For this reason, it is advisable to test the product in a small area, such as behind the ear, before application. Sometimes the irritation can be overcome by combining treatment with a low-potency topical corticosteroid.

The safety of hydroquinone in certain formulations has been questioned, however. Its use has been banned in Japan and severely restricted in South Africa. This is due to concern regarding its long-term safety with uncontrolled use and the recognition that it can contribute to the development of irreversible exogenous pigmentation, known as ochronosis. Ochronosis is primarily a risk at hydroquinone concentrations well above that available in prescription products.

DIHYDROXYACETONE

Dihydroxyacetone (DHA) is the active agent in "sunless" or "self-tanning" products. This ingredient has been available for many years; however, the ability to obtain DHA of enhanced purity accounts for the plethora of sunless tanning products on the market today.[4] Originally, DHA produced an unusual orange color when applied

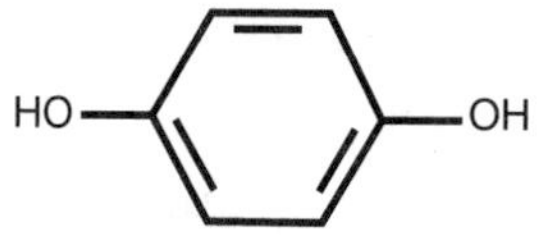

Figure 36-1 Cosmetic therapeutic agents.

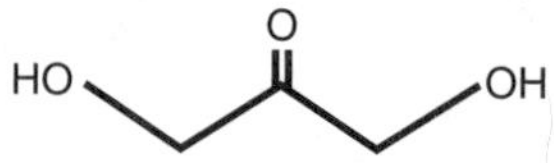

Box 36-1

Tips to Applying Self-Tanning Creams and Lotions

1. Exfoliate the skin with a polyethylene bead-containing liquid soap (Oil of Olay Daily Renewal Facewash, Age Defying Series, Procter & Gamble) before application to remove any old, dry skin that would absorb too much color.
2. Dry the skin thoroughly before application.
3. Spread an even thin coat of the self-tanning product using the palm of the hand, not the fingertips. Uneven application results in uneven staining of the skin.
4. Use less tanning cream on thicker skin areas such as the elbows and knees.
5. Wash hands immediately after application to avoid palm staining.
6. Wait 2 hours before exercising or perspiring to prevent streaking of the color.
7. Reapply the self-tanning cream every 3 to 5 days to maintain a natural color.
8. Use the entire bottle of self-tanning cream within 6 months. Older products do not work as well.
9. Remember to always apply an additional sunscreen to the self-tanning product when going outdoors.

to the skin, but now a more golden, natural tan color can be achieved.

DHA is a white, crystalline powder (see Figure 36-1), chemically characterized as a three-carbon sugar. It is stable between the pH values of 4 and 6.[5] DHA interacts with the free amino acids present in sweat and keratin. The end result of the reaction is a brown substance, mimicking a suntan in Caucasians, referred to as melanoidin.[6] Melanoidins create the orange-brown color characteristic of sunless tanning preparations. Lower amounts of keratin lead to a decreased brown color, whereas increased keratin, as is present in seborrheic keratoses and ichthyosis conditions, leads to an increased brown color. All skin can be stained with the product, including the palms and soles (Box 36-1).

Most presently available sunless tanning products contain 3% to 5% DHA, with higher concentrations used in products producing a deeper color. The deeper color, however, does not confer better sun protection. As a matter of fact, the sun protection provided by DHA is minimal, approximately a sun-protection factor (SPF) equivalent to 2, requiring an added sunscreen agent to achieve acceptable sun protection.

Sunless tanning preparations represent a safe alternative for individuals who insist on darkening their skin. The incidence of allergic reactions to DHA is low. The secret to achieving a realistic tan is careful application. Box 36-1 lists some application suggestions.

FACIAL FOUNDATIONS AND CAMOUFLAGE COSMETICS

Facial foundations and camouflage cosmetics function to add color, blend pigmentary abnormalities, and cover blemishes. The earliest cosmetic designed to cover facial blemishes was the beauty patch. These became popular in the 1600s to cover permanent facial scars left on those in Europe who survived smallpox epidemics. These were black silk or velvet pieces shaped like stars, moons, and hearts that were carefully placed about the face. Patch boxes, shallow metal boxes with a mirror in the cover, were carried everywhere to keep replacements handy should a patch fall off in public. The modern compact evolved from the facial patch box when smallpox was no longer a major health problem.

The first true facial foundation was a theatrical product used to whiten neck and arms

■ **Table 36-1**   Facial Foundations and Camouflage Cosmetics—Formulation

Type	Formulation	Advantages	Disadvantages
Water-based	Oil-in-water emulsion	Most popular type Lighter feel	May change color with wear Shorter wear Not waterproof
Oil-based	Water-in-oil emulsion	Least popular Provides moisturization Water-resistant No color change with wear	Somewhat greasy Somewhat occlusive
Oil-free	No mineral or vegetable oils, only silicone oils	Light weight, nongreasy Excellent in acne patients or oily complected patients	Not waterproof May sting on application
Water-free (anhydrous)	Oils only	Waterproof No preservatives required Excellent coverage Long wearing	Very heavy Difficult to remove Very occlusive

■ **Table 36-2**   Facial Foundations and Camouflage Cosmetics—Types

Type	Application	Comments
Shake lotion	Powder shook to mix with water	Simplest formula Short wearing Sheer coverage
Liquid	Poured from bottle	Most popular Very versatile
Mousse	Aerosolized foam sprayed from can	Least popular Sheer coverage
Cream	Dipped from jar	Thicker product Heavier coverage
Soufflé	Dipped from jar	Whipped cream Produces lighter product
Cream/Powder	Wiped from a compact	Heavy coverage Requires more application skill
Stick	Stroked from a roll-up tube	Heavy coverage Waterproof

known as "wet white" or "French White." This initial foundation consisted of face powder incorporated into a liquid vehicle. This was considered to be an improvement over simply powdering the skin due to its superior adherence to facial skin. Later, "grease paints" were developed as pigments and fillers suspended in oily vehicles. These products were difficult to wear and apply for individuals outside the theater. The first major breakthrough in facial foundations for the average woman came when Max Factor developed cake makeup, which he patented in 1936 as a powdered product removed from a compact and applied with a wet sponge. This product provided excellent coverage, created a velvety look, and added facial color.

Since that time, the variety and popularity of facial foundations have expanded tremendously. The variety in formulation and type is explored in Tables 36-1 and 36-2, respectively, while application instructions are listed in Box

36-2. Facial foundations can be a valuable adjunct in dermatologic therapy. The most popular camouflage facial foundations are the creamy products that are scooped from a jar or tin with a spatula and applied to the hand for warming. These products are the easiest to use because they exhibit a long playtime, good blending characteristics, minimal application skill, excellent coverage, and adequate wearability for most individuals.[7]

Initially, a makeup base must be selected that is closest to the patient's natural skin color. Blending usually is necessary, but no more than three colors should be combined as this produces muddy final color quality. If the patient has an underlying pigmentation problem, this counts as one color. In this case, the pink color of the wound, due to an increased vascular supply to promote healing, counts as one color. Other color abnormalities may be due to increased melanin (producing a brown color), increased hemosiderin (producing a rust color), or degenerated facial elastin (producing a yellow color).

Depending on the situation, it may be desirable to camouflage the red hues by initially applying a green undercover cosmetic and then a traditional facial foundation, thus avoiding the surgical products. If, however, the color contrast is too great, a high-coverage, surgical foundation that covers all underlying skin tones may be a better camouflaging makeup selection.

Once the closest foundation color has been selected, it may be necessary to blend in yellow, if the individual has a sallow complexion, or reds, if the patient has a ruddy complexion. All facial tones should be represented in the final foundation blend if a good color match is to be obtained. Blending is usually done by applying a small amount of the makeup to the back of the hand. This provides a good surface for blending that can be easily held up to the face to evaluate the color match and also warms the product, which allows easier mixing and application.

The final foundation color mix is then dabbed, not rubbed, over the scarred area and then applied from the central face outward into the hairline for approximately $1/4$ inch and blended over the ears and beneath the chin. It is necessary to feather the cosmetic where application ends to achieve a more natural appearance. The importance of dabbing cannot be overemphasized because scars do not contain appendageal structures, such as follicular ostia, that are necessary for good cosmetic adherence. Rubbing removes the makeup as it is applied. The cosmetic should be actually pressed into the skin and allowed to dry for 5 minutes.

After this brief drying period, the cosmetic must be set with an unpigmented, finely-ground, talc-based powder to prevent smudging, improve wearability, provide waterproof characteristics, and impart a matte finish. Camouflaging makeups are designed to be worn with this powder and do not function properly without it. The powder should be pressed, not dusted, on top of the foundation.

Lastly, shading and highlighting principles are employed to minimize the scar contour abnormalities. Unfortunately, the camouflage foundation may actually accentuate the surface irregularities of the scar and normal skin structures, such as pores and wrinkles. Depressed scars usually appear darker than the surrounding skin, even though the same color foundation has been applied, due to the presence of shadows. Thus a lighter powdered rouge is applied

Box 36-2

Facial Foundation and Camouflage Cosmetics—Application Instructions

1. Prepare the skin by cleansing.
2. Apply moisturizer, preferably with a sunscreen (Oil of Olay Daily UV Complete, Procter & Gamble), to dry areas and an astringent (Clarifying Lotion, Clinique) to oily areas to optimize facial foundation application.
3. Apply a quarter-sized amount of cosmetic to the forefinger and dab on the central forehead, nose, chin, and both cheeks.
4. Blend the foundation to cover the entire face up to the anterior hairline, to the ears, and beneath the chin.
5. Allow the foundation to set several minutes before applying other colored facial cosmetics.
6. If using a surgical foundation, apply a setting powder by pressing it into the foundation.

over the scar. If the scar were elevated, a darker powdered rouge would be applied. Lastly, a reddish powdered rouge is dusted over the central face (central forehead, nose, and chin) and upper cheeks to mimic natural color variations of the face. Unfortunately, the high-coverage surgical makeup also covers these facial landmarks, resulting in a flat, masklike face. Other colored facial cosmetics (eye shadow, eyeliner, mascara, and so on) are usually necessary to give an attractive final appearance.[8]

In general, removal of camouflaging cosmetics requires more than soap and water washing due to the waterproof nature of the product. Most companies provide an oily cleanser for cosmetic removal and then recommend soap and water cleansing of the skin. The cosmetic should only be worn when needed and thoroughly removed at bedtime.[9]

SKIN CLEANSERS

The concept of skin cleansing was first introduced 4000 years ago by the Hittites of Asia Minor who cleaned their hands with the ash of the soapwort plant suspended in water. The first modern soap-type preparation was developed about 600 BC by the Phoenicians, who saponified goat fat, water, and potassium carbonate-rich ash into a solid, waxy substance.

The first commercially marketed soap in the United States was developed in 1878 by Harvey Procter, who decided that his father's soap and candle factory should produce a delicately scented, creamy white soap to compete with imported European products. He accomplished this feat with the help of his cousin chemist, James Gamble, who made a richly lathered product called "White Soap." By accident, they discovered that whipping air into the soap solution before molding resulted in a floating soap that could not be lost in the bath. This resulted in a product known as "Ivory" soap, still manufactured today.

Soap is made by mixing a fat and an alkali to produce a fatty acid salt with detergent properties.[10-12] Additives are incorporated to adjust the alkaline pH and prevent the precipitation of calcium fatty acid salts in hard water, a phenomenon known as "soap scum." Soaps can be simplistically divided into three basic categories presented in Table 36-3. True soaps contain only soap and have an extremely alkaline pH, accounting for the irritation and drying seen with such products when used on skin with a damaged barrier. The need for more frequent, milder cleansing led to the development of new synthetic detergents.[13,14] These synthetic detergents, when formulated into bar soaps, are known as "syndets." They offer the advantage of a neutral pH and are less likely to cause skin irritation and xerosis. Sometimes synthetic detergents are combined with true soaps to yield a "combar," which combines the mildness of synthetic detergents with the superior cleansing of true soaps. Combars also have an alkaline pH. The best cleanser is formulated to leave the skin at its natural acidic pH, between 4.5 and 6.5, because long-term alterations in pH result in breakdown of the stratum corneum barrier.[15-17]

Common synthetic detergents in bar-type cleansers are sodium cocoate, sodium tallowate, sodium palm kernelate, sodium stearate, sodium palmitate, triethanolamine stearate, sodium cocoyl isethionate, sodium isethionate, sodium dodecyl benzene sulfonate, and sodium cocoglyceryl ether sulfonate. Liquid synthetic detergents include sodium laureth sulfate, cocoamido propyl betaine, lauramide DEA, sodium cocoyl isethionate, and disodium laureth sulfosuccinate. All detergents are skin irritants to a greater or lesser degree, depending on their ability to extract the intercellular lipids and destroy the stratum corneum barrier.[18-20]

■ Table 36-3   Classification of Soaps

Category	Composition	pH
True soaps	Long chain, fatty acid, alkali salts	9-10
Combars*	Alkaline soaps with a surface active agent	9-10
Syndet bars†	Synthetic detergents and fillers, contain less than 10% soap	5.5-7.0

*Combines true soap and synthetic detergents.
†Synthetic detergents.

■ **Table 36-4**   Specialty Soap Formulations

Type of Soap	Unique Ingredients
Superfatted soap	Increased oil and fat; fat ratio up to 10%
Castile soap	Olive oil used as primary fat
Cocoa butter soap	Cocoa butter used as major fat
Nut or fruit oil soap	Nut or fruit oils used as major fat
Deodorant soap	Antibacterial agents such as triclosan
French milled soap	Additives to reduce alkalinity
Floating soap	Extra air trapped during mixing process
Oatmeal soap	Ground oatmeal added (coarsely ground to produce abrasive soap, finely ground for gentle cleanser)
Acne soap	Sulfur, resorcinol, benzoyl peroxide, or salicylic acid added
Facial soap	Smaller bar size—no special ingredients
Bath soap	Larger bar size—no special ingredients
Aloe vera soap	Aloe vera added to soap—no special benefit
Vitamin E soap	Vitamin E added to soap—no special benefit
Transparent soap	Glycerin and sucrose added
Abrasive soap	Pumice, coarse oatmeal, maize meal, ground nut kernels, dried herbs, or dried flowers added
Soap-free soap	Contains synthetic detergents (Syndet bar)

Adapted from Draelos ZD: *Cosmetics in dermatology*, Edinburgh, 1995, Churchill Livingstone.

The great variety currently available in the bar cleanser market is due to specialty additives, some of which are valuable to skin care, whereas others are of marketing value only. Table 36-4 lists some of the unique attributes of the various bar cleansers.

MOISTURIZERS

Moisturizers function to retard transepidermal water loss from a damaged epidermal barrier, to soothe irritated skin, and to increase skin softness by filling the irregular spaces left by desquamating corneocytes.[21] Three mechanisms are available for rehydrating the stratum corneum—the use of occlusives, humectants, and hydrophilic matrices.[22]

Occlusives function to condition the skin by impairing evaporation of water to the atmosphere.[23] They are generally oily substances through which water cannot easily pass. Occlusive substances can be broken down into the categories listed in Table 36-5.

A dehydrated epidermis can also be conditioned through the use of humectants, which are substances that attract water, mimicking the role of the dermal glycosaminoglycans such as hyaluronic acid. Examples of topical humectants include glycerin, honey, sodium lactate, urea, propylene glycol, sorbitol, pyrrolidone carboxylic acid, gelatin, hyaluronic acid, vitamins, and some proteins. The most commonly used humectants in commercial preparations are glycerin and propylene glycol because they function both as humectants and as vehicles in many moisturizers. The amount of humectant properties provided is directly related to the concentration of the ingredient.

Topically applied humectants draw water largely from the dermis to the epidermis and rarely from the environment under conditions where the ambient humidity exceeds 70%. Water that is applied to the skin in the absence of a humectant is rapidly lost to the atmosphere; however, skin that is well hydrated after soaking retains water more efficiently if humectants are subsequently applied. Humectants may also allow the skin to feel smoother by filling holes in the stratum corneum through swelling of corneocytes.[24] However, under low humidity conditions, humectants, such as glycerin, draw

■ **Table 36-5**   Occlusive Moisturizers— Categories of Ingredients

Category	Specific Examples of Ingredients
Hydrocarbon oils and waxes	Petrolatum, mineral oil, paraffin, squalene
Silicone	Dimethicone, cyclomethicone
Vegetable oils and animal fats	Soybean oil, olive oil, lanolin
Fatty acids	Lanolin acid, stearic acid
Fatty alcohol	Lanolin alcohol, cetyl alcohol
Polyhydric alcohols	Propylene glycol
Wax esters	Lanolin, beeswax, stearyl stearate
Vegetable waxes	Carnauba, candelilla
Phospholipids	Lecithin
Sterols	Cholesterol

moisture from the skin and increase transepidermal water loss.

Lastly, hydrophilic matrices are large-molecular-weight substances that form a barrier to cutaneous water evaporation. Hyaluronic acid, a normal component of the dermal glycosaminoglycans, is a physiologic hydrophilic matrix, whereas colloidal oatmeal, which is oatmeal that has been ground to a uniform powder, is a synthetic hydrophilic matrix.

The concept of emolliency is also important because it allows the skin surface to feel smooth to the touch. Emollients can be divided into several categories—protective emollients, fatting emollients, dry emollients, and astringent emollients.[25] Protective emollients are substances, such as diisopropyl dilinoleate and isopropyl isostearate, that remain on the skin longer than average and allow the skin to feel smooth immediately on application. Fatting emollients, such as castor oil, propylene glycol, jojoba oil, isostearyl isostearate, and octyl stearate, also leave a long-lasting film on the skin but may feel greasy. Dry emollients, such as isopropyl palmitate, decyl oleate, and isostearyl alcohol, do not offer much skin protection but

produce a dry feel. Lastly, astringent or drying emollients, such as the dimethicones and cyclomethicones, isopropyl myristate, and octyl octanoate, have minimal greasy residue and can reduce the oily feel of other emollients. It is the combination of emollients and moisturizers that forms a quality skin lotion or cream.

HAIR SHAMPOOS

Shampoos are intended to remove sebum and dirt from the hair and scalp but are also designed to leave the hair manageable with body and luster[26] (see Chapter 32). Detergents are the primary sebum and dirt removal shampoo components; however, excessive removal of sebum leaves the hair dull, susceptible to static electricity, and difficult to comb. Thus careful selection and blending of detergents determines both the cleansing and cosmetic attributes of a shampoo.[27] The foaming agent is necessary to provide lather, which consumers equate with cleansing; however, the foam is largely of esthetic value. The conditioners leave the hair manageable after shampooing, but additional conditioners may be required as a separate application after the shampooing process. Thickeners, opacifiers, softeners, and fragrance are necessary for the look, feel, and smell of the shampoo but have little to do with its ability to cleanse hair. Sequestering agents prevent soap "scum" from forming on the hair, which is why shampoos and not bar soaps should be used to cleanse the hair. Soap scum can contribute to scalp pruritus and leave the hair dull and unattractive. Lastly, preservatives are necessary because most shampoos contain water that theoretically could support bacterial growth.[28]

Shampoo detergents can be chemically classified as: anionics, amphoterics, and nonionics[29] (Table 36-6). The anionics are excellent cleansers but leave the hair harsh, whereas the nonionics produce milder cleansing, leaving the hair more manageable. Amphoteric detergents are unique in that they are nonirritating to the eyes while producing mild cleansing and leaving the hair manageable. Many shampoo formulations combine detergents from the three groups to meet consumer needs. The most common detergents used in shampoos are sodium

■ Table 36-6 Shampoo Detergents[29]

Surfactant Type	Chemical Class	Characteristics
Anionics	Lauryl sulfates Laureth sulfates Sarcosines Sulfosuccinates	Deep cleansing May leave hair harsh
Amphoterics	Glycinates Propionates Betaines	Nonirritating to eyes Mild cleansing Leave hair manageable
Nonionics	Polysorbate Nonoxynols Poloxamers	Mild cleansing Leave hair manageable

laureth sulfate, sodium lauryl sulfate, tetraethylammonium (TEA) lauryl sulfate, ammonium laureth sulfate, ammonium lauryl sulfate, diethylammonium (DEA) lauryl sulfate, and sodium olefin sulfonate.[30]

HAIR PERMANENT WAVING AGENTS

Permanent waving is a method of transforming straight hair to curly hair, popular among both men and women. It requires three steps: chemical softening, rearranging, and fixing. The simplified chemistry involves the reduction of the disulfide hair shaft bonds, which is demonstrated in Box 36-3. Permanent waves are applied professionally or at home by following the basic steps listed in Box 36-4.

There are several different types of permanent waves, each employing a different waving lotion. The waving lotions consist primarily of a reducing agent in an aqueous solution with an adjusted pH. The most popular reducing agents are the thioglycolates, glycerol thioglycolates, and sulfites. Permanent waves can be simplistically classified into the following groups: alkaline, buffered alkaline, exothermic, self-regulated acid, acid, and sulfite (Table 36-7).

The majority of the permanent waves performed in hair salons are of the acid type, which

Box 36-3

Chemistry of Permanent Waving Technique*

1. Penetration of the thiol compound into the hair shaft.
2. Cleavage of the hair keratin disulfide bond (kSSk) to produce a cysteine residue (kSH) and the mixed disulfide of the thiol compound with the hair keratin (kSSR).

$$kSSk + RSH \leftrightarrow kSH + kSSR$$

3. Reaction with another thiol molecule to produce a second cysteine residue and the symmetrical disulfide of the thiol waving agent (RSSR).

$$kSSR + RSH \leftrightarrow kSH + RSSR$$

4. Rearrangement of the hair protein structure to relieve internal stress determined by curler size and hair wrapping tension.
5. Application of an oxidizing agent (as catalyst to the reaction below) to reform the disulfide cross-links.

$$kSH + HSk \leftrightarrow kSSk + H_2O$$

*Similar general chemical sequence for all types of permanents.

Box 36-4

Hair Permanent Waving Procedure[31]

1. Shampoo hair to remove dirt and sebum.
2. Section the hair into 30 to 50 areas.
3. Wind wet hair on rods with appropriate tension while placing end papers to distal hair shafts.
4. Apply waving lotion for 5 to 20 minutes to initiate the chemical reaction (see also "Chemistry of Permanent Waving Technique").
5. Perform test curl at the anterior hairline.
6. Neutralize hair twice with an oxidizing agent to reform the disulfide cross-links.
7. Dry and style hair.

are discussed later in greater detail. Acid permanent waves occur in an acidic environment with a pH of 6.5 to 7.3 and are based on thioglycolate esters such as glycerol monothioglycolate. The lower pH is an advantage because less hair shaft swelling occurs compared with

■ **Table 36-7**   Evaluation of Permanent Waving Products

Permanent Wave Type	Representative Product Names	Advantages	Disadvantages
Alkaline	Lasts So Long (Helene Curtis)	Tight, long-lasting curl produced	Harsh on hair, especially bleached or color-treated hair
Buffered alkaline	None	Tight, long-lasting curl produced	Less harsh on hair
Exothermic	Even Heat (Helene Curtis)	Produces heat for client comfort	Must be properly mixed
Self-regulated acid	Post Impressions (Helene Curtis)	Limits hair damage, leaves hair soft	Loose curl produced
Sulfite	Rave (Ogilvie)	Less odor	Loose curl produced

higher pH levels, thus hair damage is minimized. These products result in a looser, less long-lasting curl, but leave the hair soft. However, the glycerol monothioglycolate found in some acid permanent waves may cause allergic contact dermatitis in both beauticians and clients. Interestingly enough, the hair may continue to be allergenic even after all products have been thoroughly rinsed from the hair.[32]

Home permanent waves are typically lower strength than professional products to prevent the novice from inducing extreme hair damage. Thioglycolate preparations are available, in addition to sulfite permanent waves. Sulfite permanent waves do not have the characteristic odor of their thioglycolate counterparts but also cannot induce quite as tight a curl.[33]

HAIR STRAIGHTENING AGENTS

Chemical hair straightening is very similar to hair permanent waving, except that the disulfide bonds are re-formed with the hair straight rather than curved around a mandrel. Hair straightening can be accomplished with lye-based, lye-free, ammonium thioglycolate, or bisulfite creams.[34] Lye-based, or sodium hydroxide, straighteners are alkaline creams with a pH of 13. Sodium hydroxide is a caustic substance that can damage hair, produce scalp burns, and cause blindness if exposed to the eye. These products are generally restricted to professional or salon use and may contain up to 3.5% sodium hydroxide. The straightening occurs as one third of the hair cystine content is changed to lanthionine along with minor hydrolysis of the peptide bonds.[35]

Other strong alkali chemicals sometimes used in place of sodium hydroxide are guanidine hydroxide and lithium hydroxide, which are known as no-lye chemical hair straighteners. These relaxing kits contain 4% to 7% cream calcium hydroxide and liquid guanidine carbonate. The guanidine carbonate activator is then mixed into the calcium hydroxide cream to produce calcium carbonate and guanidine hydroxide, which is the active agent.

Thioglycolate straighteners are identical to permanent wave solutions except that they are formulated as thick creams, rather than lotions, to add weight and aid in holding the hair straight. They are extremely harsh on the hair, however, and the least popular of all the relaxing chemicals. The thioglycolate cream has a pH of 9.0 to 9.5, which removes the protective sebum and facilitates hair shaft penetration. Chemical burns can also occur with this straightener.[36]

The least damaging hair straightening products are the ammonium bisulfite creams. These products contain a mixture of bisulfite and sulfite in varying ratios, depending on the pH of the lotion. Many of the home chemical straightening products are of this type but produce the least permanent straightening of all the chemicals discussed. As a general rule, the chemicals that produce the greatest, longest-lasting hair straightening are also the most damaging to the hair shaft.

HAIR DYEING AGENTS

Hair coloring is an ancient tradition that was common among the ancient Persians, Hebrews, Greeks, and Romans. The use of henna, a naturally occurring plant dye, dates to the third dynasty of Egypt 4000 years ago. The Egyptians mixed the Lawsonia plant (henna) with hot water and placed the material on the head to produce an orange-red hair color. Metallic dyes containing lead acetate (obtained by dipping lead combs in sour wine) were used by Roman men to cover gray hair. Roman women, on the other hand, attempted to lighten their hair by applying lye followed by sun exposure.[37]

The modern concept of permanent hair dyeing dates to 1883 when Monnet patented a process for coloring fur using *p*-phenylenediamine and hydrogen peroxide. Feathers and hair were later dyed in 1888 and the first human application was in Paris in 1890 and in St. Louis, Missouri, in 1892. Temporary and semipermanent dyes were not developed until the 1950s when they were "borrowed" from the textile industry and incorporated into the cosmetics industry. Bleaching of the hair with hydrogen peroxide was first demonstrated at the Paris Exposition of 1867 by Thillary and Hugo. All of these products form the basis for modern hair coloring.

Pigment comprises less than 3% of the fiber mass of hair, yet is one of the most important hair cosmetic aspects. Three pigment types produce the tremendous variety of color seen in human hair: eumelanins, pheomelanins, and oxymelanins. Eumelanins are insoluble polymers accounting for the brown and black hues consisting mainly of 5,6-dihydroxyindole with lesser amounts of 5,6-dihydroxyindole-2-carboxylic acid. Pheomelanins are soluble polymers accounting for the yellow to red hues containing 10% to 12% sulfur and 1,4-benzothiazinylalanine. Eumelanin contains less sulfur than pheomelanin. A lesser pigment, known as oxymelanin, is yellow or reddish in color and probably represents bleached eumelanin pigment arising from partial oxidative cleavage of 5,6-dihydroxyindole units. Oxymelanin is distinct in that it contains no sulfur. Hair dyes attempt to mimic these pigments in reproducing a natural appearing hair color.[38,39]

Hair dyes can be divided into several types based on their formulation and permanency—gradual, temporary, semipermanent, and permanent (Table 36-8).

Gradual Hair Dyes

Gradual hair dyes, also known as metallic or progressive hair dyes, require repeated application to result in gradual darkening of the hair shaft. This product changes the hair color from gray to yellow-brown to black over a period of weeks. Hair color lightening is not possible with

■ Table 36-8　Hair Dyes

Type of Dye (Specific Product)	Mechanism of Action	Advantages	Disadvantages
Gradual (Grecian Formula, Combe)	Aqueous metallic solution	Gradually darker color production	Brittle hair produced Cannot combine with other chemical procedures
Temporary (Fancifull Rinse, Roux)	Textile dye	Easily tones or blends darker hair color	Removal in one shampooing
Semipermanent (Loving Care, Clairol)	Low molecular weight textile dye, polymer or vegetable dye	Adds highlights Can darken hair with <30% gray	Removal in 4 to 6 shampooings
Permanent (Preference, L'Oreal)	Oxidation coloring	Can lighten or darken hair color Permanent color	Possible allergenicity

this hair coloring technique. Gradual hair dyes employ water-soluble metal salts, which are deposited on the hair shaft in the form of oxides, suboxides, and sulfides. The most common metal used is lead, but silver, copper, bismuth, nickel, iron, manganese, and cobalt have also been used.[40]

Temporary Hair Dyes

Temporary hair coloring agents, also known as hair rinses, are designed to be removed in one shampooing. They are used to add a slight tint, brighten a natural shade, or improve an existing dyed shade. Their particle size is too large to penetrate through the cuticle, accounting for their temporary nature. They are based on textile dyes belonging to the following chemical classes: azo, anthraquinone, triphenylmethane, phenazinic, xanthene, or benzoquinone. These dyes are known as FDC and DC blues, greens, reds, oranges, yellows, and violets.[41]

Semipermanent Hair Dyes

Semipermanent hair coloring is designed for use on natural, unbleached hair to cover gray, add highlights, or rid hair of unwanted tones. Semipermanent hair dyes are removed in four to six shampooings due to their intermediate sized particles that can both enter and exit the hair shaft. Recently, longer lasting products within this category incorporating hydrogen peroxide have become available. The dyes are retained in the hair shaft by weak polar and Van der Waals attractive forces, thus dyestuffs with increased molecular size remain longer. The formulation of a typical semipermanent hair dye is—dyes (nitroanilines, nitrophenylenediamines, nitroaminophenols, azos, anthraquinones), alkalizing agent, solvent, surfactant, thickener, fragrance, and water. Usually, 10 to 12 dyes are mixed to obtain the desired shade.[42]

Semipermanent dyes are available as lotions, shampoos, and mousses. The shampoo-in process is most popular for home use. The dyestuff, which contains the colored molecules, is combined with an alkaline detergent shampoo to promote hair shaft swelling so that the dye can penetrate, a thickener to increase viscosity so that the product remains on the scalp, and a foam stabilizer so that the product does not run and stain facial skin. The mousse formula incorporates the dyestuff in an aerosolized foam. Both products are applied to wet, freshly shampooed hair and are rinsed in 20 to 40 minutes. Semipermanent dyes can become more permanent if applied to porous, chemically treated hair.[43]

Permanent Hair Dyes

Permanent hair coloring is so named because the dyestuff penetrates the hair shaft to the cortex and forms large color molecules that cannot be removed by shampooing. It can be used to cover gray and produce a completely new hair color, either lighter or darker than the natural hair color. Redyeing is necessary every 4 to 6 weeks, as new growth appears at the scalp.

This type of hair coloring does not contain dyes, but rather colorless dye precursors that chemically react with hydrogen peroxide inside the hair shaft to produce colored molecules. The process entails the use of primary intermediates (p-phenylenediamine, p-toluenediamine, p-aminophenol) that undergo oxidation with hydrogen peroxide. These reactive intermediates are then exposed to couplers (resorcinol, 1-naphthol, m-aminophenol, and so on) to result in a wide variety of dyes, chemically classified as indo dyes.[44]

These indo dyes can produce shades from blonde to brown to black with highlights of gold to red to orange. Variations in the concentration of hydrogen peroxide and the chemicals selected for the primary intermediates and couplers produce this color selection. Red is produced by using nitroparaphenylenediamine alone or in combination with mixtures of paraaminophenol with metaphenylenediamine, alphanaphthol, or 1,5-dihydroxynaphthalene. Yellow is produced by mixtures of orthoaminophenol, orthophenylenediamine, and nitro-orthophenylenediamine. Blue has no single oxidation dye intermediate, but is produced by combinations of p-phenylenediamine, phenylenediamine, methyltoluenediamine, or 2,4 diaminoanisol.[45]

Permanent dyeing allows hair shades to be obtained both lighter and darker than the person's original hair color. Higher concentrations of hydrogen peroxide can bleach melanin, thus the oxidizing step functions both in color production (dyeing of hair) and bleaching of melanin in hair. Boosters, such as ammonium persulfate or potassium sulfate, can be added to achieve great degrees of color lightening. The boosters must be left in contact with the hair for 1 to 2 hours for an optimal result. Nevertheless, individuals with dark hair who choose to dye their hair a light blonde color notice the appearance of reddish hues with time. The newly created blonde color molecules in the hair shaft diffuse out with grooming trauma and shampooing. This magnifies the presence of the reddish pheomelanin pigments, which cannot be thoroughly removed with the peroxide/booster system. Interestingly enough, the reddish pheomelanin pigments are more resistant to removal than brownish eumelanin pigments, for reasons that are not completely understood.

HAIR BLEACHING AGENTS

Lightening the natural color of the hair is known as "bleaching." This chemical alteration is achieved through the use of oxidizing agents at an alkaline pH. The major oxidizer employed is hydrogen peroxide, which causes oxygen to be released from the hair keratin in direct proportion to the amount of hair color lightening achieved. The concentration of the hydrogen peroxide is characterized in terms of volumes. The higher the volume of peroxide used in the bleaching process, the more dramatic the achievable hair lightening. The hydrogen peroxide solution is alkalinized to a pH between 9 and 11 by mixing with ammonia immediately before application to the hair. The chemical reaction occurs more rapidly in the presence of body heat; external heat sources are not required. Thus the hair near the scalp lightens with greater speed than the distal hair shaft.[46]

Bleaching is damaging to the hair shaft, resulting in a 2% to 3% weight loss, which promotes increased hair breakage.[47] It is estimated that 15% to 25% of the hair disulfide bonds are degraded during moderate bleaching with up to 45% of the cystine bonds broken during severe bleaching. Small amounts of the amino acids tyrosine, threonine, and methionine are also degraded. This weakening of the hair shaft is more pronounced when the hair is wet, meaning that the hair must be dried before grooming to prevent hair breakage. Many patients confuse this

increased hair breakage with hair loss. The distinction can be determined on hair pull, yielding primarily broken hairs without a terminal bulb.

Bleached hair is also more porous, readily absorbs water, performs poorly under high humidity conditions, requires a longer drying time, tangles readily, and is more susceptible to damage from further chemical processing.[48]

NAIL POLISH

Nail polish represents the primary cosmetic adornment for the nails, yet in specialized cases, it can also be of therapeutic significance in the physical thickening of the nail plate or in repairing the damaged nail plate.

Nail polish was developed in the 1920s, when it was discovered that boiled nitrocellulose could be dissolved in organic solvents, yielding a hard, glossy film after solvent evaporation. Extensive research on nitrocellulose lacquer was undertaken by the automobile industry, which found the product preferable to slow-drying oil-based paints previously used to paint cars. This technology was directly adapted to the cosmetics industry by Charles Revlon, who founded Revlon in 1932 based on his pigmented, opaque nail polish. The basic ingredients found in nail polish and their functions are displayed in Table 36-9.[49]

Specialty ingredients can be added to this basic nail polish formulation to remedy some nail problems of medical significance. Rayon or nylon fibers dissolved within the polish can provide added nail strength and plasticity when firmly adherent to the nail plate. These formulations are known as "fibered" nail polishes. Nail polish can also be used to prevent or mend onychoschizia, or lamellar splitting of the nail plate, commonly seen in mature women.

There is some concern that the use of nail polish can contribute to nail dryness and brittleness. This actually is not the case. Nail polish prevents contact of detergents with the nail, thus acting as a protectant. Furthermore, it decreases nail water vapor loss from 1.6 to 0.4 mg/cm^2/hour.[50]

Allergic contact dermatitis is seen in sensitive individuals who may develop proximal nail fold erythema and edema, fingertip tenderness and swelling, or eyelid dermatitis.[51] The North Amer-

■ **Table 36-9**   Formulation of Nail Polish[49]

Ingredient	Function
Nitrocellulose	Film-former
Toluene-sulfonamide-formaldehyde	Traditional resin—source of allergic contact dermatitis
Polyester	Hypoallergenic resin—recommended for patients with nail polish sensitivity
Dibutyl phthalate	Plasticizer—keeps polish pliable
N-butyl acetate, ethyl acetate	Solvent—evaporates, leaving film
Toluene, isopropyl alcohol	Diluent—keeps polish thin, lowers cost

ican Contact Dermatitis Group determined that 4% of positive patch tests were due to toluenesulfonamide/formaldehyde resin.[52] Even though the allergic reaction is most commonly due to wet nail enamel, Tosti and associates[53] found that 11 out of 59 patients who were patch-test positive to wet polish also reacted to the dried enamel. Allergic reactions can be severe, necessitating lost work time or rarely hospitalization.[54]

Nail polish can be tested "as is," but should be allowed to thoroughly dry, as the volatile solvent can cause an irritant reaction if not allowed to evaporate rapidly. The toluenesulfonamide/formaldehyde resin can be also tested alone in 10% petrolatum.[55] Patients who are allergic to this resin may experience no difficulty with hypoallergenic nail polishes, but allergic contact dermatitis is still a possibility.[56]

Bibliography

Baran R, Maibach HI: *Textbook of cosmetic dermatology,* London, 1998, Martin Dunitz.

Draelos ZD: *Cosmetics in dermatology,* Edinburgh, 1995, Churchill Livingstone.

O'Donoghue MN: Cosmetics and cosmetic surgery in dermatology. *Clin Dermatol* 9:201, 1991.

References

Hydroquinone
1. Jimbow K, Obatha H, Pathak M, et al: Mechanism of depigmentation of hydroquinone. *J Invest Dermatol* 62:436-449, 1974.
2. Balima LM, Graupe K: The treatment of melasma—20% azelaic acid versus 4% hydroquinone cream. *Int J Dermatol* 30:893-895, 1993.
3. Hardwick N, van Gelder LW, van der Merwe CA: Exogenous ochronosis: an epidemiological study. *Br J Dermatol* 120:229-238, 1989.

Dihydroxyacetone
4. Levy SB: Dihydroxyacetone-containing sunless or self-tanning lotions. *J Am Acad Dermatol* 27:989-993, 1992.
5. Maibach HI, Kligman AM: Dihydroxyacetone: a suntan-simulating agent. *Arch Dermatol* 82:505-597, 1960.
6. Wittgenstein E, Berry HK: Staining of skin with dihydroxyacetone. *Science* 132:894-895, 1960.

Facial Foundations/Camouflage Cosmetics

7. Schlossman ML, Feldman AJ: Fluid foundations and blush make-up. In deNavarre MG, editor: *The chemistry and manufacture of cosmetics*, ed 2, Wheaton, IL, 1988, Allured Publishing, pp 741-765.

8. Draelos ZD: Cosmetics have a positive effect on the postsurgical patient. *Cosmet Dermatol* 4:11-14, 1991.

9. Thomas RJ, Bluestein JL: Cosmetics and hairstyling as adjuvants to scar camouflage. In Thomas RJ, Richard G, editors: *Facial scars*, St. Louis, 1989, CV Mosby, pp 349-351.

Skin Cleansers

10. Willcox MJ, Crichton WP: The soap market. *Cosmet Toilet* 104:61-63, 1989.

11. Wortzman MS: Evaluation of mild skin cleansers. *Dermatol Clin* 9:35-44, 1991.

12. Jackson EM: Soap: a complex category of products. *Am J Contact Dermatitis* 5:173-175, 1994.

13. Wortzman MS, Scott RA, Wong PS, et al: Soap and detergent bar rinsability. *J Soc Cosmet Chem* 37:89-97, 1986.

14. Prottey C, Ferguson T: Factors which determine the skin irritation potential of soap and detergents. *J Soc Cosmet Chem* 26:29, 1975.

15. Wickett RR, Trobaugh CM: Personal care products. *Cosmet Toilet* 105:41-46, 1990.

16. Wilhelm KP, Freitag G, Wolff HH: Surfactant-induced skin irritation and skin repair. *J Am Acad Dermatol* 30:944-999, 1994.

17. Frosch PJ: Irritancy of soaps and detergents. In Frost P, Horwitz SN, editors: *Principles of cosmetics for the dermtologist*, St. Louis, 1982, CV Mosby, pp 5-12.

18. Mills OH, Berger RS, Baker MD: A controlled comparison of skin cleansers in photoaged skin. *J Geriatr Dermatol* 1:173-179, 1993.

19. deNavarre MG: Cleansing creams. In deNavarre MG, editor: *The chemistry and manufacture of cosmetics*, vol III, ed 2, Wheaton, IL, 1975, Allured Publishing Corporation, pp 251-264.

20. Jass HE: Cold creams. In deNavarre MG, editor: *The chemistry and manufacture of cosmetics*, vol III, ed 2, Wheaton, IL, 1975, Allured Publishing Corporation, pp 237-249.

Moisturizers

21. Goldner R: Moisturizers: a dermatologist's perspective. *J Toxicol—Cutan Ocular Toxicol* 11:193-197, 1992.

22. Boisits EK: The evaluation of moisturizing products. *Cosmet Toilet* 101:31-39, 1986.

23. Wu MS, Yee DJ, Sullivan ME: Effect of a skin moisturizer on the water distribution in human stratum corneum. *J Invest Dermatol* 81:446-448, 1983.

24. Pierard GE: What does "dry skin" mean? *Int J Dermatol* 26:167-168, 1987.

25. Elias PM: Lipids and the epidermal permeability barrier. *Arch Dermatol Res* 270:95-117, 1981.

Hair Shampoos

26. Bouillon C: Shampoos and hair conditioners. *Clin Dermatol* 6:83-92, 1988.

27. Robbins CR: Interaction of shampoo and creme rinse ingredients with human hair. In Robbins CR: *Chemical and physical behavior of human hair*, ed 2, New York, 1988, Springer-Verlag, pp 122-167.

28. Markland WR: Shampoos. In deNavarre MG, editor: *The chemistry and manufacture of cosmetics*, vol IV, ed 2, Wheaton IL, 1988, Allured Publishing, pp 1283-1312.

29. Fox C: An introduction to the formulation of shampoos. *Cosmet Toilet* 103:25-58, 1988.

30. Rieger M: Surfactants in shampoos. *Cosmet Toilet* 103:59-72, 1988.

Hair Permanent Waving Agents

31. Lee AE, Bozza JB, Huff S, de la Mettrie R: Permanent waves: an overview. *Cosmet Toilet* 103:37-56, 1988.

32. Wickett RR: Disulfide bond reduction in permanent waving. *Cosmet Toilet* 106:37-47, 1991.

33. Draelos ZK: Hair cosmetics. *Dermatol Clin* 9:19-27, 1991.

Hair Straightening Agents

34. Cannell DW: Permanent waving and hair straightening. *Clin Dermatol* 6:71-82, 1988.

35. Hsuing DY: Hair straightening. In deNavarre M, editor: *The chemistry and manufacture of cosmetics*, ed 2, Wheaton IL, 1975, Allured Publishing, p 1155.

36. Bulengo K, Bergfeld WF: Chemical and traumatic alopecia from thioglycolate in a black woman. *Cutis* 49:99-103, 1992.

Hair Dyeing Agents

37. Corbett JF: Hair coloring. *Clin Dermatol* 6:93-101, 1988.

38. Spoor HJ: Permanent hair colorants: oxidation dyes 1. Chemical technology. *Cutis* 19:424-430, 1977.

39. Corbett JF: Changing the color of hair. In Frost P, Horwitz SN, editors: *Principles of cosmetics for the dermatologist,* St. Louis, 1982, CV Mosby, pp 160-163.

40. Spoor HJ: Part II: metals. *Cutis* 19:37-40, 1977.

41. Spoor HJ: Hair dyes: temporary colorings. *Cutis* 18:341-344, 1976.

42. Spoor HJ: Semi-permanent hair color. *Cutis* 18:506-508, 1976.

43. Zviak C: Hair coloring, nonoxidation coloring. In Zviak C, editor: *The science of hair care,* New York, 1986, Marcel Dekker, pp 235-261.

44. Tucker HH: Formulation of oxidation hair dyes. *Am J Perfum Cosmet* 83:69, 1968.

45. Zviak C: Oxidation coloring. In Zviak C, editor: *The science of hair care,* New York, 1986, Marcel Dekker, pp 263-286.

Hair Bleaching Agents

46. Zviak C: Hair bleaching. In Zviak C, editor: *The science of hair care,* New York, 1986, Marcel Dekker, pp 213-233.

47. Corbett JF: Hair coloring processes. *Cosmet Toilet* 106:53-57, 1991.

48. Wall FE: Bleaches, hair colorings, and dye removers. In Balsam MS, Gershon SD, Rieger MM, et al, editors: *Cosmetics science and technology,* vol 2, ed 2, New York, 1972, Wiley-Interscience, pp 279-343.

Nail Polish

49. Wimmer EP, Scholssman ML: The history of nail polish. *Cosmet Toilet* 107:115-120, 1992.

50. Mast R: Nail products. In Whittam JH, editor: *Cosmetic safety—a primer for cosmetic scientists,* New York, 1987, Marcel Dekker, pp 265-313.

51. Scher RK: Cosmetics and ancillary preparations for the care of the nails. *J Am Acad Dermatol* 6:523-528, 1982.

52. Adams RM, Maibach HI: A five-year study of cosmetic reactions. *J Am Acad Dermatol* 13:1062-1069, 1985.

53. Tosti A, Buerra L, Vincenzi C, et al: Contact sensitization caused by toluene sulfonamide-formaldehyde resin in women who use nail cosmetics. *Am J Contact Dermatitis* 4:150, 1993.

54. Liden C, Berg M, Farm G, et al: Nail varnish allergy with far-reaching consequences. *Br J Dermatol* 128:57-62, 1993.

55. deGroot AC, Weyland JW, Nater JP, editors: *Unwanted effects of cosmetics and drugs used in dermatology,* ed 3, New York, 1994, Elsevier, p 526.

56. Shaw S: A case of contact dermatitis from hypoallergenic nail varnish. *Contact Dermatitis* 20:385, 1989.

Thomas J. Eads

Miscellaneous Topical Agents

This chapter consists of a variety of unrelated topical products prescribed and recommended by dermatologists that do not fit neatly into other chapters in this book. Only becaplermin (Regranex) and anthralin (Drithocreme, Micanol) currently require a prescription; minoxidil 2% (Rogaine) was available by prescription only until 1996, when the drug became available over-the-counter (OTC). For many of these drugs there are relatively few data on which to provide broad scientific generalizations. Nevertheless, these drugs warrant at least a brief discussion here, given significant numbers of patient questions about these products, enhanced by liberal direct-to-consumer marketing for many of the drugs in this chapter.

MINOXIDIL (ROGAINE)
Pharmacology
Minoxidil (Figure 37-1) is available in 2% and 5% topical solutions. The 2% solution contains 60% alcohol, whereas the 5% solution contains 30% alcohol.

MECHANISM OF ACTION
The specific mechanism of action is not known but does not appear to be due to vasodilation or to an antiandrogen mechanism. Minoxidil increases the duration of the anagen growth phase and gradually enlarges miniaturized hair follicles (vellus hairs) into mature terminal hairs.[1]

Clinical Uses
FDA-APPROVED INDICATION. Rogaine (2% minoxidil) was approved for prescription use by the Food and Drug Administration (FDA) in 1988. The 2% strength was approved by the FDA for OTC use in androgenetic alopecia in February 1996. The 5% strength was approved for OTC use in November 1997. The products are indicated for use in male pattern androgenetic alopecia (both concentrations) of the vertex of the scalp, and for female pattern androgenetic alopecia (2% concentration only) of the frontoparietal areas, with diffuse thinning. Minoxidil is most efficacious in the treatment of androgenetic alopecia affecting the crown area. The drug usually preserves, if not reduces, the horizontal diameter of alopecia in the crown area.[2] Studies showed that in the first 4 months of treatment, vellus hair growth constitutes much of the total hair regrowth. Thereafter terminal hair growth becomes noticeable, and these terminal hairs may increase in number up through 12 months. Therapy with minoxidil should be continued at the full twice-daily schedule indefinitely because patients who go to a daily maintenance schedule beginning at 12 months may have decreased hair counts.[2-4]

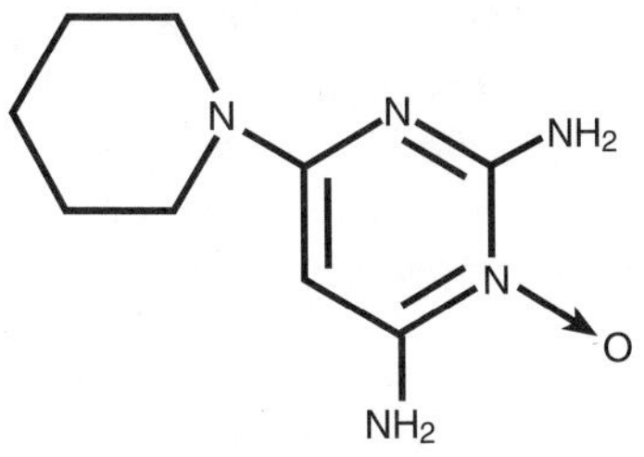

Figure 37-1   Minoxidil.

OFF-LABEL USES.   Minoxidil has been reported to have at least some efficacy in alopecia areata, congenital hypotrichosis, and loose anagen syndrome.[1]

DOSING.   All published studies evaluated Rogaine with 1 ml applied to the scalp twice a day. Therapy needs to be continued indefinitely for maintenance.

ADVERSE EFFECTS.   Irritant dermatitis and allergic contact dermatitis each occur in less than 10% of cases. Hypertrichosis of skin other than the scalp can occur if there is inadvertent application to that site. Systemic absorption is minimal. An average of 1.4% of the applied dose is absorbed. For the standard 1 ml dose, this would result in 0.28 mg of systemic absorption. If minoxidil were to be applied to the entire scalp, a systemic dose in the range of 2.4 to 5.4 mg/day might be expected.[2,5]

PREGNANCY PRESCRIBING STATUS.   Minoxidil is not recommended for pregnant or nursing women.

BECAPLERMIN (REGRANEX)
Pharmacology
Becaplermin is recombinant, human, platelet-derived growth factor-BB (PDGF-BB) and is available as a gel containing 100 µg of becaplermin per gram of gel. It is available in 2-, 7.5-, and 15-g tubes.

MECHANISM OF ACTION.   Becaplermin is biologically similar to endogenous PDGF. It promotes the chemotactic recruitment and proliferation of cells involved in wound healing. Becaplermin is thought to enhance the formation of granulation tissue, making the wound more suitable for reepithelialization.

Clinical Use
FDA-APPROVED INDICATIONS.   Becaplermin gel is indicated for the treatment of lower extremity, diabetic, neuropathic ulcers that extend into the subcutis and have an adequate blood supply. It is to be used in conjunction with a good ulcer care regimen, including debridement if necessary, pressure relief, and infection control. A review of four multicenter randomized placebo-controlled studies, with a total of 922 patients, showed becaplermin gel plus wound care to be superior to wound care alone. Three of the studies showed a statistically significant difference, whereas one study failed to establish a statistically significant difference.[6-9] Adverse reactions were similar for both treatment and placebo groups.

OFF-LABEL USES.   A phase II randomized, double-blind, placebo-controlled study showed becaplermin gel to be efficacious in the treatment of chronic full thickness pressure ulcers. In this study, patients were treated once daily with becaplermin gel. All patients received good overall wound care as well. Treatment with the gel increased the incidence of both complete healing and decreased ulcer volume at the end of the 16-week treatment period.[10]

DOSING.   Becaplermin gel is applied once daily to the ulcer in a thin continuous layer of 1/16-inch thickness. The wound is then covered with a saline-moistened dressing and left in place for 12 hours. The dressing is then removed and the gel is rinsed off with water, and another saline-moistened gauze is applied to the wound without the becaplermin underneath it[6] (Table 37-1). This two-step process is repeated daily.

ADVERSE EFFECTS.   The package insert notes that "erythematous rashes" occurred in 2% of patients on becaplermin gel, and none in the control group. Otherwise there were no local or systemic adverse reactions that occurred more frequently in the becaplermin-treated patients.[6]

PREGNANCY PRESCRIBING STATUS.   Becaplermin is classified as pregnancy category C.

■ **Table 37-1** Formula to Calculate Length of Regranex Gel in Centimeters to Be Applied Daily

Tube Size	Formula
2-g tube	(Length of ulcer × width of ulcer)/2
7.5- or 15-g tube	(Length of ulcer × width of ulcer)/4

Animal reproduction studies have not been done. It is unknown if the gel can cause any fetal harm. It is also not known if becaplermin is excreted into human milk.[6]

ANTHRALIN (DRITHOCREME, MICANOL)

Pharmacology

Drithocreme is a brand of anthralin available in a cream base with concentrations of 0.1%, 0.25%, 0.5%, and 1%. The base is composed mainly of petrolatum and water.

Micanol is a form of anthralin that is formulated in a unique delivery system. The anthralin is encapsulated in a matrix of semicrystalline monoglycerides known as crystalip. The layers of the crystalline monoglycerides protect the anthralin from oxidation and promote its stability, providing also for fewer adverse effects.[11,12]

MECHANISM OF ACTION.   Anthralin stimulates monocyte proinflammatory activity and induces extracellular generation of oxygen free radicals.[13-15] Anthralin also has anti-Langerhans' cell effects.[16]

Clinical Use

FDA-APPROVED INDICATIONS.   Anthralin is approved for the treatment of chronic plaque psoriasis. Anthralin was first synthesized over 80 years ago. The natural product, chrysarobin, comes from the South American araroba tree. Its most common use has been in the treatment of psoriasis, especially on plaques resistant to other therapies. Anthralin has been combined with ultraviolet B (UVB) phototherapy with

good results.[17] Due to staining and irritancy, anthralin has never been widely used in the United States. To overcome these adverse effects, anthralin short contact therapy became a more standard way of dosing topical anthralin (see Dosing section).

OFF-LABEL USES.   Anthralin has also been commonly used for alopecia areata. The overall safety of anthralin has made it useful in children and in adults with extensive alopecia areata, especially alopecia totalis. Growth of new hair may begin at 2 to 3 months, and approximately 25% of patients have cosmetically acceptable hair regrowth at 6 months.[18] Short contact therapy is also recommended to avoid irritation, although some degree of irritation may be necessary for a therapeutic response with alopecia areata.[1,19]

DOSING.   Short contact therapy is recommended to prevent the irritancy of the anthralin. The most common approach is to start with a lower concentration of anthralin such as 0.1%. The anthralin is left on for 10 to 20 minutes daily, and the contact time is increased weekly until the contact time is 1 hour. This approach generally reduces cutaneous irritation. Nevertheless, staining continues to be a problem. A product that contains triethanolamine (Cura-Stain) is available to reduce the irritation and staining seen with anthralin. The product is sprayed on the skin before cleaning off the anthralin and again after the removal of the material. This prevents much of the staining noted with anthralin.[12,20]

ADVERSE EFFECTS.   As previously mentioned, irritant contact dermatitis and staining of clothing, skin, hair, and nails are the most commonly observed adverse reactions seen with anthralin.

ASCORBIC ACID (VITAMIN C— CELLEX)

Pharmacology

It is difficult to stabilize ascorbic acid in a topical preparation. Cellex-C International offers several commercially available preparations, with various additives that reportedly improve

■ **Table 37-2** Representative Cellex-C Serum Products[21]

Product	Primary Ingredients
High potency serum (30 ml)	L-ascorbic acid 10%, tyrosine, zinc
Advanced-C serum (30 ml)	L-ascorbic acid 17.5%, tyrosine, zinc, resveratrol, grape seed extract, and L-ergothioneine

the stability of vitamin C in their two products (Table 37-2).

MECHANISM OF ACTION. Ascorbic acid is a necessary cofactor for the enzymes prolyl hydroxylase and lysyl hydroxylase. These enzymes are used in the formation of a stable collagen molecule and the cross-linking of collagen, respectively. UV light exposure results in the formation of free radical oxygen species and also depletes cutaneous ascorbic acid stores.

It is thought that topical ascorbic acid exerts its effect by scavenging free oxygen radicals in the aqueous compartments and by stimulating and improving collagen synthesis. Ascorbic acid does not absorb UVA/UVB and is therefore not useful as a sunscreening agent.

The addition of tyrosine and zinc to Cellex High Potency Serum has been shown to provide more than 20 times the amount of ascorbic acid found in normal skin.[22,23] The Cellex Advanced-C Serum contains resveratrol (a free radical scavenger extracted from mulberries and grapes) and L-ergothioneine (also a natural antioxidant) to further stabilize vitamin C.

Clinical Uses
INDICATIONS. Topical ascorbic acid is commonly used in the treatment of photoaged skin. A randomized, double-blind, vehicle-controlled study showed improvement in fine wrinkling, tactile roughness, coarse rhytides, skin laxity, and yellowing. Most of the clinical improvements were in tactile roughness/texture and skin hydration.[22]

DOSING. The recommended dose is 6 drops (1 ml) applied to the face daily.

ADVERSE EFFECTS. The only adverse effects reported are mild and typically resolve in the first 2 months of therapy. These minor adverse effects included stinging (55%), erythema (24%), and dry skin (<1%).[22]

PHYTONADIONE (VITAMIN K$_1$— K-Derm)
Pharmacology
Topically applied phytonadione is available as a 2% cream (K-Derm), which contains propylene glycol and parabens in the vehicle.

MECHANISM OF ACTION. The precise mechanism of topically applied phytonadione is unknown. Oral vitamin K is used to treat bleeding diatheses in patients on warfarin anticoagulation through hepatic generation of "vitamin K–dependent" clotting factors II, VII, IX, and X.

Clinical Use
INDICATIONS. Promotional literature regarding K-Derm from the S.F. Group shows dramatic results in such conditions as actinic purpura, postoperative purpura, telangiectasias, progressive pigmented purpura, and traumatic purpura. In a vehicle-controlled study in patients with actinic purpura, the K-Derm–treated areas healed significantly quicker after trauma (2.5 versus 8 days), and less purpura was noted overall. In trauma-induced purpura, the bruising cleared in 5 to 8 days in the treated bruises versus 11 to 13 days in the untreated bruises.[24]

DOSING. Apply K-Derm twice daily to affected areas. For the prevention of postoperative bruising, it is recommended that the cream be applied twice daily for 2 weeks before the procedure.

ADVERSE EFFECTS. No significant adverse reactions have been published by the S.F. Group, nor in peer-reviewed journals. It is unknown as to whether there is enough systemic absorption of the vitamin K to alter the prothrombin time or international normalized ratio (INR) of patients on warfarin anticoagulants.

VITAMIN E (MIRAK, MANY OTHERS)
Pharmacology
α-Tocopherol is the physiologically active form of vitamin E, specifically the δ fraction.

MECHANISM OF ACTION.   Vitamin E is the main lipid-soluble antioxidant for the protection of cell membranes. Vitamin E is a free radical scavenger.

Clinical Use
INDICATIONS
   Prevention of Skin Cancer.   Topical vitamin E has been effective in animals in reducing UV-induced erythema and edema. It has also been shown to reduce skin photoaging effects, skin cancer, and UV radiation–induced immunosuppression in animals. The evidence in humans has not been as clear. It may be that other antioxidants (e.g., ascorbic acid, selenium, β-carotene) in oral form are necessary to prevent tocopherol degradation.[25,26]
   Scars.   In spite of a favorable reputation, topical vitamin E has not been found to improve scar thickness or appearance.[25]
   Psoriasis.   Mirak is a new product containing vitamin E touted as being efficacious for treatment of psoriasis. The Mirak Home Care Packs consist of natural spring water, volcanic earth, and vitamin E cream. A recent placebo-controlled left-right study was done in the Netherlands to determine its efficacy. Clinical and histologic parameters were evaluated in a 6-week treatment study. The results showed that the Mirak-treated lesions had a significantly greater reduction in induration than the placebo-treated lesions. Although a reduction in desquamation and a decrease in histologic proliferation were also seen in the Mirak-treated lesions, there was not a significant difference compared with placebo-treated lesions. The conclusion was that the Mirak Home Care Packs induce a modest therapeutic effect compared with placebo. No significant adverse effects were reported.[27]

ADVERSE EFFECTS.   Follicular occlusive dermatitis has been reported.[25] Overall, adverse effects from vitamin E are quite uncommon.[27]

ALUMINUM CHLORIDE (DRYSOL, CERTAIN-DRI)
Pharmacology
Aluminum chloride has the chemical formula $AlCl_3$. This drug is available as a 20% solution in 93% anhydrous ethyl alcohol (Drysol) and a 12% solution (Certain-Dri pads and roll-on bottle).

MECHANISM OF ACTION.   Aluminum chloride reversibly inhibits eccrine gland secretion. Generally this effect persists for days and not weeks. The precise mechanism of action for this effect is unknown.

Clinical Uses
INDICATIONS.   Aluminum chloride 20% is most often used for hemostasis after minor procedures such as shave biopsies or curettage. The advantage of aluminum chloride over Monsel's solution is that it does not leave an iron residue that can persist in the dermis. The advantage of aluminum chloride over electrocautery for hemostasis is that aluminum chloride does not cause as much scarring. Aluminum chloride is useful for the treatment of palmar, plantar, and axillary hyperhidrosis.[28] Aluminum chloride has also been reported to be useful in facial and scalp hyperhidrosis.[29,30] Prevention of foot blisters while walking long distances in the heat, such as in hikers and military recruits, is an important indication for aluminum chloride.[31,32]

DOSING.   Recommendations regarding frequency of applications vary in the literature, ranging from daily applications to once weekly applications. In general it is felt that the lower concentration solutions can be applied daily. The 20% solution can be used daily initially, then tapered to thrice weekly or even once weekly as needed. The solution should be applied to completely dry skin.[28]

ADVERSE EFFECTS.   Uncommon minor reactions include irritant dermatitis, burning, or prickling sensation.[28] Significant caution should be given for use near the eye. Electrocautery should be performed only after aluminum chloride to avoid igniting this solution.

ALOE VERA

Aloe vera has extensive popular support in the lay press for a wide variety of uses. Scientific evidence supporting these uses is sparse. There have been anecdotal published reports suggesting aloe vera efficacy for acute frostbite,[33,34] lichen planus,[35] enhancement of post-dermabrasion wound healing,[36] psoriasis,[37] and venous leg ulcers.[38] Other studies failed to show any benefit in aphthous stomatitis,[39] prevention of radiation-induced skin toxicity,[40] and wound healing.[41] Allergic contact dermatitis has been reported.

Bibliography

Keller KL, Fenske NA: Uses of vitamins A, C, and E and related compounds in dermatology: a review. *J Am Acad Dermatol* 39:611-625, 1998.

Kemeny L, Ruzicka T, Braun-Falco O: Dithranol: a review of the mechanism of action in the treatment of psoriasis vulgaris. *Skin Pharmacol* 3:1-20, 1990.

Price VH: Drug therapy: treatment of hair loss. *N Engl J Med* 341:964-973, 1999.

Smiell JM, Wieman TJ, Steed DL, et al: Efficacy and safety of becaplermin in patients with non-healing, lower extremity diabetic ulcers: a combined analysis of four randomized studies. *Wound Repair Regen* 7:335-346, 1999.

References

Minoxidil

1. Price VH: Drug therapy: treatment of hair loss. *N Engl J Med* 341:964-973, 1999.
2. Katz HI, Hien NT, Prawer SE, et al: Long-term efficacy of topical minoxidil in male pattern baldness. *J Am Acad Dermatol* 16:711-718, 1987.
3. DeVillez RL: Androgenetic alopecia treated with topical minoxidil. *J Am Acad Dermatol* 16:669-672, 1987.
4. Roberts JL: Androgenetic alopecia: treatment results with topical minoxidil. *J Am Acad Dermatol* 16:705-710, 1987.
5. Franz TJ: Percutaneous absorption of minoxidil in man. *Arch Dermatol* 121:203-206, 1985.

Becaplermin

6. *Physicians' desk reference*, ed 53, Montvale, NJ, 1999, Medical Economics Co., pp 2243-2244.
7. Wieman TJ, Smiell JM, Su Y: Efficacy and safety of a topical gel formulation of recombinant human platelet derived growth factor-BB (becaplermin) in patients with chronic neuropathic diabetic ulcers: a phase III randomized placebo-controlled double-blind study. *Diabetes Care* 21:822-827, 1998.

8. Wieman TJ: Clinical efficacy of becaplermin (rhPDGF-BB) gel. Becaplermin gel studies group. *Am J Surg* 176(Suppl 2A):74S-79S, 1998.
9. Smiell JM, Wieman TJ, Steed DL, et al: Efficacy and safety of becaplermin in patients with non-healing, lower extremity diabetic ulcers: a combined analysis of four randomized studies. *Wound Rep Regen* 7:335-346, 1999.
10. Rees RS, Robson MC, Smiel JM, et al: Becaplermin gel in the treatment of pressure ulcers: a phase II randomized, double blind, placebo-controlled study. *Wound Rep Regen* 7:141-147, 1999.

Anthralin

11. Juhlin L: Nordic dithranol symposium—introduction. *Acta Derm Venereol* 192 (Suppl):5, 1992.
12. Harris DR: Old wine in new bottles: the revival of anthralin. *Cutis* 62:201-203, 1998.
13. Schmidt KN, Powda M, Packer L, et al: Antipsoriatic drug anthralin activates transcription factor NF-kappa B in murine keratinocytes. *J Immunol* 156:4514-4519, 1996.
14. Mrowietz U, Falsafi M, Schroder JM, et al: Inhibition of human monocyte functions by anthralin. *Br J Dermatol* 127:382-386, 1992.

15. Kemeny L, Ruzicka T, Braun-Falco O: Dithranol: a review of the mechanism of action in the treatment of psoriasis vulgaris. *Skin Pharmacol* 3:1-20, 1990.

16. Morhenn VB, Orenberg EK, Kaplan J, et al: Inhibition of a Langerhans' cell-mediated immune response by treatment modalities useful in psoriasis. *J Invest Dermatol* 81:23-27, 1983.

17. Carrozza P, Hausermann P, Nestle PO, et al: Clinical efficacy of narrow-band UVB (311 nm) combined with dithranol in psoriasis. An open pilot study. *Dermatology* 200:35-39, 2000.

18. Fiedler-Weiss VC, Buys CM: Evaluation of anthralin in the treatment of alopecia areata. *Arch Dermatol* 123:1491-1493, 1987.

19. Swanson NA, Mitchell AJ, Leahy MS, et al: Topical treatment of alopecia areata. *Arch Dermatol* 117:384-387, 1981.

20. Ramsay B, Lawrence CM, Shuster S, et al: Reduction of anthralin-induced inflammation by application of amines. *J Am Acad Dermatol* 22:765-772, 1990.

Ascorbic Acid

21. Cellex-C international: Company literature. www.cellex-c.com

22. Traikovich SS: Use of topical ascorbic acid and its effects on photodamaged skin topography. *Arch Otolaryngol Head Neck Surg* 125:1091-1098, 1999.

23. Halperin EC, Gaspar L, George S, et al: A double-blind, randomized prospective trial to evaluate topical vitamin C solution for the prevention of radiation dermatitis. *Int J Radiat Oncol Biol Phys* 26:413-416, 1996.

Phytonadione (Vitamin K$_1$)

24. Elson ML: Topical phytonadione (vitamin K$_1$) in the treatment of actinic and traumatic purpura. *Cosmet Dermatol* 8:25-26, 1995.

Vitamin E

25. Keller KL, Fenske NA: Uses of vitamins A, C, and E and related compounds in dermatology: a review. *J Am Acad Dermatol* 39:611-625, 1998.

26. Fuchs J: Potentials and limitations of the natural antioxidants RRR-alpha-tocopherol. L-ascorbic acid and beta-carotene in cutaneous photoprotection. *Free Radic Biol Med* 25:848-873, 1998.

27. Seyger MM, van de Kerkhof PC, van Vlijmen-Willems IM, et al: The efficacy of a new topical treatment for psoriasis. *Mirak J Eur Acad Dermatol Venereol* 11:13-18, 1998.

Aluminum Chloride

28. Anonymous: Drysol for treatment of hyperhidrosis. *Med Lett Drugs Ther* 19:20, 1977.

29. Dworin A, Sober AJ: Unilateral segmental hyperhidrosis. Response to 20% aluminum chloride solution and plastic wrap. *Arch Dermatol* 114:770-771, 1978.

30. Boyvat A, Piskin G, Erdi H: Idiopathic unilateral localized hyperhidrosis. *Acta Derm Venereol* 79:404-405, 1999.

31. Reynolds K, Darrigrand A, Roberts D, et al: Effects of an antiperspirant with emollients on foot sweat accumulation and blister formation while walking in the heat. *J Am Acad Dermatol* 33:626-630, 1995.

32. Benohanian A, Dansereau A: Influence of an antiperspirant on foot blister incidence during cross-country hiking. *J Am Acad Dermatol* 41:655-656, 1999.

Aloe Vera

33. McCauley RL, Heggers JP, Robson MC: Frostbite. Methods to minimize tissue loss. *Postgrad Med* 88(8):67-68, 73-77, 1990.

34. Heggers JP, Robson MC, Manavalen K, et al: Experimental and clinical observations on frostbite. *Ann Emerg Med* 16:1056-1062, 1987.

35. Hayes SM: Lichen planus—report of successful treatment with aloe. *Gen Dentistry* 47:268-272, 1999.

36. Fulton JE Jr: The stimulation of post dermabrasion wound healing with stabilized aloe vera gel-polyethylene oxide dressing. *J Dermatol Surg Oncol* 16:460-467, 1990.

37. Syed TA, Ahmad SA, Holt AH, et al: Management of psoriasis with aloe vera extract in a hydrophilic cream: a placebo-controlled, double blind study. *Trop Med Int Health* 1:505-509, 1996.

38. Atherton P: Aloe vera: magic or medicine? *Nurs Standards* 12:49-54, 1998.

39. Garnick JJ, Singh B, Winkley G: Effectiveness of a medicament containing silicon dioxide, aloe, and allantoin on aphthous stomatitis. *Oral Surg Oral Med Oral Pathol Oral Radiol Endodont* 86:550-556, 1998.

40. Williams MS, Burk M, Loprinzi CL, et al: Phase III double-blind evaluation of an aloe vera gel as a prophylactic agent for radiation induced skin toxicity. *Int J Rad Oncol Biol Phys* 36:345-349, 1996.

41. Rund CR: Non-conventional topical therapies for wound care. *Ostomy Wound Manage* 42:18-26, 1996.

CHAPTER 38

Mark S. Fradin

Insect Repellents

The first broad-spectrum chemical insect repellent, *N,N*-diethyl-3-methylbenzamide (DEET) (Figure 38-1), was brought to the United States market in 1957. This repellent proved to be effective against mosquitoes, ticks, biting flies, midges, chiggers, and fleas. Although these insects are mostly a source of nuisance in North America, worldwide they transmit to humans multiple bacterial, viral, protozoan, parasitic, and rickettsial diseases (Box 38-1).[1,2] Mosquitoes alone transmit disease to more than 700 million people yearly and cause 3 million deaths annually from malaria.[3]

Protection from insect bites is best achieved through the use of personal protection and habitat control. Personal protection involves avoiding infested habitats, wearing protective clothing, and applying insect repellents. Habitat control is achieved through the judicious use of chemical and biologic agents, including pesticides and insect growth regulators.

Scientific information on effective insect repellents is not readily available to consumers. The lay literature is full of anecdotal, unsupported claims of effectiveness for "natural" topical insect repellents, oral repellents, electronic repelling devices, mosquito-repelling plants, and bug "zappers." This chapter reviews the available scientific data on insect repellents and debunks some of the popular myths regarding many of the "alternative" repellents. The covered topics are summarized, grouped by efficacy, in Box 38-2.

INSECT BIOLOGY

Mosquitoes and ticks are the major vectors of arthropod-borne disease. Mosquitoes may be found all over the world, except in Antarctica. Members of the genera *Anopheles*, *Culex*, and *Aedes* most commonly bite man. More than 170 species of mosquitoes live in North America. Mosquitoes require an aquatic environment with standing water in which to develop. As a group, they adapted to complete their life cycle in a variety of habitats, including fresh water, salt water marshes, brackish water, or in water found in containers, old tires, or tree stump holes. The life cycle of the mosquito has four stages. Mosquitoes lay their eggs on the surface of still water. The eggs hatch in a few days, become larvae, change into pupae, and finally metamorphose into adult mosquitoes. Only female mosquitoes bite, requiring a blood protein meal to produce eggs.

Two families of ticks are known to be capable of transmitting pathogens to man—Ixodidae (hard ticks) and Argasidae (soft ticks). Hard ticks are so-named due to the presence of a sclerotized plate, or scutum, that covers part of their bodies. In the United States, soft ticks of the single genus *Ornithodoros* are capable of transmitting to humans the *Borrelia* spirochete that causes relapsing fever. Three genera of Ixodidae transmit disease to man—*Ixodes* (vectors for Lyme disease, babesiosis, and tick paralysis); *Dermacentor* (vectors for tularemia, Rocky Mountain

Box 38-1

Diseases Transmitted to Humans by Biting Insects[1,2]

MOSQUITOES
Eastern equine encephalitis*
St. Louis encephalitis*
Western equine encephalitis*
La Cross encephalitis*
Malaria
Yellow fever
Dengue fever
Bancroftian filariasis
Epidemic polyarthritis
Chikungunya fever

FLIES
Tularemia*
Leishmaniasis
African trypanosomiasis (sleeping sickness)
Onchocerciasis
Loa loa

CHIGGER MITES
Scrub typhus

TICKS
Lyme disease*
Rocky Mountain spotted fever*
Colorado tick fever*
Relapsing fever*
Ehrlichiosis*
Babesiosis*
Tularemia*
Tick paralysis*
Rickettsial pox*
Siberian tick typhus

FLEAS
Plague*
Murine typhus
Lice
Epidemic typhus
Relapsing fever

*May be found in the United States.

Box 38-2

Methods for Reducing the Risk of Arthropod Bites

PROVEN EFFECTIVE
Protective clothing
Screening on windows, tents
Avoidance of infested habitats
DEET-based insect repellents
Blocker repellent
Permethrin-sprayed clothing or tents
Elimination of standing water from one's home
    environment

LIMITED EFFECTIVENESS
Citronella-based repellents
Most plant-based repellents

LIMITED EFFECTIVENESS—cont'd
Skin-So-Soft Bath Oil
Citronella candles
Yard foggers

PROVEN INEFFECTIVE
Oral thiamine
Bug "zappers"
Bat houses
Blue marlin bird houses
Electronic repellers
Citronella-scented plants

spotted fever, ehrlichiosis, Colorado tick fever, and tick paralysis); and *Amblyomma* (vectors for tularemia, ehrlichiosis, and tick paralysis).[2,4] The life cycle of hard ticks takes 2 years and involves four stages of growth: the egg, six-legged larva, eight-legged immature nymph, and eight-legged sexually mature adult. Eggs hatch directly into larva, but each successive molt thereafter requires a blood meal. Most hard ticks require three hosts to complete their life cycle.

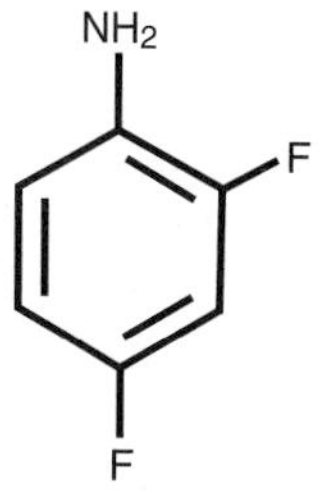

DEET

Figure 38-1   Representative insect repellent.

Larval, nymph, and adult ticks may all transmit disease during feeding. Both male and female ticks bite. Transovarial transmission enables female ticks to directly infect their offspring.

STIMULI THAT ATTRACT INSECTS

The factors involved in attracting insects to a host are complex, and not fully understood. Ticks are unable to fly or jump. They climb vegetation and "quest," waiting passively for hours or days, until they detect the vibration or carbon dioxide plume of a passing host.[5,6] Once on a host, they crawl around searching for an appropriate location on which to attach and feed.

The stimuli that attract mosquitoes to a host are much more complex.[7-12] Mosquitoes use visual, thermal, and olfactory stimuli to locate a host. Of these, olfactory cues are of greatest importance. For mosquitoes that feed during the daytime, host movement and the wearing of dark-colored clothing may initiate orientation towards an individual.[13,14] Visual stimuli appear to be important for in-flight orientation, particularly over long ranges, whereas olfactory stimuli become more important as a mosquito nears its host.

Carbon dioxide and lactic acid are the best-studied insect attractants. Carbon dioxide serves as a long-range attractant, at distances up to 36 meters.[13,15-17] At close range, skin warmth and moisture serve as attractants.[10,13,18] Volatile compounds, derived from sebum, eccrine, and apocrine sweat, or the cutaneous microflora bacterial action on these secretions, may also act as chemoattractants.[7,19,20] Anhidrotic individuals show markedly decreased attractiveness to mos-

quitoes.[7] Floral fragrances found in perfumes, lotions, soaps, and hair-care products may also attract mosquitoes.[21]

There can be significant variability in the attractiveness of different individuals to the same or different species of mosquitoes.[18,22] Men tend to be bitten by mosquitoes more readily than women,[13,23] and adults are more likely to be bitten than children.[18,22,24] Heavyset people are more likely to attract mosquitoes, perhaps due to their greater relative heat or carbon dioxide output.[25]

INSECT REPELLENTS

Despite the obvious desirability of finding an effective *oral* insect repellent, no such agent has yet been identified. There is no scientific evidence that ingesting garlic repels insects. Likewise, vitamin B_1 (thiamine), purported to be effective against mosquitoes, does not work.[26,27] Tests of over 100 ingested drugs, including other vitamins, failed to reveal any that worked well as repellents against mosquitoes.[28]

The search for the "perfect" topical repellent continues. The ideal agent would repel multiple species of biting arthropods, remain effective for at least 8 hours, cause no irritation to skin or mucous membranes, possess no systemic toxicity, be resistant to abrasion and washoff, and be greaseless and odorless. No presently available insect repellent meets all of these criteria. Efforts to find such a compound have been hampered by the multiplicity of variables that affect the inherent repellency of any chemical. Repellents do not all share a single mode of action, and different species of insects may react differently to the same repellent.[29-31]

To be effective as an insect repellent, a chemical must be volatile enough to maintain an effective repellent vapor concentration at the skin surface, but not evaporate so rapidly that it quickly loses its effectiveness. Multiple factors (Box 38-3) play a role in how effective a repellent is. These factors include the concentration, frequency, and uniformity of application, the user's activity level, the user's overall attractiveness to blood-sucking arthropods, and the number and species of the organisms trying to bite.[32] Gender may also play a role in how well a re-

Box 38-3

Factors that Affect Repellent Effectiveness[33-36]

PRODUCT-DEPENDENT

Evaporation rate from skin surface
Absorption rate from skin surface
Inherent resistance to abrasion from skin
surface
Inherent resistance to washoff from skin
surface

PRODUCT-INDEPENDENT

Environmental
Species of the biting insect
Density of the biting insects
Wind velocity
Air temperature
Wet environment (rain/water) leading to
washoff of repellent

User-dependent
Activity level of the host
User's inherent attractiveness to biting
arthropods
Frequency of repellent application
Uniformity of repellent application to the skin
Concentration of the repellent on the skin
surface
Anatomic site of repellent application

---

pellent works—DEET-based repellents seem to be less effective in women than in men.[33] The effectiveness of any repellent is reduced by abrasion from clothing; by evaporation and absorption from the skin surface; by washoff from sweat, rain, or water; or by a windy environment.[18,34-37] Each 10° C increase in ambient temperature can lead to as much as a 50% reduction in protection time, probably as a result of increased evaporation from the skin.[37] Presently available insect repellents do not "cloak" the user in a chemical veil of protection. Any untreated exposed skin can be readily bitten by hungry arthropods.[32,35]

CHEMICAL INSECT REPELLENTS

DEET

DEET (previously called *N,N*-diethyl-m-toluamide) remains the gold-standard of presently available insect repellents. DEET has been registered for use by the general public since 1957. It is a broad-spectrum repellent, effective against many species of crawling and flying insects, including mosquitoes, biting flies, midges, chiggers, fleas, and ticks.[38-43] The Environmental Protection Agency (EPA) estimates that about 30% of the United States population uses a DEET-based product every year; worldwide use exceeds 200 million people annually.[38,44] Forty years of empirical testing of more than 20,000 other compounds has not led to a more effective repellent coming to market.

FORMULATION OF AVAILABLE PRODUCTS.
In the United States, DEET is sold in concentrations from 5% to 100%, in multiple formulations, including solutions, lotions, creams, gels, aerosol and pump sprays, and impregnated towelettes (Table 38-1). EPA regulations require that the concentration of DEET in each product be disclosed on its label. Most products contain "unaltered" DEET, but two manufacturers developed extended-release formulations that made it possible to lower the repellent concentration of their products without sacrificing duration of action. 3M Company's Ultrathon proprietary polymer 33% DEET formulation, when tested under multiple different environmental/climatic field conditions, was as effective as 75% DEET, providing up to 12 hours of greater than 95% protection against mosquito bites.[45-50] (Ultrathon is presently exclusively available to the U.S. public from Travel Medicine, Inc., Northampton, MA, (800) 872-8633.) Sawyer Products' controlled-release 20% DEET lotion traps the chemical in a protein particle that slowly releases it to the skin surface, providing repellency equivalent to a standard 50% DEET preparation, lasting about 5 hours.[51]

HOW TO CHOOSE AND APPLY DEET REPELLENTS. As a general rule, higher concentrations of DEET provide longer-lasting protection. Mathematical models of the effectiveness and persistence of repellents show that the protection is proportional to the logarithm of the dose (concentration of the product). This curve tends to form a plateau at higher repellent concentrations, providing relatively less additional protection for each incremental dose of DEET over 50%.[52,53] For "casual" use therefore there is no need to use high concentrations of DEET.

■ Table 38-1   DEET-Containing Insect Repellents

Manufacturer	Product Name	Form(s)	% DEET
Sawyer Products Tampa, F (800) 940-4464	DEET Plus Sawyer Gold Sawyer 30 DEET Plus Maxi-DEET	Lotion, pump spray Lotion, pump spray Lotion Aerosol spray Solution, pump spray	17.5% 17.5% 30% 38% 100%
S.C. Johnson Wax Racine, WI (800) 558-5566	OFF! Skintastic for Kids Unscented OFF! Skintastic Unscented OFF! Fresh Scent OFF! Skintastic Unscented OFF! Unscented Deep Woods OFF! Unscented Deep Woods OFF! for Sportsmen Maximum Protection Deep Woods OFF! Deep Woods OFF! for Sportsmen	Pump spray Pump spray Lotion Lotion Aerosol spray Aerosol spray Aerosol spray Pump spray Pump spray	5% 7% 7.5% 7.5% 15% 30% 30% 100% 100%
Tender Corp. Littleton, NH (800) 258-4696	Ben's Backyard Ben's Wilderness Ben's Max 100	Lotion, pump spray Aerosol spray Lotion, pump spray	24% 27% 100%
Travel Medicine, Inc. Northampton, MA (800) 872-8633	Ultrathon	Cream	33%

United Industries Corp.
St. Louis, MO
(800) 767-9927
	Cutter Just for Kids
	Cutter Pleasant Protection with
	  Sunscreen (SPF 15)
	Cutter Unscented
	Cutter Lotion with Sunscreen SPF 15
	Cutter Backwoods Unscented
	Cutter Outdoorsman Unscented
		Pump spray
		Aerosol spray, pump
		  spray
		Aerosol spray
		Lotion
		Aerosol spray
		Aerosol spray, lotion,
		  stick
			5%
			7%
			
			10%
			10%
			23%
			30%

Wisconsin Pharmacal Co. Jackson, WI (800) 558-6614	Repel Soft Scented Repel Camp Lotion for Kids Repel Scented Repel Family Formula Repel Sportsman Formula Repel Unscented Sun Block SPF 15 Repel Sportsman Formula Repel Soft Scented Repel Family Formula Repel Classic Sportsman Formula Repel 100	Gel Lotion Pump spray Pump spray Pump spray Lotion Lotion Lotion Aerosol Aerosol Pump spray	7% 10% 18% 18% 18% 20% 20% 20% 23% 39% 100%

*Note: Some manufacturers give only the concentration of the m-isomer; others list total concentrations of all DEET isomers. Technical grade 100% DEET is 95% m-isomer and 5% other isomers.

Products with 10% to 35% DEET provide adequate protection under most conditions. The American Academy of Pediatrics currently recommends that DEET-containing repellents used on children contain no more than 10% DEET.[54]

Products with a DEET concentration over 35% are probably best reserved for circumstances in which the wearer is in an environment with a very high density of insects (e.g., a rain forest), where there is a high risk of disease transmission from insect bites, or under circumstances where there may be rapid loss of repellent from the skin surface, such as under conditions of high temperature and humidity, or rain.

Guideline for safe and effective use of insect repellents are listed in Box 38-4. Repellents may be applied directly to the skin, or to clothing, window screens, mesh insect nets, tents, or sleeping bags. Repellents should not be applied under clothing. Repellents containing DEET must be carefully applied because they can damage plastics (such as watch crystals and eyeglass frames), rayon, spandex, and painted or varnished surfaces. DEET does not damage natural fibers like wool or cotton.

Consumers applying both a DEET-based insect repellent and sunscreen should be aware that the repellent might reduce the sunscreen's effectiveness. A limited study in 14 patients, using 33% DEET repellent and SPF 15 sunscreen, revealed a mean decrease in SPF of 33.5% when the two agents were applied sequentially.[62] Combination products, in which the insect repellent and sunscreen have been formulated together, however, would be expected to provide the SPF as stated on the label.

Pharmacology of DEET

The percutaneous penetration, absorption, metabolism, and rate of excretion of DEET continues to be the subject of numerous studies.[63-69] Human studies show very variable penetration of DEET; depending on the applied dose, vehicle, anatomic site, and collection method, the reported penetration of DEET ranges from 9% to 56% of the topically applied dose.[64,68] Using human volunteers, a 1995 carefully conducted study demonstrated that the average dermal absorption of 100% DEET was 5.6%; for 15% DEET in ethanol, an average of 8.4% of the dose was absorbed.[63] Due to its lipophilic nature, DEET was rapidly absorbed within 2 hours after application and was eliminated from the plasma within 4 hours after being rinsed off the skin.[63] Absorbed DEET was metabolized completely, with 99% urinary elimi-

Box 38-4

Guidelines for Safe and Effective Use of Insect Repellents

- For casual use, choose a repellent with no more than 35% DEET. Repellents with 10% DEET or less are most appropriate for use in children.
- Use just enough repellent to lightly cover the skin; do not saturate the skin.
- Repellents should be applied only to exposed skin and clothing—do not use under clothing.
- For maximum effectiveness, apply to all exposed areas of skin.
- To apply to the face, dispense into palms, rub hands together, and then apply thin layer to face.
- Avoid contact with eyes and mouth—do not apply to children's hands to prevent possible subsequent contact with mucous membranes.
- After applying, wipe repellent from the palmar surfaces to prevent inadvertent contact with eyes, mouth, and genitals.
- Never use repellents over cuts, wounds, or inflamed, irritated, or eczematous skin.
- Do not inhale aerosol formulations or get in eyes.
- Frequent reapplication is rarely necessary, unless the repellent seems to have lost its effectiveness. Reapplication may be necessary in very hot, wet environments, due to rapid loss of repellent from the skin surface.
- Once inside, wash off treated areas with soap and water. Washing the repellent from the skin surface is particularly important under circumstances where a repellent is likely to be applied for several consecutive days.
- In tick infested areas, wear long pants, tucked into boots or socks, and long-sleeved shirts. Ticks will find it more difficult to cling to smooth, closely-woven fabrics such as nylon.[54]
- Consider spraying clothing with a permethrin-based product to prevent ticks from crawling up clothing.
- Inspect yourself and your children for ticks after leaving an infested area—most ticks require over 24 hours of attachment to transmit Lyme disease.[55]
- If found, the best method for removing a tick is to grasp it with a forceps as close to the skin surface as possible, and pull upward with steady, even pressure.[56]

Adapted from EPA Guidelines.[53]

nation, mostly within 12 hours. (Hepatic microsomal cytochrome P-450 enzymes are involved in its metabolism.[64]) Tape stripping revealed that the chemical did not accumulate in the stratum corneum nor was there evidence of systemic bioaccumulation.[63]

Toxicity of DEET

Given its use by millions of people worldwide for 40 years, DEET continues to show a remarkable safety profile. In 1980, as part of the U.S. EPA Reregistration Standard for DEET, over 30 additional animal studies were conducted to assess acute, chronic, and subchronic toxicity. There was no evidence of mutagenicity or oncogenicity, as well as no developmental, reproductive, or neurologic toxicity associated with DEET use. The results of these studies neither led to any product changes to comply with EPA safety standards nor indicated any new toxicities under normal usage.[38,70,71] The EPA's Reregistration Eligibility Decision (RED)[44] released in 1998 confirmed that the Agency believes that "normal use of DEET does not present a health concern to the general U.S. population."

Case reports of potential DEET toxicity do exist in the medical literature and are summarized in Table 38-2. Examination of this table reveals that the total number of significant cases of DEET toxicity is small (38 cases reported in the medical literature over the past four decades). Most of the associated signs and symptoms resolved without sequelae (in 30 of 38 cases). Most of these cases had long-term, excessive, or inappropriate use of DEET repellents, and the details of exposure are frequently poorly documented, making causal relationships difficult to establish. These cases show no correlation between concentration of the DEET product used and the risk of toxicity. Of the six reported deaths, three were a result of deliberate ingestion of DEET repellents.

The reports of greatest concern involve 14 cases of encephalopathy, 13 in children under the age of 8 years.[70,73-78,82] Three of these children died, one of whom had an ornithine carbamoyl transferase deficiency[74] (detected by elevated serum ammonia levels), which might have predisposed her to DEET-induced toxicity.[73] The other children recovered without sequelae. Animal studies in rats and mice show that DEET is not a selective neurotoxin.[38,66,70]

A single case of bradycardia and hypotension after "liberal" application of a DEET-based repellent has been reported in a woman 61 years of age; the symptoms resolved, without sequelae.[86] A single patient has been reported to have anaphylaxis after contact with DEET.[87] Initial repeat-insult patch tests over 21 days did not reveal any skin irritation from DEET.[38] In contrast, 12 cases of bullous contact dermatitis, confined to the antecubital fossa, were subsequently reported in military personnel who applied DEET repellent and slept with the repellent on their skin overnight.[88,91,93,94]

A 1994 study reviewed 9086 cases of DEET exposure reported to 71 poison control centers from 1985-1989.[83] Over half (54%) of these people had no symptoms at the time of the call to the poison control center. The most commonly reported symptoms related to either spraying repellent in the eyes (DEET is a known eye irritant[38]) or inhaling it. Symptoms were least likely to occur after accidental ingestion of small amounts of the repellent. Although most exposures were in children, there was no evidence that children under 6 were any more likely to develop adverse effects after use of a DEET repellent than were older individuals. No correlation was found between the severity of symptoms and age or gender of the person, or the concentration of applied DEET. Most of the exposures (88%) did not require treatment at a health care facility. Of the patients who were seen, 81% were sent home, and only 5% required hospitalization. Of the patients in whom follow-up was available, 99% of them had transient, rapidly resolving symptoms, such as eye irritation.

In summary, DEET continues to show a remarkable safety profile during 40 years of use by millions of people worldwide. Careful product choice (most often of a repellent concentration of 35% DEET or less) and application of the repellent according to EPA guidelines greatly reduce the possibility of toxicity. Conservative use of low-concentration (up to 10%) DEET products is most appropriate when applying repellents to children.

Skin-So-Soft Products

Avon's Skin-So-Soft Bath Oil received considerable media attention several years ago when it was reported by some consumers to be effective

■ Table 38-2 Reported Major Signs and Symptoms Attributed to DEET Exposure

Organ System	Clinical Presentation	# of Cases	Age/Sex	% DEET	Details of Use	Outcome	Refs.
Central nervous system	Lethargy, confusion, acute manic psychosis	1	30 yrs M	Unknown	3-week, daily, whole-body application, followed by 2-3 hours per day in a sauna	Resolved, no sequela	67
	Lethargy, headaches, ataxia, disorientation	1	6 yrs F	15%	More than 10 applications	Death (OCT heterozygote)	68, 69
	Acute encephalopathy	1	17 mos F	20%	"Frequent" over 3 weeks	Death	70
	Headaches, disorientation, ataxia, convulsions	1	5 yrs F	10%	Nightly for 3 months	Death	71
	Behavioral changes, confusion, tremors, seizures, encephalopathy	10	8 yrs or younger, 6 M 4 F	0%-95%	Concentration of DEET known in only 5/11 cases. Number of applications varies from 2 to 90. Many reports note "daily," "heavy," "frequent," or "whole body" use	Resolved, no sequela	65, 71-77
		1	29 yrs M				
	Seizures, hypotension, coma	6	1-33 yrs 4 M 2 F	47.5%-90%	Ingestion of over 50 ml of DEET	3/6 died 3/6 resolved, no sequela	78, 79
Cardiovascular	Bradycardia, hypotension	1	61 yrs F	Unknown	"Liberal" application to all exposed skin, before gardening	Resolved, no sequela	80, 81
Cutaneous/ Allergic	Anaphylaxis	1	42 yrs F	52%	Touched companion who had just applied DEET insect repellent	Resolved, no sequela	82
	Wheals	3	4 yrs M (×2)	Unknown	Urticaria developed within 10-30 minutes after application	Resolved	83-85
	Hemorrhagic bullae and erosions, confined to the antecubital fossa	12	18-20 yrs M	33%-50%	Military personnel, after applying to all exposed skin, then sleeping outdoors with repellent still on skin	9/11 resolved 2/11 scarred	86-88

as a mosquito repellent. Studies show that Skin-So-Soft Bath Oil has only a mild repellent effect.[46,95-97] Its effective half-life was found to be 30 minutes against *Aedes aegypti* mosquitoes.[95] Against *Aedes albopictus*, Skin-So-Soft Bath Oil provided 40 minutes of protection from bites, 10 times *less* effective than 12.5% DEET.[46] The limited mosquito repellent effect of Skin-So-Soft oil could be due to its fragrance, or to the presence of diisopropyl adipate and benzophenone in the formulation, both of which have some repellent activity.[98] Skin-So-Soft Bath Oil has been found to be somewhat effective against biting midges, but this effect is felt to be a result of its trapping the insects in an oily film on the skin surface.[99]

The Avon Corporation makes no claims about the Skin-So-Soft Bath Oil being an effective repellent. They currently manufacture Skin-So-Soft Bug Guard, which contains 0.10% oil of citronella as the active ingredient. In July 1999, the Avon Corporation introduced a new chemical-based insect repellent to the U.S. market, IR3535 (ethyl-3-[N-n-butyl-N-acetyl]-aminoproprionate), which can be found in Skin-So-Soft Bug Guard Plus. The limited data presently available to the public on this repellent show that while it is more effective than most botanical-based repellents, it does not match the overall efficacy of DEET.[100]

PLANT-DERIVED REPELLENTS

Literally thousands of plants have been tested as sources of insect repellents.[98,101-103] Although none of the plant-derived chemicals tested to date demonstrate the broad effectiveness and duration of DEET, a few do show repellent activity. Plants whose essential oils have been reported to have repellent activity include citronella, cedar, verbena, pennyroyal, geranium, lavender, pine, cajeput, cinnamon, rosemary, basil, thyme, allspice, garlic, and peppermint.[98,101,104-106] Unlike the synthetic insect repellents, plant-derived insect repellents have been relatively poorly studied. When tested, most of these essential oils tended to give short-lasting protection, lasting minutes to 2 hours. A summary of readily available plant-derived insect repellents is shown in Table 38-3.

Citronella

Citronella is the EPA-registered active ingredient most commonly found in "natural" or "herbal" insect repellents marketed in the United States. Oil of citronella has a lemony scent, and was originally extracted from the grass plant *Cymbopogon nardus*.

Conflicting data exist on the efficacy of citronella-based products, varying greatly depending on the study methodology, location, and species of biting insect tested. One citronella-based repellent was found to provide no repellency when tested in the laboratory against *Aedes aegypti* mosquitoes.[97] Another study of the same product, however, conducted in the field, showed an average of 88% repellency over a 2 hour exposure. The product's effectiveness was greatest within the first 40 minutes after application and then decreased with time over the remainder of the test period.[107]

In general, studies of citronella-based repellents show that they are less effective than DEET repellents. Citronella provides a shorter protection time, which may be partially overcome by frequent reapplication of the repellent. In 1997, after analyzing available data on the repellent effect of citronella, the EPA concluded that citronella-based insect repellents must contain the following statement on their labels: "For maximum repellent effectiveness of this product, repeat applications at 1 hour intervals."[108] In an attempt to prolong efficacy without requiring frequent reapplication, The All Terrain Co. (Encinitas, CA) recently released to the U.S. market a citronella-based lotion in which the essential oil is encapsulated into a beeswax matrix, which slowly releases the active ingredient to the skin surface. In laboratory testing against *Aedes aegypti*, this product provided complete protection for the first 2 hours, and 77% protection 4 hours after application.[109]

Citronella candles have been promoted as an effective way to repel mosquitoes in one's backyard. One study compared the efficacy of commercially available 3% citronella candles, 5% citronella incense, and plain candles in their ability to prevent bites by *Aedes* species mosquitoes, under field conditions.[110] Subjects near the citronella candles had 42% fewer bites than controls, who had no protection (a statistically significant difference). However, burn-

■ **Table 38-3**   Plant-Derived Insect Repellents and Permethrin Insecticide Sprays

Manufacturer	Product Name	Form(s)	Active Ingredient(s)
PLANT-DERIVED INSECT REPELLENTS			
All Terrain Co. Encinitas, CA (800) 246-7328	Herbal Armor Herbal Armor SPF 15 Herbal Armor	Lotion Lotion Pump spray	Citronella oil 12%; peppermint oil 2.5%, cedar oil 2%, lemongrass oil 1.0%, geranium oil 0.05%, in a slow-release encapsulated formula
Avon Corp. New York, NY (800) 367-2866	Skin-So-Soft: Moisturizing Suncare Plus, SPF 15 and 30 Bug Guard ± SPF 15 Bug Guard Moisturizing	Lotion Pump spray Lotion, towelettes	Citronella oil 0.05% Citronella oil 0.10% Citronella oil 0.10%
Green Ban Norway, IA (319) 446-7495	Green Ban for People Regular Double Strength	Oil Oil	Citronella Peppermint oil 5% 1% 10% 2%
Quantum, Inc. Eugene, OR (800) 448-1448	Buzz Away Buzz Away, SPF 15	Towelette, pump spray Lotion	Citronella oil 5%; oils of cedarwood, peppermint, eucalyptus, lemongrass
Tender Corp. Littleton, NH (800) 258-4696	Natrapel	Lotion, pump spray	Citronella 10%
Verdant Brands, Inc. Bloomington, MN (800) 643-8457	Blocker	Lotion, oil, pump spray	Soybean oil 2%
PERMETHRIN INSECT REPELLENTS			
Coulston Products Easton, PA (610) 253-0167	Duranon	Aerosol, pump sprays	Permethrin 0.5%
Sawyer Products Tampa, FL (800) 940-4464	Permethrin Tick Repellent	Aerosol, pump sprays	Permethrin 0.5%
United Industries Corp. St. Louis, MO (800) 767-9927	Cutter Outdoorsman Gear Guard	Aerosol spray	Permethrin 0.5%
Wisconsin Pharmacal Co. Jackson, WI (800) 558-6614	Repel Permanone	Aerosol spray	Permethrin 0.5%

ing ordinary candles was found to reduce the number of bites by 23%. There was no difference in efficacy between citronella incense and plain candles. The ability of plain candles to decrease biting may be due to their serving as a "decoy" source of warmth, moisture, and carbon dioxide.

The citrosa plant (*Pelargonium citrosum* "Van Leenii") has been marketed as being able to repel mosquitoes through the continuous release of citronella oils. Unfortunately, when tested, these plants offer no protection against bites.[111,112]

Blocker

Blocker is a "natural" repellent, which was released to the U.S. market in 1997. Blocker combines soybean oil, geranium oil, and coconut oil in a formulation that has been available in Europe for several years.[113] Studies conducted at the University of Guelph showed that this product was capable of giving over 97% protection against various *Aedes* species mosquitoes under field conditions, even after 3.5 hours of application. During the same time period, a 6.65% DEET-based spray afforded 86% protection, while Avon's Skin-So-Soft citronella-based repellent gave only 40% protection.[114] A second study showed that Blocker provided approximately 200 ± 30 minutes of complete protection from mosquito bites.[115] Blocker also provided about 10 hours of protection against biting black flies; in the same test, 20% DEET only gave 6.5 hours of complete protection.[116]

Eucalyptus

A derivative (*p*-menthane-3,8-diol, or PMD) isolated from oil of the lemon eucalyptus plant shows promise as an effective "natural" repellent.[117] This repellent has been very popular in China for years and is currently available in Europe. In field tests against anopheline mosquitoes, PMD showed repellency comparable to 50% DEET.[118] PMD required more frequent reapplication than DEET to maintain its potency but was significantly more effective than 50% citronella oil.[119,120] Release of PMD-based repellents awaits final EPA approval in the United States.

Permethrin

Pyrethrum is a powerful, rapidly-acting insecticide, originally derived from the crushed dried flowers of the daisy *Chrysanthemum cinerariifolium*.[121] Permethrin is a man-made synthetic pyrethroid. It does not repel insects, but instead works as a contact insecticide, causing nervous system toxicity, leading to death, or "knockdown," of the insect. The chemical is effective against mosquitoes, flies, ticks, fleas, human lice, and chiggers.[56,122-124] Permethrin has low mammalian toxicity, is poorly absorbed by the skin, and is rapidly metabolized by skin and blood esterases.[125]

Permethrin sprays should be applied directly to clothing, or to other fabrics (tent walls[126] or mosquito nets[127]), not to skin. The spray is nonstaining, nearly odorless, resistant to degradation by heat or sun, and maintains its potency for at least 2 weeks, even through several launderings.[122,128,129]

The combination of permethrin-treated clothing and skin application of a DEET-based repellent creates a formidable barrier against biting insects.[47,130-132] In an Alaskan field trial against mosquitoes, subjects wearing permethrin-treated uniforms and a polymer-based 35% DEET product had greater than 99.9% protection (1 bite/hour), over 8 hours; unprotected subjects were bitten an average of 1188 bites/hour.[133]

Permethrin-sprayed clothing also proved very effective against ticks. *D. occidentalis* ticks (which carry Rocky Mountain spotted fever) had 100% mortality within 3 hours of touching permethrin-treated cloth.[134] Permethrin-sprayed pants and jackets also provided 100% protection from all three life stages of *I. dammini* ticks, the vector of Lyme disease.[56] In contrast, DEET alone (applied to the skin), provided 85% repellency at the time of application. This protection deteriorated to 55% repellency at 6 hours, when tested against the lone star tick, *A. americanum*.[40] *I. scapularis* ticks, which may transmit Lyme disease, also seem to be less sensitive to the repellent effect of DEET.[39]

Permethrin-based insecticide sprays available in the United States are listed in Table 38-3. To apply to clothing, spray each side of the fabric (outdoors) for 30 to 45 seconds, just enough to moisten. Allow to dry for 2 to 4 hours before wearing.

RELATED ISSUES
Reducing Local Insect Populations

Consumers may still find advertisements for small ultrasonic electronic devices that are meant to be carried on the body and that purportedly emit sounds that are repellent to mosquitoes. Multiple studies, conducted in both the field and laboratory, show that these devices do not work.[135-137] Encouraging natural predation of insects by setting up bird or bat houses in one's backyard is also unsuccessful in reducing local mosquito populations.[138] Likewise, backyard bug "zappers," which lure and electrocute insects, are poor at reducing the local numbers of nuisance insects. One study of "zappers" showed that only 0.13% of insects killed were female (biting) mosquitoes.[139] Mosquitoes continued to be more attracted to humans than to the "zappers" themselves.[140] Pyrethrin-containing yard foggers, set off before an outdoor event, can reduce the number of insects in one's backyard for a few hours. These products should be applied before any food is brought outside and should be kept away from pets, birds, and fish ponds.

The most effective way to reduce the local population of mosquitoes is to eliminate sources of standing water such as old discarded tires, clogged gutters, planters, bird baths, or tree stump holes. Ornamental ponds may be stocked with *Gambusia* ("mosquito") fish, which eat mosquito larvae,[141] or may be treated by floating the biologic larvacide *Bacillus thuringiensis* var. *israelensis* in the water.[142,143]

Relief from Arthropod Bites

Cutaneous responses to arthropod bites range from the common localized wheal-and-flare reactions (type I hypersensitivity) to delayed bite papules (type IV hypersensitivity), rare systemic Arthus reactions, and even anaphylaxis.[144-146] Bite reactions are the result of sensitization to salivary antigens, which lead to formation of both specific immunoglobulin E (IgE) and IgG antibodies.[147-150] Immediate-type reactions are mediated by IgE, IgG, and histamine, whereas cell-mediated immunity is responsible for delayed reactions.

Several strategies exist for relieving the itch of insect bites. Topical corticosteroids can reduce the associated erythema, itching, and induration; a short, rapidly tapering course of oral prednisone can also be very effective in reducing extensive bite reactions. Applications of diphenhydramine or benzocaine (an ester-type topical anesthetic) should be avoided, due to the risk of these compounds inducing allergic contact sensitivity. Oral antihistamines can be effective in reducing the symptoms of insect bites. Cetirizine was given prophylactically in a double-blind, placebo-controlled, 2-week cross-over trial to 18 individuals who had previously experienced dramatic cutaneous reactions to mosquito bites.[151] Subjects given the active drug had a statistically significant 40% decrease in both the size of the wheal response at 15 minutes and the size of the 24-hour bite papule. The mean pruritus score, measured at 0.25, 1, 12, and 24 hours after being bitten, was 67% less than that of the untreated controls. These studies have not been done with astemizole, terfenadine, loratadine, or fexofenadine. In highly sensitized individuals, prophylactic treatment with nonsedating antihistamines may safely reduce the cutaneous reactions to arthropod bites.

After Bite, a 3.6% ammonium solution (Tender Corporation, NH), has been found to relieve the type I hypersensitivity symptoms associated with mosquito bites. In a double-blind, placebo-controlled laboratory trial, 64% of mosquito-bitten subjects experienced complete relief of symptoms after a single application of the ammonium solution; the remaining 36% of After Bite–treated subjects experienced partial relief, lasting 15 to 90 minutes after a single application. No subjects treated with placebo reported complete symptom relief.[152]

Bibliography

Curtis CF: Personal protection methods against vectors of disease. *Rev Med Vet Entomol* 80:543-553, 1992.

Fradin MS: Mosquitoes and mosquito repellents: a clinician's guide. *Ann Intern Med* 128:931-940, 1998.

Fradin MS: Protection from blood-feeding arthropods. In Auerbach PS, editor: *Wilderness medicine: management of wilderness and environmental emergencies*, ed 4, St. Louis, 2000, Mosby.

Goddard J: *Physicians guide to arthropods of medical importance*, ed 2, Boca Raton, 1996, CRC Press.

Qiu H, Jun HW, McCall JW: Pharmacokinetics, formulation, and safety of insect repellent N,N-diethyl-3-methylbenzamide (DEET): a review. *J Am Mosq Control Assoc* 14:12-27, 1998.

Spach DH, Liles WC, Campbell GL, et al: Tick-borne diseases in the United States. *N Engl J Med* 329:836-847, 1993.

References

1. McHugh CP: Arthropods: vectors of disease agents. *Lab Med* 25:429-437, 1994.
2. Goddard J: *Physician's guide to arthropods of medical importance,* ed 2, Boca Raton, 1996, CRC Press.
3. Shell ER: Resurgence of a deadly disease. *The Atlantic Monthly* 280:45-60, 1997.
4. Spach DH, Liles WC, Campbell GL, et al: Tick-borne diseases in the United States. *N Engl J Med* 329:936-947, 1993.
5. Perritt DW, Couger G, Barker RWL: Computer-controlled olfactometer system for studying behavioral responses of ticks to carbon dioxide. *J Med Entomol* 30:571-578, 1993.
6. Wilson JG, Kinzer DR, Sauer JR, et al: Chemo-attraction in the lone star tick (Acarina: Ixodidae). I. Response of different developmental stages to carbon dioxide administered via traps. *J Med Entomol* 9:245-252, 1972.
7. Maibach HI, Skinner WA, Strauss WG, et al: Factors that attract and repel mosquitoes in human skin. *JAMA* 196:263-266, 1966.
8. Curtis CF: Fact and fiction in mosquito attraction and repulsion. *Parasitology Today* 2:316-318, 1986.
9. Keystone JS: Of bites and body odour. *Lancet* 347:1423, 1996.
10. Bock GR, Cardew G, editors: *Olfaction in mosquito-host interactions,* New York, 1996, J Wiley.
11. Bowen MF: The sensory physiology of host-seeking behavior in mosquitoes. *Annu Rev Entomol* 36:139-158, 1991.
12. Davis EE, Bowen MF: Sensory physiological basis for attraction in mosquitoes. *J Am Mosq Control Assoc* 10:316-325, 1994.
13. Clements AN: The physiology of mosquitoes. Oxford, 1963, Pergamon Press.
14. Gjullin CM: Effect of clothing color on the rate of attack of *Aedes* mosquitoes. *J Econ Entomol* 40:326-327, 1947.
15. Gillies MT: The role of carbon dioxide in host-finding by mosquitoes (Diptera: Culicidae): a review. *Bull Entomol Res* 70:525-532, 1980.
16. Gillies MT, Wilkes TJ: The range of attraction of animal baits and carbon dioxide for mosquitoes. Studies in a freshwater area of West Africa. *Bull Entomol Res* 61:389-404, 1972.
17. Snow WF: The effect of a reduction in expired carbon dioxide on the attractiveness of human subjects to mosquitoes. *Bull Entomol Res* 60:43-48, 1970.
18. Khan AA: Mosquito attractants and repellents. In Shorey HH, McKelvey JJ, editors: *Chemical control of insect behavior,* New York, 1977, J Wiley, pp 305-325.
19. Schreck CE, Kline DL, Carlson DA: Mosquito attraction to substances from the skin of different humans. *J Am Mosq Control Assoc* 6:406-410, 1990.
20. Knols BG, de Jong R, Takken W: Trapping system for testing olfactory responses of the malarial mosquito *Anopheles gambia* in a wind tunnel. *Med Vet Entomol* 8:386-388, 1994.
21. Foster WA, Hancock RG: Nectar-related olfactory and visual attractants for mosquitoes. *J Am Mosq Control Assoc* 10:288-296, 1994.
22. Curtis CF, Lines JD, Ijumba J, et al: The relative efficacy of repellents against mosquito vectors of disease. *Med Vet Entomol* 1:109-119, 1987.
23. Gilbert IH, Gouck HK, Smith N: Attractiveness of men and women to *Aedes aegypti* and relative protection time obtained with DEET. *Florida Entomol* 49:53-66, 1966.
24. Muirhead-Thomson RC: The distribution of anopheline mosquito bites among different age groups. *BMJ* 1:1114-1117, 1951.
25. Port GR, Boreham PFL: The relationship of host size to feeding by mosquitoes of the *Anopheles gambiae* Giles complex (Diptera: Culicidae). *Bull Entomol Res* 70:133-144, 1980.

General Issues—Insect Repellents
26. Khan AA, Maibach HI, Strauss WG, et al: Vitamin B_1 is not a systemic mosquito repellent in man. *Trans St John's Hosp Dermatol Soc* 55:99-102, 1969.
27. Wilson CW, Mathieson DR, Jachowski LA: Ingested thiamine chloride as a mosquito repellent. *Science* 100:147, 1944.
28. Strauss WG, Maibach HI, Khan AA: Drugs and disease as mosquito repellents in man. *Am J Trop Med Hyg* 17:461-464, 1968.
29. Davis EE: Insect repellents: concepts of their mode of action relative to potential sensory mechanisms in mosquitoes (Diptera: Culicidae). *J Med Entomol* 22:237-243, 1985.

30. Rutledge LC, Collister DM, Meixsell VE, et al: Comparative sensitivity of representative mosquitoes (Diptera: Culicidae) to repellents. *J Med Entomol* 20:506-510, 1983.

31. Wright RH: Why mosquito repellents repel. *Sci Am* 233:104-111, 1975.

32. Schreck CE: Protection from blood-feeding arthropods. In Auerbach PS, editor: *Wilderness medicine: management of wilderness and environmental emergencies*, ed 3, St. Louis, 1995, Mosby, pp 813-830.

33. Golenda CF, Solberg VB, Burge R, et al: Gender-related efficacy difference to an extended duration formulation of topical N,N-diethyl-m-toluamide (DEET). *Am J Trop Med Hyg* 60:654-657, 1999.

34. Maibach HI, Akers WA, Johnson HL, et al: Insects. Topical insect repellents. *Clin Pharmacol Ther* 16:970-973, 1974.

35. Maibach HI, Khan AA, Akers WA: Use of insect repellents for maximum efficacy. *Arch Dermatol* 109:32-35, 1974.

36. Gabel ML, Spencer TS, Akers WA: Evaporation rates and protection times of mosquito repellents. *Mosq News* 36:141-146, 1976.

37. Khan AA, Maibach HI, Skidmore DL: A study of insect repellents: effect of temperature on protection time. *J Econ Entomol* 66:437-438, 1972.

DEET—Clinical Use

38. United States Environmental Protection Agency, Offices of Pesticides and Toxic Substances, Special Pesticide Review Division: *N,N-diethyl-m-toluamide (Deet) pesticide registration standard* (EPA-540/RS-81-004), Washington, DC, 1980.

39. Schreck CE, Fish D, McGovern TP: Activity of repellents applied to skin for protection against *Amblyomma americanum* and *Ixodes scapularis* ticks (Acari: Ixodidae). *J Am Mosq Control Assoc* 11:136-140, 1995.

40. Solberg VB, Klein TA, McPherson KR, et al: Field evaluation of deet and a piperidine repellent (A13-37220) against *Amblyomma americanum* (Acari: Ixodidae). *J Med Entomol* 32:870-875, 1995.

41. Frances SP: Response of a chigger, Eutrombicula hirsti (Acari: Trombiculidae) to repellent and toxicant compounds in the laboratory. *J Med Entomol* 31:628-630, 1994.

42. Mehr ZA, Rutledge LC, Inase JL: Evaluation of commercial and experimental repellents against Xenopsylla cheopis (Siphonaptera: Pulicidae). *J Med Entomol* 21:665-669, 1984.

43. Kumar S, Prakash S, Rao KM: Comparative activity of three repellents against bedbugs Cimex hemipterus (Fabr.). *Indian J Med Res* 102:20-23, 1995.

44. United States Environmental Protection Agency, Office of Pesticide Programs, Prevention, Pesticides and Toxic Substances Division: Reregistration Eligibility Decision (RED): DEET (EPA-738-F-95-010), Washington, DC, 1998.

45. Mehr ZA, Rutledge LC, Morales EL, et al: Laboratory evaluation of controlled-release insect repellent formulations. *J Am Mosq Control Assoc* 1:143-147, 1985.

46. Schreck CE, McGovern TP: Repellents and other personal protection strategies against *Aedes albopictus*. *J Am Mosq Control Assoc* 5:247-250, 1989.

47. Kline DL, Schreck CE: Personal protection afforded by controlled-release topical repellents and permethrin-treated clothing against natural populations of *Aedes taeniorhynchus*. *J Am Mosq Control Assoc* 5:77-80, 1989.

48. Gupta RK, Rutledge LC: Laboratory evaluation of controlled-release repellent formulations on human volunteers under three climatic regimens. *J Am Mosq Control Assoc* 5:52-55, 1989.

49. Schreck CE, Kline DL: Repellency of two controlled-release formulations of deet against *Anopheles quadrimaculatus* and *Aedes taeniorhynchus* mosquitoes. *J Am Mosq Control Assoc* 5:91-94, 1989.

50. Annis B: Comparison of the effectiveness of two formulations of deet against *Anopheles flavirostris*. *J Am Mosq Control Assoc* 6:430-432, 1990.

51. Feller L: Personal Communication, July 20, 1999, unpublished report, Insect repellent test report, Nomad Traveller's Store.

52. Rutledge LC, Wirtz RA, Buescher MD, et al: Mathematical models of the effectiveness and persistence of mosquito repellents. *J Am Mosq Control Assoc* 1:56-61, 1985.

53. Buescher MD, Rutledge LC, Wirtz RA: Tests of commercial repellents on human skin against *Aedes aegypti*. *Mosq News* 42:428-433, 1982.

54. Shelov SP, editor: *Caring for your baby and young child: birth to age 5*, New York, 1991, Bantam Books, p 639.

55. Office of Pesticide Programs: United States Environmental Protection Agency: Using insect repellents safely. (EPA-735/F-93-052R); 1998.

56. Schreck CE, Snoddy EL, Spielman A: Pressurized sprays of permethrin or deet on military clothing for personal protection against *Ixodes dammini* (Acari: Ixodidae). *J Med Entomol* 23:396-399, 1986.

57. Piesman J, Maupin GO, Campos EG, et al: Duration of adult female *Ixodes dammini* attachment and transmission of *Borrelia burgdorferi*, with description of a needle aspiration isolation method. *J Infect Dis* 163:895-897, 1991.

58. Piesman J: Dispersal of the Lyme disease spirochete *Borrelia burgdorferi* to salivary glands of feeding nymphal *Ixodes scapularis* (Acari: Ixodidae). *J Med Entomol* 32:519-521, 1995.

59. Piesman J, Mather TN, Sinsky RJ, et al: Duration of tick attachment and *Borrelia burgdorferi* transmission. *J Clin Microbiol* 25:557-558, 1987.

60. Sood SK, Salzman MB, Johnson BJ, et al: Duration of tick attachment as a predictor of the risk of Lyme disease in an area in which Lyme disease is endemic. *J Infect Dis* 175:996-999, 1997.

61. Needham GR: Evaluation of five popular methods for tick removal. *Pediatrics* 75:997-1002, 1985.

62. Montemarano AD, Gupta RK, Burge JR, et al: Insect repellents and the efficacy of sunscreens. *Lancet* 349:1670-1671, 1997.

63. Selim S, Hartnagel REJ, Osimitz TG, et al: Absorption, metabolism, and excretion of N,N-diethyl-m-toluamide following dermal application to human volunteers. *Fund Appl Toxicol* 25:95-100, 1995.

64. Robbins PJ, Cherniack MG: Review of the biodistribution and toxicity of the insect repellent N,N-diethyl-m-toluamide (DEET). *J Toxicol Environ Health* 18:503-525, 1986.

65. Qiu H, Jun HW, Tao J: Pharmacokinetics of insect repellent *N,N*-diethyl-*m*-toluamide in beagle dogs following intravenous and topical routes of administration. *J Pharm Sci* 86:514-516, 1997.

66. Schoenig GP, Hartnagel REJ, Osimitz TG, et al: Absorption, distribution, metabolism, and excretion of *N,N*-diethyl-*m*-toluamide in the rat. *Drug Metab Dispos* 24:156-163, 1996.

DEET Toxicity

67. Moody RP, Nadeau B: An automated *in vitro* dermal absorption procedure: III. *In vivo* and *in vitro* comparison with the insect repellent N,N-diethyl-m-toluamide in mouse, rat, guinea pig, pig, human and tissue-cultured skin. *Toxic in Vitro* 7:167-176, 1993.

68. Qiu H, Jun HW, McCall JW: Pharmacokinetics, formulation, and safety of insect repellent N,N-diethyl-3-methylbenzamide (DEET): a review. *J Am Mosq Control Assoc* 14:12-27, 1998.

69. Moody RP, Benoit FM, Riedel D, et al: Dermal absorption of the insect repellent DEET (N,N-diethyl-m-toluamide) in rats and monkeys: effect of anatomical site and multiple exposure. *J Toxicol Environ Health* 26:137-147, 1989.

70. Osimitz TG, Grothaus RH: The present safety assessment of deet. *J Am Mosq Control Assoc* 11:274-278, 1995.

71. The DEET Joint Venture Group, Chemical Specialties Manufacturers Association: Completed studies for the DEET toxicology data development program. Washington, D.C.; 1996.

72. Snyder JW, Poe RO, Stubbins JF, et al: Acute manic psychosis following the dermal application of N,N-diethyl-m-toluamide (DEET) in an adult. *Clin Toxicol* 24:429-439, 1986.

73. Heick HM, Peterson RG, Dalpe-Scott M, et al: Insect repellent, N,N-diethyl-toluamide, effect on ammonia metabolism. *Pediatrics* 82:373-376, 1988.

74. Heick HM, Shipman RT, Norman MG, et al: Reye-like syndrome associated with use of insect repellent in a presumed heterozygote for ornithine carbamoyl transferase deficiency. *J Pediatr* 97:471-473, 1980.

75. deGarbino JP, Laborde A: Toxicity of an insect repellent: N,N-diethyltoluamide. *Vet Hum Toxicol* 25:422-423, 1983.

76. Zadikoff CM: Toxic encephalopathy associated with use of insect repellant. *J Pediatr* 95:140-142, 1979.

77. Osimitz TG, Murphy JV: Neurological effects associated with use of the insect repellent N,N-diethyl-*m*-toluamide (DEET). *J Toxicol Clin Toxicol* 35:435-441, 1997.

78. Lipscomb JW, Kramer JE, Leikin JB: Seizure following brief exposure to the insect repellent N,N-diethyl-m-toluamide. *Ann Emerg Med* 21:315-317, 1992.

79. Gryboski J, Weinstein D, Ordway NK: Toxic encephalopathy apparently related to the use of an insect repellent. *N Engl J Med* 264:289-291, 1961.

80. Roland EH, Jan JE, Rigg JM: Toxic encephalopathy in a child after brief exposure to insect repellents. *Can Med Assoc J* 132:155-156, 1985.

81. Oransky S, Roseman B, Fish D, et al: Seizures temporally associated with the use of DEET insect repellent— New York and Connecticut. *MMWR Morb Mortal Wkly Rep* 38:678-680, 1989.

82. Edwards DL, Johnson E: Insect repellent-induced toxic encephalopathy in a child. *Clin Pharmacol* 6:496-498, 1987.

83. Veltri JC, Osimitz TG, Bradford DC, et al: Retrospective analysis of calls to poison control centers resulting from exposure to the insect repellent N,N-diethyl-m-toluamide (DEET) from 1985-1989. *J Toxicol Clin Toxicol* 32:1-16, 1994.

84. Tenenbein M: Severe toxic reactions and death following the ingestion of diethyltoluamide-containing insect repellents. *JAMA* 258:1509-1511, 1987.

85. Leach GJ, Russell RD, Houpt JT: Some cardiovascular effects of the insect repellent N,N-diethyl-m-toluamide (DEET). *J Toxicol Environ Health* 25:217-225, 1988.

86. Clem JR, Havemann DF, Raebel MA: Insect repellent (*N,N*-diethyl-m-toluamide) cardiovascular toxicity in an adult. *Ann Pharmacother* 27:289-293, 1993.

87. Miller JD: Anaphylaxis associated with insect repellent. *N Engl J Med* 307:1341-1342, 1982.

88. von Mayenburg J, Rakoski J: Contact urticaria to diethyltoluamide. *Contact Dermatitis* 9:171, 1994.

89. Maibach HI, Johnson HL: Contact urticaria syndrome. Contact urticaria to diethyltoluamide (immediate-type hypersensitivity). *Arch Dermatol* 111:726-730, 1975.

90. Wantke F, Focke M, Hemmer W, et al: Generalized urticaria induced by a diethyltoluamide-containing insect repellent in a child. *Contact Dermatitis* 35:186-187, 1996.

91. Amichai B, Lazarov A, Halevy S: Contact dermatitis from diethyltoluamide. *Contact Dermatitis* 30:188, 1994.

92. Reuveni H, Yagupsky P: Diethyltoluamide-containing insect repellent: adverse effects in worldwide use. *Arch Dermatol* 118:582-583, 1982.

93. McKinlay JR, Ross EV, Barrett TL: Vesiculobullous reaction to diethyltoluamide revisited. *Cutis* 62:44, 1998

94. Lamberg SI, Mulrennan JA: Bullous reaction to diethyl toluamide (DEET). Resembling a blistering insect eruption. *Arch Dermatol* 100:582-586, 1969.

Skin-So-Soft

95. Rutledge LC: Some corrections to the record on insect repellents and attractants. *J Am Mosq Control Assoc* 4:414-425, 1988.

96. Rutledge LC, Wirtz RA, Buescher MD: Repellent activity of a proprietary bath oil (Skin-So-Soft). *Mosq News* 42:557-559, 1982.

97. Chou JT, Rossignol PA, Ayres JW: Evaluation of commercial insect repellents on human skin against *Aedes aegypti* (Diptera: Culicidae). *J Med Entomol* 34:624-630, 1997.

98. King WV: Chemicals evaluated as insecticides and repellents at Orlando, Fla. *USDA Agric Handb* 69:1-397, 1954.

99. Magnon GJ, Robert LL, Kline DL, et al: Repellency of two DEET formulations and Avon Skin-So-Soft against biting midges (Diptera: Ceratopogonidae) in Honduras. *J Am Mosq Control Assoc* 7:80-82, 1991.

100. Dickens T: Personal Communication, September 5, 1999, unpublished report, Efficacy data on E. Merck 3535, 1976-1979, USDA Laboratory, Florida.

Plant-Derived Insect Repellents

101. Quarles W: Botanical mosquito repellents. *Common Sense Pest Control* 12:12-19, 1996.

102. Jacobson M, editor: *Glossary of plant-derived insect deterrents,* Boca Raton, 1990, CRC Press.

103. Sukumar K, Perich MJ, Boobar LR: Botanical derivatives in mosquito control: a review. *J Am Mosq Control Assoc* 7:210-237, 1991.

104. Grainger J, Moore C: *Natural insect repellents for pets, people and plants,* Austin, 1991, The Herb Bar.

105. Brown M, Hebert AA: Insect repellents: an overview. *J Am Acad Dermatol* 36:243-249, 1997.

106. Duke J: USDA-Agricultural Research Service Phytochemical and Ethnobotanical Databases http://www.ars-grin.gov/~ngrlsb/.

107. Surgeoner GA: Efficacy of Buzz Away Oil against spring *Aedes* spp. mosquitoes. Guelph (Ontario): Department of Environmental Biology, University of Guelph; 1995. Sponsored by Quantum, Inc.

108. United States Environmental Protection Agency, Office of Pesticide Programs, Prevention, Pesticides and Toxic Substances Division: *Reregistration eligibility decision (RED) for oil of citronella* (EPA-738-F-97-002) Washington, DC, 1997.

109. Heal JD, Surgeoner GA: Laboratory evaluation of the efficacy of All Terrain, an essential oil-based product, to repel *Aedes aegypti* mosquitoes. Department of Environmental Biology: University of Guelph; 1998. Sponsored by All Terrain Company.

110. Lindsay RL, Surgeoner GA, Heal JD, et al: Evaluation of the efficacy of 3% citronella candles and 5% citronella incense for protection against field populations of *Aedes* mosquitoes. *J Am Mosq Control Assoc* 12:293-294, 1996.

111. Matsuda BM, Surgeoner GA, Heal JD, et al: Essential oil analysis and field evaluation of the citrosa plant *"Pelargonium citrosum"* as a repellent against populations of *Aedes* mosquitoes. *J Am Mosq Control Assoc* 12:69-74, 1996.

112. Cilek JE, Schreiber ET: Failure of the "Mosquito Plant," *Pelargonium × Citrosum* 'Van Leenii,' to repel adult *Aedes albopictus* and *Culex quinquefasciatus* in Florida. *J Am Mosq Control Assoc* 10:473-476, 1994.

113. Finally, a safer insect repellent. University of California at Berkeley Wellness Letter 13:2, 1997.

114. Lindsay RL, Heal JD, Surgeoner GA: Comparative evaluation of the efficacy of Bite Blocker, Off! Skintastic, and Avon Skin-So-Soft to protect against *Aedes* species mosquitoes in Ontario. Guelph (Ontario): Department of Environmental Biology, University of Guelph; 1996. Sponsored by Chemfree Environment Inc.

115. Lindsay RL, Heal JD, Surgeoner GA: Evaluation of Bite Blocker as a repellent against spring *Aedes* spp. mosquitoes. Guelph (Ontario): Department of Environmental Biology, University of Guelph; 1996. Sponsored by Chemfree Environment Inc.

116. Lindsay RL, Surgeoner GA, Heal JD: Comparative evaluation of the efficacy of Bite Blocker and 20% DEET to repel black flies in Ontario, Canada. Guelph (Ontario): Department of Environmental Biology, University of Guelph; 1996. Sponsored by Chemfree Environment Inc.

117. Curtis CF, Lines JD, Lu Baolin L, et al: Natural and synthetic repellents. In Curtis CF, editor: *Appropriate technology in vector control*, Boca Raton, 1990, CRC Press, pp 76-89.

118. Trigg JK: Evaluation of a eucalyptus-based repellent against *Anopheles* spp. in Tanzania. *J Am Mosq Control Assoc* 12:243-246, 1996.

119. Collins DA, Brady JN, Curtis CF: Assessment of the efficacy of quwenling as a mosquito repellent. *Phytotherapy Research* 7:17-20, 1993.

120. Trigg JK, Hill N: Laboratory evaluation of a eucalyptus-based repellent against four biting arthropods. *Phytotherapy Research* 10:313-316, 1996.

121. Casida JE, Quistad GB: Pyrethrum flowers: production, chemistry, toxicology and uses. Oxford, 1995, Oxford University Press.

122. Schreck CE, Mount GA, Carlson DA: Wear and wash persistence of permethrin used as a clothing treatment for personal protection against the lone star tick (Acari: Ixodidae). *J Med Entomol* 19:143-146, 1982.

123. Lindsay RL, McAndless JM: Permethrin-treated jackets versus repellent-treated jackets and hoods for personal protection against black flies and mosquitoes. *Mosq News* 38:350-356, 1978.

124. Breeden GC, Schreck CE, Sorensen AL: Permethrin as a clothing treatment for personal protection against chigger mites (Acarina: Trombiculidae). *Am J Trop Med Hyg* 31:589-592, 1982.

125. Taplin D, Meinking TL: Pyrethrins and pyrethroids in dermatology. *Arch Dermatol* 126:213-221, 1990.

126. Schreck CE: Permethrin and dimethyl phthalate as tent fabric treatments against *Aedes aegypti*. *J Am Mosq Control Assoc* 7:533-535, 1991.

127. Lines JD, Myamba J, Curtis CF: Experimental hut trials of permethrin-impregnated mosquito nets and eave curtains against malaria vectors in Tanzania. *Med Vet Entomol* 1:37-51, 1987.

128. Schreck CE, Posey K, Smith D: Durability of permethrin as a potential clothing treatment to protect against blood-feeding arthropods. *J Econ Entomol* 71:397-400, 1978.

129. Schreck CE, Carlson DA, Weidhass DE, et al: Wear and aging tests with permethrin-treated cotton-polyester fabric. *J Econ Entomol* 73:451-453, 1980.

130. Gupta RK, Sweeney AW, Rutledge LC, et al: Effectiveness of controlled-release personal-use arthropod repellents and permethrin-impregnated clothing in the field. *J Am Mosq Control Assoc* 3:556-560, 1987.

131. Sholdt LL, Schreck CE, Qureshi A, et al: Field bioassays of permethrin-treated uniforms and a new extended duration repellent against mosquitoes in Pakistan. *J Am Mosq Control Assoc* 4:233-236, 1988.

132. Young D, Evans S: Safety and efficacy of DEET and permethrin in the prevention of arthropod attack. *Mil Med* 5:324-330, 1998.

133. Lillie TH, Schreck CE, Rahe AJ: Effectiveness of personal protection against mosquitoes in Alaska. *J Med Entomol* 25:475-478, 1988.

134. Lane RS, Anderson JR: Efficacy of permethrin as a repellent and toxicant for personal protection against the pacific coast tick and the pajaroello tick (Acari: Ixodidae and Argasidae). *J Med Entomol* 21:692-702, 1984.

Related Issues

135. Belton P: An acoustic evaluation of electronic mosquito repellers. *Mosq News* 41:751-755, 1981.

136. Lewis DJ, Fairchild WL, Leprince DJ: Evaluation of an electronic mosquito repeller. *Can Entomol* 114:699-702, 1982.

137. Foster WA, Lutes KI: Tests of ultrasonic emissions on mosquito attraction to hosts in a flight chamber. *J Am Mosq Control Assoc* 1:199-202, 1985.

138. Mitchell M: Mythical mosquito control. *Wing Beats* 3:18-20, 1992.

139. Frick TB, Tallamy DW: Density and diversity of non-target insects killed by suburban electric insect traps. *Ent News* 2:77-82, 1996.

140. Nasci RS, Harris CW, Porter CK: Failure of an insect electrocuting device to reduce mosquito biting. *Mosq News* 43:180-183, 1983.

141. Offill YA, Walton WE: Comparative efficacy of the threespine stickleback (*Gasterosteus aculeatus*) and the mosquitofish (*Gambusia affinis*) for mosquito control. *J Am Mosq Control Assoc* 15:380-390, 1999.

142. Thiery I, Hamon S: Bacterial control of mosquito larvae: investigation of stability of *Bacillus thuringiensis* var. *israelensis* and *Bacillus sphaericus* standard powders. *J Am Mosq Control Assoc* 14:472-476, 1998.

143. Su T, Mulla MS: Field evaluation of new water-dispersible granular formulations of *Bacillus thuringiensis* spp. *israelensis* and *Bacillus sphaericus* against *Culex* mosquitoes in microcosms. *J Am Mosq Control Assoc* 15:356-365, 1999.

144. McCormack DR, Salata KF, Hershey JN, et al: Mosquito bite anaphylaxis: immunotherapy with whole body extracts. *Ann Allergy Asthma Immunol* 74:39-44, 1995.

145. Reunala T, Brummer-Korvenkontio H, Palosuo T: Are we really allergic to mosquito bites? *Ann Med* 26:301-306, 1994.

146. Reunala T, Brummer-Korvenkontio H, Lappalainen P, et al: Immunology and treatment of mosquito bites. *Clin Exp Allergy* 20(Suppl 4):19-24, 1990.

147. Reunala T, Lappalainen P, Brummer-Korvenkontio H, et al: Cutaneous reactivity to mosquito bites: effect of cetirizine and development of anti-mosquito antibodies. *Clin Exp Allergy* 21:617-622, 1991.

148. Brummer-Korvenkontio H, Lappalainen P, Reunala T, et al: Immunization of rabbits with mosquito bites: immunoblot analysis of IgG anti-mosquito antibodies in rabbit and man. *Int Arch Allergy Appl Immunol* 93:14-18, 1990.

149. Peng Z, Yang M, Simons FE: Immunologic mechanisms in mosquito allergy: correlation of skin reactions with specific IgE and IgG antibodies and lymphocyte proliferation response to mosquito antigens. *Ann Allergy Asthma Immunol* 77:238-244, 1996.

150. Brummer-Korvenkontio H, Palosuo T, Francois G, et al: Characterization of *Aedes communis*, *Aedes aegypti* and *Anopheles stephensi* mosquito saliva antigens by immunoblotting. *Int Arch Allergy Appl Immunol* 112:169-174, 1997.

151. Reunala T, Brummer-Korvenkontio H, Karppinen A, et al: Treatment of mosquito bites with cetirizine. *Clin Exp Allergy* 23:72-75, 1993.

152. Zhai H, Packman EW, Maibach HI: Effectiveness of ammonium solution in relieving type I mosquito bite symptoms: a double-blind, placebo-controlled study. *Acta Derm Venereol (Stockh)* 78:297-298, 1998.

PART VIII

Injectable and Mucosal Routes of Drug Administration

CHAPTER 39

David G. Brodland
Michael J. Huether

Local Anesthetics

Local anesthetics are used daily in almost every dermatologist's practice. Whether applying a topical anesthetic to treat chronic pain or injecting the skin and subcutaneous tissue with a local anesthetic before a surgical procedure, dermatologists must be familiar with the use of these agents.

The pursuit of cost-effective care has been a major focus of concern in recent years, and local anesthetics have been responsible for allowing many traditional hospital-based procedures to be performed in a less expensive outpatient setting. More importantly, this move away from general anesthesia resulted in greater safety for patients.[1] As dermatologists continue to expand the types of procedures performed in the office, mastering the use of these medications allows them to continue providing safe and effective local anesthesia (Table 39-1).

INJECTABLE LOCAL ANESTHETICS
Lidocaine and Related Anesthetics

Local anesthetics were first used in medicine in the late 19th century. The first agent used, cocaine, was isolated in 1860 by Niemann.[2] This drug was first utilized in clinical medicine in the field of ophthalmology by Koller in 1884 as a topical anesthetic.[3] At the time, it was the only agent available and remained so until 1904 when procaine, a para-aminobenzoic acid (PABA) ester, was synthesized by Einhorn.[4] It wasn't until 1948 that an amide local anesthetic, lidocaine, was synthesized.[5] Lidocaine is now by far the most common local anesthetic in use today.

PHARMACOLOGY

Structure. Though many chemically diverse compounds have anesthetic properties, the local anesthetics used most commonly for infiltrative anesthesia are classically divided into two groups—esters (e.g., cocaine, procaine, tetracaine, benzocaine) and amides (e.g., lidocaine, mepivacaine, bupivacaine, etidocaine, prilocaine). Members of both groups have an aromatic (lipophilic) portion, an intermediate chain (ester or amide), and an amine (hydrophilic) portion[6] (Figure 39-1). Structural variations in the aromatic and amine portions affect protein binding, potency, duration of action, and other clinically relevant characteristics of use. Specifically, lipophilicity appears to be correlated with the intrinsic potency of the anesthetic. For example, bupivacaine is highly lipophilic compared with lidocaine and is also much more potent and has a longer duration of action.[7]

Absorption. Absorption of lidocaine and all injectable local anesthetics into the blood is influenced by several factors—properties of the agent, presence of a vasoconstrictor in the injected solution, site of injection, quantity of drug injected, and technique of injection. Cocaine has relatively potent vasoconstrictive properties. All other local anesthetics have varying degrees of

■ Table 39-1   Local Anesthetics

Drug	Common Trade Names	Drug Formulations
INJECTABLE ANESTHETICS		
Amide Local Anesthetics		
Bupivacaine	Marcaine, Sensoricaine	0.25% solution (*without* epinephrine)
		0.25% solution (with 1:200,000 epinephrine)
Lidocaine	Xylocaine	0.5%, 1%, 2% solution (*without* epinephrine)
		0.5%, 1%, 2% solution (with 1:100,000 epinephrine)
		0.5%, 1%, 2% solution (with 1:200,000 epinephrine)
Mepivacaine	Carbocaine	1%, 1.5%, 2%, 3% solution
Ester Local Anesthetics		
Procaine	Novocain	1% solution
TOPICAL ANESTHETICS		
Amide Local Anesthetics		
Dibucaine	Nupercainal	1% ointment
		0.5% cream
Lidocaine	Xylocaine, ELA-Max	4% cream, solution
		2% viscous solution, jelly
		2.5%, 5% ointment
		10% oral spray
Mixture of lidocaine and prilocaine	EMLA	2.5% lidocaine, 2.5% prilocaine
Ester Local Anesthetics		
Benzocaine	Solarcaine, Lanacane	20% gel, solution, aerosol
		1%-20% ointment, cream, paste
		0.5%-8% lotion
Ether Local Anesthetics		
Pramoxine	Prax, Pramagel, Caladryl	1% cream, lotion, ointment, gel
Ketone Local Anesthetics		
Dyclonine	Dyclone	0.5%, 1.0% topical solution
Antihistamines		
Diphenhydramine	Benadryl Itch Relief	1% cream
	Benadryl Injection	10 mg/ml
Doxepin	Zonalon	5% cream
Substance P Depletors		
Capsaicin	Zostrix, Capsin	0.025% cream
	Zostrix-HP	0.075% cream
VASOCONSTRICTORS		
Epinephrine	Many	1:100,000 or 1:200,000 dilution

FMLA, Eutectic mixture of local anesthesia.

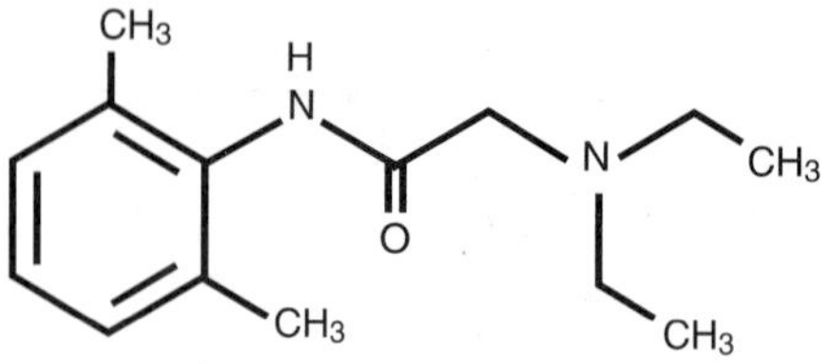

Lidocaine

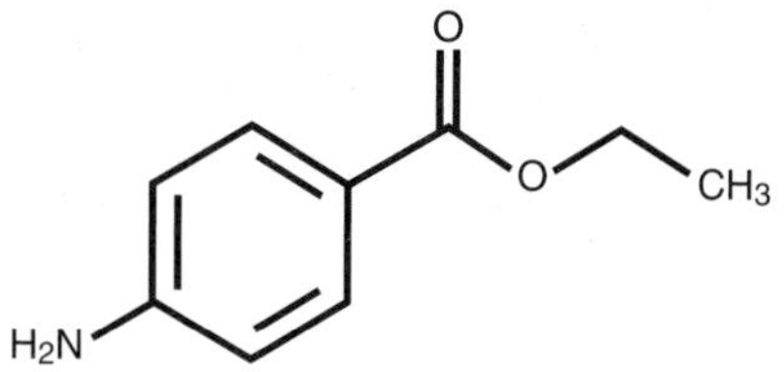

Benzocaine

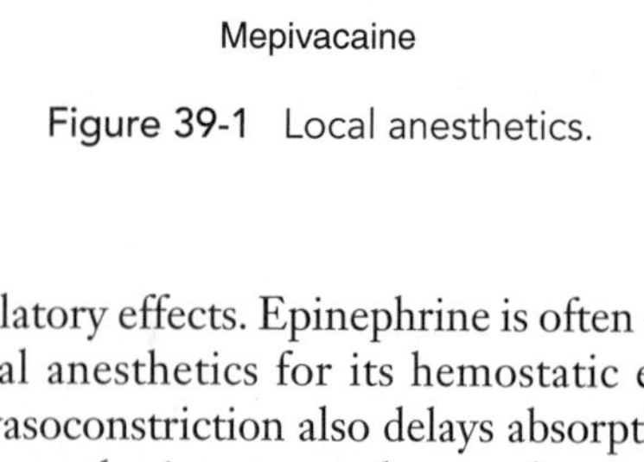

Mepivacaine

Figure 39-1 Local anesthetics.

vasodilatory effects. Epinephrine is often added to local anesthetics for its hemostatic effect. This vasoconstriction also delays absorption of these anesthetic agents, thus prolonging the anesthetic effect (Table 39-2). Without epinephrine, the approximate duration of action of lidocaine is 30 to 60 minutes. With epinephrine, this can be extended to approximately 120 to 360 minutes.[7] Skin and subcutaneous tissues of the face and scalp exhibit higher absorption than the trunk or extremities due to the increased rel-

ative density of blood vessels. Duration of anesthesia may be briefer in these highly vascularized areas. Also, if these anesthetic agents are injected too deeply, they may give inadequate anesthesia. The result is the requirement for larger volumes of local anesthetic injection, which in turn leads to increased systemic drug absorption. Incorrect infiltration technique may also lead to direct intravascular injection, risking systemic toxicity.

Bioavailability. Protein binding is a property of local anesthetics, which relates to the relative lipophilicity and hydrophobicity of the agent. Lidocaine is 60% to 80% protein bound and has an elimination half-life of 1.5 to 2.0 hours. Bupivacaine is the longest lasting local anesthetic and is 82% to 96% protein bound with an elimination half life of up to 5.0 hours.[8] Animal studies suggest that lidocaine is widely distributed in all body tissues[9]; however, each local anesthetic varies in rate and degree of penetration in various tissues and organs.

Metabolism. Amide and ester local anesthetics are metabolized differently. The amide class of local anesthetics, of which lidocaine is the prototype, is hydrolyzed by hepatic microsomal enzymes located in the endoplasmic reticulum of hepatocytes.[10] Among the amides, there is variation in rate of metabolism in the following approximate order (from fastest to slowest):[11] prilocaine > etidocaine > lidocaine > mepivacaine > bupivacaine. In patients with significant liver dysfunction, metabolism can be dramatically impaired, putting the patient at risk for systemic toxicity when relatively high volumes of local anesthetic are used. Lidocaine is specifically metabolized by hepatic microsomal enzymes of the cytochrome P-450 (CYP 3A4) system,[10] which has significant implications regarding drug interactions and is discussed later. See the Drug Interactions section for further details.

Ester local anesthetics are hydrolyzed very rapidly in the blood by pseudocholinesterase to form aromatic acids and amino alcohols. In fact, procaine has a plasma half-life of less than 1 minute.[12] Its primary metabolite is PABA, a portion of which undergoes further metabolism in the liver. Patients with pseudocholinesterase deficiency have impaired metabolism of ester anesthetics.[6]

Table 39-2   Key Pharmacologic Concepts—Commonly Used Injectable Local Anesthetics

Generic Name	Lidocaine	Bupivacaine	Mepivacaine	Procaine	Diphenhydramine
Onset of action (minutes)	<2	5	3-5	2-5	1-10
Duration of action* (minutes)	30-60 without epinephrine, 120-360 with epinephrine	120-240 without epinephrine, 180-420 with epinephrine	45-90 without epinephrine, 120-360 with epinephrine	15-60	≥30†
Relative potency	4	16	2	1	±
Protein binding (%)	60-80	82-96	60-85	5.8	80-85
Elimination half-life (hours)	1.5-2.0	1.5-5.5	1.9-3.2	0.66	2.4-9.3
Metabolism	Liver	Liver	Liver	Hydrolyzed by plasma pseudocholinesterase	Liver
Excretion	Kidney	Kidney	Kidney	Kidney	Kidney
Maximum dose	300 mg without epinephrine (4.5 mg/kg), 500 mg with epinephrine (7.0 mg/kg)	175 mg without epinephrine, 225 mg with epinephrine	400 mg	350-600 mg	None listed for tissue infiltration, IM/IV max is 400 mg/d for adults, 5 mg/kg/24 hrs for children
Special issues	Tumescent anesthesia for liposuction can be safely used at concentrations up to 55 mg/kg in the proper setting	Higher risk of cardiac toxicity at smaller doses	Has mild vasoconstrictor properties that reduce absorption		Reports of tissue necrosis, most with 5% strength; more painful injection; cautioned against this use in package insert

Adapted from McEvoy[8,77]: Physicians' desk reference, Montvale, NJ, 1999, Medical Economics Company, Inc.

IM, Intramuscular; IV, intravenous.

*May vary dramatically with concentration, location, and technique of injection.

†Possibly shorter than lidocaine.

Excretion.   Renal excretion accounts for the majority of the elimination of local anesthetics from both classes. Lidocaine's excretion is complex. The majority of the drug passes through the liver where it is metabolized, then is excreted into bile. Because very few metabolites are found in feces, it is believed that the lidocaine metabolites are then reabsorbed from the gastrointestinal tract and excreted in the urine.[13] Lidocaine metabolites represent the majority of excreted drug, with less than 10% being excreted unchanged by the kidney.[14]

Only 2% of procaine is excreted unchanged in the urine. The majority of the drug is excreted as its primary metabolite, PABA.

Mechanism of Action.   To understand the mechanism of action of local anesthetics, one must understand the normal physiology of nerve conduction. At rest, nerve axonal membranes have a transmembrane electric potential (-90 to -60 mV). This potential is maintained by an active transport sodium-potassium pump that continually pumps sodium ions into the extracellular space. Distinct sodium ion channels remain closed in this resting state, resulting in a negatively charged intracellular space (axonal cytoplasm). When a nerve is stimulated, sodium channels open, allowing the massive influx of sodium ions. This sodium influx depolarizes the membrane toward the sodium equilibrium potential ($+40$ mV), reversing the internal negative charge to a positive charge. Subsequently, sodium channels inactivate and potassium channels open, allowing the egress of potassium ions. The active transport sodium-potassium pump again restores the baseline transmembrane potential (-90 to -60 mV). It is through this process that nerve impulses are transmitted down axons and between cells.

Local anesthetics block conduction in nerves by minimizing or preventing the influx of sodium ions, thus preventing depolarization[15] (Table 39-3). This effect is thought to be mediated through induction of a conformational change in voltage-sensitive sodium channels after binding. The lipophilic portion of the drug allows penetration of the cell membrane, whereas the hydrophilic portion is thought to interact with the sodium channels on the inner surface of the cell membrane.[16]

Although local anesthetics work on all nerves, there are different propensities to block conduction, depending on nerve fiber characteristics. Among the myelinated nerves, smaller diameter fibers are more sensitive to blockade by local anesthetics.[17] Small fibers that are rele-

■ **Table 39-3**

Mechanism of Action—Commonly Used Local Anesthetics

Generic Name	Lidocaine*	Diphenhydramine	Capsaicin
Mechanism of action	Blocks nerve impulse generation and conduction by decreasing the permeability of the nerve cell membrane to Na$^+$, thus preventing depolarization[15]	Unknown, but most likely involves blocking Na$^+$ channels as with other local anesthetics[180]	Stimulation of release of substance P from sensory nerve endings; with prolonged application depletion of substance P from sensory nerve endings[154]
Therapeutic result	Type C pain and itch nerve fiber conduction blocked	Type C pain and itch nerve fiber conduction blocked	Inhibition of pain sensation
Other pharmacologic effects	Interferes with nerve conduction in other organs in which conduction occurs	Block histamine (H1) receptors, anticholinergic effects, sedative	

*And with other amide anesthetics; also applies to ester anesthetics.

vant to the dermatologist carry pain and temperature sensations (Type A, delta fibers), whereas larger and thus relatively more resistant fibers carry touch and pressure sensation (Type A, beta fibers), and the largest and most resistant fibers control proprioception and motor function (Type A, alpha fibers). Myelinated fibers are more resistant to anesthetics than unmyelinated fibers. For this reason, it is prudent to remind patients that after being anesthetized they may still feel pressure, but they should not feel pain. It is also important to remember that temporary motor paresis may occur if either high volumes of local anesthetic are used or if deep placement of the local anesthetic occurs in an area where deeper motor fibers are present under the more superficial sensory cutaneous nerves. This temporary motor paresis may be seen commonly when anesthetizing skin on the temple overlying the temporal branch of the facial nerve.

CLINICAL USE

FDA-Approved Indications.   Food and Drug Administration (FDA)–approved dermatologic indications for use of injectable local anesthetics include infiltrative anesthesia and regional nerve blocks (Table 39-4).

Infiltrative Anesthesia. Injectable local anesthetics are routinely used by dermatologists to achieve anesthesia before cutaneous surgery. Commonly used preparations are lidocaine 0.5% to 2.0% with or without epinephrine 1:100,000 or 1:200,000. The technique of infiltrative anesthesia involves injecting anesthetic directly into and surrounding the area to be treated. Papillary dermal injection is most painful and creates more tissue distortion but gives nearly instantaneous anesthesia and may be indicated in situations that require very rapid onset of anesthesia. Subcutaneous injection is the least painful plane of injection; however, this depth of injection provides less effective anesthesia for epidermal and dermal procedures unless the anesthetic is allowed to diffuse into adjacent tissue planes over several minutes. A favored method of infiltration involves injecting anesthetic slowly as the needle is advanced into the deep dermis at the junction of the subcutaneous tissue; this method strikes a balance between the previously discussed methods, allowing relatively rapid onset with less pain of injection.

Table 39-4	Lidocaine Indications and Contraindications

FDA-APPROVED INDICATIONS
Infiltrative anesthesia
Regional nerve blocks
Topical anesthesia

OFF-LABEL DERMATOLOGIC USES
Tumescent anesthesia*[30,31]
Postherpetic neuralgia[41]
Pruritus[43]

CONTRAINDICATIONS

Absolute	Relative
Hypersensitivity to lidocaine or preservatives (sulfites or parabens)	Hypersensitivity to amide anesthetics
	Pregnancy
	Significant hepatic impairment
	Significant cardiac impairment
	Myasthenia gravis
	Hyperthyroidism

PREGNANCY PRESCRIBING STATUS—CATEGORY B

---

*Well-documented clinical benefit for off-label use.

The discomfort of lidocaine injection may also be minimized by several other techniques. Pinching the skin before and during injection can decrease the pain of the initial puncture and injection. Counter stimulation, such as stretching, pressing, or rubbing, can also reduce the perceived pain of injection. Distracting the patient by conversing with them, asking questions, or asking them to wiggle their fingers or toes is often helpful as well. Using a 1-inch needle can decrease the number of punctures necessary to anesthetize a large area but may be more difficult to control. If additional punctures are required, they may be made through anesthetized skin. It is also less painful to inject from within a laceration or surgical wound edge than it is through intact skin.[18] Using a 30-gauge needle also minimizes the pain of injection,[19] but this needle size makes aspirating before injection (to confirm the extravascular location of the needle) difficult. Ice applied topically for 10 seconds affords 2 seconds of analgesia, during which time an injection of local anesthetic may be less painful. A slow rate of injection is often less painful as well.[20]

Utilization of pH-buffered lidocaine has been reported to decrease the pain of injection in controlled studies.[19] The most commonly used method for buffering is to mix 1 part sodium bicarbonate (8.4% or 1 mEq/ml) to 9 or 10 parts of 1% lidocaine with epinephrine 1:100,000.[21] This mixture is considered effective for up to 1 week at room temperature because there is a 25% or more decline in epinephrine each week when buffered.[22-24] Refrigerating the buffered solution extends the effective life of epinephrine to 2 weeks. Conversely, warming the local anesthetic to 40° C has been promoted as a means to decrease injection pain.[25,26] Adding hyaluronidase to lidocaine results in enhanced tissue dispersion of lidocaine with less tissue distortion. Hyaluronidase may also increase the pain of injection and decrease the duration of anesthesia, whereas the long-term effects on wound healing have not been evaluated.[27] It also contains thimerosal, to which patients may be allergic.[28]

Ring Block. The ring block or field block is a modification of the infiltration technique that entails surrounding the area to be anesthetized with a wall of anesthetic but not directly injecting the lesion to be biopsied or excised. This causes less tissue distortion, which in some situations offers a great advantage over the infiltrative technique. This technique may also be useful in obtaining skin biopsies for microbiologic culture. Infiltration of an anesthetic with preservatives directly into the tissue to be sampled may lead to false-negative bacterial cultures due to the antibacterial effects of the preservatives.

Regional Nerve Blocks. Regional nerve blocks are commonly used on the face, wrist, ankle, and digits. This technique is most useful when it supplants numerous injections of local infiltration necessary to treat large areas such as in facial laser resurfacing or in carbon dioxide laser destruction of large numbers of plantar warts. The anesthetic, which is commonly used at a higher concentration (2% lidocaine) for blocks, is injected in the subcutaneous fat along the course of main sensory nerves innervating the area to be treated. Although this technique can decrease the number of injections required, it typically requires more time for anesthesia to occur. The main risks associated with regional nerve block include laceration of nerve trunks, intravascular injection, and temporary motor paralysis.[29]

The most commonly used nerve block in dermatology is the digital block. Further details on the technique for this and other regional blocks are beyond the scope of this chapter.[28,29]

Off-Label Dermatologic Uses

Tumescent Anesthesia. Tumescent anesthesia, as popularized by Klein,[30] revolutionized liposuction. The tumescent technique achieves longer-lasting regional anesthesia by direct infiltration of large volumes of dilute lidocaine (0.05% or 0.1%) with epinephrine 1:1,000,000. The large volume of solution distends the subcutaneous tissue, making it firm for the advancement of liposuction cannulas. This technique modifies the pharmacokinetics of lidocaine so that absorption is delayed and peak plasma levels occur 12 to 14 hours after infiltration begins.[31] This modified pharmacokinetic profile in turn allows larger doses of lidocaine to be used for anesthesia of more extensive areas. In fact, the lidocaine dose considered safe for normal weight individuals when administered using the tumescent technique is 35 mg/kg to 50 mg/kg, and perhaps as high as 55 mg/kg.[32,33]

It has been shown that tumescent anesthesia performed alone without other anesthetic agents has an excellent safety record with no reported deaths.[34,35] However, a series of five deaths occurring in patients undergoing tumescent liposuction has been reported recently by Rao and associates.[36] In these fatalities and all reported deaths after liposuction, there has been an association with systemic anesthesia.[37] Based on this experience, the safest application of the tumescent anesthetic technique appears to be without the use of other anesthetic agents.[37]

The tumescent technique has been applied to other clinical situations in dermatology. It has been described for anesthesia before skin cancer reconstruction,[38,39] dermabrasion,[39,40] hair transplantation,[39] and scalp reduction.[39] Chiarello[41] reported using lidocaine, epinephrine, and triamcinolone for intralesional therapy of acute herpetic pain and postherpetic neuralgia using the tumescent technique.

Collagen Soft Tissue Augmentation. Lidocaine is also premixed with bovine collagen in a concentration of 0.3% to decrease the pain of injection in soft tissue augmentation.[42] In practical experience, the initial injections appear to be less painful, but when injecting into tissue adjacent to the previous injection sites, there seems to be a decrease in sensation as the lidocaine diffuses through the tissue.

Pruritus. Intravenous (IV) lidocaine has been reported as a therapeutic alternative for the treatment of severe recalcitrant pruritus.[43] In a reported case, a patient was given 100 mg of lidocaine IV after a normal electrocardiogram (EKG), and within 10 minutes, his pruritus completely resolved. Over 1 week, symptoms gradually recurred but to a level of severity that was half its initial level. After a second dose, the patient remained symptom-free for 16 days with gradual return to a level of 25% his initial symptoms. A third dose again resulted in resolution of symptoms with gradual return of pruritus. The mechanism of this prolonged effect of lidocaine on pruritus is unknown, and due to the need for intermittent dosing of the drug, the practical application of this treatment modality is limited.

Adverse Effects. Adverse effects of local anesthetics are quite uncommon given the frequent use of these agents. It is more common to experience adverse reaction related to the vasoconstrictors or the injection itself, rather than to the anesthetic. Adverse effects can be divided into toxic effects or allergic reactions and must

be differentiated from the effects of epinephrine and reactions unrelated to drug properties.

Toxic Effects. When dosage maximums are exceeded or if metabolism or excretion is impaired, blood levels of lidocaine can increase beyond safe levels. Toxic blood levels occur primarily after injection of large amounts of local anesthetics, but they have also been reported after topical application of lidocaine to mucosal surfaces, widespread dermatoses, or injured skin.[44-46] Blood levels of lidocaine correlate with distinct clinical signs and symptoms (Table 39-5) relating to toxicity primarily involving the central nervous system (CNS) and cardiovascular system.

CNS toxicity can involve any of the following: drowsiness, circumoral paresthesia, lingual paresthesia, tinnitus, nystagmus, ataxia, hallucinations, twitching, restlessness, seizures, coma, or apnea.[47] But it is important to note that the clinical signs do not necessarily progress in sequence. For example, if a large volume of lidocaine is delivered intravascularly, seizures may be the first sign of toxicity noted.[47] Complicating matters is the overlap between the signs and symptoms of lidocaine toxicity and the systemic effects of epinephrine. Anxiety, restlessness, and tremor may be due to significant systemic levels

■ **Table 39-5**   Lidocaine Blood Levels and Corresponding Signs and Symptoms of Toxicity[134]

Blood Levels	Signs and Symptoms of Toxicity
1-5 µg/ml	Increased anxiety
	Talkativeness
	Tinnitus
	Tingling and numbness of lips and tongue
	Nausea and vomiting
	Metallic taste
	Double vision
5-8 µg/ml	Nystagmus
	Muscle twitching
	Tremor
8-12 µg/ml	Seizures
	Respiratory arrest

of either drug. Given that the lidocaine dose limit has not been exceeded, these signs and symptoms can be safely assumed to be from the epinephrine. The absence of tinnitus and circumoral paresthesias also supports the diagnosis of effects due to epinephrine.

Treatment starts with recognition of the anesthetic toxicity, discontinuing further use of local anesthetics, and observing for progressive symptoms of lidocaine toxicity. If clinical signs and symptoms of toxicity suggest midrange toxic blood levels (5 to 8 μg/ml), treatment may be best accomplished by admission to the hospital for observation. Seizures are treated by the following steps: establishing an airway, delivering oxygen, administering lorazepam or diazepam, and simultaneously activating the Emergency Medical Services (EMS).

The effects of lidocaine on the cardiovascular system are due to blocking sodium channels, which leads to decreased cardiac contractility in a ratio proportional to their potency, bupivacaine being roughly four times more potent than lidocaine.[48] With lidocaine, there is a progressive deterioration with increasing blood levels going from hypotension (due to sympathetic blockade) to bradycardia and finally respiratory depression.[49] Bupivacaine toxicity may be different, with potentially fatal dysrhythmias (ventricular fibrillation) appearing as the first sign of cardiac toxicity. This may be due to the fact that bupivacaine dissociates more slowly or incompletely from the sodium channels once in the resting state.[50] Unfortunately, even though the potency of bupivacaine is roughly four times greater than lidocaine, its potential for cardiac toxicity is much higher.[48,51,52] As a rule, rare instances of cardiac toxicity require hospitalization for circulatory support.

Allergic Reactions. Allergic reactions have been estimated to make up less than 1% of all adverse reactions to local anesthetics.[53] They may be due to the anesthetic itself (true anesthetic allergy) or to preservatives such as parabens and sulfites.[54] Esters have been much more commonly shown to cause allergic reactions; this is one of the primary factors that led to a major decline in the use of ester anesthetics. Allergic reactions to amides are much more rare.[55] The two types of allergic reactions to local anesthetics are anaphylactic reactions (Type I) and delayed-type hypersensitivity reactions (Type IV). The most serious are anaphylactic reactions, which may be life threatening. These reactions are immunoglobulin E (IgE) mediated and are often heralded by urticaria, angioedema, and bronchospasm (wheezing). If these signs occur within 1 to 2 hours of anesthetic injection, they support the diagnosis of anaphylaxis.[56] A practical clue for assistance in rapidly distinguishing anaphylactic hypotension (in the absence of skin findings) from vasovagal reactions or dysrhythmias is the pulse. In anaphylaxis the patient is tachycardic, whereas in vasovagal reactions the patient is bradycardic, and finally in dysrhythmias the pulse is irregular.[56] If the patient develops signs of respiratory or hemodynamic compromise, EMS should be activated as supportive measures are instituted.

In patients who present to the office with a history of "caine" allergy, a detailed history of the previous reaction is necessary. Important information used to determine the nature of the reaction includes agents used, quantity administered, route given, presence of vasoconstrictors or preservatives, type of symptoms and signs experienced, time course, concomitant medications, past medical history, and preceding episodes.[56] This information may be more reliably obtained from the health care provider who witnessed the reaction. This physician may be able to offer alternative anesthetics, which have been used safely for that particular patient in the past. If unable to establish that the reaction was not allergic in nature, the patient should be referred for skin testing and incremental challenge. It has been suggested from limited patch-testing data that there is no cross-reaction between amides and esters.[57] The practice of simply switching classes in patients with anaphylactic reactions has been recommended by some to avoid future hypersensitivity reactions. Unfortunately, this class switching has never been proven to be safe with regard to anaphylactic reactions. Thus thorough evaluation by an allergist is recommended if the patient had a prior anaphylactic reaction.[56] If no safe local anesthetic can be determined, infiltration of injectable diphenhydramine[58,59] or saline[60] can provide reasonable local anesthesia in selected instances.

Epinephrine Effects. Although epinephrine is not a local anesthetic, its effects are often included in a discussion of local anesthetic adverse effects because they can be difficult to distinguish from one another. Transient or minor reactions frequently attributable to epinephrine include anxiety, headache, tremor, restlessness, and palpitations. Epinephrine is typically implicated as the cause of these symptoms when the total dose of anesthetic is well within the safe ranges listed in Table 39-2. These epinephrine effects may be mitigated by the use of low-dose sublingual diazepam. Epinephrine is discussed in detail later in this chapter.

Reactions Unrelated to Drug Properties. Vasovagal reactions are not due to an effect of the local anesthetic but rather to unpleasant emotional or physical stimuli. These have a characteristic pattern that includes diaphoresis, lightheadedness, bradycardia, and hypotension. Immediate measures to treat such a reaction include supine positioning with leg elevation (Trendelenburg's position), smelling salts, and a cool moist towel to the forehead. For vasovagal reactions not responding to these measures, atropine 0.4 mg delivered subcutaneously has been recommended.[61]

Local injection of nearly any substance can lead to hematoma, ecchymosis, nerve laceration, or infection, all of which may occur with the injection of local anesthetics.

Drug Interactions. Lidocaine is metabolized by the hepatic microsomal enzymes of the cytochrome CYP 3A4 system. Drugs that induce CYP 3A4 may theoretically increase lidocaine clearance and decrease lidocaine blood levels.[62] This would have no significant implications for dermatologic use because rapid clearance of systemically absorbed lidocaine would only enhance the safety profile of its use. However, CYP 3A4 inhibitors may theoretically decrease lidocaine clearance and accordingly increase lidocaine blood levels[10] (Table 39-6). A list of CYP 3A4 inhibitors was recently published.[10] The authors recommend decreasing doses of lidocaine for tumescent anesthesia (by

Table 39-6   CYP 3A4 Inhibitors Affecting Lidocaine Metabolism

Interacting Drug or Drug Category	Examples and Comments
INCREASED LEVELS OF LIDOCAINE DUE TO CYP 3A4 INHIBITORS	
Macrolide antibiotics	Erythromycin, troleandomycin >> clarithromycin
Fluoroquinolone antibiotics	Norfloxacin
Other antibiotics	Cephalosporins, doxycycline, chloramphenicol, tetracycline, metronidazole
Azole antifungal agents	Ketoconazole >> itraconazole > fluconazole
Protease inhibitors	Ritonavir, indinavir >> saquinavir, nelfinavir
Calcium channel blockers	Diltiazem, verapamil, nicardipine, nifedipine
H_2 antihistamines	Cimetidine
Corticosteroids	Methylprednisolone, dexamethasone
Diuretics	Thiazides, furosemide
Benzodiazepines	Flurazepam, midazolam, triazolam
Foods	Grapefruit juice
Antidysrhythmics	Mibefradil dihydrochloride, quinidine, amiodarone
Hormones	Danazol, thyroxine
SSRI/other antidepressants	Paroxetine, fluoxetine, fluvoxamine, sertraline, nefazodone
Miscellaneous	Methadone, pentoxifylline, propranolol, propofol, zileuton (also a CYP 1A2 inhibitor)
DECREASED LEVELS OF LIDOCAINE DUE TO CYP 3A4 INDUCTION	
Anticonvulsants	Phenytoin, phenobarbital, carbamazepine
Antituberculous agents	Rifampin, isoniazid

Data from Klein[10] and Katz[62] and *CliniSphere 2.0 CD ROM*, St. Louis, June 2000, Facts & Comparisons.

30% to 40% in females and 10% to 20% in males) when used in the presence of drugs that interfere with metabolism of lidocaine. With in-office excisional surgery or Mohs' micrographic surgery, the volume of anesthetic used rarely approaches that capable of producing toxic blood levels. However, when administering large volumes of infiltrative anesthesia, it seems prudent to incorporate dosage reductions as previously suggested in patients who are on such medications.

In addition to those listed in Table 39-6, other medications that have been reported to cause problems when given with lidocaine, either due to alteration of drug levels or by potentiating the tissue specific effect of either agent, include[62] digitalis, disopyramide, ephedrine, isosorbide dinitrate, mexiletine, pentobarbital, phenytoin, propafenone, propanone, and tocainide. In general, such case reports resulted from IV boluses of lidocaine, not after local infiltration. It should be remembered that improper injection technique can lead to inadvertent intravascular injection, effectively delivering an IV bolus of drug.

Therapeutic Guidelines. Though lidocaine is the most common local anesthetic in use today, other agents have valuable properties. Mepivacaine is very similar to lidocaine in onset and duration of anesthesia, but there is no dermatologic application for which the use of mepivacaine has clearly been shown to be advantageous. However, one study compared 0.9% saline, 1% prilocaine, 1% lidocaine, 1% mepivacaine, and 1% procaine for intradermal anesthesia and found that although all agents delivered a similar depth of anesthesia, mepivacaine was the least painful on injection.[63] Although this finding was statistically significant, the clinical significance is uncertain. Technique of injection is more important in the reduction in pain from local anesthetic injections than is the choice of local anesthetic.

Bupivacaine offers prolonged duration of anesthesia, as much as four times the duration of plain lidocaine,[64] although some feel its onset of action may be slower. This long duration of action is partially accounted for by the fact that the drug is very lipid-soluble. In general, more lipid-soluble agents are more potent, and this increased potency correlates with both CNS toxicity and cardiovascular toxicity.[7]

Mixing a rapid-onset/short-duration local anesthetic with a delayed-onset/long-duration anesthetic has been advocated by some. However, it has been shown that combining commercial preparations leads to unpredictable effectiveness,[65] which led to the conclusion that mixing agents offers no significant clinical advantages.[7] A significant trade-off of mixing two anesthetics is the inevitable dilution of the concentration of each agent being mixed, thus reducing the anesthetic potency.

Finally, in an attempt to investigate alternative, potentially advantageous methods of achieving local anesthesia, iontophoretic administration of local anesthetics has been attempted. Iontophoresis is a procedure by which electrically charged molecules are delivered into the skin by an external electric field. A small study compared 2% lidocaine with epinephrine with placebo (both delivered by iontophoresis) and found that iontophoretic delivery of the study drug resulted in decreased pain of IV cannulation after 12 minutes of iontophoresis when compared with placebo.[66] Another study showed that 30 minutes of iontophoresis using 10% lidocaine with 1:10,000 epinephrine showed earlier onset and greater degree of anesthesia when compared with eutectic mixture of local anesthesia (EMLA) applied for 30 and 60 minutes. The authors of this study noted potential problems with this iontophoresis, including lack of cost-effectiveness of the procedure, as well as problems with application to large areas of skin and application to contoured surfaces.[67]

Use of Local Anesthetics during Pregnancy. The use of local anesthetics during pregnancy should be considered cautiously but is generally acceptable. Lidocaine is classified as FDA Pregnancy Risk Category B, indicating no risk to the human fetus, despite possible animal risk; or no risk in animal studies, whereas human studies have not been performed.[68] Recommendations for use of local anesthetics in pregnancy include the following[69]: (1) avoiding use during organogenesis (15 to 56 days of gestation) when possible, (2) minimizing doses of drug delivered, (3) remaining alert for vasovagal reactions, which may occur at a higher rate during pregnancy, and (4) positioning the patient on her left side to avoid vena caval and aortic compression. Epinephrine is classified as FDA Pregnancy Risk

Category C, indicating that risk cannot be ruled out, human studies are lacking, and animal studies may or may not show risk, but benefits may justify potential risk.[68] Despite this categorization, it is felt to be unlikely that doses used in dermatologic surgery would have a significant effect over the endogenously produced epinephrine resulting from anxiety.[69] In addition, if epinephrine allows a procedure to be performed more quickly and with the use of less anesthetic, its use may be justified.[69] Although a set of general guidelines is represented, it is generally prudent to discuss the use of any medications in pregnancy with the patient's obstetrician whenever a question arises.

TOPICAL ANESTHETICS
Eutectic Lidocaine and Prilocaine Cream

Topical anesthesia has been used for many years on mucosal surfaces because of the relative ease of penetration of topical agents on mucosa. However, the keratinized stratum corneum has been a major barrier to the use of topical anesthetics on normal skin. The use of previous formulations resulted in significant dermatitis, systemic toxicity, or inadequate local analgesia.[70] EMLA represents a unique cream formulation of lidocaine and prilocaine that can deliver adequate skin analgesia. The net result is either reduction of pain from subsequent needle puncture or even replacing the need for injectable anesthesia altogether.

PHARMACOLOGY

Structure. The general structure of local anesthetics was previously described. Prilocaine, like lidocaine, is an amide local anesthetic with minor differences in the aromatic (lipophilic) portion, the intermediate chain, and the amine (hydrophilic) portions.

Absorption. The feature that makes EMLA unique is the eutectic mixture of its components, lidocaine 2.5% and prilocaine 2.5%. By mixing the crystalline forms of each in a 1:1 ratio, this combination has a lower melting point than either agent alone; this is known as a eutectic mixture.[71,72] Thus the combination is a liquid at room temperature and is subsequently able to be suspended in an oil in water emulsi-

fier.[73] It is this highly concentrated liquid combination that promotes enhanced penetration over the crystalline form of either drug individually in a cream base.[73]

The amount of EMLA systemically absorbed is directly related to the duration and surface area of application.[73] Skin blood flow, skin thickness, and presence of skin pathology lead to altered absorption but also affect the EMLA onset of action, efficacy, and duration of action.[74] Regional variation in absorption has also been noted, with faster absorption occurring on the face.[75] In patients with psoriasis or eczema, absorption is faster but duration of action is shorter.[76] Plasma levels of lidocaine and prilocaine with facial application in adults have been shown to reach a maximum by 2 to 3 hours, yet remain well below toxic levels.[75]

Bioavailability. Once absorbed, the bioavailability of both lidocaine and prilocaine is that which would be expected after any form of administration. Lidocaine was discussed previously. Prilocaine is 55% protein bound and is distributed widely throughout the body, as is lidocaine.[77]

Metabolism and Excretion. Prilocaine is metabolized by hepatic microsomes in a fashion similar to lidocaine, only at a faster rate.[78] Extra-hepatic metabolism has been suggested by animal experiments.[79] Prilocaine is excreted as metabolites via the kidney with less than 1% of the drug renally excreted unchanged.[8]

Mechanism of Action. The mechanism of action of prilocaine is similar to that of lidocaine and all amide local anesthetics as previously described.

CLINICAL USE

FDA-Approved Indications. The FDA-approved dermatologic indication for EMLA is for topical analgesia of normal intact skin[73] (Table 39-7).

Skin Surgery. If applied as directed under an occlusive dressing, such as Tegaderm or cellophane, in a quantity of 1 to 2 g/10 cm², the onset of significant analgesia occurs by approximately 60 minutes. Dermal analgesia increases for up to 3 hours if the EMLA is continuously occluded and should persist for up to 1 to 2 hours after removal of the cream.[73] Inadequate application or occlusion can contribute to inad-

Table 39-7	Eutectic Lidocaine and Prilocaine Indications and Contraindications

FDA-APPROVED INDICATIONS
Topical analgesia for use on intact skin*

OFF-LABEL USES
Mucosal analgesia[91]
Postherpetic neuralgia[102-106]
Distinction between Ehlers-Danlos syndrome
and simple hypermobility[107]
Hyperhidrosis[108]
Pruritus[109]

CONTRAINDICATIONS

Absolute	Relative
Hypersensitivity to lidocaine or prilocaine anesthetics	Mucosal application
	Application to broken skin
Congenital or idiopathic methemoglobinemia	Hypersensitivity to ester or other (nonlidocaine, nonprilocaine) amide anesthetics
Infants under 1 year of age receiving medications that induce methemoglobinemia (sulfonamides, nitroglycerin, acetaminophen, nitroprusside, phenytoin, and so on)	G-6-PD deficiency
	Significant cardiac disease
	Significant hepatic disease
	Use with class I antidysrhythmics (tocainide, mexiletine)
	Pregnancy
	Age < 1 month

PREGNANCY PRESCRIBING STATUS—CATEGORY B

*References 73, 83-85, 87, 89, 91-100, 106.

equate analgesia. For this reason, a single-unit-dose package (EMLA patch) has been developed to simplify application. Recently available in the United States, EMLA patches have been shown to be equivalent to anesthesia achieved by use of EMLA cream.[80,81] Patient instruction regarding proper use of EMLA is paramount to obtaining maximal analgesia with this product.

Depth of analgesia obtained by using EMLA is important to address in regard to skin surgery. It has been shown that the depth of analgesia increases with increasing length of application, up to a maximal depth of 5 mm. After a 90-minute application, this analgesia lasts for 30 minutes. After a 120-minute application, a 5-mm depth of analgesia lasts for 60 minutes.[82] When compared with 40% lidocaine in acid mantle ointment, EMLA was shown to induce more effective analgesia before Nd:YAG laser treatment.[83]

EMLA has been successfully used to elimi-nate pain in 61% of children when applied for 1 hour before the scalpel removal of molluscum, even in the setting of atopic dermatitis.[84,85] However, in children, it has not been shown to reduce the pain of routine vaccinations.[86]

When applied for a minimum of 2 hours, EMLA was found to be as effective as infiltrative anesthesia using lidocaine and epinephrine when split-thickness skin grafts (STSG) were harvested[87]; however, more postoperative bleeding was noted in the EMLA group, most likely due to the lack of epinephrine-induced vasoconstriction. EMLA was also compared with prilocaine injection and cryoanalgesia for skin-graft harvesting and was found to be superior to either alternative.[88]

Superficial shave excisions and punch biopsies may be possible in some patients with adequate preoperative application of EMLA. In one report evaluating excisional biopsies, curettage, and electrosurgery, EMLA was found to provide effective anesthesia in 87% of patients[89] if applied 110 to 180 minutes before surgery, using either the cream or the patch formulation. Although reports such as these are encouraging, practical experience suggests that it is not uncommon for patients to require the supplemental infiltrative anesthesia to ensure that these procedures are totally pain-free. When such supplemental injections are required, they are much better tolerated due to the degree of analgesia already achieved by use of EMLA.

EMLA has also been used for performing slit-smears for the diagnosis of Hansen's disease.[90] EMLA significantly decreased the pain of slit-smears performed on elbows and knees but disappointingly and surprisingly not on earlobes.

Genital warts have also been anesthetized successfully before punch biopsy, electrocautery destruction, and cryotherapy.[91-93]

Laser Surgery.   EMLA has been widely used as preoperative analgesia before treating port wine stains.[94,95] It is now being used for anesthesia before laser-assisted hair removal.[96]

Venipuncture.   Many studies on pain reduction with use of EMLA before venipuncture demonstrated efficacy. Statistically significant pain reduction has been shown during shorter periods of application,[97] but 45 minutes has been suggested as the minimum application time for clinically significant reduction in pain scores.[98]

Debridement of Leg Ulcers.   EMLA has also been used to achieve analgesia during leg ulcer debridement and has been shown to decrease the number of debridement sessions required to clean ulcers.[99,100] As with application to any open skin (which is not FDA-approved), consideration should be given to the possibility of increased systemic absorption of both anesthetic components of the EMLA formulation.[101]

Off-Label Dermatologic Uses

Postherpetic Neuralgia.   Postherpetic neuralgia has been treated with EMLA cream with temporary improvement of variable duration.[102-106] Although effective at once daily application, the typical large size of the area to be treated and the need for occlusion limit the routine use of EMLA in this situation.

EMLA as a Diagnostic Tool for Ehlers-Danlos Syndrome.   EMLA has been used to distinguish between patients with Ehlers-Danlos (ED) syndrome and simple hypermobility. Patients with ED syndrome, patients with simple hypermobility, and control patients were compared on their analgesic responses to EMLA.[107] Patients with ED syndrome have a significantly lower threshold to cutaneous laser stimulation and less depth of anesthesia compared with simple hypermobility patients and controls. The practical importance of this application seems limited given advances in diagnostic molecular biology methods.

Miscellaneous Dermatologic Uses.   EMLA has been used for treating hyperhidrosis[108] and has been effective in treating pruritus.[109] A wide variety of painful bullous and ulcerative dermatoses have been treated successfully with EMLA, including pemphigus vulgaris, bullous pemphigoid, lichen sclerosis, pyoderma gangrenosum, and stasis ulceration.[106] As stated previously, application to ulcerated skin is an "off-label" use.

Adverse Effects.   Adverse effects due to EMLA cream can be divided into systemic effects and local effects.

Systemic Effects—Methemoglobinemia. The most serious side effect of EMLA is methemoglobinemia. This is a unique adverse effect of prilocaine. In this condition, a metabolite of prilocaine, *O*-toluidine, is thought to cause oxidation of hemoglobin to methemoglobin.[110] This oxidized (ferric) form of hemoglobin cannot carry oxygen and makes the release of oxygen from normal ferrous hemoglobin less efficient. The final result is tissue hypoxia. An instructive case example cited in the package insert[73] is that of an infant 3 months of age who had 5 g of EMLA occluded for 5 hours on the dorsal hands and antecubital fossae. He was taking trimethoprim-sulfamethoxazole for a urinary tract infection (UTI) at the time. The patient went on to develop profound methemoglobinemia, 28% of total hemoglobin (normal methemoglobin = 0).

Patients at risk for methemoglobinemia should not use EMLA. These include patients with congenital or idiopathic methemoglobinemia and infants under the age of 12 months taking any methemoglobin-inducing agent[73] (Box 39-1).

Methemoglobinemia either spontaneously

Box 39-1

Eutectic Lidocaine and Prilocaine Cream Drug Interactions—Drugs That May Increase
the Risk of Methemoglobinemia

ANALGESICS/ANTIPYRETICS Acetaminophen Acetanilid Phenacetin	**NITRATES/RELATED DRUGS** Nitrates and nitrites Nitrofurantoin Nitroglycerin Nitroprusside
ANESTHETICS Benzocaine	**SULFONAMIDES/SULFONES** Dapsone Sulfamethoxazole Trimethoprim/sulfamethoxazole
ANTICONVULSANTS Phenobarbital Phenytoin	
ANTIMALARIAL AGENTS Chloroquine Pamaquine Primaquine Quinine	**OTHER DRUGS/CHEMICALS** Aniline dyes Naphthalene Para-aminosalicylic acid

Adapted from *Physicians' desk reference*, Montvale, NJ, 1999, Medical Economics Company, Inc.

resolves or it can be hastened by IV administration of methylene blue in severe symptomatic cases.

Other Systemic Effects. As with injectable lidocaine, the potential risk for systemic toxicity due to absorption of lidocaine or prilocaine is theoretically possible but quite unlikely.

Local Reactions. Sites treated with EMLA can experience stinging, burning, pruritus, blanching, or erythema. Allergic contact dermatitis to the prilocaine component of EMLA cream has been reported.[111,112] Patch tests for EMLA and prilocaine were positive in both patients in these reports. A previously unreported purpuric eruption occurred in five patients after a 30 to 60 minute application of EMLA cream.[113] Patch tests were negative in all patients, and it was hypothesized that the reaction was a toxic response of the vascular endothelium.

More troublesome are the reports of corneal abrasions and conjunctivitis reported in patients undergoing facial laser treatments when EMLA was applied near the eyes.[114,115] Extreme caution should be exercised in this area because the alkalinity of the product can result in a

■ **Table 39-8**   Eutectic Lidocaine and Prilocaine Cream Therapeutic Guidelines for Infants and Children[73]

Age	Body Weight	Maximum Total Dose	Maximum Application Area
1-3 months	<5 kg	1 g	10 cm²
4-12 months	5-10 kg	2 g	20 cm²
1-6 years	>10 kg	10 g	100 cm²

chemical burn, the symptoms of which may be masked at first by the anesthetic effect of the product.

Therapeutic Guidelines. Additional use instructions apply to pediatric patients.[73] Dose and area of application are recommended to be restricted in infants and children (Table 39-8).

OTHER TOPICAL LOCAL ANESTHETICS

Lidocaine

Topical lidocaine is available in topical solution, viscous solution, jelly, ointment, and spray formulations. These are all used primarily in treating cutaneous pain or pruritus. Caution should be taken in adhering to manufacturer-recommended dosing for the various preparations because systemic toxicity has been reported after topical application and was discussed previously.[44,45] Before the introduction of EMLA, 30% lidocaine was compounded in acid mantle cream for similar indications.[116] A combination of tetracaine, epinephrine (adrenaline), and cocaine, popularly known as TAC, has been extensively used in repairing pediatric lacerations. A study was published comparing EMLA to TAC for anesthesia before laceration repair in children. The results demonstrate that the EMLA group required less supplemental anesthesia to complete the procedure than the TAC group, and EMLA was therefore deemed more effective.[117]

More recently lidocaine 4% cream (ELA-Max) has been introduced. Utilizing a patented liposomal delivery system, this product has been touted in unpublished studies to provide greater pain reduction, less irritation, and erythema than EMLA.[118] At this time, there are no peer-reviewed studies that have been published to support these claims, but practical experience suggests the product is effective. It should also be noted that this product is now available without prescription.

Benzocaine

Benzocaine is a topical ester local anesthetic available in hundreds of formulations for skin and mucosal application for the temporary relief of pain and itching associated with burns, insect bites, and minor skin irritation. It is a potent sensitizer that is more likely to induce allergy if applied to broken or fissured skin, as present with a concomitant dermatitis.[119] Patients allergic to benzocaine may cross-react with other ester local anesthetics, which is supported by patch-testing data.[57] Although this appears to be true of delayed-type hypersensitivity, it has never been proven to occur with immediate, IgE-type hypersensitivity.[56] However, despite lack of specific scientific evidence, it is prudent to avoid giving systemic local anesthetics to patients with a topical sensitivity to an agent in the same class.[56]

Dyclonine

Dyclonine is a topical, ketone, local anesthetic indicated for temporary relief of pain and itching associated with postoperative wounds and mucosal anesthetic before endoscopic procedures. It has been shown to provide more pain relief than viscous lidocaine with 1% cocaine in treating radiation- and chemotherapy-induced stomatitis.[120] Dyclonine is also useful in the management of most oral ulcerative disorders by applying 0.5% solution with a cotton-tip applicator directly to involved areas every 2 to 3 hours as needed for pain. Allergic contact dermatitis to dyclonine has been reported.[121]

Other Topical Anesthetics

Pramoxine is a topical ether local anesthetic that is commonly used as a topical antipruritic agent. Dibucaine is a topical amide local anesthetic commonly used in hemorrhoidal preparations. Table 39-9 lists further information regarding topical local anesthetic agents.

CO-INJECTABLE VASOCONSTRICTORS

Epinephrine

Epinephrine (adrenaline) is most often used in dermatology as a vasoconstrictor injected with a local anesthetic. It three main purpose (1) to prolong the effect of the local anesthetic, (2) to decrease systemic absorption of the local anesthetic, and (3) to aid in hemostasis. Although other vasoconstrictors, such as phenylephrine and norepinephrine, have been previously used for these same purposes, epinephrine is the most common vasoconstrictor in use today.

PHARMACOLOGY. Epinephrine (β-[3,4-dihydroxyphenyl]-alpha-methylaminoethanol) is an endogenous catecholamine that is produced by the adrenal medulla. It is synthesized in the body from the amino acid tyrosine by a series of enzymatic steps. Both the endogenous form and the synthetic form are the levorotatory (L) isomer of the catecholamine, which is

Table 39-9 Key Pharmacologic Concepts—Commonly Used Topical Local Anesthetics

Generic Name	Lidocaine	Lidocaine and Prilocaine	Dyclonine	Capsaicin	Dibucaine	Doxepin	Benzocaine	Pramoxine
Frequency of application	q 3-4 hrs	1-3 hrs before procedure	q 2-3 hrs	3-5 times daily	q 2-4 hrs	4 times daily	prn	4 times daily
Onset of action*	<2	<60	2-10	1-2 wks	<5	<15	<5	<5
Peak effect*	2-5	120-360	2-10	4-6 wks	<5	120	<5	<5
Approximate duration of action*	30-45	60-120 after removal of occlusive dressing	<60	3-6 hrs	15-45	NA	15-45	<60
Maximum adult dose (mg)	†	NA	100	None reported with topical use	30	NA	NA	200
Special issues	Systemic toxicity reported with topical use	Only for intact skin; methemoglobinemia risk	For mucous membranes, but not conjunctiva			Indicated for use for 8 d; incidence of drowsiness ↑ if applied to >10% body surface area; allergic contact dermatitis	Maximum dose 5 g/d; methemoglobinemia is possible	

Adapted from Drug Facts and Comparisons[77]; Physicians' desk reference, Montvale, NJ, 1999, Medical Economics Company, Inc., and Breneman DL, Dunlap FE, Monroe EW, et al: J Dermatol Treat 8:161-168, 1997.

*Times given in minutes unless otherwise noted.

†Varies with the formulation.

15 times more active than the dextrorotatory (R) isomer.[8] Although epinephrine is both an α- and β-adrenergic agonist, it is the α-adrenergic properties that cause vasoconstriction.

When given subcutaneously, the vasoconstrictive effect of epinephrine takes place in 7 to 15 minutes,[122] and the duration of action is short (approximately 60 minutes).[77] Epinephrine is rapidly inactivated in tissue primarily by enzymatic transformation to metanephrine or normetanephrine.[77] These substances are then conjugated in the liver. Epinephrine also undergoes direct degradation in the liver by monoamine oxidase and catechol O-methyltransferase. Once metanephrine and normetanephrine are conjugated, they are excreted in the urine in the form of sulfates and glucuronides.[77] Either sequence results in the production of vanillylmandelic acid (VMA), which can be detected in the urine.

Mechanism of Action. Epinephrine is an α-, β[1]-, and β[2]-adrenergic agonist. Its vasoconstriction in the skin and mucous membranes is accomplished by stimulation of α-adrenergic receptors found on cutaneous vascular smooth muscle cells. Epinephrine is more effective when used with lidocaine than with bupivacaine or etidocaine because these agents already have delayed absorption due to high protein binding.

When used in higher concentrations for treating anaphylaxis, epinephrine's effect on β[1]-adrenergic receptors increases cardiac output. The β[2]-adrenergic stimulation is responsible for bronchodilation, and the α-adrenergic effects increase systemic vascular resistance, thus increasing blood pressure.

CLINICAL USE

FDA-Approved Indications. FDA-approved dermatologic indications for epinephrine are for use as a hemostatic agent, to prolong the action of local anesthetics, and to treat acute hypersensitivity reactions[77] (Table 39-10).

Hemostasis. When injected with local anesthetics, epinephrine causes vasoconstriction and helps decrease bleeding in the surgical field. It should be emphasized that the hemostatic effect of epinephrine does not become maximal until 7 to 15 minutes after injection.[122] Most commonly, it is prepackaged with the local anes-

---

Table 39-10	Epinephrine Indications and Contraindications

FDA-APPROVED INDICATIONS
Hemostasis[122,129]
Prolonging the effect of local anesthetics[77,125]
Treatment of acute allergic
   hypersensitivity[126,127]

CONTRAINDICATIONS

Absolute	Relative
Sensitivity to sodium metabisulfite	Cardiac disease: unstable angina, recent
Pheochromocytoma	myocardial infarction, recent CABG surgery,
	refractory dysrhythmias, uncontrolled
	congestive heart failure
	Uncontrolled hypertension
	Pregnancy
	Poorly controlled hyperthyroidism
	Poorly controlled diabetes mellitus
	Severe peripheral vascular disease
	Angle-closure glaucoma
	Cocaine abuse

PREGNANCY PRESCRIBING STATUS—CATEGORY C

CABG, Coronary artery bypass graft.

thetic. Some authors feel that adding epinephrine to local anesthetic just before use can decrease the pain of injection due to the higher pH of this freshly prepared solution.[29]

Epinephrine has also been used as a topical hemostatic agent. In harvesting STSG, epinephrine combined with a water-based jelly has been used as a lubricant for the dermatome, which aids in hemostasis.[123] Epinephrine in a concentration of 1:100,000 has also been combined with saline and applied with a spray bottle to STSG donor sites.[124]

Prolonging the Action of Local Anesthetics. As a direct result of vasoconstriction, the absorption of local anesthetics is delayed by using epinephrine.[125] As evident in Table 39-2, epinephrine can more than double the duration of action of local anesthetics in the skin. In the case of lidocaine, the duration of action without epinephrine is approximately 30 to 60 minutes in duration. With epinephrine, this duration is prolonged to 120 to 360 minutes. This translates into fewer injections during a relatively lengthy procedure. Another side benefit of this vasoconstriction is decreased risk of systemic toxicity.

Acute Hypersensitivity. Epinephrine is also indicated for the treatment of anaphylaxis and anaphylactoid reactions such as those due to drugs or insect stings. The dose administered in this setting is higher, 0.3 to 0.5 mg of epinephrine (1:1000) delivered subcutaneously. This dose may be repeated every 5 to 10 minutes. The treatment of anaphylaxis has been reviewed elsewhere.[126,127]

Adverse Effects

Cardiac Effects. The effect of epinephrine on the heart of healthy individuals is generally inconsequential, except for symptomatic palpitations. However, dysrhythmias and hypertension may occasionally occur with therapeutic doses or in the case of unrecognized overdosing.[77] Patients with ischemic heart disease are more susceptible to dysrhythmias and compromised coronary blood flow, due to the tachycardia and increased cardiac output caused by epinephrine.[128]

Primarily due to these potential cardiac effects, dosage maximums have been put forth in an attempt to minimize complications. There is no consensus regarding what dose is safe; it is generally recommended to use the lowest dose possible.[129] However, several authors recommend a maximum dosage of 200 μg for all patients.[130,131] Others put forth a maximum dose of 200 μg (0.2 mg) (20 ml of 1:100,000 epinephrine) for patients with heart disease and 500 μg (50 ml of 1:100,000 epinephrine) for healthy patients.[132] Still others take a more conservative approach by recommending a dosage maximum of 40 μg (0.04 mg) (4 ml of 1:100,000 epinephrine) for patients with significant cardiac disease.[130]

CNS Effects. CNS effects that may be encountered are restlessness, tremor, or headache. Other more serious complications of systemic epinephrine, including cerebral hemorrhage, hemiplegia, and subarachnoid hemorrhage, are very unlikely within dosage ranges used in dermatology.

Endocrinologic Effects. Epinephrine has also been linked to increased blood sugars and lactic acidosis in patients with diabetes mellitus.[133] Patients with pheochromocytoma or hyperthyroidism are at risk for hypertension when treated with epinephrine.[134]

Local Ischemia. Due to the vasoconstrictor effects of epinephrine, it has been traditionally taught that epinephrine should not be used with local anesthetics in areas in which its vasoconstricting effects may compromise circulation. These areas of potential risk include the nose, ear, penis, and digits. In practical experience, the ears, nose, and penis have excellent collateral flow and epinephrine may, in general, be used safely in these areas. Epinephrine may be used in small volumes for infiltrative local anesthesia of fingers and toes in patients that do not have vascular compromise. However, digital blocks using local anesthetics with epinephrine are *not* recommended, given the risk of local ischemia in a location with essentially no collateral circulation. Hemostasis in this setting is better achieved with a tourniquet. Based on a rat model and experience with norepinephrine-induced ischemia, it has been recommended that in treating digital ischemia caused by epinephrine, phentolamine may be helpful.[135]

Due to its vasoconstrictive effects, the use of epinephrine in donor sites before harvesting STSG and full-thickness skin grafts (FTSG) has been challenged. One study showed an increased risk of FTSG complications at 1-week follow-up in donor sites anesthetized with lidocaine with epinephrine but not at 6-week follow-up when compared with plain lidocaine.[136] Another study showed decreased survival of FTSG, but not STSG, when the donor site was anesthetized using lidocaine with epinephrine.[137] Although no definitive recommendation can be made, practical experience dictates that use of epinephrine in anesthetics is generally safe, but plain lidocaine can be considered for use in patients requiring these grafts who have compromised vasculature.

Drug Interactions

Beta-Blockers. Although very uncommon during dermatologic procedures,[138,139] there are case reports of malignant hypertension occurring in patients who are on noncardioselective beta-blockers, such as propranolol, after receiving epinephrine for cutaneous surgery.[140] This is thought to be due to α-adrenergic stimulation of peripheral vascular receptors while the β$_2$ receptors, which normally oppose their action, are blocked. Other commonly used nonselective beta-blockers include nadolol, timolol, and labetalol. Although the details regarding this interaction have not been worked out, it has been suggested that the infrequent nature of the occurrence with low doses of epinephrine used in dermatologic surgery makes discontinuing propranolol or other nonselective beta-blockers unnecessary.[138,139]

Tricyclic Antidepressants. Tricyclic antidepressants, such as amitriptyline and imipramine, can enhance the adverse cardiac effects of epinephrine.[141-143]

Other Medications. Antihistamines, such as chlorpheniramine and diphenhydramine, as well as thyroid replacement can potentiate the sympathomimetic effects of epinephrine.[62] Antipsychotic agents, such as haloperidol, can cause reversal of epinephrine's sympathomimetic vasopressor effects. The cardiac effects of epinephrine can be potentiated by digitalis and quinidine.[62] Table 39-11 lists epinephrine drug interactions.

Therapeutic Guidelines. Epinephrine is used in dermatologic surgery to maximize the anesthetic effect and minimize adverse effects. The optimal concentration of epinephrine has not been firmly established. A study in pigs showed that 1:200,000 dilution had similar onset of vasoconstriction, magnitude of diminished blood flow, and duration of effect when compared with 1:100,000 dilution. However, diminished effect was documented for 1:400,000 dilution.[144] In a small study of patients receiving bilateral operations, various concentrations were blindly assessed for the degree of capillary bleeding by members of the operative team. No differences were detected in the effects of varying concentrations until they were reduced past the 1:500,000 dilution.[145] Most recently, a randomized, double-blinded, prospective study helped establish that more dilute concentrations of epinephrine are effective. The onset of vasoconstriction and magnitude of diminished blood flow were compared in various dilutions of epi-

---

■ Table 39-11   Epinephrine Drug Interactions

Interacting Drug Group	Examples and Comments
POTENTIAL FOR MALIGNANT HYPERTENSION[140]	
Beta-blockers (noncardioselective)	Propranolol, nadolol, timolol, labetalol
ENHANCED SYMPATHOMIMETIC EFFECTS[143]	
Antihistamines	Chlorpheniramine, diphenhydramine
Tricyclic antidepressants	Amitriptyline, imipramine
Other drugs	Digitalis, ergotamine, quinidine, tranylcypromine, thyroxine
REVERSAL OF SYMPATHOMIMETIC EFFECTS	
Antipsychotic agents	Haloperidol

nephrine combined with 1% lidocaine. No significant differences were found between 1:400,000, 1:200,000, 1:100,000, and 1:50,000.[146] These studies suggest that smaller dilutions of epinephrine have clinically similar effects; however, its impact on systemic absorption is not discussed. The most common dilutions of epinephrine in use today are 1:100,000 and 1:200,000.

Freshly mixed lidocaine with epinephrine is touted as being less painful on injection than the premixed combination.[29] A lower pH of the premixed lidocaine and epinephrine combination is required to prevent degradation of epinephrine over time. When mixed fresh, a higher pH does not immediately degrade epinephrine and is less painful to inject. To make this solution, add 0.3 ml of 1:1,000 epinephrine to a 30 ml bottle of lidocaine.[29]

OTHER AGENTS WITH LOCAL ANESTHETIC EFFECTS
Capsaicin
Capsaicin is a naturally occurring substance that is the active agent causing the spicy taste in hot chili peppers. Hot pepper extracts have been used as food additives and as medicinal agents for centuries in countries such as Mexico, where the plants are indigenous.[147] Hot pepper extracts were used in Europe for the treatment of a painful tooth almost 150 years ago.[148] Capsaicin is formulated today as a topical lotion or cream that may be used as an adjuvant in the treatment of pain. As such, capsaicin may not be considered an anesthetic but rather a topical analgesic. As an adjuvant to the management of chronic pain, it is effective only if applied consistently and frequently over time.

PHARMACOLOGY
Structure. Capsaicin, also known as trans-8-methyl-*N*-vanillyl-6-nonenamide, is a natural alkaloid derived from plants of the Solanaceae family.

Absorption and Bioavailability. Animal studies show that after IV administration, capsaicin is distributed to the CNS and liver after 20 minutes.[149] There are no published reports of percutaneous absorption of capsaicin in human patients; however, synthetic analogs of capsaicin are being studied in animals and in ca-

daveric skin for the development of new transdermal drug delivery systems.[150,151]

Metabolism and Excretion. Capsaicin is metabolized in the liver by the cytochrome P-450 system (CYP 2E1).[152,153] Its major metabolite is dihydrocapsaicin, which is also metabolized in the liver. Dihydrocapsaicin is excreted in the urine along with its metabolites.[149]

Mechanism of Action. Topical application of capsaicin causes selective excitation of peripheral unmyelinated afferent C-fibers, which are responsible for pain[154] (see Table 39-3). This occurs by causing release of substance P, stored in synaptic vesicles, from the sensory nerve fibers, which in turn prolongs (increases) cutaneous pain transmission. With repeated applications of capsaicin, substance P is depleted, resulting in decreased pain. Recent publications have described specific capsaicin receptors expressed exclusively on small-diameter sensory neurons, which account for the selectivity of action of this agent.[155,156]

CLINICAL USE
FDA-Approved Dermatologic Indications
Postherpetic Neuralgia. One of the most common uses of capsaicin in dermatology is in treatment of postherpetic neuralgia (Table 39-12). However, the majority of published reports regarding the effectiveness of capsaicin are either uncontrolled studies or case reports.[157] One double-blinded, randomized, controlled trial of capsaicin 0.075% cream versus vehicle for postherpetic neuralgia showed that patients had improvement in pain, as measured by several different scales, with use of capsaicin.[158] Another double-blind, randomized, controlled trial showed statistically significant improvement in pain as measured by three separate pain scales. However, pain was completely or nearly completely eliminated in less than 20% of patients. One author suggests that capsaicin may be best utilized as an adjuvant in the overall approach to treatment with opioids and antidepressants because improvement with capsaicin alone is typically modest.[159]

Painful Diabetic Neuropathy. Capsaicin has been reported to improve the pain of diabetic neuropathy. One randomized, double-blind study showed a statistically significant reduction in visual analog scale assessment of pain

Table 39-12	Epinephrine Indications and Contraindications

FDA-APPROVED INDICATIONS
Postherpetic neuralgia[157-159,163]
Painful diabetic neuropathy[160-162]

OFF-LABEL DERMATOLOGIC USES
Pain Syndromes
Postmastectomy pain syndrome*[163,164]
Notalgia paresthetica[165]
Reflex sympathetic dystrophy[166]
Stump pain[167]
PUVA skin pain[168]
Burning pain[169]
Erythromelalgia[170]
Skin pain related to tumor infiltration[171]

Other Dermatoses
Psoriasis[172]
Vulvar vestibulitis[173]
Apocrine chromhidrosis[174]

CONTRAINDICATIONS

Absolute	Relative
Broken skin	Noncompliant patient

PREGNANCY PRESCRIBING STATUS—NOT APPLICABLE

PUVA, Psoralen plus ultraviolet A.
*Well-documented clinical benefits for off-label use.

at 4 weeks but not physician global assessment or categorical scales.[160] The authors believed that they could not answer the primary study questions. They mention possible confounding variables such as small study sample, short duration of treatment, or large placebo effect. The Capsaicin Study Group found a significant improvement in capsaicin-treated patients versus controls using three rating scales, although an intent-to-treat analysis showed no significant difference between study groups.[161] Also, a high placebo effect was noted, occurring in up to 58.1% of patients. The Capsaicin Study Group also found that capsaicin-treated diabetic neuropathy patients were more likely to have improvement in activities of daily living compared with placebo patients.[162]

Off-Label Dermatologic Uses.   Other reported dermatologic uses of topical capsaicin include the following: postmastectomy pain syndrome,[163,164] notalgia paresthetica,[165] reflex sympathetic dystrophy,[166] stump pain,[167] psoralen plus ultraviolet A (PUVA)–induced skin pain,[168] burning pain,[169] erythromelalgia,[170] skin pain related to tumor infiltration,[171] psoriasis,[172] vulvar vestibulitis,[173] and apocrine chromhidrosis.[174]

Adverse Effects.   Local effects are the main adverse effects of topical capsaicin. Burning sensations occur in up to 80% of patients using the product.[159] It is this burning sensation that makes it nearly impossible to blind subjects in the context of a controlled trial.[159] In addition, this same sensation increases the likelihood of patients abandoning therapy. To improve compliance, patients should be warned of significant burning and informed that this sensation diminishes with continued use over at least 1 to 2 weeks. Pruritus, erythema, coughing, and sneezing may also occur after using topical capsaicin. Patients should be cautioned to wash their hands after application to prevent inadvertent administration to uninvolved skin or mucous membranes. Other adverse effects, such as erythema and superficial erosions, can occur.[175] Capsaicin has also been shown to be toxic to keratinocytes and fibroblasts in vitro,[176] thus the application to abraded or broken skin may potentially delay wound healing.

Drug Interactions.   There are no known clinically relevant drug interactions with topical capsaicin.

Therapeutic Guidelines.   Onset of action in treating pain can be seen as soon as 1 to 2 weeks after beginning applications three to five times daily. However, the maximal analgesia may be delayed for 4 to 6 weeks,[159,177] thus an adequate therapeutic trial must last at least this duration. After each application, the effects of capsaicin last 3 to 6 hours.[175]

Antihistamines

DIPHENHYDRAMINE.   Antihistamines have long been known to have anesthetic properties.[178,179] The mechanism of action likely involves blockage of sodium channels, similar to traditional local anesthetics[180] (see Table 39-3). Injectable diphenhydramine has been advocated as an alternative to traditional local anesthetics in "caine" sensitive patients.[181,182] Recent studies in the emergency medicine literature directly compared injectable diphenhydramine with lidocaine for local anesthesia. One study was a randomized, double-blinded trial comparing diphenhydramine 1% with lidocaine 1% for local anesthesia in repairing minor lacerations in adults.[59] Diphenhydramine was found to be more painful on injection according to study participants but was found to be as effective as lidocaine in pro-

ducing local anesthesia. Another prospective, randomized, double-blind, placebo-controlled trial confirmed these findings.[58]

Although some patients can experience somnolence associated with systemic absorption of diphenhydramine, the most serious potential adverse effects of injectable diphenhydramine are due to its known tissue irritancy. For unknown reasons, several cases of tissue necrosis have been reported,[183,184] including digital necrosis resulting in amputation.[185] For these reasons, the manufacturer includes a statement in the package insert that diphenhydramine should not be used as a local anesthetic.[186] Because two of these three reports used diphenhydramine 5%, it has been suggested that necrosis may be dose-related.[58] It may prove useful to use a 1% concentration and avoid injection into areas where collateral circulation may be limited.[58] A 1% concentration is achieved by diluting a 1 ml vial containing 50 mg diphenhydramine with 4 ml sterile saline.[59]

Diphenhydramine is also marketed in several topical formulations for temporary relief of minor pain and pruritus. Unfortunately, topical diphenhydramine is also a potent sensitizer, which can result in widespread dermatitis with subsequent systemic administration of diphenhydramine or related agents.[119]

TOPICAL DOXEPIN.   Topical doxepin has been approved for short-term use in treating pruritus due to eczematous dermatitis in adults. Although it has been shown to be effective,[187,188] somnolence due to systemic absorption, local irritation, and allergic contact dermatitis[189,190] dampened the initial enthusiasm for topical doxepin.

Bibliography

Bennett RG: *Fundamentals of cutaneous surgery,* St. Louis, 1988, Mosby, pp 194-239.

Dinehart SM: Topical, local and regional anesthesia. In Wheeland RG, editor: *Cutaneous surgery,* Philadelphia, 1994, WB Saunders, pp 102-112.

Gajraj NM, Pennant JH, Watcha MF: Eutectic mixture of local anesthetics (EMLA) cream. *Anesth Analg* 78:574-583, 1994.

Grekin RC, Auletta MJ: Local anesthesia in dermatologic surgery. *J Am Acad Dermatol* 19:599-614, 1988.

Lawrence C: Drug management in skin surgery. *Drugs* 52:805-817, 1996.

Rains C, Bryson: Topical capsaicin: a review of its pharmacological properties and therapeutic potential in post-herpetic neuralgia, diabetic neuropathy and osteoarthritis. *Drugs Aging* 7:317-328, 1995.

Ritchie JM, Greene NM: Local anesthetics. In Gilman AG, Rall TW, Nies AS, et al, editors: *Goodman and Gilman's the pharmacological basis of therapeutics*, ed 8, New York, 1990, Pergamon, pp 311-331.

References

Lidocaine—Pharmacology

1. Backer CL, Tinker JH, Robertson DM, et al: Myocardial reinfarction following local anesthesia for ophthalmic surgery. *Anesth Analg* 59:257-262, 1980.
2. Wildsmith JAW, Strichartz GR: Local anaesthetic drugs—an historical perspective. *Br J Anesth* 56:937-939, 1984.
3. Fink BR: Leaves and needles: the introduction of surgical local anesthesia. *Anesthesiology* 63:77-83, 1985.
4. MacKenzie TA, Young ER: Local anesthetic update. *Anesth Prog* 40:29-34, 1993.
5. Lofgren N: *Studies on local anesthetics—Xylocaine: a new synthetic drug*, Stockholm, 1948, Haeggstroms Boktrycheri.
6. Covino BG: Local anesthesia (first of two parts). *N Engl J Med* 286:975-983, 1972.
7. Strichartz GR, Berde CB: Local anesthetics. In Miller R, editor: *Anesthesia*, New York, 1994, Churchill Livingstone, pp 489-521.
8. McEvoy GK, editor: American Hospital Formulary Service Drug Information. Bethesda: American Society of Health Systems Pharmacists, 1998.
9. Katz J: The distribution of 14C-labelled lidocaine injected intravenously in the rat. *Anesthesiology* 29:249-253, 1968.
10. Klein JA, Kassarjdian N: Lidocaine toxicity with tumescent liposuction. *Dermatol Surg* 23:1169-1174, 1997.
11. Hondeghem LM, Miller RD: Local anesthetics. In Katzung B, editor: *Basic and clinical pharmacology*, Norwalk, 1989, Appleton & Lange, p 317.
12. Reidenberg MM, James M, Dring LG: The rate of procaine hydrolysis in serum of normal subjects and diseased patients. *Clin Pharmacol Ther* 13:279-284, 1972.
13. Covino BG: Local anesthesia (second of two parts). *N Engl J Med* 286:1035-1042, 1972.
14. Beckett AH, Boyes RN, Appleton PJ: The metabolism and excretion of lignocaine in man. *J Pharm Pharmacol* 18:76S-81S, 1966.
15. Strichartz GR, Ritchie JM: The action of local anesthetics on ion channels of excitable tissues. In Strichartz G, editor: *Local anesthetics*, vol 81, Berlin, 1987, Springer-Verlag, pp 21-53.
16. Butterworth JFT, Strichartz GR: Molecular mechanism of local anesthesia: a review. *Anesthesiology* 72:711-734, 1990.
17. Gasser HS, Erlanger J: The role of fiber size in the establishment of a nerve block by pressure or cocaine. *Am J Physiol* 88:581-591, 1929.

Lidocaine—Clinical Use

18. Bartfield JM, Sokaris SJ, Raccio-Robak N: Local anesthesia for lacerations: pain of infiltration inside vs outside the wound. *Acad Emerg Med* 5:100-104, 1998.
19. Palmon SC, Lloyd AT, Kirsch JR: The effect of needle gauge and lidocaine pH on pain during intradermal injection. *Anesth Analg* 86:379-381, 1998.
20. Scarfone RJ, Jasani M, Gracely EJ: Pain of local anesthetics: rate of administration and buffering. *Ann Emerg Med* 31:36-40, 1998.
21. Martin AJ: pH adjustment area discomfort caused by the intradermal injection of lignocaine. *Anesthesia* 45:975-978, 1990.
22. Bartfield JM, Ford DT, Homer PJ: Buffered versus plain lidocaine for digital nerve block. *Ann Emerg Med* 22:216-219, 1993.
23. Stewart JH, Cole GW, Klein JA: Neutralized lidocaine with epinephrine for local anesthesia. *J Dermatol Surg Oncol* 15:1081-1083, 1989.

24. Larson PO, Ragi G, Swandby M, et al: Stability of buffered lidocaine and epinephrine used for local anesthesia. *J Dermatol Surg Oncol* 17:411-414, 1991.

25. Fialkov JA, McDougall EP: Warmed local anesthetic reduces pain of infiltration. *Ann Plast Surg* 36:11-13, 1996.

26. Colaric KB, Overton DT, Moore K: Pain reduction in lidocaine administration through buffering and warming. *Am J Emerg Med* 16:353-356, 1998.

27. Nevarre DR, Tzarnas CD: The effects of hyaluronidase on the efficacy and on the pain of administration of 1% lidocaine. *Plast Reconstr Surg* 101:365-369, 1998.

28. Dinehart SM: Topical, local, regional anesthesia. In Wheeland R, editor: *Cutaneous surgery,* Philadelphia, 1994, WB Saunders, pp 102-112.

29. Grekin RC, Auletta MJ: Local anesthesia in dermatologic surgery. *J Am Acad Dermatol* 19:599-614, 1988.

30. Klein JA: The tumescent technique for lipo-suction surgery. *Am J Cosmet Surg* 4:263-267, 1987.

31. Klein JA: The tumescent technique: anesthesia and modified liposuction technique. *Dermatol Clin* 8:425-437, 1990.

32. Klein JA: Tumescent technique for local anesthesia improves safety in large-volume liposuction. *Plast Reconstr Surg* 92:1085-1098, 1993.

33. Ostad A, Kageyama N, Moy RL: Tumescent anesthesia with a lidocaine dose of 55 mg/kg is safe for liposuction. *Dermatol Surg* 22:921-927, 1997.

34. Hanke CW, Bernstein G, Bullock S: Safety of tumescent liposuction in 15,336 patients: national survery results. *Dermatol Surg* 21:459-462, 1995.

35. Coleman WPI, Hanke CW, Lillis P, et al: Does the location of the surgery or the specialty of the physician affect malpractice claims in liposuction? *Dermatol Surg* 25:343-347, 1999.

36. Rao RB, Ely SF, Hoffman RS: Deaths related to liposuction. *N Engl J Med* 340:1471-1475, 1999.

37. Klein J: Deaths related to liposuction (letter). *N Engl J Med* 341:1001, 1999.

38. Acosta AE: Clinical parameters of tumescent anesthesia in skin cancer reconstructive surgery. *Arch Dermatol* 133:451-454, 1997.

39. Coleman WP III, Klein JA: Use of the tumescent technique for scalp surgery, dermabrasion, and soft tissue reconstruction. *J Dermatol Surg Oncol* 18:130-135, 1992.

40. Goodman G: Dermabrasion using tumescent anesthesia. *J Dermatol Surg Oncol* 20:802-807, 1994.

41. Chiarello SE: Tumescent infiltration of corticosteroids, lidocaine and epinephrine into dermatomes of acute herpetic pain or postherpetic neuralgia. *Arch Dermatol* 134:279-281, 1988.

42. Zyderm Collagen Implant package insert. Palo Alto, CA, 1995, Collagen Biomedical.

43. Fishman SM, Canaris OA, Stojanovic MP, et al: Intravenous lidocaine for treatment-resistant pruritus. *Am J Med* 102:584-585, 1997.

Lidocaine—Adverse Effects
44. Lie RL, Vermeer BJ, Edelbroek PM: Severe lidocaine intoxication by cutaneous absorption. *J Am Acad Dermatol* 23:1026-1028, 1990.

45. Mofenson HC, Caraccio TR, Miller H, et al: Lidocaine toxicity from topical mucosal application. *Clin Pediatr* 22:190-192, 1983.

46. Goodwin DP, McMeekin TO: A case of lidocaine absorption from topical administration of 40% lidocaine cream. *J Am Acad Dermatol* 41:280-281, 1999.

47. Reynolds F: Adverse effects of local anesthetics. *Br J Anaesth* 59:78-95, 1987.

48. Nath S, Haggmark S, Hohannson G, et al: Intracoronary injection of bupivacaine and lidocaine, an experimental study of cardiac rhythm, myocardial function and regional coronary artery blood flow in anaesthetised pigs. Proceedings of the Swedish Society of Anaesthetists Research Meeting. Uppsala, 1985.

49. Nancarrow C, Rutten A, Runciman W, et al: Myocardial and cerebral drug concentrations and the mechanism of death after fatal intravenous doses of lidocaine, bupivacaine, and ropivacaine in the sheep. *Anesth Analg* 69:276-283, 1989.

50. McCaughey W: Adverse effects of local anaesthetics. *Drug Saf* 7:178-189, 1992.

51. Reiz S, Nath SW: Cardiotoxicity of local anesthetic agents. *Br J Anaesth* 58:736-746, 1986.

52. Clarkson CW, Hondeghem L: Mechanism for bupivacaine depression of cardiac conduction: fast block of sodium channels during the action potential with slow recovery from block during diastole. *Anaesth* 62:396-405, 1985.

53. Schatz M, Fung DL: Anaphylactic and anaphylactoid reactions due to anesthetic agents. *Clin Rev Allergy* 4:215-227, 1986.
54. Schatz M: Skin testing and incremental challenge in the evaluation of adverse reactions. *Allergy Clin Immunol* 74:600-616, 1984.
55. Kennedy KS, Cave RH: Anaphylactic reaction to lidocaine. *Arch Otolaryngol Head Neck Surg* 112:671-673, 1986.
56. Glinert RJ, Zachary CB: Local anesthetic allergy: its recognition and avoidance. *J Dermatol Surg Oncol* 17:491-496, 1991.
57. Rothman S, Orland FJ, Flesch P: Group specificity of epidermal allergy to procaine in man. *J Invest Dermatol* 6:191-199, 1945.
58. Green SM, Rothrock SG, Gorchynski J: Validation of diphenhydramine as a dermal local anesthetic. *Ann Emerg Med* 23:1284-1289, 1994.
59. Ernst AA, Anand P, Nick T, et al: Lidocaine versus diphenhydramine for anesthesia in the repair of minor lacerations. *J Trauma* 34:354-357, 1993.
60. Wiener SG: Injectable sodium chloride as a local anesthetic for skin surgery. *Cutis* 23:242-243, 1979.
61. Fisher DA: Treatment of vasovagal reactions (letter). *J Am Acad Dermatol* 38:287-288, 1998.

Lidocaine—Drug Interactions and Therapeutic Guidelines

62. Katz HI: *Dermatologist's guide to adverse therapeutic interactions,* Philadelphia, 1997, Lippincott-Raven.
63. Prien T: Intradermal anaesthesia: comparison of several compounds. *Acta Anaesthesiol Scand* 38:805-807, 1994.
64. Fariss BL, Foresman PA, Rodeheaver GT, et al: Anesthetic properties and toxicity of bupivacaine and lidocaine for infiltration anesthesia. *J Emerg Med* 5:275-282, 1987.
65. Galindo A, Witcher T: Mixtures of local anesthetics: bupivacaine-chloroprocaine. *Anesth Analg* 59:683-685, 1980.
66. Ashburn AM, Gauthier M, Love G, et al: Iontophoretic administration of 2% lidocaine HCl and 1:100,000 epinephrine in humans. *Clin J Pain* 13:22-26, 1997.
67. Greenbaum SS, Bernstein EF: Comparison of iontophoresis of lidocaine with a eutectic mixture of lidocaine and prilocaine (EMLA) for topically administered local anesthesia. *J Dermatol Surg Oncol* 20:579-583, 1994.
68. Reed BR: Dermatologic drug use during pregnancy and lactation. *Dermatol Clin* 15:197-206, 1997.
69. Gormley DE: Cutaneous surgery and the pregnant patient. *J Am Acad Dermatol* 23:269-279, 1990.

Eutectic Mixture of Local Anesthesia (EMLA)—Pharmacology

70. Maddi R, Horrow JC, Mark JB, et al: Evaluation of a new cutaneous topical anesthesia preparation. *Reg Anaesth* 15:109-112, 1990.
71. Brodin A, Nyqvist-Mayer A, Wadsten T, et al: Phase diagram and aqueous solubility of the lidocaine-prilocaine binary system. *J Pharm Sci* 73:481-484, 1984.
72. Juhlin L, Evers H, Broberg F: A lidocaine-prilocaine cream for superficial skin surgery and painful lesions. *Acta Derm Venereol (Stockh)* 60:544-546, 1980.
73. EMLA Cream package insert. Westborough, MA, 1997, Astra USA, Inc.
74. Gajraj NM, Pennant JH, Watcha MF: Eutectic mixture of local anesthetics (EMLA) cream. *Anesth Analg* 78:574-583, 1994.
75. Juhlin L, Hagglund G, Evers H: Absorption of lidocaine and prilocaine after application of a eutectic mixture of local anesthetics (EMLA) on normal and diseased skin. *Acta Derm Venereol (Stockh)* 69:18-22, 1989.
76. Juhlin L, Rollman O: Vascular effects of a local anesthetic mixture in atopic dermatitis. *Acta Derm Venereol (Stockh)* 64:439-440, 1984.
77. *CliniSphere 2.0 CD ROM,* St. Louis, June 2000, Facts & Comparisons.
78. Eriksson E: Prilocaine. An experimental study in man of a new local anaesthetic with special regards to efficacy, toxicity, and excretion. *Acta Chirurgica Scand (Suppl)* 358:1-82, 1966.
79. Akerman B, Astrom A, Ross S, et al: Studies on the absorption, distribution and metabolism of labelled prilocaine and lidocaine in some animal species. *Acta Pharm et Toxicologica* 24:389-403, 1966.

EMLA—Clinical Use

80. Egekvist H, Bjerring P: Comparison of the analgesic effect of EMLA cream and EMLA patch on normal skin evaluated with laser-induced pain stimuli. *Acta Derm Venereol* 77:214-216, 1997.

81. Calamandrei M, Messeri A, Busoni P, et al: Comparison of two application techniques of EMLA and pain assessment in pediatric oncology patients. *Reg Anesth* 21:557-560, 1996.

82. Bjerring P, Ardendt-Nielsen L: Depth and duration of skin analgesia to needle insertion after topical application of EMLA cream. *Br J Anaesth* 64:173-177, 1990.

83. Hernandez E, Gonzalez S, Gonzalez E: Evaluation of topical anesthetics by laser-induced sensation: comparison of EMLA 5% cream and 40% lidocaine in acid mantle ointment. *Lasers Surg Med* 23:167-171, 1998.

84. der Vaard-Van Der Spek FB, Oranje AO, Lilleborg S, et al: Treatment of molluscum contagiosum using a lidocaine/prilocaine cream (EMLA) for analgesia. *J Am Acad Dermatol* 23:585-691, 1990.

85. Ronnerfalt L, Fransson J, Wahlgren CF: EMLA cream provides rapid pain relief for the curettage of molluscum contagiosum in children with atopic dermatitis without causing serious application-site reactions. *Pediatr Dermatol* 15:309-312, 1998.

86. de Waard-Van Der Spek FB, Oranje A, Mulder PG, et al: EMLA cream as a local anaesthetic in MMR vaccination. *Int J Clin Pract* 52:136, 1998.

87. Goodacre TEE, Sanders R, Watts DA, et al: Split skin grafting using topical local anaesthesia (EMLA): a comparison with infiltrated anaesthesia. *Br J Plast Surg* 41:533-538, 1988.

88. Chesany P, Raska D: Skin graft harvesting under local anesthesia. *Acta Chir Plast* 32:11-15, 1990.

89. Gupta AK, Sibbald RG: Eutectic lidocaine/prilocaine 5% cream and patch may provide satisfactory analgesia for excisional biopsy or curettage with electrosurgery of cutaneous lesions. *J Am Acad Dermatol* 35:419-423, 1996.

90. Burdick AE, Lehrer KA, Barquin L: Use of eutectic mixture of local anesthetics: an effective topical anesthetic for slit-smear testing of patients with Hansen's disease. *J Am Acad Dermatol* 37:800-802, 1997.

91. Hallen A, Ljunghall K, Wallin J: Topical anaesthesia with local anaesthetic (lidocaine and prilocaine, EMLA) cream for cautery of genital warts. *Genitourin Med* 63:36-39, 1987.

92. v d Berg GM, Lillieborg S, Stolz E: Lidocaine/prilocaine cream (EMLA) versus infiltration anaesthesia: a comparison of the analgesic efficacy for punch biopsy and electrocoagulation of genital warts in men. *Genitourin Med* 68:162-165, 1992.

93. Mansell-Gregory M, Romanowski B: Randomised double blind trial of EMLA for the control of pain related to cryotherapy in the treatment of genital HPV lesions. *Sex Transm Infect* 74:274-275, 1998.

94. Ashinoff R, Geronemus RG: Effect of topical anesthetic EMLA on the efficacy of pulsed dye laser treatment of port-wine stains. *J Dermatol Surg Oncol* 16:1008-1011, 1990.

95. Tan OT, Stafford TJ: EMLA for laser treatment of portwine stains in children. *Lasers Surg Med* 12:543-548, 1992.

96. Littler CM: Laser hair removal in a patient with hypertrichosis lanuginosa congenita. *Dermatol Surg* 23:705-707, 1997.

97. Nott MR, Peacock JL: Relief of injection pain in adults. EMLA cream for 5 minutes before venipuncture. *Anaesthesia* 45:772-774, 1990.

98. Ehrenström Reiz GME, Reiz SLA: EMLA—a eutectic mixture of local anaesthetics for topical anaesthesia. *Acta Anaesthesiol Scand* 26:596-598, 1982.

99. Holm J, Andren B, Grafford K: Pain control in the surgical debridement of leg ulcers by the use of topical lidocaine-prilocaine cream, EMLA. *Acta Derm Venereol (Stockh)* 70:132-136, 1990.

100. Lok C, Paul C, Amblard P, et al: EMLA cream as a topical anesthetic for the repeated mechanical debridement of venous leg ulcers: a double-blind, placebo-controlled study. *J Am Acad Dermatol* 40:208-213, 1999.

101. Enander Malmros I, Nilsen T, Lillieborg S: Plasma concentrations and analgesic effect of EMLA (lidocaine/prilocaine) cream for the cleansing of leg ulcers. *Acta Derm Venereol (Stockh)* 70:227-230, 1990.

102. Wheeler JG: EMLA cream and herpetic neuralgia (letter). *Med J Aust* 154:781, 1991.

103. Collins PD: EMLA cream and herpetic neuralgia (letter). *Med J Aust* 155:206-207, 1991.

104. Milligan KA, Atkinson RE, Schofield PA: Lidocaine-prilocaine cream in postherpetic neuralgia. *BMJ* 298:253, 1989.

105. Stowe PJ, Glynn C, Mino BG: A study to explore the effect of EMLA cream in postherpetic neuralgia. *Pain* 39:301-305, 1989.

106. Lycka B: Medical indications for using a topical anesthetic. *Perspect Pain Manag* 1:9-12, 1991.

107. Arendt-Nielsen L, Kaalund S, Hogsaa B, et al: The response to local anaesthetics (EMLA-cream) as a clinical test to diagnose between hypermobility and Ehlers-Danlos type III syndrome. *Scand J Rheumatol* 20:190-195, 1991.

108. Juhlin L, Hagglund G, Evers H: Inhibition of hyperhidrosis by topical application of a local anesthetic composition. *Acta Derm Venereol (Stockh)* 59:556-559, 1979.

109. Shuttleworth D, Hill S, Marks R, et al: Relief of experimentally induced pruritus with a novel eutectic mixture of local anesthetic agents. *Br J Dermatol* 119:535-540, 1988.

EMLA—Adverse Effects

110. Hjelm M, Holmdahl MH: Biochemical effects of aromatic amines. *Acta Anaesthesiol Scand* 2:99, 1965.

111. van den Hove J, Decroix J, Tennstedt D, et al: Allergic contact dermatitis from prilocaine, one of the local anaesthetics in EMLA cream. *Contact Dermatitis* 30:239, 1994.

112. Thakur BK, Murali MR: EMLA cream-induced allergic contact dermatitis: a role for prilocaine as an immunogen. *J Allergy Clin Immunol* 95:776-778, 1995.

113. de Waard-Van Der Spek FB, Oranje AP: Purpura caused by EMLA is of toxic origin. *Contact Dermatitis* 36:11-13, 1997.

114. Eaglstein NF: Chemical injury to the eye from EMLA cream during erbium laser resurfacing. *Dermatol Surg* 25:590-591, 1999.

115. McKinlay JR, Hofmeister E, Ross EV, MacAllister W: EMLA cream-induced eye injury. *Arch Dermatol* 135:855-856, 1999.

Topical Anesthetics—Lidocaine, Benzocaine, Dyclonine

116. Lubens HM, Ausdenmoore RW, Shafer AD, et al: Anesthetic patch for painful procedures such as minor operations. *Am J Dis Child* 128:192-194, 1974.

117. Zempsky WT, Karasic RB: EMLA versus TAC for topical anesthesia of extremity wounds in children. *Ann Emerg Med* 30:163-166, 1997.

118. Weiss R: New topical anesthetic beats EMLA. *Skin & Allergy News 1998* April 1, 1999.

119. Rietschel RL, Fowler J, editors: *Fisher's contact dermatitis*, Baltimore, 1995, Williams & Wilkins.

120. Carnel SB, Blakeslee DB, Oswald SG, et al: Treatment of radiation- and chemotherapy-induced stomatitis. *Otolaryngol Head Neck Surg* 102:326-330, 1990.

121. Maibach HI: Dyclonine hydrochloride, local anesthetic allergic contact dermatitis. *Contact Dermatitis* 14:114, 1986.

Epinephrine—Pharmacology and Clinical Use

122. Graham WP III: Anesthesia in cosmetic surgery. *Clin Plast Surg* 10:285-287, 1983.

123. Netscher DT, Carlyle T, Thornby J, et al: Hemostasis at skin graft donor sites: evaluation of topical agents. *Ann Plast Surg* 36:7-10, 1996.

124. Smoot EC III, Kucan JO: Epinephrine spray-bottle technique for harvesting skin grafts. *J Burn Care Rehabil* 13:221-222, 1992.

125. Todd K, Berk WA, Huang R: Effect of body locale and addition of epinephrine on the duration of action of a local anesthetic agent. *Ann Emerg Med* 21:723-726, 1992.

126. Wyatt R: Anaphylaxis. How to recognize, treat and prevent potentially fatal attacks. *Postgrad Med* 100:87-90, 1996.

127. Brown AF: Anaphylactic shock: mechanisms and treatment. *J Accid Emerg Med* 12:89-100, 1995.

Epinephrine—Adverse Effects

128. Salonen M, Forssell H, Scheinin M: Local dental anaesthesia with lidocaine and adrenaline: effects on plasma catecholamines, heart rate and blood pressure. *Int J Oral Maxillofac Surg* 17:92-94, 1988.

129. Cardiovascular disease in dental practice, Dallas, 1986, American Heart Association.

130. Malamed SF: *Handbook of local anesthesia*, ed 3, St. Louis, 1990, CV Mosby.

131. Meecham JG, Jastak JT, Donaldson D: The use of epinephrine in dentistry. *J Can Dent Assoc* 60:825-834, 1994.

132. Aikenhead AR, Smith G: *Textbook of anesthesia*, ed 2, Edinburgh, 1990, Churchill Livingstone.

133. Panacek EA, Sherman B: Lactic acidosis and insulin resistance associated with epinephrine in a patient with non-insulin dependent diabetes mellitus. *Arch Int Med* 148:1879, 1988.

134. Lawrence C: Drug management in skin surgery. *Drugs* 52:805-817, 1996.

135. Aycock BG, Hawtof DB, Moody SB: Treatment of peripheral ischemia secondary to lidocaine containing epinephrine. *Ann Plast Surg* 23:27-30, 1989.

136. Fazio MJ, Zitelli JA: Full-thickness skin grafts. Clinical observations on the impact of using epinephrine in local anesthesia of the donor sites. *Arch Dermatol* 131:691-694, 1995.

137. Wolfort S, Rorich RJ, Handren J, et al: The effect of epinephrine in local anesthesia on the survival of full- and split-thickness skin grafts: an experimental study. *Plast Reconstr Surg* 86:535-540, 1990.

Epinephrine—Drug Interactions and Therapeutic Guidelines

138. Berbaum MW, Bredle DL: Absence of significant adverse effects from low-dose subcutaneous epinephrine in dermatologic procedures. *Arch Dermatol* 133:1318-1319, 1997.

139. Dzubow LM: The interaction between propranolol and epinephrine as observed in patients undergoing Mohs' surgery. *J Am Acad Dermatol* 15:71-75, 1986.

140. Foster CA, Aston SJ: Propranolol-epinephrine interactions: a potential disaster. *Plast Reconstr Surg* 72:74-78, 1983.

141. Perusse R, Goulet J-P, Turcotte J-Y: Contraindications to vasoconstrictors in dentistry: part II. hyperthyroidism, diabetes, sulfite sensitivity, corticosteroid-dependent asthma, and pheochromocytoma. *Oral Surg Oral Med Oral Pathol* 74:687-691, 1992.

142. Perusse R, Goulet J-P, Turcotte J-Y: Contraindications to vasoconstrictors in dentistry: part I. cardiovascular disease. *Oral Surg Oral Med Oral Pathol* 74:679-686, 1992.

143. Goulet J-P, Perusse R, Turcotte J-Y: Contraindications to vasoconstrictors in dentistry: part III. pharmacologic interactions. *Oral Surg Oral Med Oral Pathol* 74:692-697, 1992.

144. Larrabee WF, Lanier BJ, Miekle D: Effect of epinephrine on local cutaneous blood flow. *Head Neck Surg* 9:287-289, 1987.

145. Grabb WC: A concentration of 1:500,000 epinephrine in a local anesthetic solution is sufficient to provide excellent hemostasis. *Plast Reconstr Surg* 63:834-835, 1979.

146. O'Malley TP, Postma GN, Holtel M, et al: Effect of local epinephrine on cutaneous blood flow in the human neck. *Laryngoscope* 105:140-143, 1995.

Capsaicin—Pharmacology

147. Lembeck F: Columbus, capsicum and capsaicin: past, present, and future. *Acta Physiol Hung* 69:265-273, 1987.

148. Rains C, Bryson HM: Topical capsaicin. A review of its pharmacological properties and therapeutic potential in post-herpetic neuralgia, diabetic neuropathy and osteoarthritis. *Drugs & Aging* 7:317-328, 1995.

149. Spina D, McKenniff MG, Coyle AJ, et al: Effect of capsaicin on PAF-induced bronchial hyperresponsiveness and pulmonary cell accumulation in the rabbit. *Br J Pharmacol* 103:1268-1274, 1991.

150. Wu PC, Fand JY, Huang YB, et al: Development and evaluation of transdermal patches of nonivamide and sodium nonivamide acetate. *Pharmazie* 52:135-138, 1997.

151. Kasting GB, Francis WR, Bowman LA, et al: Percutaneous absorption of vanilloids: in vivo and in vitro studies. *J Pharm Sci* 86:142-146, 1997.

152. Surh Y-J, Lee SS: Capsaicin, a double-edged sword: toxicity, metabolism, and chemopreventive potential. *Life Sci* 56:1845-1855, 1995.

153. Omoigui S: *The pain drugs handbook*, St. Louis, 1995, Mosby Year Book.

154. Lynn B: Capsaicin: actions on nociceptive C-fibers and therapeutic potential. *Pain* 41:61-69, 1990.

155. Biro T, Acs G, Acs P, et al: Recent advances in understanding the vanilloid receptors: a therapeutic target for treatment of pain and inflammation in skin. *J Invest Dermatol (Symp Proc)* 2:56-60, 1997.

156. Caterina MJ, Schumacher MA, Tominaga M, et al: The capsaicin receptor: a heat-activated ion channel in the main pathway. *Nature* 389:816-824, 1997.

Capsaicin—Clinical Use

157. Zhang WY, Po LW: The effectiveness of topically applied capsaicin: a meta-analysis. *Clin Pharmacol* 46:517-522, 1994.

158. Bernstein JB, Korman NJ, Bickers DR, et al: Topical capsaicin treatment of chronic postherpetic neuralgia. *J Am Acad Dermatol* 21:265-270, 1989.

159. Watson CPN: Topical capsaicin as an adjuvant analgesic. *J Pain Symptom Manage* 9:425-433, 1994.

160. Chad DA, Aronin N, Lundstrom R, et al: Does capsaicin relieve the pain of diabetic neuropathy? *Pain* 42:387-388, 1990.

161. Group TCS: Treatment of painful diabetic neuropathy with topical capsaicin. *Arch Intern Med* 151:2225-2229, 1991.

162. Group TCS: Effect of treatment with capsaicin on daily activities of patients with painful diabetic neuropathy. *Diabetes Care* 15:159-165, 1992.

163. Watson CPN, Evans RJ: The postmastectomy pain syndrome and topical capsaicin: a randomized trial. *Pain* 51:375-379, 1992.

164. Dini D, Bertelli G, Gozza A, et al: Treatment of the postmastectomy pain syndrome with topical capsaicin. *Pain* 54:223-226, 1993.

165. Wallengren J, Klinker M: Successful treatment of notalgia paresthetica with topical capsaicin: vehicle-controlled, double-blind, crossover study. *J Am Acad Dermatol* 32:287-289, 1995.

166. Cheshire WP, Snyder CR: Treatment of reflex sympathetic dystrophy with topical capsaicin—case report. *Pain* 42:307-311, 1990.

167. Rayner HC, Atkins RC, Westerman RA: Relief of local stump pain by topical capsaicin. *Lancet* 2:1276-1277, 1989.

168. Burrows NP, Norris PG: Treatment of PUVA-induced skin pain with capsaicin. *Br J Dermatol* 131:584-585, 1994.

169. Sinoff SE, Hart MB: Topical capsaicin and burning pain (letter). *Clin J Pain* 9:70-73, 1993.

170. Muhiddin KA, Gallen IW, Harries S, et al: The use of capsaicin cream in a case of erythromelalgia. *Postgrad Med J* 70:841-843, 1994.

171. Wist E, Risberg T: Topical capsaicin in treatment of hyperalgesia, allodynia and dysesthetic pain caused by malignant tumor infiltration of the skin. *Acta Oncol* 32:343, 1993.

172. Ellis CN, Berberian B, Sulica V, et al: A double-blind evaluation of topical capsaicin in pruritic psoriasis. *J Am Acad Dermatol* 29:438-442, 1993.

173. Friedrich EG: Therapeutic studies of vulvar vestibulitis. *J Reprod Med* 33:514-518, 1998.

174. Marks JG: Treatment of apocrine chromhidrosis. *J Am Acad Dermatol* 21:418-420, 1989.

175. Markovits E, Gilhar A: Capsaicin—an alternative topical treatment in pain. *Int J Derm* 36:401-404, 1997.

176. Ko F, Diaz M, Smith P, et al: Toxic effects of capsaicin on keratinocytes and fibroblasts. *J Burn Care Rehabil* 19:409-413, 1998.

177. Simone DA, Ochoa J: Early and late effects of prolonged topical capsaicin on cutaneous sensibility and neurogenic vasodilation in humans. *Pain* 47:285-294, 1991.

Antihistamines—Diphenhydramine, Doxepin

178. Landau SW, Nelson WA, Gay LN: Antihistaminic properties of local anesthetics and anesthetic properties of antihistaminic compounds. *J Allergy* 21:19, 1951.

179. Rosenthal SR, Minard D: Experiments on histamine as the chemical mediator for cutaneous pain. *J Exp Med* 70:415, 1939.

180. Clark WG, Brater DC, Johnson AR, editors: Pharmacology of local anesthesia. In *Goth's medical pharmacology*, St. Louis, 1992, Mosby Year Book, pp 397-405.

181. Rosanove R: Local anesthesia for allergic patients: the use of diphenhydramine hydrochloride as a local anaesthetic agent. *Med J Aust* 1:613, 1963.

182. Campolattaro JP, Haroldson JH: Diphenhydramine hydrochloride (Benadryl) as a local anesthetic in procaine and lidocaine sensitive patients. *Milit Med* 129:668, 1964.

183. Howard K, Conrad T, Heiser J, et al: Diphenhydramine hydrochloride as a local anesthetic: a case report. *J Am Podiatr Med Assoc* 74:240-242, 1984.

184. Dire DJ, Hogan DE: Double-blinded comparison of diphenhydramine versus lidocaine as a local anesthetic. *Ann Emerg Med* 22:1419-1422, 1993.

185. Ramsdell WM: Severe reaction to diphenhydramine (letter). *J Am Acad Dermatol* 21:1318-1320, 1989.

186. Diphenhydramine injection package insert. Morris Plains, NJ, 1996, Parke-Davis.

187. Drake LA, Millikan LE: The antipruritic effect of 5% doxepin cream in patients with eczematous dermatitis. Doxepin Study Group. *Arch Dermatol* 131:1403-1408, 1995.

188. Drake LA, Fallon JD, Sober A: Relief of pruritus in patients with atopic dermatitis after treatment with topical doxepin cream. *J Am Acad Dermatol* 31:613-616, 1994.

189. Taylor JS, Praditsuwan P, Handel D, et al: Allergic contact dermatitis from doxepin cream. One-year patch test clinic experience. *Arch Dermatol* 132:515-518, 1996.

190. Wakelin SH, Rycroft RJ: Allergic contact dermatitis from doxepin. *Contact Dermatitis* 40:214, 1999.

CHAPTER 40

Ginat Wintermeyer Mirowski

Oral Therapeutics

This chapter introduces the use of medications and the pitfalls in the management of common oral conditions and is designed to meet the needs of dermatologists, dentists, and other health care providers who care for patients with a variety of conditions that affect the oral cavity.

As in the skin, there are a limited number of reaction patterns that the mucosa can express. The differential diagnosis for these reaction patterns is often broad and varied. For example, the differential diagnosis of white lesions includes trauma (morsicatio buccarum et labiorum), lichenoid drug reaction, viral warts, dysplasia, and autoimmune reactions such as discoid lupus and lichen planus (LP).

The first step in managing mucosal diseases is to obtain a definitive diagnosis. The diagnosis may be attained by obtaining adequate biopsies for routine histology and special stains, tissues for immunohistochemical studies or cultures, and well-directed serum and laboratory studies when indicated. In addition, it is important to ascertain, by history and by physical examination, the extent of the condition in a variety of mucocutaneous areas. These areas include the vagina, esophagus, conjunctiva, nose, and skin. If the condition is limited to the oral cavity, local topical therapy can often be used exclusively. Systemic therapy is usually necessary when multiple mucosal sites are affected. If the patient has recalcitrant erosions that are localized to the buccal mucosa or to the posterior pharynx, adjunctive topical corticosteroids may enhance the systemic corticosteroid effects. In addition, adjunctive topical corticosteroids may permit a reduction in overall systemic dosing of various drugs.

REVIEW OF COMMON TERMINOLOGY

Gingivitis is an inflammation of the gums. Dental plaque is a sticky, yellow, or colorless film caused by bacteria and sloughed keratinocytes. Dental plaque contributes to gingival inflammatory reactions. Periodontitis is the condition in which the alveolar bone that supports the teeth is compromised. As gingivitis progresses, the underlying bony attachment is damaged, resulting in bone loss, loosening of the teeth, and gingival retraction. The teeth may appear longer as the roots become exposed.

EROSIVE GINGIVOSTOMATITIS

Erosive gingival condition presents as erythema, edema, tenderness, and superficial erosions on the gingivae. Patients may present to their dentist or dermatologist complaining of bleeding tender gums. The mucosal surface is eroded and friable. Attempt by the patient at maintaining good oral hygiene is compromised due to the friability and pain. A diagnostic biopsy for both hematoxylin and eosin (H&E) stain and immunofluorescence is indicated because erosive gingivae could be an oral manifestation of a blistering disorder. In erosive gingivitis, the underlying bone is intact. Severe localized bone loss suggests a neoplasm, infection, or severe immune dysregulation such as advanced human immunodeficiency virus (HIV) infection. Symmetric white reticulated striae, which are evident in the vestibules (lower third of the buccal mucosa), suggest a diagnosis of oral LP. Asymmetric white plaques on the buccal mucosa, on the moist labial mucosa, and on the dry red vermilion of the lip or the hard palate suggest the diagnosis of discoid or systemic lupus erythematosus. A complete cutaneous examination to identify characteristic lesions will potentially confirm a suspected diagnosis.

Once the diagnosis is established, the first line of therapy for less morbid oral vesiculobullous diseases, such as LP or cicatricial pemphigoid, is application of topical corticosteroids. Systemic therapy is indicated in pemphigus vulgaris and in more severe cases of LP or cicatricial pemphigus. Ointments and gel formulations are most effective for gingival disease. Cream-based products have an unpleasant taste and are less likely to adhere to wet mucosa. For ulcers on the posterior pharynx or soft and hard palate, or if the patient is unable to apply topical medication, elixirs and suspensions are very effective.

Topical Medications

Rx: Triamcinolone acetonide 0.1% gel; fluocinonide 0.05% gel, clobetasol 0.05% gel
Disp: 30-60 g
Sig: Apply a thin film to affected areas, nil per os (NPO) 30-60 minutes *or* apply to inner surface of dentures or medication trays qid and leave in place for 30 minutes.
NB*: Ointments and gel formulations are most effective for gingival disease.

Rx: Orabase (OTC)
Sig: Apply to affected area bid.
NB: Orabase is often used as a base for topical corticosteroid creams due to its improved adherence to mucosal surface. Each 7.5-g tube contains gelatin, pectin, and sodium carboxy-

methylcellulose in polyethylene and mineral oil gel. Odorless and tasteless, nonirritating, and harmless if swallowed. Gritty feeling is quite bothersome to some patients.

Rx: Triamcinolone acetonide 0.1% or 0.2% aqueous suspension (Kenalog)
Disp: 400 ml
Sig: Swish, gargle, and expectorate 5 ml qid (after meals and hs); NPO for 30 minutes after each dose.
NB: Contact time is important for maximizing efficacy. Thus instruct patients to gargle or swish for a minimum of 5-10 minutes each time. To limit systemic adverse effects, remind patients to expectorate.
Compounding instructions: Add 5 ml of 95% ethanol to a vial of triamcinolone acetonide 40 mg/ml injectable. Add nonbacteriostatic sterile water QS to 200 ml for irrigation; makes a 0.02% solution. Shake well. Expires in 6 months.

Rx: Dexamethasone elixir 0.5 mg/ml (Decadron)
Disp: 400 ml
Sig: Swish, gargle, and expectorate 5 ml qid (after meals and hs). NPO for 30 minutes after each dose.

Intralesional Corticosteroids

Rx: Triamcinolone acetonide injectable 10 mg/ml (Kenalog)
Direction: Inject using a 30-gauge needle; best used for solitary lesions recalcitrant to therapy

Systemic Medications

Rx: Prednisone 5 mg, 10 mg, 20 mg tablets
Disp: As indicated based on the patient's condition and the physician's clinical judgment
Sig: 1 mg per kg qam and taper to 5 mg qod as needed. The length of time needed to treat varies from weeks (aphthae) to months (pemphigus vulgaris or cicatricial pemphigoid) depending on the underlying disease.
NB: Insomnia, headache, irritability, weight gain, hypertension, masks fevers and unmasks diabetes; rule out (R/O) diabetes, tuberculosis (TB), osteoporosis; Obtain purified protein derivative (PPD) skin test, blood pressure (BP), bone density scan. May split dose initially to maximize antiinflammatory effects.

---

*NB, *Nota bene,* note well, alert (Latin).

Mouth Rinses

Most mouth rinses are antibacterial products that can be used as adjuncts.[1] Some are OTC (Listerine), whereas others are available by prescription such as chlorhexidine gluconate (Perio-Gard, Peridex). Pain medications (OTC) may be helpful as well. Prescription pain medications should be prescribed according to the extent and location of the conditions.

Rx: Chlorhexidine gluconate oral rinse, 0.12% (PerioGard, Peridex)
   Disp: 480 ml
   Sig: bid-qid
   NB: (11.6% alcohol, saccharin, and mint flavored). PerioGard Oral Rinse can cause staining of oral surfaces, such as tooth surfaces, restorations, and the dorsum of the tongue. Some studies note an increase in calculus formation and an alteration of taste perception.

OTC: Listerine
   Disp: 250 ml, 500 ml, 1 liter, 1.5 liters, or 1.7 liters
   Sig: Rinse full strength for 30 seconds with 20 ml ($\frac{2}{3}$ fluid ounce or 4 teaspoonfuls) bid.
   NB: May also help treat bad breath. Active ingredients: water, alcohol (26.7%), benzoic acid, poloxamer 407, and caramel. Also contains thymol 0.064%, eucalyptol 0.092%, methyl salicylate 0.060%, and menthol 0.042%.

Rx: Xylocaine 2% viscous (lidocaine)
   Disp: 100 ml
   Sig: Swish and expectorate 5 ml, 5 minutes before eating tid-qid.
   NB: Patients must be warned of the risk of aspiration due to loss of sensation (loss of gag reflex) on the soft palate and epiglottis. Risk of aspiration is reduced by applying locally with fingertip or cotton applicator.

Tips and Clinical Pearls—Erosive Gingivostomatitis

To maximize the effects of topical agents in the oral cavity, instruct the patient to be NPO for 30 to 60 minutes after use. In addition, custom acrylic "trays" can be fashioned to facilitate the delivery of corticosteroid gels to the affected gingivae (Figure 40-1). These soft trays are readily made by general dentists and are traditionally

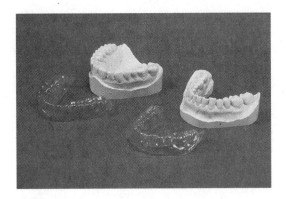

Figure 40-1   Photograph (digital) of a dental "tray."

used for delivering bleaching agents. The dentist must be made aware that the purpose of these trays is to permit longer contact of the corticosteroid and the oral mucosa, therefore acting as an occlusive agent much as Saran Wrap can be used to enhance the therapeutic effect of topical corticosteroids. With this in mind, the trays are trimmed to extend beyond the teeth and over the affected gingiva. This is counterintuitive to dentists, who usually use acidic agents in bleaching teeth and thus traditionally trim the trays at the gingival margin. Treatment with topical corticosteroids with an occlusive tray for 10 to 20 minutes two to four times daily is highly effective. Many cases of gingival LP can be managed with topical therapy alone.

Meticulous oral hygiene (brushing teeth twice daily along with daily flossing) helps limit the buildup and the inflammatory effects of plaque. Three to four visits to the dentist per year for additional oral hygiene maintenance is necessary to maximize treatment of erosive gingivostomatitis and to limit the need for long-term corticosteroids.

Pitfalls that may be encountered in patients using topical, inhaled, or systemic corticosteroids include the overgrowth of fungal organisms and the occurrence of herpes simplex virus (HSV) infections. Both of these conditions may present with an acute exacerbation of pain and decreased efficacy of the corticosteroids. Clinical evaluation is advised to assess the cause. *Candida albicans* is the most common fungus in the oral cavity. Cultures in asymptomatic adults demonstrate that it is a common oral organism (see Candidiasis treatment section). Recurrent viral infections are also common and may exacerbate discomfort in the oral cavity. Thus documenting HSV either by culture or by immunofluorescence is an indication for suppressive therapy when chronic corticosteroids are being used in oral erosive disease.

CANDIDIASIS

C. albicans is an oral commensal in as many as 40% to 65% of healthy adult mouths.[2] Thus a diagnosis of oral candidiasis cannot be made from cultures but rather requires clinical and cytologic evidence of an infection or overgrowth. Demonstration of hyphae and blastospores, from an oral smear using a potassium hydroxide (KOH) preparation, is evidence of superinfection. Early treatment of oral candidiasis is important to relieve the discomfort and to prevent systemic spread of localized disease (commonly noted in immunocompromised transplant patients). *C. albicans* is the most frequently isolated pathogen in individuals infected with HIV, accounting for almost half of all episodes of candidemia, followed by *C. tropicalis* in 20% and *C. glabrata* in approximately 10% of patients. Cultures are necessary to determine actual species affected. The innate resistance to azole antimycotic therapy of *C. glabrata* must be considered when treatment fails.

Topical Therapy

Rx: Clotrimazole (Mycelex) troches 10 mg
Disp: 70 tablets (bottles contain either 70 or 140 tablets)
Sig: Dissolve 1 tablet in mouth five times per day
NB: Tablets must be dissolved slowly in the mouth. However, these tablets contain sucrose, presenting an increased risk of developing caries with prolonged use. Fifteen percent of patients developed an elevated SGOT in clinical trials (PDR 1997). Periodic assessment of hepatic function is advisable, particularly in patients with preexisting liver disease and with long-term use (>10 to 14 days).

Rx: Clotrimazole 10 mg/ml suspension (Mycelex)
Disp: 60 ml

Sig: Swab 1-2 ml on affected areas qid, after meals and hs, NPO for 30 minutes.
Compounding instructions: Crush six 100 mg clotrimazole vaginal insert tablets, reducing to a fine powder. Add 60 ml confectioner's glycerin and mix thoroughly. Label "shake before using." The suspension is particularly useful for newborns and debilitated patients who cannot rinse.

Rx: Mycostatin pastilles 200,000 units per tablet (Nystatin)
Disp: 30 tablets
Sig: Dissolve one tablet in mouth tid.
NB: Tablets are more effective than oral suspension.

Rx: Mycostatin oral suspension, 100,000 units per ml (Nystatin)
Disp: 240 ml (12-day supply)
Sig: Gargle 400,000 units qid (after meals and hs), hold in mouth as long as possible, and expectorate. NPO for 30 minutes after each dose.
NB: The ideal target contact time is 5-10 minutes. The vehicle may contain up to 50% sucrose, possibly increasing caries risk.

Rx: Amphotericin B oral suspension 100 mg/ml (Fungizone)
Disp: 24 ml
Sig: Apply 1 ml to mouth qid or swab the oral cavity of infants and debilitated patients. NPO for 30 minutes after each dose.
NB: Use nonabsorbent swabs qid (after meals and hs). Amphotericin B is safe for swallowing. Not indicated for systemic candidiasis; works by direct contact with the oral *Candida* lesions. Therefore instruct the patient to swish and hold in mouth as long as possible before swallowing. Use a calibrated dropper for precise dosing. Yellow color of suspension may discolor the dorsal surface of the tongue. This may be used to document compliance.

Systemic Therapy

Rx: Fluconazole (Diflucan) tablets 100 mg
Disp: 15 tablets
Sig: Take 2 tablets the first day (load) and 1 tablet qd thereafter for 2 weeks.
NB: Rare hepatic toxicity, albeit unlikely with short courses of therapy. Be aware of many drug interactions (see Chapters 4 and 44).

Rx: Itraconazole (Sporanox) oral solution 10 mg/ml or 100-mg capsule

Disp: 10-14 tabs (may need to repeat). Continue for 1 week past resolution of symptoms.

Sig: 1-2 tablets PO qd with a full meal for improved absorption. Avoid concomitant antacids.

NB: Instruct patient on signs of liver dysfunction. There is no need to monitor liver function tests unless the patient reports jaundice or abdominal symptoms.

Tips and Clinical Pearls—Candidiasis

Patients who wear oral appliances, such as retainers, dentures, and partial dentures, potentially maintain a harvest of pathogenic organisms that are difficult to eradicate. Hyphae are found throughout the microscopic pores of the appliances. Thus soaking these in a dilute bleach solution (1 tsp of bleach per cup of water) for 20 minutes twice daily decreases the fungal burden and limits recurrences. In addition, antifungal powders may be applied to the inner aspect of these appliances before putting them into the mouth, for further prophylactic effects. Many oral antifungal pastilles (lozenges) also contain sugar. Therefore to improve efficacy and to limit the risk of caries, vaginal troches may be prescribed.

HYPERPIGMENTATION

Hyperpigmentation in the oral cavity may be due to internal and external pigment deposition or production. A number of medications can induce pigment deposition within the mucosa or in the bone (Tables 40-1 and 40-2).

■ Table 40-1   Common Oral Adverse Effects from Systemic Medications[3]

Oral Adverse Effect	Responsible Medications*	
Dysgeusia	Auranofin (Ridaura)	Diltiazem (Cardizem)
	Captopril (Capoten)	Ofloxacin (Floxin)
Dysphagia	Betaxolol (Kerlone)	Moricizine (Ethmozine)
	Ciprofloxacin (Cipro)	Nabumetone (Relafen)
	Clomipramine (Anafranil)	Pergolide (Permax)
	Fluvoxamine (Luvox)	Pilocarpine (Salagen)
	Foscarnet (Foscavir injection)	Pimozide (Orap)
	Ganciclovir (Cytovene)	Sertraline (Zoloft)
	Gonadotropin-releasing hormone (Lupron)	Sumatriptan (Imitrex)
		Tetracycline (Achromycin, Sumycin)
	Guanfacine (Tenex)	Venlafaxine (Effexor)
	Interferon alfa-2b (Intron A)	Zalcitabine (Hivid)
	Levodopa (Laradopa tablets)	
Gingival hyperplasia	Cyclosporine (Neoral, Sandimmune)	Mycophenolate mofetil (CellCept)
	Diltiazem (Cardizem)	Nifedipine (Adalat, Procardia)
	Interferon alfa-2b (Intron A)	Verapamil (Calan, Isoptin)
Glossodynia, sore mouth and mouth burning	Acetaminophen, butalbital, caffeine (Fioricet)	Cromolyn sodium (Gastrocrom)
		Methyldopa (Aldomet)
	Acitretin (Soriatane)	Selegiline (Eldepryl)
	Antithymocyte globulin (Thymoglobulin)	Sumatriptan (Imitrex)
		Trovafloxacin (Videx)
	Aspirin, butalbital, caffeine (Fiorinal)	Zalcitabine (Hivid)
	Clozapine (Clozaril)	
Mucosal pigmentation	Chloroquine (Aralen)	Interferon alfa-2b (Intron A)
	Hydroxychloroquine (Plaquenil)	Minocycline (Minocin, Dynacin)
Xerostomia	Acitretin (Soriatane)	Amitriptyline, chlordiazepoxide (Limbitrol)
	Acrivastine, pseudoephedrine (Semprex-D)	Amoxapine (Asendin)
	Alprazolam (Xanax)	Apraclonidine (Iopidine)

*≥1% incidence per *Physicians' desk reference.*

Continued

■ **Table 40-1** Common Oral Adverse Effects from Systemic Medications[3]—cont'd

Oral Adverse Effect	Responsible Medications*	
Xerostomia—cont'd	Bromocriptine (Parlodel)	Isotretinoin (Accutane)
	Brompheniramine, pseu-doephedrine (Bromfed cough syrup)	Leuprolide (Lupron Depot)
		Loratadine (Claritin)
	Bupropion (Wellbutrin)	Loratadine, pseudoephedrine sulfate (Claritin D)
	Butorphanol (Stadol)	Maprotiline (Ludiomil)
	Captopril (Capoten)	Moricizine (Ethmozine)
	Captopril, hydrochlorothiazide (Capozide)	Nalbuphine (Nubain)
		Nefazodone (Serzone)
	Chlorthalidone, clonidine (Combipres)	Nicardipine (Cardene)
		Nizatidine (Axid)
	Clomipramine (Anafranil)	Paroxetine (Paxil)
	Clonidine (Catapres)	Pergolide (Permax)
	Clozapine (Clozaril)	Pimozide (Orap)
	Cyclobenzaprine (Flexeril)	Propafenone (Rythmol)
	Dicyclomine (Bentyl)	Pseudoephedrine, triprolidine (Actifed)
	Disopyramide (Norpace)	Quinapril (Accupril)
	Doxazosin (Cardura)	Scopolamine—transdermal (Transderm Scop)
	Doxepin (Zonalon cream)	
	Fentanyl (Duragesic Transdermal System)	Selegiline (Eldepryl)
		Sertraline (Zoloft)
	Flumazenil (Romazicon)	Trazodone (Desyrel)
	Fluoxetine (Prozac)	Trihexyphenidyl (Artane)
	Fluvoxamine (Luvox)	Trovafloxacin (Videx)
	Guanfacine (Tenex)	Venlafaxine (Effexor)
	Hydroxyzine (Atarax)	Zolpidem (Ambien)
	Interferon alpha 2b (Intron A)	
	Ipratropium (Atrovent)	

*≥1% incidence per *Physicians' desk reference.*

Table 40-2 Chemotherapeutic Agents Associated With Mucosal Hyperpigmentation[4]

Busulfan	Linear deposition of pigment in gingiva
Fluorouracil	Patchy involvement of tongue and conjunctiva
Tegafur	Macules on lower lip and glans penis
Doxorubicin	Black pigmentation of tongue and hyperpigmented patches on buccal mucosa
Hydroxyurea	Patchy/macular hyperpigmentation of tongue and buccal mucosa
Cisplatin	Oral hyperpigmentation
Cyclophosphamide	Rare band of permanent pigmentation of gingival margin

BLACK HAIRY TONGUE

Black hairy tongue is a common asymptomatic, but unsightly, reactive condition on the dorsal surface of the tongue. Exogenous pigment is deposited on and within elongated filiform papillae. Etiologic agents include the use of broad-spectrum antibiotics, hydrogen peroxide rinses, radiation therapy, and the habitual use of tobacco and ingestion of pigmented foods and drinks (e.g., coffee, tea, and licorice). Meticulous oral hygiene, including brushing the dorsal surface of the tongue, helps control this condition.

Topical Therapy

Rx: Retin-A 0.1% gel
Disp: 15 g
Sig: Apply to dorsal surface of tongue for 5 minutes, then rinse with warm water. Brush affected area with a firm toothbrush, tongue cleaner, or tongue scraper.
NB: Tongue scrapers, such as a product called Oolitt, are mechanical devices that help to debride the superficial bacteria on the dorsal surface of the tongue. Toothbrushing is a less specific action that also helps limit the accumulation of bacteria and hyperkeratotic debris.

RECURRENT APHTHOUS ULCERS

Recurrent aphthous ulcers are the most common cause of oral ulceration. The ulcers are well circumscribed with an active erythematous halo. They may be solitary or multiple and range from 1 to 2 mm up to 1 to 2 cm. The characteristic locations include the buccal mucosa, the soft palate, the lateral and ventral tongue, and the tonsillar pillars. A biopsy is indicated to rule out a malignant or infectious process in selected persistent ulcers. The pathogenesis is unknown. Impaired cellular immunity has been implicated as a cause of larger recalcitrant ulcers.

Topical Therapy

Refer to topical agents for erosive gingivostomatitis for initial treatment. In addition a coating agent, such as sucralfate, may be helpful.[5]

Rx: Sucralfate suspension, 1 g/10 ml (Carafate suspension)
Sig: 14 fl oz

NB: Minimal gastrointestinal (GI) absorption occurs. This drug accelerates duodenal ulcer healing, due to the formation of an ulcer-adherent complex that covers and protects the ulcer.

Systemic Medications

Rx: Pentoxifylline 400-mg tablets (Trental or generic)
Disp: 90 tablets (Therapeutic trial is at least 30 days)
Sig: 1 tablet PO tid with food

Rx: Colchicine 0.6 mg tablet
Disp: 30 tabs (with one refill)
Sig: 1 tablet po bid to tid
NB: Starting at bid minimizes GI adverse effects. Use in combination with topical and systemic corticosteroids. *Adverse effects* include diarrhea, neutropenia, and male infertility. *Contraindications* include renal, gastrointestinal, cardiac, or hematologic disorders.

Rx: Thalidomide (Thalomid)
Disp: 100-300 mg/day
Sig: 200 mg PO qd for 4 weeks (due to sedation, may need to gradually increase dose to this level)
NB: Off-label use has been documented with a 55% cure rate compared with 7% cure rate in control patients.[6] In addition to its teratogenic effects, thalidomide may cause somnolence, dizziness, constipation, and peripheral neuropathy.

Tips and Clinical Pearls—Recurrent Aphthous Stomatitis

Begin treatment of recurrent aphthous ulcers with topical steroids. Gels are ideal for localized lesions in the anterior third of the mouth. When ulcers appear on the pharynx or soft palate, Decadron elixir is very effective. Localization of the ulcers is helpful in differentiating this recurrent condition from recurrent HSV in the oral cavity. Involvement of the nonkeratinizing mucosa (e.g., the labial mucosa, floor of the mouth, ventral tongue, buccal mucosa, and soft palate) suggests recurrent aphthous ulcers. On the other hand, ulcers on the hard palate, dorsal tongue, attached gingivae, or lips suggest a herpes infection.

Sodium lauryl sulfate, an emulsifying and surface cleaning agent that is used in toothpastes and mouth rinses, has been implicated in predisposing individuals to recurrent aphthous stomatitis.[7,8] However, in a double-blind, crossover clinical trial, no significant effect on the ulcer pattern was noted.[9]

ACUTE NECROTIZING ULCERATIVE GINGIVOSTOMATITIS (TRENCH MOUTH)

Acute necrotizing ulcerative gingivostomatitis (ANUG) is a common infection caused by *Treponema* organisms, *Selenomonas* organisms, fusobacterium, and *Prevotella intermedia*.[10] Characteristic punched out ulcers limited to the interdental papillae are seen. This is a condition that typically involves young adults. Precipitating events include stressful situations, such as during major school testing periods, in addition to poor oral hygiene, inadequate nutrition, and alcohol or tobacco use. Patients typically present with gingival bleeding, lymphadenopathy, fetid breath, fever, and severe gingival pain. Treatment includes optimizing oral hygiene, improving oral intake, antibiotics, professional dental cleaning, and aggressive debridement of necrotic tissues.

Systemic Medications
Rx: Penicillin V-K 250 mg
Disp: 20 tabs
Sig: 250-500 mg PO qid
NB: Dental consultation for aggressive gingival debridement to limit bone loss. Periodontal care with scaling and debridement of necrotic tissues is necessary to prevent recurrence.

Rx: Metronidazole 250 mg (Flagyl)
Disp: 28 tablets
Sig: Two PO immediately, then 1 PO qid for 7 days
NB: Use in conjunction with PerioGard mouth rinse (½ oz) two to three times daily, 30 seconds, during the acute phase. Patient may also require an analgesic. Once acute phase has subsided, patient needs dental consultation for aggressive gingival debridement (scaling/root planing and periodontal evaluation). Scaling and root planing is necessary to limit bone loss and to prevent recurrence. Patients with severe hepatic disease metabolize metronidazole slowly, and thus an adjustment on their dosing is indicated.[11]

Topical Treatment
Rx: Chlorhexidine gluconate oral rinse (see prior Rx)

MUCOSITIS (STOMATITIS)

Mucositis, or inflammation and ulceration of the oropharyngeal mucous membranes, is a frequent and painful complication of cancer chemotherapy or radiation therapy (Boxes 40-1 and 40-2). Mucositis contributes to the morbidity and the mortality of these patients, decreases the patient's quality of life, promotes viral and fungal super infections, delays cancer therapy, and compromises nutritional intake. Of the 1.2 million Americans diagnosed with cancer each year, approximately 400,000 develop oral complications associated with their treatments. Many of these problems are preventable or treatable—especially when patients, dentists, dermatologists, and oncologists work together. The therapy of mucositis is variable from hospital to hospital, and many of these therapies have not been tested in controlled settings. Thus considerable intrahospital and interhospital variability exists in mouthwash mixture components.[12]

Rx: ("Benacort-Tetrastat"; "Mary's Magic Mouthwash" at Indiana University)
Nystatin suspension 60 ml
Diphenhydramine cough syrup 180 ml
Tetracycline powder 1.5 g
Hydrocortisone powder 60 mg
Disp: 240 ml
Sig: Swish 5-10 ml up to qid. Expires in 6 months.
Compounding instructions: In a mortar, mix powders together, add a bit of syrup to make a suspension, and mix well. Add all the ingredients and stir together. Mix well on a magnetic stirrer to homogenize.

Rx: ("Xyloxylin" Sugar-free Mixture)
Diphenhydramine HCl, USP 0.14 g
Lidocaine 1% injectable 10 ml
Spearmint water 60 ml
Maalox Plus suspension QS 240 ml
Disp: 240 ml
Sig: Shake well. Swish 5-10 ml qid.

Box 40-1

Oral Complications of Cancer Treatments

Bleeding	Mucositis or stomatitis
Dysgeusia (altered taste sensation)	Necrosis of bone (osteoradionecrosis)
Dysphagia	Pain
Increased tooth decay and rampant caries	Salivary gland dysfunction or xerostomia
Jaw stiffness (trismus)	Secondary infections (viral or fungal)

Box 40-2

Chemotherapeutic Agents Associated With Stomatitis at Standard Doses[4]

MOST COMMON	**LESS COMMON—cont'd**
Bleomycin	Doxorubicin (liposomal)
Dactinomycin	Epirubicin
Daunorubicin	Floxuridine
Docetaxel	Hydroxyurea (high-dose)
Doxorubicin	Idarubicin
Edatrexate	Mechlorethamine
Fluorouracil	6-Mercaptopurine
Methotrexate	Mithramycin
Tomudex	Mitomycin
Topotecan	Paclitaxel
	Procarbazine
LESS COMMON	Tegafur
Amsacrine	6-Thioguanine
Cyclophosphamide	Vinblastine
Cytarabine	Vincristine

NB: Expires in 1 year. (Each 15 ml contains diphenhydramine 8.5 mg, lidocaine 5.25 mg, and Maalox Plus suspension 10 ml.)

Compounding instructions: Mix well together.

Rx: ("Xyloxadryl")
Lidocaine viscous 2% 100 ml
Diphenhydramine syrup 100 ml
Maalox plus suspension 100 ml
Disp: 300 ml
Sig: Shake well then swish 5-10 ml qid.
NB: Expires in 6 months. (Each 15 ml contains lidocaine viscous 2% 5 ml, diphenhydramine syrup 5 ml, and Maalox Plus suspension 5 ml.)

Compounding instructions: Mix well together.

Rx: Stomafate suspension (Methodist standard)
Sucralfate powder 24 g
Distilled water 80 ml

Diphenhydramine syrup 60 ml
Maalox Plus suspension QS 180 ml
Disp: 180 ml
Sig: Shake well, bid to qid. Refrigerate.
NB: Expires in 2 months. Each 15 ml contains sucralfate 2.0 g, diphenhydramine 12.5 mg, and Maalox Plus suspension 2.5 ml.

Compounding instructions: Mix sucralfate and water on magnetic stirrer. Add diphenhydramine syrup and mix well. Pour mixture into a graduate and QS with Maalox Plus.

Rx: ("Dr. Weisman's Philadelphia Mouthwash")
Maalox Plus suspension 90 ml
Lidocaine viscous 2% 90 ml
Diphenhydramine cough syrup 90 ml
Distilled water 180 ml
Disp: 960 ml
Sig: Shake well, bid to qid. Refrigerate.

NB: Each 5 ml contains: lidocaine 16.5 mg, Diphenhydramine 1.2 mg, and Maalox Plus suspension 3.7 ml

Compounding instructions: Mix on magnetic stirrer.

Rx: ("Radiotherapy Mixture")
Maalox Plus suspension 700 ml
Lidocaine viscous 2% 160 ml
Diphenhydramine cough syrup 100 ml
Disp: 960 ml
Sig: Shake well, bid to qid. Refrigerate.
NB: Each 5 ml contains: lidocaine 16.5 mg, diphenhydramine 1.2 mg, and Maalox Plus suspension 3.7 ml

Compounding instructions: Mix on magnetic stirrer.

XEROSTOMIA

Xerostomia (dry mouth) is a common complaint in patients with destruction or atrophy of the salivary glands. People who have dry mouth have difficulty swallowing and are very susceptible to tooth decay (carries), especially on the roots of their teeth. Saliva cleanses the tooth surfaces and neutralizes acids. Thus, saliva helps remove food, debris, and plaque from the tooth surfaces, which helps protect against oral diseases. Heavy plaque and food accumulations that tend to occur with dry mouth can also contribute to bad breath.

Some common signs and symptoms of xerostomia include a burning sensation of the tongue, impaired taste, difficulty swallowing, increased thirst, difficulty with speech or with wearing dentures, and dry, cracked lips. Xerostomia may be a result of autoimmune diseases, an end result of radiation therapy, or a consequence of trauma or the use of various medications such as decongestants, diuretics, antihypertensive medications, antidepressants, and antihistamines (see Table 40-1). In debilitated patients with a decreased chewing ability and an increase in a liquid diet and soft food intake, there is decreased stimulation of salivary flow. The lack of saliva is associated with difficulty chewing and painful swallowing, along with diminished taste and smell. In addition, mucosal erythema, increased incidence of dental carries, and salivary gland calculi are frequent complications of xerostomia.

Box 40-3

Tips for Caring for Dry Mouth

- Sip water frequently (q 2 hours) (add lemon slices or lemon juice to water)
- Chew sugar-free gum
- If appropriate, use salivary substitutes or salivary stimulants
- Minimize tobacco use (chew/smoked)
- Avoid alcohol, lemon glycerin swabs, coffee, antihistamines, anticholinergic agents, diuretics
- Suck on ice chips
- Use appropriate topical and systemic pain medications
- Maintain meticulous oral hygiene (brush twice daily, floss daily, and supplement with professional cleanings 3 to 4 times yearly)
- Suck on sugar free candy (lemon candy*)
- Rinse mouth with plain water or saline water after every meal
- Avoid eating dry, rough, or irritating foods; use liquids to soften or thin food—crackers, cereals, steaks, chips, salt, salad dressing, spicy foods
- Use fluoridated toothpaste, rinses, and water
- Exercise the jaw muscles repeatedly

*Chewing stimulates saliva secretion; citric acid in lemons stimulates saliva.

Symptomatic relief can be obtained by conservative measures and with systemic therapy (Box 40-3).

Systemic Medications

Rx: Pilocarpine (Salagen) 5 mg
Disp: 120 tablets
Sig: 1-2 tablets tid-qid, not to exceed 30 mg/day (maximum 6 tablets daily).
NB: Sweating, gastrointestinal upset, and is expensive.

Topical Anesthetics/Coating Agents

Rx: Zilactin-B (OTC)
Sig: Apply to affected area qid.
NB: Contains adhesive gel, 10% benzocaine; tannic, boric, and salicylic acids; benzyl alcohol. (Zila Pharmaceuticals: 800-922-7887)

Rx: Orabase-B (OTC)
Sig: Apply to affected area qid.
NB: Contains 20% benzocaine paste. (Colgate-Hoyt Laboratories: 800-225-3756)

Rx: Oraloe (OTC)
Sig: Apply to affected area qid.
NB: Oraloe is a freeze-dried patch containing aloe vera gel extract, benzethonium chloride, hydroxyethyl cellulose, polyvinyl-pyrrolidone, and simethicone. (Mannatech, Inc., 713-318-ALOE).

Topical Antimicrobials

Rx: Peridex or PerioGard (chlorhexidine gluconate 0.12%) oral rinse
Disp: 16 fl oz (480 ml)
Sig: Rinse with 15 ml bid (½ oz), and then expectorate. Use after breakfast and before bedtime.
NB: Warn patient about staining properties of chlorhexidine; applying medication on a cotton-tipped applicator and applying it on the ulcer helps to minimize this side effect.

Both Peridex and PerioGard contain 11.6% alcohol. Clinical effectiveness and safety have not been established in children under the age of 18.

Topical Antiinflammatory Agents

Rx: Amlexanox (Aphthasol) oral paste 5%
Disp: 5 g
Sig: Apply ¼-inch strip to mucosal ulcers qid (after meals and hs)
NB: Antiallergic medication. Wash hands immediately after applying paste. Clinical effectiveness and safety have not been established in children under the age of 18. If no improvement after 10 days should reassess (Block Pharmaceutical).

Rx: Sucralfate suspension (an aluminum salt of sucrose octasulfate)
Disp: 5 ml qid
NB: Statistically significant improvement in frequency, healing time, and pain scores associated with oral ulcers of Behçet's disease.[13] Gels taste bad and alcohol is not well tolerated. Ointments are usually better tolerated.

Bibliography

Eisen D, Lynch DP, editors: *The mouth: diagnosis and treatment,* St. Louis, 1999, Mosby.

Mirowski GW, Bettencourt JD, Hood AF: Oral infections in the immunocompromised host. *Semin Cutan Med Surg* 16:249-256, 1997.

Rogers RS III: Recurrent aphthous stomatitis: clinical characteristics and associated systemic disorders. *Semin Cutan Med Surg* 16:278-283, 1997.

Susser WS, Whitaker-Worth DL, Grant-Kels JM: Mucocutaneous reactions to chemotherapy. *J Am Acad Dermatol* 40:367-398, 1999.

Zegarelli DJ: Fungal infections of the oral cavity. *Otolaryngol Clin North Am* 26:1069-1089, 1993.

References

1. Ross NM, Charles CH, Dills SS: Long-term effects of Listerine antiseptic on dental plaque and gingivitis. *J Clin Dent* 1:92-95, 1989.

2. Zegarelli DJ: Fungal infections of the oral cavity. *Otolaryngol Clin North Am* 26:1069-1089, 1993.

3. PDR Guide to drug interactions side effects, Medical Economics, 1996.

4. Susser WS, Whitaker-Worth DL, Grant-Kels JM: Mucocutaneous reactions to chemotherapy. *J Am Acad Dermatol* 40:367-398, 1999.

5. Campisi G, Spadari F, Salvato A: Sucralfate in odontostomatology. Clinical experience. *Minerva Stomatologica* 46:297-305, 1997.

6. Jacobson JM, Greenspan JS, Spritzler J, et al: Thalidomide is an effective treatment for aphthous ulceration of the mouth and oropharynx in patients with HIV infection. *N Engl J Med* 336:1487-1493, 1997.

7. Chahine L, Sempson N, Wagoner C: The effect of sodium lauryl sulfate on recurrent aphthous ulcers: a clinical study. *Compend Cont Educ Dent* 18:1238-1240, 1997.

8. Herlofson BB, Barkvoll P: The effect of two toothpaste detergents on the frequency of recurrent aphthous ulcers. *Acta Odontologica Scand* 54:150-153, 1996.

9. Healy CM, Paterson M, Joyston-Bechal S, et al: The effect of a sodium lauryl sulfate-free dentifrice on patients with recurrent oral ulceration. *Oral Dis* 5:39-43, 1999.

10. Riviere GR, Wagoner MA, Baker-Zander SA, et al: Identification of spirochetes related to *Treponema pallidum* in necrotizing ulcerative gingivitis and chronic periodontitis. *N Engl J Med* 325:539-543, 1991.

11. Loesche WJ, Syed SA, Laughon BE, et al: The bacteriology of acute necrotizing ulcerative gingivitis. *J Periodontol* 53:223-230, 1982.

12. Mueller BA, Millheim ET, Farrington EA, et al: Mucositis management practices for hospitalized patients: national survey results. *J Pain Symptom Manage* 10:510-520, 1995.

13. Alpsoy E, Er H, Durusoy C, Yilmaz E: The use of sucralfate suspension in the treatment of oral and genital ulceration of Behçet disease: a randomized, placebo-controlled, double blind study. *Arch Dermatol* 135:529-532, 1999.

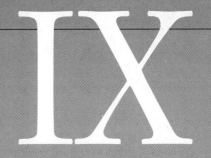

PART IX

Major Adverse Effects from Systemic Drugs

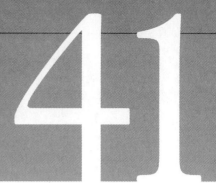

CHAPTER 41

Stephen E. Wolverton

Hepatotoxicity of Drug Therapy

The importance of drug-induced liver disease (drug hepatotoxicity) is illustrated by the following statistics[1]:

1. Drugs are estimated to be responsible for 10% of cases of hepatitis in adults.
2. Drugs are responsible for about 40% of cases of hepatitis in adults at least 50 years of age.
3. It is estimated that 25% of all cases of fulminant hepatitis are due to drugs.
4. Liver failure, when it is drug-induced on an idiosyncratic basis, is fatal 80% of the time.[2]

The vast majority of currently available systemic drugs have been reported to at least on rare occasions induce some degree of hepatotoxicity. Table 41-1 lists definitions of hepatotoxicity terms.

Several important questions must be addressed. Why is the liver a frequent site of important systemic drug reactions? Why do certain drugs induce significant hepatotoxicity on a relatively frequent basis? Why do some patients experience clinically significant hepatotoxicity from a given drug, which the vast majority of patients tolerate very well?

In this chapter, important general concepts regarding the current knowledge about drug-induced liver disease are summarized. Insightful answers to the previously mentioned questions and to many more questions are provided. The focus is on the four subsets of drug-induced liver disease that are most pertinent to practicing dermatologists, although physicians from all fields of medicine will glean principles of value to a wide variety of patients. These four subsets include (1) hepatocellular toxicity, (2) drug hypersensitivity syndrome, (3) cholestasis, and (4) steatosis progressing to fibrosis.

The ultimate motivation for writing such a chapter involves sharing principles that prevent unnecessary morbidity and rare deaths from systemic drugs while maximizing the overall safety and efficacy of important systemic drugs commonly used in dermatology. Drugs that are no longer available due to severe hepatotoxicity are listed in Table 41-2. Liver transplantations performed due to severe, irreversible liver disease induced by drugs, such as ketoconazole[3] and methotrexate,[4] are overall avoidable. Avoiding the major cost of this life-saving technology is an important goal as well.

THE LIVER AND DRUG METABOLISM

The liver concentrates many drugs while serving the major metabolic role for most drugs.[1] The overall goal of this hepatic drug metabolism is to convert pharmacologically active lipophilic

■ Table 41-1   Definitions Used in Chapter

Term	Definition
Transaminases	Collectively the enzymes AST/SGOT and ALT/SGPT
Transaminitis	Elevation of AST/SGOT or ALT/SGOT levels up to twofold above upper normal values
Toxic hepatitis	Either threefold elevation of transaminase levels, symptoms of hepatitis, or typically both
Liver failure	Severely reduced synthetic and metabolic functions of the liver
Polymorphism	Differences in enzyme activity due to genetic differences between various individuals
Enzyme variability	Differences in enzyme activity in spite of identical genotypes
Isoform	A specific CYP-450 enzyme; such as 2D6, 3A4, and so on
Idiosyncratic	Drug reactions that are unpredictable and occur independent of drug dose
Toxicity	Drug reactions that are predictable, given an adequately high dose of a few specific drugs
Neoantigens	Literally new antigens, due to covalent bonding of reactive intermediates to hepatic proteins
Steatosis	Fat deposition in the liver; subtypes microvesicular and macrovesicular
Azalides	Subset of macrolide antibiotics, including azithromycin and clarithromycin
Statins	HMG CoA reductase inhibitors such as lovastatin and atorvastatin
Threshold of concern	Laboratory test elevation above a specified level, beyond which there is increased likelihood of a more serious reaction; abnormalities of this type are almost always reversible
Critical level	Laboratory test elevation at an even greater level, beyond which there is dramatically increased likelihood of a severe reaction; lower likelihood of complete reversibility

■ Table 41-2   Some Drugs That Are No Longer Available Due to Severe Hepatotoxicity

Generic Name	Trade Name	Drug Category
Troglitazone	Rezulin	Insulin sensitizer
Zomepirac	Zomax	Nonsteroidal anti-inflammatory drug
Ticrynafen	Selacryn	Diuretic with uricosuric properties
Benoxaprofen	Oraflex	Nonsteroidal anti-inflammatory drug

hepatocyte is the central hepatic cell involved in this metabolism; it follows that the hepatocyte is the most common liver cell victimized by drug-induced liver disease. Important general concepts regarding hepatic drug metabolic systems are listed below (Box 41-1).

The human body has a complicated and intriguing system for biotransformation (conversion from lipophilic to hydrophilic molecules) and detoxification (conversion of reactive metabolic intermediates to more stable molecular compounds) of a multitude of very heterogeneous pharmaceutical molecules/drugs. These systems for biotransformation and detoxification of drugs logically evolved and developed long before all current drugs were developed. The same systems play an important role in the metabolism of a number of molecules (including steroids molecules such as corticosteroids, sex steroid, bile acids) and detoxification of various potential environmental insults (e.g., "quenching" free O_2 and superoxide radicals).

drugs into inactive hydrophilic metabolites to facilitate renal or biliary excretion. With these important functions, it should come as no surprise that the liver could be the "victim" of aberrancies in these metabolic processes. Furthermore, the

Box 41-1

Key Points About Hepatic Drug Metabolic Systems[5-8]

BASELINE PHARMACOLOGIC PRINCIPLES
- The vast majority of drugs have lipophilic properties.
- This lipophilicity is essential for drugs to effectively cross lipid membranes to arrive at the site of desired pharmacologic activity.

GENERAL GOALS OF DRUG METABOLISM
Biotransformation
- The major goal of this process is conversion of the drug from lipophilic to hydrophilic properties.
- Increased hydrophilicity is essential for drugs to be excreted by either renal or biliary routes.

Detoxification
- The overall goal is to avoid local or distant damage from reactive intermediates created during the biotransformation process.
- These reactive metabolic intermediates are usually highly electrophilic compounds that readily form covalent bonds with nearby proteins, DNA, and lipids.
- In the vast majority of patients receiving potentially hepatotoxic drugs, these detoxification systems are adequate to allow safe drug administration without risk to the liver.

PHASES OF DRUG METABOLISM
Phase I (Oxidative Reactions)
- Cytochrome P-450 enzymes—these reactions are largely accomplished by just 5 to 6 isoforms that metabolize the vast majority of drugs utilized in humans.
- Majority of reactions are oxidative, adding a hydroxyl group that provides a site for subsequent conjugation reactions.
- These oxidative reactions result in only a small increase in hydrophilicity.
- Other phase I reactions include dealkylation and halogenation.

Phase II (Conjugation Reactions)
- Enzymes involved include *N*-acetyl transferase, UDP glucuronyl transferase, and sulfotransferases.
- Major enzymes involved attach a large polar side chain to the oxidative site of the phase I reaction.
- The phase II conjugation reactions may simultaneously result in a marked increase in hydrophilicity and detoxify the reactive intermediates as well.

Increased activity of the biotransformation enzymes (due to cytochrome P-450 enzyme [CYP] inducers) can produce an increased quantity of reactive, electron scavenging, metabolic intermediates. The process of converting a pharmacologically active lipophilic drug to a reactive intermediate is known as bioactivation. Abnormalities of the detoxification systems may allow these reactive intermediates to wreak havoc locally in the liver or, through indirect mechanisms, have systemic consequences. As long as there is a reasonable balance between bioactivation and detoxification, no significant drug toxicity occurs. Spielberg and associates[9] developed the lymphocyte cytotoxicity assay as a potentially important laboratory method of assessing an individual's detoxification capacity for a limited number of drugs. The reader is encouraged to learn more about these hepatic metabolic systems from several excellent reviews.[5,6,8,10]

The question regarding the varying probability of specific individuals experiencing drug-induced liver disease can in part be answered by the presence of genetic polymorphisms in important hepatic biotransformation and detoxification enzymes (Table 41-3). The tremendous variability of enzyme activity is explained in part by distinct inheritable deoxyribonucleic acid (DNA) mutations (polymorphisms) of both phase I and phase II hepatic enzymes.[7,11] There are five CYP isoforms involved in drug-induced hepatotoxicity (CYP 1A2, 2C9, 2D6, 2E1, 3A4).[5] CYP 2C19 is not known to be responsible for producing reactive metabolites with hepatotoxic potential.

The prototype CYP enzymes with significant polymorphisms are CYP 2D6 and 2C19.[12,13]

■ Table 41-3   Phase I/Phase II Metabolic Enzymes and Detoxification Systems[5,8,11]

Enzyme Examples	Polymorphism/ Variability	Comments
PHASE I ENZYMES		
CYP 1A2*§	Variability up to ~thirtyfold	Induced by omeprazole, smoking, charbroiled meat
CYP 2C9	Variability up to ~thirtyfold	Induced by various anticonvulsants, rifampin
CYP 2C19†	Polymorphism	Is not responsible for drug-induced liver disease
CYP 2D6‡ (no inducers)	Polymorphism	10% of Caucasians have essentially no 2D6 activity
CYP 2E1§	Variability up to ~thirtyfold	Induced by ethanol, isoniazid
CYP 3A4*	Variability up to ~thirtyfold	Induced by various anticonvulsants, rifampin
PHASE II ENZYMES		
UDP glucuronyl transferases	Polymorphism	Result is glucuronidation, increased hydrophilicity
Sulfotransferases	Polymorphism	Result is sulfonation, increased hydrophilicity
N-acetyl transferase 1 and 2	Polymorphism	NAT$_2$ 50% Caucasians "slow acetylators"
DETOXIFICATION SYSTEMS		
Epoxide hydrolases	Polymorphism	Possible role in anticonvulsant hypersensitivity syndrome
Glutathione S-transferases	Polymorphism	Critical detoxification enzyme for many drugs
Free radical quenchers	Uncertain	SOD, catalase, vitamin C, vitamin E

SOD, Superoxide dismutase.
*Variability in 1A2 is assessed by metabolism of caffeine; variability in 3A4 can be assessed by erythromycin breath test or MEGX assay, studying lidocaine metabolism.
†Polymorphism in 2C19 is assessed by metabolism of S-mephenytoin (an anticonvulsant).
‡Polymorphism in 2D6 is assessed by metabolism of debrisoquine (an antidysrhythmic agent); overall fiftyfold variation in activity when comparing various individuals.
§Recent evidence suggests that there is polymorphism for these isoforms as well (see Chapter 44).

Individuals with "low activity" for CYP 2D6 may have fiftyfold less enzyme activity than individuals with the "high activity" phenotype for the same isoform. Such wide variation in activity can help explain why some individuals experience excessive and prolonged daytime sedation after a single 10-mg dose of doxepin at nighttime (a 2D6 substrate) whereas other individuals tolerate and have very little sedation with doxepin doses titrated up to 200 to 300 mg each day. By the same logic, other potentially hepatotoxic drugs that are substrates for CYP 2D6 could have excessive drug levels in patients who inherited the "low activity" phenotype. Even without genetic polymorphisms, other enzymes (such as CYP 3A4) can have significant variability (up to thirtyfold) of enzyme activity.[12]

Even more important to the topic of drug hepatotoxicity is the potential for CYP enzyme inducers to increase the enzyme activity of various CYP isoforms.[5] Such an increased activity of a given phase I oxidative enzyme increases the quantities of various reactive intermediates derived from drug substrates. The risk of drug-induced liver disease is greatest when there is an accompanying genetic (e.g., NAT_2 "slow acetylators") or acquired (decreased glutathione levels due to HIV infection) defect in phase II conjugation and detoxification systems.

Significant controversies and unanswered questions abound in this subject area. One such issue is the presence of the slow acetylator phenotype in up to 50% of Caucasians, whereas only a very small percentage of patients with this phenotype experience reactions thought to be due to this defect (e.g., drug-induced lupus erythematosus and isoniazid hepatotoxicity).[14,15] The anticonvulsant hypersensitivity syndrome has been postulated to be due to reduced activity of epoxide hydrolase, leading to increased quantities of unstable epoxide intermediates from anticonvulsants such as phenytoin, phenobarbital, and carbamazepine.[16,17] More recently this explanation has been challenged.[18]

MECHANISMS OF DRUG HEPATOTOXICITY

The most well-accepted hypothesis explaining idiosyncratic drug-induced liver disease has two components. First, there must be the presence of reactive metabolic intermediates, which are electrophilic compounds that rapidly form covalent bonds to various cellular components, if not equally rapidly detoxified. These covalent bonds result in various structural and functional changes, depending on the affected molecule (Table 41-4). These molecular components include various proteins (including the CYP isoforms), DNA, and lipids with consequences as detailed in Table 41-5. The presence of CYP inducers can significantly increase the quantities of these electrophilic reactive intermediates (Table 41-6). Second, there generally must be a defect in the cellular detoxification systems for there to be an adequate presence of these intermediates to result in significant hepatic pathology. In the absence of the CYP inducers or with normal detoxification systems, significant drug-induced liver disease from these metabolic products is distinctly uncommon.

Probably the most important component of the detoxification enzyme repertoire is the glutathione and glutathione S-transferase (GST)

system.[5] GST is an enzyme with significant polymorphism, with glutathione serving as a co-factor, and various electrophilic drug metabolites serving as GST substrates. Glutathione can be depleted in the process of electron scavenging, particularly with an unusually heavy load of reactive intermediates, such as with an acetaminophen overdose. The electron scavenging capabilities of this GST/glutathione system can be further depleted by excessive ethanol consumption, human immunodeficiency virus (HIV) infection, and malnutrition.[6,8] It stands to reason that drug hepatotoxicity, let alone drug reactions in general, is increased in these clinical settings.

Two potential outcomes are thought to occur when there are excessive quantities of reactive, electrophilic intermediates.[5,10] First is the potential for direct toxicity to neighboring cells (most notably the hepatocyte) from protein, DNA, and lipid biomembrane alterations resulting from covalent binding to these intermediates. An important final common pathway leading to cell necrosis or apoptosis is likely a disruption in calcium regulation, leading to alterations in the actin cytoskeleton and changes in cell membrane integrity.[6] Binding of fas (on the cell membrane of "damaged" hepatocytes) with fas ligand (on antigen processing cells) leading to activation of the caspase cascade and subsequent apoptosis is important pathway of cell destruction as well. Second, the covalent binding of the reactive intermediates to various proteins leads to the development of new antigens (neoantigens).[19] These neoantigens can include various CYP isoforms, which logically are "in the neighborhood" when the intermediates are created by the respective isoforms.[20,21] The end results are potentially either a direct humoral or cellular response to these neoantigens, immunologic cross-reactivity with structurally similar distant antigens, or both. Delving further into the complexities of major histocompatibility complex (MHC) molecules involved with antigen presentation, along with the uncertainties regarding the overall pathogenesis of drug-induced autoimmune disorders, is beyond the scope of this chapter. Also, given the paucity of dermatologic drugs that induce cholestasis, the mechanisms involved with this process are not discussed in this chapter (see Bibliography—Erlinger).

■ Table 41-4   Molecular Targets Involved With Drug-Induced Liver Disease[5,6]

Molecule	Consequence	Comments
Various proteins	Neoantigen formation	Reactive metabolites induce a change in structure or conformation
CYP isoforms	Neoantigen formation	CYP especially vulnerable, due to proximity to reactive metabolites
DNA	Apoptosis or necrosis	Either route results in cell death
Lipids	Loss of membrane integrity	Result of lipid peroxidation by reactive metabolites

■ Table 41-5   Cellular and Structural Targets Involved With Drug-Induced Liver Disease[5,6]

Cell or Structure	Category of Reaction	Representative Drug Etiologies
Hepatocytes	Hepatocellular necrosis	Ketoconazole, minocycline
Bile ducts, bile canaliculi	Cholestasis	Erythromycin estolate (in adults)
Endothelial cells, sinusoids	Veno-occlusive	Cyclophosphamide (very high dose)
Ito cells (fat storage cells)	Steatosis → Fibrosis	Methotrexate

■ Table 41-6   Several CYP Inducers and Inhibitors That Also Have Hepatotoxic Potential[5]

Drug	Isoform	Reaction Category
CYP INDUCERS*		
Phenytoin	Various	Hypersensitivity syndrome
Carbamazepine	Various	Hypersensitivity syndrome
Rifampin	3A4, 2C9	Hepatocellular toxicity
Isoniazid	2E1	Hepatocellular toxicity
Ethanol	2E1	Hepatocellular toxicity
CYP INHIBITORS		
Ketoconazole	3A4	Hepatocellular toxicity
Itraconazole†	3A4	Hepatocellular toxicity
Fluconazole†	2C9	Hepatocellular toxicity
Erythromycin estolate‡	3A4	Cholestasis

*In contrast with other enzyme inducers that are anticonvulsants, phenobarbital has minimal risk for hepatotoxicity.
†Itraconazole and fluconazole have far less risk for hepatocellular toxicity compared with ketoconazole.
‡Vary rare hepatotoxicity from other macrolides, including the azalide subset.

Box 41-2

Generalizations Regarding Drug-Induced Liver Disease[1,6]

MECHANISM (REGARDING PREDICTABILITY)
- The vast majority are *idiosyncratic*, which means unpredictable and without a clear relationship to drug dose
- A very small percentage are *toxic*, which means predictable and dose-dependent

TIMING
- Onset—majority occur between days 15 and 90 after the initiation of drug therapy; generally have a much more gradual onset compared with potentially serious hematologic drug reactions
- Resolution—most have a marked improvement within 15 days of drug cessation
- Above timing for hepatocellular toxicity, hypersensitivity syndrome, and cholestasis type reactions

TIMING—cont'd
- Steatosis progressing to fibrosis is much slower in onset, and more insidious in progression

REVERSIBILITY
- Most reactions are completely reversible if detected early (within days to a few weeks)
- Occasional reactions are not fully reversible if not detected early (delay of many weeks to months)
- Possible outcomes if significantly delayed diagnosis—death, liver failure requiring liver transplantation, severe fibrosis or cirrhosis, or loss of some degree of liver function indefinitely*

*In contrast to the kidneys, the liver has a tremendous reserve capacity—marked liver damage is possible before laboratory indicators of reduced liver function become abnormal.

It is worth reminding the reader of an important distinction at this point. Direct drug-induced *toxicity* to the liver merely results from excessive drug levels from very few specific drugs.[5,22] The classic biochemistry example is the effect of carbon tetrachloride on the liver. The classic pharmacologic example is an acetaminophen overdose, although pharmacologic doses of acetaminophen in the presence of a CYP 2E1 inducer (chronic excessive ethanol consumption) can produce a similar result. By definition, *toxicity* here means that virtually every individual has a reaction to carbon tetrachloride or acetaminophen given that adequately excessive quantities of these molecules are administered. In contrast, the term *idiosyncratic* suggests that only a distinct minority of individuals experience drug-induced liver disease from selected drugs and that the reaction occurs independent of drug dose. Under this heading is where the vast majority of hepatotoxicity due to drugs occurs.[6,23] What may be somewhat confusing is that the word *toxicity* is commonly used in the setting of idiosyncrasy as well. Basically, idiosyncrasy is divided into *metabolic idiosyncrasy*

(due to the local *toxic* effects of locally formed reactive intermediates) and *immunologic idiosyncrasy* (local damage from an immunologic response due to neoantigens induced by these reactive intermediates). It is with these two dichotomies in mind (toxic versus idiosyncratic reactions; metabolic idiosyncrasy versus immunologic idiosyncrasy) that the reader should progress through this chapter (Box 41-2).

RISK FACTORS FOR DRUG HEPATOTOXICITY

There are a number of factors, aside from genetic predisposition/idiosyncrasy, that help explain why some individuals react to a given medication, whereas the majority of patients do not. These factors are listed in Table 41-7. The risk factors are grouped under the headings of habits, nutrition, medical diagnoses, concomitant drugs, and demographic factors. Although the various risk factors are largely irreversible, the prudent clinician avoids certain drugs if important risk factors are present in a given pa-

■ **Table 41-7**   Risk Factors for Drug-Induced Liver Disease[1,6]

Category	Risk Factor	Explanation
Habits	Ethanol abuse	Direct toxicity, CYP 2E1 inducer, depletes glutathione
Nutrition	Malnutrition	Depletes glutathione levels
Medical diagnoses	HIV infection	Depletes glutathione levels—increased sulfonamide, dapsone reactions
	Diabetes	Increased fatty liver—increased methotrexate, retinoid toxicity
	Obesity	Increased fatty liver—increased methotrexate, retinoid toxicity
	Prior liver disease	From any etiology; major reason baseline LFTs are necessary
Concomitant drugs	CYP inducers	Increased quantities of reactive intermediates
	CYP inhibitors	Increased drug levels for substrates for a given CYP isoform
Demographic factors	Elderly patients	May be due to polypharmacy; also reduced hepatic and renal function
	Gender	Increased likelihood of certain hepatic drug reactions in females
Genetics	Various	(Multiple examples throughout chapter—see various tables/text)

tient. A classic example is the increased probability of methotrexate hepatotoxicity (steatosis → fibrosis) in the setting of one or more of the following: excessive ethanol consumption, obesity, diabetes mellitus, or renal insufficiency.[24,25] It is likely that most of the apparent reduced incidence of methotrexate-induced cirrhosis in patients with rheumatoid arthritis is due to more careful patient selection regarding methotrexate administration.[26]

There are a number of drug-specific risk factors. These include daily dose, cumulative dose, frequency of dosing, timing from drug initiation, and continuation of drug administration well after clinical or laboratory evidence of liver pathology began. Aside from a few specific examples here, the reader is encouraged to review this issue in specific chapters on azole antifungal agents (see Chapter 4), methotrexate (see Chapter 7), azathioprine (see Chapter 8), dapsone (see Chapter 11), and retinoids (see Chapter 13), to name several of the most important dermatologic agents with the potential for hepatotoxicity. Daily dose is probably a factor in retinoid hepatotoxicity,[27] whereas cumulative dose is a key determinant of

risk for methotrexate-induced liver disease.[24,25] Timing from the onset of drug administration is critical in surveillance for drugs that can cause the drug hypersensitivity syndrome (DHS), such as azathioprine,[28] dapsone,[29,30] and minocycline.[31,32] Idiosyncratic reactions to ketoconazole, albeit lacking other components of the DHS, occur in a similar timing, most notably between weeks 3 and 12 of drug administration. Frequency of drug dosing is potentially an issue with methotrexate, with inadvertent daily dosing markedly increasing drug toxicity (here the risk of pancytopenia is more likely than hepatotoxicity, however).[33]

Widespread availability of predictive testing to assess which patients are at risk for drug-induced liver disease on a genetic basis would be ideal; such testing is not widely available in clinical settings at this time.[5] Ready availability of assays for polymorphisms (such as CYP 2D6 and NAT$_2$), enzyme variability (CYP 3A4), and relative depletion of important detoxification enzyme systems (GST/glutathione detoxification system) *before* initial administration of drugs with a significant potential for hepatotoxicity would be a noble goal.

DRUG INFORMATION DISSEMINATION ISSUES

There are conceptually several more somewhat vague risk factors for drug-induced liver disease. These "risk factors" include (1) recent release of a drug (see details in the next paragragh) and (2) lack of physician or patient awareness of the potential for drug hepatotoxicity from a given drug.

It is well known that preclinical trials before the Food and Drug Administration (FDA) release of a new drug for a specific indication rarely include an adequate number of patients to detect rare idiosyncratic events. It is just not economically feasible to routinely include such a large number of patients in these preclinical trials. A good example of the consequences of the limited numbers of patients in preclinical trials is the ketoconazole hepatotoxicity story. Ketoconazole induces mild transaminase changes ("transaminitis") in 5% to 10% of patients, whereas toxic hepatitis occurs in 1 of 10,000 patients.[34] With long-term therapy, the incidence of toxic hepatitis increases to 1 of 1500. Given that preclinical trials study up to 1000 patients at the very most (typically far fewer patients are studied), the likelihood of detecting this toxic hepatitis risk before drug release was very low. The recent troglitazone (Rezulin) withdrawal from the market in the United States followed an overall similar pattern of statistics.[35,36] In addition, preclinical trials typically limit the variables studied to have the greatest chance of accurately determining whether the drug under study is truly (statistically significant) effective for the given indication in question. The number of additional drugs patients entered in the preclinical trials may take is severely limited, to limit the potential confounding variables in the study.

When the drug is released into real world clinical use, both the number of patients treated and the number of drugs these patients are receiving dramatically increase. The result can be the discovery of previously undetected, rare, idiosyncratic, drug-induced liver disease and the recognition of potentially important drug interactions. In these settings, serious liver disease and rare deaths may be detected. There are at least two "red flags," which suggest that clinicians be very cautious regarding prescribing recently released medications until substantially more real world clinical experience is gathered. These warning signs include (1) the presence of significant numbers of patients in clinical trials with mild liver function test (LFTs) elevations, namely "transaminitis," and (2) the report of even 1 to 2 deaths from drug hepatotoxicity in the studies or very soon after the drug's release. In these two settings, clinicians may either avoid prescribing the new medication or at least monitor their patients receiving the drug very carefully, especially during the first 3 to 4 months after drug therapy is initiated. Laboratory monitoring every 2 weeks (for high-risk drugs) during this initial period is generally adequate in the vast majority of cases.

Lack of physician or patient awareness of hepatotoxic risk is an important determinant of risk. Drug cessation is possible if either the patient notes symptoms of drug-induced liver disease or the physician finds abnormalities on laboratory or liver biopsy surveillance. Serious outcomes (i.e., death or the need for liver transplantation) occur primarily when the drug is continued in spite of mounting evidence of liver dysfunction.[6] Ketoconazole-related deaths occurred in this fashion.[34] Rapid dissemination of information to all physicians regarding the risk for potentially serious drug-induced liver disease for new and relatively recently released medications is ideal, albeit a very complex task. Physicians should carefully heed any "Dear Doctor" letters received from the FDA or letters from similar government agencies pertinent to physicians practicing in other countries. Academic physicians share the burden for dissemination of this important information. In turn, practicing physicians must inform their patients regarding symptoms to report and monitoring required for drugs with the potential for hepatotoxicity. It is through this multicomponent team effort that the risk of serious outcome from potentially risky, yet clinically beneficial drugs can be minimized.

CLASSIFICATION SYSTEMS

Table 41-8 lists major categories of liver toxicity due to drugs. The reader is referred primarily to the tables in this section. The ideal classification system would be based on clinical and laboratory evidence of liver disease, liver histology, and full awareness of the mechanism behind various patterns of drug-induced liver disease (Box 41-3). The reality is that adequate

■ **Table 41-8**   Major Categories of Liver Toxicity Due to Drugs[1,6]

Category	Best Diagnostic Tests	Classic Culprits	Dermatologic Drug Etiologies	Medical Drug Etiologies
Hepatocellular	AST/SGOT ALT/SGPT	Halothane	Ketoconazole Dapsone Minocycline Azathioprine Acitretin Methotrexate†	Various "statins" Flutamide Isoflurane Rifampin*
Hypersensitivity syndrome	AST/SGOT ALT/SGPT Eosinophil count	Phenytoin	Dapsone Minocycline Azathioprine Sulfonamides	Allopurinol Amox/clavulanate Phenobarbital Carbamazepine Lamotrigine
Cholestasis	Alkaline phosphatase GGT Bilirubin (conjugated)	Chlorpromazine	Erythromycin estolate TMP/SMX	Captopril Nafcillin Estrogens Rifampin‡
Steatosis → fibrosis (macrovesicular)	Liver biopsy Transaminases	Methotrexate	Etretinate (rarely) Acitretin (rarely)	Methyldopa

*Rifampin long-term use in tuberculosis creates a significant risk for hepatocellular toxicity (a nondermatologic use).
†Methotrexate occasionally induces hepatocellular toxicity, although generally mild-to-moderate severity.
‡Although rifampin more frequently induces hepatocellular toxicity; infrequently the drug causes cholestasis.

Box 41-3

Major Systems for Classifying Drug-Induced Liver Disease[1,6]

BASED ON LABORATORY TEST ABNORMALITIES (SO CALLED LIVER FUNCTION TESTS)
- Hepatocellular—primarily abnormalities in transaminase values
- Obstructive—primarily abnormalities in alkaline phosphatase, GGT, and eventually bilirubin values
- Mixed—combination of these test abnormalities (either type over time may become "mixed")

BASED ON LIVER HISTOLOGY (TO NAME A FEW)
- Steatosis—"fatty liver"; subtypes include microvesicular (pseudoalcoholic) and macrovesicular
- Fibrosis to cirrhosis—histologic evidence of abnormal fibrogenesis; cirrhosis if regenerative nodules present

BASED ON LIVER HISTOLOGY (TO NAME A FEW)—cont'd
- Granulomatous
- Veno-occlusive

BASED ON PATHOGENESIS (REGARDING PREDICTABILITY AND RELATIONSHIP TO DRUG DOSE)
- Toxic
- Idiosyncratic

SUBSETS OF IDIOSYNCRATIC REACTIONS (REALITY IS THAT THESE SUBSETS OVERLAP SIGNIFICANTLY)
- Metabolic idiosyncrasy—due primarily to local "toxic" effects of reactive intermediates
- Immunologic idiosyncrasy—due primarily to neoantigens induced by reactive intermediates

■ **Table 41-9**   Other Categories of Liver Toxicity Due to Drugs[1,6]

Category	Drug Etiologies	
Granulomatous	Diltiazem	Procainamide
	Phenytoin	Quinidine
Veno-occlusive	Cyclophosphamide (high dose)	Other intensive chemotherapy
Ischemic	Cocaine	Nicotinic acid (sustained release)
	Methylenedioxyamphetamine	
Microvesicular steatosis	Amiodarone	Valproic acid
(pseudoalcoholic)	Perhexiline	Zidovudine
	Aspirin (with Reye's syndrome)	Didanosine
	Intravenous tetracycline	
Chronic hepatitis	Methyldopa	Nitrofurantoin
	Phenytoin	Isoniazid
	Acetaminophen	Trazodone
Vascular proliferations*	Estradiol	Androgens
Direct toxicity	Acetaminophen overdose	Acetaminophen with CYP inducer

*Vascular proliferations include subcategories such as peliosis hepatis.

information about all components of this triad is rarely present. Regardless the clinician still needs to make decisions regarding the presence or absence of significant liver disease, as well as decisions regarding the magnitude of risk from continuing or restarting the drug in question with whatever laboratory information is readily available. In practice, monitoring serum LFTs, which may suggest hepatocellular or obstructive liver disease, is the basis of most clinical decision-making. Laboratory test abnormalities suggesting hepatobiliary obstruction (cholestasis) are distinctly uncommon from systemic drugs used in dermatology. A liver biopsy is routinely indicated for patients only on methotrexate therapy. (See Chapter 7 for a full discussion on the pros and cons of performing routine liver biopsies on methotrexate patients.) It is important to remind the readers that from a liver perspective the laboratory evidence for both hepatocellular toxicity and DHS patients is similar. The presence of infectious mononucleosis–like clinical findings and the characteristic pronounced eosinophilia distinguish the DHS as a distinct clinical entity. Dapsone, azathioprine, and minocycline are all capable of producing either single organ dysfunction (hepatocellular toxicity alone) or the full-blown DHS. The reader should be somewhat familiar with patterns of drug-induced liver disease that receive less emphasis in this chapter (Table 41-9).

DRUG ETIOLOGIES

Determination of the causative drug, let alone deciding if the liver disease is drug-induced at all, is a daunting task if a known, high-risk drug is not currently prescribed. More commonly the dermatologist knows when the drug being prescribed is considered to deserve careful liver monitoring. Two exceptions are worth mentioning here. One exception is regarding dapsone and azathioprine, for which virtually all physicians do careful hematologic monitoring, whereas far fewer physicians routinely check transaminase levels. Another example would be the very "delayed" discovery of the potential for minocycline to induce hepatotoxicity as an isolated finding or to induce the DHS.

In addition to drugs listed in Table 41-10, dermatologists should do at least some laboratory monitoring for liver dysfunction for additional drugs including chlorambucil, cyclophosphamide, mycophenolate mofetil, cyclosporine, isotretinoin, hydroxychloroquine, and chloroquine. Consult the individual chapters for these drugs regarding specific monitoring guidelines. Because dermatologists occasionally prescribe nonsteroidal antiinflammatory drugs (NSAIDs) for conditions such as erythema nodosum, awareness of occasional reports of drug hepatotoxicity from piroxicam (Feldene) and diclofenac (Voltaren) is important.[37-39] Pertinent to this drug

■ **Table 41-10**   Dermatologic Drugs With Significant Risk of Drug-Induced Liver Disease[1,6]

Drug Name	Category of Reaction	Less Risky Alternatives	Comments
COMMONLY USED DRUGS			
Methotrexate	Steatosis → fibrosis	Other systemic psoriasis options	Be careful regarding dose, patient selection, proper monitoring
Minocycline	Hypersensitivity syndrome	Doxycycline, tetracycline	Usually 3-12 wks into therapy, liver alone may be affected
Azathioprine	Hypersensitivity syndrome	Other immunosuppressive drugs	Usually 3-12 wks into therapy, liver alone may be affected
Dapsone	Hypersensitivity syndrome	Colchicine, sulfapyridine	Can cross-react with sulfonamides, liver alone may be affected
Sulfonamides	Hypersensitivity syndrome	Nonsulfonamide antibiotics	A rare complication with long-term therapy
Acitretin	Steatosis, hepatocellular	First-generation retinoid—isotretinoin	Serious reactions very uncommon, minor LFT changes common
LESS COMMONLY USED DRUGS			
Rifampin	Hepatocellular toxicity	Use drug only for short-term therapy	Short courses less than 7-10 d rarely problematic
Ketoconazole	Hepatocellular toxicity	Itraconazole, fluconazole, terbinafine	Short courses less than 7-10 d rarely problematic
Erythromycin estolate	Cholestasis	Other erythromycins, azalides*	Primarily in adults; not a risk with other erythromycin salts
Cimetidine	Hepatocellular toxicity	All other H_2 antagonists	A very rare complication of cimetidine
Zileuton	Hepatocellular toxicity	Zafirlukast, montelukast	LTD_4 receptor antagonists have less tendency for hepatotoxicity

*Azalides are a subset of macrolide antibiotics—include azithromycin and clarithromycin.

category is the withdrawal from the market of zomepirac (Zomax) and benoxaprofen (Oraflex) in the 1980s due to drug hepatotoxicity.[40,41]

DIAGNOSIS

There is a four step algorithm for reasonably accurate diagnosis of the etiology of any drug-induced adverse effect.

1. *Challenge* (circumstances of the original drug course).
2. *Dechallenge* (expected improvement after the drug is discontinued).

3. *Rechallenge* (*only* when it is essential to know the responsible drug with certainty *and* the reaction pattern is a relatively low-risk adverse effect).
4. *Exclusion* of other nondrug etiologies for the same adverse effect.[42,43]

Aside from mild transaminitis from potentially hepatotoxic drugs, it is not prudent to rechallenge patients who have had moderate-to-severe episodes of virtually any category of drug-induced liver disease. The risks of the rechallenge maneuver are too great to justify, given the nonlife-threatening nature of the vast majority of dermatoses treated.

The "challenge," "dechallenge," and "exclusion" steps are justifiable and essential for virtually all patients with a twofold to threefold elevation of transaminase values (Table 41-11). A drug "rechallenge" in this setting should be undertaken only after significant deliberation regarding alternative therapeutic agents *and* with very careful laboratory follow-up. When there is a onefold to twofold elevation of transaminase values ("threshold of concern"), a somewhat more liberal approach can be utilized. In this setting, it is reasonable to reduce the drug dose and follow-up the transaminase values more carefully. Above a threefold elevation of the transaminase values, it is my suggestion to stop the drug in question indefinitely unless an alternative etiology for this elevation is uncovered. This threefold elevation is how the pharmaceutical industry and FDA typically define toxic hepatitis for clinical studies. It is common for the transaminase values to rapidly increase to a tenfold to 100-fold elevation range if the responsible drug is continued in spite of elevations at or slightly above this "critical level" of a threefold elevation. Unfortunately many rechallenges or instances of drug continuation are *unintentional* in this range of laboratory abnormality due to patient noncompliance with laboratory monitoring or due to lack of physician suspicion that a drug may be responsible for the laboratory abnormality.

It is important to consider at least four other possibilities as explanations for any new onset transaminase elevations, given that the patient had no evidence of liver disease at the onset of drug therapy[1,6] (Table 41-12). These possibilities include the following:

1. Viral hepatitis—test at least for hepatitis A, B, and C; also consider cytomegalovirus (CMV) and Epstein-Barr virus (EBV)
2. Ethanol intake—the patient may not fully disclose the true amounts consumed—the MCV and GGT levels may support the role of ethanol in the process (see later discussion)
3. The presence of previously unrecognized fatty liver changes in patients who are at least moderately obese (see later discussion)
4. An interaction with the drug in question and a newly added drug from any source.

There are several pitfalls in this differential diagnosis process. One is the potential for false incrimination of ethanol in patients who are receiving drugs that alter folate metabolism, and thus, can elevate the MCV above the normal range. Likewise, GGT is a very inducible by other enzyme inducers such as anticonvulsants and rifampin. Another pitfall involves blaming the fatty liver in patients who are unlikely to be able to lose enough weight soon enough to make a significant difference in the combined effects of the drug and fatty liver to allow drug continuation long term in this clinical setting. In complicated cases in which patients approach or pass the "critical level" of threefold transaminase elevation, or if there are persistent abnormalities in the transaminase values, the clinician is encouraged to seek gastroenterologic or hepatologic consultation.

The phrase "liver function tests" is clearly a misnomer given that the most commonly used LFTs, the transaminases, merely measure hepatocyte integrity and may be elevated by abnormalities in distant organs[44,45] (see Table 41-11). Tests of hepatobiliary obstruction measure "liver function" in a sense if the intrahepatic portion of the system is abnormal but do not measure liver function if there is pathology in the extrahepatic aspects of the biliary system. Tests listed in this table that measure hepatic protein synthesis do measure one aspect of liver function; however, these tests are still not ideally specific and are abnormal only late in the disease course. Overall, the combination of laboratory tests referred to as "liver function tests" or a "liver panel" is the best available in a practical sense. More invasive tests (liver biopsy) and more complicated tests of true liver function are rarely cost-effective or practical. For most systemic drugs discussed in this chapter that are commonly prescribed by dermatologists, the combinations of serum AST/SGOT* and ALT/SGPT† remain the standard of care for laboratory surveillance. An additional diagnostic test that remains a standard of care is the periodic liver biopsy for psoriasis patients (all patients should have this test for any indication) on *long-term* methotrexate therapy (see Chapter 7).

---

*AST and SGOT are different abbreviations for the same enzyme.
†ALT and SGPT are different abbreviations for the same enzyme.

■ Table 41-11   Commonly Used Liver Function Tests[44,45]

Test Name	Comments/Limitations
TESTS FOR HEPATOCYTE INTEGRITY	
AST/SGOT	Less specific for liver than ALT/SGPT; most accurate to order both transaminases
ALT/SGPT	More specific for liver than AST/SGOT; most accurate to order both transaminases
LDH	Very nonspecific for liver; can fractionate to increase specificity
TESTS FOR HEPATOBILIARY OBSTRUCTION	
Alkaline phosphatase	Nonspecific for liver (also found in bone); can fractionate to increase specificity
γ-Glutamyl transpeptidase (GGT)	More specific for liver than alkaline phosphatase; very inducible by ethanol, drugs
Bilirubin	Later finding in setting of hepatobiliary obstruction; hemolysis gives false positives
TESTS OF HEPATIC PROTEIN SYNTHESIS	
Albumin	Very late, yet important sign of reduced liver function; nutritional influence on level
Protime/INR	Very late, yet important sign of reduced liver function
TEST FOR SEVERITY OF LIVER FAILURE	
Ammonia	Very late sign of severe, often end-stage liver disease; marker for encephalopathy risk
TEST FOR ONGOING FIBROSIS	
P3NP	False-positives from other sites of fibrosis (such as arthritis)

P3NP, Amino terminus type III procollagen peptide.

■ Table 41-12   Major Categories of Drug-Induced Liver Disease Presenting Symptoms and Diseases Mimicked[1,6]

Category	Presenting Symptoms and Signs	Diseases Mimicked
Hepatocellular toxicity	Usually asymptomatic initially; later RUQ pain, jaundice, hepatomegaly, portal hypertension	Viral hepatitis Acute alcoholic hepatitis
Hypersensitivity syndrome	Fever, fatigue, pharyngitis, morbilliform eruption, adenopathy, hepatosplenomegaly	Infectious mononucleosis, autoimmune hepatitis
Cholestasis	Usually asymptomatic initially; later pruritus, jaundice	Primary biliary cirrhosis Sclerosing cholangitis
Steatosis → Fibrosis	Asymptomatic until very late in disease course; may present with symptoms of liver failure	Chronic alcoholic hepatitis Vitamin A intoxication

RUQ, Right upper quadrant.

One additional interesting factual tidbit is the routine use of serum albumin levels by rheumatologists in monitoring patients with rheumatoid arthritis receiving long-term methotrexate therapy to help decide which patients should receive a liver biopsy.[26] Either repeated elevations of transaminase values (elevations in 5 of 9 tests performed every 6 weeks over a year's time) or albumin levels below 3.0 g/dl are the published standard of care for *that* disease in *that* specialty to indicate the need for a liver biopsy. Reduction of methotrexate protein-binding capacity with the low albumin levels provides the rationale for this guideline.

MANAGEMENT

The most basic rule in the management of significant liver complications due to systemic drugs prescribed by dermatologists (as well as physicians in all fields) is to *stop the drug* in question. An important but uncommon exception would be to consider continuing drugs that are absolutely essential to the patient's survival and that there are no suitable alternatives to replace the drug culprit. Such scenarios are distinctly uncommon in our specialty.

Systemic corticosteroids are worth considering (in the presence of the four types of drug-induced liver disease emphasized in this chapter) only for severe cutaneous features of the DHS.[6] A collaborative decision with consultants may indicate systemic corticosteroids for the occasional severe hepatic involvement of this syndrome.

Overall, the key steps of management are to (1) stop the drug in question, (2) monitor appropriate LFTs closely, (3) seek appropriate consultations, and (4) provide supportive care. Fortunately, most patients who are diagnosed early through systematic monitoring have completely reversible liver pathology. Liver transplantation is an option in management for worst-case sce-

Box 41-4

Lessons from the Past for Drugs That Are in Current Use

- *Take one's time*—Newly released drugs with any mention of a relatively high frequency of minor transaminase elevations in preclinical trials should be watched closely for 1 to 2 years after FDA release before widespread clinical use is initiated.[6]
- *Take note and stay tuned*—For drugs that have *any* early reported *deaths* from drug-induced liver disease, these deaths may be the tip of a very large "iceberg" so to speak. This was true to some extent for ketoconazole and was fully applicable to troglitazone (Rezulin). Only with much more conservative prescribing practices and very careful monitoring has ketoconazole remained available for use.
- *Do not be distracted*—Guidelines of care must be considered to be drug and disease specific. Do not be distracted by the rheumatology guidelines for methotrexate. The liver biopsy remains the standard of care for methotrexate therapy in dermatology. Recent pleas for more conservative biopsy regimens do not suggest eliminating the liver biopsy, rather merely to

consider reducing the number of biopsies required through the use of selected noninvasive tests.[46]
- *Spread the word*—In many settings of severe drug-induced liver disease, either the prescribing physician, the patient, or both were not aware of the potential risk. Both parties are important to the monitoring process. The FDA and academic physicians alike must "spread the word."
- *Be cautious with other drugs*—Newly released drugs have not stood the test of time regarding the potential for drug interactions until a couple of years after the drug's release. Always be wary of combined use of a newly released drug with *strong* CYP "inhibitors" or "inducers."
- *Stop the drug*—Most drug-induced liver deaths pertinent to dermatology came from continued use of a given drug in spite of significant clinical or laboratory markers for *serious* liver disease.[6] When in doubt, *stop the drug* in question and monitor closely until the abnormality normalizes.

narios; this expensive, life-saving technology should "never" be necessary.[3,4] Given patient awareness of key symptoms to report and systematic monitoring of the liver by established standards of care for various drugs, irreversible end-stage liver disease due to systemic drugs for dermatologic indications should be unheard of.

For less severe complications, such as mild-to-moderate transaminase elevations from onefold to twofold elevations, the clinician always has the following options (several options can be done simultaneously): (1) lower the drug dose, (2) stop the drug temporarily, (3) perform more frequent laboratory monitoring, and (4) seek consultation, even in the form of informal phone input from a trustworthy consultant. When in doubt, lean toward the conservative side of the decision making process, until the severity of the liver abnormality is clarified. All drugs discussed in this chapter can be stopped for at least 1 to 2 weeks, until the laboratory abnormality normalizes. Depending on the clinical circumstances, the drug in question may possibly be reintroduced at a lower dose with very careful laboratory follow-up.

LOOKING TO THE FUTURE— LESSONS FROM THE PAST

There is a well-quoted dictum (paraphrased a bit here)—whoever does not learn from lessons of the past is doomed to repeat the same mistakes. Detailed analysis of the events that led to the withdrawal from the market in the United States of the drugs in Table 41-2 is beyond the scope of this chapter. Box 41-4 lists a few important general principles that deal with the stories behind these drugs, along with the ketoconazole story.

Bibliography

General Overviews

Lee WM: Medical progress: drug-induced hepatotoxicity. *N Engl J Med* 333:1118-1127, 1995.

Zimmerman HJ, Ishak KG: General aspects of drug-induced liver disease. *Gastroenterol Clin North Am* 24:739-757, 1995.

General Mechanism of Hepatotoxicity

DeLeve LD, Kaplowitz N: Mechanisms of drug-induced liver disease. *Gastroenterol Clin North Am* 24:787-810, 1995.

Erlinger S: Drug-induced cholestasis. *J Hepatol* 26(Suppl 1):1-4, 1997.

Fontana RJ, Watkins PB: Genetic predisposition to drug-induced liver disease. *Gastroenterol Clin North Am* 24:811-837, 1995.

Larrey D, Pageaux GP: Genetic predisposition to drug-induced hepatotoxicity. *J Hepatol* 26(Suppl 2):12-21, 1997.

Pessayre D: Role of reactive metabolites in drug-induced hepatitis. *J Hepatol* 23(Suppl 1):16-24, 1995.

Immunology of Hepatotoxicity

Robin MA, LeRoy M, Descatoire V, et al: Plasma membrane cytochromes P450 as neoantigens and autoimmune targets in drug-induced hepatitis. *J Hepatol* 26(Suppl 1):23-30, 1997.

Van Pelt FNAM, Straub P, Manns MP: Molecular basis of drug-induced immunological liver injury. *Semin Liver Dis* 15:283-300, 1995.

References

1. Zimmerman HJ, Ishak KG: General aspects of drug-induced liver disease. *Gastroenterol Clin North Am* 24:739-757, 1995.

2. O'Grady JG, Alexander GJM, Hayllar KM, et al: Early indicators of prognosis in fulminant hepatic failure. *Gastroenterology* 97:439-445, 1989.

3. Knight TE, Shikuma CY, Knight J: Ketocona-zole-induced fulminant hepatitis necessitat-ing liver transplantation. *J Am Acad Derma-tol* 25:398-400, 1991.

4. Gilbert SC, Klintmalm G, Menter A, et al: Methotrexate-induced cirrhosis requiring liver transplantation in three patients with psoriasis. A word of caution in light of the expanding use of this "steroid sparing" agent. *Arch Intern Med* 150:889-891, 1990.

Drug Metabolism

5. Fontana RJ, Watkins PB: Genetic predisposi-tion to drug-induced liver disease. *Gastroen-terol Clin North Am* 24:811-837, 1995.

6. Lee WM: Medical progress: drug-induced hepatotoxicity. *N Engl J Med* 333:1118-1127, 1995.

7. Larrey D, Pageaux GP: Genetic predisposi-tion to drug-induced hepatotoxicity. *J Hepa-tol* 26(Suppl 2):12-21, 1997.

8. DeLeve LD, Kaplowitz N: Mechanisms of drug-induced liver disease. *Gastroenterol Clin North Am* 24:787-810, 1995.

9. Spielberg SP, Gordon GB, Blake DA, et al: In vitro analysis of idiosyncratic drug reactions. *Clin Biochem* 19:142-144, 1986.

10. Pessayre D: Role of reactive metabolites in drug-induced hepatitis. *J Hepatol* 23(Suppl 1):16-24, 1995.

11. Wormhoudt LW, Commanduer JN, Ver-meulen NP: Genetic polymorphism of hu-man n-acetyltransferase, cytochrome P-450, glutathione-S-transferase, and epoxide hy-drolase enzymes: relevance to xenobiotic metabolism and toxicity. *Crit Rev Toxicol* 29:59-124, 1999.

12. Singer MI, Shapiro LE, Shear NH: Cy-tochrome P450 3A: interactions with derma-tologic therapies. *J Am Acad Dermatol* 37:765-771, 1997.

13. Evans DA, Mahgoub A, Sloan TP, et al: A family and population study of the genetic polymorphism of debrisoquine oxidation in a white British population. *J Med Genet* 17:102-105, 1980.

14. Grant DM: Molecular genetics of the N-acetyltransferases. *Pharmacogenetics* 3:45-50, 1993.

15. Anonymous: Serious adverse reactions with sulphonamides. *FDA Drug Bull* 14:5-6, 1984.

16. Spielberg SP, Gordon GB, Blake DA, et al: Predisposition to phenytoin hepatotoxicity assessed in vitro. *N Engl J Med* 305:722-727, 1981.

17. Shear NH, Spielberg SP: Anticonvulsant hy-persensitivity syndrome: in vitro assessment of risk (cross-reactivity). *J Clin Invest* 82:1826-1832, 1988.

18. Gaedigk A, Speilberg SP, Grant DM: Charac-terization of the microsomal epoxide hydro-lase gene in patients with anticonvulsant ad-verse drug reactions. *Pharmacogenetics* 4:142-153, 1994.

Mechanisms of Hepatotoxicity

19. Van Pelt FNAM, Straub P, Manns MP: Molec-ular basis of drug-induced immunological liver injury. *Semin Liver Dis* 15:283-300, 1995.

20. Robin MA, LeRoy M, Descatoire V, et al: Plasma membrane cytochromes P450 as neoantigens and autoimmune targets in drug-induced hepatitis. *J Hepatol* 26(Suppl 1):23-30, 1997.

21. Beaune PH, Bourdi M: Autoantibodies against cytochromes P-450 in drug-induced autoimmune hepatitis. *Ann N Y Acad Sci* 685:641-645, 1993.

22. Seeff LB, Cuccherini BA, Zimmerman HJ, et al: Acetaminophen hepatotoxicity in alco-holics: a therapeutic misadventure. *Ann In-tern Med* 104:399-404, 1986.

23. Garibaldi RA, Drusin RE, Ferebee SH, et al: Isoniazid-associated hepatitis: report of an outbreak. *Am Rev Respir Dis* 106:357-365, 1972.

Risk Factors and Classification

24. Roenigk HH Jr, Auerbach R, Maibach HI, et al: Methotrexate in psoriasis: consensus con-ference. *J Am Acad Dermatol* 38:478-485, 1998.

25. Wolverton SE: Major adverse effects from systemic drugs: defining the risks. *Curr Prob Dermatol* 7:1-40, 1995.

26. Anonymous: Guideline for methotrexate drug therapy in rheumatoid arthritis. *Arthritis Rheum* 39:723-731, 1996.

27. Vahlquist A: Long-term safety of retinoid therapy. *J Am Acad Dermatol* 27:S29-33, 1992.

28. Knowles SR, Gupta AK, Shear NH, et al: Aza-thioprine hypersensitivity-like reactions—a case report and a review of the literature. *Clin Exp Dermatol* 20:353-356, 1995.

29. Prussick R, Shear NH: Dapsone hypersensi-tivity syndrome. *J Am Acad Dermatol* 35:346-349, 1996.

30. Lawrence WA, Olsen HW, Nickles DJ: Dapsone hepatitis. *Arch Intern Med* 147:175, 1987.

31. Elkayam O, Yaron M, Caspi D: Minocycline-induced autoimmune syndromes: an overview. *Semin Arthritis Rheum* 28:392-397, 1999.

32. Knowles S, Shapiro L, Shear N: Serious adverse reactions induced by minocycline: a report of 13 patients and review of the literature. *Arch Dermatol* 132:934-939, 1996.

33. Brown AM, Corrigan AB: Pancytopenia after accidental overdose of methotrexate: a complication of low-dose therapy for rheumatoid arthritis (pancytopenia). *Med J Austral* 155:493-494, 1991.

34. Lewis JH, Zimmerman HJ, Benson GD, et al: Hepatic injury associated with ketoconazole therapy: analysis of 33 cases. *Gastroenterology* 86:503-513, 1984.

Drug Etiologies and Diagnosis

35. Kohlroser J, Mathai J, Reichheld J, et al: Hepatotoxicity due to troglitazone: report of two cases and review of adverse events reported to the United States Food and Drug Administration. *Am J Gastroenterol* 95:272-276, 2000.

36. Wagenaar LJ, Kuck EM, Hoekstra JB: Troglitazone. Is it all over? *Neth J Med* 55:4-12, 1999.

37. Ramakrishna B, Viswanath N: Diclofenac-induced hepatitis: case report and literature review. *Liver* 14:83-84, 1994.

38. Schiff ER, Maddrey WC: Can we prevent nonsteroidal anti-inflammatory drug-induced hepatic failure? *Gastrointest Dis Today* 3:7-13, 1994.

39. Hepps KS, Maliha GM, Estrada R, et al: Severe cholestatic jaundice associated with piroxicam. *Gastroenterology* 101:1737-1740, 1991.

40. Fenner H: Evaluation of the efficacy and safety of NSAIDs. A new methodological approach. *Scand J Rheumatol* 80(Suppl):32-39, 1989.

41. Ross-Degnan D, Soumerai SB, Fortess EE, et al: Examining product risk in context. Market withdrawal of zomepirac as a case study. *JAMA* 270:1937-1942, 1993.

42. Kramer MS, Leventhal JM, Hutchinson TA, et al: An algorithm for the operational assessment of adverse drug reactions. I. Background, description, and instructions for use. *JAMA* 242:623-632, 1979.

43. Anonymous: Standardization of definitions and criteria of causality assessment of adverse drug reactions. *Int J Clin Pharmacol Ther Toxicol* 28:317-322, 1990.

44. Tygstrup N: Assessment of liver function: principles and practice. *J Gastroenterol Hepatol* 5:468-482, 1990.

45. Sallie R, Tredger JM, Williams R: Drugs and the liver. Part 1: testing liver function. *Biopharm Drug Dispos* 12:251-259, 1991.

46. Zachariae H: Liver biopsies and methotrexate: a time for reconsideration? *J Am Acad Dermatol* 42:531-534, 2000.

Kathleen A. Remlinger

Hematologic Toxicity of Drug Therapy

Significant hematologic toxicities from drugs used in dermatology are infrequent but potentially life-threatening adverse reactions. Avoidance of these complications is enhanced by thorough knowledge of drug metabolism, interactions, adverse effect profile, and patient factors, including the effect of age and concomitant medical diseases. Awareness of possible hematologic adverse effects and their most likely timing of occurrence can direct monitoring for toxicity. These monitoring guidelines are established for individual drugs based on the incidence of adverse reactions observed during clinical trials.

The first section of this chapter deals with general principles such as mechanisms of development of hematologic toxicities, their timing, and their predictability. The second section provides an overview of the most important specific hematologic adverse effects. The third part of the chapter reviews individual drugs, including cytotoxic agents, drugs commonly used in dermatology, and newer agents. Finally, management of hematologic toxicities is addressed.

GENERAL PRINCIPLES
Mechanisms of Hematologic Toxicities
Adverse effects from drugs may be expected or be idiosyncratic and may be secondary to direct

toxicity to cells or to immunologic reactions.[1,2] In general, toxic reactions are insidious in onset, developing over weeks to months,[2,3] although toxic hematologic reactions may be seen earlier (i.e., in days to weeks). With rechallenge, there is a latent period before onset of symptoms. On the other hand, immunoreactions appear relatively early in the course of therapy. These reactions take days to weeks to develop and once established often follow a more explosive course. Immunologic reactions recur promptly after reexposure to even small doses of the causative agent.

Cytotoxic agents are examples of drugs that commonly and predictably produce cytopenias. Most cause cell death through apoptosis.[4] Generally cytopenias from these agents represent toxic reactions that are dose-dependent and fairly predictable. A unique situation exists with azathioprine. The hematologic toxicities from this drug are determined not only by the dose of the drug but also by the level of an enzyme, thiopurine methyltransferase, that is important in the metabolism of the drug (see Azathioprine section).[5,6]

Idiosyncratic reactions from drugs also may be either toxic or immunologic. They often are related to genetic variability in metabolism of drugs, particularly from common enzyme polymorphisms.[7,8] For example, sulfonamides undergo N-acetylation as a major part of their metabolism. Over 90% of patients demonstrating hypersensitivity to sulfonamides are slow acetylators.[9] There is evidence that the hydroxylamine metabolite of sulfamethoxazole is toxic to bone marrow cells. An inherited defect in the detoxification of the hydroxylamine metabolite has been demonstrated in some patients with adverse reactions to sulfamethoxazole.[10] However, because the hypersensitivity reaction is rare compared with the number of patients who manifest the slow acetylator phenotype, other factors must be responsible.

Idiosyncratic immunoreactions account for certain adverse hematologic reactions. They are common mechanisms for drug-induced thrombocytopenia from noncytotoxic agents such as quinidine, quinine, and heparin.[11] In addition to the previously mentioned toxic mechanisms, immune mechanisms may play a role in hypersensitivity due to sulfonamides. Hydroxylamine metabolites of the sulfonamides may alter antigen presentation by cells and thus render a patient more susceptible to immunoreactions from this class of drug.[12] In some cases of drug-induced agranulocytosis, including those associated with penicillin and diclofenac use, drug-dependent antineutrophil autoantibodies have been demonstrated.[13] Overall, the mechanism for developing certain hematologic toxicities, such as neutropenia and aplastic anemia, from noncytotoxic agents is not well defined for most drugs.

Timing of Hematologic Toxicity

The type and onset of various cytopenias (e.g., agranulocytosis, aplastic anemia/pancytopenia, thrombocytopenia) from cytotoxic drugs depends on the category of drug. The cytotoxic drugs used in dermatology, especially the antimetabolites and alkylating agents, have leukopenia as their most common hematologic effect. This is because the half-life of white blood cells (WBC) is only 6 to 8 hours, compared with half-lives of 5 to 7 days and 60 days for platelets and red blood cells (RBC), respectively. A fall in the WBC count often begins 5 to 14 days after administration of a cytotoxic agent.[4] Recovery of blood counts usually starts 7 to 10 days after cessation of drug use. Drugs that are cell-cycle specific, such as the antimetabolite methotrexate, generally show earlier onset and shorter duration of myelosuppression.[14] In contrast, cytopenias

from busulfan or from the nitrosoureas, such as BCNU, occur later, typically starting 4 to 6 weeks after initiation of therapy. This applies to topical BCNU as well as to systemic BCNU.

The onset of idiosyncratic reactions is quite variable and depends on both the causative agent and the type of hematologic toxicity. These hypersensitivity reactions may be either metabolic or immunologic. The minimum time required for development of drug-induced immunocytopenias is about 6 days if the drug is administered for the first time but occurs within minutes to hours if the drug is readministered.[15]

Agranulocytosis, hemolytic anemia, and thrombocytopenia are often acute reactions occurring in the first month of therapy.[1] However, there are notable exceptions. Sulfasalazine-induced agranulocytosis generally occurs between weeks 3 and 12. Alpha-methyldopa, procainamide, and levamisole may produce autoantibodies against any of the blood cell lines after several months of therapy.[1] Also, cytopenias from these drugs may persist for months, rather than the expected several weeks, after the offending drug is stopped.

Neutropenia and thrombocytopenia are unlikely to be related to a drug if they develop more than 1 month *after* cessation of exposure to a drug (i.e., there is documentation that the blood count was normal at least 1 month after stopping the drug).[16] However, aplastic anemia can show a different time course. It sometimes occurs after months to a year or more of drug use. It may also appear 4 months, and occasionally longer, *after* cessation of the drug.[16]

Prediction of Risk for Hematologic Toxicities

Determination of the exact risk ratio for hematologic toxicity from drugs used in dermatology is difficult; however, estimates can be obtained from knowledge of pharmacogenetics and from epidemiologic studies. Some drug toxicities are dose-dependent, and others are idiosyncratic. Generally cytotoxic agents and antiviral drugs produce toxicities that are dose-dependent and follow a sigmoid-shaped curve. At low drug levels, myelosuppression may not occur. With increasing drug doses, cell death is proportional to drug concentration. With very high drug levels, the myelosuppressive effect plateaus.[4]

The incidence of idiosyncratic reactions, whether due to genetics or due to random events, can be estimated from population studies. There are several large, recently published studies of drug-related blood dyscrasias.[17-21] Our ability to extrapolate the relative risk of a drug's toxicity from these reports depends on the completeness of the reported data, the frequency of the various drugs' use, the population studied, and the ability to choose one culprit drug in those patients on multiple medications. Caution must be used in interpreting data. Studies that report the number of adverse reactions from a drug per population per year ideally should use case controls and account for the number of prescriptions written for a particular drug during the study time period. If not, the study will likely underestimate the incidence of problems from less frequently prescribed medications and overestimate the incidence from drugs prescribed frequently.

MAJOR CATEGORIES OF DRUG-INDUCED HEMATOLOGIC TOXICITY

Agranulocytosis

Agranulocytosis is defined as a neutrophil count of $<500/mm.^{3,16}$ It is often accompanied by fever, pharyngitis, dysphagia, and oral ulcerations. Mortality rate is approximately 15% (6.5% to 48%)[21,22] and is often secondary to septicemia. Concomitant renal failure is associated with a poor prognosis.[22]

Van der Klauw and associates[20] reviewed 206 cases of drug-associated agranulocytosis reported over a 20-year period (1974-1994) in the Netherlands. Among the most commonly implicated drugs were sulfasalazine and certain antibiotics, including trimethoprim-sulfamethoxazole and the penicillins (Table 42-1). Similar data come from The International Agranulocytosis and Aplastic Anemia Study, which found the annual incidence of drug-induced agranulocytosis to be 3.4 cases/10^6 patient years.[18,19] Procainamide, antithyroid drugs, and sulfasalazine were most strongly associated with agranulocytosis (Table 42-2). A Swedish study looked at drug-induced blood dyscrasias over a 10-year period (1985-1994).[17] When incidence was compared with drug sales data, drugs com-

monly associated with agranulocytosis were clozapine ($373/10^6$ patient years), sulfasalazine ($87/10^6$ patient years), and dapsone ($65/10^6$ patient years).

Aplastic Anemia (Pancytopenia)

Aplastic anemia is defined by the presence of pancytopenia (hemoglobin <10 g/dl, neutrophil count $<1500/mm^3$, and platelet count $<100,000/mm^3$) with a hypocellular marrow.[16] The International Agranulocytosis and Aplastic Anemia Study reported that 27% of their cases of aplastic anemia were likely to be drug-related.[18] Penicillamine, gold, and carbamazepine were most commonly implicated (Table 42-3). A French group compared drug use in patients with aplastic anemia with hospitalized patients and neighborhood control groups.[21] Use of gold, D-penicillamine, and colchicine was associated with high risk of aplasia. The Swedish Blood Dyscrasia study also found that 25% of their cases of aplastic anemia were probably drug-associated.[17] Trimethoprim-sulfamethoxazole had a reported risk of 13 cases/10^6 patient years. However, the authors postulated that concomitant viral disease might have played a role in the development of aplasia in some of these patients. The risk of aplastic anemia from trimethoprim-sulfamethoxazole was much lower in other studies (1.4 cases/10^6 users per 5 month period)[18] (see Sulfonamides section).

Thrombocytopenia

Thrombocytopenia is defined as a platelet count $<100,000/mm^3$.[16] In a case-control study on the incidence of drug-induced thrombocytopenia in the northeastern United States, the drugs with the highest risk were trimethoprim-sulfamethoxazole (38 cases/1 million users per week) and quinidine/quinine (26 cases/1 million users per week)[24] (Table 42-4). In a review of published case reports of drug-induced thrombocytopenia, quinidine, gold, and sulfonamides were the most commonly implicated drugs.[25] Because this was not a case-control study, no relative risk ratio could be estimated. The incidence of major bleeding was 9%, and the incidence of death was 0.8%. In the Swedish registry study, trimethoprim-sulfamethoxazole had a risk of 96 cases of thrombocytopenia per 10^6 patient years.[17] Again, the authors cautioned

■ **Table 42-1** Causes of Drug-Associated Agranulocytosis/Neutropenia

Drug	Causal Relationship Certain or Probable (number of cases)	Causal Relationship Possible (number of cases)	Total
Dipyrone	7	5	12
Mianserin*	8	2	10
Sulfasalazine†	6	1	7
Trimethoprim-sulfamethoxazole†	5	1	6
Antidysrhythmic agents	4	1	5
Penicillins†	4	1	5
Thiouracil derivatives	4	0	4
Phenylbutazone	2	2	4
Cimetidine†	1	3	4

Data from van der Klauw MM, Wilson JHP, Stricker BHCH: *Am J Hematol* 57:206-211, 1998.
*A 5-HT receptor antagonist used for migraine prophylaxis in Europe.
†Drugs used commonly in dermatology.

■ **Table 42-2** Causes of Drug-Associated Agranulocytosis

Drug	Relative Risk (95% confidence interval)*
Sulfasalazine†	207 (61-708)
Antithyroid drugs	182 (74-449)
Procainamide	163 (45-594)
Macrolides†	12 (3.6-41)
Trimethoprim-sulfamethoxazole†	10 (4-26)
Penicillin†	6.8 (1.8-26)
Allopurinol	6.7 (2.2-20)
Doxycycline†	5.8 (1.6-22)

Data from Kaufman DW, Kelly JP, Jurgelon JM, et al: *Eur J Haematol* 57(Suppl):23-30, 1996.
*Case control study. Risk is relative to no use of drug in days 1-7 before onset of agranulocytosis.
†Drugs commonly used in dermatology.

■ **Table 42-3** Drug-Associated Aplastic Anemia: Relative Risk from Drugs Used Days 29-180 Days Before Onset

Drug	Relative Risk (95% confidence interval)*
Penicillamine	49 (5.2-464)
Gold†	19 (3.6-97)
Carbamazepine	13 (3.3-54)
Allopurinol	4.6 (1.7-12)
Naproxen†	3.9 (1.6-9.7)
Butazones	3.7 (1.6-8.3)
Diclofenac	3.0 (1.3-7.0)
Indomethacin	2.8 (1.1-6.8)
Chloramphenicol	2.7 (0.8-8.7)

Data from Kaufman DW, Kelly JP, Jurgelon JM, et al: *Eur J Haematol* 57(Suppl):23-30, 1996.
*Case control study. Risk is relative to no use of drug in days 29-180 before onset of aplastic anemia.
†Drugs commonly used in dermatology.

■ **Table 42-4**   Drug-Associated
                   Thrombocytopenia:
                   Relative Risk
                   for Drugs Used 1-7
                   Days Before Onset

Drug	Relative Risk (95% confidence interval)*
Quinidine/quinine	101 (31-324)
Sulfonamides†	40 (10-162)
Dipyridamole†	14 (3.5-54)
Sulfonylureas	4.8 (1.5-16)

Data from Kaufman DW, Kelly JP, Johannes CB, et al:
Blood 82:2714-2718, 1993.
*Case-control study. Risk is relative to no use during
the week before the index day.
†Drugs commonly used in dermatology.

that concomitant viral illness might have been a
confounding factor in a number of cases. One
study found thrombocytopenia from trimethoprim-sulfamethoxazole to be twice as common
in women as in men.[26] There is no apparent
age-related predisposition.[26]

Neoplasia

The potential for induction of neoplasia is of special concern as a possible hematologic toxicity.
For most cytotoxic drugs, hematologic malignancies and cutaneous carcinomas are more likely
to occur than are other types of solid tumors. The
incidence of malignancy also depends on the
agent used. Hematologic malignancies are seen
less commonly with antimetabolites (e.g., methotrexate, azathioprine, 6-mercaptopurine
[6-MP]) than with alkylating agents because the
former do not directly interact with deoxyribonucleic acid (DNA).[27] In some instances it is
difficult to calculate the relative risk for development of malignancy because data on the potential association between a drug and neoplasm predominantly consist of individual case reports.
Also, different patient populations may have different risks despite using the same drug at similar doses. For instance, there are more reports of
lymphomas in rheumatoid arthritis patients receiving methotrexate than there are in psoriasis
patients receiving this drug.

Patients who develop a lymphoproliferative
disorder while on immunosuppressive therapy
may show regression of disease on withdrawal of
the immunosuppressive drug. This is especially
true for lymphomas demonstrating Epstein-
Barr viral genome in patients on methotrexate.[28,29] Therefore a period of watchful waiting
after cessation of the immunosuppressive
drug(s) is appropriate in this setting before deciding on the need for chemotherapy. However,
acute leukemia developing during or after immunosuppressive or cytotoxic drug use virtually
never shows spontaneous regression. These
leukemias are often associated with cytogenetic
abnormalities of chromosomes 5 or 7 and have
a very poor prognosis.[30] Treatment may be considered if clinical circumstances make this a reasonable option. Development of solid tumors in
association with drug use is discussed elsewhere
in this book.

DRUGS PRESCRIBED BY DERMATOLOGISTS—RISK OF HEMATOLOGIC TOXICITY

Box 42-1 lists various dermatologic drugs and
their potential for hematologic toxicity.

Methotrexate

Methotrexate is an antifolate antimetabolite.
Recent studies indicate a probable dissociation
between its mechanism of hematologic toxicity
and its antiinflammatory effects.[31] Methotrexate and its polyglutamate derivatives inhibit dihydrofolate reductase and thymidylate synthetase. This interference with folic acid
metabolism affects cells with rapid turnover, especially gastrointestinal mucosa and bone marrow, giving the characteristic toxicities of mucositis and cytopenias, particularly leukopenia.
Methotrexate also causes an intracellular
build-up of adenosine that may be responsible in
part for its antiinflammatory effects.[32] Prophylactic administration of folic acid 1 to 5 mg daily
may lessen toxicity, especially nausea, without
interfering with efficacy.[33,34] Alternatively, Leucovorin (folinic acid) 2.5 to 5 mg orally 24 hours
after methotrexate administration can be utilized, particularly in the presence of marked cytopenias.[25] Neither regimen has been shown

Box 42-1

Various Dermatologic Drugs—Potential for Hematologic Toxicity*

RELATIVELY HIGH-RISK DRUGS

Antimetabolites
- Methotrexate
- Azathioprine

Alkylating Agents
- Cyclophosphamide
- Chlorambucil

Other Cytotoxic/Immunosuppressive Drugs
- Hydroxyurea
- Interferons†

Sulfones and Sulfonamides
- Dapsone
- Sulfasalazine
- Trimethoprim-sulfamethoxazole

LOWER-RISK DRUGS

Other Antiinflammatory Drugs
- Antimalarials
- Colchicine
- Gold
- Penicillamine

Other Immunosuppressive Drugs
- Mycophenolate mofetil

Miscellaneous Drugs (Very Low Risk)
- Terbinafine
- Nonsteroidal antiinflammatory agents
- Antibiotics—ciprofloxacin, metronidazole, cephalosporins
- H_2 antagonists—ranitidine, cimetidine

*This represents the sequence of discussion of these drugs or drug groups in this chapter.
†Generally interferon-induced neutropenia is dose-related and is of mild-to-intermediate severity.

clearly to lessen hematologic toxicity, perhaps because myelosuppression from low-dose methotrexate is an uncommon event and studies may not have included sufficient numbers of patients to reach statistical significance. Nonetheless, because folic acid is safe and does not interfere with efficacy, it is prudent to use folic acid routinely in patients receiving methotrexate for dermatologic diseases.

Isolated thrombocytopenia from methotrexate occurs in less than 5% of rheumatologic patients.[36,37] Megaloblastic erythropoiesis is commonly seen in the bone marrow with methotrexate, but macrocytic anemia is uncommon.[38,39] There is one report of a Coombs' positive hemolytic anemia associated with methotrexate.[40] Risk of cytopenias from methotrexate is greatest in the elderly, those with renal insufficiency, and those who develop RBC macrocytosis.[37] Therefore test doses of methotrexate and careful monitoring of complete blood counts (CBCs) and renal function are especially important in these patients.

A number of drugs interact with methotrexate, and patients should be advised of specific agents to avoid. There have been several reports of severe cytopenias in patients receiving con-

comitant full dose trimethoprim-sulfamethoxazole and methotrexate, although prophylactic doses of trimethoprim-sulfamethoxazole may not cause this reaction.[41,42] Trimethoprim binds to dihydrofolate reductase, causing increased blockade of this enzyme. Sulfonamides can displace methotrexate from albumin, increasing the drug's bioavailability. If a patient develops life-threatening cytopenias on methotrexate, serum levels of the drug should be measured and Leucovorin administered at 15 mg/m² intravenously every 6 hours until the serum methotrexate level becomes undetectable. Higher doses of Leucovorin may be needed in those patients with renal insufficiency.[27]

In the 1970s Bailin[43] looked at a series of psoriasis patients treated with methotrexate and found no increase in the incidence of internal malignancies. Similar findings in psoriasis patients were described by Stern[44] and by Nyfors.[45] However, there have been increasing numbers of reports of lymphoproliferative disorders in patients taking methotrexate not only for rheumatoid arthritis or dermatomyositis but also for psoriasis.[28,29,46] Examination of peripheral lymph nodes every 3 to 6 months is advisable in patients taking methotrexate, though over 50% of the methotrexate-induced lymphomas appear in extranodal sites.[28]

Azathioprine

Azathioprine is a purine analog antimetabolite with immunosuppressive properties. It is converted to 6-MP, then subsequently metabolized by xanthine oxidase, thiopurine S-methyltransferase (TPMT), and hypoxanthine guanine phosphoribosyl transferase (HGPRT). Between 2% and 17% of patients develop hematologic toxicity, especially neutropenia.[47,48] Because cytopenias may be delayed, it is recommended that CBCs be obtained weekly for the first 4 weeks of treatment, then biweekly for the next month.[49] Severe myelosuppression may be seen in patients with homozygous TPMT deficiency, which is transmitted as an autosomal-recessive trait and is found in 0.3% of the population.[5,6,50] Approximately 11% of individuals are heterozygotes who show intermediate activity of the enzyme. Studies show inverse correlation between TPMT activity and accumulation of pharmacologically active 6-thioguanine metabolites in erythrocytes, leading to marked myelosuppression when azathioprine or 6-MP is given at conventional doses to enzyme-deficient patients.[51] Pretreatment assays for TPMT activity help predict which patients would develop severe cytopenias, who would develop cumulative toxicity, and which group might be resistant to drug effect, requiring higher drug doses because of rapid metabolism of azathioprine.[5,6]

Drug interaction between allopurinol and azathioprine or 6-MP is of particular importance.[49] Inhibition of xanthine oxidase by allopurinol greatly enhances the myelotoxicity of these two antimetabolites. Therefore if both allopurinol and azathioprine (or 6-MP) are used together, the *dose* of the antimetabolite should be *reduced* by 66% to 75%.[48,49] There are also isolated reports of neutropenia in patients taking azathioprine and captopril or azathioprine and trimethoprim-sulfamethoxazole.[52,53]

Thrombocytopenia and macrocytic anemia are seen uncommonly with azathioprine. Pure red cell aplasia, which reverses on drug withdrawal, has been recorded in several transplant patients, although rarely in dermatology patients receiving the drug.[54,55]

Azathioprine has been associated with a 1% to 8% incidence of malignancy in transplant patients who receive other immunosuppressive drugs concomitantly. Overall, when used as monotherapy in rheumatoid arthritis or multiple sclerosis, azathioprine shows only a slight increase in leukemia, lymphoma, and cutaneous squamous cell carcinomas.[56,57] There are no large studies of the risk of carcinogenicity from azathioprine in dermatology patients.

Cyclophosphamide

Cyclophosphamide is a potent immunosuppressive alkylating agent that inhibits both the induction and effector phases of the immunologic reaction. The drug particularly suppresses B cells, and also inhibits suppressor T cells more than helper T cells. Despite its efficacy, dermatologists infrequently use cyclophosphamide because of its relatively high incidence of potentially severe adverse effects. Neutropenia is seen frequently with cyclophosphamide, occurring in 29% of rheumatologic patients.[57] However, unlike the occasional permanent aplasia seen with some of the other alkylating agents, marrow suppression from cyclophosphamide is reversible. This stem-cell–sparing effect is secondary to high levels of aldehyde dehydrogenase in these cells.[58] Although thrombocytopenia may occur, cyclophosphamide is generally a platelet-sparing agent. Obesity (>20% over ideal body weight) slows the clearance of cyclophosphamide from the body.[59] However, there is no correlation between the myelosuppressive or therapeutic effects of cyclophosphamide and the drug's clearance, so presently there are no specific recommendations on adjusting drug dose in obesity.[59]

A synthetic tetrapeptide, AcSDKP (N-acetyl-ser-asp-lys-pro) has been shown to minimize hematologic toxicity when administered to mice 8 hours after treatment with cyclophosphamide.[60] Likewise, ImuVert, a *Serratia marcescens*–derived cytokine, protected rats from neutropenia when given 48 hours after cyclophosphamide.[61] Human studies may follow.

Cyclophosphamide has been associated with several neoplasms. Bladder cancer, lymphomas, acute nonlymphocytic leukemias, and myelodysplastic syndromes developed in patients receiving cyclophosphamide as a single agent.[62,63] Most unique to cyclophosphamide therapy is the risk of developing transitional cell carcinoma of the bladder.

Chlorambucil

Chlorambucil is an alkylating agent occasionally used in dermatology for treatment of Sézary syndrome, Behçet's syndrome, pyoderma gangrenosum, and vasculitis. It has few adverse reactions other than hematologic toxicity. Myelosuppression occurs and occasionally may be profound or prolonged. In treatment of patients with a high WBC count, initial doses of 6 to 10 mg/day (0.1 mg/kg/day) are used until the WBC count begins to fall. The dose then should be reduced immediately to a maintenance dose of 2 to 4 mg/day because the WBC count may continue to fall for another 10 days.[65] When treating patients with a normal WBC count, initial doses of 2 to 4 mg/day are appropriate. Weekly CBCs should be obtained during the initial 6 weeks of therapy. If the higher dose schedule is used, the WBC count should be checked twice weekly.

An increased risk of acute leukemia has been noted with chlorambucil, especially in patients with preexistent myeloproliferative disorders or malignancy.[66] Leukemia also has been seen in patients without antecedent malignancy.[67] The exact risk of chlorambucil-induced leukemias in this group is not established but is thought to be higher than expected for the general population. Use of intermittent pulse therapy, rather than daily dosing with chlorambucil, may reduce risk of neoplasia.[68]

Hydroxyurea

Hydroxyurea is a ribonucleoside reductase inhibitor that has found use in psoriasis and hypereosinophilic syndrome.[69] The drug has a low toxicity profile other than the risk of myelosuppression.[69] The WBCs are affected first and are affected to a greater extent than platelets, but neutrophils recover quickly on cessation of drug. The platelet nadir may not occur for another 7 to 10 days beyond the neutrophil nadir.[70] A progressive macrocytosis is commonly seen with chronic therapy.[69] Development of significant anemia warrants a drug holiday. The usual

dose of hydroxyurea for dermatologic diseases is 500 mg by mouth two to three times daily.[69] Most but not all studies indicate the drug has little leukemogenic potential.[69-71]

Interferons

Interferons (IFN) are naturally occurring glycoproteins that are now produced by recombinant DNA technology. IFNs have antiviral, antitumor, antiproliferative, and other immunomodulatory effects. IFN-α has been used for treatment of cutaneous T-cell lymphoma, basal cell carcinoma, squamous cell carcinoma, Kaposi's sarcoma, melanoma, condyloma acuminatum, and hemangiomas.[72,73] A flu-like syndrome is the most common side effect, seen in 98% of patients.[72] The symptoms may be mitigated by pretreatment of the patient with acetaminophen, although most patients develop tolerance to this adverse reaction. Myelosuppression occurs from inhibition of myeloid maturation.[73] It is a dose-related phenomenon that is usually mild and is reversible. Neutropenia may occur with doses as low as 3 million units. Thrombocytopenia may be seen with higher doses, especially in patients with hematologic malignancies.[73]

Dapsone

Dapsone is a sulfone used in therapy of Hansen's disease (leprosy), vasculitis, neutrophil-rich disorders, and some bullous diseases. There are three main hematologic toxicities of dapsone—hemolysis, methemoglobinemia, and agranulocytosis. Once ingested, the drug undergoes N-hydroxylation by the 3A family of hepatic cytochrome P-450 enzymes. The resultant hydroxylamines appear to be responsible for all the drug's hematologic toxicities.[74] Some of the hydroxylamines are taken up by erythrocytes and are subsequently oxidized via the glutathione pathway, resulting in disulfide byproducts that lead to unstable conformational changes in red cells. This may account for the generally mild hemolysis seen in normal individuals on dapsone.[74] Most of the disulfides subsequently are reduced to the parent drug again via glutathione reductase, which requires NADPH. Patients with glucose-6-phosphate dehydrogenase (G6PD) deficiency are unable to reduce

NADP$^+$ to NADPH at a normal rate and thus sustain brisk hemolysis from dapsone.[74] In the milder, A-type of G6PD deficiency usually seen in African-Americans, the hemolytic anemia may be marked but is self-limited because the reticulocytes produced in response to hemolysis have nearly normal levels of G6PD. In contrast, in the more severe Mediterranean type of G6PD deficiency the hemolysis is not self-limited and the offending drug must be stopped to curb the process.[75] Care is supportive with emphasis on excellent hydration. With severe hemolysis, transfusion may be necessary.

As outlined, glutathione-dependent cycling of hydroxylamine metabolites in the RBC produces methemoglobin that is again reduced to hemoglobin. Generally the methemoglobin levels remain at relatively low levels and need not be measured or treated unless the patient is symptomatic. Methemoglobinemia may be life-threatening when its level exceeds 50%.[75] Methylene blue is an effective treatment for methemoglobinemia but should not be used in G6PD-deficient patients because it causes hemolytic anemia. Cimetidine 1200 to 1600 mg/day has been shown to decrease methemoglobin levels and symptomatology in patients on chronic dapsone therapy.[76]

Dapsone-induced agranulocytosis is a relatively rare phenomenon. Population studies show an incidence of 65 cases/10^6 patient years.[17] However, the incidence may depend on the population treated. In patients with dermatitis herpetiformis the risk is reported to be as high as 1/240 to 400 patients.[77,78] Agranulocytosis is seen between weeks 3 and 12 of treatment. Patients should be warned to seek treatment immediately if they develop fever or chills, pharyngitis, dysphagia, or oral ulcerations.[79] In vitro experiments have shown that dapsone hydroxylamines may leak from erythrocytes and cause death to leukocytes, including bone marrow precursors.[80]

Some authors recommend starting dapsone at 50 mg/day and increasing the daily dose by 25 mg each week until a therapeutic effect is noted or a daily dose of 200 to 300 mg is achieved.[81] Monitoring based on likely timing of hematologic toxicities from dapsone (early occurrence of hemolysis and later risk for agranulocytosis) suggests that CBCs and reticulocyte counts be obtained weekly for the first 2 weeks of therapy, then every 2 weeks for the first 3 months of therapy. If a G6PD level is not available and therapy must be started immediately, a CBC should be obtained every 1 to 2 days for first 1 to 2 weeks and reticulocyte counts obtained at least weekly (see Chapter 11). A corrected reticulocyte count (reticulocyte index) of $\geq 3\%$ indicates an adequate marrow response for the degree of hemolysis.

(reticulocyte index = percent reticulocytes $\times$ [observed hematocrit $\div$ normal hematocrit] $\times$ 1/correction factor)*[82]

Causes for inadequate erythropoiesis, such as underlying infection, other chronic inflammatory disease, and vitamin or iron deficiency, should be sought and corrected whenever possible. Folic acid deficiency is a potential cause of inadequate reticulocyte response in chronic hemolysis because of increased requirement for the vitamin. Therefore folic acid supplementation often is given to dapsone patients to minimize chronic hemolysis.[75]

Sulfonamides

Sulfonamides have been associated with a variety of hematologic toxicities, including neutropenia, agranulocytosis, thrombocytopenia, and aplastic anemia.[17-20,22-26] Sulfasalazine has the greatest risk profile, but trimethoprim-sulfamethoxazole is also responsible for a number of toxicities.

SULFASALAZINE.

A Swedish group looked at the total number of blood dyscrasias reported with sulfonamides.[17,22] During sulfasalazine therapy, agranulocytosis occurred almost exclusively in the first 3 months of therapy. When prescription data were considered, the risk of agranulocytosis was 87/10^6 patient years (1/2400 patients in the first month of therapy, 1/700 patients during months 2 and 3, and 1/11,200 patients for months 3 through 12).[83] Mortality rate was 6.5%. After stopping the drug, 90% of patients had recovery of their WBC counts by day 15. A British study found a similar risk of

---

*Correction factor is 1 if hematocrit = 45; 1.5 if hematocrit = 35; 2 if hematocrit = 25; 2.5 if hematocrit = 15.

sulfasalazine-associated agranulocytosis, occurring in 6.8/10,000 patients (1/1470 patients) during the first 3 months of therapy.[84] The incidence of agranulocytosis was higher for patients receiving sulfasalazine for rheumatoid arthritis than for inflammatory bowel disease.[17,84] There are a few case reports on the use of granulocyte-macrophage colony–stimulating factor (GM-CSF) as treatment of drug-induced agranulocytosis,[85,86] including that from sulfasalazine.[87] Normalization of blood cell counts took 4 to 7 days. Because of lack of controls in these reports, statistical significance cannot be assigned to the apparent short recovery time with the use of hematopoietic stimulating factors.

The risk of thrombocytopenia from sulfasalazine may be higher in patients with rheumatoid arthritis than in patients receiving the drug for other diagnoses.[84] In one study of 10,000 patients on this drug, there were three cases of thrombocytopenia, all in patients treated for rheumatoid arthritis (rate of 0.8 case per 1000 patients treated for arthritis).[84] In a review of published case reports on drug-induced thrombocytopenia, sulfasalazine was implicated as the definite or probable cause in 3 out of 774 cases.[25] It was not possible to determine a relative risk of thrombocytopenia from sulfonamides because the study lacked no case controls and prescription number data. Another study reviewed 309 reports of drug-induced thrombocytopenia.[88] Six patients had received sulfasalazine.

TRIMETHOPRIM-SULFAMETHOXAZOLE.
In one series, the risk of agranulocytosis from another sulfonamide-containing drug, trimethoprim-sulfamethoxazole, was 0.6 episode per million patient days of taking the drug.[22,89] The average treatment time with trimethoprim-sulfamethoxazole before the diagnosis of agranulocytosis was 13 days.[89] Although most of the patients were taking other drugs concomitantly, in only 6% of cases were these medications previously recognized as causing agranulocytosis.

Trimethoprim-sulfamethoxazole was implicated as the definite or probable cause for 10 out of 774 cases of drug-induced thrombocytopenia in one review[25] and for 26 of 309 cases in another.[88] Trimethoprim alone was responsible for 1 case.[88] Kaufman[24] calculated the risk to be 38 cases per million users per week. The duration of thrombocytopenia from trimethoprim-sulfamethoxazole was slightly but significantly shorter when compared with that from other drugs, except quinine. Overall, there was no difference in recovery rates between those patients who had or had not received corticosteroids as treatment, although the data on corticosteroid use for sulfonamide-induced thrombocytopenia were not analyzed separately from these on other drugs. Median recovery time from thrombocytopenia was 8 days after cessation of drug therapy.[88] The mortality rate from hemorrhage was 3.6%. Despite the lack of statistical difference in recovery time, the authors recommend systemic corticosteroid use in severe symptomatic cases of drug-induced thrombocytopenia because of the difficulty of differentiating it from idiopathic thrombocytopenic purpura.

The relative risk of aplastic anemia from sulfonamides is low[18,19] to absent.[21,90] For trimethoprim-sulfamethoxazole, the incidence of pancytopenia/aplastic anemia was 1.1 case per million daily patient doses.[89] Special notice should be taken of the adverse interaction between methotrexate and trimethoprim-sulfamethoxazole, which may result in pancytopenia.[41,42] Additional hematologic toxicities from sulfonamides include hemolytic anemia[84] and pure red cell aplasia[91] from sulfasalazine. Nonhemolytic anemia (0.1 case per million daily patient doses)[89] and pure red cell aplasia[92] also have been described with trimethoprim-sulfamethoxazole.

There is not uniform agreement on whether dihydrofolate inhibition by trimethoprim or an immunologic reaction to the sulfonamide moiety is responsible for the occasional adverse hematologic reactions seen with this combination antibiotic.[26,93] Different mechanisms may be responsible in different patients with various toxicities. Drug-dependent antiplatelet antibodies are found in some patients with sulfonamide-associated thrombocytopenia.[94] However, megaloblastosis of the marrow has been seen in occasional other patients with thrombocytopenia, suggesting a trimethoprim effect.[26,95] In a study of children on trimethoprim-sulfamethoxazole, neutropenia occurred at day 10 only in patients on the antibiotic alone and not in those receiving supplemental folinic acid (20% incidence versus 0%). This again suggests interference in folic acid metabolism as a mechanism of toxicity.[96] Overall, however, studies of short-term and long-term (3 months) use of trimethoprim-sulfamethoxazole found that adverse hematologic effects were infrequent except in those patients with probable folic acid deficiency or those receiving higher than the usual dosages.[95,97-99] It is advisable to obtain a CBC with platelet count before therapy, then periodically in patients who are predisposed to folic acid deficiency (e.g., alcoholics, postpartum women). The drug should not be used in those with evidence of megaloblastic hematopoiesis, as evidenced by elevated mean corpuscular volume (MCV) or hypersegmented neutrophils, until the deficiency is treated or the megaloblastosis is found to be from an unrelated cause.[95] Trimethoprim-sulfamethoxazole should not be given to pregnant women nor in standard doses to patients on methotrexate.

Antimalarials

Antimalarials are widely used in dermatology for their antiinflammatory properties, particularly in photosensitive dermatoses. Significant hematologic effects are relatively uncommon. Patients with G6PD deficiency have brisk hemolysis with primaquine but are not at additional risk of hemolysis with the other more commonly used antimalarial agents when given standard doses.[100] Aplastic anemia occurs with quinacrine in up to 2.84 cases per 100,000, depending on the length of treatment.[101,102] In half the cases, it is preceded by a cutaneous eruption.[102] Leukopenia has been seen with all the antimalarials, occurring in 4.8% of patients on chloroquine, but less frequently in those on hydroxychloroquine. Isolated cases of agranulocytosis have been noted with all the agents, but this toxicity is rare with the exception of a newer drug, amodiaquine, which may cause agranulocytosis as frequently as 1/2000 cases.[103]

Colchicine

Colchicine inhibits cellular immunity and interferes with tubulin polymerization in leukocytes, thus acting as an immunomodulating and antiinflammatory drug.[104] It has been used in treatment of Behçet's disease, leukocytoclastic vasculitis, aphthous stomatitis, and palmoplantar pustulosis.[105] Hematologic toxicity is gener-ally associated with acute drug overdose[106] but has been described with therapeutic doses during acute[107,108] or chronic therapy.[109] The risk is higher for patients with renal or hepatic insufficiency[107,110,111] and in those patients receiving intravenous colchicine.[105,109] It is recommended that acute doses not exceed 5 mg daily.[107] After acute intoxication a transient leukocytosis may occur. With sufficiently high doses, leukocytosis is followed by pancytopenia from marrow aplasia, generally occurring between days 3 and 8. The hematologic toxicity is usually preceded by gastrointestinal and neurologic signs and symptoms and is accompanied by multiorgan failure.[106,112] Some patients develop disseminated intravascular coagulation, Heinz body hemolytic anemia, or Pelger-Huët anomaly (bilobed neutrophils).[106] When death occurs, it is generally from septicemia or hypovolemic shock.[113] Marrow recovery starts approximately 3 days after stopping the drug. Because pancytopenia does not always occur in colchicine overdose and has been occasionally described with chronic therapy, hematologic reactions from colchicine may be idiosyncratic. However, other authors attribute the hematologic effects to a direct toxicity from colchicine, which is known to accumulate in neutrophils and cause mitotic arrest.[106,107]

Gold and Penicillamine

The antirheumatic agents gold and penicillamine have been associated with aplastic anemia,[114,115] leukopenia, and thrombocytopenia.[11,15,88,116] When drug sales are considered, both gold and penicillamine have high relative risks for development of aplasia. The excess risk is 23 cases/10^6 users for gold and 60 cases/10^6 users for penicillamine (compared with occurrence of aplasia in nonusers).[18] The mortality rate is as high as 60%.[115] Treatment modalities have included chelation, immunosuppressive therapy, including antithymocyte globulin,[117] hematopoietic growth factors,[118] and bone marrow transplantation. Leukopenia is more commonly seen with gold therapy than with penicillamine.[115] Eosinophilia occurs in 5% to 40% of patients receiving gold. It may or may not be accompanied by other signs of gold toxicity.[115]

Thrombocytopenia occurs in 1% to 3% of patients receiving gold compounds.[115] It is immunomediated and may appear at any time during the course of therapy. Gold-induced thrombocytopenia is more common in patients who are HLA-DR3 positive.[116] The onset of thrombocytopenia from penicillamine is most often gradual but occasionally precipitous.[115] Generally it is reversible with cessation of the drug. Thrombotic thrombocytopenic purpura and pure red cell aplasia have also been described in association with penicillamine therapy.[115,119]

A CBC with platelet count should be obtained monthly in patients taking either gold or penicillamine. These laboratory tests should be monitored more frequently at initiation of therapy and with dose escalation.[115]

Mycophenolate Mofetil

Mycophenolate mofetil is a relatively new immunosuppressive drug that inhibits de novo purine synthesis in stimulated T cells and B cells by blocking the enzyme type II inosine monophosphate dehydrogenase.[120,121] It is approved for suppression of rejection in organ transplantation but also has been used to treat a variety of autoimmune and inflammatory skin disorders including pemphigus, pemphigoid, pyoderma gangrenosum, metastatic Crohn's disease, and psoriasis.[120,121] Adverse effects include gastrointestinal intolerance, leukopenia, anemia, thrombocytopenia, and infections.[120,121] Proliferating lymphocytes are affected more than are neutrophils because they predominantly use the de novo rather than salvage pathway for guanosine incorporation into DNA.[122] For dermatologic diseases, the usual dose of mycophenolate is 1 to 2.5 g/day in divided doses, given either as monotherapy or in combination with prednisone.[120,121]

Miscellaneous Drugs

Neutropenia may occur with the oral retinoids, but agranulocytosis is exceedingly rare.[123] Neutropenia is reversible on cessation of the drugs, although there is one report of prolonged neutropenia after use of isotretinoin for 18 weeks.[124]

Terbinafine has been associated with agranulocytosis in at least 4 patients.[125-127] The agranulocytosis occurred after 4 to 6 weeks of therapy. The estimated incidence is 1/400,000 patients.[126] The mechanism is unknown but may involve inhibition with cholesterol synthesis,

which is important in blood cell membrane formation.[127] A CBC at baseline and after 4 to 6 weeks of therapy is recommended in immunocompromised patients. Recommendations for hematologic monitoring in immunocompetent patients vary.[126,127] However, it is advisable to instruct these patients to seek immediate medical care and to obtain a CBC if they develop fever, chills, sore throat, malaise, or other signs of infection while on terbinafine.

Neutropenia has also been reported infrequently with nonsteroidal antiinflammatory agents,[129,130] ciprofloxacin,[17] systemic metronidazole,[131] cephalosporins,[3,17-20] and possibly cimetidine[132,133] and ranitidine.[20]

Thrombocytopenia is estimated to occur in 1/200,000 patients on terbinafine.[126] It may be seen rarely with thiazides,[11,23,24,88] cephalosporins,[24,88] penicillins,[24,88] rifampin,[11,24] tetracyclines,[88] ciprofloxacin,[134] retinoids,[135,136] cimetidine,[24,88] and nonsteroidal antiinflammatory agents[17,24,64,88] (see Table 42-2).

TREATMENT OF HEMATOLOGIC TOXICITIES

Reductions of drug dose should be considered for new neutropenia of 1500 to 2000/mm^3 or leukopenia of 3000 to 3500/mm^3 (Table 42-5). Cessation of the drug should be considered for new neutropenia of less than 1500/mm^3, or for thrombocytopenia of less than 100,000/mm^3. A suspect drug should definitely be stopped when the neutrophil count falls below 1000/mm^3 or the platelet count below 50,000/mm^3.[4] After recovering from the cytopenia(s), the patient can restart the drug at 50% to 75% of the previous dose, depending on the grade of toxicity encountered (Tables 42-6 and 42-7) and the seriousness of the underlying disease. Drugs that result in grades 3 to 4 toxicity should not be reused.[4] Older patients often have less marrow reserve, so for patients over 65 years of age it is prudent to begin or restart therapy with doses at the lower end of or slightly below the recommended range.

In the absence of significant cardiovascular disease, most patients tolerate a hematocrit of >26%. Transfusion of packed RBCs is indicated if the patient is symptomatic. Platelet trans-

■ **Table 42-5**   General Guidelines for Drug Discontinuation for Cytopenias*
(Cell Count per μl)

Cellular Subset	*Reduce* Drug *Dose* (at a Minimum)	Strongly Consider Discontinuing Drug	Definitely *Stop* the *Drug* in Question
White blood cells	3000-3500	2500-3000	<2500
Granulocytes	1500-2000	1000-1500	<1000
Platelets	100,000-150,000	50,000-100,000	<50,000

Data from Hande KR: Principles and pharmacology of chemotherapy. In Lee RG, Foerster J, Lukens JN, et al, editors: *Wintrobe's clinical hematology,* vol 2, ed 10, Baltimore, MD, 1999, Williams & Wilkins, p 2085.
*These are rough guidelines; each clinical scenario should be handled individually. Of particular importance is the rate of change and the timing of the change.

■ **Table 42-6**   Grades of Myelosuppression (Cell Count per μl)

Toxicity Grade	White Blood Cells	Granulocytes*	Platelets
0	≥4000	≥2000	≥100,000
1	3000-3999	1500-1999	75,000-99,000
2	2000-2999	1000-1499	50,000-74,000
3	1000-1999	500-999	25,000-49,000
4	<1000	<500	<25,000

Data from Haskell CM: Principles of cancer chemotherapy. In Haskell CM, editor: *Cancer treatment,* ed 4, Philadelphia, 1995, WB Saunders Co., p 41; Miller AB, Hoogstraten B, Staquet M, et al: *Cancer* 47:207-214, 1981.
*Granulocytes include segmented and juvenile neutrophils.

■ **Table 42-7**   Dose Adjustment Guidelines for Restarting Medications
After Recovery from Hematologic Toxicity (Cell Count per μl)

	100% Dose	75% Dose	50% Dose	Omit Dose
White blood cells	>3500	3000-3500	2500-2999	<2500
Granulocytes	>2000	1500-2000	1000-1499	<1000
Platelets	100,000	75,000-99,000	50,000-74,000	<50,000

Data from Hande KR: Principles and pharmacology of chemotherapy. In: Lee RG, Foerster J, Lukens JN, et al, editors: *Wintrobe's clinical hematology,* vol 2, ed 10, Baltimore, MD, 1999, Williams & Wilkins, p 2085.

fusions are given for a platelet count <50,000/mm³ associated with bleeding. Prophylactic platelet transfusions are given if the platelet count is less than 10,000 to 20,000/mm³.[137] Fever in a patient with an absolute neutrophil count of less than 500/mm³ is a medical emergency and should be treated immediately with broad-spectrum antibiotic coverage pending results of cultures. Recombinant human granulocyte colony–stimulating factors (G-CSF) and GM-CSF have been used to help reverse drug-induced neutropenia. These agents cause bone pain in 10% to 20% of patients. Either drug may result in cutaneous adverse effects including local injection site reactions, papular eruptions, vasculitis, and

Sweet's syndrome.[138] Both factors have been associated with sometimes fatal pulmonary infiltrates. This reaction probably occurs less often with G-CSF than with GM-CSF.[139] Because mortality is directly related to the severity and duration of neutropenia, there is rationale for the use of colony-stimulating factors in drug-induced neutropenia. However, neither cytokine has been proven to decrease the period of neutropenia or mortality outside the setting of cancer chemotherapy.[139,140] Other agents, such as intravenous gamma globulin (0.4 mg/kg/day × 5 days), also have been used to treat drug-induced immune thrombocytopenia and agranulocytosis.[15]

Acknowledgment

The author is grateful to James V. Jordan, M. D., for his insightful comments and to Paul D. Asheim for his expert typing of the manuscript.

Bibliography

Anonymous: Standardization of definitions and criteria of causality assessment of adverse drug reactions: drug-induced cytopenia. *Int J Clin Pharmacol Ther Tox* 29:75-81, 1991.

Fraiser LH, Kanekal S, Kehrer JP: Cyclophosphamide toxicity: characterizing and avoiding the problem. *Drugs* 42:781-795, 1991.

George CS, Lichtin AE: Hematologic complications of rheumatic disease therapies. *Rheum Dis Clin North Am* 23:425-437, 1997.

Spielberg SP: Pharmacogenetics and blood dyscrasias. *Eur J Haematol* 57(Suppl):93-97, 1996.

Young NS: Agranulocytosis. *JAMA* 271:935-938, 1994.

Young NS: Aplastic anaemia. *Lancet* 346:228-232, 1995.

References

General Principles

1. Heimpel H: When should the clinician suspect a drug-induced blood dyscrasia, and how should he proceed? *Eur J Haematol* 57(Suppl):11-15, 1996.

2. Young NS: Immune pathophysiology of acquired aplastic anaemia. *Eur J Haematol* 57(Suppl):55-59, 1996.

3. Young NS: Agranulocytosis. *JAMA* 271:935-938, 1994.

4. Hande KR: Principles and pharmacology of chemotherapy. In Lee RG, Foerster J, Lukens JN, et al, editors: *Wintrobe's clinical hematology*, vol 2, ed 10, Baltimore, MD, 1999, Williams & Wilkins, pp 2076-2101.

5. Snow JL, Gibson LE: The role of genetic variation in thiopurine methyltransferase activity and the efficacy and/or side effects of azathioprine therapy in dermatologic patients. *Arch Dermatol* 131:193-197, 1995.

6. Snow JL, Gibson LE: A pharmacogenetic basis for the safe and effective use of azathioprine and other thiopurine drugs in dermatologic patients. *J Am Acad Dermatol* 32:114-116, 1995.

7. Spielberg SP: Pharmacogenetics and blood dyscrasias. *Eur J Haematol* 57(Suppl):93-97, 1996.

8. Relling MV: Polymorphic drug metabolism. *Clin Pharm* 8:852-863, 1989.

9. Rieder MJ, Shear NH, Kanee A, et al: Prominence of slow acetylator phenotype among patients with sulfonamide hypersensitivity reactions. *Clin Pharmacol Ther* 49:13-17, 1991.

10. Rieder MJ, Uetrecht J, Shear NH, et al: Diagnosis of sulfonamide hypersensitivity reactions by in vitro "rechallenge" with hydroxylamine metabolites. *Ann Intern Med* 110:286-289, 1989.

11. Moss RA: Drug-induced immune thrombocytopenia. *Am J Hematol* 9:439-446, 1980.

12. Shear NH, Spielberg SP, Grant DM, et al: Differences in metabolism of sulfonamides predisposing to idiosyncratic toxicity. *Ann Intern Med* 105:179-184, 1986.

13. Salama A, Schutz B, Kiefel V, et al: Immune-mediated agranulocytosis related to drugs and their metabolites: Mode of sensitization and heterogeneity of antibodies. *Br J Haematol* 72:127-132, 1989.

14. Hoaglund HC: Hematologic complications of cancer chemotherapy. In Perry MC, editor: *The chemotherapy source book,* Baltimore, MD, 1992, Williams & Wilkins, pp 498-507.

15. Salama A, Mueller-Eckhardt C: Immune-mediated blood cell dyscrasias related to drugs. *Semin Hematol* 29:54-63, 1992.

16. Standardization of definitions and criteria of causality assessment of adverse drug reactions: Drug-induced cytopenia. *Int J Clin Pharmacol Ther Tox* 29:75-81, 1991.

17. Wiholm B-E, Emanuelsson S: Drug-related blood dyscrasias in a Swedish reporting system, 1985-1994. *Eur J Haematol* 57(Suppl):42-46, 1996.

18. Kaufman DW, Kelly JP, Jurgelon JM, et al: Drugs in the aetiology of agranulocytosis and aplastic anaemia. *Eur J Haematol* 57(Suppl):23-30, 1996.

19. Anti-infective drug use in relation to the risk of agranulocytosis and aplastic anemia: A report from the International Agranulocytosis and Aplastic Anemia Study. *Arch Intern Med* 149:1036-1040, 1989.

20. van der Klauw MM, Wilson JHP, Stricker BHC: Drug-associated agranulocytosis: 20 years of reporting in the Netherlands (1974-1994). *Am J Hematol* 57:206-211, 1998.

21. Baumelou E, Guiguet M, Mary JY, et al: Epidemiology of aplastic anemia in France: a case control study. I. Medical history and medication use. *Blood* 81:1471-1478, 1993.

Major Categories of Hematologic Toxicity

22. Keisu M, Ekman E, Wiholm B-E: Comparing risk estimates of sulphonamide-induced agranulocytosis from the Swedish Drug Monitoring System and a case-control study. *Eur J Clin Pharmacol* 43:211-214, 1992.

23. Juliá A, Olona M, Bueno J, et al: Drug-induced agranulocytosis: Prognostic factors in a series of 168 episodes. *Br J Haematol* 79:366-371, 1991.

24. Kaufman DW, Kelly JP, Johannes CB, et al: Acute thrombocytopenic purpura in relation to the use of drugs. *Blood* 82:2714-2718, 1993.

25. George JN, Raskob GE, Shah SR, et al: Drug-induced thrombocytopenia: a systematic review of published case reports. *Ann Intern Med* 129:886-890, 1998.

26. Dickson HG: Trimethoprim-sulphamethoxazole and thrombocytopenia. *Med J Austral* 2:5-7, 1978.

27. Schilsky RL: Antimetabolites. In Perry MC, editor: *The chemotherapy source book,* Baltimore, MD, 1992, Williams & Wilkins, pp 301-317.

28. Kamel OW, van de Rijn M, LeBrun DP, et al: Lymphoid neoplasms in patients with rheumatoid arthritis and dermatomyositis: Frequency of Epstein-Barr virus and other features associated with immunosuppression. *Hum Pathol* 25:638-643, 1994.

29. Salloum E, Cooper DL, Howe G, et al: Spontaneous regression of lymphoproliferative disorders in patients treated with methotrexate for rheumatoid arthritis and other rheumatic diseases. *J Clin Oncol* 14:1943-1949, 1996.

30. Le Beau MM, Albain KS, Larson RA, et al: Clinical and cytogenetic correlations in 63 patients with therapy-related myelodysplasia syndromes and acute non-lymphocytic leukemia: further evidence for characteristic abnormalities of chromosome no. 5 and 7. *J Clin Oncol* 4:325-345, 1986.

Methotrexate

31. Cronstein BN: The mechanism of action of methotrexate. *Rheum Dis Clin North Am* 23:739-755, 1997.

32. Cronstein BN, Naime D, Ostad E: The anti-inflammatory mechanism of methotrexate: Increased adenosine release at inflamed sites diminishes leukocyte accumulation in an *in vivo* model of inflammation. *J Clin Invest* 92:2675-2682, 1993.

33. Duhra P: Treatment of gastrointestinal symptoms associated with methotrexate therapy for psoriasis. *J Am Acad Dermatol* 28:466-469, 1993.

34. Morgan SL, Baggott JE, Vaughn WH, et al: Supplementation with folic acid during methotrexate therapy for rheumatoid arthritis: A double-blind, placebo-controlled trial. *Ann Intern Med* 121:833-841, 1994.

35. Shiroky JB, Neville C, Esdaile JM, et al: Low-dose methotrexate with leucovorin (folinic acid) in the management of rheumatoid arthritis: results of a multicenter randomized, double-blind, placebo-controlled trial. *Arthritis Rheum* 36:795-803, 1993.

36. Groff GD, Raddatz DA, Franck WA, et al: Hematologic abnormalities during low dose methotrexate therapy for rheumatoid arthritis (abstract). *Arthritis Rheum* 30:S41/A23, 1987.

37. Weinblatt ME, Fraser P: Elevated mean corpuscular volume as a predictor of hematologic toxicity due to methotrexate therapy. *Arthritis Rheum* 32:1592-1596, 1989.

38. Borrie P, Clark PA: Megaloblastic anaemia during methotrexate treatment of psoriasis. *BMJ* 1:1339, 1966.

39. Fulton RA: Megaloblastic anaemia and methotrexate treatment (letter). *Br J Dermatol* 114:267-268, 1986.

40. Woolley PV III, Sacher RA, Priego VM, et al: Methotrexate-induced immune haemolytic anaemia. *Br J Haematol* 54:543-552, 1983.

41. Thomas DR, Dover JS, Camp RD: Pancytopenia induced by the interaction between methotrexate and trimethoprim-sulfamethoxazole *J Am Acad Dermatol* 17:1055-1056, 1987.

42. Andersen WK, Feingold DS: Adverse drug interactions clinically important for the dermatologist. *Arch Dermatol* 131:468-473, 1995.

43. Bailin PL, Tindall JP, Roenigk HH, et al: Is methotrexate therapy for psoriasis carcinogenic? A modified retrospective-prospective analysis. *JAMA* 232:359-362, 1975.

44. Stern RS, Zierler S, Parrish JA: Methotrexate used for psoriasis and the risk of noncutaneous or cutaneous malignancy. *Cancer* 50:869-872, 1982.

45. Nyfors A, Jensen H: Frequency of malignant neoplasms in 248 long-term methotrexate-treated psoriatics. A preliminary study. *Dermatologica* 167:260-261, 1983.

46. Paul C, Le Tourneau A, Cayuela JM, et al: Epstein-Barr virus-associated lymphoproliferative disease during methotrexate therapy for psoriasis. *Arch Dermatol* 133:867-871, 1997.

Azathioprine

47. Anstey A: Azathioprine in dermatology: A review in light of advances in understanding methylation pharmacogenetics. *J R Soc Med* 88(Suppl):155P-160P, 1995.

48. Hande KR, Garrow GC: Purine antimetabolites. In Chabner BA, Longo DL, editors: *Cancer chemotherapy and biotherapy*, ed 2, Philadelphia, 1996, Lippincott-Raven Publishers, pp 235-252.

49. Rapini RP: Cytotoxic drugs in the treatment of skin disease. *Int J Dermatol* 30:313-322, 1991.

50. Yates CR, Krynetski EY, Loennechen T, et al: Molecular diagnosis of thiopurine S-methyltransferase deficiency: genetic basis for azathioprine and mercaptopurine intolerance. *Ann Intern Med* 126:608-614, 1997.

51. Lennard L, Harrington CI, Wood M, et al: Metabolism of azathioprine to 6-thioguanine nucleotides in patients with pemphigus vulgaris. *Br J Clin Pharmacol* 23:229-233, 1987.

52. Edwards CRW, Drury P, Penketh A, et al: Successful reintroduction of captopril following neutropenia. *Lancet* 1:723, 1981.

53. Bradley PP, Warden GD, Maxwell JG, et al: Neutropenia and thrombocytopenia in renal allograft recipients treated with trimethoprim-sulfamethoxazole. *Ann Intern Med* 93:560-562, 1980.

54. Thompson DF, Gales MA: Drug-induced pure red cell aplasia. *Pharmacotherapy* 16:1002-1008, 1996.

55. August PJ: Azathioprine in the treatment of eczema and actinic reticuloid (abstract). *Br J Dermatol* 107(Suppl 22):23, 1982.

56. Dutz JP, Ho VC: Immunosuppressive agents in dermatology: an update. *Dermatol Clin* 16:235-251, 1998.

57. Singh G, Fries JF, Williams CA, et al: Toxicity profiles of disease modifying antirheumatic drugs in rheumatoid arthritis. *J Rheumatol* 18:188-194, 1991.

Cyclophosphamide and Chlorambucil

58. Tew KD, Colvin M, Chabner BA: Alkylating agents. In Chabner BA, Longo DL, editors: *Cancer chemotherapy and biotherapy*, ed 2, Philadelphia, 1996, Lippincott-Raven Publishers, p 318.

59. Powis G, Reece P, Ahmann DL, et al: Effect of body weight on the pharmacokinetics of cyclophosphamide in breast cancer patients. *Cancer Chemother Pharmacol* 20:219-222, 1987.

60. Bogden AE, Carde P, de Paillette ED, et al: Amelioration of chemotherapy-induced toxicity by cotreatment with AcSDKP, a tetrapeptide inhibitor of hematopoietic stem cell proliferation. *Ann N Y Acad Sci* 628:126-139, 1991.

61. Jimenez JJ, Huang HS, Hindahl M, et al: Protection from chemotherapy-induced neutropenia by ImuVert. *Am J Med Sci* 303:83-85, 1992.

62. Baker GL, Kahl LE, Zee BC, et al: Malignancy following treatment of rheumatoid arthritis with cyclophosphamide: Long-term case-control follow-up study. *Am J Med* 83:1-9, 1987.

63. Rieche K: Carcinogenicity of antineoplastic agents in man. *Cancer Treat Rev* 11:39-67, 1984.

64. Langford CA, Klippel JH, Balow JE, et al: Use of cytotoxic agents and cyclosporine in the treatment of autoimmune disease: Part 2: inflammatory bowel disease, systemic vasculitis, and therapeutic toxicity. *Ann Intern Med* 129:49-58, 1998.

65. Clamon GH: Alkylating agents. In Perry MC, editor: *The chemotherapy source book*, Baltimore, MD, 1992, Williams & Wilkins, pp 286-300.

66. Steigbigel RT, Kim H, Potolsky A, et al: Acute myeloproliferative disorder following long-term chlorambucil therapy. *Arch Intern Med* 134:728-731, 1974.

67. Patapanian H, Graham S, Sambrook PN, et al: The oncogenicity of chlorambucil in rheumatoid arthritis. *Br J Rheumatol* 27:44-47, 1988.

68. Knopse WH: Proceedings. Bi-weekly chlorambucil treatment of chronic lymphocytic leukemia. *Cancer* 33:555-562, 1974.

Hydroxyurea and Interferons

69. Boyd AS, Neldner KH: Hydroxyurea therapy. *J Am Acad Dermatol* 25:518-524, 1991.

70. Donehower RC: Hydroxyurea. In Chabner BA, Longo DL, editors: *Cancer chemotherapy and biotherapy*, ed 2, Philadelphia, 1996, Lippincott-Raven Publishers, pp 253-261.

71. Weinfeld A, Swolin B, Westin J: Acute leukaemia after hydroxyurea in polycythemia vera and allied disorders: Prospective study of efficacy and leukaemogenicity with therapeutic implications. *Eur J Haematol* 52:134-139, 1994.

72. Stadler R: Interferons in dermatology: present-day standard. *Dermatol Clin* 16:377-398, 1998.

73. Ringenberg QS, Anderson PC: Interferons in the treatment of skin disease. *Int J Dermatol* 25:273-279, 1986.

Dapsone

74. Coleman MD: Dapsone toxicity: some current perspectives. *Gen Pharmacol* 26:1461-1467, 1995.

75. Beutler E: Glucose-6-phosphate dehydrogenase deficiency and other enzyme abnormalities. In Beutler E, Lichtman MA, Coller BS, et al, editors: *Williams hematology*, ed 5, New York, 1995, McGraw-Hill, pp 564-581.

76. Coleman MD: Dapsone: modes of action, toxicity and possible strategies for increasing patient tolerance. *Br J Dermatol* 129:507-513, 1993.

77. Machet L, Callens A, Mercier E, et al: Agranulocytose induite par la dapsone prescrite pour une dermatite herpétiforme. *Ann Dermatol Venereol* 123:328-330, 1996.

78. Hörnsten P, Keisu M, Wiholm B-E: The incidence of agranulocytosis during treatment of dermatitis herpetiformis with dapsone as reported in Sweden, 1972 through 1988. *Arch Dermatol* 126:919-922, 1990.

79. Woodbury GR, Fried W, Ertle JO, et al: Dapsone-associated agranulocytosis and severe anemia in a patient with leukocytoclastic vasculitis. *J Am Acad Dermatol* 28:781-783, 1993.

80. Coleman MD, Simpson J, Jacobus DP: Reduction of dapsone hydroxylamine to dapsone during methaemoglobin formation in human erythrocytes *in vitro* IV: implications for the development of agranulocytosis. *Biochem Pharmacol* 48:1349-1354, 1994.

81. Guzzo C, Lazarus GS, Werth VP: Dermatological pharmacology. In Gilman AG, Hardman JG, Limbird LE, et al, editors: *Goodman & Gilman's the pharmacological basis of therapeutics*, ed 9, New York, 1996, McGraw-Hill, pp 1593-1616.

82. Hillman RS, Finch CA: *Red cell manual*, ed 6, Philadelphia, 1992, F.A. Davis Company, pp 57-61.

Sulfonamides

83. Keisu M, Ekman E: Sulfasalazine associated agranulocytosis in Sweden 1972-1989: clinical features, and estimation of its incidence. *Eur J Clin Pharmacol* 43:215-218, 1992.

84. Jick H, Myers MW, Dean AD: The risk of sulfasalazine- and mesalazine-associated blood disorders. *Pharmacotherapy* 15:176-181, 1995.

85. Delannoy A, Gehenot M: Colony-stimulating factor and drug-induced agranulocytosis (letter). *Ann Intern Med* 110:942-943, 1989.

86. Palmblad J, Jonson B, Kanerud L: Treatment of drug-induced agranulocytosis with recombinant GM-CSF. *J Intern Med* 228:537-539, 1990.

87. Kuipers EJ, Vellenga E, de Wolf JT, et al: Sulfasalazine induced agranulocytosis treated with granulocyte-macrophage colony stimulating factor. *J Rheumatol* 19:621-622, 1992.

88. Pedersen-Bjergaard U, Andersen M, Hansen PB: Drug-induced thrombocytopenia: Clinical data on 309 cases and the effect of corticosteroid therapy. *Eur J Clin Pharmacol* 52:183-189, 1997.

89. Keisu M, Wiholm B-E, Palmblad J: Trimethoprim-sulphamethoxazole-associated blood dyscrasias. Ten years' experience of the Swedish spontaneous reporting system. *J Intern Med* 228:353-360, 1990.

90. Mary JY, Guiget M, Baumelou E, et al: Drug use and aplastic anaemia: the French experience. *Eur J Haematol* 57(Suppl):35-41, 1996.

91. Anttila PM, Valimaki M, Pentikainen PJ: Pure-red-cell aplasia associated with sulphasalazine but not 5-aminosalicylic acid (letter). *Lancet* 2:1006, 1985.

92. Serrate San Miguel G, Franco Comet P, Casane P, et al: Aplasia pura de la serie roja asociada a cotrimoxazole. *Med Clin (Barc)* 84:334, 1985.

93. Frisch JM: Clinical experience with adverse reactions to trimethoprim-sulfamethoxazole. *J Infect Dis* 128(Suppl):S607-S611, 1973.

94. Aster RH: Drug-induced immune thrombocytopenia: an overview of pathogenesis. *Semin Hematol* 36:2-6, 1999.

95. Co-trimoxazole and blood (editorial). *Lancet* 2:950-951, 1973.

96. Principi N, Marchisio P, Biasini A, et al: Early and late neutropenia in children treated with cotrimoxazole (trimethoprim-sulfamethoxazole). *Acta Paediatr Scand* 73:763-767, 1984.

97. Jenkins GC, Hughes DTD, Hall PC: A haematological study of patients receiving long-term treatment with trimethoprim and sulphonamide. *J Clin Pathol* 23:392-396, 1970.

98. Casey TP, Matthews JRD, Buchanan JG: Adverse haematological effects and trimethoprim-sulphamethoxazole administration. *N Z Med J* 78:433-435, 1973.

99. Herbert V: Metabolism of folic acid in man. *J Infect Dis* 128(Suppl):S601-S606, 1973.

Other Drug Categories

100. Beutler E: The hemolytic effect of primaquine and related compounds: A review. *Blood* 14:103-139, 1959.

101. Biro L, Leone N: Aplastic anemia induced by quinacrine. *Arch Dermatol* 92:574-576, 1965.

102. Schmid I, Anasetti C, Petersen FB, et al: Marrow transplantation for severe aplastic anemia associated with exposure to quinacrine. *Blut* 61:52-54, 1990.

103. Hatton CS, Peto TE, Bunch C, et al: Frequency of severe neutropenia associated with amodiaquine prophylaxis against malaria. *Lancet* 1:411-414, 1986.

104. Dallaverde E, Fan PT, Chang Y-H: Mechanism of action of colchicine. *V J Pharmacol Exp Ther* 223:197-202, 1982.

105. Sullivan TP, King LE, Boyd AS: Colchicine in dermatology. *J Am Acad Dermatol* 39:993-999, 1998.

106. Levy M, Spino M, Read SE: Colchicine: a state-of-the-art review. *Pharmacotherapy* 11:196-211, 1991.

107. Liu YK, Hymowitz R, Carroll MG: Marrow aplasia induced by colchicine. *Arthritis Rheum* 21:731-736, 1978.

108. Stanley MW, Taurog JD, Snover DC: Fatal colchicine toxicity: report of a case. *Clin Exp Rheumatol* 2:167-171, 1984.

109. Ferrannini E, Pentimone F: Marrow aplasia following colchicine treatment for gouty arthritis. *Clin Exp Rheumatol* 2:173-175, 1984.

110. Carr AA: Colchicine toxicity. *Arch Intern Med* 115:29-33, 1965.

111. Ducloux D, Schuller V, Chalopin J-M: Colchicine agranulocytosis (letter). *Nephrol Dialysis Transplant* 12:1541-1542, 1997.

112. Dodds AJ, Lawrence PJ, Biggs JC: Colchicine overdose. *Med J Aust* 2:91-92, 1978.

113. Gaultier M, Kanfer A, Bismuth C, et al: Données actuelles sur l'intoxication aiguë par la colchicine: A propos de 23 observations. *Ann Méd Interne* 120:605-618, 1969.

114. Adachi JD, Bensen WG, Ali M, et al: Gold induced aplastic anemia. *J Rheum* 12:1011-1012, 1985.

115. Chatham WW, Blackburn WD: Gold and *d*-penicillamine. In Koopman WJ, editor: *Arthritis and allied conditions. A textbook of rheumatology,* ed 13, Baltimore, MD, 1997, Williams & Wilkins, pp 655-670.

116. Adachi JD, Bensen WG, Kassam Y, et al: Gold induced thrombocytopenia: 12 cases and a review of the literature. *Semin Arthritis Rheum* 16:287-293, 1987.
117. Doney K, Storb R, Buckner CD, et al: Treatment of gold-induced aplastic anaemia with immunosuppressive therapy. *Br J Haematol* 68:469-472, 1988.
118. Brown SL, Hill ER: G-CSF in gold-induced aplastic anaemia (letter). *Ann Rheum Dis* 53:213, 1994.
119. Speth PA, Boerbooms AM, Holdrinet RS, et al: Thrombotic thrombocytopenic purpura associated with D-penicillamine treatment in rheumatoid arthritis (letter). *J Rheumatol* 9:812-813, 1982.
120. Grundmann-Kollmann M, Korting HC, Behrens S, et al: Mycophenolate mofetil: a new therapeutic option in the treatment of blistering autoimmune diseases. *J Am Acad Dermatol* 40:957-960, 1999.
121. Enk AH, Knop J: Mycophenolate is effective in the treatment of pemphigus vulgaris. *Arch Dermatol* 135:54-56, 1999.
122. Stanley JR: Therapy of pemphigus vulgaris (editorial). *Arch Dermatol* 135:76-77, 1999.

Miscellaneous Drugs

123. Windhorst DB, Nigra T: General clinical toxicology of oral retinoids. *J Am Acad Dermatol* 6:675-682, 1982.
124. Friedman SJ: Leukopenia and neutropenia associated with isotretinoin therapy (letter). *Arch Dermatol* 123:293-295, 1987.
125. Kovacs MJ, Alshammari S, Guenther L, et al: Neutropenia and pancytopenia associated with oral terbinafine (letter). *J Am Acad Dermatol* 31:806, 1994.
126. Gupta AK, Soori GS, Del Rosso JQ, et al: Severe neutropenia associated with oral terbinafine therapy. *J Am Acad Dermatol* 38:765-767, 1998.
127. Ornstein DL, Ely P: Reversible agranulocytosis associated with oral terbinafine for onychomycosis. *J Am Acad Dermatol* 39:1023-1024, 1998.
128. Lamisil (terbinafine hydrochloride) U.S. Product Monograph. Sandoz Pharmaceuticals Corporation, East Hanover, New Jersey, 1996.
129. Strom BL, Carson JL, Schinnar R, et al: Nonsteroidal anti-inflammatory drugs and neutropenia. *Arch Intern Med* 153:2119-2124, 1993.
130. Jick H, Derby LE, Garcia Rodriguez LA, et al: Nonsteroidal anti-inflammatory drugs and certain, rare, serious adverse events: a cohort study. *Pharmacotherapy* 13:212-217, 1993.
131. Smith JA: Neutropenia associated with metronidazole therapy. *Can Med Assoc J* 123:202, 1980.
132. Fitchen JH, Koeffler HP: Cimetidine and granulopoiesis: bone marrow culture studies in normal man and patients with cimetidine-associated neutropenia. *Br J Haematol* 46:361-366, 1980.
133. Strom BL, Carson JL, Schinnar R, et al: Is cimetidine associated with neutropenia? *Am J Med* 99:282-290, 1995.
134. Aydogdu I, Ozerol IH, Tayfun E, et al: Autoimmune haemolytic anaemia and thrombocytopenia associated with ciprofloxacin (letter). *Clin Lab Haematol* 19:223, 1997.
135. Naldi L, Rozzoni M, Finazzi G, et al: Etretinate therapy and thrombocytopenia (letter). *Br J Dermatol* 124:395, 1991.
136. Johnson TM, Rapini RP: Isotretinoin-induced thrombocytopenia (letter). *J Am Acad Dermatol* 17:838-839, 1987.

Treatment of Hemotologic Toxicities

137. Wandt H, Frank M, Ehninger G, et al: Safety and cost effectiveness of a 10×10^9/L trigger for prophylactic platelet transfusions compared with the traditional 20×10^9/L trigger: A prospective comparative trial in 105 patients with acute myeloid leukemia. *Blood* 91:3601-3606, 1998.
138. Asnis LA, Gaspari AA: Cutaneous reactions to recombinant cytokine therapy. *J Am Acad Dermatol* 33:393-410, 1995.
139. Demuynck H, Zachée P, Verhoef GEG, et al: Risks of rhG-CSF treatment in drug-induced agranulocytosis. *Ann Hematol* 70:143-147, 1995.
140. American Society of Clinical Oncology: Update of recommendations for the use of hematopoietic colony-stimulating factors: evidence-based clinical practice guidelines. *J Clin Oncol* 14:1957-1960, 1996.

Barbara R. Reed

Dermatologic Drugs During Pregnancy and Lactation

Treatment of many dermatologic conditions is elective. Some drugs used by the dermatologist for the patient who is pregnant or lactating may have potentially harmful effects on the mother and fetus or nursing infant. For this reason, a general reluctance exists among physicians to provide medications during pregnancy and lactation. There are, however, drugs for which use during pregnancy and lactation have no apparent contraindication. It may be of both interest and comfort to the clinician and patient to become aware of this select list of "safe" drugs.

This chapter identifies and discusses contraindications to various drugs to the extent possible with available information. When treatment with one of these drugs is essential, data must be carefully examined and evaluated so that a risk-benefit ratio may be determined, with the patient taking part in the decision-making process. A list of dermatologic medications that lack reported contraindications during pregnancy or lactation also has been compiled.

Pregnant or lactating women and their physicians face some difficult choices when dermatologic conditions arise. Many physicians choose to give no drugs during these periods, fearing legal vulnerability should a problem arise. It will be of comfort to both physician and patient to learn that some medications present minimal risk to the unborn child. A basis for intelligent decision making may be available.

Those sources available to the physician are discussed here, which may influence choice of specific drugs. Those drugs least harmful for use during pregnancy and lactation are also presented.

GENERAL PRINCIPLES
Sources for Information—Drug Use in Pregnancy and Lactation

Most physicians are aware of the Food and Drug Administration (FDA) pregnancy categories (Table 43-1) through the *Physicians' Desk Reference* (PDR).[1] However, fewer physicians are aware that there are lactation categories (Box 43-1). Revisions of FDA pregnancy categories may be forthcoming, since the categories are found to be confusing and lacking in helpful data. Additional sources of information on drug use during pregnancy and lactation are listed in Table 43-2.

Risk Related to Time of Drug Consumption

Risks from drug intake during pregnancy differ from those during the prenatal period or during lactation. Drug-related risks during pregnancy may vary with the trimester of pregnancy as well. Drugs labeled as teratogenic may put a fetus at risk for only a few weeks of pregnancy. Nevertheless, it is generally recommended that these drugs be avoided for the entire pregnancy.

■ Table 43-1 FDA Pregnancy Drug Risk Categories*

Drug Risk Category	Definition
X	• Contraindicated in pregnancy
	• There is no reason to risk use of the drug in pregnancy
D	• Positive evidence for risk to human fetus
	• *However,* benefits may outweigh risks of the drug
C	• Risk cannot be ruled out—human studies are lacking
	• Animal studies may or may not show risk
	• Potential benefits may justify potential risk
B	• No risk to human fetus despite possible animal risk
	• *Or,* no risk in animal studies and human studies have not been done
A	• Controlled studies show no fetal risk
Unrated	• No pregnancy category has been assigned

*Code of Federal Regulations: 21(part 201.57):23, 25, 1987.

Box 43-1

FDA Lactation Drug Risk Categories

DISCONTINUE	CAUTION
"A decision should be made whether to discontinue nursing or to discontinue the drug, taking into account the importance of the drug to the mother."	The label "Caution is advised if the drug is used during lactation" is used if the drug is absorbed and excreted into human breast milk and does not have known adverse reactions or tumorigenic potential.

Drugs that place a fetus or mother at risk during lactation may be different from those that affect an infant during pregnancy.

Timing—Before Conception (Contraceptive Failure)

Physicians prescribing a drug for women of childbearing age should have two concerns—(1) contraceptive failure due to medication interactions and (2) potential risk to mother and fetus caused by the drug should pregnancy occur.

Some medications have been associated with a possible risk of contraceptive failure (Table 43-3). Azathioprine[2] and nonsteroidal antiinflammatory agents (NSAIDs),[3] for example, have been associated with increased risk of contraceptive failure of the intrauterine device. Oral contraceptive failure may occur when the oral contraceptive is taken along with hepatic enzyme inducers such as griseofulvin,[4] that may increase metabolism of estrogen due to induction of hepatic microsomal enzymes.[5] Other oral medications that may reduce oral contraceptive effectiveness include rifampin,[6] which may stimulate estrogen metabolism or reduce enterohepatic circulation of estrogens, and penicillins,[7] which reduce enterohepatic circulation of estrogens. Tetracyclines[8] and sulfonamides[9] may increase breakthrough bleeding and reduce contraceptive effectiveness. Although data are sparse, pregnancy has been reported when itraconazole was used with an oral contraceptive,[10,11] suggesting that it may be a possible cause of oral contraceptive failure. However, in one study itraconazole was not found to affect plasma levels of ethinyl estradiol or norethindrone.[12] Therefore substantive data conclude that itraconazole affects hormone metabolism are absent. Both males and females should avoid methotrexate[13] if pregnancy is anticipated. A single author recommended that both males and females avoid griseofulvin,[14] but no substantiation was given.

Timing—First Trimester

During very early pregnancy, encompassing the first 2 to 2½ weeks of gestation (4 to 4½ weeks

Table 43-2 Sources for Information on Drug Use During Pregnancy and Lactation

United States Pharmacopeia Dispensing Information, Volume I (USP-DI)	• This volume, updated yearly, contains detailed information on mutagenicity, carcinogenicity, effects on fertility, teratogenicity, and lactation. • Information is available through USPC, 12601 Twinbrook Parkway, Rockville, MD 02780.
Teratogen Information Service (TERIS)	• Information generated by this group of teratologists includes a rating of exposure risk to humans of specific agents during pregnancy. • TERIS risks are rated none, unlikely, minimal, moderate, and high. • Qualifying these risks is an evaluation of data on which these risks have been based: none, poor, limited, fair, good, and excellent. • Information is available through TERIS, Department of Pediatrics, RES 207, CDMRC WJ 10, University of Washington, Seattle, WA 98195, or online at http://weber.u.washington.edu/~terisweb/ There is a nominal charge per summary.
Reproductive Toxicology Service	• This is a computer-based software or online program available by subscription. • References on the effects of drugs and physical agents on human fertility, pregnancy, and fetal development are updated regularly. • No rating system is included. • Information is available through Reproductive Toxicology Center, Columbia Hospital for Women Medical Center, 2440 M Street, NW Suite 217, Washington, DC 20037-14-4.
The American Academy of Pediatrics (AAP)	• Reviews information on effects of drugs on lactation and publishes a rating list every several years.
The World Health Organization (WHO)	• A book on lactation, available through libraries.*
Briggs et al	• A regularly updated text reviewing risks of drugs during pregnancy and lactation.†

*The WHO Working Group. Bennett PN, ed: *Drugs and human lactation*, Amsterdam, 1996, Elsevier; see also Ito S: Drug therapy for breast-feeding women. *N Engl J Med* 343:118-126, 2000.
†Briggs GG, Freeman RK, Yaffe SL: *Drugs in pregnancy and lactation*, ed 5, Baltimore, 1998, Williams and Wilkins.

Table 43-3 Medications Reportedly Associated With Contraceptive Failure

Drug	Contraceptive Drug	Proposed Mechanism
Azathioprine	Intrauterine devices	Unknown
NSAIDs	Intrauterine devices	Unknown
Griseofulvin	Oral contraceptives	Increased estrogen metabolism by hepatic microsomal enzyme induction
Rifampin	Oral contraceptives	Increased estrogen metabolism by hepatic microsomal enzyme induction *or* reduced enterohepatic circulation of estrogens
Tetracycline*	Oral contraceptives	Reduced enterohepatic circulation of estrogens
Sulfonamides*	Oral contraceptives	Reduced enterohepatic circulation of estrogens
Itraconazole*	Oral contraceptives	Unknown

*Aside from CYP enzyme inducers (griseofulvin and rifampin), other antibacterial agents and itraconazole have significant controversy regarding whether there truly is a causal role in contraceptive failure.

after the first day of the last normal menstrual cycle), cells are undifferentiated. Drugs administered during this period affect all cells equally, either killing the organism or having no effect. The net effect tends to be spontaneous abortion rather than any congenital anomalies. Animal studies reflect this finding as toxicity. Toxicity is considered as a potentially adverse outcome of pregnancy in the current FDA pregnancy categories. Human toxicity studies have not been done, due to difficulties in studying large numbers of patients using drugs in an ethical manner.

Organogenesis lasts from weeks 2 to 8 of gestation (weeks 4 to 10 after the first day of the last menstrual cycle) of the pregnancy. Differentiating cells may be affected by particular drugs and result in congenital anomalies. During this period, it is important to avoid all medications known to have possible teratogenic effects. This includes all medications listed as FDA pregnancy category X or D, as well as some drugs with other ratings or drugs that are unrated. Exceptions on an individual basis may be considered when use is essential. A list of medications that have been most clearly established as teratogenic is included in Box 43-2 and Table 43-4.

Timing—Second Trimester

In midpregnancy, maturation of various organ systems occurs. Drug metabolism by the fetus may occur at a rate different from that of the mother, with a potential effect for allowing prolonged fetal exposure to medications if fetal metabolism is slower than that of the mother. An example is maternal iodide use, which may result in fetal hypothyroidism.[15,16]

Drug excretion by the fetus into amniotic fluid also may theoretically promote prolonged exposure by virtue of skin contact with amniotic fluid or through amniotic fluid ingestion by the infant.[17] No known examples are available.

Timing—Third Trimester and Preterm

Late in pregnancy, especially near the time of delivery, nonteratogenic conditions may occur. Drugs, such as sulfonamides, which may produce kernicterus[9]; NSAIDs, which may promote persistent fetal circulation or oligohydramnios[18]; and rifampin, which has been associated with fetal hemorrhage,[6] should be avoided during this time. Maternal use of doxepin at birth may place infants at risk for respiratory depression.[19]

Timing—During Lactation

In general, use of drugs known to be teratogenic is not advised during lactation (see Box 43-2 and Table 43-4). This includes all antineoplastic agents, due to a risk of immunosuppression or possible association with carcinogenesis.

Box 43-2

Pregnancy Category X—Avoid in Pregnancy and Lactation

Acitretin	Flutamide
Estrogens	Isotretinoin
Etretinate	Methotrexate*
Finasteride	Stanozolol
Fluorouracil	Thalidomide*

*Both males and females should avoid if pregnancy is anticipated.

■ Table 43-4 Pregnancy Category D or Unrated—Drugs to Avoid in Pregnancy and Lactation

Drug	Category D	Unrated
Aspirin*	✓	
Azathioprine	✓	
Bleomycin	✓	
Colchicine	✓	
Cyclophosphamide	✓	
Griseofulvin		✓
Hydroxyurea	✓	
Mechlorethamine	✓	
Penicillamine	✓	
Potassium Iodide	✓	
Spironolactone		✓
Tetracycline	✓	

*High-dose, extended-release form should be avoided.

Many women elect to avoid exposure to all drugs, fearing some as-yet-undiscovered problem. The physician should be aware of and respectful of this wish while being able to advise patients of drugs that place them and their babies at minimal risk. Further, physicians should be mindful that treatment of some dermatologic conditions, such as onychomycosis, can be safely deferred until the completion of pregnancy and lactation.

GUIDE FOR SPECIFIC DRUG USE

Boxes 43-3 and 43-4 list drugs that are relatively safe during pregnancy and lactation.

Box 43-3

Drugs With Minimal Risk to Mother and Fetus During Pregnancy

ANALGESICS
Acetaminophen
Aspirin— low dose (avoid third trimester)
Codeine—low dose
Ibuprofen—low dose (avoid third trimester)
Meperidine—low dose
Oxycodone—low dose
Pentazocine—low dose
Propoxyphene—low dose

ANESTHETICS
Bupivicaine
Lidocaine
Lidocaine with epinephrine
Lidocaine-prilocaine
Mepivicaine

ANTIBACTERIAL AGENTS
Bacitracin—topical
Clindamycin—topical
Erythromycin (except estolate)
Erythromycin—topical
Metronidazole—topical
Mupirocin—topical
Neomycin—topical
Penicillins
Polymyxin B—topical
Sulfonamides (except third trimester)
Sulfur—topical
Sulfur with resorcinol—topical
Tetracycline—topical

ANTIFUNGAL AGENTS*
Butaconazole—topical
Ciclopirox—topical

ANTIFUNGAL AGENTS—cont'd
Clotrimazole—topical (except first trimester)
Econazole—topical (except first trimester)
Fluconazole single dose
Ketoconazole—topical
Miconazole—topical (except first trimester)
Naftifine—topical
Nystatin—oral and topical
Oxiconazole—topical
Sulconazole—topical
Terbinafine—topical
Terconazole—topical (except first trimester)
Tioconazole—topical

ANTIHISTAMINES†
Brompheniramine (except first trimester)
Cetirizine (except first trimester)
Chlorpheniramine
Cyproheptadine
Diphenhydramine
Hydroxyzine (except first trimester)

ANTIMALARIALS
Chloroquine‡

ANTIPROTOZOAL AGENTS
Metronidazole (except first trimester)

ANTISCABETIC AGENTS
Crotamiton—topical
Lindane—topical (maximum twice during pregnancy)
Malathion—topical
Permethrin—topical
Precipitated sulfur—topical

*Avoid vaginal use after membrane rupture.
†Avoid last 2 weeks of pregnancy if fetus is premature.
‡Approved for use during pregnancy only for hepatic amebiasis or malaria.   *Continued*

Box 43-3

Drugs With Minimal Risk to Mother and Fetus During Pregnancy—cont'd

ANTIVIRAL AGENTS§
Acyclovir
Famciclovir
Valacyclovir

CORTICOSTEROIDS
Oral: avoid high doses first trimester
Topical: avoid high doses long term

MISCELLANEOUS—TOPICAL ANTIACNE PRODUCTS
Benzoyl peroxide
Tretinoin (except first trimester)

MISCELLANEOUS—OTHER DRUGS
Calcipotriene—topical (low doses)
Dapsone (except close to term)
Hydroquinone—topical
Methoxsalen—topical

§Restrict use to treatment of severe herpesvirus infections.

Box 43-4

Drugs With Minimal Risk to Mother and Infant During Lactation

ANALGESICS
Acetaminophen
Codeine (low dose)
Meperidine (low dose)
Morphine (low dose)
Oxycodone (low dose)
Pentazocine (low dose)
Propoxyphene (low dose)

ANESTHETICS
Bupivacaine (low strength)
Lidocaine
Lidocaine with epinephrine
Lidocaine-prilocaine
Mepivacaine

ANTIBACTERIAL AGENTS
Bacitracin—topical
Cephalosporins
Erythromycins
Erythromycin—topical
Penicillins
Sulfur—topical
Sulfur with resorcinol—topical
Tetracycline—topical

ANTIFUNGAL AGENTS
Butoconazole—topical
Ciclopirox—topical
Clotrimazole—topical
Econazole—topical
Miconazole—topical
Naftifine—topical
Nystatin—oral and topical

ANTIFUNGAL AGENTS—cont'd
Oxiconazole—topical
Sulconazole—topical
Terbinafine—topical

ANTIHISTAMINES
(Concern for all antihistamines regarding inhibition of milk production and infantile irritability)

ANTIVIRAL AGENTS
Acyclovir
Valacyclovir

ANTISCABETIC AGENTS
Crotamiton—topical

CORTICOSTEROIDS
Oral: use prednisolone, avoid nursing for 4 hours after use
Topical: avoid use of nipple or areola

MISCELLANEOUS—TOPICAL ANTIACNE PRODUCTS
Azelaic acid
Benzoyl peroxide
Tretinoin

MISCELLANEOUS—OTHER DRUGS
Allopurinol
Calcipotriene—topical
Hydroquinone—topical
Masoprocol—topical
Methoxsalen—topical

ANALGESICS
Pregnancy
ACETAMINOPHEN. Studies to date on *aceta-minophen* (FDA pregnancy category B; TERIS* risk rated none based on good data, except at toxic levels) have not been associated with problems in humans.[20-22] Even where toxic overdoses have occurred during the first and second trimesters, most infants have been normal and there were no adverse outcomes attributable to the acetaminophen.[23] One fatality occurred in an infant whose mother took an acetaminophen overdose during the last trimester.[24] Low doses of acetaminophen are not associated with identifiable risk to the fetus during any trimester of pregnancy.

ASPIRIN. Although *aspirin* (FDA pregnancy category C, D for extended release forms; TERIS risk rated none-to-minimal based on data rated fair-to-good for occasional use of low doses of aspirin) is a known animal teratogen, studies failed to show embryotoxicity or teratogenicity in humans. Late in pregnancy, use of aspirin has been associated with neonatal and fetal hemorrhage.[25,26] There are also infrequent reports of premature closure of the ductus arteriosus,[27] postmaturity syndrome,[28] and gastroschisis.[29] Many studies show that low-dose aspirin has been successfully used to prevent fetal growth retardation, pregnancy-induced hypertension, and stillbirth.[30] On one hand, avoidance of aspirin during pregnancy has been recommended.[31] However, aspirin in low doses does not appear to be associated with teratogenic effects. Fetal or neonatal hemorrhage remains the greater concern for such low-dose aspirin therapy during the last trimester of pregnancy.

NSAIDs. *Indomethacin* (FDA unrated pregnancy category; TERIS risk for congenital malformations rated none-to-minimal based on data rated poor-to-fair; TERIS risk for premature closure of the ductus arteriosus small to moderate based on data rated fair-to-good) has been associated with oligohydramnios[17,32,33] and premature closure of the ductus arteriosus[34,35]

when used in the last trimester of pregnancy. Indomethacin has also been associated with necrotizing enterocolitis,[36] intracranial hemorrhage,[37] anuria,[38] and isolated ileal perforation.[39] Although studies have not been done on other NSAIDs, it has been recommended that all NSAIDs be avoided during the second and third trimesters.[18] Other NSAIDs include *ibuprofen* (FDA pregnancy category B; TERIS risk minimal based on data rated fair), *ketoprofen* (FDA pregnancy category B; TERIS risk unrated), and *naproxen* (FDA pregnancy category B; TERIS risk undetermined based on data rated limited). Animal studies show prolongation of gestation and delayed birth.[18] Although there are significant problems reported with use of NSAIDs during the second and third trimesters of pregnancy, use of these drugs during the first trimester has not been associated with predictable congenital anomalies.[40]

OPIOID NARCOTICS. Narcotics, such as *codeine* (FDA pregnancy category C; TERIS risk none-to-minimal based on data rated fair-to-good); *meperidine* (FDA pregnancy category C; TERIS risk rated unlikely based on data rated fair), *oxycodone* (FDA pregnancy category C; TERIS rated undetermined based on data rated poor), and *pentazocine* (FDA pregnancy category C; TERIS risk rated minimal based on data rated poor-to-fair) may be used for very short periods of time in small amounts. Use of high doses of codeine in late pregnancy, such as by addicts, has been associated with development of withdrawal symptoms in infants.[41] Respiratory malformation has been shown in humans with first-trimester use of codeine.[42] *Morphine* (FDA pregnancy category C; TERIS rating for congenital anomalies unlikely based on data rated fair-to-good; TERIS rating for neonatal neurobehavioral defects moderate based on data rated fair-to-good) is not reported to be a teratogen.[43] A single study showed an association between morphine use in mothers and inguinal hernias in children.[44] Another study showed that morphine was more likely than other drugs to produce respiratory depression in the neonate.[45] Morphine in occasional doses is not thought to cause problems in children. However, animal studies show persistent neurologic problems in offspring of animals exposed in utero,[46,47] and in

---

TERIS, Teratogen Information Service.

humans there is a significant withdrawal syndrome in infants of addicted mothers.[48] *Propoxyphene* (FDA pregnancy category C; TERIS risk rated none based on data rated good) has not been associated with an increase in congenital anomalies.[49] Risk of overdose to the infant is not known, although there have been withdrawal symptoms in infants of mothers who chronically took high doses,[50,51] and long-lasting behavioral abnormalities occurred in infants of women who chronically used propoxyphene.[52] Except for morphine, use of low doses of opioid narcotics on isolated occasions during pregnancy has not been associated with teratogenicity. The biggest risk is that of withdrawal symptoms after chronic maternal use and respiratory depression when used in high doses around the time of delivery.

Lactation
ACETAMINOPHEN. *Acetaminophen* may be used during lactation. During lactation, dose-related metabolic acidosis has been reported in an infant of a mother who had used *aspirin*. Serum salicylate level was 24 mg/dl in the infant; no maternal milk or serum salicylate levels were obtained.[53] There has been speculation as to whether the infant's salicylate level was elevated solely from consumption of breast milk.

NSAIDs. The use of *ibuprofen, ketoprofen*, and *naproxen* during lactation is controversial, with manufacturers advising against use.[54-56] In contrast, the American Academy of Pediatrics (AAP) rated use of NSAIDs as "usually compatible with lactation."[57] Use of *indomethacin* during lactation has been associated with convulsions in an infant.[58] If alternate drugs are available, they are preferable to indomethacin in both pregnancy and lactation.

OPIOID NARCOTICS. All of the opioid narcotics are excreted in low amounts in breast milk. The AAP lists *codeine, morphine*, and *propoxyphene* as compatible with breast feeding.[57] *Meperidine* has also been rated as compatible with breastfeeding in an earlier AAP publication[59] but it is not listed at all in the current AAP article.[57] *Pentazocine* and *oxycodone* have not been rated.

ANESTHETICS
Pregnancy
LOCAL ANESTHETICS. *Lidocaine* (FDA pregnancy category B; TERIS risk for local administration rated none based on data rated fair), *lidocaine with epinephrine* (FDA pregnancy category B; TERIS risk for use of therapeutic doses of epinephrine rated unlikely based on data rated fair), and *lidocaine-prilocaine* (FDA pregnancy category B; TERIS risk for local administration of prilocaine rated none based on data rated fair) have no contraindications to use during pregnancy. *Mepivacaine*[60] (FDA pregnancy category C; TERIS risk rated unlikely based on data rated limited) and *bupivacaine*[61] (FDA pregnancy category C; TERIS risk rated undetermined based on data rated limited) are for use "only if the potential benefit justifies the potential risk to the fetus" during pregnancy. In the doses used for small excisional biopsies in dermatologic practice, use of these anesthetics poses no appreciable risk to the mother or fetus.

Lactation
Lidocaine, lidocaine-prilocaine, mepivacaine, and *bupivacaine* may be used during lactation.

ANTIBIOTICS
Pregnancy
CEPHALOSPORINS. This drug family, including *cephalexin* (FDA pregnancy category B; TERIS risk rated undetermined based on data rated poor), *cefaclor* (FDA pregnancy category B; TERIS risk rated undetermined based on data rated very limited), and *cephradine* (FDA pregnancy category B; TERIS risk rated unlikely based on data rated limited-to-fair), has been reported to have a possible increase in risk of congenital defects with use during the first trimester; however, this is controversial.[63] *Cefadroxil* (FDA pregnancy category B; TERIS risk rated undetermined based on data rated very limited) use has not been associated with risk.[64] An earlier small study of women who took cephalosporins showed no increase in risk of congenital malformations.[65] No problems in the fetus have been reported after the first trimester. Until other information clarifies these findings, use of erythromycins and penicillins is prefer-

able to cephalosporins in pregnancy, especially during the first trimester.

ERYTHROMYCIN AND RELATED MACROLIDES. *Erythromycin* (FDA pregnancy category B; TERIS risk rated none based on data rated fair-to-good) has been used without reported risk, except for erythromycin estolate. *Erythromycin estolate* use has been associated with a subclinical maternal hepatotoxicity when used for longer than 3 weeks and should be avoided.[64-66] Except for estolates, erythromycins may be used during any trimester of pregnancy. Erythromycins (along with penicillins) should be considered first-choice antibiotics during pregnancy.

Azithromycin (FDA pregnancy category B; TERIS risk rated undetermined based on data rated very poor) is chemically related to erythromycin. It has not been associated with a reported risk.

Clarithromycin (FDA pregnancy category C; TERIS risk rated undetermined based on data rated none) has been associated with cardiovascular defects and fetotoxicity in animals at high doses.[67] Birth defects are diverse and may be coincidental rather than related by cause.[68] A small study has shown normal infants born to mothers who took clarithromycin.[69] Use of clarithromycin during pregnancy should be avoided pending further data.

Dirithromycin (FDA pregnancy category C; TERIS risk unrated) shows an increase in mental retardation and incomplete ossification in offspring of rats that had used the drug during pregnancy.[70] Studies in humans have not been done. Use of dirithromycin during pregnancy should be avoided pending further data.

FLUOROQUINOLONES. Drugs in this category include *ciprofloxacin, ofloxacin, levofloxacin, lomefloxacin, norfloxacin, enoxacin, trovafloxacin, sparfloxacin,* and *nalidixic acid. All* are FDA pregnancy category C. For ciprofloxacin, the TERIS risk is rated unlikely based on data rated fair. Some drugs in this class of antibacterial agents have been associated in animals with a potential risk of arthropathy,[71] but postmarketing studies failed to confirm a similar pattern in infants of mothers who have used the drug.[72-74] Because of this controversy, use of fluoroquinolones as a first-line drug during pregnancy is not advised; however, accidental administration of fluoroquinolones during pregnancy should not be an indication for abortion.[75]

PENICILLINS. Beta-lactam antibacterial agents of the penicillin family (FDA pregnancy category B; TERIS risk rated none based on data rated good) have not been associated with an increased risk of congenital anomalies. Briggs[76] stated that it is unlikely that *penicillin G, penicillin V, amoxicillin, ampicillin,* or *dicloxacillin* is teratogenic. Use of penicillins during pregnancy is not contraindicated. Penicillins (as well as erythromycins) may be considered first-line antibiotics during all trimesters of pregnancy.

SULFONAMIDES. It has been documented that sulfonamide antibiotics (FDA pregnancy category C; TERIS risk rated unlikely-to-minimal based on data rated limited-to-fair) are associated with increased risk of kernicterus and hemolysis in the newborn who is glucose-6-phosphate dehydrogenase (G6PD)-deficient.[77-78] Because it is not feasible to determine the status of G6PD deficiency in the fetus, use during late pregnancy or in the case of possible premature birth is not advised. Use during early pregnancy is not contraindicated, although other antibiotics have better data indicating no risk.

TETRACYCLINES. *Tetracyclines* (FDA pregnancy category D; TERIS risk for congenital anomalies rated none-to-minimal based on data rated fair; TERIS risk for dental anomalies rated high based on data rated excellent) are known to be a risk during the second and third trimesters because of their effects on dental staining and enamel hypoplasia.[79,80] Use of tetracycline during early pregnancy has not been associated with congenital anomalies.[81,82] *Minocycline* (FDA pregnancy category D; TERIS risk for congenital anomalies rated undetermined based on data rated very poor) and *doxycycline* (FDA pregnancy category D; TERIS risk for congenital anomalies rated unlikely based on data rated limited-to-fair; TERIS risk for dental anomalies rated undetermined based on data rated very limited) have not had reports of dental staining in infants born to mothers who used the drugs during the second or third trimesters. Because of their structural relationship to tetracycline, however, they are not advised for use during the second or third trimesters of pregnancy. Tetracyclines should also be avoided during the second and third trimesters of pregnancy.

TOPICAL ANTIBACTERIAL AGENTS.   Various topical antibacterial agents such as *erythromycin* (FDA pregnancy category B or C), *mupirocin* (FDA pregnancy category B; TERIS risk rated undetermined based on data rated none), *clindamycin* (FDA pregnancy category B; TERIS risk for oral use rated undetermined based on data rated poor, but high risk unlikely), *bacitracin* (FDA unrated pregnancy category; TERIS risk rated undetermined based on data rated none), *polymyxin B* (FDA unrated pregnancy category; TERIS risk rated undetermined based on data rated none), and *neomycin* (FDA unrated pregnancy category; TERIS risk for topical use rated none based on data rated poor-to-fair) have not been associated with teratogenicity.

Topical erythromycin and neomycin may be used during pregnancy. Use of small doses of the prescription drugs topical clindamycin and mupirocin, as well as the over-the-counter drugs bacitracin and polymyxin B, has not been associated with any risk to the fetus, though large studies have not been conducted.

Topical application of *silver sulfadiazine* (FDA pregnancy category B; TERIS risk rated unlikely based on data rated poor-to-fair) during the late third trimester is thought to pose a potential risk for kernicterus and hemorrhage in the premature infant or the infant with G6PD deficiency. Use in the third trimester is not advised by the manufacturers.[83,84]

Topical *sulfur* with or without *sodium sulfacetamide* or *resorcinol* (FDA pregnancy category C; TERIS risk rated none based on data rated poor-to-fair) has not been associated with kernicterus. The manufacturers recommend use "only if clearly needed."[85,86] Use of topical sulfur or sulfacetamide is not contraindicated during pregnancy.

Lactation
ORAL ANTIBACTERIAL AGENTS.   During lactation, oral *erythromycin, clarithromycin,*

dirithromycin, and *azithromycin* may be used with caution.[87,88] Azithromycin distribution in breast milk is not documented.[89] *Cephalosporins* may also be used with caution.[90]

Fluoroquinolones are not recommended as first-line antibiotics during lactation because of the risk of arthropathy in animals.[71]

Both oral *sulfonamides*[91] as well as topical *silver sulfadiazine*[83,84] are discouraged during lactation because of the possible risk of kernicterus to the fetus.

Systemic *tetracycline* use is controversial; the AAP states that tetracycline use is compatible with lactation,[57] and the World Health Organization (WHO) states that risk to the infant is low if antibiotic use is limited to less than 7 to 10 days.[92] However, others say that use during lactation should be avoided,[93] and there is a troublesome report of black milk with use of *minocycline* during lactation.[94] Tetracycline and derivatives should not be used routinely during lactation.

TOPICAL ANTIBACTERIAL AGENTS.   Topical *clindamycin* appears in very small amounts in milk.[95] Bloody stools have been reported in an infant whose mother was using clindamycin, although the etiology was not proven.[96] The manufacturer recommends against use during lactation,[97] although the AAP has rated oral clindamycin as compatible with lactation.[57]

Topical *erythromycins* are compatible with lactation,[98] as are topical *sulfur* preparations and topical *sodium sulfacetamide.*[85,86] The AAP has no rating for these topical drugs.

ANTIACNE PRODUCTS—TOPICAL
Pregnancy
ADAPALENE.   *Adapalene* (FDA pregnancy category C; TERIS unrated) is a topical retinoid for treatment of acne. As with other retinoids, use during pregnancy is discouraged.[99] There has been a recent report of congenital anomaly involving the eye with use of adapalene.[100] Adapalene should be avoided during pregnancy pending further information.

AZELAIC ACID.   *Azelaic acid* (FDA pregnancy category B; TERIS unrated) has not shown mutagenicity, teratogenicity, or embryotoxicity in animals.[101,102] Minimal absorption of topically applied doses occurs. Given these facts, it is unlikely that small doses of topical azelaic acid pose any risk during pregnancy.

BENZOYL PEROXIDE.   *Benzoyl peroxide* (FDA pregnancy category C; TERIS risk rated undetermined based on no data available, but states that although a small risk cannot be excluded, a high risk of congenital anomalies is unlikely) are widely available over-the-counter and as prescriptions. Although benzoyl peroxide may potentiate the carcinogenic risk of ultraviolet B (UVB) in the skin, this drug is not a carcinogen. Use during pregnancy is not contraindicated.[103,104]

METRONIDAZOLE.   Oral *metronidazole* (FDA pregnancy category B; TERIS risk of oral drug rated unlikely based on data rated good) has not been associated with congenital anomalies in humans when used orally in the first[105-107] or third[108,109] trimesters. Use of topical and vaginal metronidazole carries an "only if clearly needed" warning from the manufacturers.[110,111] There is no contraindication to use of topical metronidazole during any trimester of pregnancy.

TRETINOIN.   *Tretinoin* (FDA pregnancy category C; TERIS risk rated unlikely based on data rated fair) has been associated in case reports with teratogenicity when used during the first trimester.[112-114] A controlled study, however, failed to corroborate this risk.[115] Assuming maximal absorption, one study estimated that daily use of one gram of a 0.1% tretinoin preparation would result in serum levels of less than 15% of the vitamin A from a standard prenatal vitamin A preparation.[116] No ill effects have been reported in infants of mothers who used topical tretinoin after the first trimester of pregnancy, and one article states that topical tretinoin is a drug that may be used safely during pregnancy.[117] Because use of topical tretinoin is usually elective, and because other drugs are available for treatment of acne, topical tretinoin should be avoided during the first trimester. Use during the second and third trimesters may be considered in consultation with the woman and her obstetrician to avoid any possible confusion and misunderstanding.

Lactation

Topical *azelaic acid*[101,102] and *benzoyl peroxide*[103] have no contraindication to use during lactation. Topical *metronidazole* is unlikely to be absorbed in significant amounts to be a problem during lactation, although systemic metronidazole use is not advised.[118]

Studies of use of topical *tretinoin* during lactation in animals have shown no adverse effects.[116] The minimal amounts found in milk are not felt to be harmful to infants.[119]

ANTIFUNGAL AGENTS
Pregnancy

FLUCONAZOLE.   *Fluconazole* (FDA pregnancy category C; TERIS risk rated undetermined based on data rated very poor) in high doses has been associated with human malformations.[120,121] Teratogenicity at high doses has been reported in rodents.[122,123] Elective use of prolonged doses of fluconazole during pregnancy should be avoided during the first two trimesters of pregnancy pending further information.[124] Single-dose fluconazole does not appear to be associated with increased risk to the fetus during pregnancy.[124]

GRISEOFULVIN.   There have been several reports implicating *griseofulvin* (FDA unrated pregnancy category; TERIS risk rated undetermined based on data rated poor, with an added comment that a small risk cannot be excluded but high risk is unlikely) as a possible etiology for conjoined twins.[125,126] Animal studies show increased frequencies of fetal death, growth retardation, and skeletal anomalies, but the significance of this to humans is not known.[4] No congenital anomalies in humans other than conjoined twins have been reported. Some authors recommend that, because of this possible risk, griseofulvin use before or during early pregnancy should be avoided.[127-129]

ITRACONAZOLE.   *Itraconazole* (FDA pregnancy category C; TERIS risk rated undetermined based on data rated very poor) showed dose-related embryotoxicity and teratogenicity in rodents, thought to be due to adrenal effects.[130] Itraconazole has been used safely in a reported single pregnancy.[131] Risk of human teratogenicity with itraconazole is thought to be lowest of the systemic azole antifungal agents because in contrast with fluconazole and ketoconazole, itraconazole has little effect on steroid hormones.[132] Elective use of itraconazole during pregnancy, however, should probably be avoided pending further information.

KETOCONAZOLE. *Ketoconazole* (FDA pregnancy category C; TERIS risk rated undetermined based on data rated very poor for oral use; TERIS risk rated undetermined based on data rated none) has been associated with human[133] and animal teratogenicity and should be avoided, especially during the first trimester.[134] Ketoconazole use has been associated with impairment of progesterone secretion and prevention of implantation in rats, indicating that it may interfere with early pregnancy.[135] Ketoconazole use during the third trimester for treatment of hypercortisolism of Cushing's syndrome may be appropriate if the fetus is female.[136] Elective use of ketoconazole during pregnancy should be avoided pending further information.

NYSTATIN. *Nystatin* (FDA pregnancy category B; TERIS risk rated none based on data rated fair-to-good) is associated with no known risk to the fetus during pregnancy.[20,21] Nystatin use during all trimesters of pregnancy is not contraindicated.

TERBINAFINE. Animal studies evaluating oral *terbinafine* (FDA pregnancy category B; TERIS unrated) in pregnancy showed production of benign tumors in rats (tumorigenicity) but not fetal loss (animal toxicity).[137] Studies in humans have not been done. Although it is rated FDA pregnancy category B, the manufacturer advises against use for onychomycosis because treatment during pregnancy is elective.[138] Elective use of terbinafine during pregnancy should be avoided pending further information.

TOPICAL ANTIFUNGAL AGENTS. *Clotrimazole* (FDA pregnancy category B; TERIS risk rated unlikely based on data rated limited-to-fair, with comment that data are insufficient to state that there is no risk) used during the first trimester of pregnancy as an oral or topical treatment of vaginitis has been associated with a slightly increased risk of congenital defects in humans in one study.[139] Others note no adverse effects to the fetus.[140,141] Topical clotrimazole use after the first trimester of pregnancy and until membrane rupture has not been associated with adverse effects.

Miconazole (FDA pregnancy category C; TERIS risk for topical use rated unlikely based on data rated fair-to-good; TERIS risk for oral use rated undetermined based on data rated limited, with comment that data are insufficient to state that there is no risk) has been associated with animal fetotoxicity. Briggs states that data do not support an association between use of the drug and congenital defects.[142] Topical miconazole use after the first trimester of pregnancy and until membrane rupture has not been associated with adverse effects.

Topical *butaconazole* (FDA pregnancy category C), *ciclopirox* (FDA pregnancy category B), *ketoconazole* (FDA pregnancy category C), *naftifine* (FDA pregnancy category B), *nystatin* (FDA pregnancy category B), *oxiconazole* (FDA pregnancy category B), *sulconazole* (FDA pregnancy category C), *terbinafine* (FDA pregnancy category B), and *tioconazole* (FDA pregnancy category C) have not been studied in humans. There are no case reports associated with problems during pregnancy.

The manufacturers of *econazole* (FDA pregnancy category C),[143] *miconazole* (FDA pregnancy category B),[144] and *terconazole* (FDA pregnancy category C)[145] recommend that, during the first trimester, these products be used only when essential to the mother's welfare. Topical administration of intravaginal yeast medications is not advised close to term, as there is a risk of uterine contamination if membranes have been ruptured.[146]

Selenium sulfide (FDA pregnancy category C, for tinea versicolor; TERIS risk rated undetermined based on no data, with a comment that small risk cannot be excluded but a high risk is unlikely) should not be used by pregnant women for tinea versicolor according to the manufacturer[147] because no animal or human studies have been performed and the risk to the fetus is not known.

Lactation

SYSTEMIC ANTIFUNGAL AGENTS. The manufacturers of *fluconazole*,[122] *itraconazole*,[148] *ketoconazole*,[149] and *terbinafine*[158] recommend against use, although one reviewer states that fluconazole is "probably safe" for use during lactation.[150] No guidelines for use of *griseofulvin* are available.

TOPICAL ANTIFUNGAL AGENTS. The manufacturers of topical *ketoconazole*,[151] *terbinafine*,[152] *terconazole*,[145] and *tioconazole*[153] recommend against use of these products during lactation. *Butoconazole*,[154] *ciclopirox*,[155] *clotrimazole*,[156,157] *econazole*,[143] *miconazole*,[144] *naftifine*,[158] *oxiconazole*,[159] and *sulconazole*[160] may be used with caution during lactation. There are no published cautions against use of *nystatin*.[161]

Selenium sulfide should not be used over large areas for treatment of tinea versicolor during lactation, according to the manufacturer.[147] Selenium sulfide has been associated with suppression of lactation. The mechanism is not known.

ANTIHISTAMINES
Pregnancy

In a retrospective cohort study of 3025 infants with a birthweight of less than 1750 g, use of antihistamines during the last 2 weeks of pregnancy was associated with an increased incidence of retrolental fibroplasia.[162] The type of antihistamine was not identified.

ASTEMIZOLE.* *Astemizole* (FDA pregnancy category C; TERIS risk rated unlikely based on data rated limited-to-fair; high risk is unlikely but insufficient data to show no risk) has a very long half-life. Few problems have been documented with human use. The manufacturer recommends use only if the potential benefit justifies the potential risk to the fetus.[163] Astemizole has been listed as a drug that may be safely used during pregnancy.[103]

BROMPHENIRAMINE. *Brompheniramine* (FDA pregnancy category B; TERIS risk rated none based on data rated fair) has been associ-

---

*Currently off the market in the United States.

ated with congenital defects when used during the first trimester.[164,165] Use of brompheniramine during the second and third trimesters of pregnancy is not contraindicated.

CHLORPHENIRAMINE. There have been no studies documenting a risk of congenital malformations from *chlorpheniramine* (FDA pregnancy category B; TERIS risk rated unlikely based on data rated fair-to-good, but insufficient data to claim no risk) use during pregnancy. Use of chlorpheniramine is not contraindicated during any trimester of pregnancy.

CIMETIDINE. There is significant controversy regarding use of *cimetidine* (FDA pregnancy category C; TERIS risk rated undetermined based on data rated limited) during pregnancy. Cimetidine is a human antiandrogen, particularly at high doses. Use of this drug during pregnancies in animals has resulted in decreased weight of androgenic tissues,[165] and has been questionably associated with transient liver impairment in a single infant.[166] Pending further information, elective use of cimetidine during pregnancy should probably be avoided to obviate the theoretic risk of feminization of the fetus.[167]

CYPROHEPTADINE. *Cyproheptadine* (FDA pregnancy category B; TERIS risk rated undetermined based on data rated limited, high risk unlikely) has not been associated with problems during pregnancy.[168-170] The manufacturer reports that there is no increased risk of abnormalities when cyproheptadine is used in any of the three trimesters of pregnancy and that it should be used "only when clearly needed."[171] There are no large studies demonstrating safety.

DIPHENHYDRAMINE. *Diphenhydramine* (FDA pregnancy category B; TERIS risk rated unlikely based on data rated fair-to-good, but insufficient to state that there is no risk) has a long history of relatively uneventful use during pregnancy,[172] although it should probably be avoided during the last 2 weeks of pregnancy in case of prematurity.[173] Diphenhydramine use during pregnancy has been called "safe."[102] Many physicians consider diphenhydramine to be the antihistamine of choice for treatment of pruritus during pregnancy.

DOXEPIN. *Systemic doxepin* (FDA unrated pregnancy category; TERIS risk rated undetermined based on data rated poor) has been associated with fetal ileus,[174] as well as with cardiac problems, fetal irritability, respiratory distress, muscle spasm, and seizures in infants and should be avoided, especially close to the time of delivery.[19] Congenital malformations in humans with use in early pregnancy have not been reported. *Topical doxepin* (FDA pregnancy category B) is associated with less risk than is oral doxepin. The manufacturer states it may be used "only if clearly needed."[175] Elective use of topical doxepin in late pregnancy should be avoided.

FEXOFENADINE. The manufacturer states that the benefits should outweigh the risks for *fexofenadine* (FDA pregnancy category C; TERIS risk unrated), which has not been studied in humans during pregnancy.[176]

HYDROXYZINE. *Hydroxyzine* (FDA unrated pregnancy category; TERIS risk rated unlikely based on data rated poor-to-fair, but insufficient to state that there is no risk) is a teratogen in animals given multiples of the human dose.[177] The manufacturer of hydroxyzine contraindicates its use during pregnancy.[178] *Cetirizine* (FDA pregnancy category B; TERIS risk rated undetermined based on data rated limited-to-fair, but insufficient to state that there is no risk) is available by prescription in the United States and over-the-counter in Canada. Cetirizine is a metabolite of hydroxyzine. The manufacturer states that cetirizine should be used only if clearly needed,[179] but others say that cetirizine should not be used during the first trimester of pregnancy.[180] A small prospective study failed to demonstrate any increased risk to the fetus when hydroxyzine or cetirizine was used during pregnancy.[181] Recent studies listed hydroxyzine as a drug that may be used safely during pregnancy.[116,182,183] The most conservative position is to avoid hydroxyzine and cetirizine during the first trimester of pregnancy. Use of hydroxyzine and cetirizine during the second and third trimesters is not contraindicated, except during

the last 2 weeks of pregnancy if there is a threat of premature labor.[165]

LORATADINE. *Loratadine* (FDA pregnancy category B; TERIS risk rated undetermined based on data rated none) is chemically related to cyproheptadine. Adverse outcomes during pregnancy, including cleft palate, microtia, microphthalmia, deafness, dysmorphia, and diaphragmatic hernia, have been reported, although a clear relationship to the drug has not been established.[184] Its safety has not been established, and the manufacturer recommends use during pregnancy "only if clearly needed."[185]

TERFENADINE.* *Terfenadine* (FDA pregnancy category C; TERIS risk rated undetermined-poor, high risk unlikely) has been associated with decreased weight gain and survival of animal fetuses when used in high doses,[186] and has a possible association with polydactyly and other malformations in humans.[187] The manufacturer recommends use only if the potential benefit justifies the potential risk to the fetus.[188] Elective use of terfenadine should be avoided during pregnancy.

TRIMEPRAZINE. *Trimeprazine* (FDA unrated pregnancy category; TERIS risk unrated) has been associated with inconsistent fetal anomalies,[189,190] and its use in pregnancy is not recommended.[191] Pending further information, trimeprazine should be avoided during pregnancy.

Lactation
No antihistamines are recommended during lactation because of concern about the risk of lactation suppression and the effect on ability of the fetus to manage stress.[183]

Use of *cimetidine* is not recommended by the manufacturer[192] and USP-DI,[193] although WHO[194] classified it as safe for use during breast-feeding.

The manufacturer of *fexofenadine* states that there have been no studies of its use in lactation in humans and that the drug should be used with caution.[179]

---

*Currently off the market in the United States.

ANTIMALARIALS
Pregnancy
CHLOROQUINE AND HYDROXYCHLORO-QUINE.   Both *chloroquine* (FDA unrated pregnancy category; TERIS risk for daily dose rated minimal based on data rated poor-to-fair; TERIS risk for weekly dose rated none-to-minimal based on data rated poor-to-fair) and *hydroxychloroquine* (FDA unrated pregnancy category; TERIS risk rated undetermined based on data rated very limited, with high risk unlikely) are both accumulated in the fetal eye and retained in ocular tissue for at least 5 months.[195-197] Both carry official indications only for treatment and suppression of malaria or hepatic amebiasis.[196,197] However, some argue that the risk of flare of collagen vascular disease is also a risk for the fetus, and that continuation of antimalarials during pregnancy should be a consideration for mothers.[198-201]

QUINACRINE.   *Quinacrine* (FDA unrated pregnancy category; TERIS risk rated undetermined based on data rated very poor) has been associated with anomalies in an infant whose mother was exposed.[202] Pregnancies without adverse effects in the infant have also been reported.[203] The manufacturer advises against use during pregnancy, "except when in the judgment of the physician the benefit outweighs the possible hazard."[204]

Lactation
Use during lactation is somewhat controversial, although few reports of problems are available. WHO specifically states that *chloroquine* may be used but that *hydroxychloroquine* use during lactation should be avoided in patients with connective tissue disorders.[205] The AAP rated the risk of use of *chloroquine* and *hydroxychloroquine* as compatible with breast-feeding.[57] One author recommends that further studies be conducted before hydroxychloroquine is considered safe for use during lactation.[206]

The manufacturer of *quinacrine* provides no guidelines for use during lactation.

ANTIPROTOZOAN AGENTS
Pregnancy
ALBENDAZOLE.   *Albendazole* (FDA unrated pregnancy category; TERIS risk unrated) is teratogenic and embryotoxic in rats and rabbits. Its use in pregnant women is not recommended.[207] Pregnancy testing is recommended before use in a woman of childbearing age, and contraception should be used during the course of treatment and for 1 month thereafter.[208]

METRONIDAZOLE.   Studies evaluating *metronidazole* (FDA pregnancy category B; TERIS risk of oral drug rated none based on data rated good) found the drug to be a variable fetotoxin in animals[209,210] and carcinogenic in animals. One study in humans showed an increased incidence of malformations in infants born to mothers exposed to oral metronidazole during the first trimester of pregnancy, although no pattern of abnormality was found.[211] Manufacturers vary on recommendations for use of oral metronidazole during pregnancy; one manufacturer[118] advised against use of oral metronidazole during the first trimester, while another[212] advised that the same drug may be used "only if clearly needed."

Recent studies have not confirmed teratogenic risk of metronidazole in humans.[106-109,213] This new information is in contrast to that of previous authors who recommended avoidance of metronidazole during the first trimester of pregnancy.[214]

PENTAMIDINE.   *Pentamidine* (FDA pregnancy category C; TERIS risk rated undetermined based on data rated very poor) showed embryotoxicity and delayed ossification in rats.[215] Aerosolized pentamidine is also controversial, although this form of administration results in minimal delivery of drug to the fetus.[216] The manufacturer recommends use only if clearly needed.[217] Use of pentamidine during pregnancy is controversial.[218]

THIABENDAZOLE.   *Thiabendazole* (FDA pregnancy category C; TERIS risk rated undetermined based on data rated poor) has been associated with cleft palate in rats given high doses in olive oil but not in the aqueous preparation.[219] Topical thiabendazole is probably absorbed. No studies in humans are available, and the manufacturer recommends use of oral thiabendazole only if risk to the fetus justifies the potential benefit to the mother.[220]

Lactation

Use of *albendazole* in lactation has not been associated with risk,[212] although one of its metabolites is carcinogenic in animals.[221] Dermatologic use of albendazole during lactation should be avoided pending further information.

During lactation, use of systemic *metronidazole* is not recommended because of its carcinogenicity in animals. The AAP lists the risk of systemic metronidazole as unknown, but possibly of concern, and recommends that after a single dose of metronidazole, breast-feeding should be postponed for 12 to 24 hours to allow excretion of the drug.[57] Use of *pentamidine* during lactation is not recommended.[215,217]

The manufacturer recommends that *thiabendazole* be discontinued during lactation[220]; however, no reported problems with use of systemic or topical thiabendazole during lactation in humans have been encountered.

ANTISCABETICS

Pregnancy

CROTAMITON. *Crotamiton* (FDA pregnancy category C; TERIS risk rated undetermined based on data rated none) absorption in humans has not been studied. The manufacturer advises that because animal studies have not been done and risk is not fully understood, crotamiton should be used "only if clearly needed."[222] Adverse effects from use of crotamiton during pregnancy have not been reported.

IVERMECTIN. *Ivermectin* (FDA pregnancy category C; TERIS risk unrated) is teratogenic in animals at high doses.[223] One study has shown no significant increase in congenital anomalies when ivermectin was given during pregnancy.[224] Its use for treatment of scabies is not FDA-approved. Pending further studies, ivermectin should be avoided during pregnancy.

LINDANE. Use of *lindane* (FDA pregnancy category B; TERIS risk rated undetermined based on data rated poor, with high risk unlikely, but a substantial risk with doses high enough to be toxic to the pregnant woman) has been both discouraged[225-226] and, more recently, recommended.[227-229] In high doses in animal studies it

produced testicular degeneration.[230] In addition, lindane may be mildly estrogenic.[231] Misuse of the product or use on traumatized or otherwise abnormal skin is thought to be responsible for adverse occurrences.[232] Careful use of lindane is not contraindicated by the manufacturer[233]; lindane should be used for no longer than the label advises and no more than twice during a pregnancy.[234] Briggs[235] suggests that because of the potential toxicity of lindane, pyrethrins (such as permethrin) are recommended.

PERMETHRIN. Topical *permethrin* (FDA pregnancy category B; TERIS risk rated undetermined on data rated very poor and no indication that there is a high risk of congenital anomalies) has been recommended as the preferred treatment for scabies and lice during pregnancy.[236,237] Animal studies have not shown evidence of teratogenicity.[238] Permethrin is poorly absorbed.[239] Adverse reports are minimal considering the extensive use of permethrin.[240] The manufacturer recommends that permethrin be used "only if clearly needed."[241]

PRECIPITATED SULFUR. This time-honored topical therapy has been associated with fatalities after use in animals and humans, as reported by Rasmussen.[227] In this report, *sulfur* was applied to abraded skin. Given its relative ineffectiveness, use of other antiscabetic medications during pregnancy is preferable.

Lactation

Crotamiton has no documented problems during lactation. No information is available for *precipitated sulfur.*

Ivermectin is excreted in milk and has been used in large populations in third-world countries without identifiable problems for the infant.[224,242]

The manufacturers of *lindane* state that it is unlikely that amounts of lindane sufficient to cause serious adverse reactions are absorbed, but that breast-feeding should be avoided for 4 days if there is concern.[233] Others recommend avoidance of breast-feeding for 2 days.[234] Briggs[235] states that the amount of medication actually delivered to the infant during breast-feeding may be clinically insignificant.

Permethrin is an animal tumorigen; the

manufacturer recommends against breast-feeding while the mother is using the medication.[241]

ANTIVIRAL AGENTS
Pregnancy
ACYCLOVIR.   *Acyclovir* (FDA pregnancy category C; TERIS risk of topical acyclovir rated undetermined based on limited data, and the risk of systemic acyclovir is unlikely on data rated fair-to-good) is not teratogenic in animals but causes fetal death, growth retardation, and malformations in rats at maternotoxic doses.[243,244] Use in human pregnancies has not been associated with adverse fetal effects.[245,246] The manufacturer states that acyclovir should not be used in pregnancy unless the potential benefit justifies the potential risk to infants.[247] Briggs[248] states that there are insufficient data available to establish the safety of this medication, and that acyclovir use for disseminated herpes simplex virus (HSV) infections has been helpful in reducing mortality for these conditions, but that use for recurrent HSV infections is not as convincing an indication. Except near term or in cases of severe systemic involvement, acyclovir is not necessary to use during pregnancy.

FAMCICLOVIR.   *Famciclovir* (FDA pregnancy category B; TERIS risk unrated) has not shown teratogenicity in animals but causes benign tumors in rats. The manufacturer states it is to be used only if clearly needed.[249]

VALACYCLOVIR.   *Valacyclovir* (FDA pregnancy category B; TERIS risk unrated), the prodrug of acyclovir, has not been associated with teratogenicity in animals. Uneventful use during human pregnancy has been reported by the manufacturer, who recommends use only if potential benefit to the mother justifies the potential risk to the infant.[250] Guidelines for use of acyclovir should be followed.

Lactation
Famciclovir is a rat tumorigen and the manufacturer advises discontinuation of the medication during lactation.[249] The manufacturers of *acyclovir* and *valacyclovir* recommend that the drugs be used with caution during lactation.[247,250] The

AAP rated acyclovir as compatible with breast-feeding.[57]

CORTICOSTEROIDS
Pregnancy
SYSTEMIC CORTICOSTEROIDS.   The use of systemic *corticosteroids* (FDA pregnancy category C; TERIS risk rated unlikely based on data rated poor-to-fair) in animal studies during pregnancy has been associated with an increased risk of cleft palate, placental insufficiency, spontaneous abortion, and growth retardation in utero.[251,252] In humans, no teratogenic effects or serious problems are observed with use of low doses of systemic corticosteroids, but use of high doses is associated with a potential risk of growth suppression, inhibition of endogenous steroids, and steroid problems in infants.[253] Congenital cataracts have been reported in an infant whose mother received prednisone throughout pregnancy.[254] One small study concluded that the risk of use of corticosteroids during pregnancy was so low as to be undetectable, although the incidence of cleft palate was higher than would have been expected.[255] Some authors stated that the risk of teratogenicity of corticosteroids is so low as to be undetectable.[256,257,263] Prednisone in doses of 10 mg/day or less are, pending further data, not contraindicated during pregnancy.[258] However, there is concern that systemic corticosteroids given in doses of 10 mg/day throughout pregnancy may be associated with low birthweight,[259,260] and that low birthweight may be associated with later development of hypertension and cardiovascular mortality.[261]

Use of prednisone in doses of 40 to 80 mg/day for short periods of time has not increased the risk of congenital anomalies, except in cases in which antiphospholipid abnormalities presented a confounding factor.[262]

TOPICAL CORTICOSTEROIDS.   Topical *corticosteroids* (FDA pregnancy category C; TERIS risk rated unlikely based on data rated poor-to-fair) utilized during pregnancy are not thought to be associated with significant risk to the fetus. Manufacturers of the more potent topical corticosteroids issue a warning against their use in large amounts, extensively, or for protracted periods in pregnant patients or in those planning to become pregnant.[263-267] There was a report of intrauterine growth retardation in the infant of a mother who used the equivalent of 40 mg of triamcinolone daily through topical application.[268] In general, use of topical corticosteroids for limited periods of time has not been associated with congenital anomalies. Pregnant women who use large amounts of topical corticosteroid preparations over extensive parts of the body should be warned of the possibility of low birthweight babies.

Lactation

Use of *systemic corticosteroids* does not appear to affect the blood chemistry or infection rate of nursing infants.[253,269] If therapy is long-term, or if corticosteroids are required in doses exceeding 20 mg/day, it has been advised that prednisolone rather than *prednisone* be used. Nursing should be delayed for 3 to 4 hours after a dose to minimize exposure of the infant to the drug.[270] Corticosteroid use during lactation has been called "safe."[271] Despite this, one manufacturer contraindicates use of its product, *prednisolone*, during lactation.[272] Most prednisone products are generic, and information from the manufacturers is not included in the PDR. The AAP rated corticosteroid use as compatible with breast-feeding.[57]

Topical corticosteroids should not be applied to the breasts before nursing. There is a report of hypertension in an infant whose mother was applying topical steroids to the nipple.[273]

MISCELLANEOUS DRUGS
Anthralin

Anthralin (FDA pregnancy category C; TERIS risk rated undetermined based on data rated none, high risk unlikely) has not been studied in humans or animals during pregnancy. Anthralin is known to have tumorigenic and cocarcinogenic potential.[274] Manufacturers recommend use "only if clearly needed" during pregnancy and recommend against use during lactation.[275,276] Use during pregnancy and lactation is without support in the literature.

Calcipotriene

Calcipotriene (FDA pregnancy category C; TERIS risk rated undetermined based on data

rated very poor, with a high risk unlikely when used in recommended doses) is a vitamin D analog. Studies in animals given high oral doses of vitamin D showed skeletal abnormalities.[277] With topical use, fetal toxicity was not seen until maternal toxicity was approached. During lactation, no problems have been identified.

Clofazimine

Clofazimine (FDA unrated pregnancy category; TERIS risk rated minimal based on data rated poor-to-fair) has been associated with skin discoloration in infants up to 1 year of age whose mother used the drug during pregnancy[278] and lactation.[279] No human anomalies attributable to clofazimine have been observed.[280]

Coal Tar

Coal tar (FDA pregnancy category C; TERIS risk rated undetermined based on data rated none, high risk unlikely) is a known carcinogen and mutagen.[281] Use of the shampoo has been associated with uptake of coal tar.[282] No studies have been done in humans. The manufacturer advises that pregnant women "seek the advice of a health professional."[283] No information on use during lactation is available. Use of coal tar as a first-line therapy during pregnancy and lactation should be avoided pending further information.

Cyclosporine

Cyclosporine (FDA pregnancy category C; TERIS risk rated minimal based on data rated fair for malformations and small-to-moderate based on data rated fair for intrauterine growth retardation) is embryotoxic, fetotoxic, and carcinogenic in some animal studies[284,285] but not in others.[286] Use in humans has been associated with congenital anomalies in 2 of 154 cases in one study[287] as well as an increased risk of premature births in other reports.[288,289] A number of successful pregnancies with cyclosporine have been noted.[290-293] Briggs[294] states that use of cyclosporine during pregnancy poses no major risk to the developing fetus.

Use of *cyclosporine* during lactation is not recommended because of the risk of nephrotoxicity, hypertension, and malignancy in infants.[295] The AAP recommends against use in breast-feeding, citing possible immunosuppression, unknown effect on growth, or association with carcinogenesis.[57]

Dapsone

Dapsone (FDA pregnancy category C; TERIS risk rated undetermined based on data rated very limited) has been used in pregnant women for treatment of leprosy.[296] The safety of dapsone during pregnancy for leprosy and dermatitis herpetiformis is supported in the literature.[297-299] Briggs[300] states that use of dapsone during pregnancy poses no major risk to the fetus. Stopping therapy during the last month of pregnancy may minimize a theoretic risk of neonatal kernicterus.[301] During lactation, use of dapsone is controversial. WHO[302] and the manufacturer advise against use[303]; however, the AAP rated its use as "usually compatible."[57]

Gold

Gold (FDA pregnancy category C; TERIS risk rated undetermined based on data rated limited) administered to animals has been associated with congenital abnormalities and gastroschisis.[304,305] Studies in humans have not shown significant effects, and normal infants have been born to mothers who used gold.[306-308] Gold has been recommended as the antirheumatic drug of least risk during pregnancy.[309] Use of gold during lactation is controversial; the manufacturers recommend against use because of risk to the infant.[310,311] The AAP listed gold as usually compatible with breast-feeding.[57]

Hydroquinone

Topical *hydroquinone* (FDA pregnancy category C; TERIS risk rated undetermined based on data rated very poor; high risk unlikely) has no specific contraindications for use during pregnancy or lactation, although the manufacturer states that safety during pregnancy has not been established.[312]

Imiquimod

Topical *imiquimod* (FDA pregnancy category B; TERIS risk not listed) has been demonstrated to produce reduced pup weights and delayed ossification in rats at maternotoxic doses.[313] Distribution in human milk has not been demonstrated. The AAP has no rating.

Interferons

Alfa 2b *interferons* (FDA pregnancy category C; TERIS risk rated undetermined based on data rated very poor) are used for treatment of condyloma acuminatum. Use of high doses of interferons for treatment of malignant neoplasms has been associated with fetotoxic effects in humans.[314,315] However, the doses used for treatment of warts (one million IU per lesion 3 times per week for 3 weeks for one to five lesions) is much lower than the dose for treatment of malignancies (10 to 20 million IU subcutaneously 3 to 5 times per week). Normal pregnancies with use of high-dose interferons have been reported.[316] Use of interferon for elective treatment of warts during pregnancy is not advisable. Manufacturers advise against use during lactation.[317-321]

Methoxsalen

Methoxsalen (FDA pregnancy category C; TERIS risk rated unlikely based on data rated poor-to-fair; data insufficient to state no risk) has not been studied in animals. Several studies reported no problems in infants whose mother or father had been treated with oral methoxsalen and UVA in the periconceptional period or early pregnancy.[322-324] One study included pregnancies that occurred 1 or more years after treatment and did not identify any increased risk of harm to the fetus[326]; however, these studies were small. It has been suggested that women who become pregnant during or after psoralen plus ultraviolet A (PUVA) treatment should be offered prenatal karyotyping to rule out the possibility of chromosomal abnormalities.[327] During lactation, the manufacturer advises against use of oral methoxsalen but states that topical methoxsalen may be "used with caution."[225]

Minoxidil

Topical *minoxidil* (FDA pregnancy category C; TERIS risk rated undetermined based on data rated poor) has been associated with transient hypertrichosis after oral use.[326,327] Cardiac and other anomalies have also been reported, although the number of pregnancies is too small to determine a direct causal effect.[328] The manufacturer recommends that the medication not be used in pregnant and lactating women.[329] Others recommended that pregnancy be delayed until 1 month after discontinuation of topical minoxidil.[330] The AAP rates minoxidil as being compatible with breast-feeding.[57]

Pentoxifylline

Pentoxifylline (FDA pregnancy category C; TERIS risk rated undetermined based on data rated poor; high risk unlikely) has been associated with a possible increased risk of cardiovascular and other defects.[331] The manufacturer recommends use only if clearly needed during pregnancy and recommends against use during lactation.[332]

Podophyllum

Topical *podophyllum* (FDA pregnancy category C; TERIS risk rated undetermined based on data rated poor) is cytotoxic and teratogenic. TERIS comments that a high risk of congenital anomalies is unlikely, as long as topical application is limited to a small area. Use of podophyllum on large areas may be associated with substantial risk. Data on teratogenicity are not conclusive, but podophyllum use should be avoided because of the potential risk of myelotoxicity and neurotoxicity to the mother.[333] Use during any trimester of pregnancy is not recommended.[334] The manufacturer recommends against use during pregnancy and lactation.[335]

SUMMARY

1. The physician should determine whether a woman of childbearing age is pregnant before prescribing any medication. If she is not currently pregnant, she must be told to disclose her pregnancy as early as possible when it occurs because of possible risk to herself or the baby.
2. If a woman is already pregnant it is important to determine her estimated date of conception and current trimester of pregnancy. Risks of drugs vary according to trimester of pregnancy.
3. If a woman is not pregnant and is being given a medication that will place her at high risk for problems during early pregnancy (e.g., methotrexate, isotretinoin), she should be extensively counseled about the risk to herself and her fetus. In addition, she should have regular pregnancy testing before and during her treatment course.
4. If a woman is already pregnant and has indications for a medication that places herself or her fetus at risk, her physician should review her actual risk from the previously mentioned sources. TERIS and Briggs are especially helpful in delineating this risk. It is recommended that the physician document the discussion of risk with the patient.
5. Where there is minimal risk of a drug whose use is optional, discussion with the patient and her primary care physician(s) before prescription is advised. The dermatologist should anticipate that a primary care physician might have a personal bias towards or against the use of specific drugs during pregnancy or lactation.
6. Breast-feeding also affects which drugs may be prescribed. Some drugs that cannot be used during pregnancy may be used during lactation, whereas other drugs that may be used during pregnancy should be avoided during lactation.
7. For drug use during lactation, controversy among several sources regarding risk may exist. Best sources include the AAP and WHO.
8. If a manufacturer publishes a contraindication for use of a drug during pregnancy or lactation and use of this drug is optional, the drug should be used only under exceptional clinical circumstances in which the overall health of the mother is at significant risk, and after a risk-benefit conversation with the patient and her obstetrician or pediatrician has been documented.

References

1. *Physicians' desk reference*, Montvale, NJ, 1998, Medical Economics Data Production Company.
2. Zerner J, Doil KL, Drewry J, et al: Intrauterine contraceptive device failures in renal transplant patients. *J Reprod Med* 26:99-102, 1981.

3. Papiernik E, Rozenbaum H, Amblard P, et al: Intra-uterine device failure: relation with drug use. *Eur J Obstet Gynecol Reprod Biol* 32:205-212, 1989.

4. Griseofulvin, systemic. In *USP-DI. Drug information for the health care professional,* vol 1, Taunton, MA, 1998, Rand McNally, pp 1527-1529.

5. *USP-DI. Drug information for the health care professional,* vol 1, Taunton, MA, 1995, Rand McNally, pp 1258-1266.

6. Rifampin, systemic. In *USP-DI. Drug information for the health care professional,* vol 1, Taunton, MA, 1998, Rand McNally, pp 2509-2516.

7. Penicillins, systemic. In *USP-DI. Drug information for the health care professional,* vol 1, Taunton, MA, 1998, Rand McNally, pp 2253-2275.

8. Tetracyclines, systemic. In *USP-DI. Drug information for the health care professional,* vol 1, Taunton, MA, 1998, Rand McNally, pp 2801-2810.

9. Sulfonamides, systemic. In *USP-DI Drug information for the health care professional,* vol 1, Taunton, MA, 1998, Rand McNally, pp 2681-2686.

10. Pillans PI, Sparrow MJ: Pregnancy associated with a combined oral contraceptive and itraconazole. *N Z Med J* 106:436, 1993.

11. Hingston GR: Pregnancy associated with a combined oral contraceptive and itraconazole. *N Z Med J* 8:106:528, 1993.

12. Van de Velde V, DeCoster R, Doolaege R, et al: No indication of decrease in plasma levels of oral contraceptives after 15 days itraconazole administration in premenopausal women. *Aust J Dermatol* 38(Suppl):283, 1997.

13. Methotrexate Product Information, Seattle, WA, Immunex Corporation, 1998.

14. Vallance P: Drugs and the fetus. *BMJ* 312(7038):1053-1054, 1995.

15. Wolff J: Iodide goiter and the pharmacologic effects of excess iodide. *Am J Med* 47:101-124, 1969.

16. Mehta PS, Mehta SJ, Vorherr H: Congenital iodide goiter and hypothyroidism: a review. *Obstet Gynecol Surv* 38:237-247, 1983.

17. Livezey GT, Rayburn DR: Principles of perinatal pharmacology. In WF Rayburn, FP Zuspan, editors: *Drug therapy in obstetrics and gynecology,* ed 3, St. Louis, 1992, Mosby-Year Book, p 3.

18. Anti-inflammatory drugs, nonsteroidal, systemic. In *USP-DI. Drug information for the health care professional,* vol 1, Taunton, MA, 1998, Rand McNally, pp 376-422.

19. Antidepressants, tricyclic, systemic. In *USP-DI. Drug information for the health care professional,* vol 1, Taunton, MA, 1998, Rand McNally, pp 260-272.

20. Jick H, Holmes LB, Hunter JR et al: First trimester drug use and congenital disorders. *JAMA* 246:343-346, 1981.

21. Aselton PA, Jick H, Milunsky A, et al: First trimester drug use and congenital disorders. *Obstet Gynecol* 65:451-455, 1985.

22. Heinonen OP, Slone D, Shapiro S: *Birth Defects and Drugs in Pregnancy,* Littleton, MA, 1977, John Wright-PSG, pp 286-288, 434.

23. Riggs BS, Bronstein AC, Kulig K, et al: Acute acetaminophen overdose during pregnancy. *Obstet Gynecol* 74:247-253, 1989.

24. Wang PH, Yang MJ, Lee WL, et al: Acetaminophen poisoning in late pregnancy. A case report. *J Reprod Med* 42(6):367-371, 1997.

25. Stuart MJ, Gross SJ, Elrad H, et al: Effects of acetylsalicylic-acid ingestion on maternal and neonatal hemostasis. *N Engl J Med* 307:909-912, 1982.

26. Rumack CM, Guggenheim MA, Rumack BH, et al: Neonatal intracranial hemorrhage and maternal use of aspirin. *Obstet Gynecol* 58:52s-56s, 1981.

27. Levin DL, Fixler DE, Morriss FC, et al: Morphologic analysis of the pulmonary vascular bed in infants exposed in utero to prostaglandin synthetase inhibitors. *H Pediatr* 478-483, 1978.

28. Collins B, Turner G: Salicylates and pregnancy. Letter to the editor. *Lancet* 2:1494, 1973.

29. Martinez-Frias ML, Rodriguez-Pinilla E, Prieto L: Prenatal exposure to salicylates and gastroschisis: a case-control study. *Teratology* 56:241-243, 1997.

30. Romero R, Lockwood C, Oyarzun E, et al: Toxemia: new concepts in an old disease. *Semin Perinatol* 12:302-323, 1988.

31. Briggs GG, Freeman RK, Yaffe SL: *Drugs in pregnancy and lactation,* ed 5, Baltimore, MD, 1998, Williams and Wilkins, pp 73-81.

32. Moise KJ Jr: Indomethacin therapy in the treatment of symptomatic polyhydramnios. *Clin Obstet Gynecol* 34:310-318, 1991.

33. Moise KJ Jr: Polyhydramnios: Problems and treatment. *Semin Perinatol* 17(3):197-209, 1993b.

34. Eronen M, Pesonen E, Kurki T, et al: The effects of indomethacin and a beta-sympathomimetic agent on the fetal ductus arteriosus during treatment of premature labor: a randomized double-blind study. *Am J Obstet Gynecol* 164:141-146, 1991.

35. Moise KJ Jr: Effect of advancing gestational age on the frequency of fetal ductal constriction in association with maternal indomethacin use. *Am J Obstet Gynecol* 168:1350-1353, 1993a.

36. Major CA, Lewis DF, Harding JA, et al: Tocolysis with indomethacin increases the incidence of necrotizing enterocolitis in the low-birth-weight neonate. *Am J Obstet Gynecol* 170:102-106, 1994.

37. Norton ME, Merrill J, Cooper BAB, et al: Neonatal complications after the administration of indomethacin for preterm labor. *N Engl J Med* 329:1602-1607, 1993.

38. van der Heijden BJ, Carlus C, Narcy F, et al: Persistent anuria, neonatal death, and renal microcystic lesions after prenatal exposure to indomethacin. *Am J Obstet Gynecol* 171:617-623, 1994.

39. Fejgin MD, Delpino ML, Bidiwala KS: Isolated small bowel perforation following intrauterine treatment with indomethacin. *Am J Perinatol* 11(4):295-296, 1994.

40. Briggs GG, Freeman RK, Yaffe SL: *Drugs in pregnancy and lactation,* ed 5, Baltimore, MD, 1998, Williams and Wilkins, pp 524-526, 757-758.

41. Mangurten H, Benawra R: Neonatal codeine withdrawal in infants of nonaddicted mothers. *Pediatrics* 65:159-160, 1980.

42. Briggs GG, Freeman RK, Yaffe SL: *Drugs in pregnancy and lactation,* ed 5, Baltimore, MD, 1998, Williams and Wilkins, pp 254-255.

43. Mellin GW: Drugs in the first trimester of pregnancy and fetal life of *Homo sapiens. Am J Obstet Gynecol* 90:1169-1180, 1964.

44. Heinonen OP, Slone D, Shapiro S: *Birth defects and drugs in pregnancy,* Littleton, MA, 1977, Publishing Sciences Group, p 484.

45. Campbell C, Phillips OC, Frazier TM: Analgesia during labor: a comparison of pentobarbital, meperidine, and morphine. *Obstet Gynecol* 17:714-718, 1961.

46. Geber WF, Schramm LC: Congenital malformations of the central nervous system produced by narcotic analgesics in the hamster. *Am J Obstet Gynecol* 123:705-713, 1975.

47. Geber WF: Effects of central nervous system active and nonactive drugs on the fetal central nervous system. *Neurotoxicology* 1:585-593, 1977.

48. Levy M, Spino M: Neonatal withdrawal syndrome: associated drugs and pharmacologic management. *Pharmacotherapy* 13(3):202-211, 1993.

49. Heinonen OP, Slone D, Shapiro S: *Birth defects and drugs in pregnancy,* Littleton, MA, 1977, John Wright-PSG, pp 287-288, 294, 434, 471, 484.

50. Quillian WW II, Dunn CA: Neonatal drug withdrawal from propoxyphene. *JAMA* 235(19):2128, 1976.

51. Tyson HK: Neonatal withdrawal symptoms associated with maternal use of propoxyphene hydrochloride (Darvon). *J Pediatr* 85(5):684-685, 1974.

52. Saillenfait AM, Vannier B: Methodological proposal in behavioural teratogenicity testing: Assessment of propoxyphene, chlorpromazine, and vitamin A as positive controls. *Teratology* 37:185-199, 1988.

53. Clark JH, Wilson WG: A 16-day-old breastfed infant with metabolic acidosis caused by salicylate. *Clin Pediatr* 20:53-54, 1981.

54. Motrin Product Information, Fort Washington, PA, McNeil PPC, Inc, 1998.

55. Orudis/Oruvail Product Information, Philadelphia, PA, Wyeth-Ayerst Laboratories Inc., 1997.

56. Naprosyn Product Information, Nutley, NJ: Roche Laboratories, Inc., 1995.

57. American Academy of Pediatrics Committee on Drugs. Transfer of drugs and other chemicals into human milk. *Pediatrics* 93:137-150, 1994.

58. Fairhead FW: Convulsions in a breast-fed infant after maternal indomethacin. *Lancet* 2:576, 1978.

59. American Academy of Pediatrics Committee on Drugs. The transfer of drugs and other chemicals into human breast milk. *Pediatrics* 72:375-383, 1983.

60. Carbocaine Product Information, Sanofi Winthrop Pharmaceuticals, New York, NY, 1996.

61. Marcaine Product Information, Sanofi Winthrop Pharmaceuticals, New York, NY, 1996.

62. Briggs GG, Freeman RK, Yaffe SL: *Drugs in pregnancy and lactation*, ed 5, Baltimore, MD, 1998, Williams and Wilkins, pp 151-152, 172-173, 175-176.

63. Briggs GG, Freeman RK, Yaffe SL: *Drugs in pregnancy and lactation*, ed 5, Baltimore, MD, 1998, Williams and Wilkins, pp 152-153.

64. Landers DV, Green JR, Sweet RL: Antibiotic use during pregnancy and the postpartum period. *Clin Obstet Gynecol* 26:391-406, 1983.

65. Sullivan D, Csuka ME, Blanchard B: Erythromycin ethinylsuccinate hepatotoxicity. *JAMA* 243:1074, 1980.

66. Gribble MJ, Chow AW: Erythromycin. *Med Clin North Am* 66:79-89, 1982.

67. Biaxin Product Information, North Chicago, IL, Abbott Laboratories, 1997.

68. Briggs GG, Freeman RK, Yaffe SL: *Drugs in pregnancy and lactation*, ed 5, Baltimore, MD, 1998, Williams and Wilkins, pp. 219-220.

69. Schick B, Hom M, Librizzi A, et al: Pregnancy outcome following exposure to clarithromycin. Abstract. Organization of Teratology Information Services Salt Lake City. May 2-4, 1996.

70. Dirithromycin, systemic. In *USP-DI. Drug information for the health care professional*, vol 1, ed 15, Taunton, MA, 1998, The US Pharmacopeial Convention, pp 1230-1232.

71. Fluoroquinolones-systemic. In *USP-DI. Drug information for the health care professional*, vol 1, ed 15, Taunton, MA, 1998, The US Pharmacopeial Convention, pp 1458-1465.

72. Pastuszak A, Andreou R, Schick B, et al: New postmarketing surveillance data supports a lack of association between quinolone use in pregnancy and fetal and neonatal complications. *Reprod Toxicol* 9(6):584, 1995.

73. Schaefer C, Amoura-Elefant E, Vial T, et al: Pregnancy outcome after prenatal quinolone exposure. Evaluation of a case registry of the European Network of Teratology Information Services (ENTIS). *Eur J Obstet Gynaecol Reprod Biol* 69(2):83-89, 1996.

74. Loebstein R, Addis A, Ho E, et al: Pregnancy outcome following gestational exposure to fluoroquinolones: a multicenter prospective controlled study. *Antimicrob Agents Chemother* 42(6):1336-1339, 1998.

75. Briggs GG, Freeman RK, Yaffe SL: *Drugs in pregnancy and lactation*, ed 5, Baltimore, MD, 1998, Williams and Wilkins, pp 210-211.

76. Briggs GG, Freeman RK, Yaffe SL: *Drugs in pregnancy and lactation*, ed 5, Baltimore, MD, 1998, Williams and Wilkins, pp 52, 60-62, 323-324, 826-830.

77. Stirrat GM: Prescribing problems in the second half of pregnancy and during lactation. *Obstet Gynecol Surv* 1:311-317, 1976.

78. Pomerance JJ, Yaffe SJ: Maternal medication and its effect on the fetus. *Curr Probl Pediatr* 4:1-60, 1973.

79. Toaff R, Ravid R: Tetracyclines and the teeth. *Lancet* 2:281-282, 1962.

80. Cohlan SQ: Tetracycline staining of teeth. *Teratology* 15:127-130, 1977.

81. Heinonen OP, Slone D, Shapiro S: *Birth defects and drugs in pregnancy*, Littleton, MA, 1977, Publishing Sciences Group Inc.

82. Czeizel AE, Rockenbauer M: Teratogenic study of doxycycline. *Obstet Gynecol* 89(4):524-528, 1997.

83. Silvadene Product Information, Kansas City, MO, 1995, Hoechst Marion Merrell Dow.

84. SSD Product Information, Lincolnshire, IL, Boots Pharmaceutical, 1993.

85. Novacet Product Information, Mount Olive, NJ, Knoll Laboratories, 1995.

86. Sulfacet-R Product Information, Collegeville, PA, Dermik Laboratories, Inc., 1996.

87. Erythromycins, systemic. In *USP-DI. Drug information for the health care professional*, vol 1, Taunton, MA, 1998, Rand McNally, pp 1340-1347.

88. Zithromax Product Information, New York, NY, Pfizer Labs Division, Pfizer, Inc., 1996.

89. Azithromycin, systemic. In *USP-DI. Drug information for the health care professional*, vol 1, Taunton, MA, 1998, Rand McNally, pp 477-479.

90. Cephalosporins, systemic. In *USP-DI. Drug information for the health care professional*, vol 1, Taunton, MA, 1998, Rand McNally, pp 744-770.

91. Hepburn JS, Paxson NF, Rogers AN. Secretion of ingested sulfanilamide in breast milk and in the urine of the infant. *J Biol Chem* 123:liv-lv, 1938.

92. The WHO Working Group. Bennett PN, editor: *Drugs and human lactation*, Amsterdam, 1996, Elsevier, pp 135-136.

93. Tetracyclines, systemic. In *USP-DI. Drug information for the health care professional,* vol 1, Taunton, MA, 1998, Rand McNally, pp 2801-2812.

94. Hunt MJ, Salisbury EL, Grace J, et al: Black breast milk due to minocycline therapy, *Br J Dermatol* 134(5):943-944, 1996.

95. Clindamycin, topical: In *USP-DI. Drug information for the health care professional,* vol 1, Taunton, MA, 1998, Rand McNally, 847-849.

96. Mann CF: Clindamycin and breast-feeding. *Pediatrics* 66:1030-1031, 1980.

97. Cleocin T Product Information, Kalamazoo, MI, The Upjohn Company, 1995.

98. Erythromycins, topical. In *USP-DI. Drug information for the health care professional,* vol 1, Taunton, MA, 1998, Rand McNally, pp 1337-1339.

99. Differin Product Information, Fort Worth, TX, Galderma Laboratories Inc., 1996.

100. Autret E, Berjot M, Jonville-Bera AP, et al: Anophthalmia and agenesis of optic chiasma associated with adapalene gel in early pregnancy. *Lancet* 350(9074):339, 1997.

101. Nazzaro-Porro M: Azelaic acid, *J Am Acad Dermatol* 17:1033-1041, 1987.

102. Azelex Product Information, Irvine, CA, Allergan Inc., 1997.

103. Benzoyl peroxides, topical. In *USP-DI. Drug information for the health care professional,* vol 1, Taunton, MA, 1998, Rand McNally, pp 549-552.

104. Rothman KE, Pochi P: Use of oral and topical agents for acne in pregnancy. *J Am Acad Dermatol* 19:431-435, 1988.

105. Burtin P, Taddio A, Ariburnu O, et al: Safety of metronidazole in pregnancy: a meta-analysis. *Am J Obstet Gynecol* 172:525-529, 1995.

106. Correa-Villasenor A, Ferencz C, Loffredo C, et al: Variation in epidemiologic characteristics for subgroups of membranous ventricular septal defects. *Teratology* 53(2):93, 1996.

107. Caro-Paton T, Carvajal A, de Diego IM, et al: Is metronidazole teratogenic? A meta-analysis. *Br J Clin Pharmacol* 44:179-182, 1997.

108. Norman K, Pattinson RD, de Souza J, et al: Ampicillin and metronidazole treatment in preterm labour: a multicentre, randomized controlled trial. *Br J Obstet Gynaecol* 101:404-408, 1994.

109. Svare J, Langhoff-Roos J, Andersen LF, et al: Ampicillin-metronidazole treatment in idiopathic preterm labour: a randomized controlled multicentre trial. *Br J Obstet Gynaecol* 104:892-897, 1997.

110. Metrogel-Vaginal Product Information, St. Paul, MN, 3M Pharmaceuticals, 1997.

111. Metrogel Product Information, Fort Worth, TX, Galderma Laboratories, Inc., 1995.

112. Willhite CC, Sharma RP, Allen PV, et al: Percutaneous retinoid absorption and embryotoxicity. *J Invest Dermatol* 95:523-529, 1990.

113. Camera G, Pregliasco P: Ear malformation in baby born to mother using tretinoin cream (letter). *Lancet* 339:687, 1992.

114. Lipson AH, Collins F, Webster WS: Multiple congenital defects associated with maternal use of topical tretinoin. *Lancet* 341:1352-1353, 1993.

115. Jick SS, Terris BZ, Jick H: First trimester topical tretinoin and congenital disorders. *Lancet* 341(8854):1181-1182, 1993.

116. Zbinden G: Investigations on the toxicity of tretinoin administered systemically to animals. *Acta Derm Venereol (Stockh)* 74(Suppl):36-40, 1975.

117. Koren G, Pastuszak A, Ito S: Drugs in pregnancy. *N Engl J Med* 338(16):1128-1137, 1998.

118. Flagyl Product Information, Chicago, IL, G.D. Searle and Co., 1997.

119. Briggs GG, Freeman RK, Yaffe SL: *Drugs in pregnancy and lactation,* ed 5, Baltimore, MD, 1998, Williams and Wilkins, pp 1045-1049.

120. Lee BE, Feinberg M, Abraham JJ et al: Congenital malformations in an infant born to a woman treated with fluconazole. *Pediatr Infect Dis J* 11:1062-1064, 1992.

121. Pursley TJ, Blomquist IK, Abraham J, et al: Fluconazole-induced congenital anomalies in three infants. *Clin Infect Dis* 22(2):336-340, 1996.

122. Diflucan Product Information, New York, NY, Pfizer Inc., 1997.

123. Mastroiacovo P, Mazzone T, Botto LD, et al: Prospective assessment of pregnancy outcomes after first-trimester exposure to fluconazole. *Am J Obstet Gynecol* 175(6):1645-1650, 1996.

124. Briggs GG, Freeman RK, Yaffe SL: *Drugs in pregnancy and lactation,* ed 5, Baltimore, MD, 1998, Williams and Wilkins, pp 436-439.

125. Rosa FW, Hernandez C, Carlo WA: Griseofulvin teratology. *Lancet* 1:171, 1987.

126. Metneki J, Czeizel A: Griseofulvin teratology including two thoracopagus conjoined twins. *Lancet* 1:1042, 1987.

127. Gris-Peg Product Information, Irvine, CA, Allergan Inc., 1994.

128. Grifulvin V Product Information, Raritan, NJ, Ortho Pharmaceutical Corporation, 1997.

129. Fulvicin P/G Product Information, Kenilworth, NJ, Schering Corporation, 1996.

130. van Cauteren H, Lampo A, Vandenberghe J, et al: Safety aspects of oral antifungal agents. *Br J Clin Pract Symp Suppl* 71:47-49, 1990.

131. Chotmongkol V, Sookprasert A: Itraconazole in cryptococcal meningitis in pregnancy: a case report. *J Med Assoc Thai* 75:606-608, 1992.

132. Antifungals, azole, systemic. In *USP-DI. Drug information for the health care professional*, vol 1, Taunton, MA, 1998, Rand McNally, pp 291-299.

133. Lind J: Limb malformations in a case of hydrops fetalis with ketoconazole use during pregnancy. *Arch Gynecol* 235(Suppl):398, 1985.

134. Buttar HS, Moffatt JH, Bura C: Pregnancy outcome in ketoconazole-treated rats and mice. *Teratology* 39:444, 1989.

135. Weisinger EC, Mayerhofer S, Wenish C, et al: Fluconazole in *Candida albicans* sepsis during pregnancy: case report and review of the literature. *Infection* 24(3):263-266, 1996.

136. Amado JA, Pesauera C, Gonzalez EM et al: Successful treatment with ketoconazole of Cushing's syndrome in pregnancy. *Postgrad Med J* 66:221-223, 1990.

137. Terbinafine-systemic. In *USP-DI. Drug information for the health care professional*, vol 1, Taunton, MA, 1998, Rand McNally, pp 2787-2790.

138. Lamisil Product Information, Summit, NJ, Novartis Pharmaceuticals, 1997.

139. Rosa FW, Baum C, Shaw M: Pregnancy outcomes after first-trimester vaginitis drug therapy. *Obstet Gynecol* 69:751-755, 1987.

140. Antifungals, azole, vaginal. In *USP-DI. Drug information for the health care professional*, vol 1, Taunton, MA, 1998, Rand McNally, pp 291-299.

141. Briggs GG, Freeman RK, Yaffe SL: *Drugs in pregnancy and lactation*, ed 5, Baltimore, MD, 1998, Williams and Wilkins, pp 235-236.

142. Briggs GG, Freeman RK, Yaffe SL: *Drugs in pregnancy and lactation*, ed 5, Baltimore, MD, 1998, Williams and Wilkins, pp 728-729.

143. Spectazole Product Information, Raritan, NJ, Ortho Pharmaceutical Corporation, 1994.

144. Monistat Cream Product Information, Raritan, NJ, Ortho Pharmaceutical Corporation, 1995.

145. Terazol Product Information, Raritan, NJ, Ortho Pharmaceutical Corporation, 1991.

146. Berkowitz RL, Capriotti EA, Cote JR, et al: *Handbook for prescribing medications during pregnancy*, ed 2, Boston/Toronto, 1986, Little, Brown, and Co, p 54.

147. Selsun Product Information, Columbus, OH, Ross Laboratories, 1998.

148. Sporanox Product Information. Titusville, NJ, Janssen Pharmaceutica, 1997.

149. Nizoral Tablet Product Information, Titusville, NJ, Janssen Pharmaceutica, 1996.

150. Briggs GG, Freeman RK, Yaffe SL: *Drugs in pregnancy and lactation*, ed 5, Baltimore, MD, 1998, Williams and Wilkins, pp 436-439.

151. Nizoral Cream Product Information, Titusville, NJ, Janssen Pharmaceutica, 1996.

152. Lamisil Cream Product Information, Summit, NJ, Novartis Pharmaceuticals, 1997.

153. Vagistat Product Information, New York, NY, Bristol-Myers Products, 1998.

154. Femstat Product Information, Palo Alto, CA, Syntex Laboratories Inc., 1988.

155. Loprox Product Information, Orlando, FL, Hoechst-Roussel Pharmaceuticals Inc., 1996.

156. Lotrimin Product Information, Kenilworth, NJ, Schering Corporation, 1994.

157. Mycelex G Product Information, Elkhart, IN, Miles Inc., 1992.

158. Naftin Product Information, Irvine, CA, Allergan Inc., 1996.

159. Oxistat Product Information, Research Triangle Park, NC, Glaxo Pharmaceuticals, 1998.

160. Exelderm Product Information, Buffalo, NY, Westwood-Squibb Pharmaceuticals, Inc., 1998.

161. Nystatin USP Product Information, Minneapolis, MN, Paddock Laboratories, Inc., 1995.

162. Briggs GG, Freeman RK, Yaffe SL: *Drugs in pregnancy and lactation*, ed 5, Baltimore, MD, 1998, Williams and Wilkins, pp 115-116.

163. Hismanal Product Information, Titusville, NJ, Janssen Pharmaceuticals, 1997.

164. Heinonen OP, Slone D, Shapiro S: *Birth defects and drugs in pregnancy,* Littleton, MA, 1977, Publishing Sciences Group, p 437.

165. Vigersky RA, Mehlman I, Glass CR, et al: Treatment of hirsute women with cimetidine: a preliminary report. *N Engl J Med* 301:1042, 1980.

166. Sawyer D, Conner CS, Scalley R: Cimetidine: adverse reactions and acute toxicity. *Am J Hosp Pharm* 38:188-197, 1981.

167. Briggs GG, Freeman RK, Yaffe SL: *Drugs in pregnancy and lactation,* ed 5, Baltimore, MD, 1998, Williams and Wilkins, pp 206-209.

168. Sadovsky R, Pfeifer Y, Polishuk WZ, et al: A trial of cyproheptadine in habitual abortion. *Isr J Med Sci* 8:623-625, 1972.

169. Kasperlik-Zaluska A, Migdalska B, Hartwig B, et al: Two pregnancies in a woman with Cushing's syndrome treated with cyproheptadine. *Br J Obstet Gynaecol* 87:1171-1173, 1980.

170. Khir ASM, How J: Successful pregnancy after cyproheptadine treatment for Cushing's disease. *Eur J Obstet Gynecol Reprod Biol* 13:343-347, 1981.

171. Periactin Product Information, West Point, PA, Merck & Co., Inc., 1997.

172. Lione A, Scialli AR: The developmental toxicity of the H-1 histamine antagonists. *Reproductive Toxicology* 10:247-255, 1996.

173. Briggs GG, Freeman RK, Yaffe SL: *Drugs in pregnancy and lactation,* ed 5, Baltimore, MD, 1998, Williams and Wilkins, pp 343-346.

174. Falterman CG, Richardson CJ: Small left colon syndrome associated with maternal ingestion of psychoactive drugs. *J Pediatr* 97:308-310, 1980.

175. Zonalon Product Information, Lincolnshire, IL, GenDerm, 1998.

176. Allegra Product Information, Kansas City, MO, Hoechst Marion Roussel, 1996.

177. Briggs GG, Freeman RK, Yaffe SL: *Drugs in pregnancy and lactation,* ed 5, Baltimore, MD, 1998, Williams and Wilkins, pp 520-521.

178. Atarax Product Information, East Hanover, NJ, Roerig Division of Pfizer, Inc., 1993.

179. Zyrtec Product Information, New York, NY, Pfizer Inc., 1997.

180. Antihistamines, systemic. In *USP-DI. Drug information for the health care professional,* vol 1, Taunton, MA, 1998, Rand McNally, pp 315-333.

181. Einarson A, Bailey B, Jung G, et al: Prospective controlled study of hydroxyzine and cetirizine in pregnancy. *Ann Allergy Asthma Immunol* 78(2):183-186, 1997.

182. Koren G, Pastuszak A, Ito S: Drugs in pregnancy. *N Engl J Med* 338(126):1128-1137, 1998.

183. Einarson A, Bailey B, Jung G, et al: Prospective controlled study of hydroxyzine and cetirizine in pregnancy. *Ann Allergy Asthma Immunol* 78(2):183-186, 1997.

184. Briggs GG, Freeman RK, Yaffe SL: *Drugs in pregnancy and lactation,* ed 5, Baltimore, MD, 1998, Williams and Wilkins, pp 628-629.

185. Claritin Tablet Information, Kenilworth, NJ, Schering Corporation, 1996.

186. Woodward JK: Pharmacology and toxicology of nonclassical antihistamines. *Cutis* 42:5-9, 1988.

187. Briggs GG, Freeman RK, Yaffe SL: *Drugs in pregnancy and lactation,* ed 5, Baltimore, MD, 1998, Williams and Wilkins, pp 1008-1009.

188. Seldane Product Information, Kansas City, MO, Hoechst Marion Rousell, 1993.

189. Rumeau-Rouquette C, Goujard J, Huel G: Possible teratogenic effect of phenothiazines in human beings. *Teratology* 15:57-64, 1977.

190. Heinonen OP, Slone D, Shapiro S: *Birth defects and drugs in pregnancy,* Littleton, MA, 1983, John Wright-PSG, pp 323, 347.

191. Temaril Product Information, Irvine, CA, Allergan Herbert, 1991.

192. Tagamet Product Information, Philadelphia, PA, SmithKline Beecham Pharmaceuticals, 1997.

193. Histamine H2 receptor antagonists-systemic. In *USP-DI. Drug information for the health care professional,* vol 1, Taunton, MA, 1998, Rand McNally, pp 1579-1589.

194. The WHO Working Group. Bennett PN, editor: *Drugs and human lactation.* Amsterdam, 1996, Elsevier, pp 316-317.

195. Lindquist NG, Sjostrand SE, Ullberg S: Accumulation of chorioretinotoxic drugs in the foetal eye. *Acta Pharmaceutica Toxicol (Copenhagen)* 28:64, 1970.

196. Plaquenil Product Information, New York, Sanofi Pharmaceuticals, 1998.

197. Aralen Product Information, New York, Sanofi Pharmaceuticals, 1998.

198. Buchanan NM, Toubi E, Khamashta MA, et al: Hydroxychloroquine and lupus pregnancy: review of a series of 36 cases. *Ann Rheum Dis* 55(7):486-488, 1996.

199. Parke AL, Rothfield NF: Antimalarial drugs in pregnancy—the North American experience. *Lupus* 5(Suppl 1):S67-S69, 1996.

200. Parke A, West B: Hydroxychloroquine in pregnant patients with systemic lupus erythematosus. *J Rheumatol* 10:1715-1718, 1996.

201. Khamashta MA, Buchanan NM, Hughes GR: The use of hydroxychloroquine in lupus pregnancy: the British experience. *Lupus* 5(Suppl 1):S65-S66, 1996.

202. Vevera J, Zatloukal F: Case of congenital malformation probably produced by atabrine taken early in pregnancy. *Cesk Pediatr* 19:211-212, 1964; In Nishumra H, Tanimura T, editors: *Clinical aspects of the teratogenicity of drugs,* New York, 1976, American Elsevier, p 145.

203. Humphreys F, Marks JM: Mepacrine and pregnancy. *Br J Dermatol* 118:452, 1988.

204. Atabrine Product Information, New York, NY, Sanofi-Winthrop Pharmaceuticals, Inc., 1994.

205. The WHO Working Group. Bennett PN, editor: *Drugs and human lactation,* Amsterdam, 1996, Elsevier, pp 375-376.

206. Parke AL: Antimalarial drugs, pregnancy and lactation. *Lupus* 2(Suppl 1):S21-S23, 1993.

207. Auer H, Kollaritsch H, Juptner J, et al: Albendazole and pregnancy. *Appl Parasitol* 35(2):146-147, 1994.

208. Albenza Product Information, SmithKline Beecham Pharmaceuticals, Philadelphia, PA, 1997.

209. Bost RG: Metronidazole: toxicology and teratology. In Fiegold SM, editor: *Metronidazole: proceedings of the international metronidazole conference 1976,* New York, 1977, Excerpta Medica, pp 112-118.

210. Roe FJC: Toxicologic evaluation of metronidazole with particular reference to carcinogenic, mutagenic, and teratogenic potential. *Surgery* 93:158-164, 1983.

211. Peterson WF, Stauch JE, Ryder CD: Metronidazole in pregnancy. *Am J Obstet Gynecol* 94:243-249, 1966.

212. Protostat Product Information, Raritan, NJ, Ortho Pharmaceutical Corporation, 1992.

213. Czeizel AE, Rockenbauer M: A population based case-control teratologic study of oral metronidazole treatment during pregnancy. *Br J Obstet Gynaecol* 105(3):322-327, 1998.

214. Chow AW, Jewesson PJ: Pharmacokinetics and safety of antimicrobial agents during pregnancy. *Rev Infect Dis* 7:287-313, 1985.

215. Pentamidine, systemic. In *USP-DI. Drug information for the health care professional,* vol 1, Taunton, MA, 1998, Rand McNally, pp 2286-2289.

216. Briggs GG, Freeman RK, Yaffe SL: *Drugs in pregnancy and lactation,* ed 5, Baltimore, MD, 1998, Williams and Wilkins, pp 830-832.

217. Pentam Product Information, Deerfield, IL, Fujisawa USA, Inc., 1992.

218. Briggs GG, Freeman RK, Yaffe SL: *Drugs in pregnancy and lactation,* ed 5, Baltimore, MD, 1998, Williams and Wilkins, pp 830-832.

219. Thiabendazole, systemic. In *USP-DI. Drug information for the health care professional,* vol 1, Taunton, MA, Rand McNally, pp 2820-2823.

220. Mintezol Product Information, West Point, PA, Merck and Co.,1997.

221. Delatour P, Parisk RC, Gyurik RJ: Albendazole: a comparison of relay embryotoxicity of individual products. *Ann Rech Vet* 12:159-167, 1981.

222. Eurax Product Information, Buffalo, NY, Westwood-Squibb Pharmaceuticals, Inc., 1998.

223. Stromectol Product Information, West Point, PA, Merck and Co., Inc., 1997.

224. Pacque M, Munoz B, Poetschke G, et al: Pregnancy outcome after inadvertent ivermectin treatment during community-based distribution. *Lancet* 336(8729):1486-1489, 1990.

225. Hurwitz S: Scabies in babies. *Am J Dis Child* 126:226-228, 1973.

226. Pramanik AK, Hansen RC: Transcutaneous gamma benzene hexachloride absorption and toxicity in infants and children. *Arch Dermatol* 115:1224-1225, 1979.

227. Rasmussen JE: The problem of lindane. *J Am Acad Dermatol* 5:507-516, 1981.

228. Rasmussen JE: Lindane, a prudent approach. *Arch Dermatol* 123:1008-1009, 1987.

229. Shacter B: Treatment of scabies and pediculosis with lindane preparations: an evaluation. *J Am Acad Dermatol* 5:517-527, 1981.

230. Chowdhury AR, Gautam AK, Bhatnagar VK: Lindane-induced changes in morphology and lipids profile of testes in rats. *Biomed Biochim Acta* 49:1059-1065, 1990.

231. Lee B, Broth P: Scabies: transcutaneous poisoning during treatment. *Pediatrics* 59:643, 1977.

232. Friedman SJ: Lindane neurotoxic reaction in nonbullous congenital ichthyosiform erythroderma. *Arch Dermatol* 123:1056-1058, 1987.

233. Kwell Product Information. Humacao, Puerto Rico, Reedco, Inc., 1997.

234. Lindane, topical. In *USP-DI. Drug information for the health care professional*, vol 1, Taunton, MA, 1998, Rand McNally, pp 1876-1879.

235. Briggs GG, Freeman RK, Yaffe SL: *Drugs in pregnancy and lactation*, ed 5, Baltimore, MD, 1998, Williams and Wilkins, pp 613-614.

236. Altschuler DZ, Kenney LR: Pediculocide performance, profit, and the public health. *Arch Dermatol* 122:259-261, 1986.

237. Haustein U, Hlawa B: Treatment of scabies with permethrin versus lindane and benzyl benzoate. *Acta Derm Venereol* 69:348-351, 1986.

238. Miyamoto J: Degradation, metabolism and toxicity of synthetic pyrethroids. *Environ Health Persp* 14:15-28, 1976.

239. Frantz TJ, Lehman PA, Franz SF, et al: Comparative percutaneous absorption of lindane and permethrin. *Arch Dermatol* 132:901-905, 1996.

240. Meinking TL, Taplin D: Safety of permethrin vs. lindane for the treatment of scabies. *Arch Dermatol* 132:959-962, 1996.

241. Elimite Product Information, Irvine, CA, Allergan, 1997.

242. Ogbuikiri J, Ozumba B, Okonkwo P: Ivermectin levels in human breast milk. *Eur J Clin Pharmaceut* 46:81-90, 1994.

243. Chahoud I, Stahlmann R, Bochert G, et al: Gross structural defects in rats after acyclovir application on day 10 of gestation. *Arch Toxicol* 62:8-14, 1988.

244. Stahlmann R, Klug S, Lwendowski C, et al: Prenatal toxicity of acyclovir in rats. *Arch Toxicol* 61:468-479, 1988.

245. Andrews EB, Tilson HH, Hurn BAL, et al: Acyclovir in pregnancy registry. An observational epidemiologic approach. *Am J Med* 85(Suppl 2A):123-128, 1988.

246. Andrews EB, Yankaskas BC, Cordero JF, et al: Acyclovir in pregnancy registry: six years' experience. *Obstet Gynecol* 79:7-13, 1992.

247. Zovirax Product Information. Research Triangle Park, NC, Glaxo Wellcome Co., 1997.

248. Briggs GG, Freeman RK, Yaffe SJ: *Drugs in pregnancy and lactation*, ed 5, Baltimore, MD, 1998, Williams and Wilkins, pp 12-18.

249. Famvir Product Information, Philadelphia, PA, SmithKline Beecham Pharmaceuticals, 1998.

250. Valtrex Product Information, Research Triangle Park, NC, Glaxo Wellcome Co., 1997.

251. Walker BE: Cleft palate produced in mice by human-equivalent dosage with triamcinolone. *Science* 149:862-863, 1965.

252. Gandelman R, Rosenthal C: Deleterious effects of prenatal prednisolone exposure upon morphological and behavioral development of mice. *Teratology* 24:293-301, 1981.

253. Corticosteroids/corticotropin-glucocorticoid effects-systemic. In *USP-DI. Drug information for the health care professional*, vol 1, Taunton, MA, 1998, Rand McNally, pp 952-978.

254. Kraus AM: Congenital cataract and maternal steroid ingestion. *J Pediatr Ophthalmol* 12:107-108, 1975.

255. Fraser F, Sajoo A: Teratogenic potential of corticosteroids in humans. *Teratology* 51(1):45-46, 1995.

256. Czeizel AE, Rockenbauer M: Population-based case-control study of teratogenic potential of corticosteroids. *Teratology* 56(5):335-340, 1997.

257. Briggs GG, Freeman RK, Yaffe SL: *Drugs in pregnancy and lactation*, ed 5, Baltimore, MD, 1998, Williams and Wilkins, pp 884-886.

258. Caldwell JR, Furst DE: The efficacy and safety of low-dose corticosteroids for rheumatoid arthritis. *Semin Arthritis Rheum* 21:1-11, 1991.

259. Reinisch JM, Simon NF, Karow WG, et al: Prenatal exposure to prednisone in human and animals retards intrauterine growth. *Science* 202:436-438, 1978.

260. Smith KD, Steingerger E, Rodriguez L: Prednisone therapy and birth weight. *Science* 296:96-97, 1979.

261. Langley-Evans SC: Intrauterine programming of hypertension by glucocorticoids. *Life Sciences* 60:1213-1221, 1997.

262. Lockshin MD, Druzin ML, Qamar T: Prednisone does not prevent fetal death in women with antiphospholipid antibody. *Am J Obstet Gynecol* 160:439-443, 1989.

263. Cormax Product Information, Teaneck, NJ, Oclassen Pharmaceuticals, 1996.

264. Diprolene Product Information, Kenbough, NJ, Schering Pharmaceuticals, 1997.

265. Psorcon Product Information, Kalamazoo, MI, Upjohn Pharmaceuticals, 1997.

266. Temovate Product Information, Research Triangle Park, NC, Glaxo Wellcome, 1996.

267. Ultravate Product Information, Buffalo, NY, Westwood-Squibb Pharmaceuticals, 1997.

268. Katz FH, Thorp JM Jr, Bowes WA Jr: Severe symmetric intrauterine growth retardation associated with the topical use of triamcinolone. *Am J Obstet Gynecol* 162:396-397, 1990.

269. Ost L, Wettrell G, Bjorkhem I, et al: Prednisolone excretion in human milk. *J Pediatr* 106:1008-1011, 1985.

270. Anderson PO: Corticosteroid use by breast-feeding mothers. *Clin Pharm* 6:445, 1987.

271. Rayburn WF: Glucocorticoid therapy for rheumatic diseases: maternal, fetal, and breast-feeding considerations. *Am J Reprod Immunol* 28(3-4):138-140, 1992.

272. Hydeltra-T.B.A. Product Information. West Point, PA, Merck & Co., Inc., 1997.

273. De Stefano P, Bongo C, Borgna-Pignatti C, et al: Factitious hypertension with mineralocorticoid excess in an infant. *Helv Paediatr Acta* 38:185-189, 1983.

274. Baturay N, Trombetta L: Cocarcinogenic and tumor-promoting capabilities of anthralin. *Arch Dermatol Res* 280(7):443-450, 1988.

275. Drithocreme Product Information, Collegeville, PA, Dermik Laboratories, Inc., 1998.

276. Micanol Product Information, Tampa, FL, Bioglan Pharmaceuticals, 1996.

277. Calcipotriene topical. In *USP-DI. Drug information for the health care professional,* vol 1, Taunton, MA, 1998, Rand McNally, pp 672-675.

278. Farb H, West DP, Pedvis-Leftick A: Clofazimine in pregnancy complicated by leprosy. *Obstet Gynecol* 59:122-123, 1982.

279. Browne SG, Hogerzeil LM: "B663" in the treatment of leprosy. Preliminary report of a pilot trial. *Lepr Rev* 33:6-10, 1962.

280. Briggs GG, Freeman RK, Yaffe SL: *Drugs in pregnancy and lactation,* ed 5, Baltimore, MD, 1998, Williams and Wilkins, pp 224-225.

281. Sarto F, Zordan M, Tomanin R; et al: Chromosomal alterations in peripheral blood lymphocytes, urinary mutagenicity and excretion of polycyclic aromatic hydrocarbons in six psoriatic patients undergoing coal tar therapy. *Carcinogenesis* 10(2):329-334, 1989.

282. VanSchooten FJ, Moonen EJ, Rhijnsburger E, et al: Dermal uptake of polycyclic aromatic hydrocarbons after hairwash with coal-tar shampoo (letter) (see comments). *Lancet* 26;344(8935):1505-1506, 1994. Comment in *Lancet* 4;345(8945):326, 1995.

283. Fototar Product Information, Costa Mesa, CA, ICN Pharmaceuticals, Inc., 1996.

284. Cyclosporine-systemic. In *USP-DI. Drug information for the health care professional,* vol 1, Taunton, MA, 1998, Rand McNally, pp 1098-1102.

285. Sangalli L, Bortolotti A, Passerini F, et al: Placental transfer, tissue distribution, and pharmacokinetics of cyclosporine in the pregnant rabbit. *Drug Metab Dispos* 18:102-106, 1990.

286. Ryffel B, Donatsch P, Madorin M, et al: Toxicological evaluation of cyclosporin A. *Arch Toxicol* 53:107-141, 1983.

287. Armenti VT, Ahlswede KM, Ahlswede BA: National transplantation pregnancy registry—outcomes of 154 pregnancies in cyclosporine-treated female kidney transplant recipients. *Transplantation* 57:502-506, 1994.

288. Armenti VT, Ahlswede KM, Ahlswede BA, et al: Variables affecting birthweight and graft survival in 197 pregnancies in cyclosporine-treated kidney transplant recipients. *Transplantation* 59:476-479, 1995.

289. Radomski JS, Ahlswede BA, Jarrell BE, et al: Outcomes of 500 pregnancies in 335 female kidney, liver, and heart transplant recipients. *Transplant Proc* 27:1089-1090, 1995.

290. Burrows D, O'Neil T, Sorrells T: Successful twin pregnancy after renal transplant maintained on cyclosporine A immunosuppression. *Obstet Gynecol* 1988 72(3 Pt 2):459-461, 1995.

291. Burrows DA, O'Neil TJ, Sorrells TL, et al: Cyclosporin A in a pregnant patient affected with systemic lupus erythematosus. *Rheumatol Int* 12(2):77-81, 1992.

292. Ostensen M: Treatment with immunosuppressive and disease modifying drugs during pregnancy and lactation. *Am J Reprod Immunol* 28(3-4):148-152, 1992.

293. Hussein MM, Mooij JM, Roujouleh H: Cyclosporine in the treatment of lupus nephritis including two patients treated during pregnancy. *Clin Nephrol* 40(3):160-163, 1993.

294. Briggs GG, Freeman RK, Yaffe SL: *Drugs in pregnancy and lactation,* ed 5, Baltimore, MD, 1998, Williams and Wilkins, pp 279-281.

295. Sandimmune Product Information, Summit, NJ, Novartis Pharmaceuticals, 1997.

296. Maurus JN: Hansen's disease in pregnancy. *Obstet Gynecol* 52:22-25, 1978.

297. Tuffanelli DL: Successful pregnancy in a patient with dermatitis herpetiformis treated with low-dose dapsone. *Arch Dermatol* 118:876, 1982.

298. Kahn G: Dapsone is safe during pregnancy. *J Am Acad Dermatol* 13:838-839, 1985.

299. Dapsone, systemic. In *USP-DI. Drug information for the health care professional,* vol 1, Taunton, MA, 1998, Rand McNally, pp 1126-1128.

300. Briggs GG, Freeman RK, Yaffe SL: *Drugs in pregnancy and lactation,* ed 5, Baltimore, MD, 1998, Williams and Wilkins, pp 296-300.

301. Thornton YS, Gowe ET: Neonatal hyperbilirubinemia after treatment of maternal leprosy. *S Med J* 82:668, 1989.

302. The WHO Working Group, Bennett PN, editor: Drugs and Human Lactation. Amsterdam, 1996, Elsevier, pp 139-140.

303. Dapsone Product Information, Princeton, NJ, Jacobus Pharmaceutical Co. Inc., 1997.

304. Szabo KT, Guenriero J, Kang YJ: The effect of gold-containing compounds on pregnant rats and their fetuses. *Vet Pathol* 15(Suppl 5):89, 1978.

305. Szabo KT, DiFebbo ME, Phelan DG: The effects of gold-containing compounds on pregnant rabbits and their fetuses. *Drug Intell Clin Pharm* 16:482-483, 1982.

306. Miyamoto T, Mijaya S, Horiuchi Y, et al: Gold therapy in bronchial asthma—special emphasis upon blood levels of gold and its teratogenicity. *Nippon Naika Gakai Zasshi* 63:1190-1197, 1974.

307. Tarp U, Graudal H: A follow-up study of children exposed to gold compounds in utero. *Arthritis Rheum* 16:777-778, 1985.

308. Briggs GG, Freeman RK, Yaffe SL: *Drugs in pregnancy and lactation,* ed 5, Baltimore, MD, 1998, Williams and Wilkins, pp 490-492.

309. Needs CJ, Brooks PM: Antirheumatic medication in pregnancy. *Br J Rheumatol* 24:291-297, 1985.

310. Solganol Product Information, Kenilworth, NJ, Schering Corporation, 1997.

311. Myochrisine Product Information, West Point, PA, Merck and Co., Inc., 1994.

312. Melanex Topical Solution Product Information, Los Angeles, CA, Neutrogena Dermatologics, 1995.

313. Imiquimod. In *USP DI. Drug information for the health care professional,* pp 1110-1111, August 1998.

314. Frieden IJ, Reese V, Cohen D: PHACE syndrome. The association of posterior fossa brain malformations, hemangiomas, arterial anomalies, coarctation of the aorta and cardiac defects, and eye abnormalities. *Arch Dermatol* 132(3):307-311, 1996.

315. Faulds D, Benfield P: Interferon beta-1b in multiple sclerosis. An initial review of its rationale for use and therapeutic potential. *Clin Immunother* 1:79-87, 1994.

316. Baer MR: Normal full-term pregnancy in a patient with chronic myelogenous leukemia treated with alpha-interferon (letter). *Am J Hematol* 37:66, 1991.

317. Betaseron Product Information, Richmond, CA, Berlex Laboratories, 1996.

318. Avonex Product Information, Cambridge, MA, Biogen Inc., 1998.

319. Alferon Product Information, Norwalk, CT, The Purdue Frederick Company, 1997.

320. Roferon Product Information, Nutley, NJ, Roche Pharmaceuticals, 1997.

321. Intron Product Information, Kenilworth, NJ, Schering Corporation, 1997.

322. Stern RS, Lange R: Outcomes of pregnancies among women and partners of men with a history of exposure to methoxsalen photochemotherapy (PUVA) for the treatment of psoriasis. *Arch Dermatol* 127:347-350, 1991.

323. Gunnarskog JG, Kallen AJB, Lindelop BG, et al: Psoralen photochemotherapy and pregnancy. *Arch Dermatol* 129:320-323, 1993.

324. Garbis H, Elefant E, Bertolotti E, et al: Pregnancy outcome after periconceptional and first-trimester exposure to methoxsalen photochemotherapy. *Arch Dermatol* 131:492-493, 1995.

325. Oxsoralen Lotion Product Information, Costa Mesa, CA, ICN Pharmaceuticals, Inc., 1996.

326. Rosa FW, Indanpaan-Heikkila J, Asanti R, et al: Fetal minoxidil exposure. *Pediatrics* 80:120, 1987.

327. Kaler S, Patrinos M, Lambert G, et al: Hypertrichosis and congenital anomalies associated with maternal use of minoxidil. *Pediatrics* 79(3):434-436, 1987.

328. Briggs GG, Freeman RK, Yaffe SL: *Drugs in pregnancy and lactation,* ed 5, Baltimore, MD, 1998, Williams and Wilkins, pp 737-739.

329. Rogaine Topical Solution Product Information, Kalamazoo, MI, The Upjohn Company, 1997.

330. Carlson TG, Geenstra ES: Toxocologic studies with the hypotensive agent minoxidil. *Toxicol Appl Pharmacol* 39:1-11, 1977.

331. Briggs GG, Freeman RK, Yaffe SL: *Drugs in pregnancy and lactation,* ed 5, Baltimore, MD, 1998, Williams and Wilkins, p 836.

332. Trental Product Information, Somerville, NJ, Hoechst-Roussell Pharmaceuticals Inc., 1995.

333. Briggs GG, Freeman RK, Yaffe SL: *Drugs in pregnancy and lactation,* ed 5, Baltimore, MD, 1998, Williams and Wilkins, pp 877-878.

334. Podophyllum, topical. In *USP DI. Drug information for the health care professional,* vol 1, Taunton, MA, 1998, Rand McNally, pp 2371-2373.

335. Condylox Product Information, Teaneck, NJ, Oclassen Pharmaceuticals, Inc., 1997.

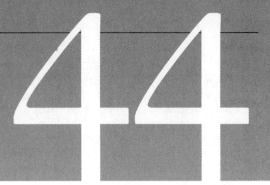
Lori E. Shapiro
Neil H. Shear

Drug Interactions

Patients and physicians are often concerned about the risk of using multiple drugs simultaneously. Drug interactions may lead to adverse outcomes; however, most patients receiving drugs with significant potential for interactions do not manifest clinically significant adverse outcomes. It is important to be aware of situations in which the patient is truly at risk.[1] Adverse drug interactions may lead to increased toxicity, decreased efficacy, or both.[2] Although it is impossible to remember all drug interactions, knowledge of the interactive properties of drugs can help prevent serious adverse drug interactions. Nonprescription drugs, herbal or alternative medicines, and foods (e.g., grapefruit juice) may be implicated in drug interactions. Prediction of drug interactions is possible when those agents that are likely to produce alterations in drug metabolism via inhibition or induction of the cytochrome P-450 (CYP) system are recognized. Many of these drug combinations can be administered safely with appropriate dosage adjustments or by substitution with another member of the drug class with less potential for drug interactions.

Increased risk of drug-induced toxicity or therapeutic failure can result when a new drug is added to a therapeutic regimen. The drugs of interest can be grouped into two categories—"accomplices" and "bullets."[3] Accomplice drugs are those drugs that help other drugs become more dangerous or less effective. Commonly used synonyms for accomplice drugs are "inhibitors" or "inducers." Bullet drugs directly cause morbidity and sometimes mortality because of increased toxicity or decreased efficacy. Commonly used synonyms for bullet drugs are "targets" or "substrates."

Drug interactions involve either a pharmacokinetic or pharmacodynamic mechanism.[4] In pharmacokinetic interactions, one drug alters the rate or degree of absorption, distribution from binding sites, hepatic metabolism, or excretion of another drug. Pharmacodynamic interactions occur when one drug induces a change in another, usually by synergistic effects, without altering its plasma level, or occur when drugs compete for binding to a receptor directly related to the pharmacologic response.

Most relevant drug interactions in dermatology have a pharmacokinetic mechanism, and recent studies suggest that the most clinically important drug interactions involve hepatic drug biotransformation pathways catalyzed by the CYP family of enzymes. Many of the drug interactions of particular relevance to dermatologists involve the CYP 3A4 isoenzymes. Knowledge of the interactive potential of various drugs can help prevent serious adverse drug interactions.[5] The most important "accomplice" drugs interfere with drug absorption, distribution, and elimination, as well as metabolism. Foods, such as grapefruit juice, are also important accomplices to consider.

Important bullet drugs for dermatologists include dermatologic therapies such as certain nonsedating H_1 antihistamines, cyclosporine, methotrexate, azathioprine, and certain antimicrobial agents. Commonly prescribed nondermatologic treatments, such as digitalis, warfarin, oral contraceptives, quinidine, and cisapride, can also be bullets. All dermatologists should be familiar with this list of bullet drugs and their respective accomplices.

POTENTIAL CONSEQUENCES OF DRUG-DRUG INTERACTIONS

Pharmacokinetically based mechanisms of drug interactions can be understood in terms of causing the metabolism or excretion of a drug to be unusually slow or fast.[6] The major consequence is either a high or low plasma and tissue level of the drug.

If the metabolism of the drug is impeded due to enzyme inhibition, a high plasma level may result. Subsequently, there may be increased pharmacologic activity, which may or may not be a problem depending on the therapeutic index of the drug. However, not only may the desired effect be enhanced but also any undesirable side effects. If activation of a prodrug is inhibited, then a reduced level of therapeutic effectiveness might be expected. Also when the major pathway of drug metabolism of a drug is partially or completely blocked, alternative pathways may become more favorable, which may be a problem if the secondary pathway leads to biotransformation to a toxic product. Furthermore, the increased level of a drug due to inhibition of the CYP enzymes involved in its oxidation may lead to inhibition of another CYP isoform.

When levels of various CYP isoforms or any other enzyme are induced, the major concern is a lack of therapeutic effectiveness. Alternatively, a prodrug could be activated too rapidly and a dangerously high level of the active drug could result.

THE ASSESSMENT OF RISK IN THE CLINICAL OUTCOME OF DRUG INTERACTIONS

The clinical importance of specific drug interactions is often either overestimated or underestimated, as these assessments are largely based on clinical experience in using the particular drug combination.[7] The clinical outcome of most drug interactions is highly situational. Most patients who receive drugs with the potential for interactions do not develop adverse effects. Emphasis should be placed on those factors that increase or decrease the risk to a given patient.

To prevent or detect drug interactions, the physician needs to identify risk factors in the individual patient. Some patient groups are more likely than others to develop adverse events caused by drug interactions (Box 44-1). Risk factors are listed and grouped by category in this box.[8]

The elderly frequently experience drug interactions as a result of physiologic changes that accompany the aging process and the types of drugs that older patients receive.[9] Polypharmacy, which is common in the elderly, makes them particularly susceptible. Various medications may impair pathways of drug elimination by interfering with drug metabolism, thus increasing the likelihood of adverse drug reactions. Alterations due to advanced age, including changes in drug-protein binding and drug distribution in tissue, may promote drug interactions.

Patients with acquired immunodeficiency syndrome (AIDS) have a higher rate of adverse drug reactions. In some instances, this may relate to phenotypic changes in drug metabolism, which can vary with AIDS progression.[10]

A major source of interindividual differences in drug metabolism are genetic polymorphisms, which are inherited significant variations in the activity of drug metabolizing enzymes. These polymorphisms exist for various CYP isoforms and N-acetyltransferase (Table 44-1). There are also interethnic differences in drug metabolism, differences in the expression of CYP isoforms and glucuronyltransferases, as well as different frequencies of genetic polymorphisms.[11] Several of these genetic polymorphisms are now well studied at the epidemiologic, protein, and deoxyribonucleic acid

Box 44-1

Patient Risk Factors for Drug Interactions

MULTIPLE MEDICATIONS
- Polypharmacy demographic risk factors
- Female gender
- Extremes of age (very young and elderly)

MAJOR ORGAN DYSFUNCTION (ESPECIALLY MULTIPLE ORGANS)
- Liver dysfunction
- Renal dysfunction
- Congestive heart failure

METABOLIC AND ENDOCRINE RISK FACTORS
- Obesity
- Hypothyroidism
- Hypoproteinemia

PHARMACOGENETIC RISK FACTORS
- Slow acetylator phenotype
- Other genetic polymorphisms (see text)

OTHER MEDICAL ISSUES
- Hypothermia
- Hypotension
- Dehydration

Adapted from Andersen W, Feingold D: *Arch Dermatol* 131:468-473, 1995.

■ **Table 44-1** Influences on the Activity of Various Cytochrome Isoforms

	1A2	2C9/19	2D6	2E1	3A4
Nutrition	+			+	+
Smoking	+				
Alcohol				+	
Drugs	+	+	+		+
Environmental factors	+			+	+
Genetics		+	+		

Adapted from Rendic S, DiCarlo FJ: *Drug Metab Rev* 29:413-580, 1997.

(DNA) levels. In some cases, it is possible to determine an individual's genotype.[12] Further details on genetic polymorphisms are discussed later.

Disease states can either predispose a patient or protect a patient from the adverse effects of a drug interaction. The disease state itself may directly affect the outcome of the interaction. The disease state may dictate the way in which a drug is used and this subsequently affects the outcome. When a drug has more than one therapeutic action, an interacting drug may affect the action of another drug when it is used to treat one disease but not when it is used to treat another disease. This is known as pharmacologic selectivity.

An example of intrinsic effects of disease states includes when epinephrine is given to patients receiving noncardioselective β-adrenergic blockers and results in hypertension in patients who do not have anaphylaxis. The same β-blockers inhibit the pressor response of epinephrine in patients with anaphylaxis.[13]

An example of a disease-dependent drug interaction is the concomitant use of nonsteroidal antiinflammatory drugs (NSAIDs) and methotrexate. Available evidence indicates that the risk of this combination is considerably greater in patients receiving methotrexate for cancer (i.e., in large doses) compared with patients receiving lower dosages for psoriasis.[14]

Gender-related differences in pharmacokinetics may cause variations in drug absorption, gastric emptying, and distribution based on percent of adipose tissue.[15] Gender-related differences in receptor density and sensitivity, enzyme activity (CYP 2D6), and underlying disease activities also contribute to pharmacokinetic variation. This variability causes confusion as tables and lists outlining potentially interacting agents can vary between different sources. The effect of obesity on metabolism is cytochrome-specific. Obesity decreases the activity of CYP 3A4 and increases the activity of CYP 2E1.[16]

The medications that are most likely to be involved in drug interactions must also be evaluated. Interactions occur with drugs that have a narrow margin of safety, thus a narrow therapeutic index. Drugs with the potential for such serious interactions include warfarin, monoamine oxidase inhibitors, and cyclosporine.

ABSORPTION

Drug interactions in the gastrointestinal (GI) tract can result in decreased absorption. This decrease reduces the bioavailability or the amount of drug available to the systemic circulation and results in subtherapeutic serum concentrations (Table 44-2). The mechanisms of most drug interactions that alter absorption involve the formation of drug complexes that reduce absorption, alterations in the gastric pH, or changes in GI motility that alter transit time.[17]

Common drugs that form complexes with other drugs include antacids, sucralfate, and cholesterol-binding resins. A significant interaction occurs between multivalent cations such as the tetracyclines and fluoroquinolone antibiotics. There is an 85% reduction in the absorption of ciprofloxacin when ingested 5 to 10 minutes after a dose of an aluminum hydroxide/magnesium hydroxide antacid.[18] Alendronate, the new bisphosphonate for the prevention and treatment of osteoporosis, forms complexes with many drugs, thereby further decreasing its already low oral absorption.

Drugs that increase gastric pH, such as proton pump inhibitors, antacids, and H_2 antihistamines, may reduce the absorption of drugs

■ Table 44-2   Drug Interactions that Increase Risk of "Bullet" Drug Toxicity[2,3]

Mechanism	"Bullet" Drugs	"Accomplice" Drugs	Time Course
Competitive inhibition of CYP 3A4	Cisapride Cyclosporine Dapsone H_1 antihistamines • Astemizole • Terfenadine Macrolides • Erythromycin	Antidepressants • Fluoxetine • Nefazadone Azole antifungals • Ketoconazole • Itraconazole • Fluconazole Grapefruit juice HIV-1 protease inhibitors • Indinavir • Ritonavir Macrolides • Clarithromycin • Erythromycin Quinine	Rapid
Reduced metabolic clearance	Azathioprine Methotrexate	Allopurinol Salicylates	Rapid
Displacement from plasma proteins	Methotrexate	NSAIDs Salicylates Sulfonamides	Rapid
Reduced renal elimination	Methotrexate	NSAIDs Penicillins Probenecid Salicylates Sulfonamides	Rapid
Synergy	Methotrexate Isotretin Acitretin Serotonin reuptake inhibitors	Retinoids Sulfonamides Tetracyclines Alcohol Monoamine oxidase inhibitors	Variable

such as ketoconazole and itraconazole, which are absorbed best in an acidic environment.[19] Drugs that affect GI motility, such as anticholinergic agents and cisapride, may decrease the rate of absorption but not the extent of absorption. An overall reduction in the extent of drug absorption has more clinical significance.[1]

Some drugs may interfere with the enterohepatic recirculation of a bullet drug. When the bullet drug is excreted into the GI tract, the accomplice drug can bind to it and prevent its reabsorption back into the systemic circulation. The bound bullet drug is excreted in the feces, thereby effectively shortening its half-life by reducing the total absorption. An example of this is the concurrent administration of warfarin and cholestyramine. The half-life of warfarin is shortened by oral cholestyramine.

DISTRIBUTION

Drugs that are highly protein bound (>90%) may cause drug interactions based on alterations in drug distribution. When one drug displaces another from plasma protein-binding sites, the free serum concentration of the displaced drug is increased and its pharmacologic effect increases. However, the unbound fraction of the drug is not only more available to sites of action but is also more readily eliminated. Any enhanced pharmacologic effect occurs only transiently because of a compensatory increase in elimination, and the clinical effect of displacement interactions is usually negligible. Therefore these interactions involving drug displacement from binding proteins tend to be self-limiting. Typically the pharmacologic activity of the displaced drug is increased for a few days. This is followed by return of the pharmacologic response back to the previous unbound serum concentration even if the concomitant therapy is continued. Therefore it is safe to say that if a patient does not manifest an adverse event from the combination therapy in the first week or so of administration, an adverse event probably will not occur. In practice, protein-binding displacement interactions do not produce clinically important changes in drug response unless the drug also has a limited distribution in the body, is slowly eliminated, or has

a low therapeutic index.[1] For this reason, protein-binding displacement interactions may assume greater importance when the displacing accomplice drug also reduced the elimination of the bullet (target or substrate) drug. A good example of this principle involves interactions with NSAIDs and methotrexate.

Medications that are most susceptible to interactions based on changes in drug distribution involving displacement from binding proteins include warfarin, sulfonamides, and phenytoin.[9]

METABOLISM

The most clinically relevant drug interactions are caused by alterations in drug metabolism (Table 44-3). When drugs are administered, they are metabolized through a series of reactions to enhance drug hydrophilicity (water solubility) and facilitate drug excretion. These drug biotransformation reactions are grouped into two categories—phase I and phase II. Phase I reactions involve intramolecular changes, such as oxidation, reduction, and hydrolysis, that make the drug somewhat more polar. Phase II reactions are conjugation reactions in which an endogenous substance combines the functional group derived from phase I reactions to produce a highly polar drug conjugate that can be readily eliminated. Examples of these phase II reactions include glucuronidation and sulfonation.

The metabolic products are often less active than the parent drugs or may even be inactive. More commonly the metabolite is inactive. However, some metabolites may have enhanced activity or toxic effects including roles of these metabolites in carcinogenesis, mutagenesis, or teratogenesis.[20] Therefore biotransformation may include both detoxification and toxification processes. An example of this principle would be cyclophosphamide. This drug is actually a prodrug that is metabolized to phosphoramide mustard (the active form of the drug) and to a second metabolite, acrolein, which induces bladder toxicity.

The most important organ of biotransformation is the liver, although other organs (e.g., the small intestine and lung) can contribute to overall drug metabolism, depending on the route of administration. Drug-metabolizing en-

■ **Table 44-3**   Drug Interactions that Reduce Efficacy of "Bullet" Drug Toxicity

Mechanism	Bullet Drugs	Accomplice Drugs	Time Course
Reduced gastrointestinal absorption	Azole antifungals • Itraconazole • Ketoconazole Tetracycline Dapsone	Antacids Didanosine H₂ antihistamines Proton pump inhibitors Divalent cations • Calcium • Magnesium	Rapid
Induction of CYP 3A4	Calcineurin inhibitors • Cyclosporine • Tacrolimus Oral contraceptives Prednisone Warfarin	Anticonvulsants • Carbamazepine • Phenytoin • Phenobarbital Antituberculous agents • Isoniazid • Rifampin Dexamethasone Griseofulvin	1 to 2 weeks
Antagonistic effects	Epinephrine Cyproheptadine	β-Blockers SSRI antidepressants • Fluoxetine • Paroxetine	Rapid

zymes include the CYP mixed-function oxidases, thiopurine methyltransferase, *N*-acetyltransferase, epoxide hydrolases, and glutathione synthetase.[21]

CYTOCHROME P-450 ENZYMES

The CYP enzymes are the most important drug-metabolizing enzymes. They are present in the endoplasmic reticulum of many types of cells but are at highest concentration in hepatocytes.[22] These heme-containing proteins exist as gene superfamilies, with the encoded isoforms exhibiting distinct but overlapping substrate specificities and isoform-specific regulatory and pharmacogenetic properties.[23] The enzymes were given their name because under reactive conditions their complexes with carbon monoxide display an easily detected absorbance maximum at 450 nm. In general, CYP enzymes with greater than 40% homology are included in the same family, and those with greater than 55% sequence identity are included in the same subfamily.[24] An Arabic number is used to designate individual enzymes

within a subfamily. The enzymes were numbered in the order in which they were identified. More than 500 CYP enzymes have now been identified, with 18 of 74 families existing in mammals. Twenty subfamilies have been mapped in the human genome. Families 1 to 3 contribute substantially to drug and nondrug xenobiotic metabolism, whereas the remainder are important in the metabolism and/or biosynthesis of endogenous compounds such as bile acids, eicosanoids, retinoids, and steroids.[25]

The use of recombinant DNA technology provides an unlimited source of CYP enzymes for studying structure and function. It is now relatively straightforward to use in vitro studies to determine which CYP isoforms oxidize a particular drug and which drugs can inhibit or induce oxidation reactions catalyzed by this isoform. The major limitation of in vitro approaches is that the most optimal therapeutic concentration of a new drug and of its primary metabolites or its concentration in a given tissue is not precisely known.[20,26]

It is also possible to do logical in vivo studies to test the relevance of in vitro findings.[6] Individuals known to have high or low activity in a particular CYP isoform (determined by the use of other noninvasive assays) can be examined with regard to the pharmacokinetics of the new drug to see if there is a match. This match refers to correlation between in vivo pharmacokinetic studies and in vitro testing of the patient's CYP isoform. In certain cases, inducers or inhibitors of a specific CYP isoform can be given safely to study volunteers to verify that a CYP enzyme is involved in metabolizing the drug. Also, the drug under consideration can be given to study volunteers to determine if the study drug affects the pharmacokinetics of other drugs through enzyme induction or inhibition.

Emphasis on drug safety is increasing, as newly developed drugs become more potent. The Food and Drug Administration (FDA) now requires in vitro information on the CYP isoforms involved in the oxidation of a drug early in the development process. The in vitro information comes from studies using liver microsome fractions or hepatocyte cultures that cover both phase I and phase II reactions to permit quantitative prediction of the various metabolic pathways. The increasing availability of specific antibodies and selective substrates and inhibitors for each major CYP enzyme provides the tools for initial studies. The in vitro information can be used to guide the more expensive in vivo studies. In particular, potential adverse drug interactions due to pharmacokinetics can be predicted, and the number of in vivo interaction studies can be minimized.[24] The preclinical studies of drug metabolism should determine the metabolic pathways, the enzyme systems responsible, whether a genetic polymorphism is involved, whether the drug is an inducer or inhibitor, and what the possible drug interactions are. The in vitro procedures may be used to select from a series of potential candidates in terms of which will least likely cause problems with drug-drug interactions. The major known human CYP isoforms can also use the in vitro studies as a guide in predicting bioavailability by screening candidate drugs for resistance to oxidation.

Knowledge of the substrates, inhibitors, and inducers of these enzymes assists in predicting clinically significant drug interactions. Fortunately, the metabolism of most drugs can be ac-

counted for by a relatively small subset of the CYP isoforms. It is thought that over 90% of human drug oxidation can be attributed to six enzymes (isoforms): CYP 1A2, 2C9/10, 2C19, 2D6, 2E1 and 3A4.[27] One third to one half of drug metabolism can be attributed to CYP 3A4. This statistic indicates the greater likelihood of drug-drug interactions involving CYP 3A4. The concept that most drug oxidation reactions are catalyzed primarily by a small number of CYP enzymes is important in that approaches to identifying drug-drug interactions become more feasible, both in vitro and in vivo. Deciding what is clinically relevant is a challenging, relatively new field of investigation.[28]

Using in vitro tests that focus on cytochrome enzymes alone to predict clinical interactions may not always be reliable for three reasons. First, it is not always possible to know the therapeutic concentration of a new drug and of its primary metabolites in specific tissues.[26] Second, there are a large number of pathways and interactions, and it is impossible to test them all. Third, even the demonstration of an in vitro effect does not tell physicians whether the effect is likely to occur in clinical practice (i.e., the clinical significance of an in vitro interaction is unknown). Until clinical data demonstrate the presence or absence of a clinically significant interaction, dosage adjustments are premature.[29] Multiple clinical reports of interactions are the best evidence that concurrent use of two drugs may have an adverse outcome.

Each CYP isoform can oxidize several drugs and have wide substrate specificity. A drug may have a very high affinity for one particular CYP. Under physiologic conditions, this CYP isoform almost exclusively catalyzes the drug's oxidation. Many commonly used drugs have been identified as substrates for specific CYP subfamilies.[30] Examples would include cyclosporine and finasteride, which are substrates of CYP 3A4.

The enzyme CYP 1A2 partially catalyzes theophylline, warfarin, and caffeine metabolism (Box 44-2). Fluoroquinolone antibiotics (e.g., ciprofloxacin) and macrolide antibiotics (e.g., erythromycin) inhibit CYP 1A2. Drugs such as phenytoin, phenobarbital, omeprazole, and cigarette smoke increase (induce) this isoform's activity.

CYP 2C9 has substrates that include phenytoin, warfarin, and tolbutamide. Fluconazole in-

Box 44-2

CYP 1A2 Substrates and Selected Accomplices (Inhibitors and Inducers)

SUBSTRATE	**INHIBITORS—cont'd**
Tricyclic Antidepressants	*Other Drugs*
Amitriptyline	Ticlopidine
Clomipramine	
Desipramine	*HIV-1 Protease Inhibitors*
Imipramine	Ritonavir
Other Drugs	*Proton Pump Inhibitors*
Caffeine	Omeprazole
Tacrine	
Theophylline	**INDUCERS**
Warfarin	*Anticonvulsants*
Zileuton	Barbiturates
	Phenytoin
INHIBITORS	
Azole Antifungal Agents	*Antituberculous Agents*
Ketoconazole	Rifampin
Fluoroquinolones	*Foods and Habits*
Ciprofloxacin	Brussels sprouts
Norfloxacin	Cabbage
	Charbroiled foods
H₂ Antihistamines	Cigarette smoking
Cimetidine	
Macrolides	
Clarithromycin	
Erythromycin	

hibits 2C9, which is relevant to dermatologists[31] (Box 44-3). Rarely, a genetic defect for 2C9 is present.[20]

The enzyme CYP 2D6 mediates the metabolism of substrate psychotropic drugs such as amitriptyline, desipramine, nortriptyline, and cocaine, as well as cardiac drugs such as debrisoquine, metoprolol, encainaide, flecainide, and propafenone (Box 44-4). The gene encoding this enzyme exhibits a polymorphism that leads to clinical phenotypes showing either "extensive" or "poor" drug metabolism. CYP 2D6 activity can vary more than 1000-fold due to genetic polymorphism.[32] Much of the unpredictability of patient tolerance to doxepin for pruritus relates to CYP 2D6 polymorphism. The SSRI type of antidepressants are inhibitors of CYP 2D6, potentially leading to significant increased risk of excessive sedation or even cardiotoxicity when coprescribed with doxepin. The drugs haloperidol and quinidine also inhibit CYP 2D6.[33]

Members of the CYP 3A4 subfamily are the most abundant of the human cytochromes, accounting for up to 70% of GI (hepatic and GI epithelium) cytochromes. CYP 3A4 is also located in the placenta, uterus, kidney, lung, and fetus. This subfamily is the major metabolizing isoform for many of the drugs prescribed by dermatologists. The most important CYP isoform is 3A4. Recent data suggest that CYP 3A5 isoform may also be of clinical importance. This isoform is found in 20% to 30% of adult livers and is expressed in the stomach. In the intestinal tract, CYP enzymes are present in the crypt cells, but the highest concentration is in the en-

Box 44-3

CYP 2C9 Substrates and Selected Accomplices (Inhibitors and Inducers)

SUBSTRATES
Antibacterial Agents
Sulfonamides

Anticonvulsants
Phenytoin
Valproic acid

HMG CoA Reductase Inhibitors
Fluvastatin

NSAIDs
Diclofenac
Ibuprofen
Piroxicam

Tricyclic Antidepressants
Amitriptyline

Other Drugs
Losartan
Warfarin

INHIBITORS
Antibacterial Agents
Sulfonamides
Trimethoprim

Antidysrhythmics
Amiodarone

INHIBITORS—cont'd
Azole Antifungal Agents
Fluconazole
Ketoconazole

H2 Antihistamines
Cimetidine

HIV-1 Protease Inhibitors
Ritonavir

Proton Pump Inhibitors
Omeprazole

SSRI Antidepressants
Fluvoxamine

INDUCERS
Anticonvulsants
Barbiturates
Carbamazepine

Antituberculous Agents
Rifampin

Other Drugs
Ethanol

---

terocytes (GI epithelial cells) at the tips of the villi. Enterocyte CYP 3A4 can cause significant first pass metabolism of up to 50% of orally administered cyclosporine.[34]

There is significant interindividual variability in the metabolic activity of CYP 3A4 isoforms. The extent of variability may be as much as twentyfold or more.[24] Factors reported to influence the activity and level of CYP 3A4 include nutritional, drug, and environmental. Population studies to date suggest the unimodal ("bell-shaped curve") distribution of CYP 3A4 activity. The individual degree of CYP 3A4 activity may have clinical relevance. Patients with low rates of dapsone hydroxylation, presumably reflecting low CYP 3A4 activity, were found to have a 5.4-fold higher incidence of aggressive bladder cancer, suggesting a protective role for CYP 3A4.[35]

Successful application of information on CYP isoforms to prevent drug interactions and improve the therapeutic risk:benefit ratios can occur only if the specific enzyme that is responsible for the metabolism of a drug is known. An enhanced understanding of the way in which CYP enzymes metabolize drugs can improve drug therapy in a variety of ways. Drug interactions should be more predictable based on the knowledge of which compounds induce and inhibit specific CYP enzymes.[33]

Box 44-4

CYP 2D6 Substrates and Selected Accomplices (Inhibitors and Inducers)

SUBSTRATES

Analgesics
Codeine
Dextromethorphan
Meperidine
Morphine

Antidysrhythmics
Encainide
Flecainide
Mexiletine
Propafenone

Antipsychotic Agents
Clozapine
Haloperidol
Pimozide
Risperidone

β-Blockers
Metoprolol
Propranolol

Miscellaneous Antidepressants
Trazodone
Venlafaxine

SSRI Antidepressants
Fluoxetine
Paroxetine

Tricyclic Antidepressants
Amitriptyline
Clomipramine
Desipramine
Doxepin

INHIBITORS
Allylamine Antifungals
Terbinafine

INHIBITORS—cont'd
Antidysrhythmics
Amiodarone
Propafenone
Quinidine

Antipsychotic Agents
Haloperidol
Thioridazine

H_2 Antihistamines
Cimetidine

SSRI Antidepressants
Fluoxetine
Paroxetine
Sertraline

Tricyclic Antidepressants
Clomipramine
Desipramine

HIV-1 Protease Inhibitors
Ritonavir

INDUCERS
Anticonvulsants
Carbamazepine
Phenobarbital
Phenytoin

Antituberculous Agents
Isoniazid
Rifampin

Induction of Cytochrome P-450 3A4

Many enzymes involved in drug biotransformation are able to increase in amount and activity in response to substances known as inducers. It usually takes at least a week before the effects of maximal enzyme induction are manifest. The rapidity of the onset of enzyme induction depends on the half-life of the enzyme-inducing drug. The elimination of a drug substrate is enhanced by specific enzyme inducers, typically resulting in a reduction of the pharmacologic response for the more rapidly metabolized drug.

Box 44-5

CYP 3A4 Selected Inhibitors and Inducers ("Accomplices")

INHIBITORS
Antibiotics
Clarithromycin*
Erythromycin*
Metronidazole
Norfloxacin
Quinupristin and dalfopristin (Synercid)
Troleandomycin

Azole Antifungals
Fluconazole* (> 200 mg/d)
Itraconazole*
Ketoconazole*

Calcium Channel Blockers
Diltiazem
Nifedipine
Verapamil

HIV-1 Protease Inhibitors
Indinavir*
Nelfinavir
Ritonavir*
Saquinavir

SSRI Antidepressants
Fluoxetine
Fluvoxamine
Paroxetine
Sertraline

INHIBITORS—cont'd
Other Inhibitors
Amiodarone
Antiprogestins
Cannabinoids
Cimetidine
Grapefruit juice
Interferon-γ
Quinine
Tacrolimus

INDUCERS
Anticonvulsants
Carbamazepine
Ethosuximide
Phenobarbital
Phenytoin
Primidone

Antituberculous Agents
Isoniazid
Rifampin

Other Inducers
Dexamethasone
Griseofulvin
Nefazadone

*These drugs are particularly potent inhibitors of CYP 3A4 and can lead to clinically important drug interactions.

The onset and cessation of enzyme induction are gradual because the induction phase depends on the accumulation of the particular inducing agent and subsequent synthesis of new enzyme, whereas cessation of enzyme induction depends on elimination of the inducer and decay of the increased enzyme levels.

Rifampin is one of the most potent inducers of CYP 3A4 and induces this cytochrome isoform more rapidly than enzyme inducers with longer half-lives. Other inducers of this isoform include anticonvulsants, dexamethasone, and griseofulvin[36] (Boxes 44-5 and 44-6). In general, enzyme induction appears to be dose-dependent, with larger doses of a given enzyme inducer producing a greater degree of enzyme induction.[37] Due to high interpatient variability and differences in susceptibility of various bullet (substrate) drugs, it is difficult to predict what dose of the inducer will produce what degree of enzyme induction in a given patient. This variability is influenced by age, genetics, concurrent therapy with more than one inducer, concurrent therapy with an enzyme inhibitor, and the presence of liver disease.[37]

The effect of CYP 3A4 induction may be an increase in hepatic metabolism. In the setting of concomitant administration of rifampin and oral contraceptives, rifampin may enhance estrogen metabolism and explain why women

Box 44-6

CYP 3A4 Substrates ("Bullet" Drugs)

ANTIBACTERIAL AGENTS
Erythromycin
Rifampin

ANTIDYSRHYTHMICS
Amiodarone
Digoxin
Lidocaine
Propafenone
Quinidine

ANTICONVULSANTS
Carbamazepine
Ethosuximide

ANTIDEPRESSANTS
Amitriptyline
Doxepin
Imipramine
Sertraline

BENZODIAZEPINES
Alprazolam
Diazepam
Midazolam
Triazolam

CALCIUM CHANNEL BLOCKERS
Amlodipine
Diltiazem
Felodipine
Isradipine
Nifedipine
Verapamil

CANCER CHEMOTHERAPY
Busulfan
Cyclophosphamide
Docetaxel
Doxorubicin
Etoposide
Isofosfamide
Paclitaxel
Tamoxifen
Vinblastine
Vincristine

H₁ ANTIHISTAMINES
Astemizole
Fexofenadine
Loratadine
Terfenadine

HIV-1 PROTEASE INHIBITORS
Indinavir
Nelfinavir
Ritonavir
Saquinavir

HMG CoA REDUCTASE INHIBITORS
Atorvastatin
Lovastatin
Pravastatin
Simvastatin

IMMUNOSUPPRESSIVE DRUGS
Corticosteroids
Cyclophosphamide
Cyclosporine
Tacrolimus

PROTON PUMP INHIBITORS
Omeprazole

MISCELLANEOUS DRUGS
Acetaminophen
Cisapride
Codeine
Dapsone
Enalapril
Estrogens
Flutamide
Losartan
Oral contraceptives
Pimozide
Retinoic acid
Sildenafil (Viagra)
Theophylline
Warfarin
Zileuton

treated with this combination of therapy may experience oral contraceptive failure.[38]

Accomplice drugs that function as inducers of CYP 3A4 may enhance metabolism of a CYP 3A4 substrate to active metabolites with the potential for enhanced toxicity. The alkylating agent cyclophosphamide is a prodrug that requires metabolic activation to phosphoramide mustards for its therapeutic effect. Unfortunately, metabolic activation also leads to the formation of acrolein, which causes the bladder toxicity seen with this medication.[39]

Inhibition of Cytochrome P-450 3A4

The inhibition of drug metabolism is the most important mechanism for drug interactions because it can lead to an increase in plasma drug concentration, an increased drug response, and resultant toxicity. Inhibition of drug metabolism begins within the first one or two doses of the inhibitor (accomplice) and is maximal when a steady state concentration of the inhibitor is achieved (see Boxes 44-5 and 44-6).

Inhibitory interactions can be either competitive or noncompetitive. An example of competitive inhibition involves the tight binding of accomplice drugs (CYP 3A4 inhibitors), such as ketoconazole, cimetidine, and erythromycin, to the heme moiety of the CYP-450 isozyme. As long as the accomplice drug (enzyme inhibitor in this case) occupies this specific site of the CYP 3A4 isoform, the bullet drug (substrate) cannot be biotransformed.[40] As the concentration of the inhibiting drug increases, the degree of saturation of the specific isoenzyme system is increased. When the enzyme system is saturated, further metabolic activity by that enzyme system is limited. At that point, a patient becomes the equivalent of a poor metabolizer and concentrations of coprescribed medications begin to rise. The extent of inhibition of one drug by another depends on the affinity each compound has for the CYP isoform. Competitive inhibition depends on the affinity of the substrate for the enzyme being inhibited, the concentration of substrate required for inhibition, and the half-life of the inhibitor drug. The onset and cessation of enzyme inhibition are dependent on the half-life and time to steady state of the accomplice (inhibitor) drug. For example, acute ethanol ingestion and cimetidine both in-

dependently inhibit CYP 1A2 drug metabolism within 24 hours of a single dose. In contrast, amiodarone (which inhibits CYP 2C9) may not effectively inhibit this enzyme for months due to its long half-life.[41] Generally the time frame for most enzyme inhibitors to have their initial effect is within several days.

The significance of an elevated plasma level of a particular drug is determined largely by the therapeutic index of the drug. Therefore when considering the potential clinical relevance of an interaction, one must exercise more caution with drugs that have a narrow therapeutic index.

There is a growing amount of published literature on the relative inhibitory potential of different drugs on the various CYP isoenzymes using both in vitro and in vivo techniques. However, there is not a simple one-to-one correlation of isoform activity to the final metabolic fate of a specific drug. In reality, multiple isoforms are often involved in metabolizing drugs.[42] There are limitations to the concept of enzyme specificity that at its extreme supposes that each xenobiotic has an enzyme uniquely devoted to its metabolism. In fact, several enzymes may be involved in the metabolism of a particular drug, and a single enzyme may preferentially metabolize many drugs.[43] Because of the complexity of the CYP system and the uncertainty of how an experimental model applies to clinical scenarios, much of the practical clinical information comes from case reports. The clearance of many drugs involves multiple enzyme pathways. Therefore a potential drug interaction does not necessarily mean that the combination always results in a significant interaction. As an example, warfarin is listed as a CYP 1A2 substrate, but the CYP 2C9 family accounts for 85% of its clearance.[44] CYP 3A4 also has a relatively minor role in warfarin metabolism. The clinician needs to be consistently aware of potential interactions when prescribing multiple medications, especially when prescribing drugs with a relatively high risk of interactions through various cytochrome pathways.

Noncompetitive inhibition is less common and occurs when the enzyme is destroyed, inactivated, or changed by the accomplice such that it can no longer metabolize the original substrate. Spironolactone forms suicidal, reactive, intermediate metabolites that inactivate CYP

3A4.[45] The antiprogestins mifepristone, lilopristone, and onapristone are oxidized to reactive species capable of inactivating their metabolizing enzyme, CYP 3A4.[46] These drugs are a relatively new class of agents with promise in the treatment of some forms of breast and prostate cancer, meningioma, uterine leiomyoma, endometriosis, and as contraceptive agents.

DRUG INTERACTION RISKS BY DRUG CATEGORY

Table 44-4 lists drug categories in which there are variable risks for drug interactions involving metabolism.

Antihistamines
Terfenadine (Seldane) has been removed from the market due to its serious cardiovascular drug interactions. Its active acid metabolite, fexofenadine (Allegra), has taken the parent drug's place and is devoid of the potential for fatal drug interactions.[47] Terfenadine was reported in 1990 to cause QT prolongation and torsades de pointes when given with ketoconazole.[48] Serum concentrations of terfenadine were excessive and

concentrations of its main metabolite were reduced, suggesting inhibition of metabolism. Similar cardiotoxicity had been reported with terfenadine overdose, and it was concluded that ketoconazole inhibition of terfenadine metabolism led to cardiotoxic levels of terfenadine. Subsequently, six healthy volunteers were given terfenadine, and after a steady state concentration was achieved, ketoconazole was added.[49] Excessive levels of terfenadine were measured with concomitant prolongation of the QT interval on the electrocardiogram. This interaction was not clearly defined nor appreciated until 11 years after terfenadine was first marketed.

Similar interactions with nonsedating H_1 antihistamines have been described with itraconazole, ketoconazole, and fluconazole, the latter when given in doses above 200 mg/day.[50] Erythromycin and clarithromycin also can cause QT prolongation in combination with certain nonsedating H_1 antihistamines. Data on significant drug interactions with antidepressants and antihistamines are less clear. However, caution should be exercised in the concomitant administration of selective serotonin reuptake inhibitors (SSRIs) such as fluoxetine, fluvoxamine, and sertraline, as well as nefazodone, with nonse-

■ **Table 44-4**   Drug Categories in which There Are Variable Risks for Drug Interactions Involving Metabolism

Drug Class	Drugs with *Greater* Potential for Interactions	Drugs with *Less* Potential for Interactions
Macrolides	Clarithromycin Erythromycin	Azithromycin
Nonsedating H_1 antihistamines	Astemizole Terfenadine	Loratadine Cetirizine Fexofenadine
Fluoroquinolones	Ciprofloxacin Enoxacin	Levofloxacin Lomefloxacin Ofloxacin
H_2 antihistamines	Cimetidine	Famotidine Nizatidine Ranitidine
HIV-1 protease inhibitors	Ritonavir Indinavir	Saquinavir Nelfinavir
HMG CoA reductase inhibitors	Simvastatin Lovastatin Atorvastatin Cerivastatin	Pravastatin Fluvastatin

dating H_1 antihistamines. Tricyclic antidepressants should be used cautiously as they have a propensity to cause dysrhythmias. Grapefruit juice caused QT prolongation in patients ingesting 240 ml in combination with terfenadine 60 mg twice daily.[51,52] Astemizole undergoes extensive metabolism to active metabolites and, like terfenadine, the parent drug is potentially cardiotoxic with high plasma levels.

To minimize the risk of severe interactions, alternative nonsedating antihistamines, such as cetirizine, fexofenadine, and loratadine, can be prescribed. Azithromycin would be the macrolide of choice in combination with these antihistamines. Paroxetine and venlafaxine can be used safely as alternatives to SSRI antidepressants with higher risk for interactions such as fluoxetine, fluvoxamine, and sertraline.

Azole Antifungals

The azole antifungal agents include the original imidazoles, such as ketoconazole, in addition to the two newer triazoles, itraconazole and fluconazole. In particular, itraconazole requires an acid milieu for absorption, such that concomitant antacids, H_2 antihistamines, proton pump inhibitors (such as omeprazole), and didanosine significantly reduce absorption.

Among the systemic azole antifungals, ketoconazole has been shown in vitro to be the strongest inhibitor of CYP 3A4. However, in vivo plasma-free concentrations of fluconazole are 10 times greater, so in vivo interactions at enzymatic sites are similar to those seen with ketoconazole. This potential for CYP 3A4 inhibition by fluconazole primarily occurs with doses greater than 200 mg/day. The drug substrates metabolized via these enzymes that can lead to moderate-to-severe drug interactions are phenytoin, warfarin, cisapride, and cyclosporine. Phenytoin concentrations were significantly increased 48 hours after fluconazole administration resulting from a 33% decrease in the clearance of phenytoin.[53] When the azole antifungals (especially ketoconazole and itraconazole) are administered with cyclosporine, the concentrations of the latter are increased, requiring monitoring of cyclosporine levels. Similarly, frequent monitoring of the international normalized ratio (INR) is required for patients on warfarin who require therapy with an azole antifungal. The azole antifungals (most importantly fluconazole) reportedly increase the anticoagulant effects of warfarin by twofold to threefold.

Torsades de pointes, prolonged QT interval, and death have been reported in patients receiving azole antifungals and cisapride, as well as in patients on azole antifungals and astemizole or terfenadine.[47-49] This is due to elevated levels of cisapride in the former, and of astemizole or terfenadine in the latter, all of which are cardiotoxic.

Azole antifungals interfere with the metabolism of benzodiazepines, such as triazolam and midazolam, leading to increased levels and excessive sedation. There is also decreased metabolism of HMG-CoA reductase inhibitors, leading to increased drug levels and rhabdomyolysis. There is decreased metabolism of tacrolimus and indinavir as well.

Peripheral edema from an interaction between nifedipine and itraconazole has been reported. It was suspected that itraconazole, an accomplice drug, could inhibit the metabolism of this calcium channel blocker, a bullet drug. This resulted in an increased serum nifedipine concentration and leg edema. This hypothesis was confirmed by obtaining serum levels of nifedipine, itraconazole, and hydroxy-itraconazole, the active metabolite of itraconazole, before and after the administration of itraconazole.[54] The authors recommended that patients receiving azole antifungals and calcium channel blockers be monitored for side effects, such as leg edema and hypotension, because of the increased serum concentration of the calcium channel blocker.

Itraconazole is an inhibitor of CYP 3A4, whereas fluconazole inhibits CYP 2C9 significantly more than its minimal inhibitory role of CYP 3A4. Fluconazole (and not itraconazole) interacts with losartan, an angiotensin converting enzyme inhibitor used as an antihypertensive agent. Fluconazole inhibits the metabolism of losartan to the active metabolite E-3174.[31] The clinical significance of this interaction remains unclear, but the possibility of a reduced therapeutic effect of losartan should be kept in mind.

In contrast with the triazole antifungals, terbinafine is an allylamine that does not inhibit CYP 3A4.[55] This antifungal may be a viable therapeutic option in patients on concomitant therapy with high likelihood of drug interactions with the antifungal agents that are triazoles.

Allylamine Antifungals

Terbinafine (Lamisil) is an orally active allylamine antifungal used in the treatment of dermatophytoses in Canada since 1993. At least seven CYP enzymes are involved in terbinafine metabolism. Recombinant human CYPs predict that CYP 2C9, CYP 1A2, and CYP 3A4 may be the most important for total metabolism.[56]

There are 3 levels of activity of CYP 2D6 in the population: poor metabolizers (PM), extensive metabolizers (EM), and ultra rapid metabolizers. EM status is by far the most common and is considered "normal." About 7.5% of white American and European populations and less than 2% of Asian and Black Americans are PMs. Inhibition of CYP 2D6 would make individuals who have active enzyme (extensive metabolizers) into poor metabolizers while they were receiving terbinafine, and possibly for weeks after stopping the drug. This inhibition can cause two problems. First, there is an accumulation of parent drug that can result in dose-dependent drug toxicity, and second, there can be reduced formation of active metabolites that can result in loss of efficacy.[57]

There are CYP 2D6 mutations in the population (greater than 17) and the most common allele is designated CYP 2D6*1A. Nonactive alleles vary among ethnic populations. Investigations reveal that drug effects may be different on different alleles. For now, terbinafine appears to be a potent inhibitor of CYP 2D6, so clinicians should be aware of potential interactions. The area of greatest concern because of possible severity and common use would be bradycardia from excess beta-blockade (e.g., propranolol) or from accumulation of donepezil.[58] Codeine can lose its analgesic effect because the active metabolite, morphine, is not formed when CYP 2D6 activity is low.[59] In the case of terbinafine, the reported drug interactions associated with the inhibition of the CYP 2D6 pathway include nortriptyline.[60]

What is the impact on clinical practice? This remains unknown but should change the information that patients are given when this drug is prescribed. Although terbinafine (Lamisil) has been on the market for 6 years, clinicians are still learning fundamental information about its metabolism.

Cimetidine

Cimetidine can produce significant inhibition of CYP 1A2, 2C9, 2D6, and 3A4. Of these isoforms, clinically significant inhibition is most important with CYP 3A4 and 1A2. In contrast, other H_2 antihistamines (e.g., ranitidine, nizatidine, and famotidine) do not produce significant inhibition of these CYP isoforms. There is concern because this medication is available over-the-counter in the United States. Its use by dermatologists increased in the therapy of verruca vulgaris. Examples of clinically relevant interactions with cimetidine include theophylline, aminophylline, metoprolol, nifedipine, and quinidine.[61] The interaction involving β-blockers metoprolol and propranolol results in significant sinus bradycardia and hypotension. Therefore dosage adjustments may need to be made if these agents are administered together. Atenolol and nadolol have not been shown to interact with cimetidine. When the clinical scenario allows, alternative H_2 antihistamines previously mentioned without interaction potential can be substituted for cimetidine.

Cyclosporine

Numerous drug interactions with cyclosporine surfaced that are associated with its metabolism and presystemic metabolism by the CYP 3A4 enzyme in the liver and intestine, respectively. It is thought that GI tract metabolism may explain its erratic absorption. In fact, CYP 3A4 inhibitors have been administered intentionally to improve the bioavailability of cyclosporine and reduce dosing requirements. Ketoconazole 200 to 400 mg/day can decrease the daily dose of cyclosporine by 60% to 80%.[62]

Diltiazem decreases cyclosporine dosing by as much as 30%.[63] Enzyme inhibitory effects due to grapefruit juice have been variable. Other drugs that alter cyclosporine concentrations via CYP 3A4 inhibition include verapamil, nicardipine, fluconazole, itraconazole, ketoconazole, erythromycin, clarithromycin, and tacrolimus.[61] Conversely, CYP 3A4 inducers, such as rifampin, phenytoin, carbamazepine, and phenobarbital, may significantly decrease cyclosporine concentrations. Cyclosporine trough levels, signs of toxicity, and adequate immunosuppressive response should be monitored when these inhibitors or inducers are combined with cyclosporine.

Grapefruit Juice

Grapefruit juice interactions are of potential clinical relevance in the individual patient for a wide range of drugs. Grapefruit juice elevates serum concentrations of cyclosporine, certain calcium channel blockers, and other CYP 3A4 substrates by competing for the same metabolic pathway.[64] The mechanisms of grapefruit juice interactions are exclusively pharmacokinetic in nature. The effect is mediated mainly by the inhibition of CYP 3A4 in the small intestinal wall by either fresh or frozen grapefruit juice.[64] This results in a diminished first pass metabolism with higher bioavailability and increased maximal plasma concentrations of drug substrates of this enzyme. The effect is most pronounced in drugs with high first-pass degradation such as felodipine, nifedipine, saquinavir, cyclosporine, midazolam, triazolam, terazosin, ethinyl estradiol, 17-β-estradiol, prednisone, and the HMG-CoA reductase inhibitors lovastatin and simvastatin.[66,67]

It is not yet clear which component in grapefruit juice is to blame. Bergamottin, a furocoumarin compound, is thought to be the major factor for this CYP 3A4 enzyme inhibition, with a minor role attributable to flavonoids such as naringenin and quercetin.[68] Bergamottin (6,7-dihydroxybergamottin) has CYP 3A4 inhibition potential equal to, or stronger than, the prototypical CYP 3A4 inhibitor, ketoconazole.[69]

Even a change in the brand or batch of grapefruit juice may influence the grapefruit juice/drug interaction to an unpredictable degree because grapefruit juice is a natural product that is not standardized in composition. Similar interactions have not been seen with other citrus fruit juices such as orange juice. Lack of 6,7-dihydroxybergamottin in orange juice probably accounts for the absence of CYP inhibitory effects.[70]

The idea of using grapefruit juice as a cost-cutting measure has been used in patients on concomitant cyclosporine therapy.[71] Because grapefruit juice inhibits the metabolism of cyclosporine, combining the two would lower the required daily dose of cyclosporine, hence reducing drug costs of this expensive immunosuppressive agent. Recent studies demonstrate that grapefruit juice increases the bioavailability of saquinavir without affecting its clearance, suggesting that inhibition of intestinal CYP 3A4 may represent a way to enhance effectiveness without increasing the dose.[72]

It is recommended that patients refrain from ingesting grapefruit juice when taking a drug that is extensively metabolized by the CYP 3A4 pathway, unless the absence of a potential interaction has been documented. Many hospital dietary services have removed grapefruit juice as an option from inpatient menus to reduce the risk of drug interactions.

Herbal Remedies

Herbal medicines have become a popular therapy. They are often perceived as being "natural" and therefore harmless. Many of our current drugs including digitalis, atropine, and narcotic derivatives have been derived from plants. Little is known about the relative safety of herbal therapies compared with prescription drugs. Because of underreporting of interactions and the fact that the trend towards increasing herbal remedy use is recent, present knowledge represents the tip of the iceberg. It is estimated that 80% of the world's population rely primarily on traditional medicines using plant extracts or their active ingredients.

The interactions of phytomedicines with prescription medications are underresearched.[73] Because herbs are not sold as drugs, no proof of efficacy or warnings about side effects are required. When a drug is prescribed the dosage and quality of the substance are assured. No such standardization or quality control exists for herbal preparations. Contamination, mislabeling, and misidentification of herbs are also problems. Some patients do not know what they are taking, as they may purchase a product whose ingredients are listed in a foreign language only.

Either inactivation or enhancement of pharmacologic activity is possible.[73] For example, concomitant administration of phenytoin and the Ayurvedic remedy shankhapushpi has been reported to lead to reduced phenytoin concentration and loss of seizure control.[74] There has been a case report of increased anticoagulation in a patient on warfarin who used Chinese herbal drugs.[75] A crossover trial with healthy volunteers ingesting Chinese herbs containing glycyrrhizin demonstrated altered prednisolone pharmacokinetics.[76] Serious side effects such as bone marrow depression, hypertension, and dysrhythmias developed in 13 patients who took herbal therapies that were mail ordered from Hong Kong. Analysis of the pills revealed the presence of prednisone, indomethacin, and lead.[77] The Canadian Drug Reaction Monitoring Program received reports of adverse reactions to certain Chinese herbal preparations that contain heavy metals such as arsenic, mercury, lead, and cadmium.[78] Commonly used herbs that may cause dermatitis include aloe, chamomile, garlic, and ginseng.[79]

When taking a history of medications, it is important to ask specifically about prescription, nonprescription, and herbal therapies. Advise patients to tell you if they are taking herbal remedies so you can monitor for side effects. Warn pregnant patients not to take herbs unless their safety can be assured.

HMG CoA Reductase Inhibitors

Although dermatologists may not prescribe these medications, their use by primary physicians and various specialists is widespread. Coadministration of itraconazole with lovastatin and simvastatin is contraindicated. Itraconazole inhibits the metabolism of lovastatin, resulting in significantly increased concentrations of lovastatin, which has been associated with rhabdomyolysis.[80-82] Itraconazole may also inhibit the metabolism of simvastatin.[83] The use of atorvastatin and cerivastatin with CYP 3A4 inhibitors is not recommended because these drugs are also metabolized by the hepatic CYP 3A4.[84,85] Fluvastatin is metabolized via CYP 2C9[86] and therefore is not likely to result in clinically significant drug interactions when used in combination with CYP 3A4 inhibitors.[87] Fluvastatin is an inhibitor of CYP 2C9.[88] The metabolism of pravastatin is minimally influenced by CYP 3A4 and thus is also a safe alternative.[83]

Macrolide Antibiotics

When a macrolide and a nonsedating antihistamine are required, azithromycin should be used because this macrolide does not produce significant inhibition of CYP 3A4.[89] As with the interaction involving the nonsedating antihistamines, azithromycin should be used in combination with cisapride if a macrolide is required. When erythromycin is prescribed to a patient on long-term warfarin, there is a risk of increased plasma warfarin with increased anticoagulation and hemorrhage. This occurs because warfarin in relatively small quantities is a CYP 3A4 substrate and erythromycin a potent inhibitor.

Pimozide

Pimozide is a psychotropic drug with narrow neurologic and cardiac therapeutic range. It is a recognized treatment for delusions of parasitosis. Pimozide is oxidized by two CYP isoforms, CYP 3A4 and CYP 1A2, with the former being the responsible isoform at therapeutically relevant pimozide concentrations.[90] Although the contribution of CYP 1A2 appears marginal, this isoform may assume a greater role if the activity of CYP 3A4 is very low. Therefore a greater risk of adverse effects is expected when pimozide is prescribed simultaneously with various metabolic inhibitors of these two CYP pathways. These include the azole antifungals and macrolide antibiotics that are inhibitors of CYP 3A4. Furthermore, pimozide interactions may occur when used in combination with fluvoxamine or fluoroquinolones (e.g., ciprofloxacin, enoxacin, and norfloxacin) that inhibit 1A2. The risk of concomitant administration of CYP 3A4 inhibitors with pimozide is highlighted by a recent report of fatal cardiac dysrhythmia in patients taking pimozide and clarithromycin.[91]

There may be reduced efficacy of pimozide in the presence of inducers of CYP 3A4, such as rifampin and carbamazepine, and smokers may require higher pimozide doses because of higher CYP 1A2 activity. These influences may explain the interindividual variability in pimozide pharmacokinetics.

Pimozide is an inhibitor of CYP 2D6 without being a substrate of this isoform. This may be caused by mechanism-based inhibition or by accumulation of an inhibitory metabolite. Identifying potential risk factors that could modulate the efficacy and toxicity of pimozide is important to optimize the safe use of this drug.

Protease Inhibitors

Ritonavir, indinavir, saquinavir, and nelfinavir are all substrates and inhibitors of CYP 3A4, whereas ritonavir also inhibits CYP 2D6.[92] Ritonavir and indinavir are the most significant 3A4 inhibitors, although saquinavir and nelfinavir are less potent inhibitors. Of these antiretroviral agents, ritonavir is the most potent inhibitor, having inhibitory potency slightly less than ketoconazole.[93] Ritonavir may also induce CYP 3A4 and 1A2, leading to autoinduction of its own metabolism and that of other agents like theophylline, a CYP 1A2 substrate. Any drug metabolized via 3A4 could interact with any of these protease inhibitors. Likewise, a variety of drugs that induce the CYP 3A4 isozyme could lead to a decrease in the serum concentrations of the protease inhibitors. These agents are likely to be prescribed in combination with nucleosides and several other drugs used to treat infections in patients with AIDS. Nucleoside drugs do not have any important CYP-mediated interactions.

Human immunodeficiency virus (HIV)-1 protease inhibitors should be prescribed cautiously in combination with drugs primarily metabolized by the 3A4 system and those metabolized by the 2D6 system (ritonavir only). Concurrent administration should be accompanied by clinical monitoring for enhanced side effects that may result in dosage adjustments in some patients. Nelfinavir and saquinavir appear to have the least interaction potential of these HIV-1 protease inhibitors.

GENETIC POLYMORPHISMS

Each of the isoenzymes of the P-450 system is under genetic control. Because of genetic polymorphism, different individuals have varying levels of activity for several of these CYP isoforms.[92] Genetic polymorphism means that within a normal population, certain individuals have a fully functional enzyme whereas other individuals have reduced or essentially no enzyme activity. Individuals with genetically determined low levels of enzyme activity are referred to as *poor metabolizers*. Individuals who have a fully functional enzyme are known as *extensive metabolizers*. There are yet others who have more than the usual levels of enzyme activity; they are referred to as *ultra-rapid metabolizers*. Still others have partially functional enzymes and are *slower metabolizers* than normal. These factors account, in part, for the extremely wide range in blood levels of drugs, such as tricyclic antidepressants, across various individuals receiving the same dose. This represents an example of genetic polymorphism in the CYP 2D6 pathway.[57]

Poor metabolizers have been demonstrated to show higher than normal plasma levels of several drugs and may be at increased risk of adverse effects.[94] Poor metabolizers may have a larger response and be at greater risk of toxicity than extensive metabolizers for drugs that are highly dependent on clearance to an inactive metabolite by the particular isoform.

Not all CYP isoforms exhibit this genetic polymorphism. Those isoforms demonstrating significant polymorphism include CYP 1A2, 219, 2D6, and 2E1. Ethnic differences exist with regard to the percentage of a population who are extensive or poor metabolizers. Approximately 5% to 10% of North Americans and 1% of Asians lack CYP 2D6 activity.[57] Codeine is an ineffective analgesic until it is metabolized to morphine, the activate metabolite. Because this process is facilitated by CYP 2D6, poor metabolizers do not respond well to codeine.

The 2C family consists of isoforms 2C9, 2C10, 2C19, and others. Cytochrome 2C19 exhibits genetic polymorphism, with 20% of Asians and African-Americans and 3% to 5% of Caucasians reported to be poor metabolizers.

In one study, 12% of subjects were found to be slow 1A2 metabolizers and about 40% were found to be fast metabolizers.[95]

Poor metabolizers can be identified through drug challenge testing using debrisoquine sulfate for the CYP 2D6 system, mephenytoin for the CYP 2C19 system, and caffeine for the CYP 1A2 system.[95] These tests are not routinely used in clinical practice, and there are no clinical parameters that are useful in predicting the metabolizing status of a given individual.

Pharmacogenetic variation can also occur in other drug metabolizing enzymes. Pertinent to dermatologists, the enzyme thiopurine

S-methyltransferase (TPMT) is important in the metabolism of azathioprine and 6-mercaptopurine to nontoxic metabolites.[96] There is a 0.3% rate of homozygous deficiency of this enzyme, putting these patients at great risk for toxicity, especially myelosuppression.[96] Conversely, 88% of the population is homozygous dominant for the active TPMT enzyme and may therefore require doses greater than the recommended dose of 1 to 2 mg/kg/day to achieve therapeutic success. Determination of the patient's TPMT level provides information *a priori* that allows individualization of azathioprine dosing, thereby minimizing toxicity and maximizing efficacy.

PHARMACODYNAMIC MECHANISMS OF DRUG INTERACTIONS

Pharmacodynamic interactions can occur from an antagonistic or synergistic drug effect. The synergistic effects can occur with the therapeutic or adverse effects of the drug.

Antagonistic Effects

Interactions through antagonistic effects can occur when two drugs used in an individual patient have opposing end organ results. Antagonistic effects can arise when a patient taking a β-blocker develops anaphylaxis and may be refractory to the therapeutic effects of epinephrine. A recent meta-analysis of randomized controlled trials studied the efficacy of folic acid and folinic acid in reducing methotrexate-induced gastrointestinal toxicity in patients with rheumatoid arthritis.[97] The review shows a reduction of 80% in mucosal and gastrointestinal side effects in patients receiving low-dose (<5 mg/week) folic acid. On the flip side, there are no indications so far that folic acid may alter the efficacy of methotrexate. No major differences in disease activity between placebo and folic acid at low or high dosages were found. When prescribing antagonistic medications, one must realize the potential for reduced efficacy of the intended medication. Clinical studies should help define these issues as in the case of concomitant methotrexate and folic acid.

Synergistic Effects

Interactions through synergistic effects can occur when two drugs used in an individual patient share the same target organ for toxicity. Synergistic effects can occur when retinoids and methotrexate are both prescribed for the same patient because of each drug's potential to cause hepatotoxicity. Similarly, when retinoids and tetracycline antibiotics are coprescribed, the risk of the development of pseudotumor cerebri is increased compared with when either drug is used as a single agent. When methotrexate and sulfonamides are coprescribed, methotrexate may induce folate deficiency-causing, sulfonamide-induced, megaloblastic anemia.[98] It is important to consider synergistic effects when counseling patients regarding new medications, particularly because many over-the-counter drugs may act synergistically such as ethanol and acetylsalicylic acid.

SUMMARY

Dealing with and avoiding potential drug interactions is a significant challenge in the clinical setting. New information continues to appear rapidly, but dermatologists must be fully aware of the interaction potential for the drugs they prescribe. Box 44-5 highlights particularly potent inhibitors and Table 44-4 highlights therapeutic choices to help minimize the risk of serious drug interactions. The clarification of the role that various CYP-450 enzymes have in drug metabolism helped clinicians understand the mechanism of clinically important interactions. Over time, this understanding will lead to clearer recommendations and guidelines for drugs that have significant interaction potential. Because the best evidence for clinically relevant drug interactions comes from case reports, prescribing physicians can have a major impact. Observations of drug interactions should be confirmed, if possible, by serum drug concentrations. Then they should be reported to regulatory bodies and submitted to journals. By understanding the mechanisms behind drug interactions and staying alert for toxicities, clinicians can help make drug therapy safer and reduce the fear of drug interactions.

Bibliography

Anastasio G, Cornell K, Menscer D: Drug interactions: keeping it straight. *Am Fam Phys* 56:883-894, 1997.

Andersen W, Feingold D: Adverse drug interactions clinically important for the dermatologist. *Arch Dermatol* 131:468-473, 1995.

Anonymous: Drug interactions. *Med Lett Drugs Ther* 41:61-62, 1999.

Barranco VP: Clinically significant drug interactions in dermatology. *J Am Acad Dermatol* 38:599-612, 1998.

Gupta AK, Katz HI, Shear NH: Drug interactions with itraconazole, fluconazole and terbinafine and their management. *J Am Acad Dermatol* 41:237-249, 1999.

Michalets E: Update: clinically significant cytochrome P450 drug interactions. *Pharmacotherapy* 18:84-112, 1998.

Quinn DI, Day RO: Drug interactions of clinical importance: an updated guide. *Drug Saf* 12:393-396, 1995.

Singer MI, Shapiro LE, Shear NH: Cytochrome P450 3A: interactions with dermatologic therapies. *J Am Acad Dermatol* 37:765-771, 1997.

Wormhoudt LW, Commanduer JN, Vermeulen NP: Genetic polymorphism of human n-acetyltransferase, cytochrome P-450, glutathione-S-transferase, and epoxide hydrolase enzymes: relevance to xenobiotic metabolism and toxicity. *Crit Rev Toxicol* 29:59-124, 1999.

References

Introduction

1. Hansten PD: Drug interactions. *Drug Interactions Newsletter* 893-906, 1996.
2. Shapiro LE, Singer MI, Shear NH: Pharmacokinetic mechanisms of drug-drug and drug-food interactions in dermatology. *Curr Opin Dermatol* 4:25-31, 1997.
3. Singer MI, Shapiro LE, Shear NH: Cytochrome P450 3A: interactions with dermatologic therapies. *J Am Acad Dermatol* 37:765-771, 1997.
4. Tatro DS: *Drug interaction facts*, St. Louis, 1996, Facts & Comparisons.
5. Shapiro LE, Singer MI, Shear NH: Pharmacokinetic mechanisms of drug-drug and drug-food interactions in dermatology. *Curr Opin Dermatol* 4:25-31, 1997.
6. Guengerich FP: Role of cytochrome p450 enzymes in drug-drug interactions. *Adv Pharmacol* 43:7-35, 1997.
7. Hansten PD, Horn JR: The assessment of risk in the clinical outcome of drug interactions. *Appl Ther* 481-497, 1997.

Assessment of Risk in Clinical Outcome

8. Andersen W, Feingold D: Adverse drug interactions clinically important for the dermatologist. *Arch Dermatol* 131:468-473, 1995.
9. Montamat SC, Cusack BJ, Vestal RE: Management of drug therapy in the elderly. *N Engl J Med* 321:303-309, 1989.

10. Lee BL, Wong D, Benowitz HL, et al: Altered patterns of drug metabolism in patients with acquired immunodeficiency syndrome. *Clin Pharmacol Ther* 53:529-535, 1993.
11. Kalow W, Goedde H, Agarwal D: *Ethnic differences in reactions to drugs and xenobiotics*, New York, 1986, AR Liss.
12. Brly F, Marez D, Sabbagh N, et al: An efficient strategy for detection of known and new mutations of the CYP 2D6 gene using single stand conformation polymorphism analysis. *Pharmacogenetics* 5:373-384, 1995.
13. Toogood J: Beta blocker therapy and the risk of anaphylaxis. *Can Med Assoc J* 136:929, 1987.
14. Tugwell P, Bennett K, Bell M, et al: Methotrexate in rheumatoid arthritis: indications, contraindications, efficacy and safety. *Ann Intern Med* 107:358, 1987.
15. Thurmann PA, Hompesch BC: Influence of gender on the pharmacokinetics and pharmacodynamics of drugs. *Int J Clin Pharmacol Ther* 36:586-590, 1998.
16. Kotlyar M, Carson SW: Effects of obesity on the cytochrome P450 enzyme system. *Int J Clin Pharmacol Ther* 37:8-19, 1999.

Absorption, Distribution, Metabolism

17. Anastasio G, Cornell K, Menscer D: Drug interactions: keeping it straight. *Am Fam Phys* 56:883-894, 1997.

18. Marchbanks C: Drug-drug interactions with fluoroquinolones. *Pharmacotherapy* 13:23-25, 1993.

19. Bodey GP: Azole antifungal drugs. *Clin Infect Dis* 14:5161-5169, 1992.

20. Meyer U: Overview of enzymes of drug metabolism. *J Pharmacokin Biopharm* 24:449-459, 1996.

21. Riddick DS: Drug biotransformation. In Kalant H, Toschlau W, editors: *Principles of medical pharmacology,* ed 6, New York, 1996, Oxford University Press.

Cytochrome P-450 Enzymes

22. Watkins PB: Drug metabolism by cytochromes P450 in the liver and small bowel. *Gastroenterol Clin North Am* 21:511-526, 1992.

23. Birkett DJ, Mackenqie PI, Veronese ME, et al: In vitro approaches can predict human drug metabolism. *Trends Pharmacol Sci* 14:292-294, 1993.

24. Rendic S, DiCarlo FJ: Human cytochrome P450 enzymes. *Drug Metab Rev* 29:413-580, 1997.

25. Nelson DR, Doymans L, Kamataki T, et al: P450 superfamily: update on new sequences, gene mapping, accession numbers and nomenclature. *Pharmacogenetics* 6:1-42, 1996.

26. Drug Interactions. *Med Lett Drug Ther* 41:61-62, 1999.

27. Guengerich FP: Human cytochrome p450 enzymes. In Ortiz de Montellano PR, editor: *Cytochrome P450,* ed 2, New York, 1995, Plenum, pp 473-535.

28. Shapiro LE, Shear NH: Drug-drug interactions: How scared should we be? (editorial) *Can Med Assoc J* 161:1266-1267, 1999.

29. Ford N, Sonnichsen D: Clinically significant cytochrome P-450 drug interactions—a comment. *Pharmacotherapy* 18:890-891, 1998.

30. Kerremans A: Cytochrome P450 isoenzymes—importance for the internist. *Netherlands J Med* 48:237-243, 1996.

31. Gupta AK, Katz HI, Shear NH: Drug interactions with itraconazole, fluconazole and terbinafine and their management. *J Am Acad Dermatol* 41:237-249, 1999.

32. Touw DJ: Clinical implications of genetic polymorphisms and drug interactions mediated by cytochrome P-450 enzymes. *Drug Metab Drug Interact* 14:55-82, 1997.

33. Slaughter RL, Edwards DF: Recent advances: the cytochrome P450 enzymes. *Ann Pharmacother* 29:619-624, 1995.

34. Quinn DI, Day RO: Drug interactions of clinical importance: an updated guide. *Drug Saf* 12:393-396, 1995.

35. Fleming CM, Persad R, Kaisary A, et al: Low activity of dapsone *N*-hydroxylation as a susceptibility risk factor in aggressive bladder cancer. *Pharmacogenetics* 4:199-207, 1994.

Cytochrome P-450 Inducers and Inhibitors

36. Tatro DS: *Drug interaction facts,* St. Louis, 1997, Facts and Comparisons.

37. Hansten PD: Pharmacokinetic drug interaction mechanisms and clinical characteristics. *Appl Ther* 499-517, 1997.

38. Shenfield G: Oral contraceptives: are drug interactions of clinical significance? *Drug Saf* 32:114-116, 1993.

39. Park BK, Pirmohamed M, Kitteringham N: The role of cytochrome P450 enzymes in hepatic and extrahepatic human drug toxicity. *Pharmacol Ther* 68:385-424, 1995.

40. Virani A, Mailis A, Shapiro LE, et al: Drug interactions in human neuropathic pain pharmacotherapy. *Pain* 73:3-13, 1997.

41. Heimark LD, Wienkers L, Dunze K, et al: The mechanism of the interaction between amiodarone and warfarin in humans. *Clin Pharmacol Ther* 51:398-407, 1992.

42. Goldberg R: The P-450 system. *Arch Fam Med* 5:406-412, 1996.

43. Jefferson J: Drug interactions—friend or foe? *J Clin Psychiatry* 59(Suppl 4):37-47, 1998.

44. Rettie AE, Korzekwa KR, Kunze KL, et al: Hydroxylation of warfarin by human cDNA-depressed cytochrome P450: a role for P450 2C9 in the etiology of (s)-warfarin-drug interactions. *Chem Res Toxicol* 5:54-59, 1992.

45. Jang GR, Benet LZ: Antiprogestin-mediated inactivation of cyctochrome P450 3A4. *Pharmacology* 56:150-157, 1998.

46. Anonymous: Fexofenadine. *Med Lett Drugs Ther* 38:95-96, 1996.

Antihistamines

47. Monahan BP, Ferguson CL, Kelleavy ES, et al: Torsades de pointes occurring in association with terfenadine use. *JAMA* 264:2788-2790, 1990.

48. Honig PK, Worthan DC, Zamani K, et al: Terfenadine-ketoconazole interaction: pharmacokinetic and electrocardiographic consequences. *JAMA* 269:1513-1518, 1993.

49. Cantilena LR, Sorrels S, Wiley T, et al: Flu-conazole alters terfenadine pharmacokinetics and electrocardiographic pharmacodynamics (abstract). *Clin Pharmacol Ther* 57:185, 1995.

50. Anonymous: Grapefruit juice interactions with drugs. *Med Lett Drugs Ther* 37:73-74, 1995.

51. Benton R, Honig P, Zamani K, et al: Grapefruit juice alters terfenadine pharmacokinetics, resulting in prolongation of repolarization on the electrocardiogram. *Clin Pharmacol Ther* 59:383-388, 1996.

Azole and Allylamine Antifungals

52. Touchette MA, Chandrasekar PH, Milad MA, et al: Contrasting effects of fluconazole and ketoconazole on phenytoin and testosterone disposition in man. *Br J Clin Pharmacol* 34:75-78, 1992.

53. Tailor S, Gupta A, Walder S, et al: Peripheral edema due to nifedipine-itraconazole interaction: a case report. *Arch Dermatol* 132:350-352, 1996.

54. Kaukonen KM, Olkkola KT, Neuvonen PJ: Fluconazole but not itraconazole decreased the metabolism of losartan to E-3174. *Eur J Clin Pharmacol* 53:445-449, 1998.

55. First MR, Schroeder TJ, Michael A, et al: Cyclosporine-ketoconazole interactions. Long-term follow-up and preliminary results of a randomized trial. *Transplantation* 55:1000-1004, 1993.

56. Vickers AEM, Sinclair JR, Zollinger M, et al: Multiple cytochrome P-450s involved in the metabolism of terbinafine suggest a limited potential for drug-drug interactions. *Drug Metab Dispos* 27:1029-1038, 1999.

57. Wormhoudt LW, Commanduer JN, Vermeulen NP: Genetic polymorphism of human n-acetyltransferase, cytochrome P-450, glutathione-S-transferase, and epoxide hydrolase enzymes: relevance to xenobiotic metabolism and toxicity. *Crit Rev Toxicol* 29:59-129, 1999.

58. Barner EL, Gray SL: Donepezil use in Alzheimer disease. *Ann Pharmacother* 32:70-77, 1999.

59. Tseng CY, Wang SL, Lai MD, et al: Formation of morphine from codeine in Chinese subjects of different CYP 2D6 genotypes. *Clin Pharmacol Ther* 60:177-182, 1996.

60. Van der Kuy PH, Hooymans PM: Nortriptyline intoxication induced by terbinafine. *BMJ* 316:441, 1998.

61. Michalets E: Update: clinically significant cytochrome P450 drug interactions. *Pharmacotherapy* 18:84-112, 1998.

Cyclosporine

62. Gomez D, Wacher VJ, Tomlanovich SJ, et al: The effects of ketoconazole on the intestinal metabolism and bioavailability of cyclosporine. *Clin Pharmacol Ther* 58:15-19, 1995.

63. Shennib H, Auger JL: Diltiazem improves cyclosporine dosage in cystic fibrosis lung transplant recipients. *J Heart Lung Transpl* 10:292-296, 1994.

Grapefruit Juice

64. Fuhr U: Drug interactions with grapefruit juice. *Drug Saf* 18:251-272, 1998.

65. Roller L: Drugs and grapefruit juice (letter). *Clin Pharmacol Ther* 1:87, 1998.

66. Kantola T, Kivisto KT, Neuvonen PJ: Grapefruit juice greatly increases serum concentrations of lovastatin and lovastatin acid. *Clin Pharmacol Ther* 63:397-402, 1998.

67. Schmiedlin-Ren P, Edwards DJ, Fitzsimmons ME, et al: Mechanisms of enhanced oral bioavailability of CYP 3A4 substrates by grapefruit juice constituents. Decreased enterocyte CYP 3A4 concentration and mechanism-based inactivation by furanocoumarins. *Drug Metab Dispos* 25:1228-1233, 1997.

68. Fukuda K, Ohta T, Oshima Y, et al: Specific CYP 3A4 inhibitors in grapefruit juice: furocoumarin dimers as components of drug interaction. *Pharmacogenetics* 7:391-396, 1997.

69. Edwards DJ, Bellevue FH, Woster PM: Identification of 6,7-dihydroxybergamottin, a cytochrome P450 inhibitor, in grapefruit juice. *Drug Metab Dispos* 24:1287-1290, 1996.

70. Hollander AA, van der Woude FJ, Cohen AF: Effect of grapefruit juice on blood cyclosporin concentration (letter). *Lancet* 346:123, 1995.

71. Kupferchmidt HH, Fattinger KE, Ha HR, et al: Grapefruit juice enhances the bioavailability of the HIV protease inhibitor saquinavir in man. *Br J Clin Pharmacol* 45:355-359, 1998.

Herbal Remedies

72. Ernst E: Harmless herbs? A review of the recent literature. *Am J Med* 104:170-178, 1998.

73. De Smet PAGM, D'Arcy PF: Drug interactions with herbal and other non-orthodox remedies. In D'Arcy PF, editor: *Mechanisms of drug interactions*, Berlin, 1996, Springer.

74. Dandekar P, Chandra RS, Dalvi SS, et al: Analysis of a clinically important interaction between phenytoin and shankhapushpi, an Ayurvedic preparation. *J Ethnopharmacol* 35:285-288, 1992.

75. Tam LS, Chan TYK, Leung WK, et al: Warfarin interactions with Chinese traditional medicines: danshen and methyl salicylate medicated oil. *Aust N Z J Med* 25:258, 1995.

76. Homma M, Oka K, Ikeshima K, et al: Different effects of traditional Chinese medicines containing similar herbal constituents on prednisolone pharmacokinetics. *J Pharm Pharmacol* 47:687-692, 1995.

77. Goldman JA, Myerson G: Chinese herbal medicine: camouflaged prescription anti-inflammatory drugs, corticosteroids, and lead. *Arthritis Rheum* 34:1207, 1991.

78. Canadian Adverse Drug Reaction Monitoring Program. Herbal preparations:

79. Borins M: The dangers of using herbs. *Postgrad Med* 104:91-99, 1998.

HMG CoA Reductase Inhibitors

80. Neuvonen PJ, Jalava K-M: Itraconazole drastically increases plasma concentrations of lovastatin and lovastatin acid. *Clin Pharmacol Ther* 60:54-61, 1996.

81. Lees RS, Lees AM: Rhabdomyolysis from the coadministration of lovastatin and the antifungal agent itraconazole (letter). *N Engl J Med* 333:664-665, 1995.

82. Horn M: Coadministration of itraconazole with hypolipidemic agents may induce rhabdomyolysis in healthy individuals (letter). *Arch Dermatol* 132:1254, 1996.

83. Neuvonen PJ, Kantola T, Kivisto KT: Simvastatin but not pravastatin is very susceptible to interaction with the CYP 3A4 inhibitor itraconazole. *Clin Pharmacol Ther* 63:332-341, 1998.

84. Desager JP, Orsmans Y: Clinical pharmacokinetics of 3-hydroxy-3-methylglutaryl-coenzyme A reductase inhibitors. *Clin Pharmacokinet* 31:348-371, 1996.

85. Boberg M, Angerbauer R, Fey P, et al: Metabolism of cerivastatin by human liver microsomes in vitro. Characterization of primary metabolic pathways and of cytochrome P450 isozymes involved. *Drug Metab Dispos* 25:321-331, 1997.

86. Fischer V, Johanson L, Heitz F, et al: The 3-hydroxy-3-methylglutaryl coenzyme A reductase inhibitor fluvastatin: effect on human cytochrome P-450 and implications for metabolic drug interactions. *Drug Metab Dispos* 27:410-416, 1999.

87. Kantola T, Kivisto KT, Neuvonen PJ: Differential effects of itraconazole on fluvastatin and lovastatin pharmacokinetics. *Eur J Clin Pharmacol* 52:A134, 1997.

88. Meadowcroft AM, Williamson KM, Patterson JH, et al: The effects of fluvastatin, a CYP 2C9 inhibitor, on losartan pharmacokinetics in healthy volunteers. *J Clin Pharmacol* 39:418-424, 1999.

Other Drug Categories

89. McKindley D, Dufresne R: Current knowledge of the cytochrome P-450 isozyme system: can we predict clinically important drug interactions? *Med Health* 81:38-42, 1998.

90. Desta Z, Kerbusch T, Soukhova N, et al: Identification and characterization of human cytochrome P450 isoforms interacting with pimozide. *J Pharmacol Exp Ther* 285:428-437, 1998.

91. Flockhart DA, Richard E, Woosley RL, et al: Metabolic interaction between clarithromycin and pimozide may result in cardiac toxicity. *Clin Pharmacol Ther* 59:189A, 1996.

92. Deeks SG, Smith M, Holodniy M, et al: HIV-1 protease inhibitors. *JAMA* 277:145-153, 1997.

93. von Moltke LL, Greenblatt DJ, Grassi JM, et al: Protease inhibitor as inhibitors of human cytochromes P450: high risk associated with ritonavir. *J Clin Pharmacol* 38:106-111, 1998.

Genetic Polymorphisms and Pharmacodynamic Mechanisms

94. Daly AK: Molecular basis of polymorphic drug metabolism. *J Molec Med* 73:539-553, 1995.

95. Butler M, Lang N, Young J, et al: Determination of CYP 1A2 and NAT2 phenotypes in human populations by analysis of caffeine urinary metabolites. *Pharmacogenetics* 2:116-127, 1992.

96. Snow J, Gibson L: A pharmacogenetic basis for the safe and effective use of azathioprine and other thiopurine drugs in dermatologic patients. *J Am Acad Dermatol* 32:114-116, 1995.

97. Ortiz Z, Shea B, Suarez-Almazor ME, et al: The efficacy of folic acid and folinic acid in reducing methotrexate gastrointestinal toxicity in rheumatoid arthritis. A meta-analysis of randomized controlled trials. *J Rheumatol* 25:36-43, 1998.

98. Barranco VP: Clinically significant drug interactions in dermatology. *J Am Acad Dermatol* 38:599-612, 1998.

CHAPTER 45

Sandra R. Knowles

Neil H. Shear

Drug Hypersensitivity Syndromes

Dermatologists prescribe a wide spectrum of medications encompassing topical corticosteroids and antimicrobials to systemic medications such as dapsone, methotrexate, and cyclosporine. Each class of drugs is associated with its own adverse reaction profile, ranging from common and relatively benign reactions (e.g., mild gastrointestinal reactions) to rare but potentially serious reactions. This chapter highlights some of the more common drug reaction syndromes encountered by a dermatologist, including the drug hypersensitivity syndrome (DHS), drug-induced lupus (DIL), serum sickness–like reaction (SSRI), and acute generalized exanthematous pustulosis (AGEP) (Box 45-1).

DRUG HYPERSENSITIVITY SYNDROME

DHS, which is characterized by a triad of fever, skin eruption, and internal organ involvement, has been well described for a number of drugs, including anticonvulsants, sulfonamide antibiotics, dapsone, minocycline, and allopurinol[1,2] (Box 45-2). Although this reaction has been estimated to occur between 1 in 1000 and 1 in 10,000 exposures, its true incidence is unknown because of variable presentation and inaccurate reporting.[3,4] DHS occurs most frequently on first exposure to the drug, with initial symptoms starting 2 to 6 weeks after exposure to the drug (Table 45-1). In patients with a history of DHS, reexposure to the offending agent may cause development of symptoms within 1 day. DHS is not related to dose or serum concentration of the drug.[5]

A mild to high fever ranging from 38° to 40° C and malaise, which can be accompanied by pharyngitis and cervical lymphadenopathy, are the presenting symptoms in most patients. Atypical lymphocytosis with a subsequent prominent eosinophilia may occur during the initial phases of the reaction in many patients.[1] A generalized exanthem occurs in approximately 85% of patients and usually occurs simultaneously with the appearance of the fever or shortly after. Skin manifestations can range from an exanthematous eruption to more serious eruptions such as exfoliative dermatitis. Liver abnormalities, presenting as elevated transaminases, alkaline phosphatase, prothrombin time, and bilirubin, are present in approximately 50% of patients; in some patients, development of severe hepatitis with jaundice may occur.[6] Other organs, such as the kidney (interstitial nephritis, vasculitis), central nervous system (encephalitis, aseptic meningitis), or the lungs (interstitial pneumonitis, res-

Box 45-1

Drug Hypersensitivity Syndromes

Drug hypersensitivity syndrome (DHS)
Serum sickness–like reactions (SSLR)
Drug-induced lupus (DIL)
Acute generalized exanthematous pustulosis
   (AGEP)
Severe cutaneous adverse reactions (SCAR)
   Erythema multiforme major (EMm)
   Stevens-Johnson syndrome (SJS)
   Toxic epidermal necrolysis (TEN)
Drug-induced systemic inflammatory response
   syndrome (SIRS)

Box 45-2

Medications Associated With Drug Hypersensitivity Syndrome

ANTICONVULSANTS
Carbamazepine
Lamotrigine
Phenobarbital
Phenytoin

ANTIRETROVIRAL AGENTS
Indinavir
Nevirapine

SULFONAMIDES AND RELATED DRUGS
Dapsone
Sulfasalazine
Sulfonamide antibiotics

OTHER ANTIBACTERIAL AGENTS
Minocycline
Nitrofurantoin

MISCELLANEOUS DRUGS
Allopurinol

Box 45-3

Medications Associated With Drug-induced Pseudolymphoma

Amitriptyline   Cyclosporine
Allopurinol   Diltiazem
Atenolol   Phenytoin
Carbamazepine

piratory distress syndrome, vasculitis), may less commonly be involved. A small subgroup of patients may become hypothyroid as part of an autoimmune thyroiditis within 2 months of initiation of symptoms.[7] This is characterized by a low thyroxine level, an elevated level of thyroid-stimulating hormone, and autoantibodies, including antimicrosomal antibodies.

Pseudolymphoma

Although some clinicians use the term *drug-induced pseudolymphoma* interchangeably with *DHS*, pseudolymphoma applies only to patients who have both clinical and histologic features suggestive of lymphoma. The drug eruption is subacute, usually composed of single or multiple nodules, with no accompanying systemic signs.[8] It is not considered a premalignant state. The syndrome occurs after 1 week to 2 years of exposure to the drug (Box 45-3).[9] The symptoms and physical findings generally resolve within 7 to 14 days of drug discontinuation. Histopathologically, two types of pseudolymphomas are distinguished—T-cell pseudolymphoma (band-like pattern that simulates mycosis fungoides) and B-cell pseudolymphoma (nodular pattern). Management of drug-induced pseudolymphoma often involves no treatment other than withdrawal of the offending agent. Complete blood cell count and serum chemistries are usually within normal limits. Long-term follow-up is necessary to rule out the possibility of pseudo-pseudolymphoma.[10]

Anticonvulsants

The DHS has been associated with the aromatic anticonvulsants, namely phenytoin, phenobarbital, and carbamazepine.[6] It has been suggested that the formation of toxic metabolites by phenytoin, carbamazepine, and phenobarbital may play a pivotal role in the development of DHS.[11] Phenytoin, carbamazepine, and phenobarbital are metabolized by cytochrome P-450 (CYP) to chemically reactive metabolites, although the specific metabolite is unknown. This

Table 45-1 Clinical Features of Drug Hypersensitivity Syndrome, Serum Sickness–like Reaction, Pseudolymphoma, and Systemic Inflammatory Response Syndrome

Syndrome	Cutaneous Features	Onset of Symptoms	Fever	Internal Organ Involvement	Arthralgia	Lymphad-enopathy
Drug hypersensitivity syndrome	Exanthem Exfoliative dermatitis Pustular eruptions Erythema multiforme/ Stevens-Johnson syndrome/toxic epidermal necrolysis	2-6 weeks	Present	Present	Absent	Present
Pseudolymphoma	Single or multiple papulonodules	6 months	Absent	Absent	Absent	Present*
Serum sickness–like reaction	Urticaria Exanthem	7-14 days	Present	Absent	Present	Present
Drug-induced systemic inflammatory re-sponse syndrome	Present or absent If present, usually a generalized, erythematous rash	Hours to weeks (mean 14 days)	Present (may have rigors and hypotension)	Absent or present	Absent or present	Absent

*Biopsy shows atypical hyperplasia simulating malignancy.

metabolite is thought to be detoxified by epoxide hydroxylases; however, if detoxification is defective, the toxic metabolite may act as a hapten and initiate an immunoresponse, causing cell necrosis directly or indirectly via pathways leading to apoptosis.

In one study,[11] 75% of a series of patients with anticonvulsant DHS to one aromatic anticonvulsant showed in vitro cross-reactivity to the other two. In addition, in vitro testing showed that there is a familial occurrence of hypersensitivity to anticonvulsants.[11] Although lamotrigine is not an aromatic anticonvulsant, there have been several reports documenting a DHS associated with its use as well.[12-14]

Sulfonamide Antibiotics

Sulfonamide antibiotics have also been reported to cause DHS in susceptible individuals.[15] The primary metabolic pathway for sulfonamides involves acetylation to a nontoxic metabolite, followed by renal excretion. An alternative metabolic pathway, quantitatively more important in slow acetylators, involves the CYP mixed-function oxidase system. These enzymes can transform the parent compound to reactive metabolites, namely hydroxylamines and nitroso compounds that produce cytotoxicity independent of preformed drug-specific antibody.[16] In most individuals, detoxification of the metabolite occurs. However, in patients who are unable to detoxify this metabolite (e.g., glutathione deficient), development of DHS may occur.[17] The detoxification defect is present in 2% of the population, but only 1 in 10,000 people manifest symptoms of DHS. However, the patient's sibling(s) and other first-degree relatives are at an increased risk (perhaps 1 in 4) of having a similar defect. Other aromatic amines, such as procainamide, dapsone, and acebutolol, are metabolized to similar compounds, and clinicians recommend avoidance of these drugs in patients who develop symptoms compatible with a sulfonamide DHS because of the potential for cross-reactivity. However, cross-reactivity with sulfonamides should not occur with related drugs that are not aromatic amines (e.g., sulfonylureas, thiazide diuretics, furosemide, acetazolamide).

Dapsone

There are several reports of dapsone-induced DHS, also known as the sulfone syndrome,[18,19] with a variety of dermatologic conditions, including leprosy, dermatitis herpetiformis, acne vulgaris, psoriasis, and lupus erythematosus. Dapsone-induced DHS usually occurs 4 or more weeks after initiation of therapy and is typified by fever, rash, and hepatitis.[18]

Dapsone is metabolized primarily via two pathways—N-acetylation and N-hydroxylation. N-acetylation is mediated by N-acetyltransferase type 2, whereas N-hydroxylation is mediated primarily by CYP 3A4. Reactive intermediate metabolites produced by N-hydroxylation, such as hydroxylamines, are formed that can induce hemolytic anemia and methemoglobinemia. In addition, these reactive metabolites are involved in the pathogenesis of dapsone-induced DHS.[18] Cimetidine, an inhibitor of CYP 3A4, has been shown to reduce the formation of the toxic hydroxylamine metabolites of dapsone in vitro but does not affect acetylation of dapsone.[20] Subsequent studies showed that long-term (at least 3 months) concurrent cimetidine results in increased plasma dapsone levels, without an increase in hemolysis, and reduced methemoglobinemia.[21] Whether or not concurrent use of dapsone and cimetidine also reduces the incidence of dapsone hypersensitivity syndrome is unknown.

Minocycline

DHS has also been associated with minocycline,[2] usually occurring 2 to 4 weeks after therapy is started. The pathogenesis of minocycline-induced DHS is unknown; however, minocycline metabolism may generate an iminoquinone derivative, which is a reactive metabolite. Neither tetracycline nor doxycycline contains the amino acid side chain that has the potential to form a reactive metabolite; this may support the medical experience that neither tetracycline nor doxycycline is associated with DHS.[22] However, certainty regarding the absence of cross-reactivity between minocycline and other tetracyclines is lacking; therefore caution is advised regarding administration of other tetracyclines in patients who develop a DHS after minocycline.

Differential Diagnosis

The differential diagnosis of DHS includes other cutaneous drug reactions, acute viral infections (e.g., Epstein-Barr virus, hepatitis virus, influenza virus, cytomegalovirus), lymphoma, and idiopathic hypereosinophilic syndrome. After DHS has been recognized by the symptom complex of fever, rash, and lymphadenopathy, there are a minimum number of laboratory tests (Box 45-4) that help to evaluate internal organ involvement, which may be asymptomatic. Liver transaminases, complete blood count, and urinalysis and serum creatinine should be performed at the initial evaluation. In addition, the clinician should be guided by the presence of symptoms, which may suggest specific internal organ involvement (e.g., respiratory symptoms). Thyroid function tests should be measured and repeated in 2 to 3 months. A skin biopsy may be helpful if the patient has a blistering or a pustular eruption. Unfortunately, diagnostic or confirmatory tests to establish drug causation are not readily available. An in vitro test using a mouse hepatic microsomal system is used for research purposes to evaluate patients who develop DHS.[11,23] Oral rechallenges are not recommended due to the severity of the DHS reactions.

Treatment

Although the role of corticosteroids is controversial, most clinicians would elect to start prednisone at a dose of 1 to 2 mg/kg/day if symptoms are severe. Antihistamines or topical corticosteroids can also be used to alleviate symptoms. Because the risk of DHS is substantially increased in first-degree relatives of patients who had DHS reactions, counseling of family members is a crucial part of the assessment of this syndrome.[11]

Box 45-4

Management of Patients With Drug Hypersensitivity Syndrome

1. Discontinue the offending drug
2. Obtain the following laboratory tests:
   a. At presentation
   - Complete blood count and differential
   - Liver function tests
   - Urinalysis (including microscopic)
   - Serum creatinine
   - Other tests may be needed, depending on the symptom presentation (e.g., chest radiograph for respiratory symptoms)
   - Baseline thyroid function tests (e.g., TSH)
   b. At <3 weeks
   - Repeat abnormal tests and investigate/treat as medically appropriate
   c. At 3 weeks
   - Repeat blood work/investigations as clinically warranted
   - Monitor for exacerbation of fever, rash
   d. At 3 months
   - TSH
   - Review warnings about cross-reacting drugs and risk of family members
3. Skin biopsy indicated if blistering or pustular eruption
4. Antihistamines or topical corticosteroids to treat patient's symptoms
5. Assess the need for systemic corticosteroid therapy

TSH, Thyroid-stimulating hormone.

SERUM SICKNESS AND SERUM SICKNESS–LIKE REACTIONS

Serum sickness is a clinical syndrome characterized by fever, lymphadenopathy, arthralgias, cutaneous eruptions, gastrointestinal disturbances, and malaise and is often associated with proteinuria, without evidence of glomerulonephritis.[24] It was first described with the injection of foreign proteins such as equine antitoxins, snake and spider antivenins, antilymphocyte globulins, and streptokinase. Serum sickness is mediated by the tissue deposition of circulating immunocomplexes, the activation of complement, and the ensuing inflammatory response.

In contrast, serum sickness–like reactions (SSLRs) are defined by the presence of fever, rash (usually urticarial), and arthralgias occurring 1 to 3 weeks after drug initiation. Other findings, such as lymphadenopathy and eosinophilia, may also be present. However, immunocomplexes, hypocomplementemia, vasculitis, and renal lesions are absent in SSLRs (see Table 45-1).

Epidemiologic studies in children suggest that the risk of SSLRs is greater with cefaclor as compared to other antibiotic therapy, including other cephalosporins.[34,35] The overall incidence rate of cefaclor SSLRs has been estimated to be approximately 0.024% to 0.2% per course of cefaclor prescribed. Although the pathogenesis is unknown, it has been postulated that in genetically susceptible hosts, a reactive cefaclor metabolite is generated during its metabolism that may bind with tissue proteins and elicit an inflammatory response manifesting as SSLR.[36]

Other drugs that have recently been implicated in the causation of SSLRs include minocycline[2,25] and cefaprozil[26] (Box 45-5). The incidence rates for these drugs are unknown.

Treatment

Discontinuation of the culprit drug and symptomatic treatment with antihistamines and topical corticosteroids are recommended in patients with SSLR. A short course of oral corticosteroids may be required in patients with more severe symptoms. The drug causing the SSLR should be avoided in the future. For cefaclor and cefprozil, the risk of cross-reaction with other beta-lactam antibiotics is small and the further administration of another cephalosporin is usually well tolerated.[37] However, some clinicians recommend that all beta-lactam drugs should be avoided in patients who experience SSLR from cefaclor.[38] No information is available regarding cross-reactivity among the tetracycline antibiotics in patients with minocycline SSLR.

Box 45-5

Medications Associated With Serum Sickness–like Reaction[25-33]

ANTIBACTERIAL AGENTS
Cefaclor
Cefprozil
Ciprofloxacin
Minocycline
Penicillins
Sulfonamides

ANTICONVULSANTS
Carbamazepine
Phenytoin

ANTIFUNGAL AGENTS
Itraconazole

SSRI ANTIDEPRESSANTS
Fluoxetine

DRUG-INDUCED LUPUS

Drug-induced lupus (DIL) is characterized by frequent musculoskeletal complaints, fever, weight loss, pleuropulmonary involvement in more than half of patients, and rarely, renal, neurologic, or vasculitic involvement. Most patients have no cutaneous findings of lupus erythematosus. A positive antinuclear antibody (ANA) titer with a homogeneous pattern is the most common serologic abnormality. Importantly, only a minority of patients who develop a positive antinuclear antibody titer related to drug ingestion develop clinical disease compatible with DIL. DIL should be suspected in patients who do not have a history of idiopathic lupus erythematosus, who develop antinuclear antibodies and at least one clinical feature of lupus erythematosus after an appropriate duration of drug treatment, and whose symptoms resolve after discontinuation of the drug.[39] In general, the onset of symptoms and serologic changes may be more than 1 year after starting therapy.

A number of drugs, including procainamide, hydralazine, chlorpromazine, isoniazid, methyldopa, and penicillamine, have been implicated in DIL. However, recently there have been numerous cases of DIL in association with minocycline.[2,40,41]

Most cases associated with minocycline have been reported in young adult females who were using minocycline for acne an average of 2 years after the initiation of drug therapy.[2] The symptoms are usually of acute onset including malaise, fever, polyarthralgia, and rarely, rash. The rash can be urticarial as well as erythematous or vasculitic.[41] Arthritis is often present, affecting both small and large joints.

Laboratory findings include variable white cell counts from leukopenia to leukocytosis, high erythrocyte sedimentation rates, and positive ANA, with titers as high as 1:1600.[40] Liver transaminases (ALT and AST) may be elevated up to 10 times normal.[40] Box 45-6 lists monitoring recommendations for patients on long-term minocycline therapy.

A positive ANA with a homogeneous pattern is the most common serologic abnormality in DIL. Although antihistone antibodies are seen in up to 95% of DIL, they are not specific for

Box 45-6

General Recommendations for Patients on Minocycline

1. Minocycline should be avoided in patients with SLE or in those with a history of SLE in a first-degree relative.
2. Relative contraindications to the use of minocycline include the presence of underlying hepatic or renal disease.
3. No routine baseline or periodic laboratory monitoring is indicated.
4. Antinuclear antibody and hepatic transaminase levels should be monitored only in patients receiving chronic minocycline therapy who develop relevant symptoms.
5. Appropriate laboratory monitoring (see Table 45-2) should be done for patients who develop DHS or SSLR.
6. Any patient with a serious adverse reaction such as DHS, SSLR, or DIL should be advised to avoid the entire class of tetracycline antibiotics (see text).

SLE, Systemic lupus erythematosus.

the syndrome and are found in 50% to 80% of patients with idiopathic lupus erythematosus.[42] In contrast with idiopathic lupus erythematosus, antibodies against deoxyribonucleic acid (DNA) are typically absent.[43] Several patients with DIL attributed to minocycline had positive antineutrophil cytoplasmic antibodies, which may be directed against myeloperoxidase or elastase.[41,44] Although the relation of these antibodies to the pathogenesis of the disease is unknown, it has been suggested that the neutrophil enzyme myeloperoxidase is involved in the metabolism of drugs that can induce lupus. For example, in one study comparing the serology of DIL with idiopathic lupus erythematosus, all six patients (100%) with hydralazine-induced lupus had antimyeloperoxidase antibodies versus 21% with idiopathic lupus erythematosus.[45]

In general, seroconversion from a negative to a positive ANA titer alone is not a sufficient reason to discontinue treatment with a drug. However, once DIL is suspected, treatment with the drug believed to be responsible should be stopped immediately. Symptoms of DIL are usually self-limiting once treatment with the of-

fending drug has been discontinued and generally resolve in 4 to 6 weeks; however, the ANA may remain positive for 6 to 12 months. Rechallenge may result in recurrence of symptoms.[40,41] Nonsteroidal antiinflammatory drugs (NSAIDs) can be used for symptomatic treatment of musculoskeletal complaints. Short courses of prednisone may be necessary in severe cases.[46] It is important to recognize minocycline as a possible cause of DIL because many patients are young and female, the usual population with idiopathic lupus erythematosus.

ACUTE GENERALIZED EXANTHEMATOUS PUSTULOSIS

AGEP is characterized by a fever above 38° C and a cutaneous eruption with nonfollicular sterile pustules on an edematous erythematous background.[47] The interval between drug administration and the onset of the eruption can vary from 2 days to 2 to 3 weeks. A long interval probably indicates primary sensitization and the shorter interval may be related to an unintentional reexposure.[47] The onset is usually abrupt, with the eruption starting on the face and spreading to the trunk and lower limbs. Two weeks later, generalized desquamation occurs. Some patients may present with additional skin lesions, including petechial purpura, erythema multiforme–like target lesions, vesicles, or blisters.[48] Characteristic laboratory findings include leukocytosis, which is usually neutrophilic. The spongiform pustule is the major histologic feature of AGEP; papillary dermal edema, polymorphous perivascular infiltrates with eosinophils, leukocytoclastic vasculitis, and necrotic keratinocytes may also be evident.[48]

AGEP is most commonly associated with beta-lactam and macrolide antibiotic usage,[48] although many other drugs have been implicated, including calcium channel blockers and analgesics (Box 45-7). There have been several reported cases of terbinafine-induced AGEP.[49,50] Differential diagnosis includes pustular psoriasis, DHS with pustulation, and Sneddon-Wilkinson disease.

Discontinuation of therapy is usually the extent of treatment necessary in most patients. However, the use of systemic corticosteroids may be indicated in some patients, depending

Box 45-7

Medications Associated With Acute Generalized Exanthematous Pustulosis

ANTICONVULSANTS
Carbamazepine
Phenytoin

ANTIFUNGAL AGENTS
Itraconazole
Terbinafine

ANTIMALARIAL AGENTS
Hydroxychloroquine

CALCIUM CHANNEL BLOCKERS
Diltiazem
Nifedipine

BETA-LACTAM ANTIBIOTICS
Amoxicillin
Cefaclor
Cefuroxime
Cephalexin
Penicillin

MACROLIDE ANTIBIOTICS
Azithromycin
Erythromycin
Spiramycin

OTHER ANTIBIOTICS
Ciprofloxacin
Doxycycline
Isoniazid
Streptomycin
Sulfonamides

OTHER DRUGS
Acetaminophen
Allopurinol
Diclofenac
Furosemide

MERCURY

on the extent of the reaction.[51,52] Readministration of the suspected drug is not recommended because recurrence of lesions usually occurs within hours of drug administration.[47,53]

Patch testing has been used to aid in the diagnosis of AGEP,[49,54,55] usually producing an isomorphic pustular reaction with subcorneal pustules on the biopsy specimen. The tests are often positive within 6 hours.[47]

SEVERE CUTANEOUS ADVERSE REACTIONS—ERYTHEMA MULTIFORME MAJOR, STEVENS-JOHNSON SYNDROME, TOXIC EPIDERMAL NECROLYSIS

Severe cutaneous adverse reactions, which may represent variants of the same disease process, encompass a spectrum from the less serious erythema multiforme major (EMm) to more serious reactions such as Stevens-Johnson syndrome (SJS) and toxic epidermal necrolysis (TEN). Differentiation among the three patterns depends on the nature of the skin lesions and extent of body surface area involvement. The more severe forms of TEN have a greater percentage of body surface area of epidermal detachment. Target lesions tend to change from the classic, raised, three-ringed-iris lesion to a more purpuric or erythematous two-ringed lesion (Table 45-2). Clinically, each of these reaction patterns is characterized by the presence of the triad of mucous membrane erosions, target lesions, and epidermal necrosis with skin detachment.[56] The more severe the reaction, the more likely it is that it has been drug-induced. A large percentage of EMm/SJS cases are not drug related and may develop after a variety of other predisposing factors, including infections, neoplasia, and autoimmune diseases. The most frequent drugs cited as causes for EMm, SJS, or TEN are the anticonvulsants, antibiotics (e.g., sulfonamides), allopurinol, and NSAIDs (e.g., piroxicam).[57]

The pathogenesis of severe cutaneous adverse drug reactions (ADRs) is unknown, although a metabolic basis has been hypothesized.[11] Sulfonamides and anticonvulsants, which are the two groups of drugs most frequently as-

■ **Table 45-2** Classification and Characteristics of Severe Cutaneous Adverse Reactions

Classification	Erythema Multiforme Major	Stevens-Johnson Syndrome	Toxic Epidermal Necrolysis
Epidermal detachment (% of body surface area)	<10	<10	>30
Typical targets	Yes	No	No
Atypical targets	Flat	Flat	Flat
Macules	No	Yes	Yes
Mucous membrane involvement	Yes	Yes	Yes
Severity	+	++	+++
Likelihood of drug etiology	+	++	+++

+, Low; ++, moderate; +++, high.

sociated with SJS and TEN, are metabolized to toxic metabolites that are subsequently detoxified in most individuals. However, in predisposed patients with a genetic defect, the metabolite may bind covalently to proteins. In some of these patients, the metabolite-protein adducts may trigger an immunoresponse that may lead to cutaneous ADRs.[58]

To rule out concurrent internal organ involvement, complete blood counts, liver enzymes, and chest x-rays should be performed. Treatment of EMm, SJS, and TEN includes discontinuation of a suspected drug and supportive measures, such as careful wound care, hydration, and nutritional support.[59,60] The use of corticosteroids in SJS and TEN is controversial. Some clinicians believe corticosteroids may be beneficial when administered early in the disease and at relatively high dosage.[61] However, other authors suggest that corticosteroids do not shorten the recovery time and may increase the risk of complications including secondary infections (potentially leading to sepsis) and gastrointestinal bleeding.[59,62] Uncontrolled studies showed that plasmapheresis[63] and human intravenous immunoglobulin (IVIg) may be beneficial.[64] In a pilot study, 10 patients with clinically and histologically confirmed TEN were treated with IVIg at doses ranging from 0.2 to 0.75 g/kg of body weight per day for 4 consecutive days. Disease progression was rapidly reversed and outcome was favorable in all cases. Patients who have developed a severe cutaneous adverse re-

action (i.e., EMm, SJS, TEN) should not be rechallenged with the drug nor undergo desensitization with the medication.

DRUG-INDUCED SYSTEMIC INFLAMMATORY RESPONSE SYNDROME

The systemic inflammatory response syndrome (SIRS) is defined by two or more of the following: fever (>38.5° C), tachypnea (>20 breaths/minute), tachycardia (>90 beats/minute), and leukocytosis (>12,000 cells/mm^3 or >10% immature forms).[65] Azathioprine-induced SIRS has been described in the literature.[66,67] In these patients, a fever with or without gastrointestinal symptoms most commonly develops within hours or weeks after initiation of the azathioprine. Because the initial reaction is often misdiagnosed as an infection, a rechallenge is mistakenly carried out. On azathioprine rechallenge, the reaction is generally more severe and on many occasions life-threatening. In addition, the "rechallenge" reaction usually manifests itself more rapidly than the initial episode. Dermatologic eruptions (usually a generalized erythematous rash), hepatotoxicity, and nephritis have also been reported.

The mechanism is unknown but may relate to sudden mediator or cytokine release. Sepsis-like reactions (i.e., fever, hypotension, oliguria) may result from increased production of cytokines such as tumor necrosis factor (TNF).

Box 45-8

Steps in Evaluating a Suspected Adverse Drug Reaction[61]

Clinical diagnosis of the reaction
- Not related to causality assessment, for example, diagnosis is not an "amoxicillin rash" but rather the description of the skin eruption

Analysis of drug exposure
- Prescription drugs
- Nonprescription medications
- Herbal or holistic therapies

Differential diagnosis
- Consider nondrug and other drug causes

Literature search
- Include medical journals, textbooks, pharmaceutical manufacturers

Confirmation
- Rechallenge—in vivo (oral,* skin testing, patch testing) and in vitro

Confirmation—cont'd
- Dechallenge—discontinuation of the medication and resolution of the reaction

Advice to the patient
- Include drug involved in the reaction, patient's predisposition to possible recurrence on exposure to the drug, potential cross-reaction to other drugs, genetic predisposition of family members, if applicable
- Enrollment in the MedicAlert program

Reporting to licensing authorities and/or manufacturer

*In vivo oral rechallenge should be performed <u>only</u> for relatively low-risk drug reaction pattern.

Other postulated mechanisms for these reactions include immunologic (e.g., immunoglobulin E [IgE]-mediated) or idiosyncratic.[66]

Because of the potential severity of the reaction on rechallenge, any patient who experiences fever, hypotension, arthralgias, severe nausea and vomiting, or leukocytosis while on azathioprine should not be rechallenged with either azathioprine or 6-mercaptopurine.

GENERAL DISCUSSION

Drug reaction syndromes are often a challenging management problem. A systematic, stepwise approach for the diagnosis of drug reactions can help to untangle complicated clinical scenarios with exposure to multiple agents[68,69] (Box 45-8). Dermatologists must be able to recognize drug reaction syndromes such as AGEP, DHS, SSLR, and DIL. All alternatives in the differential diagnosis for each specific syndrome need to be considered. A careful and complete drug history is essential; this includes, but is not limited to, all new drugs started within the preceding 6 weeks, over-the-counter preparations, and herbal/naturopathic remedies. The fourth step in the diagnosis of an adverse drug reaction is to determine the probability that each possible drug may have caused the reaction pattern observed. When serious drug reaction syndromes are considered, then even a low likelihood of causation should be respected and the drug should be avoided in the future.

Bibliography

Bastuji-Garin S, Rzany B, Stern R, et al: Clinical classification of cases of toxic epidermal necrolysis, Stevens-Johnson syndrome, and erythema multiforme. *Arch Dermatol* 129:92-96, 1993.

Bocquet H, Bagot M, Roujeau J: Drug-induced pseudolymphoma and drug hypersensitivity syndrome (drug rash with eosinophilia and systemic symptoms: DRESS). *Semin Cutan Med Surg* 15:250-257, 1996.

Elkayam O, Yaron M, Caspi D: Minocycline-induced autoimmune syndromes: an overview. *Sem Arthritis Rheum* 28:392-397, 1999.

Rieder M: In vivo and in vitro testing for adverse drug reactions. *Ped Clin North Am* 44:93-111, 1997.

Roujeau JC, Stern R: Severe adverse cutaneous reactions to drugs. *N Engl J Med* 331:1272-1285, 1994.

Rubin RL: Etiology and mechanisms of drug-induced lupus. *Curr Opin Rheumatol* 11:357-363, 1999.

Schlienger RG, Shear NH: Antiepileptic drug hypersensitivity syndrome. *Epilepsia* 39(Suppl 7):S3-7, 1998.

Shear N: Diagnosing cutaneous adverse reactions to drugs. *Arch Dermatol* 126:94-97, 1990.

References

Drug Hypersensitivity Syndrome

1. Roujeau JC, Stern R: Severe adverse cutaneous reactions to drugs. *N Engl J Med* 331:1272-1285, 1994.

2. Knowles S, Shapiro L, Shear N: Serious adverse reactions induced by minocycline: a report of 13 patients and review of the literature. *Arch Dermatol* 132:934-939, 1996.

3. Tennis P, Stern R: Risk of serious cutaneous disorders after initiation of use of phenytoin, carbamazepine, or sodium valproate: a record linkage study. *Neurology* 49:542-546, 1997.

4. Gennis M, Vemuri R, Burns E, et al: Familial occurrence of hypersensitivity to phenytoin. *Am J Med* 91:631-634, 1991.

5. Morkunas A, Miller M: Anticonvulsant hypersensitivity syndrome. *Medical Toxicology* 13:727-739, 1997.

6. Vittorio C, Muglia J: Anticonvulsant hypersensitivity syndrome. *Arch Intern Med* 155:2285-2290, 1995.

7. Gupta A, Eggo M, Uetrecht J, et al: Drug-induced hypothyroidism: the thyroid as a target organ in hypersensitivity reactions to anticonvulsants and sulfonamides. *Clin Pharmacol Ther* 51:56-67, 1992.

8. Callot V, Roujeau J, Bagot M, et al: Drug-induced pseudolymphoma and hypersensitivity syndrome: two different clinical entities. *Arch Dermatol* 123:1315-1321, 1996.

9. Schreiber M, McGregor J: Pseudolymphoma syndrome. *Arch Derm* 97:297-300, 1968.

10. Sinnige H, Boender C, Kuypers E, et al: Carbamazepine-induced pseudolymphoma and immune dysregulation. *J Intern Med* 227:355-358, 1990.

11. Shear N, Spielberg S: Anticonvulsant hypersensitivity syndrome, in vitro assessment of risk. *J Clin Invest* 82:1826-1832, 1988.

12. Chaffin J, Davis S: Suspected lamotrigine-induced toxic epidermal necrolysis. *Ann Pharmacother* 31:720-723, 1997.

13. Wadelius M, Karlsson T, Wadelius C, et al: Lamotrigine and toxic epidermal necrolysis. *Lancet* 348:1041, 1996.

14. Schlienger R, Knowles S, Shear N: Lamotrigine-associated anticonvulsant hypersensitivity syndrome. *Neurology* 51:1172-1175, 1998.

15. Epstein M, Wright J: Severe multisystem disease caused by trimethoprim-sulfamethoxazole: possible role of an in vitro lymphocyte assay. *J Allergy Clin Immunol* 86:416-417, 1990.

16. Cribb A, Spielberg S: Sulfamethoxazole is metabolized to the hydroxylamine in humans. *Clin Pharmacol Ther* 51:522-526, 1992.

17. Shear N, Spielberg S, Grant D, et al: Differences in metabolism of sulfonamides predisposing to idiosyncratic toxicity. *Ann Intern Med* 105:179-187, 1986.

18. Prussick R, Shear N: Dapsone hypersensitivity syndrome. *J Am Acad Dermatol* 35:346-349, 1996.

19. McKenna K, Robinson J: The dapsone hypersensitivity syndrome occurring in a patient with dermatitis herpetiformis. *Br J Dermatol* 137:646-663, 1997.

20. Coleman M, Scott A, Breckenridge A, et al: The use of cimetidine as a selective inhibitor of dapsone N-hydroxylation in man. *Br J Clin Pharmacol* 30:761-767, 1990.

21. Rhodes L, Tingle M, Park B, et al: Cimetidine improves the therapeutic/toxic ratio of dapsone in patients on chronic dapsone therapy. *Br J Dermatol* 132:257-262, 1995.

22. Shapiro L, Knowles S, Shear N: Comparative safety and risk management of tetracycline, doxycycline and minocycline. *Arch Dermatol* 133:1224-1230, 1997.

23. Rieder M: In vivo and in vitro testing for adverse drug reactions. *Ped Clin North Am* 44:93-111, 1997.

Serum Sickness–like Reaction

24. Lawley T, Bielory L, Gascon P, et al: A prospective clinical and immunologic analysis of patients with serum sickness. *N Engl J Med* 311:1407-1413, 1984.

25. Harel L, Amir J, Livni E et al: Serum-sickness like reaction associated with minocycline therapy in adolescents. *Ann Pharmacother* 30:481-483, 1996.

26. Lowery N, Kearns GL, Young RA, et al: Serum sickness-like reactions associated with cefprozil therapy. *J Pediatr* 125:325-328, 1994.

27. Stricker BH, Tijssen JG: Serum sickness-like reactions to cefaclor. *J Clin Epidemiol* 45:1177-1184, 1992.

28. Platt R, Dreis MW, Kennedy DL, et al: Serum sickness-like reactions to amoxicillin, cefaclor, cephalexin and trimethoprim-sulfamethoxazole. *J Infect Dis* 158:474-476, 1988.

29. Shapiro LE, Knowles SR, Shear NH: Fluoxetine-induced serum sickness-like reaction. *Ann Pharmacother* 31:927, 1997.

30. Slama TG: Serum sickness-like illness associated with ciprofloxacin. *Antimicrob Agents Chemother* 34:904-905, 1990.

31. Igarashi M, Bando Y, Shimanuki K, et al: Immunosuppressive factors detected during convalescence in a patient with severe serum sickness induced by carbamazepine. *Int Arch Allergy Immunol* 100:378-381, 1993.

32. Menitove JE, Rassiga AL, McLaren GD, et al: Antigranulocyte antibodies and deranged immune function associated with phenytoin-induced serum sickness. *Am J Hematol* 10:277-284, 1981.

33. Park H, Knowles S, Shear NH: Serum sickness-like reaction to itraconazole. *Ann Pharmacother* 32:1249, 1998.

34. Heckbert S, Stryker W, Coltin K, et al: Serum sickness in children after antibiotic exposure: estimates of occurrence and morbidity in a Health Maintenance Organization population. *Am J Epidemiol* 132:336-342, 1990.

35. Stricker B, Vandenbroek J, Keuning J, et al: Cholestatic hepatitis due to antibacterial combination of amoxicillin and clavulanic acid (Augmentin). *Dig Dis Sci* 34:1576-1580, 1989.

36. Kearns G, Wheeler J, Childress S, et al: Serum sickness-like reactions to cefaclor: role of hepatic metabolism and individual susceptibility. *J Pediatr* 125:805-811, 1994.

37. Vial T, Pont J, Pham E, et al: Cefaclor-associated serum sickness-like disease: eight cases and review of the literature. *Ann Pharmacother* 26:910-914, 1992.

38. Grammer L: Cefaclor serum sickness. *JAMA* 275:1152-1153, 1996.

Drug-Induced Lupus

39. Hess E: Drug-related lupus. *N Engl J Med* 318:1460-1462, 1988.

40. Gough A, Chapman S, Wagstaff K, et al: Minocycline-induced autoimmune hepatitis and systemic lupus erythematosus-like syndrome. *BMJ* 312:169-172, 1996.

41. Akin E, Miller L, Tucker L: Minocycline-induced lupus in adolescents. *Pediatrics* 926-928, 1997.

42. Gioud M, Kaci M, Monier J: Histone antibodies in systemic lupus erythematosus: a possible diagnostic tool. *Arthritis Rheum* 25:407-413, 1982.

43. Yung R, Richardson B: Drug-induced lupus. *Rheum Dis Clin North Am* 20:61-86, 1994.

44. Gaffney K, Merry P: Antineutrophil cytoplasmic antibody-positive polyarthritis associated with minocycline therapy. *Br J Rheumatol* 35:1326-1336, 1996.

45. Nassberger L, Sjoholm A, Jonsson H, et al: Autoantibodies against neutrophil cytoplasm components in systemic lupus erythematosus and in hydralazine-induced lupus. *Clin Exp Immunol* 81:380-383, 1990.

46. Masson C, Chevailler A, Pascaretti C, et al: Minocycline related lupus. *J Rheumatol* 23:2160-2161, 1996.

Acute Generalized Exanthematous Pustulosis

47. Beylot C, Doutre M, Beylot-Barry M: Acute generalized exanthematous pustulosis. *Semin Cutan Med Surg* 15:244-249, 1996.

48. Roujeau J, Bioulac-Sage P, Bourseau C, et al: Acute generalized exanthematous pustulosis: analysis of 63 cases. *Arch Dermatol* 127:1333-1338, 1991.

49. Kempinaire A, De Raeve L, Merckx M, et al: Terfinabine-induced acute generalized exanthematous pustulosis confirmed by a positive patch-test result. *J Am Acad Dermatol* 37:653-655, 1997.

50. Dupin N, Gorin I, Djien V, et al: Acute generalized exanthematous pustulosis induced by terbinafine. *Arch Dermatol* 132:1253-1254, 1996.

51. Vicente-Callja J, Aguirre AN, Crespo V, et al: Acute generalized exanthematous pustulosis due to diltiazem: confirmation by patch testing. *Br J Dermatol* 137:837-839, 1997.

52. Demitsu T, AYamada, Tusui K, et al: Acute generalized exanthematous pustulosis induced by dexamethasone injection. *Dermatology* 193:56-58, 1996.

53. Park Y, Kim J, Kim C: Acute generalized exanthematous pustulosis induced by itraconazole. *J Am Acad Dermatol* 36:794-796, 1997.

54. Moreau A, Dompmartin A: Drug-induced acute generalized exanthematous pustulosis with positive patch tests. *Int J Dermatol* 34:263-266, 1995.

55. Dewerdt S, Vaillant L, Machet L, et al: Acute generalized exanthematous pustulosis induced by lansoprazole. *Acta Derm Venereol (Stockh)* 77:250, 1997.

Erythema Multiforme/Stevens-Johnson Syndrome/Toxic Epidermal Necrolysis

56. Bastuji-Garin S, Rzany B, Stern R, et al: Clinical classification of cases of toxic epidermal necrolysis, Stevens-Johnson syndrome, and erythema multiforme. *Arch Dermatol* 129:92-96, 1993.

57. Roujeau J, Kelly J, Naldi L, et al: Medication use and the risk of Stevens-Johnson syndrome or toxic epidermal necrolysis. *N Engl J Med* 333:1600-1607, 1995.

58. Wolkenstein P, Charue D, Laurent P, et al: Metabolic predisposition to cutaneous adverse drug reactions. *Arch Dermatol* 131:544-551, 1995.

59. Barone C, Bianchi M, Lee B, et al: Treatment of toxic epidermal necrolysis and Stevens-Johnson syndrome in children. *J Oral Maxillofac Surg* 51:264-268, 1993.

60. Fine J: Management of acquired bullous skin diseases. *N Engl J Med* 333:1475-1484, 1995.

61. Patterson R, Miller M, Kaplan M, et al: Effectiveness of early therapy with corticosteroids in Stevens-Johnson syndrome: experience with 41 cases and a hypothesis regarding pathogenesis. *Ann Allergy* 73:27-34, 1994.

62. Prendville J, Hebert A, Greenwald M, et al: Management of Stevens-Johnson syndrome and toxic epidermal necrolysis in children. *J Pediatr* 115:881-887, 1989.

63. Chaidemenos G, Chrysomallis FK, Mourellou O, et al: Plasmapheresis in toxic epidermal necrolysis. *Int J Dermatol* 36:218-221, 1997.

64. Viard I, Wehrli P, Bullani R, et al: Inhibition of toxic epidermal necrolysis by blockade of CD95 with human intravenous immunoglobulin. *Science* 282:490-493, 1998.

Drug-Induced Systemic Inflammatory Response Syndrome

65. Opal S: Sepsis. In Dale D, Federman D, editors: *Scientific American medicine*, vol II, New York, 1998, Scientific American, Inc.

66. Knowles S, Gupta A, Shear N, et al: Azathioprine hypersensitivity-like reactions: a case report and a review of the literature. *Clin Exp Dermatol* 20:353-356, 1995.

67. Wilson B: Azathioprine hypersensitivity mimicking sepsis in a patient with Crohn's disease. *Clin Infectious Dis* 17:940-941, 1993.

General Discussion

68. Shear N: Diagnosing cutaneous adverse reactions to drugs. *Arch Dermatol* 126:94-97, 1990.

69. Bocquet H, Bagot M, Roujeau J: Drug-induced pseudolymphoma and drug hypersensitivity syndrome (drug rash with eosinophilia and systemic symptoms: DRESS). *Semin Cutan Med Surg* 15:250-257, 1996.

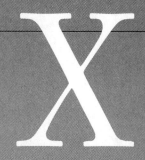

Special Pharmacology and Therapeutic Topics

CHAPTER 46

Marc Alan Darst
Crystal S. Blankenship

Pharmacoeconomics

Pharmacoeconomics is the branch of health economics that examines the costs and benefits of drug therapy. Pharmacoeconomics seeks to find the least expensive means by which to produce the most beneficial outcome. To make a rational decision about the use of a specific treatment, one must look beyond the direct acquisition cost of a pharmaceutical by examining its impact on total health resource utilization. Along with beneficial effects, pharmaceuticals may cause various negative effects, many of which are unpredictable. Pharmacoeconomics considers the value of a medicine to be its ability to improve the total cost of care without negatively affecting quality. A pharmacoeconomic analysis defines an explicit set of criteria that takes this value into account to yield a recommendation for spending limited resources.[1] More than just determining the acquisition cost of a drug, pharmacoeconomic evaluations identify how a particular pharmaceutical agent may produce a positive outcome that lowers total healthcare costs.[2]

The four major forms of analysis used in economic evaluation are (1) cost-minimization, (2) cost-benefit, (3) cost-effectiveness, and (4) cost-utility. Each analysis is useful in its own way, but none is all-inclusive and each has its own indications and limitations. This chapter reviews the four types of analyses; examines their applications, strengths, and limitations; and covers a variety of pharmacoeconomic topics of interest to the clinician today.

COST-MINIMIZATION ANALYSIS

Cost-minimization compares the cost of two or more interventions with outcomes or consequences that are assumed or demonstrated to be equivalent based on an objective review of clinical outcomes literature. Because the objective is to identify the least expensive alternative, the outcomes themselves are not assigned a monetary valuation. The evaluation does not consider patient preferences, drug allergies, or other mitigating circumstances. In reality, it is difficult to demonstrate that all therapeutic alternatives have equal outcomes; therefore this type of analysis is of limited use. Cost-minimization comparisons are usually between different dosing routes (e.g., intravenous [IV] versus by mouth [PO] routes of administration for the same medicine), dosing regimens (e.g., q6h versus q8h for the same drug), or therapeutic equivalents (e.g., doxycycline versus tetracycline).[1] To perform an accurate analysis, all costs of the drug's administration must be included. This includes expenses that are difficult to measure, such as nursing time, as well as other costs borne by the patient. Simply add all the costs of each therapy being considered and compare the totals. The lowest total is the least expensive (minimal cost) therapy.

COST-BENEFIT ANALYSIS

Cost-benefit analysis compares the cost of a therapy with its benefit, expressing each in monetary terms. As in business, the goal is to achieve the highest return on an investment. A key assumption of this analysis is that there exist finite resources to fund the intervention or project.[3] To perform this analysis, a monetary value must be assigned to the outcomes, such as the dollar value of a life saved, a year of life lengthened, or the morbidity avoided by applying the therapy. This tool allows comparison of multiple therapies or interventions with various outcomes. Researchers can compare total costs of different therapies or analyze the incremental benefit of selecting one therapy over another. To make the comparison, calculate both the benefits per patient as well as the costs per patient. Multiply each by the total number of patients to determine total benefits and total costs. Armed with these data, three different numbers may be calculated—(1) benefit-to-cost ratio (total benefits ÷ total costs), (2) net benefit (total benefits − total costs), and (3) return on investment (net benefit ÷ total costs). When comparing therapies, the one with the highest net benefit is not always the alternative with the highest return on investment. The therapy with the highest net benefit is generally the preferred therapy,[1] unless resources are insufficient to implement it. Then, the therapy with the highest return on investment is the preferred choice.

COST-EFFECTIVENESS ANALYSIS

Cost-effectiveness analysis examines the ratio of the cost of therapy to the outcome. Outcomes are expressed in physical or natural units such as lives saved or diseases prevented. Results are expressed as financial units per result (e.g., dollars per lives saved). This analysis assumes that the outcome is worthwhile, thus it does not necessarily lead to cost reduction, but instead to the cost-efficient achievement of the desired result.[1] A therapy with lower overall effectiveness may be preferred over

Table 46-1   Oral Drug Therapies for Pustular Acne

	Drug A	Drug B
Acquisition cost of therapy (acquisition cost plus treatment of adverse effects)	$120	$180
Adverse effects (skin peeling, rash, nausea)	10%	15%
Effectiveness (% reduction in pustules after 6 months)	85%	95%
Cost-effectiveness ratio (cost/effectiveness)	141	189

Adapted from Gibson G: Understanding and implementing the economics of pharmacoeconomics. *Manag Care Med* 37:9-24, 1995.

a more effective therapy if the more effective choice costs more to achieve its results. Other costs of therapy, such as treatment of side effects, must be included in this analysis. Simply take the total cost of the therapy and divide by the effectiveness of the therapy. The therapy with the lower cost-effectiveness ratio is the better choice.

Table 46-1 represents the following example. A staff model HMO formulary includes Drug A for the oral treatment of pustular acne. A member of the dermatology department requests that a new drug, Drug B, be added to your formulary. To analyze the request, data were obtained.

The new Drug B is less cost-effective than Drug A, as demonstrated by a higher cost-effectiveness ratio. Thus it may be excluded from the formulary, or restricted only to use after Drug A failure. A more thorough analysis could include the cost of drug failures (money wasted on therapy that did not work) and determination of specific patient populations in which Drug B would be preferred.

COST-UTILITY ANALYSIS

The cost-utility analysis is unique because it considers the patient's preferences and the morbidity of suffering and pain.[1] This analysis is similar to the cost-effectiveness analysis except that the outcomes are adjusted for patient preferences, or utility.[3] Outcomes are expressed in terms of *Quality-Adjusted Life Years* (QALY), which is the number of years life is extended by a treatment multiplied by the utility rating of the quality of life of those years. If the quality of life yielded by the intervention is less than perfect, the amount of debilitation is assigned a utility rating between 0 (death) and 1.0 (normal health), which is then multiplied by the number of years to generate the QALY figure. If there is a state regarded as conceptually worse than death, it is assigned a negative number. For example, when an intervention yields 1 more year of normal life, it has a value of 1 QALY. Expressing results in QALY identifies the difference between two life-extending treatments. This type of analysis is limited by the difficulty of defining the units of outcome measure, as the utility index rating is subjective and usually determined by polling a healthy general populace. Thus the values may not reflect the views of actual patients.[4] Gill and Feinstein[5] suggest assigning the rating by polling patients and asking their opinion of their quality of life after the treatment, then generating the index. Several tools have been developed to measure the utility variable. These include the EuroQol©,[6] the Quality of Well Being (QWB) scale,[7] and the Mark Health Utilities Index (Mark HUI-III).[8,9]

For example, suppose there are two fictitious therapies for mycosis fungoides. As indicated by Table 46-2, the obvious choice is Ther-

■ **Table 46-2**   Two Fictitious Therapies for Mycosis Fungoides

	Therapy 1	Therapy 2
Total cost of therapy	$20,000	8500
Increased life (expectancy	10 yrs	6 yrs
Utility ratio (0.0 to 1.0)	0.8	0.5
QALY added (life expectancy × utility ratio)	8	3
Cost-utility ratio (cost per QALY added)	2500	2833

Adapted from Gibson G: Understanding and implementing the economics of pharmacoeconomics. *Manag Care Med* 37:9-24, 1995.

apy 1. If the cost-utility ratios are similar, it may be prudent to encourage the patient to choose the path taken.

"FORGOTTEN" AND INDIRECT COSTS OF THERAPY

The term *indirect cost* can be confusing. Strictly speaking, there are only two types of cost—direct and indirect. Larson[10] points out that a direct cost is any cost that involves a monetary exchange. Thus costs that at first glance might appear to be indirect are actually direct costs. Clinicians like to call these the "forgotten" costs of therapy. Some forgotten costs include nursing staff time needed to educate the patient about the therapy and its administration and the cost of supplies such as tubing and administration sets. Others include laboratory tests, or in the case of methotrexate, periodic liver biopsies, as well as treatment of any biopsy complications. Too frequently, the only direct cost included in an analysis is that of drug acquisition. When considering all the costs of the therapy, drug acquisition price may be the least expensive portion of therapy. Also, drug acquisition cost varies depending on perspective—average wholesale price (AWP), cost to the institution, or cost to the patient. Indirect costs do not involve an exchange of money, but can be considered lost opportunity costs such as the cost to the patient of time away from work, time away from family, and transportation costs.[10] Indirect costs are usually too difficult to generalize to include in the analysis but should be part of the decision-making process when discussing possible therapies with the patient. In short, although clinicians often consider only the acquisition cost of the therapies prescribed, when constructing analyses such as these, they must be careful to ensure that appropriate forgotten and indirect costs are included.

For example, examine total costs of therapy for two different diseases, mycosis fungoides (cutaneous T-cell lymphoma) and psoriasis. The treatment of both overlaps in the use of ultraviolet B (UVB) phototherapy and psoralen plus ultraviolet A (PUVA) therapy, which have no laboratory monitoring costs. Both diseases have various medical treatments as shown in Tables 46-3 and 46-4. Some of these other treatments have significant laboratory monitoring require-

Table 46-3   Psoriasis Systemic Therapy Cost Comparison—Costs per Year

Therapy	Dose or Frequency	Medication Cost	Monitoring Cost	Phototherapy Cost	Office Visits Cost	Total Cost per Year
UVB phototherapy	Twice weekly	None	None	708.75	233.00	941.75
Maintenance (UVB)	Twice monthly	None	None	252	189.00	441.00
PUVA phototherapy	Twice weekly	141.50*	211.00	757.35	233.00	1342.85
Maintenance (PUVA)	Twice monthly	94.35	55.00	505.05	189.00	843.40
Acitretin	25 mg daily	3573.96	677.52	None	422.00	4547.48
(Soriatane)	50 mg daily	6845.64	677.52	None	422.00	7945.16
Methotrexate	7.5 mg weekly	372.84	1210.75	None	422.00	1879.59
	15 mg weekly	662.52	1210.75	None	422.00	2169.27
Cyclosporine	200 mg daily	4489.44	1531.02	None	989.00	7009.46
(Neoral)	300 mg daily	6977.16	1531.02	None	989.00	9497.18

MONITORING GUIDELINES—FACTORS USED TO DETERMINE COST

UVB—none

PUVA—twice yearly eye examinations, once yearly fundus photos, no other monitoring

Soriatane (acitretin)—triglycerides, cholesterol, SGOT, CBC—initially monthly, eventually every 3 months

Methotrexate—CBC, SGOT—initially every 2 weeks, eventually every 2 months, plus 1 liver biopsy

Neoral (cyclosporine)—CBC, BUN, creatinine, triglycerides, cholesterol, SGOT, uric acid, potassium, magnesium—initially every 2 weeks, then every month

OFFICE VISITS

UVB and PUVA—monthly during induction phase (3 months), every 3 months during maintenance phase

Soriatane (acitretin)—every month initially (3 months), then every 3 months

Methotrexate—every month initially (3 months), then every 3 months

Neoral (cyclosporine)—every 2 weeks for 1-2 months, then monthly

CPT codes: 99203 = $107, 99213 = $63, 11100 (punch biopsy) = $108, fundus photos = $76.

*PUVA phototherapy medication cost calculated based on 30 mg Oxsoralen Ultra dose.

Table 46-4 Mycosis Fungoides Systemic Therapy Cost Comparison—Cost per Year

Therapy	Dose or Frequency	Medication Cost	Monitoring Cost	Phototherapy or Radiation Cost	Office Visits Cost	Total Cost per Year
UVB phototherapy	Twice weekly	None	None	708.75	233.00	941.75
Maintenance (UVB)	Twice monthly	None	None	252.00	189.00	441.00
PUVA phototherapy	Twice weekly	141.50*	211.00	757.35	233.00	1342.85
Maintenance (PUVA)	Twice monthly	94.35	55.00	505.05	189.00	843.40
Nitrogen mustard	Daily 10% body	388.73	None	None	422.00	810.73
	Daily 100% body	3887.30	None	None	422.00	4309.30
Bexarotene	150 mg daily	7262.88	742.81	None	485.00	8490.69
(Targretin)	300 mg daily	14,489.82	742.81	None	485.00	15,717.63
	450 mg daily	21,716.76	742.81	None	485.00	22,944.57
Electron beam	One course†	None	None	20,000.00	252.00	20,252.00

MONITORING GUIDELINES—FACTORS USED TO DETERMINE COST

UVB—none
PUVA—twice yearly eye examinations, once yearly fundus photos, no other monitoring
Nitrogen mustard—no laboratory monitoring
Targretin (bexarotene)— CBC, SGOT, triglycerides, cholesterol, TSH (all but TSH every 2 weeks initially, then every month)
Electron beam—no laboratory monitoring

OFFICE VISITS

UVB and PUVA—monthly during induction phase (3 months), every 3 months during maintenance phase
Soriatane (acitretin)—every month initially (3 months), then every 3 months
Nitrogen mustard—every month initially (3 months), then every 3 months
Targretin (bexarotene)—every month initially (3 months), then every 2 months
Electron beam—weekly visits included for 10 weeks, then follow q 2 months (alternating with dermatologist) for year 1, q 3 months for year 2, then q 6 months for years 3-5
CPT codes: 99203 = $107, 99213 = $63, 11100 (punch biopsy) = $108, fundus photos = $76.

*PUVA phototherapy medication cost calculated based on 30 mg Oxsoralen Ultra dose.
†One course of electron beam therapy = $20,000 (including the professional fees and hospital charges).

ments as detailed in the guidelines below each table.

ANALYZING THE ANALYSES

Each of the previous analyses has inherent strengths and weaknesses. The type of data you wish extracted determines the type of analysis chosen.

Cost-minimization is used when clinicians wish to choose the least expensive alternative between two therapies deemed adequate or equal. It does not identify the most beneficial therapy, nor does it take into account patient preferences or adverse reactions.

Cost-benefit is used to compare the total costs of programs, interventions, or therapies with multiple outcomes. It can also be used to aid in determination of fund allocation.[11] The drawback to this analysis is that because the costs and benefits must both be expressed in the same terms, a monetary value must be attached to all possible outcomes. This raises an ethical dilemma, as the assignment of such values is subjective and affected by cultural bias.

Cost-effectiveness is the most commonly used analysis because of its objectivity.[12] It is used when the desired outcome has been identified and the most cost-efficient way to achieve that one outcome is sought. Its advantage over the cost-benefit analysis is that outcomes are expressed in natural units (lives saved, and so on), not monetary units. The drawback is that because the results must be measured on a common scale, it does not allow for comparisons between totally different areas of medicine with different outcomes, even if either outcome would be satisfactory.[13] Therapy can be specifically tailored to various patient populations based on the therapy's cost-effectiveness ratio in each cohort. Many data sources are available to assist in making these comparisons, notably the Regenstrief Medical Record System at Indiana University Medical Center, a large databank focusing primarily on outpatient care.[14] Many other databases are listed in the literature.[14-16]

Cost-utility analysis is the most ethical method to evaluate therapies because it seeks to balance patient preferences against the financial burdens of providing the care. However, the political climate within some institutions may create barriers to using this method. Many institutions review departmental budgets in a vacuum. This rewards minimizing the individual departments' drug expenditures and discourages use of costlier drug therapies that may actually reduce overall costs.[17]

All pharmacoeconomic analyses are based on assumptions and best guesses. To assess the extent to which the results depend on key assumptions, a sensitivity analysis should be performed. After identifying the key points in the therapy's decision tree, the assumptions are varied and the calculations repeated.[4] Factors, such as rate of side effects, variation in response to therapy, or fixed overhead expenses, may be varied. By determining the point at which the outcomes change, the degree of confidence one may have in the results is obtained.[4] The types of analysis are thoroughly addressed in the literature and may include one-way, multi-way, and threshold analysis.[18] Researchers use ranges of values for sensitivity analyses.[12] This approach gives a range of values over which the pharmacoeconomic analysis is valid. An analysis in which many values can be varied and still generate a similar conclusion is considered a "robust" study.[19]

Two of the controversies surrounding the field of pharmacoeconomics are the sources and accuracy of data. There is much variability in the quality of data available to use in the analyses. Inpatient data may be gleaned from discharge summaries, Current Procedural Terminology (CPT) and Diagnosis Related Group (DRG) records, and registration data. Care must be exercised in utilizing such databases because none of the inpatient data is easily interpreted and may reflect bias of the institution that provided it. Each source of data should be analyzed carefully and its limitations taken into account when constructing a model for analysis. These problems may include lack of accuracy in diagnosis, coding errors, or failure to completely list all the patients' comorbid conditions.[20] Before basing a far-reaching decision on data obtained from either a purchased or internally generated database, one must exercise due diligence in ascertaining that the data meet the requirements of the study and that the data are as reliable as possible.

HOW ARE PHARMACOECONOMIC ANALYSES USED?

Any group that has a formulary should review pharmacoeconomic data as part of the evaluation of a new agent for formulary addition. The group may use internal or published data for calculations. It should also analyze the circumstances under which the drug should be used to obtain maximum benefit. For example, a hospital may find that one dose a day of a more expensive medication such as levofloxacin (Levaquin) may be the most efficient method to treat community-acquired pneumonia, but another multiple drug regimen would be better to treat the pathogens in nursing home–acquired pneumonia. Formulary restrictions may be based on this type of analysis. For example, some insurance companies may deny payment for oral medications for onychomycosis, such as itraconazole (Sporanox) or terbinafine (Lamisil), unless the patient failed standard initial therapy and has pain from the condition. A more restrictive formulary may regard any antifungal therapy as not clinically indicated unless the patient has a systemic fungal infection.

Currently, prescribing is both an empiric process as well as a negotiation with the patient and insurers about their preference of regimens. As more analyses are published, physician groups will be able to assemble protocols to guide their therapies in accordance with pharmacoeconomic principles. Currently, many insurance companies developed clinical treatment pathways that they are happy to distribute to physicians caring for their customers. Because clinical pharmacists, who have reputations to protect, often develop these guidelines, physicians can place a fair amount of trust in them. However, the guidelines are obviously subject to the biases of the company that developed them.

When examining pharmaceutical company–sponsored trials, there is potential for bias in the design, analysis, and interpretation of the data. The raw data may be manipulated by analyzing clinically insignificant attributes of the drug that make it appear better than its competitors. Because manufacturers generally retain approval options over publication rights of sponsored research, studies that show unfavor-able results may never be submitted for publication. Friedberg and associates[21] found a statistically significant difference in the conclusions of published pharmacoeconomic studies when sponsored by pharmaceutical manufacturers versus nonprofit organizations. In fact, unfavorable conclusions were reached in 38% of trials sponsored by the nonprofit organizations compared with only 5% of those sponsored by manufacturers.[21] Pharmaceutical companies have limited resources and thus must use them to develop the most promising drugs. As pointed out by Gagnon,[22] negative economic findings may result in termination of a drug's development. In 1991, De Masi and co-workers[23] published data showing that the cost of development for every new medicine developed in 1987 was $230.8 million. The Boston Consulting Group found that by 1990 that figure had risen to $500 million.[24] Table 46-5 illustrates the rising costs of a representative sample of drugs over the past decade.

Not only are many of the prices of established drugs rising each year, but also new drug prices continue to increase. Table 46-6 illustrates a survey of the retail cost of several recently released drugs.

Drug prices have been rising by 12% per year since 1993,[25] reaching 17% by 1999.[26] This trend is likely to continue, especially with the advent of Wall Street becoming heavily involved with drugs earlier in their inception and development. In the past, pharmaceutical companies developed drugs with a goal in mind or took providential discoveries from pure science researchers and further developed them into usable products. Now, drug companies often buy technologies from universities then bring the drugs to market, thus bypassing several years of bench work for the company. Investment analysts and investment bankers alike keep a close eye on these developments, trying to predict which companies will have the next "billion dollar drug" such as Prozac (fluoxetine). With this indirect pressure on the pharmaceutical companies, there is a distinct possibility that drugs with borderline or negligible profitability, such as the so-called orphan drugs, will not be brought to market.

Physicians have a general ethical obligation to help control costs for patients. Over the next

■ Table 46-5   Cost Comparison of Commonly Used Systemic Drugs

Drug	Trade Name	Size	AWP 1990	AWP 1995	AWP 2000	Retail 2000*
Isotretinoin	Accutane	40 mg	$2.84	$4.45	$7.32	$7.94
Etretinate	Tegison	25 mg	$2.17	$3.08	N/A	N/A
Acitretin	Soriatane	25 mg	N/A	N/A	$8.99	$9.93
Methotrexate	Methotrexate	2.5 mg	$2.88	$3.81	$1.66	$1.98
Azathioprine	Imuran	50 mg	$.79	$1.18	$1.46	$1.50
Cyclosporine	Neoral	100 mg	$4.07†	$5.29†	$6.11	$6.29
Ciprofloxacin	Cipro	500 mg	$2.36	$3.13	$4.15	$4.40
Azithromycin	Zithromax	250 mg	$6.50 (1992)	$4.83	$5.40	$6.84
Acyclovir	Zovirax	200 mg	$.67	$1.11	$1.31	$1.45
Fluconazole	Diflucan	200 mg	$9.00	$9.00	$9.78	$12.31
Methoxsalen	Oxsoralen Ultra	10 mg	N/A	$4.22	$6.16	$6.25

*Average price per tablet/capsule for one hospital pharmacy and two retail pharmacies surveyed in the Indianapolis, Indiana area.
†These 1990 and 1995 prices represent the Sandimmune formulation of cyclosporine.

■ Table 46-6   Some Recently Released Medications Used in Dermatology and Rheumatology

Generic Name	Trade Name	Typical Dose	Cost 2000 AWP
Denileukin diftitox	Ontak	150 µg/ml (2-ml vial)	$992.50/vial
Etanercept	Enbrel	25-mg vial	$141.49/vial
Leflunomide	Arava	10 mg	$8.16
Leflunomide	Arava	20 mg	$8.16
Bexarotene	Targretin	75 mg	$10.25
Thalidomide	Thalomid	50 mg	$7.84

century, there will be a limited number of dollars available for health care. Physicians owe it to patients and society to define the best treatments that will minimize the morbidity to the patient while at the same time not wasting valuable economic resources.

PHARMACEUTICAL PRICING

There are three basic patterns of pricing strategy that drug companies use in setting retail prices for their products. These may be described as (1) linear, (2) parity (flat), and (3) logarithmic. *Linear* pricing occurs when a drug's price rises in a linear relationship to its dose. For example, the price of a 10-day supply of Drug A may be $4 at 250 mg qid, $8 at 500 mg qid, and $16 at 1000 mg qid. *Logarithmic* pricing occurs when the price per milligram of increasing doses changes, but not in a linear relationship to the dose. For example, the price of 4 mg of methylprednisolone (Medrol) is $0.83 and 16 mg is $1.81. *Parity* pricing occurs when the price of a drug is the same for all doses. For example, the price of Arava (leflunomide) is the same for the 10-mg and 20-mg doses. Figure 46-1 illustrates the dose-price relationships of these three pricing methods.

Each of these pricing strategies is chosen as a result of the drug company's market research and their goal in capturing a portion of the marketplace. The logarithmic method may simply represent savings generated by packaging larger

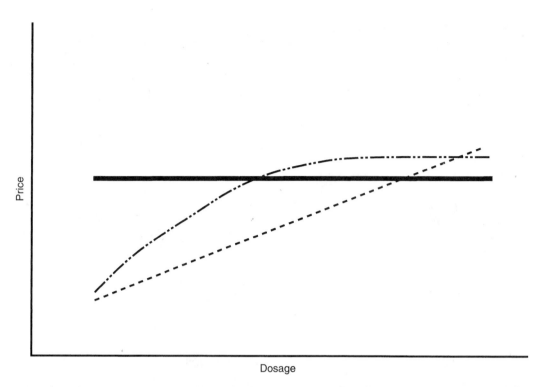

Figure 46-1   Three models of drug pricing. *Dotted line*, logarithmic; *dashed line*, parity; *solid line*, linear.

amounts of the drug because it costs the company basically the same amount to package each of the strengths. The only difference is the cost of the raw materials, which in the case of interferon may be quite high but for hydrocortisone may be quite low. The parity pricing method is effective if the company wishes to capture more market share based on price or to help retain customers who require higher doses of the medication. The linear pricing strategy may demonstrate that the raw product is quite expensive or that the company is in the market early and wishes to maximize their profits.

AVERAGE WHOLESALE PRICE

The traditional measurement of pharmaceutical pricing is the AWP. This price actually has no relation to the wholesale price paid by pharmacies. The AWP is a price set arbitrarily by the individual pharmaceutical companies,[27] much as the Manufacturer's Suggested Retail Price (MSRP) is set on an automobile. In light of this, one might ask if it is appropriate for the phar-

maceutical companies to insist on comparing drugs based on the AWP.

The pharmacist's acquisition price is a generally discounted price determined by volume contracting with drug companies or wholesalers. The typical retail markup on drugs in a recent survey prepared for the U.S. Congress demonstrates that for Long Island, New York residents, Medicare patients paid an average of 129% more than so-called preferred customers (large insurance companies who purchase huge volumes of pharmaceuticals). This high volume allows the insurers to dictate the amount pharmacies are reimbursed for items dispensed.[28] If the pharmacy declines, the insurer takes its business to a competing pharmacy. Carroll[29] found that for pharmacies to survive financially, they must be reimbursed a minimum of AWP minus 15% plus a $6.95 filling fee. However, most insurance companies reimburse pharmacies between 10% and 15% below AWP plus a filling fee (~$2.00). This comes out to less than Carroll's figure; thus pharmacies have to cost-shift to those patients who pay full retail price. The average pharmacy today breaks even or loses money on prescription drugs. They are forced to rely on sales of nutritional supplements, dry goods, liquor, and tobacco to make up for their losses on pharmaceutical sales to realize any profits. Unfortunately, even though physicians would undoubtedly prefer to use the most economically appropriate drugs for their patients, there is currently no comprehensive source of accurate drug prices.[30]

WHOLESALE ACQUISITION COST

Pharmaceutical manufacturers are required to sell their drugs at the same cost to all their retail pharmacy and wholesale customers. This is regulated by the Robinson-Patman Act, part of the Clayton Antitrust Act.[31] Recently, large mail-order pharmacy houses and pharmacy benefit management firms have become popular with insurers. Patients are required to mail in 60 to 90 day prescriptions of their chronic medications to these warehouses. Due to a loophole in the law, these firms are able to purchase pharmaceuticals at a deep discount. Because their acquisition cost is much lower than the retail pharmacies, they can charge the insurer less than the neighborhood pharmacy and still make a profit. This practice is currently the subject of nationwide litigation by retail pharmacists.[32]

PHARMACEUTICAL MANUFACTURER COSTS

The pharmaceutical industry is a research and development (R&D) industry. This industry traditionally contained two types of pharmaceutical companies—research-based and nonresearch-based. The traditional view of a pharmaceutical company is one that researches and develops a drug, then markets it commercially. Nonresearch-based companies may buy rights to market older drugs from the research companies or manufacture older drugs as generics. This distinction is blurring as research companies buy products from other companies. Generic manufacturers also perform limited research to prove their product is equivalent to the brand drug.

The pharmaceutical industry is expected to spend $24,031,700,000 on R&D in the year 2000. Overall, a pharmaceutical company plows 1 out of every 5 dollars back into R&D to develop new drugs,[33] of which only 3 out of 10 make enough money to pay for their own R&D costs.[34]

PHARMACEUTICAL PATIENT ASSISTANCE PROGRAMS

To their credit, most pharmaceutical companies recognize that many individuals are forced to choose between food, rent, or medicine and have instituted various patient assistance programs. These programs usually require the physician's office to assist the patient in applying for benefits. The paperwork varies from fairly simple to very complex. A classic example is the Roche Pharmaceuticals indigent patient program supplying isotretinoin without cost to selected indigent patients with severe acne vulgaris. Some companies mail the drugs to the physician's office for the patient to pick up, whereas others send them directly to the patient. Some programs have strict income limits that the patient must meet before consideration. A complete list of these programs may be downloaded from http://www.phrma.org/patients. The physician should seriously consider whether he or she wants to become involved in the process of patient assistance programs as they may take significant staff time for which there is no reimbursement.

GENERICS AND SUBSTITUTION

A number of well-known pharmaceuticals had their patents expired recently, allowing generic companies to seek Food and Drug Administration (FDA) approval for their production and marketing. The recent generic availability of cyclosporine, which was previously only marketed as Neoral, is an example relevant to dermatology. Until a few years ago, insurance companies and patients assumed the physician knew the best drug for the patient and paid for the brand-name product. As the price of pharmaceuticals rose, insurance companies, patients, and hospitals began looking at ways to minimize pharmacy costs. The market was ripe for competition, which came in the form of generic drugs. Formerly, physicians considered generics to contain impurities or be subject to manufacturing deficiencies or to be less efficacious. Over the past 20 years, both the public and physicians began to regard them as merely less expensive substitutes for the name-brand compounds.

WHY IS PHARMACOECONOMICS IMPORTANT TO CLINICIANS?

Pharmacoeconomics impacts physicians every day. Many ways are unseen such as decisions by pharmaceutical companies regarding the drugs to develop or discontinue. Others, such as formulary restrictions, are apparent daily.

In this chapter, an overview of the four most common forms of analysis and their strengths and limitations was given. The importance of including proper indirect costs has been stressed.

Several examples of pharmacoeconomics applications were described, as well as factors affecting the pricing of pharmaceuticals. Hopefully, this chapter stimulates the reader to do further reading in the area. More than that, it will hopefully prompt the reader to become involved in the drug evaluation process whenever possible such as serving on the pharmacy and therapeutics committee at local hospitals. At the very least, it should give a better foundation for evaluation of the information presented by the pharmaceutical company representatives who visit the office.

As long as physicians remain ignorant of what pharmacoeconomics is and what information it can and cannot provide, they are at the mercy of those who would present data and provide the conclusions they think should be drawn. Physicians owe it to themselves and their patients to learn more about this field so they may be better advocates for their patients' care.

Bibliography

Bootman JL, Townsend RJ, McGhan WF: Introduction to pharmacoeconomics. In Bootman JL, Townsende RJ, McGhan WF, editors: *Principles of pharmacoeconomics*, ed 2, Cincinnati, 1996, Harvey Whitney, pp 5-18.

Gagnon, JP: A primer on pharmacoeconomics. *Manag Care Med* 37:11-18, 1995.

Gibson G: Understanding and implementing the economics of pharmacoeconomics. *Manag Care Med* 37:9-24, 1995.

Luks-Golger D, Caspi A: The ABC's of pharmacoeconomic research. *Pharm Ther* 25:88-90, 2000.

Reeder CE: Overview of pharmacoeconomics and pharmaceutical outcomes evaluations. *Am J Health Syst Pharm* 52(19 Suppl 4):S5-8, 1995.

Walley T, Haycox A: Pharmacoeconomics: basic concepts and terminology. *Br J Clin Pharmacol* 43:343-348, 1997.

References

1. Gibson G: Understanding and implementing the economics of pharmacoeconomics. *Manag Care Med* 37:9-24, 1995.
2. Luks-Golger D, Caspi A: The ABC's of pharmacoeconomic research. *Pharm Ther* 25:88-90, 2000.
3. Reeder CE: Overview of pharmacoeconomics and pharmaceutical outcomes evaluations. *Am J Health Syst Pharm* 52(19 suppl 4):S5-8, 1995.
4. Jolicoeur LM, Jones-Grizzle AJ, Boyer JG: Guidelines for performing a pharmacoeconomic analysis. *Am J Hosp Pharm* 49:1741-1747, 1992.
5. Gill TM, Feinstein AR: Critical appraisal of the quality of life measurements. *JAMA* 262:619-626, 1989.
6. EuroQol Group: EuroQol—a new facility for the measurement of health related quality of life. *Health Pol* 16:199-208, 1990.

7. Kaplan RM, Bush JW, Bern CC: Health status: types of validity and the index of well-being. *Health Serv Res* 11:478-527, 1976.

8. Feeny DH, Furlong W, Barr RD, et al: A comprehensive multiattribute system for classifying the health status of survivors of childhood cancer. *J Clin Oncol* 10:923-928, 1992.

9. Feeny DH, Leiper A, Barr RD, et al: The comprehensive assessment of health status in survivors of childhood cancer: application to high-risk acute lymphoblastic leukemia. *Br J Cancer* 67:1047-1052, 1993.

10. Larson LN: Cost determination and analysis. In Bootman JL, Townsend RJ, McGhan WF, editors: *Principles of pharmacoeconomics,* ed 2, Cincinnati, 1996, Harvey Whitney, pp 45-59.

11. Bootman JL, Townsend RJ, McGhan WF: Introduction to pharmacoeconomics. In Bootman JL, Townsend RJ, McGhan WF, editors: *Principles of pharmacoeconomics,* ed 2, Cincinnati, 1996, Harvey Whitney, pp 5-18.

12. Gagnon JP: A primer on pharmacoeconomics. *Manag Care Med* 37:11-18, 1995.

13. Walley T, Haycox A: Pharmacoeconomics: basic concepts and terminology. *Br J Clin Pharmacol* 43:343-348, 1997.

14. Else BA, Armstrong EP, Cox ER: Data sources for pharmacoeconomic and health services research. *Am J Health-Syst Pharm* 54:2601-2608, 1997.

15. Paul JE, Tilson HH: Use and opportunities for administrative data bases in pharmacoeconomic research. In Spilker B: *Quality of life and pharmacoeconomics in clinical trials,* ed. 2, Philadelphia, 1996, Spilker, pp 1165-1172.

16. Edinberg S, McCormick KA: Databases— their use in developing clinical guidelines and estimating the cost impact of guideline implementation. *JAHIMA* 67:24-30, 1996.

17. Brixner DI: Outcomes research, pharmacoeconomics and the pharmaceutical industry. *J Man Care Pharm* 2:48-52, 1996.

18. Sanchez L: Applied pharmacoeconomics: evaluation and use of pharmacoeconomic data from the literature. *Am J Health-Syst Pharm* 56:1630-1637, 1999.

19. Mosdell KW: Primary literature documents. In Mosdell KW, Kier KL, Stanovich FE, editors: *Drug information: a guide for pharmacists,* Stamford, 1996, Appleton & Lange, pp 67-88.

20. Gandhi SJ, Salmon JW, Kong SX, et al: Administrative databases and outcomes assessment: an overview of issues and potential utility. *J Man Care Pharm* 5:215-222, 1999.

21. Friedberg M, Saffran B, Stinson TJ, et al: Evaluations of conflict of interest in economic analyses of new drugs used in oncology. *JAMA* 282:1453-1457, 1999.

22. Gagnon JP: Sources of bias in economic analysis of new drugs (comment, letter). JAMA 283:1423, 2000.

23. DiMasi JA, Hansen RW, Grabowski HG, et al: Cost of innovation in the pharmaceutical industry. *J Health Econ* 10:107-142, 1991.

24. PhRMA Facts, http://www.phrma.org/facts/phfacts/12_99a.html, December 1999.

25. Cauchon D: High prices force tough decisions. *USA Today* Nov 10, 1999, pp 10A.

26. Zimmerman R: Drug Spending Soared 17.4% During 1999, pp A3 and A6. *Wall Street Journal,* June 27, 2000.

27. Prepared by the staff of the Health and Human Services Department for the President of the United States. Report to the President: Prescription drug coverage, spending, utilization and prices. http://aspe.hhs.gov/health/reports/drugstudy/index.htm. April 2000.

28. Anonymous: Prescription drug pricing on Long Island: Companies profit at the expense of older Americans. July 26, 1999. Their phone number is 202-225-5051. http://www.house.gov/carolynmccarthy/

29. Carroll NV: Estimating a reasonable reimbursement from community pharmacies in third-party programs. *Manag Care Interface* 12:73-76, 79-80, 1999.

30. Kolassa M: Guidance for clinicians in discerning and comparing the price of pharmaceutical agents. *J Pain Sympt Man* 9:235-243, 1994.

31. The relevant provisions are set forth in sections 2(a)-(f) of the Clayton Act, 15 U.S.C. 13(a)-(f); references to the Robinson-Patman Act in the text therefore are intended to be to section 2 of the Clayton Act, as amended by the Robinson-Patman Act.

32. McMains MB: Personal correspondence. July 2000 (Professor of Food and Drug Law, Indiana University School of Law at Indianapolis).

33. PhRMA Annual Survey and Standard and Poor's Compustat, McGraw-Hill, 1999, Philadelphia.

34. Grabowski H, Vernon J: Returns to R&D on new drug introduction in the 1980s. *J Health Econ* 13(4):383-406, 1994.

CHAPTER 47

Stephen E. Wolverton
Marshall Kapp

Informed Consent and Risk Management

Any chapter on the subject of informed consent addresses a panoply of complex historical, ethical, and medicolegal principles. The actual risk of incurring legal liability from failure to inform a patient about the risks of a given procedure or medication is relatively small but important. In addition to legal considerations, this chapter emphasizes the ethical and medical principles from which informed consent derives its meaning. The communication process that constitutes informed consent is discussed. It is important to realize from the outset that physician-patient communication, and not merely a signature on a form, is the basis of informed consent. In reality, most informed consent in medical practices occurs in the absence of any patient signature on a consent form.

This chapter covers the historical evolution of informed consent in the United States, underlying ethical perspectives, and resulting basic legal principles. In addition, the formal components of informed consent are addressed, and a brief overview of medicolegal risk management in dermatology is presented.

HISTORICAL PERSPECTIVE

Informed consent as it is known today was first initiated in 1767 in English Common Law, which addressed the right to give or withhold permission for medical care.[1] In 1914, Judge Cardozo addressed informed consent in a case of alleged assault and battery by a physician against a patient. He recorded that "every human being of adult years and of sound mind has the right to determine what shall be done with his body."[2] The Nuremberg Code, which followed the War Crimes Trials in 1947, was the first major document to spell out and refer to informed consent as a dictum of medical care.[3] The actual term *informed consent* was first used by the courts in 1957 (Box 47-1).[4]

The "professional standard" ("reasonable physician" standard) for informing patients was first described in 1960 in a landmark malpractice case in Kansas.[5] In 1962, the U.S. Food and Drug Administration (FDA) was authorized to establish and enforce standards to be used by drug investigators. Informed consent was determined to be a central requirement for these studies. The "material risk standard" ("reasonable patient" standard) was first enunciated in 1972 in the *Canterbury v. Spence* case.[6] The professional standard and the material risk standard are explained in detail later.

The medicolegal concept of informed consent continues to evolve today. The practitioner is advised to become familiar with the statutes

Box 47-1

Time Line for Important Laws and Decisions Regarding Informed Consent

1767   English Common Law addressed right to give or withhold permission for medical care.

1914   Judge Cardozo ruling regarding "battery" in *Schloendorff v. Society of New York Hospitals.*

1947   Nuremberg Code lays foundation for current basis of informed consent for medical care and research.

1957   First use of the phrase "informed consent" by courts in *Salgo v. Leland Stanford Board of Trustees* ruling.

1960   "Professional standard" established for information provided to patients in *Natanson v. Kline.*

1962   FDA authorized to establish and enforce standards for drug investigation—informed consent established a central requirement.

1972   "Material-risk standard" established for information provided to patients in *Canterbury v. Spence.*

and judicial decisions pertaining to informed consent in the state where he or she practices. In addition, practice standards that are developed by various specialties will increasingly affect informed consent in the future.

ETHICAL PERSPECTIVE

The principle of informed consent reflects the basic ethical responsibility to respect the personal autonomy of the patient. The goal is to have the decision to use a given medication or to undergo a surgical procedure made by the person most directly affected by the consequences of that decision, namely the patient.[7] Ideally, this allows more intelligent and rational decision making.

Several important potential medical benefits may be achieved through truly informed consent. A greater sense of partnership and active mutual participation within the patient-physician relationship may be achieved. Over-

all, there should be more openness and less authoritarianism in this relationship. Increased compliance and greater assistance from the patient in ongoing surveillance may be achieved. In addition, professional self-scrutiny with respect to medical decisions is encouraged.

In most cases, thorough provision of information to a patient for a medical decision is good medical practice, is sound legally, and is sound ethically.[8] Ethically, the concept of autonomy embraces the right to receive information and act on it, giving or withholding consent.

BASIC LEGAL PRINCIPLES

Several important general legal principles need to be understood before the specific components of informed consent are addressed. As stated before, the physician should become familiar with the statutes and judicial precedent directly dealing with informed consent in his or her own jurisdiction.

The physician ultimately has legal responsibility for both the process and the outcome of medical therapy, even though many associated medical personnel may be involved with this therapy. With this principle in mind, ensuring the adequacy of informed consent can never be delegated to medical students or to nurses. In addition, one cannot relegate the informed consent dialogue to a pamphlet or to another source of information. The aforementioned personnel and information sources can, however, serve important complementary and reinforcement roles in the communication process.

"Express consent" is the explicit communication of consent by words or writing.[7] The greater the risk of the medical intervention, the more advisable it is to obtain express consent. "Implied consent" is more commonly operant in medical interventions. In many situations involving little risk or intrusiveness, the patient's actions may imply concurrence or consent. "Implied consent" is not an exception to the informed consent doctrine but rather is one form of indicating consent.

Litigation based on total lack of consent—namely, unauthorized touching of the patient ("battery")—is distinctly uncommon today. Inadequate explanation of a procedure or of medication risks may constitute negligence. Liability may be incurred for inadequate communication, even in instances when the quality of care and the outcome are otherwise fine.

It is important to address the setting in which informed consent occurs to properly delineate the extent of communication and documentation that is necessary. Investigative drug research has rigid guidelines mandated by federal regulations.[9] Detailed consent forms are central to investigative work in the pharmaceutical industry.

The legal rules for prescribing FDA-approved medications with significant adverse effects are less clear-cut. As a general principle, the use of an approved drug for an off-label ("unapproved") indication requires more detailed information in the informed consent process than when the same drug is prescribed for FDA-approved indications. (See Components of Informed Consent section for further discussion on the adequacy of information presented.)

A majority of prescriptions for systemic drugs used in dermatology are actually for unapproved (off-label) indications. The approval by the FDA actually constitutes approval for *labeling* by the manufacturer, which thus limits the types of claims that the manufacturer can make in advertising and in package inserts regarding the drug.[10] An FDA-approved indication documents that there is sufficient information presented to the FDA by the pharmaceutical firm to establish efficacy and safety for the particular indication. If the drug is too risky overall, it is taken off the market. There are many rare diseases for which it is unrealistic to attempt to gather adequate information to obtain a specific FDA indication. It is not economically sound for older, off-patent drugs to receive the investigational scrutiny necessary to get FDA approval for a different indication. It is both medically acceptable and legal to use approved drugs for unapproved indications when there are clinical data to support this use. The Federal Food, Drug and Cosmetics Act clearly states that the FDA has authority to regulate only drugs and not physicians.

In medical and legal terms, the risks of therapy should be proportional to the risks of the disease being treated. Dermatologic conditions, such as toxic epidermal necrolysis and pemphi-gus vulgaris, are examples of serious diseases that can for selected patients justify potentially risky treatments, in contrast with many other less serious conditions treated by dermatologists. Good medicine sometimes requires the taking of calculated risks, with the consent of the patient, to achieve important medical results.[11] The location of one's practice, whether in an academic setting or in private practice, may dictate the level of risk from systemic drug therapy that is justifiable. Medications with a very high degree of risk are used more commonly in the academic setting.

Signed informed consent forms usually are legally required only in research protocols.[12] For clinical practice, the Joint Commission on Accreditation of Healthcare Organizations (JCAHO) requires consent forms primarily for surgical procedures.[13] JCAHO accreditation is a means of qualifying for reimbursement from third-party payers for medical services.

The consent form, even if not legally required, documents that at least some communication took place. Aside from the aforementioned surgical settings, the means of documenting that informed consent occurred is secondary in importance to the communication process. The documentation for most systemic drugs used in dermatology requires only chart notations that discussion about medication risks, benefits, limitations, and alternatives occurred. An important exception is the use of isotretinoin by women of childbearing potential, for which pharmaceutical company–provided information packets and informed consent forms remain the standard of practice.

COMPONENTS OF INFORMED CONSENT

There are three important components of informed consent.[14] First, the consent must be "voluntary"; patients should be able to exercise their free power of choice without the intervention of any element of force, fraud, deceit, duress, or other ulterior forms of constraint or coercion. Second, the patient's agreement should be truly informed. Third, the capacity or "competence" of the patient who agrees to a procedure or a medication is essential. It is important

Box 47-2

General Components of an Adequate Informed Consent Discussion

1. The diagnosis or diagnostic possibilities
2. The nature and purpose of the proposed intervention (surgical or medical)
   a. Reasonably foreseeable risks that may occur
   b. Potential benefits of the therapy and the likelihood that these benefits will occur
   c. Limitations of the proposed intervention
3. Alternatives to the proposed intervention, including the alternative of no therapy[16]
4. The physician's advice regarding the therapeutic options
5. Time for questions and clarification

to know whether the patient is mentally able to think rationally about personal medical care.

There exists a split in the law concerning how much information the physician must communicate to the patient.[7] The professional standard ("reasonable physician" standard, "community" standard, majority rule) is the standard of communication in most jurisdictions. Under this standard, the information that must be presented is what a reasonable, prudent physician would disclose under similar circumstances. In a minority of jurisdictions, the material risk standard ("reasonable patient" standard, minority rule, "prudent person" standard) is used to determine the amount of information presented. In this case, the amount of information that a reasonable patient in the same situation would want and need to know to make a knowledgeable decision is the basis of risk disclosure. Potential advantages of the material risk standard include enhanced communication, better consumer awareness of health issues, potentially less litigation, and improved quality of medical care.[7] In perhaps one or two states, a "subjective" or "individual patient" standard may still be used. Under that standard, instead of an average or a reasonable patient's information needs used as the basis of disclosure, the information provided should be what that particular patient would need to know in that particular set of circumstances.

Short of full disclosure of every known or foreseeable risk, the standards just discussed still rely on an individual physician's determination for disclosure of risk according to the severity or frequency of a given risk. The greater the frequency of the risk materializing and, in particular, the greater the severity of the risk, the more important the disclosure of this risk before the medical intervention takes place.

Box 47-2 lists general components that must be included in the informed consent discussion.[15]

SYSTEMIC DRUGS AND INFORMED CONSENT

Adequate discussion before prescribing systemic drugs with a significant potential risk for adverse effects can be divided into discussions of the risks of the drug and of the patient's role in surveillance necessary to detect these adverse effects. It is important to educate the patient about the common and serious adverse effects that may occur with the medication. This discussion should include means of detecting the adverse effects, as well as appropriate intervention should any of these adverse effects occur. In addition, the necessity of surveillance measures, including laboratory tests, special examinations, and other tests to monitor the therapy, is important to communicate to the patient. This previous list of items that are needed for informed consent can form the basis for this discussion.

Documentation of physician-patient communication is essential. There is a hierarchy of documentation options that are appropriate for different clinical situations. A patient-signed consent form with a witness's signature is necessary both in investigative drug research and for unusually risky medications. This form should be specific to the drug being studied or prescribed. An alternative to the consent form would be a progress note documenting the informed consent discussion, with a patient's signature under this note. With most systemic drugs used in dermatology, the physician should document that a discussion on risks, benefits, limitations, and alternatives took place. In addition, the notation may include the proposed surveillance for adverse effects. In this scenario, only a physician's signature is necessary on the note in the medical record. With drugs that present minimal risk of adverse effects, extensive chart documentation is generally not essential, although some written notation is advisable.

The witness's signature merely documents that it appears to the witness that the consent is voluntary and the patient is competent. To sign, it may not be necessary for the witness to observe the full information presentation. The witness should not be a physician associated with the physician prescribing the medication.

OPTIMIZING PATIENT UNDERSTANDING

Important issues regarding a patient's assimilation of the information provided about risks of a specific systemic drug include an understanding of this discussion at the time it takes place, as well as long-term memory effects. Various measures can be used to improve the patient's understanding and long-term retention of information.[17,18] These measures include providing written materials, asking the patient to restate in his or her own words the information just presented, and using multiple channels of communication (verbal and visual). Repetition of key points is also helpful. Material that is organized into categories is more likely to be retained as well.

Information should be provided in as nonpressured and empathetic a way as possible.[7] Discussion should take place in clear, nontechnical, and understandable language. The clinician should consider the values and the sociologic characteristics of a particular patient. The discussion should allow time for questions in an open fashion. Having family members present may aid in the communication process and in long-term retention of information.[19]

CIRCUMSTANCES NOT REQUIRING INFORMED CONSENT[20]

An important exception to the principle of informed consent is any condition that requires emergency treatment, such that the condition presents the risk of death or serious disability if the treatment is not given immediately. The principle of "therapeutic privilege" is applicable in these few cases when, in the physician's opinion, withholding information is in the best interest of a particular patient because disclosure of information would be very likely to result in imminent and serious harm to the patient. In addition, risks that are commonly known by the public need not be disclosed. Finally, the "defense of waiver" occurs when the patient voluntarily and knowingly relinquishes the right to informed consent. These circumstances are not commonly applicable to the use of systemic drugs in dermatology.

A more complicated but relevant area is the process of informed consent for minors.[21] The most prudent principle is to include parents in decisions involving minors regarding any therapy that has a significant potential risk. However, some exceptions exist. An "emancipated minor" is defined as a fully self-supporting person living on his or her own. A "mature minor" is defined as a person, usually 15 to 17 years of age, with a degree of maturity that renders him or her capable of understanding information and rationally giving consent to nonrisky therapy. In both of these exceptions, minor therapeutic decisions may be made by the physician and the patient in the absence of parental consent. Otherwise, parental participation in therapeutic decisions for which there are significant risks is generally the most conservative, safest approach to take.

MEDICOLEGAL RISK MANAGEMENT

Successful negligence lawsuits predicated *solely* on the *failure* of the physician *to obtain informed consent* are quite uncommon. To succeed, a plaintiff would need to establish the elements listed in Box 47-3.

Most successful malpractice claims involve proof of *substandard performance in patient care* rather than or in addition to proof of lack of informed consent. Nevertheless, reasons beyond legal theory alone dictate the need for informed consent.

Several general provider behaviors and patient characteristics increase the risk of mal-

Box 47-3

Elements of a Successful Malpractice Lawsuit Regarding Failure of Informed Consent

1. A reasonably foreseeable risk was not disclosed by the physician, and the adverse outcome actually occurred.
2. This "materialized risk" resulted in injury to the patient.
3. The therapy would not have been accepted by the patient if he or she had been adequately informed of the risk.

practice suits. Physicians' behaviors such as poor communication, impersonal care, lack of empathetic listening to patients' complaints and concerns, and personality conflicts have all been deemed as important factors contributing to patient dissatisfaction.[22,23] At the same time the physician should be careful in dealing with patients who have unrealistic expectations or who have a psychologic disturbance.

DERMATOLOGIC MALPRACTICE STUDIES

There is only one study for which the data (at least through the 1980s) address successful malpractice litigation involving dermatologists. In this study, Hollabaugh and colleagues[24] surveyed academic dermatologic programs in the United States, evaluating malpractice litigation from the 1960s through the 1980s. Of 58 lawsuits reported, 10 involved systemic drugs in dermatologic settings. Adverse effects from glucocorticosteroids, methotrexate, dapsone, and antibiotics (trimethoprim-sulfamethoxazole and tetracycline) were involved.

Other important reasons for malpractice litigation in this study included surgical complications.[25] It is generally agreed that the increasing participation of dermatologists in cosmetic and complicated surgical procedures will increase the risk of malpractice litigation. One can predict that the increasing use of systemic therapy with significant risk of adverse effects may also increase the physician's potential liability.

There is significant information regarding the primary reasons for malpractice litigation that can be obtained directly from medical malpractice insurers.

SUMMARY

Few medical interventions are totally devoid of potential adverse effects and resultant potential for medicolegal liability. There are numerous important clinical indications for systemic drugs used in dermatology from which patients may benefit, albeit with varying degrees of risk. Two important areas of malpractice defense include development of a good physician-patient relationship and familiarity with typical malpractice problems encountered by physicians. Compassionate, open, and empathetic interchange with the patients, although not foolproof, is a critical element of medicolegal risk management. Careful assessment of areas with high medicolegal risks, measures undertaken to minimize these risks, and surveillance by patient and physician for early detection of important adverse effects are all critical to optimal use of systemic drugs in dermatology. Thorough understanding and use of the principles of informed consent are essential to optimizing the risk-benefit ratio for these drugs.

Bibliography

Gittler GJ, Goldstein EJC: The elements of medical malpractice: an overview. *Clin Infect Dis* 23:1152-1155, 1996.

Kapp MB: *Geriatrics and the law,* ed 3, New York, 1999, Springer, pp 13-40.

Liang BA: *Health law and policy: a survival guide to medicolegal issues for practitioners,* Boston, 2000, Butterworth Heinemann, pp 29-44.

Wagner RF Jr, Torres A, Proper S: Informed consent and informed refusal. *Dermatol Surg* 21:551-559, 1995.

References

1. Faden RR, Beauchamp T: *A history and theory of informed consent,* New York, 1986, Oxford University Press.
2. *Schloendorff v. Society of New York Hospitals,* 211 N.Y. 125, 105 N.E. 2d 92 (1914).
3. Nuremberg Code. Reprinted in Brody BA: *The ethics of biomedical research: an international perspective,* New York, 1998, Oxford University Press, p 213.
4. *Salgo v. Leland Stanford Board of Trustees,* 154 Cal. App.2d 560, 578, 317 P.2d 170 (1957).
5. *Natanson v. Kline,* 186 Kan. 393, 350 P.2d 1093 (1960).
6. *Canterbury v. Spence,* 464 F.2d 772 (D.C. Cir. 1972).
7. Kapp MB: *Geriatrics and the law,* ed 3, New York, 1999, Springer, pp 13-40.
8. American Medical Association, Council on Ethical and Judicial Affairs: Code of Medical Ethics: Current Opinions with Annotations. Chicago: Author, 1998-1999 ed, pp 134-135.
9. 45 Code of Federal Regulations Part 46.
10. Curran WJ, Hall MA, Bobinski MA, Orentlicher D: *Health care law and ethics,* ed 5, New York, 1998, Aspen Law & Business, p 962.
11. Weisbard AJ: Defensive law: a new perspective on informed consent. *Arch Intern Med* 146:860-861, 1986.
12. 45 Code of Federal Regulations Part 46.117.
13. Joint Commission on Accreditation of Healthcare Organizations: comprehensive Accreditation Manual for Hospitals. Chicago, Author, 1999.
14. Rozovsky FA: *Consent to treatment: a practical guide,* ed 2, Gaithersburg, MD, 1997, Aspen Publishers.
15. Appelbaum PS, Lidz CS, Meisel A: *Informed consent: legal theory and clinical practice,* New York, 1987, Oxford University Press.
16. Shriner DL, Wagner RF, Weedn VW, et al: Informed consent and risk management in dermatology: to what extent do dermatologists disclose alternative and treatment options to their patients? *J Contemp Health Law Policy* 8:137-162, 1992.
17. Barry MJ, Fowler FJ Jr, Mulley AG Jr, et al: Patient reactions to a program designed to facilitate patient participation in treatment decisions for benign prostatic hyperplasia. *Med Care* 33:771-782, 1995.
18. Krynski MD, Tymchuk AJ, Ouslander JG: How informed can consent be? New light on comprehension among elderly people making decisions about enteral tube feeding. *Gerontologist* 34:36-43, 1994.
19. Pratt CC, Jones L, Shin H, Walker AJ: Decision making among single older women and their caregiving daughters. *Gerontologist* 29:792-797, 1989.
20. Furrow BR, Greaney TL, Johnson SH, et al: *Health law,* St. Paul, MN, 1995, West Publishing Company, pp 281-284.
21. Holder AR: Minors' rights to consent to medical care. *JAMA* 257:3400-3402, 1987.
22. Levinson W: Physician-patient communication: a key to malpractice prevention. *JAMA* 272:1619-1620, 1994.
23. Levinson W, Roter DL, Mullooly JP, et al: Physician-patient communication: the relationship with malpractice claims among primary care physicians and surgeons. *JAMA* 277:553-559, 1997.
24. Hollabaugh ES, Wagner RF, Weedn VW, et al: Patient personal injury litigation against dermatology residency programs in the United States, 1964-1988: implications for future risk-management programs in dermatology and dermatologic surgery. *Arch Dermatol* 126:619-622, 1990.

CHAPTER 48

William H. Eaglstein

FDA Drug Approval Process

The United States Food and Drug Administration (FDA) is the federal agency charged with regulating all of our foods, drugs, medical devices, biologics, and cosmetics. Although the lay public assumes that physicians know a great deal about the FDA, physicians receive little education about the FDA in medical school, residency, or postgraduate training. This lack of education may be in part because many FDA issues deal largely with legal or social policy. However, science and medical research information is fundamental to carrying out the FDA missions, and the agency's policies have a tremendous impact on public health and on the practice of medicine, since the FDA regulatory jurisdiction is estimated to encompass an enormous 25 cents of every dollar Americans spend.

The FDA is part of the Department of Health and Human Services, which is in the executive branch of the federal government. Thus the FDA commissioner is appointed by the president, with the advice and consent of the Congress. Until the recent imposition of "user fees," the FDA budget for the drug approval process was almost totally derived from Congress, which also has oversight responsibility for the FDA. This year the FDA estimates it will spend $156 million on new drug evaluation, with more than 1200 people involved throughout the agency. This total more than triples the $47 million spent in 1992 before the user fees were instituted. Overall, the fiscal year 1998 FDA budget was $1,076.8 million (including $151.7 million in prescription drug user fees) with 9144 employees. Clearly, the budget is too small with too few employees to actively make decisions affecting 25% of the gross national product, with the system depending a great deal on voluntary self-regulation.

This chapter focuses primarily on the approval process for prescription drugs, although much of the information is also applicable to biologics and devices. The FDA role in regulating foods, over-the-counter (OTC) medicines, and cosmetics is discussed only briefly.

THE FEDERAL FOOD, DRUG, AND COSMETIC ACT OF 1938

The first federal law governing food, drugs, and cosmetics was enacted in 1938 (Table 48-1). Considerable credit for the passage of the Federal Food, Drug, and Cosmetic Act of 1938 is given to the author Sinclair Lewis, whose books describing conditions in the meat packing industry led to public outrage and the eventual congressional action. Physicians, however, were also active in promoting and creating federal standards. Before the 1938 act, there were no federal standards regarding drug safety or efficacy. This was the era of "snake oil" and elixirs. However, the original act only required that drugs be proved safe. It was assumed that doctors and patients would work out which drugs were effective and that market forces would as-

■ **Table 48-1** Timeline for Major Pharmaceutical Legislation in the United States

Year	Legislation Regulating Pharmaceutical Industry
1938	Food, Drug, and Cosmetic Act
1962	Kefauver-Harris Drug Amendments
1983	Orphan Drug Act
1984	Drug Price Competition and Patent Term Restoration Act
1992	Prescription Drug User Fee Act
1997	Food and Drug Modernization Act (FADMA)

■ **Table 48-2** FDA-Approval Process

Development Activities	Years (Average)
Laboratory and animal studies	6.5*
File IND with FDA	
Clinical studies (phases)	
I Pharmacologic profile	1.5
II Safety and limited efficacy	2
III Extensive trials	3.5
File NDA with FDA	
FDA review and approval	1.5
	TOTAL: 15 years

IND, Investigative new drug; *NDA,* new drug application.
*Patent usually issued relatively early in this time period.

sure the success of only efficacious drugs. The current high cost of drug development has led some to call for a reversion to this standard by approving all safe drugs and allowing clinical experience and market forces to pick out those indications for which the drugs are truly effective.

Although thalidomide was never approved by the FDA and was never sold in the United States, the birth defects caused by the drug alarmed the American population so much that Congress passed a comprehensive FDA reform bill. In 1962, the Kefauver-Harris Drug Amendment added the requirement that drugs also be proved effective before they could be marketed. Since then, all potential drugs must be proved both safe and effective before approval for marketing (premarket approval).

To satisfy these requirements, sponsors (usually pharmaceutical companies) test drugs by a variety of methods that include bioassays, animal models, and finally human trials (Table 48-2). The process is costly (from $200 million to $500 million) and takes about 15 years (which is double the time needed in 1964). The wide range in development costs reflects not only the variations inherent in the type of drug and the sponsor's efficiency, but also the variety of accounting methodologies. For example, the cost of "losers" (drugs that fail at some point in the development process) are typically added to the costs of developing the "winners." Other factors

accounting for the wide range of development costs include whether the cited cost is in pre-tax or after-tax dollars and whether there is inclusion of lost interest income on the dollars invested in the development process.

PHASE I TO PHASE IV TESTING

For every 5000 pharmaceutical compounds evaluated or screened, five reach the stage of clinical trials and only about one of these five actually reach the market after FDA approval. Of those compounds reaching clinical trials, 70% pass Phase I, 33% pass Phase II, 27% pass Phase III, and 20% (1 in 5) receive an approved new drug application (NDA). The sponsors conduct and pay for those studies needed to prove safety and efficacy. The FDA evaluates and judges the testing results but rarely does drug testing. However, the FDA is involved in the sponsor's test plans, especially in allowing human testing. Since potential new drugs have not been proved safe and effective, they may not be given as therapy. The sponsor may give the investigational drug to patients for evaluation (testing) only after submitting an investigative new drug (IND) exemption.

FDA guidelines for human testing divide the premarket testing process into three phases. In Phase I, patients or healthy volunteers receive the drug to study its safety along with metabolic and pharmacologic profiles. Usually, Phase I testing involves 20 to 80 subjects, and the safety testing is general, as well as specific, depending on the toxicities detected in animal studies. Phase I will give enough pharmacokinetic and pharmacologic information to allow the design of controlled clinical studies used in Phase II.

In Phase II studies, the drug is tested for safety and efficacy in limited numbers, usually several hundred patients. Often, dose-ranging studies are conducted as part of Phase II. Phase III studies involve larger numbers of patients, usually several hundred to several thousand, most often in randomized-controlled trials (RCT), to evaluate efficacy and safety in a larger, well-controlled setting. Phase III will also provide sufficient data to allow development of a benefit-to-risk relationship and development of a label. The FDA considers any written, printed, or graphic material that is affixed to or appears on a drug or its package to be a "label." Labeling is required on all drugs while in interstate commerce or held for sale after shipment or delivery in interstate commerce. Each word of a drug's label has been scrutinized and often negotiated by both the FDA and the sponsor. The Physicians' Desk Reference is largely a collection of drug labels. Use of a drug for a condition, or in a manner not described on the label, gives rise to the phrase, "off-label use."

For totally new drugs, or new molecular entities (NMEs), efficacy and safety must be demonstrated in at least two RCTs. In RCTs, patients receive either the drug being tested (the "active" drug) or the control drug (frequently a placebo). Usually RCTs are double-blinded, which means that neither the patients nor the investigators know which agent, active or control, a given patient is receiving. All human (and animal) testing is approved by institutional review boards (IRBs) at each investigative site.

At the end of Phase III testing, a new drug has usually been received by 1000 to 3000 patients. Given these numbers, it is not surprising that adverse effects are often not discovered until a drug has been on the market for several years. Overall, 51% of approved drugs have serious adverse effects not detected before FDA approval. It is interesting to note that some other countries (unlike the United States) have the postmarketing safety monitoring done by a separate organization from the organization that gives initial approval to a drug. For example, in the United Kingdom, drug approval and safety monitoring processes are entirely separate. The safety monitoring unit may order changes in product labeling or the outright withdrawal of a marketed drug. France has a well-developed network of regional pharmacovigilance centers, a national database for practitioners, and a drug safety journal.

Occasionally, the FDA approves a drug but requires additional studies or reporting. These studies are referred to as postmarket, or Phase IV, studies. When a drug appears to offer significant advantage over current therapy for serious or life-threatening disease, it may be given accelerated development and review status. Accelerated review may reduce the review time to as little as 6 months before final drug approval.

NEW DRUG APPLICATION

Ordinarily, after completing Phase III testing, the sponsor submits all results as part of the request for premarket approval. The average NDA contains about 100,000 pages of information. In the future, the FDA plans to receive this information electronically. Evaluating the large volume of data, including animal, toxicologic, and human testing information, does not usually begin until a completed application is submitted. By this time, large sums of money and a great deal of effort have been put into the process by the sponsor. By the 1980s, the average time needed for the FDA to evaluate a submission had become 29 months. The Prescription Drug User Fee Act of 1992 was passed to address this problem. By requiring sponsors to pay the FDA a fee ("users fee") to have their mandated studies evaluated, this law designated money with which the FDA hired 600 new staff, mostly aimed at drug review, and reduced the time required for evaluation of NDAs to between 12 and 18 months. The Prescription Drug User Fee Act was renewed in 1997 for a second 5 years.

FDA ADVISORY PANELS

After reaching decisions on a drug's safety, efficacy, and the "benefit-to-risk ratio," the FDA often asks for advice from its standing, or ad hoc, advisory panels, which are composed of experts who are not full-time government employees. These panels usually consist of physicians, scientists, and statisticians who are special government employees for the time they serve, which is usually 1 to 2 days, once or twice a year. The panel members individually review the written information before their formal public meeting. At the FDA Advisory Panel meeting, participants hear from the sponsor, the FDA, and other interested parties. The panels are convened to answer specific questions posed by the FDA about the drug application. The questions almost always include the broad issue of whether the sponsor has demonstrated safety and efficacy for the intended use. The FDA is not required to follow the advice from the advisory panels but usually does. The panel conclusions are often mentioned in the popular press, leading patients to the misunderstanding that a new drug has been approved and is on the market. FDA Advisory Panels are not required for all new drugs.

OFF-LABEL DRUG USE

Traditionally, once a drug was approved, it could only be marketed and promoted for the disease indication for which it was studied (intended use). Other uses are called "off-label" uses because the FDA-approved written instructions and information ("label") are based on information just for uses that were formally studied. Off-label treatment is fully legal and is commonly used. For example, most pediatric treatments are off-label because few drugs have been developed and studied in populations of children. Even changing the total dosage or frequency of giving a drug can make its use off-label. Many of the combination chemotherapy regimens used in oncology have not been approved by the FDA, are not described on the label, and are considered off-label. Examples of off-label uses common in dermatology include Botox for wrinkles, cyclosporine for atopic dermatitis, and pentoxifylline for venous ulcers. Congress has been clear in its intent that the FDA not interfere with the practice of medicine. As long as the physician is prescribing an approved drug for an off-label use to help the

well-being of an individual patient and has a reasonable scientific basis for expecting success, the off-label use is appropriate within the context of the practice of medicine. Such therapy may be referred to as innovative therapy. It should be noted that on occasion sponsors do seek label changes, and toward that end, appropriate studies are submitted to the FDA for approval. FDA approval for methotrexate use in psoriasis patients is an example pertinent to dermatology.

In 1998, the Food and Drug Modernization Act (FADMA) of 1997 was changed, allowing pharmaceutical companies to promote (teach about and recommend to physicians) off-label uses of an approved drug. Such off-label use promotion is allowed only if there is significant published data supporting the drug's off-label use as both safe and effective and showing that the sponsor is committed to conducting further studies of the drug for the off-label use. In addition to the changes on promotion of off-label uses, the new law has allowed companies to advertise directly to consumers for approved prescription drugs.

GENERIC DRUG USE

When patents expire on the brand-name or pioneer drugs, generic formulations become available, often for a much lower cost. Originally, generics were produced and sold by so-called generic drug companies. Recently, generic drugs have also been manufactured (and marketed by) the brand name producers. Generic drugs must also be approved by the FDA before being marketed. As noted earlier, to secure FDA marketing approval, the pioneer drug must be shown to be safe and effective in clinical trials. However, after marketing, the pioneer drugs are often reformulated. The FDA standard for reformulated pioneer drugs must be shown to be bioequivalent to the pioneer formulation. Bioequivalence is assumed to equal therapeutic equivalence. Bioequivalence is demonstrated by showing similar peak serum concentrations and area under the curve values after a single oral dose of the generic or reformulated drug. Topical drugs usually do not have significant serum value. The FDA proposed a new standard of bioequivalence related to the concentration of the active drug in the stratum corneum. Generic topical products with formulations identical to the brand name or that have clinical trial proof of safety and efficacy are also approvable. No serious therapeutic differences between brand name originals and FDA-approved generics have been reported.

SPECIAL DRUG APPROVAL CATEGORIES

Treating patients with drugs that are under investigation but not approved for marketing in the United States for any indication is complicated. Regulations developed since the acquired immunodeficiency syndrome (AIDS) epidemic make it possible for patients to "import" non-approved drugs for personal use under a physician's care. "Compassionate use" or treatment INDs (as compared to study INDs) are typically limited to patients who have received the test drug under protocol and who still need it after completion of the protocol study. Drugs sold as a treatment IND are priced to recover only "costs" rather than to achieve a profit.

Many other laws have indirect but important general effects on the drug development and approval process. For example, since proving safety and efficacy is so time-consuming, the Drug Price Competition and Patent Restoration Act of 1984 gives the sponsor back some of the patent protection time consumed with meeting the premarket approval requirements. Similarly, the Orphan Drug Act of 1983 offers tax and other incentives to encourage companies to prove the safety and efficacy of drugs whose potential market (number of potential patients) is too small to recover their drug development costs.

RELATED ISSUES

It is important to recognize that the approval processes for devices, biologics, and OTC drugs are similar but somewhat different than the process for prescription drugs. For example,

OTC drug status is dependent on a much higher level of safety and a need for patients to be able to independently recognize when the drug is indicated. Furthermore, physicians should recognize that there is not an FDA regulatory process for surgery.

It should also be noted the FDA process is considerably different from the drug regulatory process used in many other countries. For example, in some countries a nongovernmental organization evaluates the data and submits a recommendation, which the government usually accepts. In other countries, safety data are required. However, the FDA processes are highly regarded by other countries, some of which use a United States FDA approval as the basis for their own country's approval of a given drug. The FDA is proud of the fairly low number of approved drugs that are subsequently recalled or taken off of the market. For example, from 1970 to 1992, a total of 56 drugs were withdrawn from the U.K., U.S., German, and French markets, but only 9 of the drugs were withdrawn from the United States. However, between September 1997 and September 1998, 5 drugs were taken off the market, prompting concern that the agency was too focused on fast approval. A recently published FDA analysis of the FDA's rate of withdrawal shows 3.2% from 1979 to 1983, 3.5% from 1988 to 1989, 1.6% from 1989 to 1993, and 1.2% from 1994 to 1998. From 1987 to 1997, only 6 drugs were pulled off the U.S. market after approval. This analysis tends to refute the idea that faster approvals led to reduced drug safety. On the other hand, critics often lament the "drug-lag" that results in many drugs being available in other countries significantly before release in the United States. Finally, it is important to recognize that the laws governing the drug-approval process are drafted to meet broad public health and social policy considerations. The regulations that are developed to implement these laws quickly become complicated and are constantly fine-tuned to meet new circumstances and specific situations.

Bibliography

Bioequivalence of generics. *Med Lett Drugs Ther* 41:47-50, 1999.

FDA Drug Review: Postapproval Risks, 1976-1985. Washington, DC, US General Accounting Office; April 26, 1990. GAO/PEMD-90-15.

FDA's Fiscal Year 1999 Justification of Estimates for Appropriation Committee and Performance Plan. Internet address: FDA.gov/co/oms/ofm/budget99cj.htm.

FDA New Drug Development and Review. Internet address: FDA.gov/cder/handbook/index.htm.

Food and Drug Law Institute: Seventy-fifth anniversary volume of food and drug law. Washington, DC, 1984. Library of Congress Catalog Card Number: 84-080030.

Friedman MA, Woodcock J, Lumpkin MM, et al: The safety of newly approved medicines. Do recent market removals mean there is a problem? *JAMA* 281(18):1728-1734, 1999.

In deference of the FDA (editorial). *Lancet* 346: 981, 1995.

Moore TJ, Psaty BM, Furberg CD: Time to act on drug safety. *JAMA* 279:1571-1573, 1998.

New Drug Approvals. Internet address: Pharma.org

Torres A: The use of food and drug administration-approved medications for unlabeled (off-label) uses. The legal and ethical implications. *Arch Dermatol* 130:32-36, 1994.

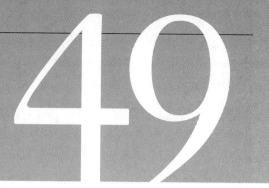

CHAPTER 49

Saqib J. Bashir
Howard I. Maibach

Topical Drug Testing

Topical drugs and topical delivery systems must be tested before they can be accepted for general human use. Adverse effects can occur localized to the skin, systemic organs, or both. The extent of required testing varies with the ingredients and the target population of the product.

Novel agents must be tested rigorously; no assumptions can be made regarding their safety with regard to topical or systemic effects, such as reproductive toxicity and carcinogenesis. In the United States, new drug development is overseen by the Food and Drug Administration (FDA). After animal testing, an Investigational New Drug (IND) application is submitted to the FDA, which must be approved before clinical studies can begin. Compounds with therapeutic potential must demonstrate safety and efficacy in these preclinical studies. Toxicologic and pharmacologic testing usually include determination of the lethal dose in three different species and pathologic studies for organ toxicity. Drug metabolism and excretion are also determined. If the FDA approves these data, clinical studies on humans in controlled trials may begin. After phase III studies have been completed, a New Drug Application (NDA) may be submitted to the FDA. If the NDA is accepted, the new product can be marketed. All favorable and unfavorable data must be submitted. Approval depends on whether the drug is safe and effective, whether it can be manufactured consistently, and whether the drug's benefits outweigh the risks of its use. (For a more complete discussion on this FDA approval process see Chapter 48.)

Evaluation of a topical drug delivery system encompasses both the drug(s) and the components of the delivery system. The FDA can categorize these systems either as a new medicinal product or as a new dosage form. If the drug is a new active substance, a full toxicology profile is necessary (e.g., carcinogenic and mutagenic assays). The testing requirements may be reduced when the system includes compounds that are marketed in other dosage forms. Topical delivery systems must also be tested for their ability to cause irritant and allergic contact dermatitis. An evaluation plan for transdermal systems is described by Prevo and associates.[1]

PERCUTANEOUS ABSORPTION
Systemic Adverse Reactions to Topical Compounds

Systemic adverse reactions to topically applied compounds (percutaneous toxicity) are an important aspect of topical drug safety. Although adverse skin reactions may be readily attributed to topical substances, systemic effects may go unnoticed or unattributed to the topical drug. Therefore case reports are rare and methodologic scientific testing is necessary to ensure the safety of topical preparations. In particular, the precise conditions and doses that cause adverse reactions require elucidation.

Percutaneous toxicity is dependent on percutaneous absorption (PCA). Therefore the factors that modulate a drug's skin penetrative properties may also modulate the toxicity of the substance, especially if a dose-response relationship is present (see Dermatopharmacokinetics section). This section considers the systemic effects that have been associated with topical drug use and the methods by which they can be predicted.

Forms of Percutaneous Toxicity

Percutanous toxicity can be acute or chronic, may affect reproduction, induce carcinogenesis, or cause a drug interaction. These effects may be related to the drug itself, its metabolites (which can be formed in the skin or distally), or to the vehicle or other excipients.

ACUTE TOXICITY

Anaphylactic Reactions. Acute systemic toxicity can be exemplified by immediate type (Type I) hypersensitivity reactions, which can occur within minutes of topical drug administration. Some recent cases are described here.

Saryan and colleagues[2] report anaphylaxis to bacitracin ointment that had been applied to the skin abrasions of a motorcycle accident victim who subsequently developed anaphylactic shock. Subsequent prick tests were positive to the bacitracin ointment but were negative to Xylocaine and a cleansing solution that had also been administered. Lin and co-workers[3] also reported anaphylaxis to bacitracin after its application to an excoriated area of a tinea pedis–infected foot. The patient experienced local and subsequently generalized pruritus, followed by anaphylaxis and cardiorespiratory arrest. After recovery, enzyme-linked immunosorbent assay (ELISA), Prausnitz-Küstner (P-K) testing on a Rhesus monkey, and basophil histamine release assays were performed. Skin testing was not performed because of the near fatal episode. The P-K test was positive (1:8 dilution); however, the ELISA and basophil histamine release test results were negative. Perhaps the negative test results occurred because bacitracin may act as a hapten, requiring a protein carrier, which is absent in the in vitro assays. However, the passive transfer of the immediate-type, hypersensitivity reaction to the Rhesus monkey suggests that immunoglobulin E (IgE) to baci-

tracin was formed. This group also suggests that a break in the skin barrier may be necessary for anaphylaxis to occur, which is consistent with this and other previously described cases.

Erel and associates[4] described a further example of anaphylaxis to a topical drug. Skin prick testing was performed on two patients who experienced anaphylaxis to rifamycin SV. P-K testing was also performed on one patient's spouse to test for passive transfer of IgE. Both patients tested positive to the drug but negative to the other constituents of Rifocine (Gruppo Lepetit, Italy) and were also negative to common aeroallergens and latex. These findings suggest that Rifamycin induced the IgE-mediated, immediate hypersensitivity reaction.

Anaphylaxis is a serious, acute adverse effect of topical drug administration in some patients. These cases, among others,[5-8] demonstrate that anaphylaxis can occur in topical preparations that are in widespread use, without any perceived need for resuscitation equipment. Therefore the dangers to the patient are increased if physicians are not aware of the potential for any topically applied substance to theoretically cause anaphylaxis in any patient, however rare.

Nonimmunologic Acute Toxicity. Substances that rapidly diffuse through the skin to reach target organs can mediate nonimmunologic toxicity. Examples of such chemicals include chemical warfare agents such as nerve gases and pesticides.

CHRONIC TOXICITY.
Chronic toxicity to topically applied drugs may occur with repeated exposure. This may depend on physiologic clearance of the drug between doses and the total drug dose itself. If a sufficient amount of the drug accumulates, this may cause toxicity at target organs, whereas a rapidly cleared toxic compound may have no effect or an effect that may be delayed for many years. Factors affecting drug clearance, such as age or hepatic or renal pathology, may further contribute to the drug's toxicity.

Topical corticosteroids demonstrate an example of potential chronic systemic toxicity that is related to the dose, duration of therapy, and site of application.[9]

Reproductive Toxicity. Reproductive toxicity, considered in its entirety, may affect both males and females. Exposure to toxic compounds at any stage in reproductive life can result in diminished fertility of the parents or in fetal abnormalities.

Infertility may be caused by many factors, including abnormal germ cell formation and disorders of the menstrual cycle, libido, fertilization, and implantation. Teratogenesis, abortion, perinatal death, functional abnormalities, growth retardation, or cancer may be caused by several mechanisms, including chromosomal abnormalities contributed by either parent, maternal hormonal disturbances, and direct and indirect fetal exposure to chemicals in pregnancy.[10]

Many orally administered drugs are well known to affect reproduction by the previously mentioned means. However, there are few reports demonstrating that topically applied substances can have the same effects.[11,12] For the majority of chemicals, blood levels after topical exposure are much lower than with oral exposure, and therefore the risks of any toxicity are considered lower. However, dermal exposure often circumvents first-pass hepatic metabolism—a feature that is exploited in transdermal drug delivery. Such drug delivery systems are an increasingly fashionable method of delivering drugs for systemic therapy. There is therefore a risk of reproductive harm if high blood levels of a toxic compound are achieved because "first-pass" hepatic metabolism is avoided.

The lack of data for percutaneously administered substances is not considered by Barlow[10] to be a drawback, if oral animal testing has been performed and the percutaneous bioavailability of the drug can be calculated. With these data, an estimate of the safety of the compound can be made. However, animal data are not always easily extrapolated to humans. Although many compounds that affect human reproduction have quantitatively similar effects in animals, humans are much more sensitive to certain substances, for example, alcohol and thalidomide.

Retinoids are a class of drugs extensively used in dermatology practice that are known to be orally teratogenic.[13] However, the teratogenicity of topically administered retinoids, in their current form and at routine doses, is much debated. Schaefer and Zesch[14] demonstrated that locally high concentrations of all-*trans*-retinoic acid (RA) could be found in the epidermis, with low concentrations in the dermis. Kemper and colleagues[15] showed no alteration in the endogenous plasma levels of all-*trans*-RA after topical administration. In one study, investigators applied a gel 13-*cis*-RA formulation and found no increase in endogenous plasma levels for either 13-*cis*-RA or all-*trans*-RA.[16] These investigations suggest that any risk is very low. Jick and co-workers[17] performed a retrospective case control study, comparing 215 topical retinoid patients who had delivered live or stillborn infants to 430 age-matched nonexposed controls. All of the treated group became pregnant within 4 months of receiving a prescription for topical tretinoin, or had obtained a prescription in the first trimester. The relative risk of a treated patient having a baby with a major congenital abnormality was 0.7% (CI 0.2 to 2.3), suggesting that topical tretinoin was not associated with major congenital disorders. However, Martínez-Frías and Rodriguez-Pinilla[18] argue that the Jick study[17] is inconclusive, as the authors did not establish whether those prescribed the topical tretinoin actually used it, and how much they really utilized. Further, they also contend that studies attempting to establish the safety of topical tretinoin to date are too small to detect an increase in birth defects, when the average frequency in "normal" circumstances is 1.5/1000 births. In a study of a few hundred people, small increases in frequency may remain unnoticed. Weight is given to this argument. Also, Doran and Cunningham,[19] in their detailed review, suggest that, although current normal therapeutic use of topical retinoids appears to be low risk, newer synthetic retinoids with higher potency may pose a greater risk, even with low plasma drug levels.

Carcinogenesis and Photocarcinogenesis. Few data describe the carcinogenic potential of topical drugs in humans. Human case reports, epidemiologic data, animal testing studies, and experimental systems for testing deoxyribonucleic acid (DNA) mutations are methods by which topical drugs can be tested. However, interpreting the relevance to humans can be difficult, especially if different methods yield different results.

The WHO International Agency for Research on Skin Cancer[20] compiled data on the carcinogenic properties of dithranol, which is used to treat psoriasis. Dithranol (anthraline) was a tumor-promoting agent in mouse skin after initiation with either 7,12-dimethylbenz anthracene or urethane. Tumors included squamous cell carcinomas and papillomas. Mice initiated with urethane also developed lymphomas when treated with dithranol. However, no case reports or epidemiologic data regarding human tumors were available to the working group. Other experimental systems, such as assessing DNA point mutations in *Salmonella typhimurium* (Ames mutagenicity assay) and *Saccharomyces cerevisiae*, yielded negative or weakly positive results. The varying results between models highlight the difficulty in assessing the carcinogenic potential of topical drugs in humans.

Photocarcinogenesis that is due to ultraviolet irradiation may be enhanced by substances that are not necessarily known to be tumor promoters. No single standard assay defines a substance's photocarcinogenic ability, but several methods are described by Forbes.[21] Photocarcinogens include 5- or 8-methoxypsoralen, coal tar pitch, and *trans*-RA. The clinical relevance of the latter for humans remains *sub judice*.

Animal Models of Systemic Toxicity

There are two main approaches to the animal study of systemic toxicity—the dose-response approach and the fixed-dose approach. The former is better suited to the study of new substances about which little or no information is known, whereas the latter is more suitable if some prior toxicologic information exists.[22]

DOSE-RESPONSE APPROACH.   The lethal dose in 50% of test animals (LD_{50}) is determined by different routes of administration in one or more species. Percutaneous toxicity can be assessed by applying series of graded doses to the test animals. Body weight, signs of toxicity, mortality, and gross pathology are the parameters usually assessed. Oral toxicity may also be assessed to provide data for drug abuse or misuse, and inhalation toxicity is useful for drugs in aerosol form. Acute and cumulative toxic effects are also evaluated using graded doses. Similarly, the pharmacokinetics are also established. A "no effect" level in the most sensitive and relevant species to humans is established, to which a safety factor is added to allow for a margin of error in the human dose.

FIXED-DOSE APPROACH.   This is a more rapid method that tests for the *absence* of systemic effects at a dose that is magnitudes higher than the anticipated human dose. Based on the mode and site of application, dose and duration of use, and previously established toxicologic data, the safety (rather than the toxicity of a drug) can be tested in a particular setting.

Dermatopharmacokinetics

As previously stated, percutaneous toxicity depends on the ability of the toxic substance to penetrate the skin (percutaneous penetration). Kligman[23] states that the skin should be regarded as a "potential portal of entry," rather than as a barrier when considering toxicity to topical compounds.

This section considers some physical, physiologic, and chemical properties that affect percutaneous penetration and also some experimental methodology.

DOSE-RESPONSE RELATIONSHIPS.   Percutaneous penetration occurs in a dose-response manner—the percent dose and mass absorbed (μg) vary with the concentration of drug applied to the skin (μg/cm^2), although the efficiency of absorption decreases at increased doses.[24] The degree of drug absorbed can be expressed as a flux (μg/cm^2/hr), which importantly considers the time dimension in the equation. As the duration of the exposure determines the total amount of absorbed drug, the duration of exposure also has a bearing on toxicity. If one is able to remove the drug from the skin rapidly, toxicity may be avoided.

MULTIPLE DOSING AND PENETRATION ENHANCERS.   Repeated applications of a drug to the same site can increase percutaneous penetration to deliver more drug than a single, high dose equal in the cumulative amount delivered.[25] In this in vivo study, volunteers were given three administrations of hydrocortisone in 1 day to the same skin site and also a single administration of the equivalent dose 2 to 3 weeks later at an adjacent skin site. The multiple-dose regimen approximately doubled the amount of hydrocortisone absorbed, whether the vehicle was acetone or cream.

Laurocapram (1-dodecylazacycloheptan-2-one) is an enhancer of percutaneous penetration of drugs. This chemical is thought to act by partitioning the skin into lipid bilayers and thereby disrupting structure.[26] Wester and colleagues[27] demonstrated that repeated daily application of laurocapram cream in humans (washing the site after each dose) resulted in an increase in the amount of laurocapram absorbed after each dose, until a steady state was eventually achieved (day 8). Szolar-Platzer and associates[28] demonstrated the ability of laurocapram to enhance the percutaneous penetration of the surfactant sodium lauryl sulfate in vitro. Therefore laurocapram can enhance both its own absorption and that of other compounds with repeated dosing. The presence of percutaneous enhancers, such as laurocapram, may therefore increase the ability of a compound to cause adverse affects, both locally and systemically.

Hewitt[29] studied the comparative bioavailability of diclofenac sodium lotion compared with an aqueous solution after topical application to viable human skin in vitro. In addition, the difference between a single dose and multiple doses (8 times) was also determined. An in vitro flow-through diffusion cell system was employed, using radiolabeled diclofenac sodium. The single-dose study showed no statistic difference between diclofenac delivered in lotion or an aqueous solution; however, the lotion delivered significantly greater doses of diclofenac in the multiple dosing regimen. The authors conclude that a constituent of the lotion (dimethylsulfoxide) enhances human skin absorption of diclofenac when used in a multidose regimen but not after a single dose.

SURFACE AREA.   The skin ratio of skin surface area to body volume may affect the toxicity of a compound. Young children have a relatively large surface area to volume ratio. Young children therefore are at greater risk of percutaneous toxicity than an obese adult, who has a smaller surface area to body volume ratio.[23] It may therefore be beneficial to know the physical characteristics of the target patients to predict and avoid toxicity, although in many settings this may not be possible.

In patients with widespread skin disease or during an acute exacerbation, the surface area covered by the drug may be much greater than in normal use. Therefore doses of topical drugs significantly higher than average should be tested when topical drug safety is assessed. Some

patients, having already received a prescription, may increase the dose several-fold during a flare, potentially increasing the risk of toxicity. Also, physicians prescribing higher than normal amounts of various topical products in a difficult case should be aware of the potential of toxicity from increased percutaneous penetration.

SKIN SITE.   Regional differences in permeability of the skin depend on the thickness of intact stratum corneum. According to Feldmann and Maibach[30] the highest total absorption of hydrocortisone is from the scrotum, followed by the forehead, head, scalp, back, forearms, palms, and plantar surfaces in decreasing order.

The application site for drug use is important in study design. It is important (when known) that the study site be the body site of intended topical use, even if this is not the most convenient site to study. In clinical therapy, patients should also be told to avoid applying a drug on a particular skin site if increased absorption is likely to lead to increased toxicity.

AGE AND MENOPAUSE.   Oriba and coworkers[31] studied the PCA of hydrocortisone and testosterone that was applied to the vulvar and ventral forearm regions of premenopausal and postmenopausal women. The effect of age on PCA was measured using the menopause as a time point. PCA of hydrocortisone was significantly greater in vulvar skin than forearm skin in both premenopausal and postmenopausal women. Absorption of hydrocortisone by vulvar skin of premenopausal women was significantly greater than in postmenopausal women. The ventral forearm skin of premenopausal women tended to show increased absorption compared with postmenopausal women, but statistical significance was not reached. These results provide evidence that the skin barrier integrity to hydrocortisone may increase with age. However, the PCA of testosterone was significantly increased on the vulva compared with the arm only in postmenopausal women. No significant differences in the PCA of testosterone in vulvar or forearm skin were observed between the two age groups. Therefore age and site may alter penetration profiles selectively.

SKIN INTEGRITY.   Wilhelm and associates[32] investigated the effect of sodium lauryl sulfate

(SLS)–induced skin irritation on the PCA of radiolabeled hydrocortisone, indomethacin, ibuprofen, and acitretin in the hairless guinea pig. Utilizing several techniques, including skin biopsy, tape stripping, and collection of excreta, they determined the systemic absorption. In the tape stripping method, cells adhered to the tape are dispersed with an organic solvent, such as methanol or ethanol, before scintillation. They demonstrated that systemic absorption of topically applied drugs, evaluated by urinary and fecal excretion in SLS-irritated skin, was significantly increased for hydrocortisone (factor 2.6) followed by ibuprofen (1.9 times) and indomethacin (1.6 times) but not increased for acitretin.

However, drug concentrations in the viable epidermis and dermis (measured by tape stripping) were 70% lower in SLS-irritated than normal skin for hydrocortisone but not different for ibuprofen, indomethacin, and acitretin. Thus the influence of the state of the skin (irritant dermatitis versus healthy) on percutaneous penetration was different for diverse drugs in this model.

RACE.   Lotte and colleagues[33] investigated the effect of race on the PCA of some organic compounds in vivo. Black, Caucasian, and Asian subjects were exposed to radiolabeled benzoic acid, caffeine, and acetylsalicylic acid topically for 30 minutes and the ^{14}C-labeled chemical. PCA was determined by both urinary excretion and the tape stripping technique. No statistic difference was found in PCA of benzoic acid, caffeine, or acetylsalicylic acid in these races.

OCCLUSION.   Occlusion of a topically applied compound can increase the amount that penetrates the skin.[34] Occluding the application site may decrease evaporation and surface loss of the drug and increase the hydration of the skin, promoting PCA.

PERCUTANEOUS ABSORPTION MODELS. Skin's accessibility greatly facilitates its pharmacologic study. In addition to traditional techniques of blood and excreta examination, methods such as tape stripping, skin washing, bioengineering methods, skin biopsy, and hair, sweat, and sebum collection allow detailed investigation. Each parameter allows different aspects of the drug's behavior in skin to be assessed together to give an overview of skin pharmacokinetics and pharmacodynamics. In addition to human in vivo assays, there are also animal and in vitro assays with cadaveric skin.

Plasma levels of topically applied substances are usually below assay detection level; therefore radiolabeled drugs can be used to provide an indirect measure of concentration. The amount of radioactivity excreted in urine and feces is then determined. One pitfall of this method is that the skin may metabolize the compound into a substance that is not cleared by the measured route. A calculation is described by Wester and Maibach[32] to attempt to adjust for this. Stripping layers of stratum corneum with adhesive cellophane tape allows the amount of drug in the stratum corneum to be assayed. This can be done using radiolabeled compounds or by an assay for chemical content such as high performance liquid chromatography. Some advantages of this technique are that one can assay for drug concentration against time, with short or long intervals, and many test sites can be utilized in one subject. Similarly, sweat and sebum are relatively easy to collect and can be analyzed with similar methods. Wester and Maibach[26] provide an example of integrated dermatopharmacokinetics in man. They studied the PCA of ^{14}C-1 radiolabeled isofenphos (a pesticide) in human volunteers in vivo and in vitro with human cadaver skin. In the in vivo section of the study, they utilized wash techniques to determine the evaporation of the compound from the skin, tape-stripping data to demonstrate that there was no residual isofenphos in the stratum corneum, and urinary excretion data to determine the total percentage dose absorbed. This was followed by the in vitro diffusion studies on cadaveric skin, which allowed the authors to compare the effectiveness of in vitro modeling in predicting human experience.

Summary of Percutaneous Absorption
This section demonstrates the complexity of PCA. Several major influences on absorption have been listed, which exemplify a common theme that each variable can influence the absorption of different drugs with diverse results. It is unwise to generalize when considering der-

matopharmacokinetics. Topical drug testing must therefore be targeted carefully at the population that will use the product.

DERMATOTOXICOLOGY

A given drug's potential for skin irritation and allergy, photo-induced effects, and immediate hypersensitivity reactions are important factors that can determine whether an individual patient will comply with a topical drug regimen, and indeed whether a particular formulation will be licensed for use. This importance is reflected with the many assays that help predict these reactions and the constant drive to improve these testing methods. This section discusses these skin reactions and outlines some experimental models to give an overview of the field.

Irritant Dermatitis

ACUTE IRRITANT DERMATITIS.   Topical irritants, with sufficient potency and dose, can cause acute skin irritation, independent of constitutional susceptibility. This form of irritation is often the result of a single accidental exposure to a strong irritant. Novel compounds may be tested for their potential to cause acute irritant dermatitis by the Draize rabbit test, which is accepted as a standard test by several governmental agencies.

The Draize model[35] and its modifications are commonly used to assay skin irritation using albino rabbits. The procedure adopted in the U.S. Federal Hazardous Substance Act (FHSA) is described in Tables 49-1 and 49-2.[36-38] Table 49-3 compares this method with some other modifications of the Draize model.[38]

Draize utilized the scoring system shown in Table 49-2 to calculate the Primary Irritation Index (PII). This index is calculated by averaging both the erythema scores and the edema scores of all sites tested (both abraded and nonabraded sites). These two averages are then added together to give the PII value. A value of <2 is considered nonirritating, 2 to 5 mildly irritating, and >5 severely irritating. A value of at least 5 defines an irritant by Consumer Product Safety Commission (CPSC) standards. Subsequent laboratory and clinical experience demonstrated that the value judgements (i.e., nonirritating, mildly irritating, severely irritating) proposed by Draize require clinical judgement and perspective. The PII index should not be viewed in an absolute sense. Many materials irritating to the rabbit may be well tolerated by human skin.

■ Table 49-1   Draize-FHSA Model[37,38]

Number of Animals	6 Albino Rabbits (clipped)
Test sites	2 × 1 in² sites on dorsum One site intact, the other abraded (e.g., with hypodermic needle)
Test materials	Applied undiluted to both test sites Liquids: 0.5 ml Solids/semisolids: 0.5 g
Occlusion	1-in² surgical gauze over each test site Rubberized cloth over entire trunk
Occlusion period	24 hrs
Assessment	24 and 72 hrs Visual scoring system

■ Table 49-2   Draize-FHSA Scoring System[37,38]

	Score
ERYTHEMA AND ESCHAR FORMATION	
No erythema	0
Very slight erythema (barely perceptible)	1
Well-defined erythema	2
Moderate-to-severe erythema	3
Severe erythema ("beet red") to slight eschar formation (injuries in depth)	4
EDEMA FORMATION	
No edema	0
Very slight edema (barely perceptible)	1
Slight edema (edges of area well defined by definite raising)	2
Moderate edema (raised >1 mm)	3
Severe edema (raised >1 mm and extending beyond the area of exposure)	4

■ **Table 49-3**   Examples of Modified Draize Irritation Method[38]

	Draize	FHSA	DOT	FIFRA	OECD
Number of animals	3	6	6	6	6
Abrasion/intact	Both	Both	Intact	2 of each	Intact
Dose liquids	0.5 ml undiluted	0.5 ml undiluted	0.5 ml	0.5 ml undiluted	0.5 ml
Dose solids	0.5 g in solvent	0.5 g in solvent	0.5 g	0.5 g moistened	0.5 g moistened
Exposure period (hr)	24	24	4	4	4
Examination (hr)	24, 72	24, 72	4, 48	0.5, 1, 24, 48, 72	0.5, 1, 24, 48, 72
Removal of test materials	Not specified	Not specified	Skin washed	Skin wiped	Skin washed
Excluded from testing	—	—	—	Toxic materials pH ≤ 2 or ≥ 11.5	Toxic materials pH ≤ 2 or ≥ 11.5

FHSA, Federal Hazardous Substance Act; *DOT,* Department of Transportation; *FIFRA,* Federal Insecticide, Fungicide, and Rodenticide Act; *OECD,* Organization for Economic Cooperation and Development.

Although the Draize scoring system does not include vesiculation, ulceration, and severe eschar formation, all of the Draize-type tests are used to evaluate corrosion (skin necrosis after a chemical insult) as well as irritation. When severe and potentially irreversible reactions occur, the test sites are further observed on days 7 and 14, or even later if necessary.

Modifications to the Draize assay attempted to improve its prediction of human experience. The model is criticized for inadequately differentiating between mild and moderate irritants. However, it serves well in hazard identification, often overpredicting the severity of human skin reactions.[38] Therefore Draize assays for topical irritancy continue to be recommended by regulatory bodies.

CUMULATIVE IRRITATION.   Frequent exposure to an acute irritant may lead to the onset of cumulative irritant dermatitis, which may become chronic. The classic signs are erythema and increasing dryness, followed by hyperkeratosis with frequent cracking and occasional erythema. Both animal and human models have been used to predict cumulative irritation.

The repeat application patch test is one example of an animal assay that was developed to

rank the irritant potential of products. Putative irritants are applied under occlusion to the same site for 3 to 21 days. The degree of occlusion influences percutaneous penetration, which may in turn influence the sensitivity of the test. Patches used vary from Draize type gauze dressings to metal chambers. Therefore a reference irritant material is often included in the test to help standardize interpretation of the results. Various animal species have been used, such as the guinea pig and the rabbit.[39,40] Wahlberg[40] measured skinfold thickness with Harpenden calipers to assess the edema-producing capacity of chemicals in guinea pigs. This model demonstrated clear, dose-response relationships and discriminating power, except for acids and alkalis, where no change in skinfold thickness was found.

Human models present data that is species specific. Two different teams of investigators[39,41] described a cumulative irritation assay, which has become known as the "21-day," cumulative irritation assay. The purpose of the test is to screen new formulas before marketing. A 1-inch square of Webril is saturated with liquid or with 0.5 g of viscous substances and applied to the surface of the pad to be applied to the skin. The patch is applied to the upper back and sealed with occlusive tape. The patch is removed after 24 hours, and then reapplied after examination of the test site. This is repeated for 21 days and the Irritant Dose 50 can then be calculated.

Modifications have been made to this method. The chamber scarification test (see below) was developed to predict the effect of repeated applications of a potential irritant to damaged skin, rather than testing only for irritancy to healthy skin. The cumulative patch test previously described failed to predict adverse reactions to skin damaged by acne or shaving, or in sensitive areas such as the face.[42]

The chamber scarification test was developed[43,44] to test the irritant potential of products on damaged skin. Six to eight 1-mm sites on the volar forearm were scratched eight times with a 30-gauge needle, without causing bleeding. Four scratches were parallel and the other four were perpendicular to these. Duhring chambers, containing 0.1 g of test material (e.g., ointments, creams, or powders), are then placed over the test sites. For liquids, a fitted pad saturated with 0.1 ml of the material tested may be used. Chambers containing fresh materials are reapplied daily for 3 days. The sites are evaluated by visual scoring 30 minutes after removal of the final set of chambers. A scarification index may be calculated if both normal and scarified skin is tested, to reflect the relative degree of irritation between compromised and intact skin. This index is the score of scarified sites divided by the score of intact sites. However, the relationship of this assay to routine use of substances on damaged skin remains to be established. Another compromised skin model, the arm immersion model of compromised skin, is described later.

PHOTOIRRITATION.   Photoirritation, which is induced by photoactive chemicals, requires ultraviolet (UV) radiation in the test process. This requirement discriminates this photoirritation from the standard mechanism of chemical irritation. The UV region of the electromagnetic spectrum usually activates photochemicals, although visible light (e.g., 5-aminolevulinic acid) may also cause photoirritation.[45] Photoactive chemicals may reach the skin by either systemic or topical routes and may also be the metabolite of a nonphotoactive substance.

Photoirritation occurs when a photoactive chemical enters the viable elements of the skin, either percutaneously or systemically, and becomes excited by UV irradiation penetrating the skin. The photo-excited drug (e.g., chlorpromazine) may transfer its energy to oxygen, producing cytotoxic, oxygen-free radicals. Alternatively, as in the case of psoralens, oxygen radicals are not necessary to produce phototoxic effects.

Clinically, these effects are seen as erythema, vesiculation or bullae, increased skin temperature, and pruritus, followed by long-lasting hyperpigmentation. The full sequence of these morphologic features may not always be present.

Photoirrants encompass a wide range of topical and oral substances, examples of which are listed in Table 49-4. Methods for testing photoirritation have been described in humans and animals such as the mouse, rabbit, and guinea pig. Marzulli and Maibach[45,46] describe a method for testing topical photoirritation. The test chemical (0.05 ml) is applied to the skin and is irradiated after 5 minutes for a period of 25 to 40 minutes, from a distance of 8 to 10 cm. In animals, the skin is examined for erythema and edema at 1 hours, 5 hours, 24 hours, and 7 days. In humans, bullae and vesiculation may be seen, and hyperpigmentation may occur some time later. Positive controls using a psoralen and negative controls with only a vehicle are employed for comparison.

Animal models of phototoxicity testing are reviewed in detail by Lambert and colleagues.[47]

Allergic Contact Dermatitis

Allergic contact dermatitis can be predicted by many experimental assays. Traditional animal assays are numerous,[48] and one example is outlined here. The general principles of the assays are the same—to monitor the development of allergic contact dermatitis in an exposure after an induction of allergy. However, the variations in routes of administration, skin conditions, occlusion, and other factors result in varying sensitivity and specificity. Other assays include human assays; novel techniques, such as the murine local lymph node assay, are described later.

Mathematic models may also provide information regarding the likelihood of a particular molecule causing allergy. Termed *quantita-*

■ **Table 49-4** Examples of Photoirritants[45]

TOPICAL PHOTOIRRITANTS

Dyes	Anthraquinone, disperse blue 35, eosin, methylene blue, rose bengal, toluidine blue, cadmium sulfide in tattoos
Fragrances	Oil of bergamot
Furocoumarins	Angelicin, bergapten, psoralen, 8-methoxypsoralen, 4,5',8-trimethylpsoralen
Plant products	Celery, figs, limes, bogweed, parsnips, fennel, dill
Coal tar components	Acridine, anthracene, benzopyrene, creosote, phenanthrene, pitch, pyridine

SYSTEMIC PHOTOIRRITANTS

Antibiotics	Griseofulvin, nalidixic acid, sulfanilamide, tetracyclines
Chemotherapeutics	Dacarbazine, 5-fluorouracil, vinblastine
Drugs—other	Amiodarone, chlorpromazine, chloroquine, tolbutamide
Diuretics	Hydrochlorothiazide, furosemide
NSAIDs	Benoxaprofen, naproxen, piroxicam
Porphyrins	Hematoporphyrin
Psoralens	8-methoxypsoralen, 5-methoxypsoralen

NSAIDs, Nonsteroidal antiinflammatory drugs.

tive structural analysis relationships (QSAR), these models are based on databases of reported allergens. Given a sufficiently large database of chemical structures, the likelihood of a particular functional group or combinations of functional groups causing allergy may be predicted.[49] Although the field of QSAR allergic contact dermatitis is young and the database is small and not completely validated, its predictive power is impressive.

GUINEA PIG MAXIMIZATION TEST.[50,51] In this assay, 20 test and 10 to 20 control guinea pigs are used. The induction process is in two phases—intradermal injections on day 0 and a 48-hour occlusive patch on day 7 (boosting). This is followed by a challenge test on day 21.

Challenge reactions are examined at 24 and 48 hours after removal of the patch and scored according to a standard rating scale. Control animals are treated similarly to the test animals, except no test substance is applied. Kligman and Basketter[52] recommend in their critique of the test that one control group should receive only FCA, as this substance lowers the skin's irritant threshold. Without this control, irritant reactions may be interpreted erroneously as allergic reactions, when the skin is challenged with the "nonirritating" concentration identified in pre-

liminary irritation studies. Further, the control group should be exposed to an irritant stimulus comparable in intensity to that of the test substance (e.g., SLS). The purpose of this is to control for the "excited skin syndrome," which may cause one or more false-positive results. Individual rechallenge tests should also be performed to rule out false-positive reactions in this setting. Truly allergic reactions last for several weeks, whereas nonspecific irritation diminishes after 2 to 3 days. Rechallenging is performed weekly on the contralateral flank.

THE LOCAL LYMPH NODE ASSAY. The murine local lymph node assay (LLNA) measures the activity of injected [^{3}H]-methylthymidine in the lymph nodes draining a topical test site.[53] This is thought to reflect the clonal expansion of T-lymphocytes in these nodes during induction sensitization.

The test substance is applied topically to the dorsum of both ears, in a vehicle determined by the solubility of the test material. After 5 days, [^{3}H]-methylthymidine is injected intravenously into both the test and control mice, which are then sacrificed 5 hours later. The auricular lymph nodes are then excised, and the [^{3}H]-methylthymidine count is measured by β-scintillation. A count three times greater than

Method—Guinea Pig Maximization Test

Day 0: Paired intradermal injections (0.1 ml each) into the clipped and shaved shoulder region.

Inject each of the following:
- Freund's Complete Adjuvant (FCA)
- Test article in vehicle (e.g., water, paraffin oil, propylene glycol)
- Mixture of dissolved or suspended test article with FCA (1:1)

Day 7: Topical occlusive patch applied for 48 hours over shoulder (clipped on Day 6).
- Concentration applied should be moderately irritating
- If substance is nonirritating, then pretreat region with 10% SLS on Day 6 freshly after clipping

Day 21: Challenge test is performed on a 4-cm² area on the left flank.
- Shave test region
- Apply nonirritating concentrations (e.g., via Finn chamber)
- Apply occluded vehicle for control

Day 28: Rechallenge/cross-test at contralateral flank weekly.

the control group is considered consistent with sensitization.

PHOTOALLERGIC DERMATITIS. The study of photoallergic dermatitis was stimulated by an outbreak of contact photoallergy caused by antimicrobial halogenated salicyanilides in soap.[54] The photomaximization test[55] was developed as a predictive model, consisting of an exaggerated cutaneous exposure to a chemical and UV light. The goal is to determine whether photosensitization can be induced in a subject, resulting in an allergic response with subsequent exposure to both the chemical and UV light. Given that the energy of the photons acting on a photoallergen to allow a given chemical to sensitize may be specific, a broad spectrum of UV irradiation should be used when testing novel compounds. Xenon arc simulators (solar simulators) are lamps that produce a spectrum similar to sunlight and are utilized in this assay. A 5% concentration of test agent is applied to the skin using tuberculin syringes (10 μl/cm²) and oc-

cluded with nonwoven cotton cloth, which is secured with clear, occlusive tape. After 24 hours, the patches are removed and the sites are exposed to three minimal erythema doses (MEDs) from the solar simulator. (The MED is the lowest dose that produces minimal, uniform erythema with a clear border at the test site and is determined before the study is begun.) After a 48-hour rest period, during which the sites were left open, another occlusive application is made to the same site. This test site is again irradiated with three MEDs 24 hours after reapplication. The sequence is repeated for a total of six exposures over a 3-week period.

After a 10- to 14-day rest, a single challenge exposure is made to a fresh test site. A 1% test agent is applied for 24 hours under occlusion, followed by a challenge of 4.0 J/cm² of UVA. Controls included an irradiated, vehicle-treated site and a nonirradiated site of chemical exposure to reveal the presence of contact sensitization. The reactions are evaluated at 24 and 48 hours postirradiation for erythema, edema, or vesiculation, which if absent in control sites signifies the induction of photoallergy.[56]

Contact Urticaria Syndrome

Contact urticaria syndrome (CUS), an immediate-type, hypersensitivity reaction, follows within minutes to an hour after contact with an eliciting substance. First described by Maibach and Johnson,[57] the syndrome consists of a spectrum ranging from local erythema and edema, accompanied by itching, burning, and tingling, to extracutaneous effects such as bronchial asthma and anaphylaxis. Generally, the syndrome can be divided into nonimmunologic and immunologic etiologies, although in some cases the mechanism is not known.

NONIMMUNOLOGIC CONTACT URTICARIA. The guinea pig ear swelling test is used as a rapid, quantitative assay for nonimmunologic contact urticaria. The guinea pig ear mimics human skin in several respects, including the morphology of the reaction, timing of the maximal response, and concentration required to elicit the reaction. The response to an eliciting substance is measured by the change in ear lobe thickness, caused by edema, after topical drug administration. The response varies with concentration in both humans and in this model and reaches a maximum of a 100% increase in thickness about 40 to 50 minutes postapplication, depending on the vehicle. Testing in human patients is usually performed as an open test on the back or on the dorsal or ventral forearm. There is, however, variation in skin sites, such that testing should be performed on the site where the substance is to be typically applied. In addition to visual scoring, bioengineering techniques, such as laser Doppler flowmetry and chromametry, help to more precisely quantify human responses. Performing dilution series can identify a threshold concentration at which CUS is elicited for a particular substance in a particular subject.[58]

IMMUNOLOGIC CONTACT URTICARIA. Laurema and Maibach[59] discussed a potential model for immunologic contact urticaria. Mice are sensitized to trimellitic anhydride (TMA), which is a low molecular weight hapten (192 Da). The mice are sensitized in a two-step process of application of TMA to their shaved, tape-stripped trunks. One week after the second dosing, a TMA was applied to the ears of the mice, resulting in a swelling peaking at 1 hour and a second phase peaking at 24 hours. However, an early onset of ear swelling can also be seen in nonsensitized mice, suggesting a nonimmunologic component. Diphenhydramine and betamethasone dipropionate both attenuate the swelling response. Although this may be a potential model to study immunologic contact urticaria, the authors believe further studies are required.

Study Design

DISEASE MODELS. The quality of in vitro, animal, and human disease models has a direct bearing on the results obtained in any testing process. One cannot assume that all diseases that exist in man also coexist in animals. Animal diseases that do occur in nature may have many similarities and dissimilarities with their human "equivalents." Furthermore, similar morphology does not imply similar pathology or pathogenesis. Therefore tests performed on animals may not have adequate human relevance in the study of a given disease process or therapeutics. In vitro models have the advantage that their design can be manipulated to suit the chosen conditions as closely as possible. However, extrapolation of the data to humans is again difficult. Additionally, the behavior of tissue in vitro may differ from that in vivo, given that in vitro conditions can never truly be physiologic.

Human experimental studies provide data that are species relevant and also allow the careful investigator to make the study relevant to site, race, dose, underlying health, age, and other factors that make up the reality of the general use of topical drugs and cosmetics. However, the use of human subjects is potentially dangerous and should be undertaken with caution.

Psoriasis is a disease that has been extensively modeled by in vitro, animal, and human methods and therefore provides insights into testing methods.[60] The basis of psoriasiform models is their ability to simulate clinical psoriasis histologically. The normal structure of the mouse tail consists of scale areas, which are parakeratotic and lack a granular layer, similar to human psoriasis. The mouse tail also contains hinge areas, which are orthokeratotic and have a granular layer, similar to normal human skin. These histologic features form the basis of the mouse tail test, in which oral, topical, or subcutaneous drugs can be administered, with the aim of inducing orthokeratosis and the formation of a granular cell layer in the scale region. The efficacy of putative therapeutic agents can be assessed, utilizing histologic end points that serve as surrogate clinical end points. This model (and its modified version) have been used to test many antipsoriatic drugs. In the modified mouse tail test, dithranol 3% induced 85% orthokeratosis, and retinoic acid 1% induced 86.4% orthokeratosis. However, in these models, the mouse skin is in its normal state, whereas the human skin is in a pathologic state. Therefore this model cannot be used to detect drugs that modify the pathogenesis of the disease but only to detect a change in disease expression.

Other animal models also exist. Genetic mutations in mice resulted in their expression of psoriasiform disease. Two examples are the flaky skin mouse *(fsm)* model and the chronic proliferative dermatitis mouse *(cpdm)* model, which are both histologically similar to human psoriasis. Xenographic models have also been employed in psoriasis studies, which allow the investigator to study human tissue without the complications of using people. Psoriatic skin from human punch biopsies has been transplanted into athymic (nude) mice and retains some psoriasiform features. However, the rate of DNA synthesis falls markedly, suggesting that the maintenance of the xenograft depends on host (human) factors.

This change in the behavior of explants also affects in vitro modeling of psoriasis. Keratinocyte cultures from patients with psoriasis do not differ in their proliferation and differentiation markers from normal skin as they do in vivo. It may be that other cells or nonskin factors are essential for maintenance of the psoriasis phenotype in vivo.

Human models are required to test data obtained from animal studies. In the study of psoriasis a skin tape stripping model induces ornithine decarboxylase (ODC), which is the rate limiting enzyme in the formation of polyamines that are elevated in psoriasis. This biochemical model has been used to study protein kinase C inhibitors and cyclosporine. However, one inhibitor (sphingosine) caused epidermal necrolysis, illustrating the dangers of drug testing in humans. In another model, ultrasound analysis of human plaques pretreatment and posttreatment can be used to quantify drug effect, in an accurate, objective, and noninvasive manner.

Laurema and Maibach[61] reviewed a microplaque assay, which is a micromodel of plaque psoriasis. The principle of the assay is that several different topical agents can be applied to the same plaque in discrete areas. The application can either be under occlusion (with 15 mm between each application site) or an open application. Efficacy can be assessed by clinical scoring, laser Doppler measurement of superficial blood flow, ultrasound measurement of skin thickness, and histologically. This is a patient-based human model, capable of yielding the directly relevant information.

These examples of psoriasis models illustrate the diverse approaches to disease modeling and that results can vary between models and species. Each model has its advantages and disadvantages, which should be considered in both study design and interpretation of data.

PAIRED COMPARISON STUDIES. This form of study is particularly useful, as subjects act as their own control, reducing intersubject variation. Subjects who have symmetrically distributed disease can be tested on one side of the body in comparison to the other side. Healthy volunteers can have test sites and control sites, rather than using a different population for control.

BIOENGINEERING METHODS. Despite the investigator's skill, subjective assessment of erythema, edema, and other visual parameters may be confounded by interobserver and intraobserver variation. Although the eye may be more sensitive than current spectroscopy and chromametric techniques, the reproducibility and increased statistic power of such data may provide greater benefit. A combination of techniques, such as transepidermal water loss, capacitance, ultrasound, laser Doppler flowmetry, spectroscopy, and chromametric analysis, in addition to skilled observation may increase the precision of the tests. Andersen and Maibach[48] compared various bioengineering techniques, finding that clinically indistinguishable reactions induced significantly different changes in barrier function and vascular status. An outline describing a variety of these techniques is provided by Patil and associates.[38]

RANDOMIZED CLINICAL TRIALS. Once deemed safe to be tested on humans, new topical products and delivery systems must be subject to randomized clinical trials. Careful selection of the target population, with strict inclusion and exclusion criteria, will provide meaningful data on the safety (and efficacy) of a product in general use. Randomization is essential to exclude selection bias at every level, from skin site, if multiple sites are used, to selection of treatment and control groups. Ideally, the same subject could serve as his or her own control for many topical studies; however, systemic toxicity studies require the selection of a random, matched control group. Although blinding may be difficult for topical studies, it does help reduce observer bias and can be relatively easily employed in systemic studies. Another source of potential error is the interpretation of subjective data, which can lead to interobserver variation, intraobserver variation, and other forms of bias such as number bias (where the investigator may have a subconscious preference for one number over another). Therefore it is helpful to qualify relatively subjective data with more precise objective data, utilizing appropriate bioengineering methods previously described.

Randomized trials often reveal findings data that are not generated by smaller studies. Previously unforeseen adverse effects may arise. In addition, adverse effects that were thought to be significant may actually be rare when examined in a larger population.

SUMMARY

Many aspects of topical drug testing have been presented in this chapter. Unwanted effects can range from local to systemic and from minor to fatal. A variety of methods have been described that are useful in the predictive testing of these effects. However, the difficulties in applying models to a clinical setting have also been demonstrated, emphasizing both the complexity and the importance of topical drug testing.

Bibliography

Bashir SJ, Maibach HI: Methods for testing the irritation and sensitization methods for drugs and enhancers. In Kydonieus AF, Wille JJ, editors: *Biochemical modulation of skin reactions,* Boca Raton, FL, 1999, CRC Press, pp 45-60.

Bashir SJ, Maibach HI: Quantitative structure analysis relationships in the prediction of skin sensitization potential. In Kydonieus AF, Wille JJ, editors: *Biochemical modulation of skin reactions,* Boca Raton, FL, 1999, CRC Press, pp 61-64.

Combes RD: Mutagenicity. In Elsner P, Merck HF, Maibach HI, editors: *Cosmetics: controlled efficacy studies and regulation,* Berlin, 1999, Springer, pp 291-308.

Prevo ME, Cormier M, Matriano J: Developing a toxicology evaluation plan for a transdermal delivery systems. In Marzulli FN, Maibach HI, editors: *Dermatotoxicology methods: the laboratory worker's vade mecum,* Washington, DC, 1998, Taylor & Francis, pp 75-88.

Surber C, Smith EW, Schwarb FP, et al: Drug concentration in the skin. In Bronough RL, Maibach HI, editors: *Percutaneous absorption: drugs—cosmetics—mechanisms—methodology,* ed 3, New York, 1999, Marcel Dekker, pp 347-374.

References

1. Prevo ME, Cormier M, Matriano J: Developing a toxicology evaluation plan for transdermal delivery systems. In Marzulli FN, Maibach HI, editors: *Dermatotoxicology methods: the laboratory worker's vade mecum,* Washington, 1998, Taylor & Francis, pp 75-88.

2. Saryan JA, Dammin TC, Bouras AE: Anaphylaxis to topical bacitracin zinc ointment. *Am J Emerg Med* 16:512-513, 1998.

3. Lin FL, Woodmansee D, Patterson R: Near-fatal anaphylaxis to topical bacitracin ointment. *J Allergy Clin Immunol* 101:136-137, 1998.

4. Erel F, Karaayvaz M, Deveci M, et al: Severe anaphylaxis from rifamycin SV. *Ann Allergy Asthma Immunol* 81:257-260, 1998.

5. Knowles SR, Shear NH: Anaphylaxis from bacitracin and polymyxin B (Polysporin) ointment. *Int J Dermatol* 34:572-573, 1995.

6. Cardot E, Tillie-Leblond I, Jeannin P, et al: Anaphylactic reaction to local administration of rifamycin SV. *J Allergy Clin Immunol* 95: 1-7, 1995.

7. Conraads VM, Jorens PG, Ebo DG, et al: Coronary artery spasm complicating anaphylaxis secondary to skin disinfectant. *Chest* 113:1417-1419, 1998.

8. Torricelli R, Wüthrich B: Life-threatening anaphylactic shock due to skin application of chlorhexidine (letter). *Clin Exp Allergy* 26:112, 1996.

9. Mills CM, Marks R: Side effects of topical glucocorticoids. *Curr Probl Dermatol* 21:122-131, 1993.

10. Barlow SM: Reproductive hazards from chemicals absorbed through the skin. In Marzulli FN, Maibach HI, editors: *Dermatotoxicology,* ed 5, Washington, 1996, Taylor & Francis, pp 283-288.

11. Camera G, Pregliasco P: Ear malformation in baby born to mother using tretinoin cream. *Lancet* 339:687, 1992.

12. Lipson A, Collins FWW: Multiple congenital defects associated with maternal use of topical tretinoin. *Lancet* 341:22, 1993.

13. Rosa RW: Teratogenicity of isotretinoin. *Lancet* 2:513, 1983.

14. Schaefer H, Zesch A: Penetration of vitamin A acid into human skin. *Acta Dermatol Venereol (Stockh)* 74(Suppl):50-55, 1975.

15. Kemper C, Holland ML, Thorne EG, et al: Percutaneous absorption of ^{3}H-tretinoin following long-term administration of topical tretinoin. *Dermatologica* 181:351, 1990.

16. Jensen BK, McGann BA, Kachevsky BS, et al: The negligible systemic availability of retinoids with multiple and excessive topical application of isotretinoin 00.5% geo (Isotrex) in patients with acne vulgaris. *J Am Acad Dermatol* 24:425-428, 1991.

17. Jick SS, Terris BZ, Jick H: First trimester tretinoin and congenital disorders. *Lancet* 341:1181-1182, 1993.

18. Martínez-Frías ML, Rodriguez-Pinilla E: First-trimester exposure to topical tretinoin: its safety is not warranted (letter). *Teratology* 60:5, 1999.

19. Doran TI, Cunningham WJ: Retinoids and their mechanisms of toxicity. In Marzulli FN, Maibach HI, editors: *Dermatotoxicology,* ed 5, Washington, 1996, Taylor & Francis, pp 289-298.

20. IARC monographs on the evaluation of carcinogenic risks to humans. Some miscellaneous pharmaceutical substances. International Agency for Research on Cancer: Secretariat of the World Organization, 0250-9555, v13, 75-82, 1990.

21. Forbes PD: Carcinogenesis and photocarcinogenesis test models. In Marzulli FN, Maibach HI, editors: *Dermatotoxicology,* ed 5, Washington, 1996, Taylor & Francis, pp 535-544.

22. Foster GV Jr: Animal models to assess systemic effects. In Kligman AM, Leyden JJ, editors: *Safety and efficacy of topical drugs and cosmetics,* New York, 1980, Grune & Stratton, pp 99-118.

23. Kligman AM: Systemic toxicity. In Kligman AM, Leyden JJ, editors: *Safety and efficacy of topical drugs and cosmetics,* New York, 1980, Grune & Stratton, pp 239-248.

24. Wester RC, Maibach HI: Percutaneous absorption in humans. In Marzulli FN, Maibach HI, editors: *Dermatotoxicology methods: the laboratory worker's vade mecum,* Washington, 1998, Taylor & Francis, pp 15-28.

25. Wester RC, Melendres J, Logan F, et al: Triple therapy: multiple dosing enhances hydrocortisone percutaneous absorption in vivo in humans. In Smith E, Maibach HI, editors: *Percutaneous penetration enhancers,* Boca Raton, FL, 1995, CRC Press, pp 343-349.

26. Wester RC, Maibach HI: Percutaneous absorption. In Marzulli FN, Maibach HI, editors: *Dermatotoxicology,* ed 5, Washington, 1996, Taylor & Francis, pp 35-48.

27. Wester RC, Melendres J, Sedik L, et al: Percutaneous absorption of azone following single and multiple dosing in human volunteers. *J Pharm Sci* 83:124-125, 1994.

28. Szolar-Platzer C, Patil S, Maibach HI: Effect of topical laurocapram (Azone) on the *in vitro* percutaneous permeation of sodium lauryl sulfate using human skin. *Acta Derm Venereol* 76:182-185, 1996.

29. Hewitt PG, Poblete N, Wester RC, et al: In vitro cutaneous disposition of a topical diclofenac lotion in human skin: effect of a multi-dose regimen. *Pharm Res* 15:988-992, 1998.

30. Feldmann RJ, Maibach HI: Regional variation in percutaneous penetration of 14C cortisol in man. *J Invest Dermatol* 48:181, 1967.

31. Oriba HA, Bucks DA, Maibach HI: Percutaneous absorption of hydrocortisone and testosterone on the vulva and forearm: effect of the menopause and site. *Br J Dermatol* 134:229-233, 1996.

32. Wilhelm KP, Surber C, Maibach HI: Effect of sodium lauryl sulfate-induced skin irritation on in vivo percutaneous penetration of four drugs. *J Invest Dermatol* 97:927-932, 1991.

33. Lotte C, Wester RC, Rougier A, et al: Racial differences in the in vivo percutaneous absorption of some organic compounds: a comparison between black, Caucasian and Asian subjects. *Arch Dermatol Res* 284:456-459, 1993.

34. Bucks D, Maibach HI: Occlusion does not uniformly enhance penetration in vivo. In Bronough RL, Maibach HI, editors: *Percutaneous absorption: drugs—cosmetics—mechanisms—methodology,* ed 3, New York, 1999, Marcel Dekker, pp 81-106.

35. Draize TH, Woodland G, Calvery HO: Methods for the study of irritation and toxicity of substances applied to the skin and mucus membranes. *J Pharmacol Exp Ther* 82:377-390, 1944.

36. Code of Federal Regulations. Office of the Federal Registrar, National Archive of Records. General Services Administration, 1985, title 16, parts 1500.40-1500.42.

37. Patrick E, Maibach HI: Comparison of the time course, dose response and mediators of chemically induced skin irritation in three species. In Frosch PJ, Dooms-Goosens A, Lachapelle JM, et al, editors: *Current topics in contact dermatitis,* New York, 1989, Springer-Verlag, pp 399-402.

38. Patil SM, Patrick E, Maibach HI: Animal, human and in vitro test methods for predicting skin irritation. In Marzulli FN, Maibach HI, editors: *Dermatotoxicology methods: the laboratory worker's vade mecum,* Washington, 1998, Taylor & Francis, pp 89-104.

39. Phillip, L, Steinberg M, Maibach HI, et al: A comparison of rabbit and human skin responses to certain irritants. *Toxicol Appl Pharmacol* 21:369-382, 1972.

40. Wahlberg JE: Measurement of skin fold thickness in the guinea pig. Assessment of edema-inducing capacity of cutting fluids acids, alkalis, formalin and dimethyl sulfoxide. *Contact Dermatitis* 28:141-145, 1993.

41. Lanmnan BM, Elvers WB, Howard CS: The role of human patch testing in a product development program. In Proceedings Joint Conference on Cosmetic Sciences, Washington, DC, 1968, Toilet Goods Association, pp 135-145.

42. Battista CW, Rieger MM: Some problems of predictive testing. *J Soc Cosmet Chem* 22:349-359, 1971.

43. Frosch PJ, Kligman AM: The chamber scarification test for irritancy. *Contact Dermatitis* 2:314-324, 1976.

44. Frosch PJ, Kligman AM: The chamber scarification test for testing the irritancy of topically applied substances. In Drill VA, Lazar P, editors: *Cutaneous toxicity,* New York, 1977, Academic Press, p 150.

45. Marzulli FN, Maibach HI: Photoirritation (phototoxicity, phototoxic dermatitis). In Marzulli FN, Maibach HI, editors: *Dermatotoxicology,* ed 5, Washington, 1996, Taylor & Francis, pp 231-238.

46. Marzulli FN, Maibach HI: Perfume phototoxicity. *J Soc Cosmet Chem* 21:686-715, 1970.

47. Lambert LA, Wamer WG, Kornhauser A: Animal models for phototoxicity testing. In Marzulli FN, Maibach HI, editors: *Dermatotoxicology,* ed 5, Washington, 1996, Taylor & Francis, pp 515-530.

48. Anderson KE, Maibach HI: Guinea pig sensitization assays: an overview. *Curr Probl Dermatol* 14:263-290, 1985.

49. Hostnek JJ: Structure-activity relationships in contact sensitization. In Marzulli FN, Maibach HI, editors: *Dermatotoxicology methods: the laboratory worker's vade mecum,* Washington, 1998, Taylor & Francis, pp 115-120.

50. Magnusson B, Kligman AM: The identification of contact allergens by animal assay, the guinea pig maximization test. *J Invest Dermatol* 52:268-276, 1969.

51. Magnusson B, Kligman AM: Allergic contact dermatitis in the guinea pig. Springfield, IL, 1970, Charles C Thomas.

52. Kligman AM, Basketter DA: A critical commentary and updating of the guinea pig maximization test. *Contact Dermatitis* 32:129-134, 1995.

53. Kimber I: The local lymph node assay. In Marzulli FN, Maibach HI, editors: *Dermatotoxicology methods: the laboratory worker's vade mecum,* Washington, 1998, Taylor & Francis, pp 145-152.

54. Wilkinson DS: Photodermatitis due to tetrachlorosalicylanilide. *Br J Dermatol* 73:213-219, 1961.

55. Kaidbey KH, Kligman AM: Photomaximization test for identifying photallergic contact sensitizers. *Contact Dermatitis* 6:161-169, 1980.

56. Kaidbey K: The evaluation of photoallergic contact sensitizers in humans. In Marzulli FN, Maibach HI, editors: *Dermatotoxicology methods: the laboratory worker's vade mecum,* Washington, 1998, Taylor & Francis, pp 251-258.

57. Maibach HI, Johnson HL: Contact urticaria syndrome: contact urticaria to diethyltoluamide (immediate type hypersensitivity). *Arch Dermatol* 112:1289-1291, 1975.

58. Lahti A: Nonimmunologic contact urticaria. In Amin S, Lahti A, Maibach HI, editors: *Contact urticaria syndrome,* Boca Raton, FL, 1997, CRC Press, pp 5-10.

59. Lauremma A., Maibach HI: Model for immunologic contact urticaria. In Amin S, Lahti A, Maibach HI, editors: *Contact urticaria syndrome,* Boca Raton, FL, 1997, CRC Press, pp 27-32.

60. Bashir SJ, Maibach HI: Pharmacological models for psoriasis syndromes. In Roenigk HH Jr, Maibach HI, editors: *Psoriasis,* ed 3, New York, 1998, Marcel Dekker, pp 715-726.

61. Lauremma AI, Maibach HI: Psoriasis small plaque assay for assessment of topical drug activity. In Roenigk HH Jr, Maibach HI, editors: *Psoriasis,* ed 3, New York, 1998, Marcel Dekker, pp 727-730.

Kenneth B. Gordon
Dennis P. West

Biologic Therapy in Dermatology

With the advent of recombinant deoxyribonucleic acid (DNA) technology, coupled with advances in microbiology and immunology, the field of biologic therapy is expanding rapidly. "Biologic therapies" are defined as proteins that are produced in vitro and made through recombinant DNA techniques. Biologic therapies are now used in clinical practice in many specialties, with dermatology being a primary focus for the development of new agents. In particular, psoriasis has been a target for the development of several new biologic immune modulators. In this chapter the principles that govern the development of these new biologics that have potential as significant new therapies for the treatment of skin disease are reviewed. Emphasis is given to psoriasis, both as an immunologic disease model and as an example of how several biologic therapies impacted this disorder in clinical studies to date.

TYPES OF BIOLOGIC AGENTS

The concept of biologic therapy is not new. Biologic agents are protein drugs designed to imitate or inhibit the actions of naturally occurring proteins. The most familiar biologic therapy to physicians is insulin, which for the past two

decades has been made with the use of recombinant DNA technology for use in patients with diabetes mellitus. In addition, the administration of genetically engineered growth factors has been of significant importance in oncology.[1] Also, genetically engineered immunomodulating biologic agents have been used in solid organ transplantation since the development of antithymocyte globulin and OKT3 for prevention of transplant rejection.[2,3] Drugs used for these earlier studies, including OKT3[4,5] and anti-cluster of differentiation (CD)4 monoclonal antibodies,[6] were also investigated in dermatologic conditions. Thus the concept of biologic agents for the treatment of human disease is well established.

Biologic therapies being developed in dermatology are primarily immunomodulating agents that are designed to alter the immune responses that are the basis for cutaneous diseases such as psoriasis and atopic dermatitis. These agents fall into three basic categories (1) recombinant human cytokines, (2) humanized monoclonal antibodies, and (3) molecular receptors that can bind target molecules.

Recombinant human cytokines are proteins produced in vitro after the genetic sequence of the cytokine has been inserted into a cell line to make large quantities of the protein. These recombinant cytokines can then be given to patients in intravenous, intramuscular, or subcutaneous forms. These agents are capable of duplicating the normal physiologic function of various cytokines.[7,8]

Humanized monoclonal antibodies are the most popular form of biologic therapy in clinical development. Antibodies are proteins that have two components. One component is the fraction antibody binding (Fab) portion that specifically recognizes and binds to part of a target protein. This target could be a cell surface molecule important in disease development or an extracellular protein, such as a cytokine, which may alter the course of the disease. The second component, the fraction crystallizable (Fc) portion, is the part of the antibody that is relatively constant and is recognized by Fc receptors on many cells. The difficulty in designing molecules for therapeutic use is that antibodies with an Fab portion that recognize the

therapeutic human target must be developed in other animals. The human immune system is unlikely to create an immune response against normal human proteins, outside of pathologic conditions such as autoimmune diseases. However, the Fc portions of the molecule derived from a mouse or rabbit will be viewed by the human immune system as a foreign invader and with a physiologic attempt to eliminate this animal-derived protein. To overcome this problem, recombinant DNA technology is used to produce molecules having an Fc fragment that mimics a normal human antibody while maintaining the Fab fraction (the less immunogenic fraction) made by other species.[9-11] These molecules can then be produced in large quantities by various types of cell lines.[12] An example of this type of molecular design is the anti-CD11a molecule (Genentech Corporation) used in the treatment of psoriasis (Figure 50-1, *A*). One interesting variation of this principle is the devel-

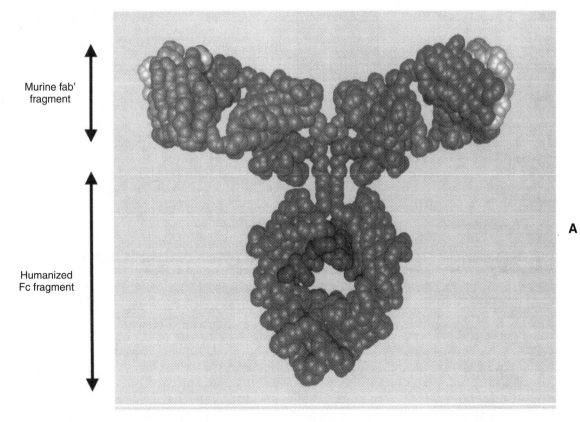

Murine fab' fragment

Humanized Fc fragment

A

Figure 50-1   A, Three-dimensional structure of anti-CD11a molecule demonstrating murine Fab fraction and humanized Fc fraction of IgG. *(Courtesy of Patricia Walicke, M.D., Ph.D., Genentech Corporation.)*

Continued

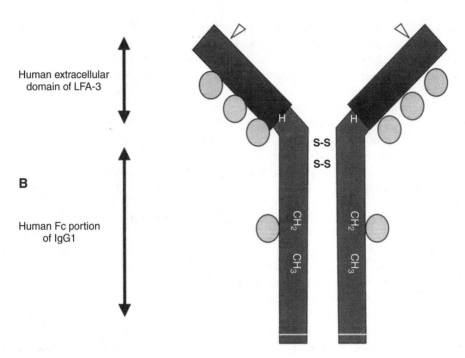

Figure 50-1, cont'd   B, Schematic of LFA-3/TIP molecule demonstrating the extracellular domain of human LFA-3 bound to the Fc portion of human IgG1. *(Courtesy of Daniel Magilavy, M.D., Biogen Corporation.)*

opment of a mouse that produces fully human antibodies, thus eliminating the need to genetically engineer a murine antibody.[13] This technology has been used to create a human antibody against the human IL-8 molecule (Abgenix Corporation).[14]

Another type of biologic therapy is a variation on the use of humanized monoclonal antibodies. Instead of using the Fab portion of a monoclonal antibody developed in an animal, this type of agent uses the natural binding site of the cell surface receptor of the target protein or cytokine to inhibit the target protein.[11] These receptors are often attached to the Fc portion of human immunoglobulin G (IgG) to capitalize on the relatively long half-life of IgG. The drug half-life can therefore be extended and the protein will not be viewed as foreign by the patient's immune system. Because these receptor-based agents use the binding site of the targeted protein, it is possible that cellular signaling events may take place and potentially lead to a different range of activities compared with those seen with the monoclonal antibody approach. One example of a humanized receptor fusion protein is the

lymphocytic function–associated antigen (LFA)-3/TIP molecule (Biogen) used in the treatment of psoriasis (Figure 50-1, *B*).

ADVERSE EFFECTS FROM BIOLOGIC THERAPIES

Unlike nonbiologic therapies, which often have multiple effects on various organ systems, the biologic therapies are targeted to the immune system. Thus if designed properly, the adverse effect profile of biologic agents should be relatively limited. Moreover, the likelihood of drug interactions or metabolic effects often seen with nonbiologic systemic drugs is minimized because biologic therapies mimic naturally occurring proteins and are metabolized similarly to other serum proteins.

Because the biologic medications in development for psoriasis are immunomodulating agents, a primary concern is the potential for immunosuppression. A medication that inhibits T-cell activity by any mechanism can potentially increase patient susceptibility to infections (most commonly viral infections) and the development or exacerbation of certain malignancies.[15] Although one study that measured antibody responses in the context of a biologic agent did show a decrease in T cell–directed antibody production,[16] preliminary studies have not substantiated that the immunosuppressive effects of these medications are clinically significant. Widespread clinical use of these agents will establish the clinical significance of any biologic therapy–induced immunosuppression. Importantly, it is very unlikely that biologic agents will induce a greater degree of immunosuppression than traditional immunosuppresant medications used in dermatology, including corticosteroids, methotrexate, and cyclosporine.

The second major concern of biologic therapy relates to a constellation of symptoms induced by an early biologic therapy, OKT3. The "cytokine release syndrome" consists of fever, headache, abdominal discomfort, and hypotension (which can be severe).[17] This syndrome is believed to be due to OKT3-induced transient activation of T cells through its receptor the CD3 molecule,[18] with subsequent release of large amounts of the cytokines tumor necrosis factor (TNF)-α and interferon (IFN)-γ.[19,20] This reaction is somewhat specific for drugs that may activate T cells in this manner and should not be a significant effect seen with biologic medications that do not act through this specific receptor. Moreover, medications that target and inhibit the CD3 receptor may be designed to decrease the likelihood and severity of cytokine release syndrome.[21,22] Importantly, most of the newer biologic agents do not induce the cytokine release syndrome. Other symptoms, including headache and "flu-like" symptoms, are commonly seen, but these symptoms are generally mild and rarely lead to a discontinuation of therapy.

In the case of recombinant cytokine therapy, it is clear that genetically engineered cytokines have effects similar to naturally occurring proteins.[1] These effects can include transient flu-like symptoms or other short-term cytokine-induced hypersensitivity reactions. However, chronic use of these proteins may have the potential to induce other types of immune dysfunction.[23]

STRATEGIES FOR BIOLOGIC THERAPIES—THE PSORIASIS MODEL

To understand the pharmacologic design and clinical use of these medications, it is helpful to develop a model for the various strategies used in their development. Because psoriasis is presently a major target for biologic therapy, it is helpful to understand the immunology of psoriasis and to understand how immunologic responses might be modified by biologic therapies.

It is generally accepted that psoriasis is an immunologically mediated disease.[24] Significantly, the activity of specific T cells is necessary for induction and propagation of this disease. The centrality of T cells in psoriasis is illustrated by the efficacy of cyclosporine[25,26] for patients with psoriasis, and by animal models demonstrating that activated T cells are able to induce psoriatic plaques.[27]

Immunologic steps in the development of psoriasis are shown in Figure 50-2. The first step is activation of T cells. This activation step requires two different cellular signals that are accomplished through cell-cell interactions between surface proteins on T cells and antigen presenting cells (APC) such as dendritic cells or macrophages (Table 50-1). The "first signal" is the interaction of the T-cell receptor with antigen presented by the APC. Cell surface proteins important to this first signal are listed in Table 50-1. The "second signal" is also called "co-stimulation" and is delivered by a number of surface interactions,[28,29] which likely have slightly different activities.[30,31] Both of these signals are necessary for the initial activation of T cells in psoriasis (Figure 50-3).

Once T cells are activated, they must transit from lymph nodes and the circulation into skin. Specific cell surface proteins on T cells and the vascular endothelium including selectins, integrins, and other adhesion molecules mediate this movement. The best known of these cellular interactions is the relationship between LFA-1 on T cells and intracellular adhesion molecule (ICAM)-1 on endothelial cells. Once in the skin, activated T cells secrete various cytokines that induce the pathologic changes of psoriasis.[32] Cytokines are proteins that are secreted by immune cells and bind to very specific receptors on

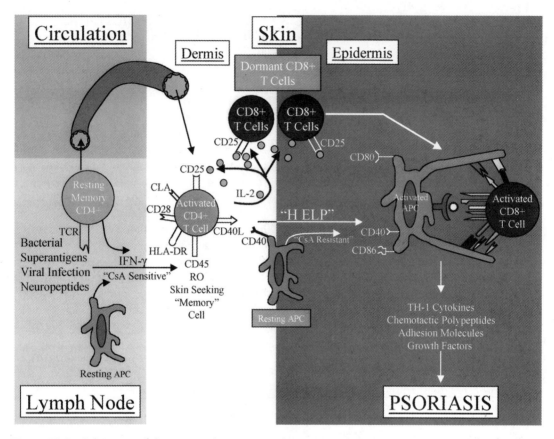

Figure 50-2 Schematic of the immunologic events that govern the initiation and maintenance of psoriasis. *(Nickoloff BJ: Arch Dermatol 135:1104-1110, 1999.)*

■ **Table 50-1   Abbreviations Used in this Chapter**

Anti-CD11a	Monoclonal antibody toward the alpha chain (CD11a) of LFA-1	IL-4	Interleukin-4
		IL-8	Interleukin-8
APC	Antigen presenting cells	IL-10	Interleukin-10
CD2	Cluster of differentiation 2	LFA-1	Lymphocytic function-associated antigen-1
CD3	Cluster of differentiation 3		
CD4	Cluster of differentiation 4	LFA-3	Lymphocytic function-associated antigen-3
CD28	Cluster of differentiation 28		
CTCL	Cutaneous T-cell lymphoma	LFA-3/TIP	Recombinantly-engineered LFA-3/ IgG1 human fusion protein
DAB	Beta subunit of diphtheria toxin		
Fab	Fraction antibody binding	MHC	Major histocompatibility complex
Fc	Fraction crystallizable	PASI	Psoriasis Activity and Severity Index
ICAM	Intercellular adhesion molecule		
ICAM-1	Intercellular adhesion molecule-1	Th1	T helper cells type 1
IFN-α	Interferon alpha	Th2	T helper cells type 2
IFN-γ	Interferon gamma	TNF-α	Tumor necrosis factor alpha
IL-2	Interleukin-2		
IL-2/DAB	Interleukin-2 *combined with* diphtheria toxin beta subunit		

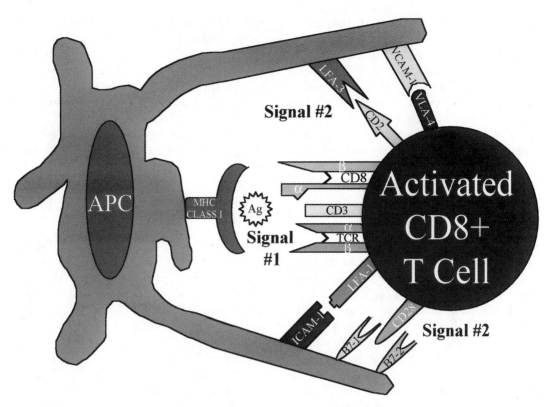

Figure 50-3 Schematic of the cell-cell interactions between an antigen presenting cell (APC) and T cell needed for the stimulation of T cells. Each of these interactions could be a target for biologic therapy. *(Nickoloff BJ:* Arch Dermatol *135:1104-1110, 1999.)*

the cell surface, influencing keratinocytes and other cells to produce the pathology of psoriasis.[33] The specific cytokine profile in psoriasis is known as a T helper cell type 1 (Th1) response[34]; this subset of T cells produces primarily IFN-γ and interleukin (IL)-2.[35] Other local cells, including keratinocytes and local neutrophils, are induced to produce other cytokines, including TNF-α[36,37] and IL-8,[38,39] which are thought to be important in the pathophysiology of psoriasis. All of these cytokines are important in the development of psoriasis and represent possible targets of biologic therapies.

This simplification of the immunology of psoriasis assists in understanding strategies for immunomodulation with biologic therapy. These strategies may be categorized into four basic "strategies": (1) elimination of activated T cells, (2) inhibition of T-cell activation, (3) induction of immune deviation, and (4) inhibition of cytokines. Although the discussion in the next sec-

tion is primarily directed towards psoriasis, the concepts can be applied to a wide variety of immunologically mediated skin diseases.

Strategies for Biologic Therapy of Psoriasis

The basic "strategies" for reducing or eliminating the role of T cells in inducing psoriasis are expanded in the following sections. Although these approaches are central to the treatment of psoriasis, they can be applied to a wide variety of immune-mediated dermatoses.

STRATEGY 1—ELIMINATION OF ACTI-VATED T CELLS.   The most direct method for eliminating the T-cell activity required for psoriasis is to remove the offending T cells. Biologic therapies can be designed to specifically attach to surface markers on activated T cells and eliminate these cells specifically. For example, activated T cells are the primary cells that express high levels of the high affinity IL-2 receptor and also express high levels of important surface markers (such as CD2)[40] involved in co-stimulation. A biologic agent designed to attach to these T cell–specific molecules could be used to induce apoptosis in activated T cells and thus down-regulate the immune response of psoriasis. This could be accomplished by internalization of a "cellular poison" attached to the biologic molecule or through cellular signaling.[41] This strategy was used in the development of denileukin diftitox (Ontak, Ligand Pharmaceuticals), one of the first biologic therapies to show efficacy in psoriasis.[42] Denileukin diftitox is a genetically engineered molecule, which combines the binding site of IL-2 with the β-subunit of diphtheria toxin. When IL-2 binds to its receptor as expressed on T cells, the receptor and the agent are internalized into the cell. When this molecule is internalized, the diphtheria toxin is released and kills the offending cell.[43] Elimination of the activated T cells that drive psoriasis may provide significant advantages over other forms of therapy. Most importantly, it could induce more lasting remissions of the disease because it takes time to repopulate the epidermis and dermis with activated T cells. Some data suggest that the selectivity of agents using this strategy might extend to selective elimination of Th1 cells that are most active in psoriasis.[44] A potential weakness in this strategy is that despite the relative selectivity, T cells not related to psoriasis may also be eliminated, thereby giving these agents a generalized immunosuppressive effect.

STRATEGY 2—INHIBITION OF T-CELL ACTIVATION.   A second strategy employed by biologic agents has been to block the initiation of T-cell activity. Because T cells remain active after stimulation for about 14 days, it is clear that T cells must continuously be reactivated for the persistence of psoriatic plaques. For both the initial stimulation of new T cells and restimulation of recently activated T cells, the APC–T cell interaction requires both signal 1 and signal 2. Biologic therapies have been developed to block almost all of the well-defined APC–T cell interactions including (signal 1) major histocompatibility complex (MHC)/CD3 or MHC/CD4 and (signal 2) B7/CD28, ICAM-1/LFA-1,

and LFA-3/CD2. If these molecules are successful in blocking these interactions, they could effectively reduce the immune response that is driving psoriasis. One potentially important aspect of this strategy may be the blockade of T-cell migration into the skin. Because many of the same molecules intrinsic to the APC–T cell interaction also govern T-cell migration into the skin (most notably ICAM-1 and LFA-1), it may be possible to treat psoriasis and other immunologic disease states by inhibiting migration of these cells to the skin through blockade with various biologic therapies (Table 50-2).

STRATEGY 3—INDUCTION OF IMMUNE DEVIATION.   A third technique used in biologic therapy is immune deviation.[45] In contrast to the previous mechanisms that use an antibody or receptor to block T-cell function, this strategy utilizes a cytokine to influence the activity of pathogenic T cells.[46] This strategy exploits the dual population of T cells that drive immune-mediated diseases such as psoriasis. T cells in psoriasis primarily secrete Th1 cytokines, IFN-γ and IL-2. These cytokines induce release of other cytokines, such as TNF-α, which in turn have a significant role in the pathology of psoriasis. T helper cell type 2 (Th2) cytokines, such as IL-4, IL-10,[47] and IL-11,[48,49] act to down-regulate Th1 T cells.[50,51] Thus administration of Th2 cytokines should theoretically down-regulate the Th1 cytokines and inhibit formation and persistence of psoriatic plaques. Both

■ **Table 50-2**   Immunologic Components of Signal 1 and Signal 2

	Antigen Presenting Cell	T cell
Signal 1	MHC-antigen complex	T-cell receptor CD3
	MHC-I	CD8
	MHC-II	CD4
Signal 2	B7-1 or B7-2	CD28
	ICAM-1	LFA-1
	LFA-3	CD2
	CD40	CD40 ligand

IL-10[52,53] and IL-11[49,54] have been studied for treatment of psoriasis.

STRATEGY 4—INHIBITION OF CYTOKINES.

A fourth strategy that can be exploited by biologic therapy is the elimination of cytokines, which may be important in the development of psoriasis.[55] Cytokines have significant effector functions in psoriasis, but may be eliminated after release by T cells or other immunologically active cells with a role in psoriasis. It might be possible to alter the course of psoriasis by binding these cytokines and eliminating their biologic activity. For example, IL-8 is produced by keratinocytes and neutrophils in large quantities in psoriasis.[56] IL-8 is a chemokine, a molecule that attracts immune cells into psoriatic skin[38] and may play a role in the development of the proliferative vasculature typically found in psoriasis.[57] As a result, binding of IL-8 with biologic therapies could inhibit chemotaxis of the immune cells that induce psoriasis. Other cytokines that might be amenable to this strategy would be IFN-α and TNF-γ.[58,59]

BIOLOGIC THERAPY FOR PSORIASIS

Because much of the information on biologic agents for psoriasis is theoretic, it is helpful to use a few clinical examples to illustrate this discussion. Selected biologic agents in clinical development for psoriasis are listed in Table 50-3. Two biologic agents are in their final stages of testing for use in psoriasis, LFA-3/TIP (Biogen) and anti-CD11a (Genentech). These two agents are briefly reviewed to demonstrate the rationale behind their efficacy in psoriasis. It is important to note that these two agents, though seemingly quite similar, may utilize different biologic strategies that potentially result in subtle, though important, differences in clinical outcome.

LFA-3/TIP

One of the main co-stimulatory signals for T cells is binding of LFA-3 from an APC to CD2 on activated T cells. LFA-3/TIP is a genetically engineered protein that attaches the binding site of LFA-3 to the constant region of a human IgG

(Figure 50-1, *B*). This molecule binds to CD2 on the surface of T cells through the LFA-3 portion, thereby blocking activity of this molecule. The complex is relatively protected from the immunologic responses of the patient because the majority of the molecule appears to the immune system as a normal human antibody. LFA-3/TIP was originally designed to work via blockade of the co-stimulatory signal as described in strategy 2. However, it has been shown in early studies that treatment with this drug decreases the numbers of activated or memory T cells[61] in the circulation and thus might also work by strategy 1, with elimination of the T cells that are driving psoriasis.

In early trials, approximately 60% of the patients treated with LFA-3/TIP showed greater than 50% improvement in the Psoriasis Activity and Severity Index (PASI) and 33% showed at least a 75% improvement in PASI in the optimal dose range. The mean decrease in PASI was 53%. Patients also tolerated this medication with few adverse effects; there was not a significant increase in clinically important infections.[60] Importantly, patients who cleared or almost cleared, based on physicians' global assessment, remained clear for a mean of almost 8 months. These data suggest that the elimination of potentially active T cells might induce longer-term remissions than those from traditional systemic therapy in psoriasis. The potential for LFA-3/TIP–prolonged remissions in psoriasis is a significant advantage for this biologic therapy. However, it is also possible that the relative immunosuppression induced by the elimination of memory or activated T cells would recover more slowly, compared with the recovery if these populations of T cells were simply inhibited by the drug.

Anti-CD11a

CD11a is part of the complex of surface molecules that make up LFA-1, the primary binding site for ICAM-1. The LFA-1/ICAM-1 interaction has an important role in both co-stimulation of activated T cells for migration of various immune cells into the skin. The anti-CD11a molecule is a humanized monoclonal antibody that blocks this LFA-1/ICAM-1 interaction.[16] Thus this molecule should work at the activation and migration phase of T-cell activity in

Table 50-3   Selected Biologic Agents for Psoriasis

Immunologic Name	Brand Name	Generic Name	Company	Molecular Design	Proposed Mechanism	References
STRATEGY 1						
LFA-3/TIP	Amevive		Biogen	Immunoglobulin/receptor fusion protein	Binds to CD2 to block co-stimulation. May also eliminate memory and activated T cells	56, 57
IL-2/DAB	Ontak	Denileukin diftitox	Ligand Pharmaceuticals	Cytokine/toxin fusion protein	Introduces β-subunit of diphtheria toxin into activated T cells, eliminates activated T cells	
Anti-CD3a (HuM291)	Nuvion	Visilizumab	Protein Design Labs	Humanized monoclonal antibody	Binds to activated T cells and induces apoptosis	19, 58
STRATEGY 2						
Anti-CD11a			Genentech/Xoma (United States) LLC	Humanized monoclonal antibody	Blocks LFA-1/ICAM-1 interactions, inhibiting co-stimulation and T cell migration into skin	13, 59
Anti-B7-1			IDEC Pharmaceuticals	Humanized monoclonal antibody	Blocks B7/CD28 interaction and inhibits co-stimulation	60
Anti-CD25	Zenapax	Daclizumab	Protein Design Labs	Humanized monoclonal antibody	Blocks IL-2 receptor and potential T cell growth	61-64
CTLA-4/Ig			Bristol-Myers/Squibb	Immunoglobulin/receptor fusion protein	Binds to B7 and blocks co-stimulation	65

Agent	Brand name	Generic name	Manufacturer	Type	Mechanism	References
STRATEGY 3						
rIL-10				Recombinant cytokine	Induces Th2 type differentiation in activated T cells	48, 66, 67
rIL-11	Neumega	Oprelvekin	Genetics Institute	Recombinant cytokine	Induces Th2 type differentiation in activated T cells	45, 50
STRATEGY 4						
Anti-IL-8 (ABX-0204)			Abgenix	Human monoclonal antibody	Blocks activity of IL-8, inhibiting immune cell migration into the skin and angiogenesis	11
Anti-TNF-α	Remicade	Infliximab	Centocor	Humanized monoclonal antibody	Binds to and blocks activity of TNF-α, decreasing immune activity	55, 68
Anti-TNF-α	Embrel	Etanercept	Immunex	Immunoglobulin/receptor fusion protein	Binds to and blocks activity of TNF-α, decreasing immune activity	69

DAB, β-Subunit of diphtheria toxin.

psoriasis, thus strategy 2. Unlike LFA-3/TIP, there is no evidence of elimination of pathogenic T cells. Though activated T cells are viable, this inhibition of activation and migration of T cells results in immunosuppression similar to that achieved by LFA-3/TIP. However, it follows that anti-CD11a therapy would not likely produce prolonged remission of psoriatic activity.

Clinical trials of anti-CD11a have shown significant promise with this medication. There is an approximately 60% reduction of PASI scores in patients treated with this medication. In the optimal dose group, 62% of patients had a greater than 50% decrease in PASI while 30% had a decrease of greater than 75%. In addition, there has been no increase in clinically significant infections. Other adverse effects include headache and flu-like symptoms, which seem to lessen with continued administration of the medication.[63]

OTHER POTENTIAL INDICATIONS FOR BIOLOGIC THERAPY IN DERMATOLOGY

Psoriasis has been the primary focus in the development of biologic therapy for cutaneous diseases because this dermatosis affects a relatively large percentage of the population, has a well-established immunologic pathogenesis, and lacks definitive treatment for patients with severe disease. However, a number of other skin diseases are also appropriate targets for biologic therapy.

Atopic Dermatitis
Analogous to psoriasis, atopic dermatitis is primarily a T cell–mediated disease that should respond to T cell–directed biologic therapies. In contrast to psoriasis, atopic dermatitis is primarily a Th2-mediated disease. The primary strategy for biologic therapy for atopic dermatitis has been induction of immune deviation (strategy 3) by treatment with recombinant IFN-γ. This strategy has shown mixed results in clinical trials and is not as well advanced as biologic therapy for psoriasis.[74-78]

Cutaneous T-Cell Lymphoma
Cutaneous T-cell lymphoma (CTCL) is a malignant proliferation of immune cells that migrate to the skin. This condition should be amenable to treatment with strategy 1, the elimination of the offending T cells; in this case the goal of therapy is elimination of the malignant T-cell clone. Biologic therapy using this strategy is in commercial use as denileukin diftitox in the treatment of CTCL. Similar to its use in psoriasis, denileukin diftitox is internalized into activated T cells expressing the high affinity IL-2 receptor, including the malignant T cells in CTCL. This internalization and subsequent release of diphtheria toxin kills the offending malignant cell.[79-81]

SUMMARY

Biologic therapy in dermatology is emerging as an important approach to treatment. Various biologic therapies are being established as viable alternatives in the treatment of a wide variety of immune-mediated and malignant conditions of the skin. Biologic therapy holds the promise of incorporating new insights, regarding the pathophysiology of cutaneous diseases combined with rationally designed drugs using basic immune principles, to treat these conditions in a safe and effective manner.

Bibliograpy

Bonifati C, Ameglio F: Cytokines in psoriasis. *Int J Dermatol* 38:241-251, 1999.

McNiece IK: New cytokines and their clinical application. *Cancer Treat Res* 101:389-405, 1999.

Nickoloff BJ: The immunologic and genetic basis of psoriasis. *Arch Dermatol* 135:1104-1110, 1999.

Vial T, Descotes J: Immune-mediated side-effects of cytokines in humans. *Toxicology* 105:31-57, 1995.

References

Types of Biologic Agents

1. Crawford J, Foote M, Morstyn G: Hematopoietic growth factors in cancer chemotherapy. *Cancer Chemother Biol Response Modif* 18:250-267, 1999.
2. Carrier M, Jenicek M, Pelletier LC: Value of monoclonal antibody OKT3 in solid organ transplantation: a meta-analysis. *Transplant Proc* 24:2586-2591, 1992.
3. Chatenoud L, Bach JF: Selective immunosuppression with anti-T cell monoclonal antibodies. *Clin Nephrol* 38(Suppl 1):S53-S60, 1992.
4. Berger CL, Kung P, Goldstein G, et al: Use of Orthoclone monoclonal antibodies in the study of selected dermatologic conditions. *Int J Immunopharmacol* 3:275-282, 1981.
5. Weinshenker BG, Bass BH, Ebers GC, et al: Remission of psoriatic lesions with muromonab-CD3 (orthoclone OKT3) treatment. *J Am Acad Dermatol* 20:1132-1133, 1989.
6. Rizova H, Nicolas JF, Morel P, et al: The effect of anti-CD4 monoclonal antibody treatment on immunopathological changes in psoriatic skin. *J Dermatol Sci* 7:1-13, 1994.
7. McNiece IK: New cytokines and their clinical application. *Cancer Treat Res* 101:389-405, 1999.
8. Schuh JC, Morrissey PJ: Development of a recombinant growth factor and fusion protein: lessons from GM-CSF. *Toxicol Pathol* 27:72-77, 1999.
9. Stigbrand T, Ahlstrom KR, Sundstrom B, et al: Alternative technologies to generate monoclonal antibodies. *Acta Oncol* 32:841-844, 1993.
10. Choy EH: Clinical pharmacology and therapeutic potential of monoclonal antibody treatment in rheumatoid arthritis. *Drugs Aging* 12:139-148, 1998.
11. Parren PW: Preparation of genetically engineered monoclonal antibodies for human immunotherapy. *Hum Antibodies Hybridomas* 3:137-145, 1992.
12. Neri D, Petrul H, Roncucci G: Engineering recombinant antibodies for immunotherapy. *Cell Biophys* 27:47-61, 1995.
13. Bruggemann M, Neuberger MS: Strategies for expressing human antibody repertoires in transgenic mice. *Immunol Today* 17:391-397, 1996.
14. Lohner ME, Krueger JG, Gottlieb A, et al: Clinical trials of a fully human anti-IL-8 antibody for the treatment of psoriasis (abstract). *Br J Dermatol* 141:989, 1999.

Adverse Effects

15. Dunn DL: Problems related to immunosuppression. Infection and malignancy occurring after solid organ transplantation. *Crit Care Clin* 6:955-977, 1990.
16. Gottlieb A, Krueger JG, Bright R, et al: Effects of administration of a single dose of a humanized monoclonal antibody to CD11a on the immunobiology and clinical activity of psoriasis. *J Am Acad Dermatol* 42:428-435, 2000.
17. Norman DJ, Chatenoud L, Cohen D, et al: Consensus statement regarding OKT3-induced cytokine-release syndrome and human antimouse antibodies. *Transplant Proc* 25:89-92, 1993.
18. Vossen AC, Tibbe GJ, Kroos MJ, et al: Fc receptor binding of anti-CD3 monoclonal antibodies is not essential for immunosuppression, but triggers cytokine-related side effects. *Eur J Immunol* 25:1492-1496, 1995.
19. Chatenoud L, Ferran C, Legendre C, et al: In vivo cell activation following OKT3 administration. Systemic cytokine release and modulation by corticosteroids. *Transplantation* 49:697-702, 1990.
20. Gaston RS, Deierhoi MH, Patterson T, et al: OKT3 first-dose reaction: association with T cell subsets and cytokine release. *Kidney Int* 39:141-148, 1991.
21. Cole MS, Anasetti C, Tso JY: Human IgG2 variants of chimeric anti-CD3 are nonmitogenic to T cells. *J Immunol* 159:3613-3621, 1997.
22. Cole MS, Stellrecht KE, Shi JD, et al: HuM291, a humanized anti-CD3 antibody, is immunosuppressive to T cells while exhibiting reduced mitogenicity in vitro. *Transplantation* 68:563-571, 1999.
23. Vial T, Descotes J: Immune-mediated side-effects of cytokines in humans. *Toxicology* 105:31-57, 1995.

Strategies for Biologic Therapies— the Psoriasis Model

24. Nickoloff BJ: The immunologic and genetic basis of psoriasis. *Arch Dermatol* 135:1104-1110, 1999.

25. Lebwohl M, Ellis C, Gottlieb A, et al: Cyclosporine consensus conference: with emphasis on the treatment of psoriasis (see comments). *J Am Acad Dermatol* 39:464-475, 1998.

26. Mozzanica N, Pigatto PD, Finzi AF: Cyclosporin in psoriasis: pathophysiology and experimental data. *Dermatology* 187(Suppl 1):3-7, 1993.

27. Wrone-Smith T, Nickoloff BJ: Dermal injection of immunocytes induces psoriasis (see comments). *J Clin Invest* 98:1878-1887, 1996.

28. Damle NK, Klussman K, Linsley PS, et al: Differential costimulatory effects of adhesion molecules B7, ICAM-1, LFA-3, and VCAM-1 on resting and antigen-primed CD4+ T lymphocytes. *J Immunol* 148:1985-1992, 1992.

29. Geppert TD, Lipsky PE: Activation of T lymphocytes by immobilized monoclonal antibodies to CD3. Regulatory influences of monoclonal antibodies to additional T cell surface determinants. *J Clin Invest* 81:1497-1505, 1988.

30. Parra E, Wingren AG, Hedlund G, et al: Costimulation of human CD4+ T lymphocytes with B7 and lymphocyte function-associated antigen-3 results in distinct cell activation profiles. *J Immunol* 153:2479-2487, 1994.

31. Wingren AG, Parra E, Varga M, et al: T cell activation pathways: B7, LFA-3, and ICAM-1 shape unique T cell profiles. *Crit Rev Immunol* 15:235-253, 1995.

32. Bonifati C, Ameglio F: Cytokines in psoriasis. *Int J Dermatol* 38:241-251, 1999.

33. Bata-Csorgo Z, Hammerberg C, Voorhees JJ, et al: Intralesional T-lymphocyte activation as a mediator of psoriatic epidermal hyperplasia. *J Invest Dermatol* 105:89S-94S, 1995.

34. Schlaak JF, Buslau M, Jochum W, et al: T cells involved in psoriasis vulgaris belong to the Th1 subset. *J Invest Dermatol* 102:145-149, 1994.

35. Ferenczi K, Burack L, Pope M, et al: CD69, HLA-DR and the IL-2R identify persistently activated T cells in psoriasis vulgaris lesional skin: blood and skin comparisons by flow cytometry. *J Autoimmun* 14:63-78, 2000.

36. Ettehadi P, Greaves MW, Wallach D, et al: Elevated tumor necrosis factor-alpha (TNF-alpha) biological activity in psoriatic skin lesions. *Clin Exp Immunol* 96:146-151, 1994.

37. Mussi A, Bonifati C, Carducci M, et al: Serum TNF-alpha levels correlate with disease severity and are reduced by effective therapy in plaque-type psoriasis. *J Biol Regul Homeost Agents* 11:115-118, 1997.

38. Barker JN, Jones ML, Mitra RS, et al: Modulation of keratinocyte-derived interleukin-8 which is chemotactic for neutrophils and T lymphocytes. *Am J Pathol* 139:869-876, 1991.

39. Biasi D, Carletto A, Caramaschi P, et al: Neutrophil functions and IL-8 in psoriatic arthritis and in cutaneous psoriasis. *Inflammation* 22:533-543, 1998.

Four Specific Strategies for Biologic Therapy

40. Schraven B, Samstag Y, Altevogt P, et al: Association of CD2 and CD45 on human T lymphocytes. *Nature* 345:71-74, 1990.

41. Panchal RG: Novel therapeutic strategies to selectively kill cancer cells. *Biochem Pharmacol* 55:247-252, 1998.

42. Gottlieb SL, Gilleaudeau P, Johnson R, et al: Response of psoriasis to a lymphocyte-selective toxin (DAB389IL-2) suggests a primary immune, but not keratinocyte, pathogenic basis. *Nat Med* 1:442-447, 1995.

43. Waters CA, Snider CE, Itoh K, et al: DAB486IL-2 (IL-2 toxin) selectively inactivates high-affinity IL-2 receptor-bearing human peripheral blood mononuclear cells. *Ann N Y Acad Sci* 636:403-405, 1991.

44. Reinke P, Schwinzer H, Hoflich C, et al: Selective in vivo deletion of alloactivated TH1 cells by OKT3 monoclonal antibody in acute rejection. *Immunol Lett* 57:151-153, 1997.

45. Finkelman FD: Relationships among antigen presentation, cytokines, immune deviation, and autoimmune disease (comment). *J Exp Med* 182:279-282, 1995.

46. Ruuls SR, Sedgwick JD: Cytokine-directed therapies in multiple sclerosis and experimental autoimmune encephalomyelitis. *Immunol Cell Biol* 76:65-73, 1998.

47. Seifert M, Sterry W, Effenberger E, et al: The antipsoriatic activity of IL-10 is rather caused by effects on peripheral blood cells than by a direct effect on human keratinocytes. *Arch Dermatol Res* 292:164-172, 2000.

48. Schwertschlag US, Trepicchio WL, Dykstra KH, et al: Hematopoietic, immunomodulatory and epithelial effects of interleukin-11. *Leukemia* 13:1307-1315, 1999.

49. Trepicchio WL, Ozawa M, Walters IB, et al: IL-11 is an immune-modulatory cytokine which downregulates IL-12, type 1 cytokines, and multiple inflammation-associated genes in patients with psoriasis (abstract). *Br J Dermatol* 141:976, 2000.

50. Adorini L, Trembleau S: Immune deviation towards Th2 inhibits Th-1-mediated autoimmune diabetes. *Biochem Soc Trans* 25:625-629, 1997.

51. Asadullah K, Sabat R, Wiese A, et al: Interleukin-10 in cutaneous disorders: implications for its pathophysiological importance and therapeutic use. *Arch Dermatol Res* 291:628-636, 1999.

52. Asadullah K, Docke WD, Ebeling M, et al: Interleukin 10 treatment of psoriasis: clinical results of a phase 2 trial. *Arch Dermatol* 135:187-192, 1999.

53. Asadullah K, Sterry W, Ebeling M, et al: Clinical and immunological effects of IL-10 therapy in psoriasis (abstract). *Br J Dermatol* 141:989, 1999.

54. Trepicchio WL, Ozawa M, Walters IB, et al: Interleukin-11 therapy selectively downregulates type I cytokine proinflammatory pathways in psoriasis lesions (published erratum appears in *J Clin Invest* 105(3):396, 2000). *J Clin Invest* 104:1527-1537, 1999.

55. Kemeny L, Michel G, Dobozy A, et al: Cytokine system as potential target for antipsoriatic therapy. *Exp Dermatol* 3:1-8, 1994.

56. Sticherling M, Sautier W, Schroder JM, et al: Interleukin-8 plays its role at local level in psoriasis vulgaris. *Acta Derm Venereol* 79:4-8, 1999.

57. Nickoloff BJ, Mitra RS, Varani J, et al: Aberrant production of interleukin-8 and thrombospondin-1 by psoriatic keratinocytes mediates angiogenesis. *Am J Pathol* 144:820-828, 1994.

58. Feldman M, Taylor P, Paleolog E, et al: Anti-TNF alpha therapy is useful in rheumatoid arthritis and Crohn's disease: analysis of the mechanism of action predicts utility in other diseases. *Transplant Proc* 30:4126-4127, 1998.

59. Oh CJ, Das KM, Gottlieb AB: Treatment with anti-tumor necrosis factor alpha (TNF-alpha) monoclonal antibody dramatically decreases the clinical activity of psoriasis lesions. *J Am Acad Dermatol* 42:829-830, 2000.

LFA-3/TIP and Anti-CD11a

60. Krueger G: Phase II trial results of Amevive (LFA3TIP) in patients with chronic plaque psoriasis (abstract). *Br J Dermatol* 141:979, 1999.

61. Magilavy D, Kruger GG: The response of chronic plaque psoriasis to Amevive (LFA3TIP) and the selective suppression of peripheral memory/effector T cells (CD45RO+) versus naive T cells (CD45RA+) is linked to serum levels of LFA3TIP (abstract). *J Invest Dermatol* 114:776, 2000.

62. Hsu DH, Shi JD, Homola M, et al: A humanized anti-CD3 antibody, HuM291, with low mitogenic activity, mediates complete and reversible T-cell depletion in chimpanzees. *Transplantation* 68:545-554, 1999.

63. Gottlieb A, Miller B, Chaudhari U, et al: Clinical and histologic effects of subcutaneously administered anti-CD11a (hu1124) in patients with psoriasis (abstract). *J Invest Dermatol* 114:840, 2000.

Other Biologic Therapies Under Investigation

64. Gottlieb A, Abdulghani A, Totoritis R, et al: Results of a single-dose, dose-escalating trial of an anti-B7 monoclonal antibody (IDEC-114) in patients with psoriasis (abstract). *J Invest Dermatol* 114:840, 2000.

65. Beniaminovitz A, Itescu S, Lietz K, et al: Prevention of rejection in cardiac transplantation by blockade of the interleukin-2 receptor with a monoclonal antibody (see comments). *N Engl J Med* 342:613-619, 2000.

66. Ekberg H, Backman L, Tufveson G, et al: Zenapax (daclizumab) reduces the incidence of acute rejection episodes and improves patient survival following renal transplantation. No 14874 and No 14393 Zenapax Study Groups. *Transplant Proc* 31:267-268, 1999.

67. Przepiorka D, Kernan NA, Ippoliti C, et al: Daclizumab, a humanized anti-interleukin-2 receptor alpha chain antibody, for treatment of acute graft-versus-host disease. *Blood* 95:83-89, 2000.

68. Vincenti F, Nashan B, Light S: Daclizumab: outcome of phase III trials and mechanism of action. Double therapy and the triple therapy study groups. *Transplant Proc* 30:2155-2158, 1998.

69. Abrams JR, Lebwohl MG, Guzzo CA, et al: CTLA4Ig-mediated blockade of T-cell costimulation in patients with psoriasis vulgaris. *J Clin Invest* 103:1243-1252, 1999.

70. Asadullah K, Sterry W, Stephanek K, et al: IL-10 is a key cytokine in psoriasis. Proof of principle by IL-10 therapy: a new therapeutic approach. *J Clin Invest* 101:783-794, 1998.

71. Reich K, Hilmes D, Middel P, et al: Treatment of psoriasis with interleukin-10 downregulates the epidermal interleukin-8/CXC-2 pathway (abstract). *Br J Dermatol* 141:980, 1999.

72. Markham A, Lamb HM: Infliximab: a review of its use in the management of rheumatoid arthritis *Drugs* 59:1341-1359, 2000.

73. Weinblatt ME, Kremer JM, Bankhurst AD, et al: A trial of etanercept, a recombinant tumor necrosis factor receptor:Fc fusion protein, in patients with rheumatoid arthritis receiving methotrexate (see comments). *N Engl J Med* 340:253-259, 1999.

Biologic Therapy for Atopic Dermatitis

74. Boguniewicz M, Jaffe HS, Izu A, et al: Recombinant gamma interferon in treatment of patients with atopic dermatitis and elevated IgE levels. *Am J Med* 88:365-370, 1990.

75. Hanifin JM, Schneider LC, Leung DY, et al: Recombinant interferon gamma therapy for atopic dermatitis. *J Am Acad Dermatol* 28:189-197, 1993.

76. Reinhold U, Kukel S, Brzoska J, et al: Systemic interferon gamma treatment in severe atopic dermatitis. *J Am Acad Dermatol* 29:58-63, 1993.

77. Musial J, Milewski M, Undas A, et al: Interferon-gamma in the treatment of atopic dermatitis: influence on T-cell activation. *Allergy* 50:520-523, 1995.

78. Jang IG, Yang JK, Lee HJ, et al: Clinical improvement and immunohistochemical findings in severe atopic dermatitis treated with interferon gamma. *J Am Acad Dermatol* 42:1033-1040, 2000.

Biologic Therapy for CTCL

79. Hesketh P, Caguioa P, Koh H, et al: Clinical activity of a cytotoxic fusion protein in the treatment of cutaneous T-cell lymphoma. *J Clin Oncol* 11:1682-1690, 1993.

80. Foss FM, Borkowski TA, Gilliom M, et al: Chimeric fusion protein toxin DAB486IL-2 in advanced mycosis fungoides and the Sézary syndrome: correlation of activity and interleukin-2 receptor expression in a phase II study. *Blood* 84:1765-1774, 1994.

81. Kuzel TM, Rosen ST, Gordon LI, et al: Phase I trial of the diphtheria toxin/interleukin-2 fusion protein DAB486IL-2: efficacy in mycosis fungoides and other non-Hodgkin's lymphomas. *Leuk Lymphoma* 11:369-377, 1993.

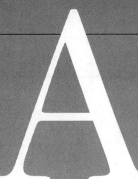

Systemic Drug Costs

Generic	Trade	Dose	AWP Generic	Pricing Method	AWP Trade	Pricing Method
PENICILLINS						
Penicillin V	Pen Vee K, V-cillin K	250 mg	0.17	A	0.06	C
		500 mg	0.13		0.09	
Amoxicillin	Amoxil, Polymox	250 mg	0.22	C	0.08	D
		500 mg	0.39		0.32	
Dicloxacillin	Dynapen	250 mg	0.54	B	0.38	C
		500 mg	1.15		0.66	
Amoxicillin/clavulanate	Augmentin	500 mg	—	n/a	3.56	C
		875 mg	—		4.75	
CEPHALOSPORINS						
Cephalexin	Keflex, Keftabs	250 mg	0.54	B	1.58	B
		500 mg	1.07		3.11	
Cephradine	Velosef, Anspor	250 mg	0.55	D	0.89	B
		500 mg	1.31		1.75	
Cefadroxil	Duracef, Ultracef	500 mg	3.31	n/a	2.77	D
		1000 mg	—		7.14	
Cefaclor	Ceclor, Extended release	250 mg	2.01	n/a	1.19	D
		375 mg	—		4.00	
Loracarbef	Lorabid (pulvules)	200 mg	—	n/a	4.00	C
		400 mg	—		5.00	
Cefprozil	Cefzil	250 mg	—	n/a	3.30	B
		500 mg	—		6.54	
Cefuroxime axetil	Ceftin	250 mg	—	n/a	7.08	C
		500 mg	—		7.43	
Cefpodoxime proxetil	Vantin	100 mg	—	n/a	3.05	C
		200 mg	—		4.03	
Ceftibutin	Cedax	400 mg	—	n/a	7.42	n/a
Cefixime	Suprax	200 mg	—	n/a	3.75	B
		400 mg	—		7.35	

A special acknowledgment to Crystal S. Blankenship, Kristen Hummer, Sonya J. Keinath, and Andrea K. LaRoche for their work on this appendix.

AWP, Average wholesale price; *A*, unity: price same regardless of drug dose (within 5% range); *B*, linear: price per mg same regardless of drug dose (within 5% range); *C*, logarithmic: price per mg least with larger doses; *D*, inverse: price per mg least with lower doses.

Continued

Generic	Trade	Dose	AWP Generic	Pricing Method	AWP Trade	Pricing Method
MACROLIDES						
Azithromycin	Zithromax	250 mg	—	n/a	6.76	B
		600 mg	—		16.21	
Clarithromycin	Biaxin	250 mg	—	n/a	3.52	A
		500 mg	—		3.52	
Erythromycin base	Eryc	250 mg	0.26	n/a	0.52	A
	E-mycin	333 mg	—		0.51	
Erythromycin estolate	Ilosone	250 mg	0.32	n/a	0.32	n/a
Erythromycin ethyl succinate	EES	400 mg	0.28	n/a	0.24	n/a
FLUOROQUINOLONES						
Ciprofloxacin	Cipro	500 mg	—	n/a	4.15	A
		750 mg	—		4.15	
Levofloxacin	Levoquin	250 mg	—	n/a	7.31	C
		500 mg	—		8.54	
Sparfloxacin	Zagam	200 mg	—	n/a	6.69	n/a
Enoxacin	Pentrex	200 mg	—	n/a	3.27	C
		400 mg	—		3.43	
Gatifloxacin	Tequin	200 mg	—	n/a	7.03	A
		400 mg	—		7.03	
Lomefloxacin	Maxaquin	400 mg	—	n/a	6.94	n/a
Moxefloxacin	Avelox	400 mg	—	n/a	8.71	n/a
Norfloxacin	Noroxin	400 mg	—	n/a	3.81	n/a
Ofloxacin	Floxin	200 mg	—	n/a	3.94	C
		400 mg	—		4.95	
TETRACYCLINES						
Tetracycline	Sumycin	250 mg	0.08	C	0.06	B
		500 mg	0.13		0.11	
Minocycline	Minocin, Dynacin	50 mg	1.39	C	2.09	C
		100 mg	1.87		3.48	
Doxycycline hyclate	Vibramycin, Vibratabs	50 mg	2.69	A	2.28	C
		100 mg	2.59		4.09	
Doxycycline monohydrate	Monodox	50 mg	—	n/a	1.22	C
		100 mg	—		1.92	
OTHER ANTIBACTERIAL AGENTS						
Rifampin	Rifadin, Rimactane	150 mg	1.34	C	1.90	A
		300 mg	2.18		1.93	
Trimethoprim/ sulfamethoxazole	Septra DS Bactrim DS	160 mg/ 800 mg	0.37	n/a	1.29	n/a
					1.03	
Clindamycin	Cleocin	150 mg	0.78	n/a	1.79	B
		300 mg	—		3.56	

AWP, Average wholesale price; *A*, unity: price same regardless of drug dose (within 5% range); *B*, linear: price per mg same regardless of drug dose (within 5% range); *C*, logarithmic: price per mg least with larger doses; *D*, inverse: price per mg least with lower doses.

Generic	Trade	Dose	AWP Generic	Pricing Method	AWP Trade	Pricing Method
ANTIFUNGAL AGENTS						
Terbinafine	Lamisil	250 mg	—	n/a	7.65	n/a
Itraconazole	Sporanox	100 mg	—		7.07	n/a
Fluconazole	Diflucan	150 mg	—	n/a	11.89	C
		200 mg	—		12.22	
Griseofluvin	Gris-PEG	125 mg	0.34	C	0.58	B
		250 mg	0.61		1.08	
(ultramicrosize)	Fulvicin P/G	165 mg	—	n/a	0.78	C
		330 mg	0.80		1.34	
(microsize)	Grifulvin V	250 mg	—	n/a	—	n/a
		500 mg	1.32		1.41	
Ketoconazole	Nizoral	200 mg	3.01	n/a	3.51	n/a
ANTIVIRAL AGENTS						
Acyclovir	Zovirax	400 mg	0.35	D	2.92	C
		800 mg	3.80		5.39	
Valacyclovir	Valtrex	500 mg	—	n/a	3.44	n/a
Famciclovir	Famvir	125 mg	—	n/a	3.02	C
		500 mg			7.03	
CORTICOSTEROIDS						
Oral						
Prednisone	Deltasone	5 mg	0.10	B	0.06	A
		20 mg	0.16		0.07	
Prednisolone	None	5 mg	0.09	n/a	—	n/a
Methylprednisolone	Medrol	4 mg	0.69	n/a	0.83	C
		16 mg	—		1.81	
Intramuscular						
Triamcinolone diacetate	Aristocort	25 mg/ml	—	n/a	4.06	n/a
Triamcinolone acetonide	Kenalog	10 mg/ml	—	n/a	1.53	C
		40 mg/ml	2.99		5.86	
IMMUNOSUPPRESSANTS						
Methotrexate						
Methotrexate	None	2.5 mg	3.06	n/a	—	n/a
	Rheumatrex (pack of 3)	2.5 mg	—	n/a	4.47	n/a
	None	25 mg/ml	5.78	n/a	—	n/a
Azathioprine and Related Drugs						
Azathioprine	Imuran	50 mg	1.31	n/a	1.46	n/a
6-thioguanine	Thioguanine	40 mg	—	n/a	??	

Continued

Generic	Trade	Dose	AWP Generic	Pricing Method	AWP Trade	Pricing Method
IMMUNOSUPPRESSANTS—cont'd						
Cytotoxic Agents						
Cyclophosphamide	Cytoxan	25 mg	—	n/a	2.23	C
		50 mg	—		4.09	
Chlorambucil	Leukeran	2 mg	—	n/a	1.58	n/a
Hydroxyurea	Hydrea	500 mg	1.29	n/a	1.42	n/a
Mycophenolate mofetil	CellCept*	250 mg	—	n/a	2.25	B
		500 mg	—		4.50	
Cyclosporine and Related Drugs						
Cyclosporine	Neoral	25 mg	1.38	B	1.53	B
		100 mg	5.50		6.10	
Sirolimus	Rapamune (1 mg/ml)	1 ml	—	n/a	6.85	B
		2 ml	—		13.70	
		5 ml	—		34.25	
Tacrolimus	Prograf	1 mg	—	n/a	2.86	B
		5 mg	—		14.31	
DAPSONE AND RELATED DRUGS						
Dapsone	None	25 mg	0.28	A	—	n/a
		100 mg	0.28		—	
Sulfapyridine		500 mg	32.60†	n/a	—	n/a
Sulfasalazine	Azulfidine	500 mg	0.15	n/a	0.29	n/a
	Azulfidine Entabs	500 mg	—		0.35	n/a
ANTIMALARIAL AGENTS						
Hydroxychloroquine	Plaquenil	200 mg	1.05	n/a	1.42	n/a
Chloroquine	None	250 mg	0.81	n/a	—	n/a
	Aralen	500 mg	—		4.50	A
	Aralen (pack of 6)	500 mg	—		4.33	
Quinacrine	Atabrine	100 mg	??		??	
RETINOIDS						
Isotretinoin	Accutane	20 mg	—	n/a	6.31	C
		40 mg	—		7.33	
Acitretin	Soriatane	10 mg	—	n/a	6.84	C
		25 mg	—		9.00	
Bexarotene	Targretin	75 mg	—	n/a	10.25	n/a
PSORALENS						
Methoxsalen	Oxsoralen Ultra	10 mg	—	n/a	4.16	n/a
	8-MOP	10 mg	??		—	
	Oxsoralen Lotion 1%	30 ml	—	n/a	113.03	n/a
Trioxsalen	Trisoralen	5 mg	—	n/a	2.74	n/a

AWP, Average wholesale price; *A*, unity: price same regardless of drug dose (within 5% range); *B*, linear: price per mg same regardless of drug dose (within 5% range); *C*, logarithmic: price per mg least with larger doses; *D*, inverse: price per mg least with lower doses.

*200 mg/ml liquid also available ($1.80/ml).

†Only price available was for bulk powder 100 grams.

Generic	Trade	Dose	AWP Generic	Pricing Method	AWP Trade	Pricing Method
IINTERFERONS						
Interferon α-2$_b$	Intron A	3 million IU	—	n/a	35.63	B
		5 million IU	—		59.38	
Interferon α-2$_a$	Roferon A	3 million IU	—	n/a	34.97	B
		6 million IU	—		69.91	
Interferon α-N$_3$	Alferon N	5 million IU	—	n/a	165.41	n/a
Interferon-γ	Actimmune	3 million IU	—	n/a	210.00	n/a
ANTIHISTAMINES						
First-Generation H$_1$ Antihistamines (Sedating)						
Diphenhydramine	Benadryl	25 mg	0.08	D	0.17	D
		50 mg	0.42		0.51	
Cyproheptadine	Periactin	4 mg	0.01	n/a	0.47	
Promethazine	Phenergan	25 mg	0.23	C	0.48	C
		50 mg	0.11		0.69	
Chlorpheniramine	Chlor-Trimeton	4 mg	0.01	D	0.18	C
		12 mg (ER)	0.12		0.42	
Hydroxyzine	Atarax, Vistaril	25 mg	0.10	C	0.94	C
		50 mg	0.15		1.17	
Second-Generation H$_1$ Antihistamines (Less-Sedating)						
Loratadine	Claritin	10 mg	—	n/a	2.69	n/a
Cetirizine	Zyrtec	5 mg	—	n/a	1.85	C
		10 mg	—		2.32	
Fexofenadine	Allegra	60 mg	—	n/a	1.16	n/a
Other Antihistamines						
Doxepin	Sinequan	10 mg	0.25	C	0.39	C
		25 mg	0.30		0.51	
Cromolyn sodium	Gastrocrom	100 mg/ 5 ml	—	n/a	1.88	n/a
ANTIANDROGENS AND ANDROGEN INHIBITORS						
Antiandrogens						
Spironolactone	Aldactone	25 mg	0.25	D	0.46	C
		50 mg	0.71		0.85	
Flutamide	Eulexin	250 mg	—	n/a	2.03	n/a
Cimetidine	Tagamet	200 mg	0.81	C	0.26	D
		400 mg	1.25		1.91	
Androgen Inhibitors						
Finasteride	Propecia	1 mg	—	n/a	1.56	C
	Proscar	5 mg	—		2.28	

Continued

Generic	Trade	Dose	AWP Generic	Pricing Method	AWP Trade	Pricing Method
ANXIOLYTIC AND ANTIPSYCHOTIC AGENTS						
Anxiolytic Agents						
Alprazolam	Xanax	0.25 mg	0.58	C	0.86	C
		0.5 mg	0.70		1.07	
Buspirone	Buspar (Dividose)	10 mg	1.54	n/a	1.39	C
		30 mg	—		3.74	
Antipsychotic Agents						
Pimozide	Oral	2 mg	—	n/a	0.80	n/a
Risperidone	Risperdal	1 mg	—	n/a	2.43	C
		3 mg	—		4.78	
Olanzapine	Zyprexa	5 mg	—	n/a	5.53	C
		10 mg	—		8.40	
Quetiapine	Seroquel	100 mg	—	n/a	2.29	B
		200 mg	—		4.50	
SSRI ANTIDEPRESSSANTS						
Fluoxetine	Prozac	10 mg	—	n/a	2.52	A
		20 mg	—		2.59	
Paroxetine	Paxil	20 mg	—	n/a	2.23	A
		30 mg	—		2.30	
Sertraline	Zoloft	25 mg	—	n/a	2.20	A
		50 mg	—		2.27	
Fluvoxamine	Luvox	25 mg	—	n/a	2.20	A
		50 mg	—		2.31	
Citalopram	Celexa	20 mg	—	n/a	1.93	A
		40 mg	—		2.02	
OTHER ANTIDEPRESSANTS						
Doxepin	Sinequan	10 mg	0.27	C	0.40	C
		25 mg	0.33		0.51	
Amitriptyline	Elavil	10 mg	0.10	C	0.22	C
		25 mg	0.13		0.44	

AWP, Average wholesale price; *A*, unity: price same regardless of drug dose (within 5% range); *B*, linear: price per mg same regardless of drug dose (within 5% range); *C*, logarithmic: price per mg least with larger doses; *D*, inverse: price per mg least with lower doses.
‡Supply has been extremely limited over past 2 years. Cost varies highly with market availability.

Generic	Trade	Dose	AWP Generic	Pricing Method	AWP Trade	Pricing Method
OTHER ANTIDEPRESSANTS—cont'd						
Bupropion	Wellbutrin	75 mg	—	n/a	0.80	C
		100 mg	—		1.05	
	Wellbutrin SR	100 mg	—	n/a	1.30	C
		150 mg	—		1.40	
Venlafaxine	Effexor	37.5 mg	—	n/a	1.12	C
		75 mg	—		1.22	
	Effexor SR	37.5 mg	—	n/a	2.00	C
		75 mg	—		2.25	
Nefazodone	Serzone	100 mg	—	n/a	1.15	A
		200 mg	—		1.15	
NEW USES OF OLDER DRUGS—UPDATE						
Colchicine	None	0.6 mg	0.14	n/a	—	n/a
Nicotinamide	None	100 mg	0.02	C	—	
		500 mg	0.06			
Auranofin	Ridaura	3 mg	—	n/a	1.79	n/a
Potassium iodide	None	Powder	0.07/g	n/a	—	n/a
	(solution)	1 g/ml	0.13		—	
Danazol		200 mg	2.10	n/a	3.56	n/a
Stanozolol	Winstrol	2 mg	—	n/a	0.77	n/a
MISCELLANEOUS SYSTEMIC DRUGS						
Thalidomide	Thalomid	50 mg	—	n/a	7.84	n/a
Clofazimine	Lamprene	50 mg	—	n/a	0.17	n/a
Immunoglobulin‡	Various	6 g vial	28.72	n/a	—	n/a
		12 g vial	—		—	
Penicillamine	Cupramine	250 mg	—	n/a	1.06	n/a
Glycopyrrolate	Robinul	1 mg	—	n/a	0.63	C
	Robinul Forte	2 mg	—		1.00	
Biotin	None	0.3 mg	0.04	n/a	—	n/a

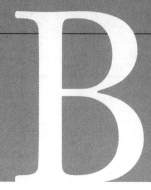

Topical Drug Costs

Generic	Trade	Size	AWP Generic	Pricing Method	AWP Trade	Pricing Method
TOPICAL ANTIBACTERIAL AGENTS: WOUND CARE						
Bacitracin	Bacitracin ointment	30 g	—		5.03	n/a
(above) +	Polysporin ointment	15 g	3.00	C	3.67	C
polymyxin B		30 g	4.70		5.76	
(above) + neomycin	Neosporin ointment	30 g	2.55	n/a	—	
Gentamicin	Garamycin cream	15 g	3.98	D	21.34	n/a
		30 g	9.50		—	
		15 g	4.63	D	21.34	n/a
		30 g	12.17		—	
Mupirocin	Bactroban ointment	15 g	—		21.85	C
		30 g	—		39.45	
Silver sulfadiazine	Silvadene cream	20 g	3.67	C	5.30	C
		85 g	10.31		15.60	
		400 g	30.38		37.44	
TOPICAL ANTIBACTERIAL AGENTS: ACNE AND ROSACEA PRODUCTS						
Clindamycin	Cleocin T solution	60 ml	18.84	n/a	34.94	n/a
	Cleocin T gel	30 g	—		30.76	C
		60 g	—		55.41	
	Cleocin T lotion	60 ml	—		42.80	n/a
Metronidazole	Metrogel (0.75%)	45 g	—		41.81	n/a
	Metrocream	45 g	—		41.81	n/a
	Metrolotion	59 ml	—		44.19	n/a
	Noritate cream (1%)	30 g	—		40.01	n/a
Azalaic acid	Azelex cream	30 g	—		35.44	n/a
Benzoyl peroxide	Benzac W gel (10%)	60 g	15.10	C	16.69	C
		90 g	20.05		22.13	
	Desquam X gel (10%)	45 g	7.75	D	12.70	C
		90 g	18.52		22.50	
Erythromycin*	Benzamycin gel	23.3 g	—		42.52	B
		46.6 g	—		81.16	
	Erygel (2%)	30 g	—		29.94	B
		60 g	—		56.30	

A special acknowledgment to Crystal S. Blankenship, Kristen Hummer, Sonya J. Keinath, Andrea K. LaRoche, Heather Klinge, and Jessica Boyce for their work on this appendix.
AWP, Average wholesale price; A, unity: price same regardless of drug dose (within 5% range); B, linear: price per mg same regardless of drug dose (within 5% range); C, logarithmic: price per mg least with larger doses; D, inverse: price per mg least with lower doses.
*Combination of 3% erythromycin and 5% benzoyl peroxide.

Generic	Trade	Size	AWP Generic	Pricing Method	AWP Trade	Pricing Method
TOPICAL ANTIFUNGAL AGENTS						
Ketoconazole	Nizoral cream	30 g	—		29.34	C
		60 g	—		44.58	
	Nizoral shampoo	120 ml	—		21.56	n/a
Miconazole	Monistat Derm cream	15 g	—		16.62	C
		30 g	—		27.90	
Oxiconazole	Oxistat cream	30 g	—		28.73	C
		60 g	—		43.55	
	Oxistat lotion	30 ml	—		26.84	n/a
Naftifine	Naftin cream	30 g	—		36.65	C
		60 g	—		56.80	
	Naftin gel	20 g	—		28.78	C
		60 g	—		57.82	
Terbinafine	Lamisil cream	15 g	—		32.61	C
		30 g	—		58.40	
	Lamisil spray	30 ml	—		62.21	n/a
Butenafine	Mentax cream	15 g	—		29.56	C
		30 g	—		52.97	
Ciclopirox	Loprox cream	15 g	—		13.04	C
		30 g	—		23.31	
	Loprox lotion	30 g	—		25.64	B
		60 g	—		48.83	
TOPICAL ANTIVIRAL AGENTS						
Acyclovir	Zovirax cream	15 g	—		47.80	n/a
Penciclovir	Denavir cream	15 g	—		22.90	n/a
Imiquimod	Aldara cream	12 pkt	—		124.80	n/a
Podofilox	Condylox ?gel/sol.	3.5 g	—		92.18	n/a
TOPICAL ANTIPARASITIC AGENTS						
Permethrin	Elimite cream (5%)	60 g	25.31	n/a	26.25	n/a
	Nix (1%)	60 ml	—		9.20	
Lindane	Kwell lotion	60 ml	12.15	n/a	16.38	C
		480 ml	—		51.39	
	Kwell shampoo	60 ml	—		11.91	C
		480 ml	—		65.65	
Crotamiton	Eurax cream	60 g	—		12.72	n/a
	Eurax lotion	60 ml	—		13.56	n/a
Malathion 0.5%	Ovide	59 ml	—		31.25	n/a
TOPICAL CORTICOSTEROIDS						
Low Potency						
Hydrocortisone (2.5%)	Cream	30 g	10.22	C	—	
		120 g	16.50		—	
		454 g	70.52		—	
	Ointment	30 g	8.84	C	—	
		454 g	69.27		—	
Desonide	DesOwen cream	15 g	9.76	C	16.50	C
		60 g	26.11		42.56	
	DesOwen ointment	15 g	10.56	C	16.50	C
		60 g	28.47		42.56	

Continued

Generic	Trade	Size	AWP Generic	Pricing Method	AWP Trade	Pricing Method
TOPICAL CORTICOSTEROIDS—cont'd						
Intermediate Potency						
Fluocinolone (0.025%)	Synalar cream	15 g	2.91	C	17.96	C
		60 g	5.02		42.20	
	Synalar ointment	15 g	4.58	C	17.96	C
		60 g	9.32		42.20	
Triamcinolone acetonide (0.1%)	Kenalog cream	15 g	3.65	C	14.17	C
		80 g	5.94		41.78	
		454 g	20.69		—	
	Kenalog ointment	15 g	3.07	C	14.16	n/a
		80 g	6.29		—	
		454 g	17.94		—	
Hydrocortisone butyrate (0.1%)	Locoid cream	15 g	—		17.42	C
		45 g	—		36.05	
	Locoid ointment	15 g	—		17.42	C
		45 g	—		36.05	
Hydrocortisone valerate	Westcort cream	15 g	13.58	C	16.69	C
		60 g	33.90		41.64	
	Westcort ointment	15 g	13.81	C	16.69	C
		60 g	34.46		41.64	
High Potency						
Amcinonide (0.1%)	Cyclocort cream	30 g	—		27.00	C
		60 g	—		45.39	
	Cyclocort ointment	30 g	—		27.00	C
		60 g	—		45.39	
Desoximetasone	Topicort cream (0.25%)	15 g	15.99	C	21.24	C
		60 g	36.58		51.01	
	Topicort ointment (0.25%)	15 g	16.84	C	21.05	C
		60 g	40.52		50.63	
Flucinonide	Lidex cream	30 g	14.56	C	29.87	C
		60 g	22.59		50.07	
	Lidex ointment	30 g	23.82	C	29.87	C
		60 g	38.19		50.07	
Betamethasone dipropion	Diprosone cream	15 g	7.73	C	25.97	C
		45 g	12.97		47.63	
	Diprosone ointment	15 g	8.67	C	25.97	C
		45 g	13.00		47.63	
Super Potency						
Halobetasol	Ultravate cream	15 g	—		27.25	C
		50 g	—		65.57	
	Ultravate ointment	15 g	—		27.25	C
		50 g	—		65.57	
Clobetasol	Temovate cream	15 g	21.45	C	25.86	C
		45 g	43.20		52.06	
	Temovate ointment	15 g	20.09	C	25.86	C
		45 g	40.46		52.06	

AWP, Average wholesale price; *A*, unity: price same regardless of drug dose (within 5% range); *B*, linear: price per mg same regardless of drug dose (within 5% range); *C*, logarithmic: price per mg least with larger doses; *D*, inverse: price per mg least with lower doses.

TOPICAL RETINOIDS

Generic	Trade	Size	AWP Generic	Pricing Method	AWP Trade	Pricing Method
Tretinoin	Retin-A cream (0.25%)	20 g	27.53	C	32.04	C
		45 g	52.17		60.66	
	Retin-A cream (0.05%)	20 g	31.07	C	35.94	C
		45 g	58.26		67.38	
	Retin-A gel (0.01%)	15 g	—		27.96	C
		45 g	—		66.00	
	Retin-A gel (0.025%)	15 g	—		28.50	C
		45 g	—		66.54	
Tretinoin	Avita cream (0.025%)	20 g	—		30.08	C
		45 g	—		56.25	
	Avita gel (0.025%)	20 g	—		33.38	C
		45 g	—		62.10	
Tretinoin	Retin-A Micro gel (0.1%)	20 g	—		35.34	C
		45 g	—		66.84	
Adapalene	Differin gel (0.1%)	15 g	—		27.31	C
		45 g	—		64.38	
Tazarotene	Tazarac gel (0.05%)	30 g	—		60.00	B
		100 g	—		200.00	
	Tazarac gel (0.1%)	30 g	—		63.75	B
		100 g	—		212.50	

TOPICAL CHEMOTHERAPEUTIC AGENTS

Generic	Trade	Size	AWP Generic	Pricing Method	AWP Trade	Pricing Method
5-fluorouracil	Efudex cream (5%)	25 g	—		102.13	n/a
	Efudex solution (2%)	10 ml	—		71.44	n/a
	Solution (5%)	10 ml	—		102.13	n/a
	Fluoroplex cream (1%)	30 g	—		55.25	n/a
	Fluoroplex solution (5%)	30 ml	—		55.25	n/a

ALPHA-HYDROXY ACID PRODUCTS AND AGENTS FOR HYPERKERATOSIS

Generic	Trade	Size	AWP Generic	Pricing Method	AWP Trade	Pricing Method
Lactic acid 12%	Lac-Hydrin cream	140 g	—		35.75	C
		385 g	—		46.80	
	Lac-Hydrin cream	225 g	—		34.14	C
		400 g	—		53.75	
Salicylic acid	Keralyt gel	30 g	—		8.32	n/a
Urea	Carmol cream (40%)	30 g	—		20.84	C
		90 g	—		37.66	
	Ultra Mide 25 cream	105 g	—		9.60	C
	Lotion (25%)	240 ml	—		15.50	

TOPICAL VITAMIN D$_3$

Generic	Trade	Size	AWP Generic	Pricing Method	AWP Trade	Pricing Method
Calcipotriene	Dovonex cream	30 g	—		46.73	B
		60 g	—		92.64	
	Dovonex ointment	30 g	—		46.73	B
		60 g	—		92.64	
	Dovonex solution	60 ml	—		89.08	n/a

Continued

Generic	Trade	Size	AWP Generic	Pricing Method	AWP Trade	Pricing Method
LOCAL ANESTHETICS: INJECTABLE						
Lidocaine (with epinephrine)	Xylocaine (1%)	20 ml	3.07	C	2.32	C
		50 ml	5.20		5.28	
Bupivacaine (with epinephrine)	Marcaine (0.25%)	30 ml	10.38	B	8.67	C
		50 ml	16.98		11.64	
	Marcaine (0.5%)	30 ml	11.26	C	9.42	C
		50 ml	15.11		12.68	
Mepivacaine (with epinephrine)	Carbocaine (1%)	30 ml	12.12	C	—	
		50 ml	14.84		—	
	Carbocaine (2%)	20 ml	13.61	C	—	
		50 ml	20.34		—	
LOCAL ANESTHETICS: TOPICAL						
Lidocaine/prilocaine	EMLA cream	30 g	—		45.12	n/a
Pramoxine	Prax lotion (1%)	15 ml	—		4.42	C
		120 ml	—		11.04	
Doxepin	Zonalon cream (5%)	30 g	—		23.57	C
		45 g	—		31.82	
Capsaicin	Zostrix cream (0.025%)	20 g	8.69	C	—	
		60 g	9.25		11.94	n/a
	Zostrix cream (0.075%)	30 g	10.33	A	7.98	B
		60 g	10.97		16.20	
ORAL PRODUCTS IN TYPICAL CHAPTERS						
Ivermectin	Stromectol	3 mg	—		4.99	B
		6 mg	—		9.97	
Thiabendazole	Mintezol tablets	500 mg	—		1.16	n/a
	Mintezol suspension	120 ml	—		24.14	n/a

AWP, Average wholesale price; *A,* unity: price same regardless of drug dose (within 5% range); *B,* linear: price per mg same regardless of drug dose (within 5% range); *C,* logarithmic: price per mg least with larger doses; *D,* inverse: price per mg least with lower doses.
EMLA, Eutectic mixture local anesthetic (2.5% lidocaine, 2.5% prilocaine).

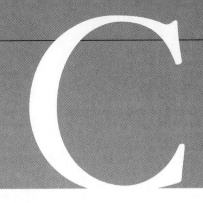
Representative Costs of Laboratory Tests for Monitoring Therapy

Laboratory Test	Hospital A	Hospital B	Private A	Average
GENERAL CHEMISTRIES				
SMA-12/Chem-12	42.85	42.25	39.00	41.37
LIVER FUNCTION				
SGOT/AST	25.00	21.25	31.00	25.75
SGPT/ALT	25.00	21.25	31.00	25.75
RENAL FUNCTION				
BUN	25.00	19.00	31.00	25.00
Creatinine	25.00	23.25	31.00	26.42
Urinalysis	38.25	20.25	31.00	29.83
HEMATOLOGY				
CBC	28.75	29.75	31.00	29.83
CBC with differential platelets	35.00	32.75	31.00	32.92
G6PD level	91.00	51.75	87.00	76.58
Reticulocyte count	32.50	18.00	32.00	27.50
PREGNANCY				
Serum β-HCG	54.25	41.25	53.00	49.50
Urine β-HCG	37.00	17.00	64.00	39.33
LIPID				
Triglycerides	30.75	23.25	31.00	28.22
Cholesterol	30.75	16.00	31.00	25.92
HDL-cholesterol	42.50	20.25	59.00	40.58
MISCELLANEOUS				
Potassium	25.00	19.00	31.00	25.00
Uric acid	30.75	23.25	31.00	28.33
Magnesium	40.50	30.75	41.00	37.50
TSH	93.25	58.25	100.00	83.83

INDEX